Selected Papers on

Tissue Optics

Applications in Medical Diagnostics and Therapy

Books in SPIE's Milestone Series
Brian J. Thompson, Series Editor

Forthcoming

SPIE Milestone Series
Volume MS 102

Selected Papers on
Tissue Optics
Applications in Medical Diagnostics and Therapy

Valery V. Tuchin, *Editor*
Saratov State University
Saratov Branch of the Mechanical
  Engineering Institute of the
  Russian Academy of Sciences

Brian J. Thompson
General Editor, SPIE Milestone Series

SPIE Optical Engineering Press

A Publication of SPIE—The International Society for Optical Engineering
Bellingham, Washington USA

Library of Congress Cataloging-in Publication Data

Selected papers on tissue optics: applications in medical diagnostics and therapy / Valery
  V. Tuchin, editor.
        p. cm. — (SPIE milestone series ; v. MS 102)
    "A publication of SPIE—The International Society for Optical Engineering."
    Includes index.
    ISBN 0-8194-1695-9 (hardbound)
    1. Tissues—Optical properties—Congresses. I. Tuchin, V.V. (Valeri̇̌ Viktorovich) II.
Series.
    [DNLM: 1. Scattering, Radiation—collected works. 2. Light—collected works. 3.
Lasers—collected works. 4. Diagnostic Imaging—collected works. QC427.4 S464
1994]
    QH642.S45 1994
    611'.018—dc20
    for Library of Congress   94-28511
                                                                            CIP

ISBN 0-8194-1695-9

Published by
SPIE—The International Society for Optical Engineering
P.O. Box 10, Bellingham, Washington 98227-0010 USA
Telephone 206/676-3290 (Pacific Time) • Fax 206/647-1445

This book is a compilation of outstanding papers selected from the world literature on
optical and optoelectronic science, engineering, and technology. SPIE Optical
Engineering Press acknowledges with appreciation the authors and publishers who have
given their permission to reprint material included in this volume. An earnest effort has
been made to contact the copyright holders of all papers reproduced herein.

Printed in the United States of America

Introduction to the Series

There is no substitute for reading the original papers on any subject even if that subject is mature enough to be critically written up in a textbook or a monograph. Reading a well-written book only serves as a further stimulus to drive the reader to seek the original publications. The problems are, which papers, and in what order?

As a serious student of a field, do you really have to search through all the material for yourself, and read the good with the not-so-good, the important with the not-so-important, and the milestone papers with the merely pedestrian offerings? The answer to all these questions is usually yes, unless the authors of the textbooks or monographs that you study have been very selective in their choices of references and bibliographic listings. Even in that all-too-rare circumstance, the reader is then faced with finding the original publications, many of which may be in obscure or not widely held journals.

From time to time and in many disparate fields, volumes appear that are collections of reprints that represent the milestone papers in the particular field. Some of theses volumes have been produced for specific topics in optical science, but as yet no systematic set of volumes has been produced that covers connected areas of optical science and engineering.

The editors of each individual volume in the series have been chosen for their deep knowledge of the world literature in their fields; hence, the selection of reprints chosen for each book has been made with authority and care.

On behalf of SPIE, I thank the individual editors for their diligence, and we all hope that you, the reader, will find these volumes invaluable additions to your own working library.

Brian J. Thompson
University of Rochester

Selected Papers on
Tissue Optics
Applications in Medical Diagnostics and Therapy

Contents

Preface

Tissue optics as a growing field of modern science is of great interest to scientists, engineers, and medical doctors, who are developing new methods and instruments for optical and laser medicine. Tissue optics has been characterized by such very important applications as biomedical diagnostics and light dosimetry in phototherapy. This Milestone volume presents selected key reprints and a bibliography of additional references on optics of different biotissues and bioliquids, including skin, eye, and dental tissues, brain, muscle, blood, etc. The papers discuss fundamentals, experimental techniques, and applications of tissue optics: light propagation in tissues, CW, time- and frequency-domain approaches, photothermal and tissue optics modification effects, optical polarization anisotropy of tissues and ensembles of mammalian cells, coherent light scattering effects, principles of speckle-field formation and interferometry, tissue and blood absorption spectroscopy, optical imaging and tomography, phototherapy, and light dosimetry.

During the past 25 years numerous conferences have taken place that demonstrate new achievements in tissue optics and laser medical diagnostics and therapy. The Proceedings of these conferences, plus monographs, books of selected papers, special issues of journals, and some review articles on tissue optics and applications are cited in a bibliography of additional references following this preface (p. xix).

The extensive literature on tissue optics and its applications in biomedicine made the selection of papers to include herein a difficult task. Thus, the editor decided to limit his attention to the papers that, in his opinion, are needed by many scientists, engineers, and medical doctors who are designing and using optical and laser diagnostic and therapeutic methods and instruments in their practical work.

In preparing this Milestone volume, the editor has selected a few well-known review articles that may help the reader to obtain an overview of the topic. Most of the papers reprinted here have a maximal citation rating for the past 10 years, but also included are some excellent papers that were published more recently, whose citation index, the editor hopes, will be equally great in a few years. In order to reflect some historical aspects, to show seminal works and other important but lengthy papers, and to signify the wide range of possible directions of investigations and applications of tissue optics, included in the bibliography of additional references (cited chronologically) is a selection of interesting papers that can be useful not only for scientists, engineers, and medical doctors but also for students and teachers.

For the most part, the selected papers were originally published in peer-reviewed journals, with only a few of them taken from book chapters or conference proceedings; these latter were included only if they were seminal works with a great citation index or recently published, pioneering works, and then only if corresponding peer-reviewed articles were not available. The collection is divided into five sections, which will be discussed individually.

Section One: Introduction

Britton Chance's general review of developments of the classical optical method in cell and tissue spectroscopy begins the volume (p. 3). The paper was selected not only because the author, in selecting his topic, has "chosen to bridge the past and the present with a biophysical theme that is just as viable now as it was in the past," but also because the author is a man who did so much for the development of tissue optics.

Akira Ishimaru, a world renowned specialist in light scattering by turbid media, reviewed the mathematical descriptions of the propagation and scattering characteristics of light in turbid materials, such as tissues (p. 17); this review should be very useful to the reader interested in the basic physical concepts of tissue optics.

Finally, a short overview by Leon Goldman, a person so famous in the field of laser medicine that he has the Medical Excellence Award named after him, shows the new trends in dermatological microscopy and medical instrumentation for early clinical diagnostics (p. 23).

Section Two: Optics of Tissues with Strong Scattering

Continuous wave scattering

Here we present papers describing the optics of such strongly scattering tissues as the skin, blood vessel wall, muscle, dental tissue, etc. [Anderson and Parrish (p. 29), van Gemert and coworkers (p. 85), Al'tshuler and Grisimov (p. 159), and Keijzer and coworkers (p. 108)]. These descriptions include both different tissue models—one-, two-, and three-dimensional and one-, two-, and multilayer—and different fruitful approaches to light distribution analysis in tissues, based on the radiative transfer theory, the theory of photon random walk, and the usage of the Monte Carlo simulation method [Groenhuis and coworkers (pp. 36 and 43), Wilson and Adam (p. 48), Yoon and coworkers (p. 55), Nossal and coworkers (p. 68), Profio (p. 78), and Yaroslavsky and Tuchin (p. 115)].

A large group of the reprints represents experimental and inverse modeling techniques for tissue scattering and absorption coefficients and anisotropy factor measurements: collimated light and integrating sphere spectrophotometry, scattering light differential angular measurements, Kubelka-Munk formalism, the adding-doubling method, and condensed Monte-Carlo simulations [Groenhuis and coworkers (pp. 36 and 43), Marchesini and coworkers (p. 94), Graaff and coworkers (p. 120), and Prahl and coworkers (p. 149)]. A review by Cheong and coworkers (p. 129) gives up-to-date information about the optical properties of many tissues. A tissue refractive index measurement technique and data for some mammalian tissues are also presented [Bolin and coworkers (p. 101)]. The paper by Schmitt and coworkers (p. 164) shows the importance of polarization effects for light propagation in a multiply scattering medium.

Time-domain approach

This collection of papers, by Patterson, Chance, and Wilson (p. 186), Cui, Wang, and Chance (p. 208), Delpy and coworkers (p. 176), Yoo, Liu, and Alfano (p. 199), Jacques (p. 192), Ferrari and coworkers (p. 211), and Das, Yoo, and Alfano (p. 220) illustrates the prospects for time-resolved backscattering spectroscopy of tissues. The reader may find here analytical and numerical descriptions of the short pulse propagation of light in random media, studies of photon migration depth in tissues, descriptions of different time-gating measuring methods and instruments, and experimental data for tissue optical parameters.

Frequency-domain approach

This novel field of tissue optics investigations is represented by fundamental papers on photon density waves propagation and their refraction, diffraction, and interference in a strongly scattering medium with absorption [Fishkin and coworkers (p. 233), O'Leary and coworkers (p. 279), Boas and coworkers (p. 295), Fishkin and Gratton (p. 299), Svaasand and coworkers (p. 313), and Schmitt and coworkers (p. 283)]. Another group of papers describes the theoretical base and experimental techniques for optical parameter determination: application of the random walk theory (Gandjbakhche and coworkers, p. 244), diffusion (Arridge and coworkers, p. 246), and more rigorous (Yaroslavsky and Tuchin, p. 274) approximations, experimental methods, and data (Lakowicz and Berndt, p. 223, and Patterson and coworkers, p. 230).

Thermal and tissue optical properties modification effects

Three papers devoted to different aspects of soft and hard tissue laser heating under nonablating conditions begin this subsection [Jacques and Prahl (p. 322), van Gemert and Welch (p. 332), and Sagi and coworkers (p. 349)]. The paper by Ivanov and coworkers (p. 357) describes some soft tissue optical properties modification effects caused by compression, squeezing, and puncture. Human aorta optical properties modification effects caused by laser irradiation, dehydration, and thermal damage are analyzed by Schwarzmaier and coworkers (p. 363) and by Çilesiz and Welch (p. 368).

Optics of blood

Different aspects of blood optics are discussed here: diffuse reflectance and transmittance, blood components absorption and refraction spectra, changes of blood optical properties in the process of its motion, and light scattering polarization features of erythrocyte ensembles and separate leukocytes [Reynolds and coworkers (p. 380), Steinke and Shepherd (p. 389), Shumilina (p. 399),

Lindberg and Öberg (p. 400), Korolevich and coworkers (p. 405), and de Grooth and coworkers (p. 409)].

Section Three: Eye Tissue Optics

This section presents papers developing the concept of weakly scattering tissues, which are extremely transparent due to scatterers ordering and turbid due to scatterers disordering. The mammalian eye front segment tissues, such as the cornea, the sclera, and the crystalline lens, may be described using this concept. The reader has the opportunity to become acquainted with physical and mathematical models of transparent and turbid cornea and crystalline lens in the papers by Benedek (p. 417), Bettelheim and Ali (p. 432), Farrell and coworkers (p. 439), Tuchin and coworkers (p. 448), and Vérétout and coworkers (p. 452).

Section Four: Coherent Light Scattering by Biotissues

The first three papers in this section describe laser speckle phenomenon and its positive and negative aspects in the application to medical diagnostics, including blood flow monitoring in the skin, internal organs, and ocular fundus [Ruth (p. 471), Aizu and Asakura (p. 479), and Briers (p. 494)]. The next two papers, by Latina and coworkers (p. 501) and Dhadwal and coworkers (p. 510), reflect modern directions in quasi-elastic light scattering applications in biomedicine: for early detection of cataractogenesis in a human eye lens. The paper by Artal and Navarro (p. 516) shows the use of speckle interferometry in investigations of optical properties of posterior eye segment tissues, the living human fovea.

High-resolution low-coherence light interferometry applied to nondiffusive eye tissues and highly scattering arterial wall tissue is described by Fercher and coworkers (p. 519) and by Clivaz and coworkers (p. 526). Another aspect of coherent light capabilities is demonstrated in the paper by Masters on the quantitative analysis of human corneal endothelial cell patterns using the Fourier transform method (p. 529). The final three papers here, by Spears and coworkers (p. 537), Toida and coworkers (p. 549), and Beuthan and coworkers (p. 551), illustrate the possibilities of coherent light techniques in image detection in highly scattering tissues.

Section Five: Applications in Diagnostics and Therapy

Because of the numerous original papers on this intensively developing topic, two review articles are presented, by Sevik and coworkers (p. 559) and Tuchin (p. 621), that summarize many original works and give the main directions of optical diagnostics and therapy developments. In addition to these review papers, a few recently published papers are included. The papers by Ferrari and coworkers (p. 581), Anderson (p. 587), and Kopola and coworkers (p. 593) illustrate the possibilities of clinical applications of light diagnostic techniques and appropriate instruments. The papers by Andersson-Engels and coworkers (p. 598), French and coworkers (p. 601), and Barbour and coworkers (p. 607) show perspectives of tissue optical imaging and tomography. The final three papers, by Marijnissen and Star (p. 639), Svaasand and coworkers (p. 647), and Jacques (p. 655), give information about the principles of light delivery and light dosimetry during laser-induced photodynamic and hyperthermic therapy of tumors.

Bibliography of Additional References

As noted above, this collection of reprints is accompanied by a list of selected references that provide additional background and perspective for readers who want to go beyond the papers selected for this volume. The list is sorted into the same categories as the reprints, but the last section has additional subheadings showing the main directions of tissue optics applications.

It should be noted that some excellent papers on tissue optics and applications were included in previous Milestones: *Selected Papers on Quasielastic Light Scattering by Macromolecular, Supramolecular, and Fluid Systems,* edited by Benjamin Chu, and *Selected Papers on Photodynamic Therapy,* edited by David Kessel. Both books are cited in the bibliography additional references.

It also should be noted that two very powerful optical technologies for medical science and applications, fluorescence and Raman spectroscopy, are not presented in this Milestone volume owing to the extensive publications on these topics (some monographs, proceedings, and review articles are cited in the bibliography of additional references). Perhaps a future Milestone volume on Biotissue Spectroscopy might include fluorescence, Raman, photothermal, and some other very powerful techniques of tissue investigations, or perhaps papers on biotissue spectroscopy will be selected for inclusion in possible future Milestone volumes on Fluorescence and Raman Spectroscopy Methods.

Acknowledgments

I am grateful to Milestone Series Editor Brian J. Thompson and my colleagues, especially Drs. Alexander Priezzhev, Sergey Utz, and Il'ja Yaroslavsky, for providing valuable advice during the paper selection process, the authors for sending me copies of their reprints, and Nina Lakodina, Dixie Cheek, and my students Igor Meglinsky and Vladimir Kukavsky for help in the preparation of this volume.

In conclusion it is important to say that the final responsibility for the selection rests with this volume editor, who encourages himself that his look from Russia on the world problems will be supported.

Valery V. Tuchin
Saratov State University
Saratov Branch of Mechanical
Engineering Institute of
Russian Academy of Sciences
September 1994

Bibliography of Additional References

Proceedings, Monographs, Reprint Books, Journal Special Issues, and Selected Review Articles

L. Goldman, R.J. Rockwell, *Lasers in Medicine* (Gordon and Breach, 1971).

D. Sliney, M. Wolbarsht, *Safety with Lasers and Other Optical Sources* (Plenum, 1980).

Lasers in Biology and Medicine, F. Hillenkamp, R. Pratesi, and C.A. Sacchi, eds. (Plenum, 1980).

Bioengineering and the Skin, M.A. Hingham, ed. (Kluwer, Boston, 1981).

Biological Events Probed by Ultra-Fast Laser Spectroscopy, R. Alfano, ed. (Academic, New York, 1982).

The Science of Photomedicine, J.D. Regan and J.A. Parrish, eds., (Plenum, 1982).

Biomedical Applications of Laser Light Scattering, D.B. Sattelle, W.I. Lee, and B.R. Ware, eds. (Elsevier, Amsterdam, 1982).

P.R. Carey, *Biomedical Application of Raman and Resonance Raman Spectroscopy* (Academic, New York, 1982).

Optics and Biomedical Sciences, G. van Bally and P. Greguss, eds. (Springer-Verlag, 1982).

F.S. Parker, *Applications of Infrared, Raman, and Resonance Raman Spectroscopy in Biochemistry* (Plenum, 1983).

K. Arnt, J. Noe, and S. Rosen, *Cutaneous Laser Therapy, Principles and Methods* (Wiley, 1983).

S.M. Donn, L.R. Kuhns, *Pediatric Transillumination* (Year Book Medical, Chicago, 1983).

Porphyrin Photosensitization, D. Kessel and T.J. Dougherty, eds. (Plenum, 1983).

Porphyrin Localization and Treatment of Tumors, D.R. Doiron and C.J. Gomer, eds. (Alan R. Liss, 1984).

Special Issue on Lasers in Biology and Medicine, IEEE J. Quantum Electron. 20, 1342-1532 (1984).

The Ocular Lens: Structure, Function, and Pathology, H. Maisel, ed. (Dekker, 1985).

Photodynamic Therapy of Tumors and Other Disease, G. Jori and C. Perria, eds. (Libreria Progetto, Padova, 1985).

V.S. Letokhov, "Laser biology and medicine," Nature 316, 325-330 (1985).

J.L. Boulnois, "Photophysical processes in recent medical laser developments: a review," Lasers Med. Sci. 1, 41-46 (1986).

Information Processing in Medical Imaging, S.L. Bacharack, ed. (Martinus Nijhoff, 1986).

Photobiology of the Skin and the Eye, E.M. Jackson, ed. (Dekker, 1986).

J.R. Lakowicz, *Principles of Fluorescence Spectroscopy* (Plenum, 1986).

Special Issue on Lasers in Biology and Medicine, IEEE J. Quantum Electron. 23, 1701-1855 (1987).

Biological Applications of Raman Spectroscopy, T.G. Spiro, ed. (Wiley, Vols. 1 and 2, 1987; Vol. 3, 1988).

Laser Scattering Spectroscopy of Biomedical Objects, J. Stepanek, P. Auzenbacher, and B. Sedlacek, eds., Studies in Physics and Theoretical Chemistry Vol. 45 (Elsevier, Amsterdam, 1987).

Lasers in de Geneeskunde, M.J.C. van Gemert and T.A. Boon, eds. (Samson Stafleu Alphen aan den Rijn, Brussels, 1987).

Light in Biology and Medicine, Vol. 1, R.H. Douglas, J. Moan, and F. Doll'Acqua, eds. (Plenum, 1988).

Y. Ozaki, "Medical application of Raman spectroscopy," Appl. Spectrosc. Rev. 24, 259-312 (1988).

Photodynamic Therapy of Neoplastic Disease, D. Kessel, ed. (CRC Press, Cleveland, 1989).

Photodynamic Therapy: Mechanisms, T.J. Dougherty, ed., Proc. SPIE Vol. 1065 (1989).

Dosimetry of Laser Radiation in Medicine and Biology, G. Muller and D.H. Sliney, eds., SPIE Inst. Ser. Vol. IS5 (1989).

Special Issue on Tissue Optics, L.E. Preuss and A.E. Profio, eds., Appl. Opt. 28, 2207-2357 (1989).

Photon Migration in Tissues, B. Chance, ed. (Plenum, 1989).

A.V. Priezzhev, V.V. Tuchin, L.P. Shubochkin, *Laser Diagnostics in Biology and Medicine* (Nauka, Moscow, 1989).

Advances in Photochemotherapy, T. Hasan, ed., Proc. SPIE Vol. 997 (1989).

Thermal and Optical Interactions with Biological and Related Composite Materials, M.J. Berry and G. Harpole, eds., Proc. SPIE Vol. 1064 (1989).

Radiation Measurement in Photobiology, B.L. Diffey, ed. (Academic, New York, 1989).

E.A. Chernitskii and E.I. Slobozhanina, *Spectral Luminescence Analysis in Medicine* (Nauka, Minsk, 1989).

F.A. Duck, *Physical Properties of Tissue: A Comprehensive Reference Book* (Academic, London, 1990).

Special Issue on Lasers in Medicine and Biology, R. Birngruber, S.N.R. Bruck, and J. Isner, eds., IEEE J. Quantum Electron. 26(12), (1990).

Noninvasive Diagnostic Techniques in Ophthalmology, B.R. Masters, ed. (Springer-Verlag, 1990).

Oxygen Transport to Tissue XII, J. Piper et al., eds. (Plenum, 1990).

Confocal Microscopy, T. Wilson, ed. (Academic, London, 1990).

J.B. Pawley, *Handbook on Biological Confocal Microscopy* (Plenum, 1990).

Laser Applications in Life Sciences, S.A. Akhmanov, M.Yu. Poroshina, N.I. Koroteev, and B.N. Toleutaev, eds., Proc. SPIE Vol. 1403 (2 vols), (1990).

1st International Confernce on Lasers and Medicine, V.I. Konov, G. Muller, and A.M. Prokhorov, eds., Proc. SPIE Vol. 1353 (1990).

Proceedings of the 2nd Plenary Workshop on Tumor Therapy, Lasers Med. Sci. 5(2), (1990).

Selected Papers on Quasielastic Light Scattering by Macromolecular, Supramolecular, and Fluid Systems, B. Chu, ed., SPIE Milestone Ser. Vol. MS12 (1990).

Time-Resolved Laser Spectroscopy in Biochemistry II, J.R. Lacowicz, ed., Proc. SPIE Vol. 1204 (2 vols), (1990).

Biomedical Optics 1991 Proceedings (Los Angeles):

Optical Fibers in Medicine VI, A. Katzir, ed., Proc. SPIE Vol. 1420;

Lasers in Urology, Laparoscopy, and General Surgery, J.J. Pietra-fitta, R.W. Steiner, G.M. Watson, eds., Proc. SPIE Vol. 1421;

Lasers in Dermatology and Tissue Welding, O.T. Tan, J.V. White, and R.A. White, eds., Proc. SPIE Vol. 1422;

Ophthalmic Techniques, C.A. Puliafito, ed., Proc. SPIE Vol. 1423;

Laser-Tissue Interaction II, S.L. Jacques, ed., Proc. SPIE Vol. 1427;

Holography, Interferometry, and Optical Pattern Recognition in Biomedicine, H. Podbielska, ed., Proc. SPIE Vol. 1429.

Encyclopedia of Human Biology, Vol. 5 (Academic, 1991).

Laser Doppler Blood Flowmetry, A.P. Shepherd and P.A. Oberg, eds. (Kluwer, Boston, 1991).

Laser Non-Surgical Medicine: New Challenges for an Old Application, L. Goldman, ed. (Technomic, Lancaster, PA, 1991).

Bioptics: Optics in Biomedicine and Environmental Sciences, O.D. Soares and A.V. Scheggi, eds., Proc. SPIE Vol. 1524 (1991).

Laser in Dermatology, R. Steiner, R. Kaufman, M. Landthaler, and O. Braun-Falco, eds. (Springer-Verlag, 1991).

Laser Systems for Photobiology and Photomedicine, A.N. Chester, S. Martellucci, and A.M. Scheggi, eds. (Plenum, 1991).

Biomedical Optics 1992 Proceedings (Los Angeles):

Time-Resolved Laser Spectroscopy in Biochemistry III, J.R. Lako-wicz, ed., Proc. SPIE Vol. 1640;

Physiological Monitoring and Early Detection Diagnostic Methods, T.S. Mang, ed., Proc. SPIE Vol. 1641;

Diagnostic and Therapeutic Cardiovascular Interventions II, G.S. Abela, ed., Proc. SPIE Vol. 1642;

Laser Surgery: Advanced Characterization, Therapeutics, and Systems III, R.R. Anderson, ed., Proc. SPIE Vol. 1643;

Ophthalmic Technologies II, J. Parel, ed., Proc. SPIE Vol. 1644;

Optical Methods for Tumor Treatment and Detection: Mechanisms and Techniques in Photodynamic Therapy, T.J. Dougherty, ed., Proc. SPIE Vol. 1645;

Laser-Tissue Interaction III, S.L. Jacques, ed., Proc. SPIE Vol. 1646;

Holography, Interferometry, and Optical Pattern Recognition in Biomedicine II, H. Podbielska, ed., Proc. SPIE Vol. 1647;

Fiber Optic Medical and Fluorescent Sensors and Applications, D.R. Hansmann, F.P. Milanovich, G.G. Vurek, and D.R. Walt, eds., Proc. SPIE Vol. 1648;

Optical Fibers in Medicine VII, A. Katzir, ed., Proc. SPIE Vol. 1649;

Medical Lasers and Systems, S.D. Harman and D.M. Harris, eds., Proc. SPIE Vol. 1650.

Quantitative Spectroscopy in Tissue, K. Frank and M. Kessler, eds. (pmi-Verlag, Frankfurt am Main, 1992).

The Formation, Handling, and Evalution of Medical Images, A.T. Pokropek and M.A. Viergever, eds., NATO ASI Series F (Springer-Verlag, 1992).

Oxygen Transport to Tissue XIII, T.K. Goldstrich et al., eds. (Plenum, 1992).

Tissue Optics, A.J. Welch and M.C.J. van Gemert, eds. (Academic, New York, 1992).

Photodynamic Therapy: Basic Principles and Clinical Applications, B.W. Henderson and T.J. Dougherty, eds. (Dekker, 1992).

Optical Methods of Biomedical Diagnostics and Therapy, V.V. Tuchin, ed., Proc. SPIE Vol. 1981 (1992).

Laser Study of Macroscopic Biosystems, J.E.I. Korppi-Tommola, ed., Proc. SPIE Vol. 1922 (1992).

Special Sections on Biomedical Optics, A. Katzir, ed., Opt. Eng. 31(7), 1399-1486 (July 1992), and 32(2), 216-367 (Feb. 1993).

V.V. Tuchin, "Laser and fiber optics in biomedicine," Laser Phys. 3(4), 767-820, and 3(5), 925-950 (1993).

V.V. Tuchin, *Laser and Fiber Optics in Biomedicine* (Saratov State University Publ., Saratov-Inotec-Progress Publ., Moscow, 1993, floppy-disk edition).

Principles and Practice of Ophthalmology: Basic Sciences, D.M. Albert and F.A. Jakobiec, eds. (W.B. Saunders, Philadelphia, 1993).

Medical Optical Tomography: Functional Imaging and Monitoring, G. Müller, B. Chance, R. Alfano. S. Arridge, J. Beuthan, E. Gratton, M. Kaschke, B. Masters, S. Svanberg, P. van der Zee, eds., SPIE Inst. Ser. Vol. IS11 (1993).

Biomedical Optics 1993 Proceedings (Los Angeles):

Lasers in Otolaryngology, Dermatology, and Tissue Welding, R.R. Anderson, L.S. Bass, S.M. Shapshay, J.V. White, R.A. White, eds., Proc. SPIE Vol. 1876 (1993);

Ophthalmic Technologies III, A. Katzir, J. Parel, Q. Ren, eds., Proc. SPIE Vol. 1877 (1993);

Diagnostic and Therapeutic Cardiovascular Interventions III, G.S. Abela, ed., Proc. SPIE Vol. 1878 (1993);

Lasers in Urology, Gynecology, and General Surgery, C.J. Daly, W.S. Grundfest, D E Johnson, R J. Lanzafame, R W. Steiner, Y. Tadir, G.M. Watson, eds., Proc. SPIE Vol. 1879 (1993);

Lasers in Orthopedic, Dental, and Veterinary Medicine II, D. Gal, S.J. O'Brien, C.T. Vangsness, J.M. White, H.A. Wigdor, eds., Proc. SPIE Vol. 1880 (1993);

Optical Methods for Tumor Treatment and Detection: Mechanisms and Techniques in Photodynamic Therapy II, T.J. Dougherty, ed., Proc. SPIE Vol. 1881 (1993);

Laser-Tissue Interaction IV, S.L. Jacques, A. Katzir, eds., Proc. SPIE Vol. 1882 (1993);

Low-Energy Laser Effects on Biological Systems, M. Belkin, A. Katzir, M. Schwartz, eds., Proc. SPIE Vol. 1883 (1993);

Static and Dynamic Light Scattering in Medicine and Biology, R.J. Nossal, R. Pecora, A.V. Priezzhev, eds., Proc. SPIE Vol. 1884 (1993);

Advances in Fluorescence Sensing Technology, J.R. Lakowicz, R.B. Thompson, eds., Proc. SPIE Vol. 1885 (1993);

Fiber Optic Sensors in Medical Diagnostics, F.P. Milanovich, ed., Proc. SPIE Vol. 1886 (1993);

Physiological Imaging, Spectroscopy, and Early Detection Diagnostic Methods, R.L. Barbour, M.J. Carvlin, eds., Proc. SPIE Vol. 1887 (1993);

Photon Migration and Imaging in Random Media and Tissues, R.R. Alfano, B. Chance, eds., Proc. SPIE Vol. 1888 (1993);

Holography, Interferometry, and Optical Pattern Recognition in Biomedicine III, H. Podbielska, ed., Proc. SPIE Vol. 1889 (1993);

Biomolecular Spectroscopy III, H.H. Mantsch, L.A. Nafie, eds., Proc. SPIE Vol. 1890 (1993).

Biomedical Optics Europe 1993 Proceedings (Budapest):

Laser Interaction with Hard and Soft Tissue, H. Albrecht, R.W. Steiner, L.O. Svaasand, and M.J. van Gemert, eds., Proc. SPIE

Vol. 2077;

Photodynamic Therapy of Cancer, G. Jori, J. Moan, and W.M. Star, eds., Proc. SPIE Vol. 2078;

Laser Applications in Ophthalmology, S.T. Melamed, ed., Proc. SPIE Vol. 2079;

Dental Applications of Lasers, G.B. Altshuler and R. Hibst, eds., Proc. SPIE Vol. 2080;

Optical Biopsy, R. Cubeddu, S. Svanberg, and H. van den Bergh, eds., Proc. SPIE Vol. 2081;

Quantification and Localization Using Diffuse Photons in a Highly Scattering Medium, B. Chance, D.T. Delpy, M. Ferrari, V.V. Tuchin, and M.J. van Gemert, eds., Proc. SPIE Vol. 2082;

Microscopies, Holography, and Interferometry in Biomedicine, A.F. Fercher, A. Lewis, H. Podbielska, H. Schneckenburger, and T. Wilson, eds., Proc. SPIE Vol. 2083;

Biomedical Optoelectronic Devices and Systems, N.I. Croitoru and R. Pratesi, eds., Proc. SPIE Vol. 2084;

Biomedical and Medical Sensors, O.S. Wolfbeis, ed., Proc. SPIE Vol. 2085;

Medical Applications of Lasers, K. Atsumi, C. Borst, F.W. Cross, H.J. Geschwind, D. Jocham, J. kvasnicka, H.H. Scherer, M.A. Trelles, and E. Unsoeld, eds., Proc. SPIE Vol. 2086.

Cell and Biotissue Optics: Applications in Laser Diagnostics and Therapy, V.V. Tuchin, ed., Proc. SPIE Vol. 2100 (1993).

Imaging of Brain Function and Metabolism, U. Dirnagl et al., eds. (Plenum, 1993).

Proceedings of the International Society on Oxygen Transport to Tissue (Mainz, Germany, 1992), P. Baupel, ed. (Plenum, 1993).

Selected Papers on Photodynamic Therapy, D. Kessel, ed., SPIE Milestone Ser. Vol. MS82 (1993).

Special Issue on Photon Migration in Tissue and Biomedical Applications of Lasers, M. Motamedi, ed., Appl. Opt. 32(4), 367-434 (February 1, 1993).

Biomedical Optics 1994 Proceedings (Los Angeles):

Ophthalmic Technologies IV, J. Parel, Q. Ren, eds., Proc. SPIE Vol. 2126 (1994);

Lasers in Surgery: Advanced Characterization, Therapeutics, and Systems IV, R.R. Anderson, ed., Proc. SPIE Vol. 2128 (1994);

Lasers in Urology, D.E. Johnson, R.W. Steiner, G.M. Watson, eds., Proc. SPIE Vol. 2129 (1994);

Diagnostic and Therapeutic Cardiovascular Interventions IV, G.S. Abela, ed., Proc. SPIE Vol. 2130 (1994);

Clinical Applications of Modern Imaging Technology II, L.J. Cerullo, K.S. Heiferman, H. Liu, H. Podbielska, A.O. Wist, L.J. Zamorano, eds., Proc. SPIE Vol. 2132 (1994);

Optical Methods for Tumor Treatment and Detection: Mechanisms and Techniques in Photodynamic Therapy III, T.J. Dougherty, ed., Proc. SPIE Vol. 2133 (1994);

Laser-Tissue Interaction V, S.L. Jacques, ed., Proc. SPIE Vol. 2134A (1994);

Ultraviolet Radiation Hazards, M. Belkin, D.H. Sliney, eds., Proc. SPIE Vol. 2134B (1994);

Advances in Laser and Light Spectroscopy to Diagnose Cancer and Other Diseases, R.R. Alfano, ed., Proc. SPIE Vol. 2135 (1994);

Biochemical Diagnostic Instrumentation, R.F. Bonner, G.E. Cohn, T.M. Laue, A.V. Priezzhev, eds., Proc. SPIE Vol. 2136 (1994).

Selected Papers

Optics of Tissues with Strong Scattering

Continuous wave scattering

"Spectral transmission and reflectance of excised human skin," J.D. Hardy, H.T. Hammel, D. Murgatroyd, J. Appl. Physiol. 9, 257-264 (1956).

"Penetration of epidermis by ultraviolet rays," M.A. Everett, E. Yeargers, R.M. Sayre, R.L. Olsen, Photochem. Photobiol. 5, 533-542 (1966).

"A note on the theory of backscattering of light by living tissue," R.L. Longini, R. Zdrojkowski, IEEE Trans. Biomed. Eng. BME-15, 4-10 (1968).

"Quantitative evaluation of reflection spectra of living tissue," R. Wodick, D.W. Lubbers, Z. Hoppe-Seylers, Physiol. Chem. 335, 583-594 (1974).

"Measurements on the depth penetration of light (0.35-1.0 μm) in tissue," J. Eichler, J. Knof, H. Lenz, Rad. Environ. Biophys. 14, 239-242 (1977).

"Analysis of diffuse reflectance from a two layer tissue model," S. Takatani, M.D. Graham, IEEE Trans. Biomed. Eng. BME-26, 656-664 (1979).

"A theoretical and experimental study of light absorption and scattering by in vivo skin," J.B. Dawson, B.J. Barker, D.J. Ellis, E. Grassam, J.A. Cotterill, G.W. Fisher, J.W. Feather, Phys. Med. Biol. 25, 695-709 (1980).

"Melanin, a unique biological absorber," M.L. Wolbarsht, A.W. Walsh, G. George, Appl. Opt. 20, 2184-2186 (1981).

"Analytical modeling for the optical properties of the skin with in vitro and in vivo applications," S. Wan, R.R. Anderson, J.A. Parrish, Photochem. Photobiol. 34, 493-499 (1981).

"Optical properties of human skin," R.R. Anderson, J.A. Parrish, in The Science of Photomedicine, J.D. Regan and J.A. Parrish, eds., 147-194 (Plenum, 1982).

"A mathematical model for ultraviolet optics in skin," B.L. Diffey, Phys. Med. Biol. 28, 647-657 (1983).

"Forward scattering properties of human epidermal layers," W.A.G. Bruls, J.C. van der Leun, Photochem. Photobiol. 40, 231-242 (1984).

"A portable instrument for quantifying erythema induced by UV radiation," B.L. Diffey, R.J. Oliver, P.M. Farr, Brit. J. Dermatol. 111, 663-672 (1984).

"Spectroscopic characteristics of human melanin in vivo," N. Kollias, A.H. Baqer, J. Invest. Dermatol. 85, 593-601 (1985).

"Optical properties of human blood vessel wall and plaque," M.J.C. van Gemert, R. Verdaasdonk, E.G. Stassen, G.A.C.M. Schets, G.H.M. Gijsbers, J.J. Bonnier, Laser Surg. Med. 5, 235-237 (1985).

"Penetration of unfocused laser light into the skin," P.J. Kolari, Dermatol. Res. 277, 342-344 (1985).

"A theory of diffuse light scattering by lungs," J.P. Butler, S. Suzuki, E.H. Oldmixon, F.G. Hoppin, J. Appl. Physiol. 58, 89-96 (1985).

"Light scattering by lungs correlates with stereologic measurements," S. Suzuki, J.P. Butler, E.H. Oldmixon, F.G. Hoppin, J. Appl. Physiol. 58, 97-104 (1985).

"Spectroscopic characteristics of rat skeletal and cardiac tissues in the visible and near-infrared region," M. Tamura, A. Seiyama, O. Hazeki, Adv. Exp. Med. Biol. 215, 297-300 (1986).

"Absorption mechanisms of human melanin in the visible, 400-720 nm," N. Kollias, A.H. Baqer, J. Invest. Dermatol. 89, 384-388 (1987).

"A study of the three-dimensional distribution of light (632.8 nm) in tissue," F.P. Bolin, L.E. Preuss, R.C. Taylor, T.S. Sandu, IEEE J.

Quantum. Electron. QE-23, 1734-1738 (1987).

"Quantitative evaluation of optical reflection spectra of blood-free perfused guinea pig brain using a nonlinear multicomponent analysis," U. Heiurich, J. Hoffmann, D.W. Lubbers, Pflugers Arch. 409, 152-157 (1987).

"Practical models for light distribution in laser irradiated tissue," A.J. Welch, G. Yoon, M.J.C. van Gemert, Laser Surg. Med. 6, 488-493 (1987).

"Relations between the Kubelka-Munk and the transport equation models for anisotropic scattering," M.J.C. van Gemert, W.M. Star, Lasers Life Sci. 1, 287-298 (1987).

"Tissue optics for slab geometry in the diffusion approximation," M.J.C. van Gemert, A.J. Welch, W.M. Star, M. Motamedi, W.F. Cheong, Lasers Med. Sci. 2, 295-302 (1987).

"Angular dependence of the He-Ne laser light scattering by human dermis," S.L. Jacques, C.A. Alter, S.A. Prahl, Lasers Life. Sci. 1, 309-333 (1987).

"Model for photon migration in turbid biological media," R.F. Bonner, R. Nossal, S. Havlin, G.H. Weiss, J. Opt. Soc. Am. A4, 423-432 (1987).

"Indirect versus direct techniques for the measurement of the optical properties of tissues," B.C. Wilson, M.S. Patterson, S.T. Flock, Photochem. Photobiol. 46. 601-608 (1987).

"Total attenuation coefficients and scattering phase functions of tissues and phantom materials at 633 nm," S.F. Flock, B.C. Wilson, M.S. Patterson, Med. Phys. 14, 835-841 (1987).

"Determination of absorption and scattering coefficients from diffuse transmission measurement," G. Yoon, W.F. Cheong, A.J. Welch, Lasers Surg. Med. 7, 71-77 (1987).

"Light propagation in human tissues: the physical origin of the inhomogeneous scattering mechanisms," W.E. Blumberg, Biophys. J. 51, 288a-295a (1987).

"Simulation of the point spread function for light in tissue by a Monte Carlo method," P. van der Zee, D.T. Delpy, Adv. Exp. Med. Biol. 215, 179-192 (1987).

"Computed point spread functions for light in tissue," P. van der Zee, D.T. Delpy, Adv. Exp. Med. Biol. 222, 191-197 (1988).

"Optics of tissue in multi-layer slab geometry," M.J.C. van Gemert, G.A.C.M. Schets, M.S. Bishop et al., Lasers Life Sci. 2, 1-18 (1988).

"Spectral properties of human atherosclerotic blood vessel walls," A.A. Oraevsky, V.S. Letokhov, S.E. Ragimov, V.G. Omel'yanenko, A.A. Belyaev, B.V. Shekhonin, R.S. Akchurin, Lasers Life Sci. 2, 275-288 (1988).

"Measurement of rat brain spectra," B. Hagihara, N. Okutani, M. Nishioka, N. Negayama, W. Ohtani, S. Takamura, K. Oka, Adv. Exp. Med. Biol. 222, 351-357 (1988).

"Optical diffusion in layered media," M. Keijzer, W.M. Star, P.R.M. Storchi, Appl. Opt. 27, 1820-1824 (1988).

"Optical propagation in tissue with anisotropic scattering,," M.R. Arnfield, J. Tulip, M.S. McPhee, IEEE Trans. Biomed. Eng. BME-35, 372-381 (1988).

"Light dosimetry in optical phantoms and in tissues: I. Multiple flux and transport theory," W.M. Star, J.P.A. Marijnissen, M.J.C. van Gemert, Phys. Med. Biol. 33, 437-454 (1988).

"Reflection and transmission of light from the esophagus: The influence of incident angle," N.S. Nishioka, S.L. Jacques, J.M. Richter, R.R. Anderson, Gastroenterology 94, 1180-1185 (1988).

"Statistics of penetration depth of photons reemitted from irradiated tissue," G.H. Weiss, R. Nossal, R.F. Bonner, J. Mod. Opt. 36, 349-359 (1989).

"Approximate theory of photon migration in a two-layer medium," H. Taitelbaum, S. Havlin, G.H. Weiss, Appl. Opt. 28, 2245-2249 (1989).

"Applications of the 1-D diffusion approximation to the optics of tissues

and tissue phantoms," J.L. Karagiannes, Z. Zhang, B. Grossweiner, L.I. Grossweiner, Appl. Opt. 28, 2311-2317 (1989).

"Comparing the P3-approximation with diffusion theory and with Monte Carlo calculations of light propagation in a slab geometry," W.M. Star, in Dosimetry of Laser Radiation in Medicine and Biology, SPIE Inst. Ser. IS5, 146-154 (1989).

"The spectral dependence of the optical properties of the human brain," H.J.C.M. Sterenborg, M.J.C. van Gemert, W. Kamphorst, J.G. Wolbers, W. Hogervorst, Lasers Med. Sci. 4, 221-227 (1989).

"A Monte Carlo model of light propagation in tissue," S.A. Prahl, M. Keijzer, S.L. Jacques, A.J. Welch, in Dosimetry of Laser Radiation in Medicine and Biology, SPIE Inst. Ser. IS5, 102-113 (1989).

"Optics of tissue," L.O. Svaasand, C.J. Gomer, in Dosimetry of Laser Radiation in Medicine and Biology, SPIE Inst. Ser. IS5, 114-132 (1989).

"Optical properties of rat liver between 350 and 2200 nm," P. Parsa, S.L. Jacques, N.S. Nishioka, Appl. Opt. 28, 2325-2330 (1989).

"Light propagation parameters of anisotropically scattering media, based on a rigorous solution of the transport equation," R. Graaff, J.G. Aarnoudse, F.F.M. de Mul, H.W. Jentink, Appl. Opt. 28, 2273-2279 (1989).

"Influence of pathlength on remote optical sensing of properties of biological tissue," R. Nossal, R.F. Bonner, G.H. Weiss, Appl. Opt. 28, 2238-2244 (1989).

"Optical radiation interaction with living tissue," M. Seyfried, in Radiation Measurement in Photobiology (Academic, UK, 1989).

"Monte Carlo modeling of light propagation in highly scattering tissue 1: Model predictions and comparison with diffusion theory," S.T. Flock, M.S. Patterson, B.C. Wilson, D.R. Wyman, IEEE Trans. Biomed. Eng. BME-36, 1162-1168 (1989).

"Monte Carlo modeling of light propagation in highly scattering tissue 2: comparison with measurements in phantoms," S.T. Flock, B.C. Wilson, M.S. Patterson, IEEE Trans. Biomed. Eng. BME-36, 1169-1173 (1989).

"Similarity relations for the interaction parameters in radiation transport," D.R. Wyman, M.S. Patterson, B.C. Wilson, Appl. Opt. 28, 5243-5349 (1989).

"Accuracies of the diffusion approximation and its similarity relations for laser irradiated biological media," G. Yoon, S.A. Prahl, A.J. Welch, Appl. Opt. 28, 2250-2255 (1989).

"Measurements and calculations of the energy fluence rate in a scattering and absorbing phantom at 633 nm," C.J.M. Moes, M.J.C. van Gemert, W.M. Star, J.P.A. Marijnissen, S.A. Prahl, Appl. Opt. 28, 2292-2296 (1989).

"In vitro optical properties of human and canine brain and urinary bladder tissues at 633 nm," R. Splinter, W.F. Cheong, M.J.C. van Gemert, A.J. Welch, Lasers Surg. Med. 9,37-41 (1989).

"Multilayer model of photon diffusion in skin," J.M. Schmitt, G.X. Zhou, E.C. Walker, R.T. Wall, J. Opt. Soc. Am. A7, 2141-2153 (1990).

"An investigation of factors affecting the accuracy of in vivo measurements of skin pigments by reflectance spectrophotometry," M. Hajizadeh-Safar, J.W. Feather, J.B. Dawson, Phys. Med. Biol. 35, 1301-1305 (1990).

"Noninvasive computerized analysis of skin chromophores in vivo by reflectance spectroscopy," P.H. Anderson, P. Bjerring, Photodermatol. Photoimmunol. Photomed. 7, 249-257 (1990).

"Transmission measurements on various tissue samples between 1064 and 2000 nm," D. Blanc, M.J. Colles, Lasers Med. Sci. 5, 71-75 (1990).

"Optical properties of normal and diseased human breast tissues in the visible and near infrared," V.G. Peters, D.R. Wyman, M.S. Patterson, G.L. Frank, Phys. Med. Biol. 35, 1317-1334 (1990).

"Optical reflectance and transmittance of tissues: Principles and applications," B.C. Wilson, S.L. Jacques, IEEE J. Quantum

Electron. QE-26, 2186-2199 (1990).

"Gaussian beam spread in biological tissues," L.I. Grossweiner, J.L. Karagiannes, P.W. Johnson, Z. Zhang, Appl. Opt. 29, 379-383 (1990).

"Investigation of skin by ultraviolet remittance spectroscopy," K.F. Kolmel, B. Sennhenn, K. Giese, Brit. J. Dermatol. 122, 209-216 (1990).

"Effect of waveguide light propagation in the human tooth," G.B. Altshuler, V.N. Grisimov, Sov. Biophys. Dokl. AN SSSR 310(5), 1245-1248 (1990) (in Russian).

"Angular dependence of He-Ne laser light scattering by bovine and human dentine," J.R. Zijp, J.J. ten Bosch, Arch. Oral. Biol. 36, 283-289 (1991).

"Optical attenuation characteristics of breast tissues at visible and near-infrared wavelengths," H. Key, E.R. Davies, P.C. Jackson, P.N. Wells, Phys. Med. Biol. 36, 579-590 (1991).

"Monte Carlo modelling of light propagation in breast tissue," H. Key, E.R. Davies, P.C. Jackson, P.N. Wells, Phys. Med. Biol. 36, 591-602 (1991).

"Estimation of optical parameters in a living tissue by solving the inverse problem of the multiflux radiative transfer," L. Fukshansky, N. Fukshansky-Kazarinova, A.M. Remisowsky, Appl. Opt. 30, 3145-3153 (1991).

"Determination of macroscopic optical properties of multilayer random media by remote sensing," R.L. Barbour, H.L. Graber, R. Aronson, J. Lubowsky, in Time-Resolved Spectroscopy and Imaging of Tissues, Proc. SPIE 1431, 52-62 (1991).

"Human tooth as an optical device," G. Altshuler, A. Belikov, A. Erofeev, I. Vitiaz, in Holography, Interferometry, and Optical Pattern Recognition in Biomedicine, Proc. SPIE 1429, 95-104 (1991).

"The propagation of optical radiation in tissue. 1. Models of radiation transport and their application," M.S. Patterson, B.C. Wilson, D.R. Wyman, Lasers Med. Sci. 6, 155-168 (1991).

"The propagation of optical radiation in tissue. 2. Optical properties of tissue and resulting fluence distribution," M.S. Patterson, B.S. Wilson, D.R. Wyman, Lasers Med. Sci. 6, 379-390 (1991).

"In vivo measurement of the optical interaction coefficients of human tumours at 630 nm," I. Driver, C.P. Lowdell, D.V. Ash, Phys. Med. Biol. 36, 805-813 (1991).

"In vivo measurements of laser irradiation in human tissue by small isotropic detector," I. Melnik, R. Steiner, Lasermedizin 8, 73-77 (1992).

"Monte Carlo modeling of light transport in tissues," S.L. Jacques, in Tissue Optics, A.J. Welch and M.J.C. van Gemert, eds. (Academic, 1992).

"Measurements of argon laser light attenuation in the skin 'in vivo' using a unique animal model," Z.F. Gourgouliatos, A.J. Welch, K.R. Diller, Lasers Med. Sci. 7, 63-71 (1992).

"The relationship of surface reflectance measurements to optical properties of layered biological media," W. Cui, L.E. Ostrander, IEEE Trans. Biomed. Eng. BME-39, 194-201 (1992).

"A diffusion theory model of spatially resolved, steady-state diffuse reflectance for the noninvasive determination of tissue optical properties in vivo," T.J. Farrel, M.S. Patterson, B. Wilson, Med. Phys. 19, 881-888 (1992).

"The use of a neural network to determine tissue optical properties from spatially resolved diffuse reflectance measurements," T.J. Farrel, B.C. Wilson, M.S. Patterson, Phys. Med. Biol. 37, 2281-2286 (1992).

"Two integrating spheres with an intervening scattering sample," J.W. Pickering, C.J.M. Moes, H.J.C.M. Sterenborg, S.A. Prahl, M.J.C. van Gemert, J. Opt. Soc. Am. 9, 621-631 (1992).

"Measurements of optical tissue properties using integrating sphere technique," A. Roggan, O. Minet, C. Schroder, G. Muller, in Medical Optical Tomography: Functional Imaging and Monitoring,

SPIE Inst. Ser. IS11, 149-165 (1993).

"Double-integrating sphere system for measuring the optical properties of tissue," J.M. Pickering, S.A. Prahl, N. van Wieringen, J.F. Beek, H.J.C. Sterenborg, M.J.C. van Gemert, Appl. Opt. 32, 399-410 (1993).

"Optical properties of human dermis in vitro and in vivo," R. Graaff, A.C.M. Dassel, M.H. Koelink et al., Appl. Opt. 32, 435-447 (1993).

"Similarity relations for anisotropic scattering in absorbing media," R. Graaff, J.G. Aarnoudse, F.F.M. de Mul, H.W. Jentink, Opt. Eng. 32, 244-252 (1993).

Time-domain approach

"Picosecond laser stereometry light scattering measurements on biological material," J.L. Martin, Y. LeCarpentier, A. Antonetti, G. Grillon, Med. Biol. Eng. Comput. 18, 250-252 (1980).

"Femtosecond optical ranging in biological systems," J.G. Fujimoto, S. DeSilvestri, E.P. Ippen, C.A. Puliafito, R. Margolis, A. Oseroff, Opt. Lett. 11, 150-152 (1986).

"Time resolved propagation of ultrashort laser pulses within turbid tissues," S.L. Jacques, Appl. Opt. 28, 2223-2229 (1989).

"Dynamic effect of weak localization on the light scattering from random media using ultrafast laser technology," K.M. Yoo, Y. Takiguchi, R.R. Alfano, Appl. Opt. 28, 2343-2349 (1989).

"Time dynamics of photon migration in semiopaque random media," P.P. Ho, P. Baldeck, K.S. Wong, K.M. Yoo, D. Lee, R.R. Alfano, Appl. Opt. 28, 2304-2310 (1989).

"When does the diffusion approximation fail to describe photon transport in random media," K.M. Yoo, F. Liu, R.R. Alfano, Phys. Rev. Lett. 64, 2647-2650 (1990).

"Coherent backscattering of light from biological tissues," K.M. Yoo, G.C. Tang, R.R. Alfano, Appl. Opt. 29, 3237-3239 (1990).

"Determination of the scattering and absorption lengths from temporal profile of a backscattered pulse," K.M. Yoo, R.R. Alfano, Opt. Lett. 15, 276-278 (1990).

"Monte Carlo simulation of light transmission through living tissues," Y. Hasegawa, Y. Yamada, M. Tamura, Y. Nomura, Appl. Opt. 30, 4515-4520 (1991).

"Time-resolved reflectance spectroscopy," S.L. Jacques, S.T. Flock, in Future Trends in Biomedicine Applications of Lasers, Proc. SPIE 1525, 35-40 (1991).

"Boundary conditions for a model of photon migration in a turbid medium," D. Ben-Avraham, H. Taitelbaum, G.H. Weiss, Lasers Life Sci. 4, 29-36 (1991).

"Effects of optical constants on time-gated transillumination of tissue and tissue-like media," S. Andersson-Engels, R. Berg, S. Svanberg, J. Photochem. Photobiol. B: Biol. 16, 155-167 (1992).

"Picosecond time of flight measurement of living tissue: time resolved Beer-Lambert law," Y. Nomura, M. Tamura, in Oxygen Transport to Tissue XIII, T.K. Goldstich et al., eds. (Plenum, 1992).

"Quantitative measurement of optical absorbance by time-resolved spectroscopy," Y. Yamashita, K. Ohta, T. Hayakawa, in Quantitative Spectroscopy in Tissue, K. Frank and M. Kessler, eds., Chap. 8, 98-104 (pmi-Verlag, Frankfurt am Main, 1992).

"Spectral optical density measurement of small particles and breast tissues," B.B. Das, K.M. Yoo, F. Liu, R.R. Alfano, J. Cleary, R. Prudente, E. Celmer, Appl. Opt. 32, 549-553 (1993).

"Pulse transmission and imaging through biological tissues," F. Liu, K.M. Yoo, R.R. Alfano, Appl. Opt. 32, 554-558 (1993).

"Light distribution from ultrashort laser pulses in tissue: a simulation study," H.J. Schmitt, V. Blazek, E. Gaelings, U. Haberland, in Quantification and Localization Using Diffused Photons in a Highly Scattering Medium, Proc. SPIE 2082, 114-122 (1993).

Frequency-domain approach

"Detection and localization of absorbers in scattering media using frequency-domain principles," K.W. Berndt, J.R. Lakowicz, in Time-Resolved Spectroscopy and Imaging of Tissues, Proc. SPIE 1431, 149-160 (1991).

"Principles of phase-resolved optical instruments," S.L. Jacques, in Future Trends in Biomedical Applications of Lasers, Proc. SPIE 1525, 143-153 (1991).

"Diffraction of intensity modulated light in strongly scattering media in the presence of a 'semi-infinite' absorbing or reflecting plane bounded by a straight edge," J.B. Fishkin, E. Gratton, in Time-Resolved Laser Spectroscopy in Biochemistry III, Proc. SPIE 1640, 362-367 (1992).

"A laser heterodyning detector for frequency-domain ultrafast spectroscopy," K. Berland, E. Gratton, M. van de Ven, in Time-Resolved Laser Spectroscopy in Biochemistry III, Proc. SPIE 1640, 370-378 (1992).

"Spatial localization of absorbing bodies by interfering diffusive photon-density waves," A. Knuttel, J.M. Schmitt, J.R. Knutson, Appl. Opt. 32, 381-389 (1993).

"Properties of photon density waves in multiple-scattering media," B.J. Tromberg, L.O. Svaasand, T.T. Tsay, R.C. Haskell, Appl. Opt. 32, 607-616 (1993).

"Effect of local absorption changes on phase shift measurement using phase modulation spectroscopy," W. Cui, L.E. Ostrander, in Photon Migration and Imaging in Random Media and Tissues, Proc. SPIE 1888, 289-296 (1993).

Thermal and tissue optical properties modification effects

"On increasing of laser and other radiation transmission through soft opaque physical and biological media," G.A. Askar'yan, Sov. J. Quantum Electr. 9, 1379-1383 (1982).

"Erythema and melanogenesis action spectra of normal human skin," J.A. Parrish, K.P. Jaenicke, R.R. Anderson, Photochem. Photobiol. 36, 187-191 (1982).

"Thermal response of laser irradiated biological tissues," A.J. Welch, IEEE J. Quantum Electr. QE-20, 1471-1480 (1984).

"The change in light reflection of the retina during therapeutic laser-photocoagulation," W. Weinberg, R. Birngruber, B. Lorentz, IEEE J. Quantum Electr. QE-20, 1481-1489 (1984).

"Investigation of the erythema effectiveness curve with tunable lasers," A. Anders, P. Aufmuth, E.-M. Bottger, H. Tronnier, Dermatosen in Beruf und Umwelt. 32, 166-170 (1984).

"Thermal and optical properties of living tissue: Application to laser induced hyperthermia," L.O. Svaasand, T. Boerslid, M. Oeveraasen, Lasers Surg. Med. 5, 589-602 (1985).

"Effect of photosensitizer concentration in tissue on the penetration depth of photoactivating light," B.C. Wilson, M.S. Patterson, D.M. Burns, Lasers Med. Sci. 1, 235-244 (1986).

"A review of the complex phenomena that result when a laser heats living tissue," R.C. McCord, Lasers and Applications 5, 61-65 (1986).

"Different lasers for angioplasty: thermooptical comparison,," N.P. Furzikov, IEEE J. Quantum Electr. QE-23, 1751-1755 (1987).

"Photobleaching of photofrin II as a means of eliminating skin photosensitivity," D.G. Boyle, W.R. Potter, Photochem. Photobiol. 46, 997-1001 (1987).

"About changes of radiation reflection coefficient of layered biotissues during laser coagulation," V.K. Pustovalov, I.A. Khorungii, Sov. J. Quantum Electr. 14, 1718-1720 (1987).

"Change in epidermal transmission due to UV-induced hyperplasia in hairless mice: a first approximation of the action spectra," H.J.C.M. Sterenborg, J.C. van der Leun, Photodermatology, 5, 71-82 (1988).

"Changes in birefringence as markers of thermal damage in tissues," S. Thomsen, J.A. Pearce, W.-F. Cheong, IEEE Trans. Biomed. Eng. BME-36, 1174-1179 (1989).

"Light and temperature distribution in laser irradiated tissue, the influence of anisotropic scattering and refractive index," M. Motamedi, S. Rastegar, G. LaCarpentier, A.J. Welch, Appl. Opt. 28, 2230-2237 (1989).

"Optothermal mathematical model and experimental studies for laser irradiation of arteries in the presence of blood flow," D. Decker-Dunn, D.A. Christensen, W. Mackie, J. Fox, G.M. Vincent, Appl. Opt 28, 2263-2272 (1989).

"Heat generation in laser irradiated tissue," A.J. Welch, J.A. Pearce, K.R. Diller, G. Yoon, W.-F. Cheong, ASME J. Biomech. Eng. 111, 62-68 (1989).

"A theoretical study of the effect of optical properties in laser ablation of tissue," S. Rastegar, M. Motamedi, A.J. Welch, L.J. Hayes, IEEE Trans. Biomed. Eng. BME-36, 1180-1187 (1989).

"A model for optical and thermal analysis of laser balloon angioplasty," W.-F. Cheong, A.J. Welch, IEEE Trans. Biomed. Eng. BME-36, 1233-1243 (1989).

"Physics of thermal processes in laser-tissue interaction," A.L. McKenzie, Phys. Med. Biol. 35, 1175-1209 (1990).

"Thermally induced optical property changes in myocardium at 1.06 μm," G.J. Derbyshire, D.K. Bogen, M. Unger, Lasers Sur. Med. 10, 28-34 (1990).

"Reflectance as an indirect measurement of the extent of laser-induced coagulation," Y. Yang, M.S. Markov, H.G. Rylander, W.S. Weinberg, A.J. Welch, IEEE Trans. Biomed. Eng. BME-37, 466-473 (1990).

"Optical properties of normal, diseased, and photocoagulated myocardium at the Nd:YAG wavelength," R. Splinter, R.H. Svenson, L. Littmann, J.R. Tuntelder, C.H. Chuang, G.P. Tatsis, H. Thompson, Lasers Surg. Med. 11, 117-124 (1991).

"Photoablation," K. Dorschel, G. Muller, in Future Trends in Biomedical Applications of Lasers, Proc. SPIE 1525, 253-279 (1991).

"Monte Carlo modelling of light transport in tissue: The effect of laser coagulation on light distributions," M. Essenpreis, P. van der Zee, T.N. Mills, in Bioptics: Optics in Biomedicine and Environmental Sciences, Proc. SPIE 1524, 122-137 (1991).

"The implication of photobleaching for photodynamic therapy," L.O. Svaasand, W. Potter, in Photodynamic Therapy: Basic Principles and Clinical Aspects, B. Henderson and T.J. Dougherty, eds. (Dekker, 1992).

"Role of temperature dependence of optical properties in laser irradiation of biological tissue," S. Rastegar, B.M. Kim, S.L. Jacques, in Laser-Tissue Interaction III, Proc. SPIE 1646, 228-235 (1992).

"Effect of dehydration on optical properties of tissue," F. Chambettaz, F. Marquis-Weible, R.P. Salathe, in Laser-Tissue Interaction III, Proc. SPIE 1646, 383-390 (1992).

"Temperature distribution in biotissues under CW low-intensity laser irradiation," A.N. Yakunin, Yu.N. Scherbakov, V.V. Tuchin, S.R. Utz, I.V. Yaroslavsky, in Laser-Tissue Interaction III, Proc. SPIE 1646, 161-171 (1992).

"Heating of biological tissue by laser irradiation:temperature distribution during laser ablation," A. Sagi, A. Avidor-Zehavi, A. Shitzer, M. Gerstmann, S. Akselrod, A. Katzir, Opt. Eng. 31, 1425-1431 (1992).

"Dynamic optical property changes: implications for reflectance feedback control of photocoagulation," M.R. Jerath, C.M. Gardner, H.G. Rylander III, A.J. Welch, J. Photochem. Photobiol. B: Biol. 16, 113-126 (1992).

"Changes in the optical properties (at 632.8 nm) of slowly heated myocardium," J.W. Pickering, S. Bosman, P. Posthumus et al., Appl. Opt. 32, 367-371 (1993).

"Computer simulation of surface temperature profiles during CO laser irradiation of human enamel," D. Yu, J.L. Fox, J. Hsu, G.L. Powell, W.I. Higuchi, Opt. Eng. 32, 298-305 (1993).

"Computer simulations for the irradiation planning of laser induced thermotherapy," A. Roggan, G. Muller, Med. Tech. 4, 18-24 (1993).

Optics of blood

"Optical transmission and reflection by blood," R.J. Zdrojkowski, N.R. Pisharoty, IEEE Trans. Biomed. Eng. BME-17, 122-128 (1970).

"Optical diffusion in blood," C.C. Johnson, IEEE Trans. Biomed. Eng. BME-17, 129-134 (1970).

"Transport calculations for light scattering in blood," G.D. Pederson, N.J. McCormick, L.O. Reynolds, Biophys. J. 16, 199-207 (1976).

"The theory of the back scattering of light by blood," G. Eason, A. Veitch, R. Nisbeth, F. Turnbull, J. Phys. D 11, 1463-1479 (1978).

"Recovery of the absorption spectra of oxy- and deoxyhemoglobin from the coefficients of diffuse transmission and reflection coefficients of whole blood," G.S. Dubova, A.Ya. Khairullina, S.F. Shumilina, J. Appl. Spectrosc. 36, 66-71 (1982).

"Precise method of determining blood oxygen content," V.S. Bondarenko, G.S. Dubova, E.A. Mishurov, A.Ya. Khairullina, S.F. Shumilina, Biomed. Eng. 17, 9-12 (1983).

"Optical properties of thin layers of bovine serum albumin, gamma-globulin, and hemoglobin," H. Arwin, Appl. Spectr. 40, 313-318 (1986).

"Diffuse reflectance of whole blood:model for diverging light beam," J.M. Steinke, A.P. Shepherd, IEEE Trans. Biomed. Eng. BME-34, 826-834 (1987).

"Comparison of Mie theory and the light scattering of red blood cells," J.M. Steinke, A.P. Shepherd, Appl. Opt. 27, 4027-4033 (1988).

"Four-parameter white blood cell differential counting based on light scattering measurements," L.W.H.M. Terstappen, B.G. de Grooth, K. Visscher, F.A. van Kouterik, J. Greve, Cytometry 9, 39-43 (1988).

"Flow-cytometric light scattering measurement of red blood cell volume and hemoglobin concentration," D.H. Tycko, M.H. Metz, E.A. Epstein, A. Grinbaum, Appl. Opt. 29, 1355-1365 (1990).

"Absorption and multiple scattering by suspensions of aligned red blood cells," V.S. Lee, L. Tarrasenko, J. Opt. Soc. Am. A8, 1135-1141 (1991).

Eye Tissue Optics

"The physical basis for transparency of the crystalline lens," S. Trokel, Invest. Ophthal. Vis. Sci. 1, 493-500 (1962).

"On the transparency of the storm in the mammalian cornea," T. Feuk, IEEE Trans. Biomed. Eng. BME-17, 186-190 (1970).

"Light scattering in the cornea," R.W. Hart, R.A. Farrell, J. Opt. Soc. Am. 59, 766-774 (1969).

"The transparency of the mammalian cornea," J.L. Cox, R.A. Farrell, R.W. Hart, M.E. Langham, J. Physiol. 210, 601-616 (1970).

"Spectral studies on normal and cataracts intact human lenses," R.B. Kurzel, M.L. Wolbarsht, B.S. Yamanashi, Exp. Eye. Res. 17, 65-72(1973).

"Transparency of pair-related, random distributions of small scatterers, with applications to the cornea," V. Twersky, J. Opt. Soc. Am. 65, 524-530 (1975).

"Quantitative verification of the existence of high molecular weight protein aggregates in the intact normal human lens by light-scattering spectroscopy," I.A. Jedziniak, D.F. Nicoli, H. Barain, G.B. Benedek, Invest. Ophthal. Vis. Sci. 17, 51-57 (1978).

"Fundus reflectometry: a step toward optimization," R. Birngruber, V.P. Gabel, F. Hillenkamp, Mod. Probl. Ophthal. 18, 383-390 (1979).

"Structural implications of small-angle light scattering from cornea," R.L. McCally, R.A. Farrell, Exp. Eye Res. 34, 99-113 (1982).

"Short-range order of crystalline proteins accounts for eye lens transparency," M. Delaye, A. Tardieu, Nature 302, 415-417 (1983).

"Measurement of refractive index in an intact crystalline lens," W.C.W. Campbell, Vision Research 24, 409-415 (1984).

"A new method of measuring in viva the lens transmittance, and study of lens scatter, fluorescence and transmittance," R.C. Zeimer, J.M. Noth, Ophthalmic Res. 16, 246-255 (1984).

"Physical basis of lens transparency," F.A. Bettelheim, in The Ocular Lens: Structure, Function and Pathology, H. Maisel, ed., 265-300, (Dekker, 1985).

"Spectroscopic studies on human lens crystalline," J.N. Liang, U.P. Audley, L.T. Chylack, Jr., Biochim. Biophys. Acta, 832, 197-203 (1985).

"Effects of fibril orientations on light scattering in the cornea," D.E. Freund, R.L. McCally, R.A. Farrell, J. Opt. Soc. Am. A3, 1970-1982 (1986).

"Polarization characteristics of human cornea," I.L. Maksimova, V.V. Tuchin, L.P. Shubochkin, Opt. Spectrosc. USSR 60, 801-806 (1986).

"Laser light scattering by anisotropic binary biological objects (eye medium treatment)," V.V. Tuchin, L.P. Shubochkin, I.L. Maksimova, in Laser Scattering Spectroscopy of Biological Objects, Studies in Physics and Theoretical Chemistry Vol. 45, 611-620 (1987).

"Multiple scattering in the cornea," T.B. Smith, J. Modern Optics 35, 93-101 (1988).

"Light scattering matrix of the eye lens," I.L. Maksimova, V.V. Tuchin, L.P. Shubochkin, Opt. Spectrosc. USSR 65, 615-620 (1988).

"Eye lens proteins and transparency: from light transmission theory to solution x-ray structural analysis," A. Tardieu, M. Delaye, Ann. Rev. Biophys. Biophys. Chem. 17, 47-70 (1988).

"Light scattering from cornea and corneal transparency," R.L. McCally, R.A. Farrell, in Noninvasive Diagnostic Techniques in Ophthalmology, B. Masters, ed., 189-210 (Springer-Verlag, 1990).

"Quantitative photoacoustic spectroscopy of cataractous human lenses," U. Bernini, R. Reccia, P. Russo, J. Photochem. Photobiol. B: Biol. 4, 407-417 (1990).

"The photophysics and photobiology of the eye," J. Dillon, J. Photochem. Photobiol. B: Biol. 10,23-40 (1991).

"IR spectra of lens crystalline," J. Rozyczka, A. Gutsze, Lens Eye Toxic. Res. 8, 217-228 (1991).

"Transmission of the normal and cataractous lenses," A. Bielski, T. Robaczewski, J. Wolnikowski, L. Bieganowski, Lens Eye Toxic. Res. 8, 101-108 (1991).

"Relationships between human cataracts and environmental radiant energy. Cataract formation, light scattering and fluorescence," S. Zigman, G. Sutliff, M. Rounds, Lens Eye Toxic. Res. 8, 259-280 (1991).

"Photon correlation spectroscopy of light scattered by eye lenses in in viva conditions," M. van Laethem, B. Babusiaux, A. Nee tens, J. Clauwaert, Biophys. J. 59, 433-444 (1991).

"Evaluating cataract development with Scheimpflug camera," O. Hockwin, K. Sasaki, S. Lerman, in Noninvasive Diagnostic Techniques in Ophthalmology, B.R. Masters, ed., 281-318 (Springer-Verlag, 1990).

"Scanning laser polarimetry of the retinal nerve fiber layer," A.W. Dreher, K. Reiter, in Polarization Analysis and Measurement, Proc. SPIE 1746, 34-41 (1992).

"Hierarchical structure and light scattering in the cornea,," R.A. Farrell, D.E. Freund, R.L. McCally, Mat. Res. Soc. Symp. Proc. 255, 233-246 (1992).

"Objectified measurements of eye lens transparency in a volunteer group of advanced age, carried out over a period of 3.5 years results of a Scheimpflug-photographic study," U. Muller-Breitenkamp, H. Laser, O. Hockwin, Ophthal. Res. 24, 40-46 (1992).

"Refractive index and axial distance measurements in 3-D microscopy," T.D. Visser, J.L. Oud, G.J. Brakenhoff, Optik 90, 17-19 (1992).

Coherent Light Scattering by Biotissues

"Vibration measurement of the human ear drum in vivo," O.J. Lokberg, K. Hognoen, O.M. Holje, Appl. Opt. 18, 763-765 (1979).

"Surface roughness of acid-etched and demoralized bovine enamel measured by a laser speckle method," R.A.J. Groenhuis, W.L. Jongebloed, J.J. ten Bosch, Caries Res. 14, 333-340 (1980).

"Speckle techniques for use in biology and medicine," O.J. Lokberg, in Optics in Biomedical Sciences, G. van Bally and P. Greguss, eds., 144-153 (Springer-Verlag, 1982).

"Surface roughness of a dental amalgam via laser scattering test," R.N. Konishi, J.Q. Whitley, R.P. Kusy, Dent. Mater. 1, 55-57 (1985).

"Optical quality of the eye lens surface from roughness and diffusion measurements," R. Navarro, J.A. Mendez-Morales, J. Santamaria, J. Opt. Soc. Am. 3, 228-234 (1986).

"Determination of the point-spread function of human eyes using a hybrid optical-digital method," J. Santamaria, P. Artal, J. Bescos, J. Opt. Soc. Am. A4, 1109-1114 (1987).

"Cellular Vibration and Motility in the Organ of Corti," international team for ear research, directors S.M. Khanna and R. Dandliker; head of research J.-F. Willemin, Acta Oto-Laryngologica, Suppl. 467 (Almqvist and Wiksell Periodical Co., Stockholm, 1989).

"Confocal microscopy of ocular tissue," B.R. Masters, in Confocal Microscopy, T. Wilson, ed., 305-324 (Academic, London, 1990).

"Fourier transform method for statistical evaluation of corneal endothelial morphology," B.R. Masters, in Noninvasive Diagnostic Techniques in Ophthalmology, B.R. Masters, ed., 122-141 (Spring-Verlag, 1990).

"Electronic holography and speckle methods for imaging through tissue using femtosecond gated pulses," E. Leith, H. Chen, Y. Chen, D. Dilworth, J. Lopez, R. Masri, J. Rudd, J. Valdmanis, Appl. Opt. 30, 4204-4210 (1991).

"Speckles, and speckle techniques for bio-medical applications," O.J. Lokberg. in Bioptics: Optics in Biomedicine and Environmental Sciences, Proc. SPIE 1524, 35-47 (1991).

"Strukturanalyse der hautoberfache durch computergestutzte laser-profilometrie," R. Saur, U. Schramm, R. Steinhoff, H.H. Wolff, Der Hautarzt 42, 499-506 (1991).

"Tissue perfusion monitoring and imaging by coherent lightscattering," G. Nilsson, A. Jakobsson, K.W. Wardell, in Bioptics: Optics in Biomedicine and Environmental Sciences, Proc. SPIE 1524, 90-109 (1991).

"Some applications of holographic interferometry in biomechanics," J. Ebbeni, in Bioptics: Optics in Biomedicine and Environmental Sciences, Proc. SPIE 1524, 75-82 (1991).

"Micron-resolution ranging of cornea anterior chamber by optical reflectometry," D. Huang, J. Wang, C.P. Lin, C.A. Puliafito, J.G. Fujimoto, Lasers Surg. Med. 11, 419-425 (1991).

"Optic measurement of the axial eye length by laser Doppler interferometry," C.K. Hitzenberger, Invest. Vis. Sci. 32, 616-624 (1991).

"Corneal thickness measurement by low-coherence interferometry," C.K. Hitzenberger, Appl. Opt. 31, 6637-6642 (1992).

"Quantitative holographic studies in biomedicine," R.J. Pryputniewicz, in Holography, Interferometry, and Optical Pattern Recognition in Biomedicine II, Proc. SPIE 1647, 206-214 (1992).

"Confocal microscopy of the in situ crystalline lens," B.R. Masters, J. Microscopy 165, Pt. 1, 159-167 (1992).

"Surface roughness measurements of dental fillings by optical methods," M. Bouchard, M. Doucet, G. April, in Holography, Interferometry, and Optical Pattern Recognition in Biomedicine II, Proc. SPIE 1647, 137-147 (1992).

"High-speed optical coherence domain reflectometry," E.A. Swanson, D. Huang, M.R. Hee, J.G. Fujimoto, C.P. Lin, C.A. Puliafito, Opt. Lett. 17, 151-153 (1992).

"Stress-induced rigidification of erythrocytes as determined by laser diffraction and image analysis," G. Wolf, R. Bayer, D. Ostuni, Opt. Eng. 37, 1475-1481 (1992).

"3-D living cell imaging with high spatial and time resolutions," V.P. Tychinsky, A.V. Tavrov, D.O. Shepelsky, T.V. Vyshenskaja, in Holography, Interferometry, and Optical Pattern Recognition in Biomedicine II, Proc. SPIE. 1647, 96-100 (1992).

"High-resolution coherent tomography," K. Dorschel, B. Messer, O. Minet, G. Muller, in Medical Optical Tomography: Functional Imaging and Monitoring, SPIE Inst. Ser. IS11, 348-354 (1993).

"Holographic studies of the dynamic and structural characteristics of biological objects," O.V. Angelsky, P.P. Maksimyak, Opt. Eng. 32, 267-270 (1993).

"Noncontact determination of skin blood flow using the laser speckle method: application to patients with peripheral arterial occlusive disease (PAOD) and to type-1 diabetics," B. Ruth, J. Schmand, D. Abendorth, Lasers Surg. Med. 13, 179-188 (1993).

"Speckle pattern statistics analysis in human skin structure investigations," D.A. Zimnyakov, S.A. Lepestkin, I.I. Polyakov, V.V. Tuchin, S.R. Utz, in Quantification and Localization Using Diffused Photons in a Highly Scattering Media, Proc. SPIE 2082, 98-106 (1993).

"Speckle interferometry for biotissue vibration measurement," S.S. Ul'yanov, V.P. Ryabukho, V.V. Tuchin, Opt. Eng. 33, 908-914 (1994).

Applications in Diagnostics and Therapy

Photothermal spectroscopy

"Pulsed photothermal radiometry of human artery," F.H. Long, T.F. Deutsch, IEEE J. Quantum Electr. 23, 1821-1826 (1987).

"Measurement of the optical and thermal properties of biliary calculi using pulsed photothermal radiometry," F.H. Long, N.S. Nishioka, T.F. Deutsch, Lasers Surg. Med. 7, 461-466 (1987).

"Pulsed photothermal radiometry for depth profiling of layered media," F.H. Long, R.R. Anderson, T.F. Deutsch, Appl. Phys. Lett. 51, 2076-2078 (1987).

"Pulsed photothermal radiometry in turbid media: internal reflection of backscattered radiation strongly influences optical dosimetry," R.R.

Anderson, H. Beck, U. Bruggemann, W. Farinelli, S.L. Jacques, J.A. Parrish, Appl. Opt. 28, 2256-2262 (1989).

"Opto-thermal in vivo monitoring of sunscreens on skin," R.E. Imhof, C.J. Whitters, D.J.S. Birch, Phys. Med. Biol. 35, 95-102 (1990).

Tissue and blood absorption and scattering spectroscopy

"Determination of the distribution function of erythrocytes according to size by the spectral transparency method," A.Ya. Khairullina, S.F. Shumilina, J. Appl. Spectrosc. 19, 1078-1083 (1973).

"Determination of the absorption spectra of hemoglobin by light-scattering methods," G.S. Dubova, A.Ya. Khairullina, S.F. Shumilina, J. Appl. Spectrosc. 27, 1444-1450 (1977).

"Noninvasive infrared monitoring of cerebral and myocardial oxygen sufficiency and circulatory parameters," F.F. Jobsis, Science 198, 1264-1267 (1977).

"Spectrophotometric monitoring of arterial oxygen saturation in the fingertip," I. Yoshiya, Y. Simada, K. Tanaka, Med. Biol. Eng. Comput. 18, 27-32 (1980).

"The determination of oxygen percentage in whole blood," A.Ya. Khairullina, Vestsyi Akad. Navuk BSSR, Ser. Fiz.-Mat. Navuk N 6, 72-76 (1984).

"Noninvasive monitoring of cerebral oxygenation in preterm infants: preliminary observations," J.E. Brazy, D.V. Lewis, M.H. Mitnick, F.F. Jobsis, Pediatrics 75, 217-225 (1985).

"Non-invasive optical methods for the study of cerebral metabolism in the human newborn: a technique for the future?," P.A. Rea, J. Crowe, Y. Wickramasinghe, P. Rolfe, J. Med. End. Technol. 9, 160-166 (1985).

"An integrated circuit-based optical sensor for in vivo measurement of blood oxygenation," J.M. Schmitt, J.D. Meindl, F.G. Nihm, IEEE Trans. Biomed. Eng. BME-33, 98-107 (1986).

"Quantification of cerebral oxygenation and hemodynamics in sick newborn infants by near infrared spectrophotometry," J.C. Wyatt, M. Cope, D.T. Delpy, S. Wray, E.O.R. Reynolds, Lancet 2, 1063-1066 (1986).

"Role of light scattering in whole blood oximetry," J.M. Steinke, A.P. Shepherd, IEEE Trans. Biomed. Eng. BME-33, 294-301 (1986).

"Reflectance measurements of hematocrit and oxyhemoglobin saturation," J.M. Steinke, A.P. Shepherd, Am. J. Physiol. 253, H147-153 (1987).

"Near infrared spectrophotometric monitoring of hemoglobin and cytochrome aa$_3$ in situ," O. Hazeki, A. Seiyama, M. Tamura, Adv. Exp. Med. Biol. 215, 283-290 (1987).

"Comparison of time-resolved and unresolved measurements of deoxyhemoglobin in brain," B. Chance, J.S. Leigh, H. Miyake, D.S. Smith, S. Nioka, R. Greenfeld, M. Finander, K. Kaufmann, W. Levy, M. Young, P. Cohen, H. Yoshioka, R. Boretsky, Proc. Natl. Acad. Sci. USA 85, 4971-4975 (1988).

"Time-resolved spectroscopy of hemoglobin and myoglobin in resting and ischemic muscles," B. Chance, S. Nioka, J. Kent, K. McCully, M. Fountain, R. Greenfeld, G. Holtom, Anal. Biochem. 174, 698-707 (1988).

"Noninvasive pulse oximetry utilizing skin reflectance photoplethysmography," Y. Mendelson, B.D. Ochs, IEEE Trans. Biomed. Eng. BME-35, 798-805 (1988).

"A near-infrared spectrophotometric method for studying brain O_2 in man during +Gz acceleration," D.H. Glaister, F.F. Jobsis, J. Aerospace Med. 59, 199-207 (1988).

"Methods of quantitating cerebral near infrared spectroscopy data," M. Cope, D.T. Delpy, E.O.R. Reynolds, S. Wray, J. Wyatt, P. van der Zee, Adv. Exp. Med. Biol. 222, 183-189 (1988).

"Characterization of the near infrared absorption spectra of cytochrome aa$_3$ and haemoglobin for non-invasive monitoring of cerebral oxygenation," S. Wray, M. Cope, D.T. Delpy, J.S. Wyatt, E.O.R.

Reynolds, Biochim. Biophys. Acta 33, 184-192 (1988).

"Effects of crying on cerebral blood volume and cytochrome aa$_3$," J.E. Brazy, J. Pediatr. 112, 457-461 (1988).

"Near infrared monitoring of human skeletal muscle oxygenation during forearm ischemia," N.B. Hampson, C. Piantadosi, J. Appl. Physiol. 64, 2449-2457 (1988).

"A miniature hybrid reflection type optical sensor for measurement of hemoglobin content and oxygen saturation of whole blood," S. Takatani, H. Noda, H. Takano, T. Akutsu, IEEE Trans. Biomed. Eng. BME-35, 187-198 (1988).

"Non-invasive determination of venous hemoglobin saturation in the dog by derivative near infrared spectroscopy," M. Ferrari, D.A. Wilson, D.F. Hanley, J.F. Hartman, R.J. Traystman, M.C. Rogers, Am. J. Physiol. 256, H1493-H1499 (1989).

"Non-invasive detection of skeletal muscle underperfusion with near-infrared spectroscopy in patients with heart failure," J.R. Wilson, D.M. Mancini, K. McCully, N. Ferraro, V. Lanoce, B. Chance, Circulation 80, 1668-1674 (1989).

"Cerebral oxygen availability by NIR spectroscopy during transient hypoxia in humans," N.B. Hampson, E.M. Camporesi, B.W. Stolp, R.E. Moon, J.E. Shook, J.A. Grebel, C.A. Piantadosi, J. Appl. Physiol. 69, 907-913 (1990).

"In situ monitoring of organs," K. Frank, M. Kessler, K. Appelbaum, J. Zundorf, H.-P. Albrecht, G. Siebenhaar, in Handbook of Critical Care, Chap. 8, 145-159 (Little, Brown, and Co., 1990).

"Effects of indomethacin on cerebral haemodynamics and oxygen delivery investigated by near infrared spectroscopy in very preterm infants," A.D. Edwards, J.S. Wyatt, C.E. Richardson, A. Potter, M. Cope, D.T. Delpy, E.O.R. Reynolds, Lancet 2, 1491-1495 (1990).

"Simple photon diffusion analysis of the effects of multiple scattering on pulse oximetry," J.M. Schmitt, IEEE Trans. Biomed. Eng. BME-38, 1194-1203 (1991).

"Noninvasive cerebral optical spectroscopy for monitoring cerebral oxygen delivery and hemodynamics," P.W. McCormick, M. Stewart, M.G. Goetting et al., Crit. Care. Med. 19, 89-97 (1991).

"Skeletal muscle oxygenation monitoring by near infrared spectroscopy," R.A. De Blasi, E. Quaglia, M. Ferrari, Biochem. Int. 25, 241-248 (1991).

"Response of cerebral blood volume to changes in arterial carbon dioxide tension in preterm and term infants," J.S. Wyatt, A.D. Edwards, M. Cope, D.T. Delpy, D.C. McCormick, A. Potter, E.O.R. Reynolds, Pediatr. Res. 29, 553-557 (1991).

"Skin reflectance pulse oximetry in vivo measurements from the forearm and calf," Y. Mendelson, M.J. McGinn, J. Clin. Monit. 7, 7-12 (1991).

"The detection of cytochrome oxydase heme iron and copper absorption in the blood-perfused and blood-free brain in normoxia and hypoxia," H. Miyake, S. Nioka, A. Zaman, D.S. Smith, B. Chance, Anal. Biochem. 192, 149-155 (1991).

"Effects of hypoxemia and bradycardia on neonatal cerebral haemodynamics," L.N. Livera, S.A. Spencer, M.S. Thorniley, Y.A. Wickramasinghe, P. Rolfe, Arch. Child. 66, 376-380 (1991).

"Evaluation of a new reflectance pulse oximeter for clinical applications," Y. Shimada, K. Nakashima, Y. Furiwara, T. Komatsu, M. Kawanishi, J. Takezawa, S. Takatani, Med. Biol. Eng. Comput. 29, 557-561 (1991).

"Absorption spectra of human fetal and adult oxyhemoglobin, de-oxyhemoglobin, carboxyhemoglobin, and methemoglobin," W.G. Zijlstra, A. Buursma, W.P. Meeuwsen-van der Roest, Clin. Chem. 37, 1633-1638 (1991).

"Fetal monitoring with pulse oximetry," N. Johnson, V.A. Johnson, J. Fisher, B. Jobbings, J. Bannister, R.J. Lilford, Brit. J. Obst. Gynec. 98, 36-41 (1991).

"Oxygen consumption of human skeletal muscle by near infrared spectroscopy during tourniquet-induced ishaemia in maximal voluntary contraction," R.A. De Blasi, M. Cope, M. Ferrari, Adv. Exp. Med. Biol. 317, 771-777 (1992).

"Spectrophotometric measurements of haemoglobin saturation and concentration in skin during the tuberculin reaction in normal human subjects," D.K. Harrison, S.D. Evans, N.C. Abbot, J.S. Beck, P.T. McCollum, Clin. Phys. Physiol. Measur. 13, 349-363 (1992).

"Experimental and clinical evaluation of a noninvasive reflectance pulse oximeter sensor," S. Takatani, C. Davies, N. Sakakibara, A. Zurick, E. Kraenzler, L.R. Golding, G.P. Noon, Y. Nose, M.E. DeBakey, J. Clin. Monit. 8, 257-266 (1992).

"Recovery from exercise-induced desaturation in the quadriceps muscle of elite competitive rowers," B. Chance, M.T. Dait, C. Zhang, T. Hamaoka, K. Hagerman, Am. J. Physiol. 262, 766-775 (1992).

"Cognition-activated low-frequency modulation of light absorption in human brain," B. Chance, Z. Zhuang, C. UnAh, C. Alter, L. Lipton, Proc. Natl. Acad. Sci. USA. Neurobiology. 90, 3770-3774 (1993).

"Diagnostic potentials of laser nephelometry of aggregating erythrocytes suspension," N.N. Firsov, A.V. Priezzhev, O.M. Ryaboshapka, I.V. Sirko, in *Laser Study of Macroscopic Biosystems*, Proc. SPIE 1922, 133-144 (1993).

Optical imaging and tomography

"Transillumination as an aid in the diagnosis of breast lesions," M. Cutler, Surg. Gynecol. Obstetr. 48, 721-729 (1929).

"Diaphanography: A method for evaluation of the female breast," B. Ohlsson, J. Gundersen, D.-M. Nilsson, World J. Surg. 4, 701-705 (1980).

"Methods of breast imaging," C.H. Jones, Phys. Med. Biol. 27, 463-499 (1982).

"Transillumination of breast tissues: Factors governing optimal imaging of lesions," D.J. Watmough, Radiology 147, 89-92 (1983).

"Fundamental studies of image diagnosis by visual lights," M. Kaneko, S. Goto, T.M. Fukaya, H.M. Isoda, T. Hayashi, T. Hayakawa, Y. Yamashita, Med. Imag. Technol. 28, 83-84 (1984).

"A simulation method for the study of laser transillumination of biological tissues," J.M. Maarek, G. Jarry, B. de Losnac, A. Lansiart, B.M. Hung, Ann. Biomed. Eng. 12, 281-284 (1984).

"Diaphanography in the diagnosis of breast cancer," B. Drexler, J.L. Davis, G. Schofield, Radiology 157, 393-400 (1985).

"Spectral transmittance and contrast in breast diaphanography," A. Ertefai, A.E. Profio, Med. Phys. 12, 393-400 (1985).

"In vivo measurement of breast composition using optical spectroscopy," R.L. Egan, P.A. Dulan, H.F. Staddart, Contemporary Surg. 30 53-57 (1987).

"Contrast in diaphanography of the breast," G.A. Navarro, A.E. Profio, Med. Phys. 15, 181-187 (1988).

"Scientific basis of breast diaphanography," A.E. Profio, G.A. Navarro, O.W. Sartorius, Med. Phys. 16, 60-65 (1989).

"Transillumination imaging performance: a time -of-flight imaging system," J.C. Hebden, R.A. Kruger, Med. Phys. 17, 351-356 (1990).

"Breast cancer diagnosis by laser transmission photo-scanning with spectro-analysis (Rep 4)," P. He, M. Kaneko, M. Takai et al., Radiat. Med. 8, 1-5 (1990).

"Breast biopsy analysis by spectroscopic imaging," C.H. Barlow, D.H. Burns, J.B. Callis, in Photon Migration in Tissues, B. Chance, ed., 111-119 (Plenum, 1990).

"Image reconstruction of the interior of bodies that diffuse radiation," J.R. Singer, F.A. Grunbaum, P. Kohn, J.P. Zubelli, Science 248, 990-993 (1990).

"Diffuse tomography," F.A. Grunbaum, P. Kohn, G.A. Latham, J.R. Singer, J.P. Zubelli, in Time-Resolved Spectroscopy and Imaging of Tissues, Proc. SPIE 1431, 232-238 (1991).

"Image processing of human corneal endothelium based on a learning network," W. Zhang, A. Hasegawa, K. Itoh, Y. Ichioka, Appl. Opt. 30, 4211-4217 (1991).

"The first demonstration of laser computed tomography achieved by coherent detection imaging method for biomedical applications," M. Toida, T. Ichimura, H. Inaba, IEICE Trans E 74, 1692-1694 (1991).

"Photons for prompt tumor detection," R.R. Alfano, P.P. Ho, K.M. Yoo, Physics World 5, 37-40 (1991).

"Imaging through a scattering wall using absorption," K.M. Yoo, F. Liu, R.R. Alfano, Opt. Lett. 16, 1068-1070 (1991).

"Imaging object hidden in highly scattering media using femtosecond second harmonic generation cross-correlation time-gating," K.M. Yoo, Q. Xing, R.R. Alfano, Opt. Lett. 16, 1019-1021 (1991).

"Ballistic 2-D imaging through scattering walls using an ultrafast optical Kerr gate," L. Wang, P.P. Ho, C. Liu, G. Zhang, R.R. Alfano, Science 253, 769-771 (1991).

"A time-of-flight breast imaging system: spatial resolution performance," J.C. Hebden, R.A. Kruger, in Time-Resolved Spectroscopy and Imaging of Tissues, in Time-Resolved Spectroscopy and Imaging of Tissues, Proc. SPIE 1431, 225-231 (1991).

"Time resolved imaging through a highly scattering medium," J.C. Hebden, R.A. Kruger, K.S. Wong, Appl. Opt. 30, 788-794 (1991).

"Reconstruction methods for infra-red absorption imaging," S.R. Arridge, P. van der Zee, M. Cope, D.T. Delpy, in Time-Resolved Spectroscopy and Imaging of Tissues, Proc. SPIE 1431, 204-215 (1991).

"Application of transport theory to infrared medical imaging," R. Aronson, R.L. Barbour, J. Lubowsky, H. Graber, in Operation Theory: Adv. and Appl. 51, 64-75 (Birkhauser Verlag, Basel, 1991).

"Photon dynamics in tissue imaging," B. Chance, J. Haselgrove, N.-G. Wang, M.B. Maris, E. Sevick, in Future Trends in Biomedical Applications of Lasers, Proc. SPIE 1525, 68-82 (1991).

"Frequency domain imaging using array detectors: present status and prospects," C.G. Morgan, J.G. Murray, A.C. Mitchell, in Future Trends in Biomedical Applications of Lasers, Proc. SPIE 1525, 83-90 (1991).

"Two- and three-dimensional visualization of the living cornea and ocular lens," B.R. Masters, Machine Vis. Appl. 4, 227-232 (1991).

"Optical coherence tomography," D. Huang, E.A. Swanson, C.P. Lin, J.S. Schuman, W.G. Stinson, W. Chang, M.R. Hee, T. Flotte, K. Gregory, C.A. Puliafito, J.G. Fujimoto, Science, 254, 1178-1181 (1991).

"Two-dimensional coherent detection imaging in multiple scattering media based on the directional resolution capability of the optical heterodyne method," M. Toida, M. Kondo, T. Ichimura, H. Inaba, Appl. Phys. B52, 391-394 (1991).

"Optical coherence tomography," D. Huang, E.A. Swanson, C.P. Lin, J.S. Schuman, W.G. Stinson, W. Chang, M.R. Hee, T. Flotte, K. Gregory, C.A. Puliafito, J.G. Fujimoto, Science, 254, 1178-1181 (1991).

"Two-dimensional coherent detection imaging in multiple scattering media based on the directional resolution capability of the optical heterodyne method," M. Toida, M. Kondo, T. Ichimura, H. Inaba, Appl. Phys. B52, 391-394 (1991).

"Time-dependent optical spectroscopy and imaging for biomedical applications," B.C. Wilson, E.M. Sevick, M.S. Patterson, B. Chance, Proc. IEEE, 80, 918-930, (1992).

"Evaluating the spatial resolution performance of a time resolved optical imaging system," J.C. Hebden, Med. Phys. 19, 1081-1087 (1992).

"Investigation of the nonlinear aspects of imaging through a highly scattering medium," J.C. Haselgrove, N.G. Wang, B. Chance, Med. Phys. 19, 17-23 (1992).

"Imaging through scattering media with holography," E. Leith, C. Chen, H. Chen, Y. Chen, D. Dilworth, J. Lopez, J. Rudd, P.-C. Sun, J. Valdmanis, G. Vossler, J. Opt. Soc. Am. A9, 1148-1153 (1992).

"Imaging of a translucent object hidden in a highly scattering medium from the early portion of the diffuse component of a transmitted ultrafast laser pulse," K.M. Yoo, B.B. Das, R.R. Alfano, Opt. Lett. 17, 958-960 (1992).

"Relation between light scanning and the histologic and mammographic appearance of malignant breast tumors," O. Jarlman et al., Acta Radiologica 33, 63-68 (1992).

"Diagnostic accuracy of light scanning and mammography in women with dense breast," O. Jarlman et al., Acta Radiologica 33, 69-71 (1992).

"Frequency domain imaging of absorbers obscured by scattering," E.M. Sevick, J.R. Lakowicz, H. Szmacinski, K. Nowaczyk, M.L. Johnson, J. Photochem. Photobiol. B: Biol. 16, 169-185 (1992).

"Evaluation of steady-state, time- and frequency-domain data for the problem of optical diffusion tomography," H.L. Graber, R.L. Barbour, J. Lubowsky, R. Aranson, B.B. Das, K.M. Yoo, R.R. Alfano, in Physiological Monitoring and Early Detection Diagnostic Methods, Proc. SPIE 1641, 6-20 (1992).

"Simulation of time-resolved optical computer tomography imaging," Y. Yamada, Y. Hasegawa, H. Maki, Opt. Eng. 32, 634-641 (1993).

"Laser tomography of heterogeneous scattering media using spatial and temporal resolution," G. Jarry, J.P. Lefebvre, S. Debray, J. Pevez, Med. Biol. Eng. Comput. 31, 157-164 (1993).

"Optical time-of-flight and absorbance imaging of biological media," D. Benaron, D. Stevenson, Science 259, 1463-1466 (1993).

"Spatial resolution in photon diffusion imaging from measurements of time-resolved transmittance," H. Wabnitz, R. Willenbrock, J. Neukammer, U. Sukowski, H. Rinneberg, in Photon Migration and Imaging in Random Media and Tissues, Proc. SPIE 1888, 48-61 (1993).

"A novel approach to laser tomography," E. Gratton, W.W. Mantulin, M.J. van de Ven, J.B. Fishkin, M. Maris, B. Chance, Bioimaging 1, 40-46 (1993).

"Time-resolved transillumination of turbid media," G. Mitic, J. Kolzer, J. Otto, E. Plies, G. Solkner, W. Zinth, in Quantification and Localization Using Diffused Photons in a Highly Scattering Medium, Proc. SPIE 2082, 26-32 (1993).

"Time-resolved optical tomography," J.C. Hebden, K.S. Wong, Appl. Opt. 32, 372-380 (1993).

"Ophthalmic diagnostics using optical coherence tomography," J.A. Izatt, M.R. Hee, D. Huang, J.G. Fujimoto, E.A. Swanson, C.P. Lin, J.S. Schuman, C.A. Puliafito, in Ophthalmic Technologies III, Proc. SPIE 1877, 136-144 (1993).

"Femtosecond transillumination optical coherence tomography," M.R. Hee, J.A. Izatt, J.M. Jacobson, J.G. Fujimoto, E.A. Swanson, Opt. Lett. 18, 950-952 (1993).

"In vivo optical coherence tomography in ophthalmology," A.F. Fercher, C.K. Hitzenberger, W. Drexler, G. Kamp, I. Strasser, H.C. Li, in Medical Optical Tomography: Functional Imaging and Monitoring, SPIE Inst. Ser. IS11, 355-370 (1993).

"Three-dimensional confocal microscopy and visualization of the in situ cornea," B.R. Masters, M.A. Farmer, Comput. Med. Imag. Graph. 17, 211-219 (1993).

"Real-time scanning slit confocal microscopy of the in-vivo human cornea," B.R. Masters, A.A. Thaer, Appl. Opt. 33, 695-701 (1994).

Phototherapy and light dosimetry

"New concepts in therapeutic photomedicine: photochemistry optical targeting and the therapeutic window," J.A. Parrish, J. Invest. Dermatol. 77, 45-50 (1981).

"Dosimetry considerations in phototherapy," A.E. Profio, D.R. Doiron, Med. Phys. 8, 190-196 (1981).

"Laser photomedicine," J.A. Parrish, T.F. Deutsch, IEEE J. Quantum Electr. QE-20, 1386-1396 (1984).

"Photodynamic and photohyperthermic response of malignant tumors," L.O. Svaasand, Med. Phys. 12, 455-461 (1985).

"Instrumentation and light dosimetry for intra-operative photodynamic therapy (PDT) of malignant brain tumors," B.C. Wilson, P.J. Muller, J.C. Yanch, Phys. Med. Biol. 31, 125-133 (1986).

"Optical dosimetry in photodynamic therapy," L.I. Grossweiner, Lasers Surg. Med. 6, 462-466 (1986).

"Dose measurements in photodynamic therapy of cancer," A.E. Profio, D.R. Doiron, Lasers Surg. Med. 7, 1-5 (1987).

"Treatment system for whole bladder wall photodynamic therapy with in vivo monitoring and control of light dose rate and dose," J.P.A. Marijnissen, H. Jansen, W.M. Star, J. Urol. 142, 1351-1357 (1989).

"Spatial light distribution in tumors: Phantom measurements," P. Lenz, Med. Phys. 16, 326-332 (1989).

"New approaches to local destruction of tumours-interstitial laser hyperthermia and photodynamic therapy," S.G. Bown, in Future Trends in Biomedical Applications of Lasers, Proc. SPIE 1525, 325-330 (1991).

"The history of photochemotherapy," R. Roelandts, Photodermat. Photoimmunol. Photomed. 8, 184-189 (1991).

"The role of skin optics in diagnostic and therapeutic uses of lasers," S.L. Jacques, in Lasers in Dermatology, R. Steiner et al., eds., 1-21, Springer-Verlag (1991).

"Light delivery and optical dosimetry in photodynamic therapy of solid tumors," W.M. Star, B.C. Wilson, M.S. Patterson, in Photodynamic Therapy: Basic Principles and Clinical Applications, B.W. Henderson and T.J. Dougherty, eds., 335-368 (Dekker, 1992).

Section One
Introduction

Reprinted with permission from *Annual Review of Biophysics and Biophysical Chemistry,* Vol. 20, pp. 1-28 (1991). ©1991 Annual Reviews, Inc.

OPTICAL METHOD

Britton Chance

Department of Biochemistry and Biophysics, University of Pennsylvania, Philadelphia, Pennsylvania 19104

KEY WORDS: tissue spectrophotometry, tissue imaging, time-resolved spectroscopy, photon migration in tissues

CONTENTS

INTRODUCTION

In selecting my topic, I have chosen to bridge the past and the present with a biophysical theme that is just as viable now as it was in the past.

For this reason, I have chosen the term *Optical Method,* coined by Otto Warburg (138–140) in the 1930s. Many other subjects are left for another time, such as rapid reactions, enzyme substrate compounds, mathematical modeling, NMR studies, and so on. Nevertheless, this prefatory chapter takes the form of a general review of developments of the classical optical method in optical spectroscopy, beginning with and proceeding through its application to organelles and tissue spectroscopy. Cell and tissue fluorometry in vivo and in the freeze-trapped state led to two- and three-dimensional imaging of localized biochemical events. The new field of time-resolved spectroscopy for quantitation of pigment concentration and for imaging is also described.

DEVELOPMENTS THROUGH WORLD WAR II

The optical method is the most robust and best-surviving method of biophysics. It was functional at the outset; spectroscopic studies of Mac-Munn's histohemins (94), Tyndall's dual-beam infrared spectrophotometer (132), Keilin's microspectroscope and then Warburg's "optischertest—optical test" (138–140) were used to detect substrate phosphorylation by measuring the change in absorption at 334 nm that resulted from reduction of pyridine nucleotide. The Warburg spectrophotometer was a masterpiece of optical and mechanical technology of the 1930s. The device measured over a remarkably wide range from the UV to the visible region. In 1934, a duplicate was constructed for Hugo Theorell's laboratory in Stockholm, where I had the chance to study the quality of the design and its execution. I am not aware of examples manufactured elsewhere. Th. Bucher made this instrument much more practical (11, 12).

A parallel development was the pre-war effort of Beckman to build a precision spectrophotometer based upon Cary's quartz monochromator and DuBridge's electrometer. Another method was R. W. Wood's ingenious dual grating spectrophotometer. None of these approaches addressed the problem of tissue spectrophotometry, the pioneer of which was Glenn Millikan (102–104), who adopted Tyndall's (132) principle of the differential galvanometer. By scribing a line in the photovoltaic cell and applying yellow and green filters to the two halves, he was able to measure hemoglobin and myoglobin deoxygenation in the stimulated or ischemic cat soleus muscle. During the war years, he and Pappenheimer (106) showed that red light was more suitable for detecting hemoglobin deoxygenation in the ear lobe using the aviation medicine oximater—the precursor of our pulse oximeters.

Just before World War II, I was able to improve the speed of spectro-

THE POST-WAR YEARS: INSTRUMENTATION DEVELOPMENTS

Spectroscopy of Suspended Cells and Organelles

As World War II ended and the 28 volumes on radar technology were completed (29), I undertook the design and construction of a spectrophotometer that would perform reliably in the observation of cytochromes in suspensions of cells and in organelles (21). This technology began with Keilin's microspectroscope (72) in which he took advantage of the fact that visible light propagated fairly well through suspensions of yeast cells and bacteria that were rich in cytochromes. Many researchers were interested in employing photoelectric spectrophotometry for this purpose, and indeed Glenn Millikan (102–104) pioneered these developments when he showed that some light was propagated through living muscle using a simple dual-wavelength system.

Single-Beam Spectrophotometry

Other workers of importance generally used single-beam spectrophotometry. Bauman (9) was a pre-war investigator, whilst Arvanitaki & Chalazonitis (2) employed microspectroscopy in the post-war interval. Caspersson (16–18) and his colleagues, particularly Bo Thorell (129), exploited the single-beam method for microspectroscopy, particularly of hemoglobin. Lundegardh (93), a pioneer in flame photometry, applied single-beam spectroscopic techniques to bundles of plant roots with originality and enthusiasm, but could not compensate for very large, non-specific changes that occurred in the plant roots during translocation of ions. His bent was so mechanically inclined that he ingeniously zero set the recorder pen, making a mechanical slide for the chart paper rather than inserting a potentiometer. Although the technique generally worked well, some obvious problems were implicit in the method, particularly in the study of the time course of redox changes that in particular cases were found to differ at the α and γ bands of clearly recognized heme proteins such as cytochrome c. Nevertheless, he profited by placing the detector close to the root bundle. Lou Duysens (48) thoughtfully analyzed light absorption of chlorophyll in leaves and pointed to the "self absorption error" in stacked pigments. He, too, developed a sensitive single-beam method. However, dual- and split-beam technologies proved to be superior for scattering material.

The Dual-Wavelength Spectrophotometer

It was quite natural for me, having been a student of Millikan's (102–104) and having constructed a differential colorimeter for rapid reactions used

photometry about 10^3-fold by using the photo-emissive phototube, first made of CsO on Ag and then of Sb cathodes. Not surprisingly, the spectrophotometric apparatus I employed in my first rapid-flow apparatus followed Millikan's design of a dual-wavelength system (19). In fact, my spectrophotometer was a three-wavelength system operating differentially between 430 and 400 nm. At the same time it admitted light to a third detector for measuring in the 630-nm region to detect the reaction product. So it indeed was a three-channel, dual-wavelength spectrophotometer; one channel was differential, and the others single ended. The integral feature of this colorimeter was the first feedback circuit for stabilizing the lamp voltage so that very sensitive single- and double-beam operation was possible. It performed remarkably and could detect submicromolar concentrations of peroxidase with electronic bandwidths of over 100 Hz. Using a six-inch-diameter iron sewer pipe as a necessary magnetic shield, I built what may have been the first cathode-ray oscilloscope used in biochemistry (with the supervision of J. P. Hervey) to record flow studies in sub-millisecond reaction times. For example, the first stopped-flow recordings from 50 ms onwards with a timing error of 10 ms were used to study bioluminescent flashes in 1940 [but compare Q. H. Gibson on the origins of this most useful method (55)]. This sensitivity and speed also allowed continuous and stop-flow studies of the correlations between the kinetics of what is now termed peroxidase compound II and the overall reaction leading to malachite green formation. These studies linked the Michaelis-Menten hypothesis for overall kinetics with those of a functional enzyme-substrate intermediate. These links were quantified by mechanical differential analyzer solutions of the nonlinear differential equations that represent the theory (20).

The precision of low-noise and drift amplifiers in the microvolt range improved greatly during the war years 1941–1946 by the Precision Circuitry Group (29) of the MIT Radiation Lab, which was responsible for the design and construction of all the range-measuring equipment for the many radars produced by the remarkable laboratory, from the well known anti-aircraft radar SCR 584 to the precision offset bombing computer (AOPA44). The radar circuits required the development of several pulse circuits and specialized computers. The general use of microvolt chopper amplifiers and phase detectors (143, see also 29) used by Keithly (Grass Instruments, etc) was of especial importance in precision circuit development. Other developments became part of the new electronics technology, e.g. subminiature circuit assemblies. The electron multiplier phototubes (PMTs) were used as wide band noise generators for jamming circuits and thus put into high-volume production in a form that generated pure "shot noise" and had minimal ion feedback noise.

4

in pre- and post-war studies, to undertake on my return from Theorell's and Keilin's laboratories the development of a spectrophotometer for the study of Keilin's & Hartree's heart muscle particles (74), a research area that had been up to that point almost the exclusive domain of the Cambridge laboratory. It was decided at the outset that the instrument had to be able to scan in wavelength to verify by quantitative spectrophotometry the positions of the absorption bands that Keilin studied with the microspectroscope (72). Second, the work of Lundegaard (93) led to the recognition that the light-scattering properties were unlikely to be constant during the study. The optical geometry itself was a problem because most configurations place the sample near the light source and attempt to collect scattered light at the entrance slit of the monochromator. An instrument was made so that the single sample illuminated by white light was, through a mirror system, imaged onto the entrance slits of two quartz monochromators. Such an attempt was doomed by the small aperture of the Carey design quartz monochromator sold by the Beckman Company. R. W. Wood designed a double-replica grating $f = 35$ spectrophotometer that was put into small-scale production as a commercial colorimeter [see review by Kasten (70, 71)]. This instrument would have been a better choice, but its wavelength range was restricted, the stray light was not precisely determined, and its availability was limited. Without a doubt, the design was well ahead of Cary's ultra conservative design but lacked adjustable slits that could have afforded the variable resolution necessary for resolving cytochrome absorption bands effectively in the visible and near-UV regions.

The obvious next step was to illuminate the two monochromators from the same light source and to combine these wavelengths upon the sample. However, because the highly scattering samples commingled the light from the two monochromators, the proper solution was to time-share the two wavelengths upon a single sample at an appropriate high frequency (60 Hz initially and later 200 Hz), thus achieving phase encoding and allowing the use of phase demodulation circuits. Indeed, World War II experiences with the Brown vibrating reed "chopper" and the appropriate sensitive phase detectors soon provided a system that had adequate spectral resolution and photoelectric sensitivity to cover the necessary range from 320 to 605 nm with a spectral interval of 1–2 nm. A reactant sensitivity of submicromolar amounts of cytochromes with a response time of 20 ms was obtained. A key to this study was, however, the adoption of an optical geometry between sample and detector that was the antithesis of the commercial instruments of that time. Even now, the detector is too removed from the sample to avoid collecting scattered light. In our apparatus, the detector nearly touched the sample and gathered much of the

scattered light, as W. W. Slater (122) also found. For this simple reason, few of the commercial instruments of that time, or indeed of this time, are appropriate for spectrophotometry of turbid materials. This problem was also involved in a contemporary development of Slater & Holton (121) using a British instrument. The dual-wavelength method has undergone few significant changes of technology since then, although the performance has been significantly improved by the employment of a $f = 3.5$ grating monochromator with WI Tungston-iodine lamps or narrow-band interference filters that are rapidly rotated between the light source and the sample, a configuration used early on by Butler & Norris (13, 14), and adopted by us as well.

Several companies all over the world have manufactured this instrument or their perception of it; no patent was applied for because, at that time, the Vice-President of Medical Affairs of the University of Pennsylvania, Dr. A. N. Richards, felt that all medical research should be in the public domain. This is a far cry from the present attitude, and it certainly led to a Spartan existence at the University of Pennsylvania.

The instrument was put to work in the summer of 1954 and immediately produced both controversial and consistent results with respect to Keilin's findings (73, 74). Perhaps the most important result was the clear demonstration of the 552 band in the Keilin & Hartree (74) heart muscle preparation, which was to become known as cytochrome c_1, but had been termed by Keilin & Slater (75) as cytochrome e.[1] But more important was the problem of the sluggish cytochrome b of the Keilin & Hartree (74) preparation, which led me to conclude that the Keilin & Hartree (74) preparation was significantly denatured and that an understanding of the respiratory chain would only come from studying mitochondria directly. This time was exciting in mitochondriology because Lehninger (89), Lardy (88), and Lipmann (92) [to say nothing of D. E. Green's "cyclophorase" preparation (59)] were all attempting to produce material that had achieved the theoretical P : O values of Ochoa (105) and Lehninger (89).

Prominent among the results was the detection of the strong absorption band of NADH in yeast cells that responded characteristically to oxidizing and reducing substrates. These results, presented in a lecture in Germany (42), appeared to significantly stimulate a field of redox chemistry at the substrate level, a topic that would soon be proposed by Klingenberg (76).

In the early 1950s, Gene Kennedy visited Philadelphia in order to test Fritz Lipmann's idea that uncouplers evoked a different cytochrome system. The study was carried out in the hottest part of the summer,

[1]The manuscripts of these findings sent to the Molteno Institute for criticism received, after due delay, the admonition to the young scientist, "never send unpublished works."

and the dual-wavelength apparatus was located in D. W. Bronk's "Physiology Laboratory"—shielded rooms that had little or no ventilation. The mitochondria rapidly died of overheat, as nearly did Gene Kennedy. In late 1953, Al Lehninger, and in 1954, Henry Lardy, Ron Williams, and I prepared a stable guinea pig- and rat-liver mitochondria to measure for the first time spectroscopic and oximetric responses to initiation and cessation of respiration in the controlled and activated states of mitochondria (42). The redox repercussions of these rate changes allowed us to identify the five states of mitochondrial activity, which have subsequently been useful in the elucidation of metabolic control phenomena (23). The fact that cross-over points for the activation of phosphorylation could be identified at the three points in the respiratory chain structurally identified with NADH dehydrogenase, cytochromes bc_1, and the aa_3 transmembrane macromolecules, set the stage for a wild goose chase to find the intermediates that controlled the respiration. On the other hand, it focused attention upon these three components as being not only biochemically different, as found by D. E. Green and others, but also functionally different in their response to the energy coupling process.

The dual-wavelength method also allowed an early study of the kinetics of reduction and oxidation of the components of the respiratory chain of intact mitochondria in many eukaryote and prokaryote cells. These studies afforded evidence for a reaction sequence that was based on Eric Ball's (4) attempts to determine redox potentials and the effects of site selective inhibitors, and/or solubilization and reconstitution of the members of the chain. In fact, the flow apparatus development was improved from the design that had been found appropriate for the peroxidase intermediate and was redesigned to yield a large cross-sectional area of the sample. In 1955, the new flow apparatus was used to study the cytochrome reaction sequence in intact yeast cells at subzero temperatures using methanol as a cryoprotectant. In fact, the parallel studies of mitochondria in their natural state in the eukaryote yeast cell and as isolated from mammalian organs gave credibility to these preparations. My first paper using the optical method in studies of the oxidation of a component of cytocrome b in the presence of antimycin a was submitted to the Paris IUB Congress for verbal presentation in 1952. However, the paper was never presented; the Chairman of the session, Professor E. C. Slater, read a telegram to the President of the Congress regretting the author's inability to present the paper on account of "participatory obligations to the US Olympic Team." However, opportunities to present the data on yeast cells were afforded at the famous McCollum/Pratt Symposium in 1954, and by the presentation of a Harvey Lecture in 1953 (22).

The Split-Beam Spectrophotometer

SPECTRA OF CYTOCHROMES IN CELL SUSPENSIONS A parallel development to the dual-wavelength spectrophotometer was the "split-beam" spectrophotometer in which two samples were employed, usually one in the oxidized and the other in the reduced state. The spectrophotometer scanned the difference between the two and regulated the baseline by maintaining a constant signal throughout one sample by means of feedback of that particular signal to regulate the dynode voltage of the detector photomultiplier. This device was engineered by C. C. Yang (147–149) and turned out to be a workhorse for the many microbiologists and metabolic biochemists who came to the laboratory. One of the important discoveries obtained with this instrument was that of Lucile Smith & Aristid Lindenmayer who obtained the difference spectrum in yeast cells of what was later termed P_{450} (123). A similar observation was made in mitochondrial suspensions by G. R. Williams (42). This work was followed up diligently on a tissue-distribution basis by Garfinkel (52) and in detail by Klingenberg (76) and many others. At the same time, Lucile Smith satisfied her curiosity for the CO compounds of microorganisms by using this instrument on a variety of most interesting bacteria. Out of these studies came a better understanding of the distribution of cytochromes aa_3, a_1, and the discovery of what was to be termed cytochrome o (39). R. W. Estabrook perfected the low temperature spectroscopic technique and quantified the "low temperature enhancement factors" in incisive studies of cytochromes and P_{450} (49). The so-called "Yang machine," was independently invented by Lenart Akerman in Bo Thorell's laboratory in Sweden (40, 110, 129), who sold the patent on this device to the Beckman Instrument Corporation.[2] In any case, the split-beam principle with dynode feedback control became the paragon of many commercial instruments and, indeed, served as the workhorse of this laboratory in many forms that led to a computer-controlled version put together by J. Sorge.

Developments of optical technology important for tissue studies emerged from the laboratory of Dr. D. W. Lubbers (63, 67, 90). The rapid-scan spectrophotometer was the first of its kind and achieved at an early date a performance in rapid recording unexcelled by any similar instruments because of the galvanometer-driven scanning mechanism. This instrument was far too expensive for many laboratories, but enabled a pioneer study of the scattering properties of tissues and the appropriate algorithms for correction of spectral distortions.

Other methods for compensating for scattered light were the opal-glass

[2] Beckman waited approximately a decade to put this excellent principle on the market, presumably because it would have cut sales of the then dinosauer Beckman model DU.

method of Shibata (119), who put a diffuser in front of the detector and achieved good results.

CROSS ILLUMINATION STUDIES The split beam instrument, however, was not very resistant to cross illumination because of the dynode control circuit. A cross-illumination leak would severely offset the baseline. For this reason, most of the photolysis recombination studies were done using the dual-wavelength method, which intrinsically rejected the common-mode effects of cross illumination. Furthermore, it employed only one sample, and thus ensured that the signals at both wavelengths would receive equal photolysis signals. The intrinsic common-mode rejection of the dual-wavelength system resulted from the fact that the light flashes were time shared on a single detector with AC coupling, allowing the system to reject leakage of the photolysis light. Thus, the availability of the dual-wavelength method sensitive to submicromolar concentration of cytochromes with a reasonable time resolution, together with an efficient sample chamber allowing operation at subzero temperatures, afforded an instrument suitable for many problems of photobiology, in addition to permitting a resolution of other vexing problems of that time.

The work of Warburg on *Atmungsferment* (136, 137, 141) critically depended upon the photolysis of the cytochrome a_3 CO compound, whilst Keilin & Hartree (74) could not photodissociate the CO compound of their cytochrome oxidase preparation. Even with the dual-wavelength method, a good cross-filter methodology was needed in which one filter admitted the photolysis light and the other filter admitted the measuring light, the two filters affording mutually exclusive transmission. The favored design was to measure in the region of the Soret band and to illuminate in the region of the alpha band. An appropriate light source turned out to be the carbon arc available from A. J. Rawson's photokymographs, which provided for me, and indeed for Otto Warburg as well, high intensities of red light. This apparatus allowed one to observe at 430 nm the disappearance of this band through intense illumination in the region of the alpha band of cytochrome oxidase CO. With this method, one could not only demonstrate the photolysis and recombination of cytochrome oxidase CO, but also calibrate the values of the extinction coefficient using similar studies of carboxymyoglobin of known characteristics. Thus these extinction coefficients could be compared with those of Warburg with excellent precision and thereby afford not only qualitative, but quantitative, data to show that the cytochrome aa_3 present in yeast cells, isolated mitochondria, etc, had the same characteristics as Warburg's *Atmungsferment*. While these results came too late to be of concern to either Warburg or Keilin at that time, they certainly extended the utility of Warburg's excel-

lent action spectra and furthermore told us that photolysis recombination kinetics can be of great value in the studies of pigments of unknown function, as indeed was taken up in the study of P_{450} by Estabrook & Cooper (49).

The crossed illumination technology developed for the investigation of the CO compounds led to the study of cytochrome kinetics in plants and bacteria at room temperature and verified their photooxidation. L. Smith & M. Baltscheffsky (124) conducted very early studies of this type.

LOW-TEMPERATURE STUDIES The use of cross illumination techniques at low temperatures was more important than at room temperature. Not only was dissociability of cytochrome oxidase-CO at temperatures of −100°C and below clearly demonstrated, but the photodissociability of carboxymyoglobin and hemoglobin was explored (37). Biphasic recombination had already been observed in the 1960s (37). The logical extension of these studies, at liquid helium temperatures, was taken up by Frauenfelder (3) and as a result of observed nonexponential kinetics in recombination, trapped substates were postulated. We (151) explored the selection of substate population by optical pumping. Currently, this is the method of choice for studying a particular set of "slowly recombining species." The study is ongoing in several laboratories at the present time as attested by the active discussions at a recent symposium (51).

FLASH ACTIVATION—THE COMING OF THE LASER The xenon flash lamp had been used in the classical adaptation of Roughton's single-flash ligand-exchange methodology of 1926 by Quentin Gibson (55) and several collaborators, particularly Colin Greenwood (56). However, the time resolution of the xenon flash method is limited by the long exponential decay of the flash, and the advent of the ruby laser signaled a great extension of the time resolution of the flash method. In our laboratory, Schleyer set up a ruby laser (36) and investigated several photochemical reaction kinetics, and DeVault (46, 47) reached the millisecond region at liquid nitrogen temperatures to find that the oxidation rate of cytochrome c in the reaction center of chromatium is temperature independent. Further studies at liquid helium temperature verified this observation, and, for the first time, a truly temperature-independent reaction in the biological system was demonstrated. This independence was ascribed to a quantum mechanical electron tunneling process from cytochrome c to the light-activated reaction center. A simple theory was put forward that led to a calculation of the tunneling distance between cytochrome c and the reaction center of 28 Å (46, 47). Interestingly enough, the X-ray crystallographic study of the reaction-center cytochrome c complex as determined by Michel et al for *Rhodopseudomonas viridis* (101) and by the Los Angeles group for *Rhodobacter* *sphaeroides* (1) gave distances within the experimental error of our initial tunneling calculation. These natural tunneling reactions are much faster than those exhibited by the ruthenium model systems and, perhaps, represent nature's adaptation of appropriate energy barriers to an optimal tunneling process. Thus, the quest of the Warburg/Keilin discrepancy opened in our laboratory and that of many others a whole field of low-temperature kinetic studies in respiratory and photosynthetic systems.

EXPERIMENTAL RESULTS

Photochemical Action Spectra

The Warburg method itself was vastly improved by Leroy Castor who undertook the measurement oxygen uptake with the platinum micro-electrode, which had been well exploited by Bronk and his colleagues, and used by us to determine the ADP/O values of suspensions of mitochondria (42). In this case, focusing a bright spot of monochromatic light on a drop of CO-inhibited cells of a suspension of organelles with an appropriate CO/O_2 ratio afforded large changes of respiration in the drop as measured by the platinum microelectrode. This method yielded important information clarifying Warburg's data on cytochromes a_3, a_1, and $a_2(d)$ and led to the discovery of the protoporphyrin IX-like cytochrome oxidase (cytochrome *o*) that turned out to be an energy-conserving quinol oxidase in many types of cells.

Fluorometry of NADH in Mitochondria and Muscle

The study of other intracellular fluorochromes was reviewed by F. Kasten (70, 71), who has himself contributed to the application of various fluorescence methods in cytochemistry. Two different French groups, led by E. Derrien, J. Turchini, and A. Policard (111), carried out fluorescence microscopic observations of porphyrins in the 1920s. Turchini showed that in different organs and tissues, porphyrin autofluorescence varied according to functional differences. Policard studied fluorescing tissue porphyrins and used Wood's filter to investigate the effects of UV-micro-beam irradiation of mitochondria. However, the study of redox states and kinetics of NADH in living cells originated in the observation of O. Warburg (138–140) in which the solution of NADH excited in the near UV fluoresced at 460 nm and thus could readily be detected in vitro. Duysens obtained fluorescence emission from yeast cells (48), and my studies in Theorell's laboratory with Herrick Baltscheffsky not only identified the strong fluorescence with mitochondrial NADH (340-nm excitation and 460-nm emission) but also verified that the five redox states of mitochondria found using the dual-wavelength optical spectroscopic

method corresponded to five different relative levels of fluorescence intensity (26). In particular, the ADP-activated state 4-to-state 3 transition caused NADH oxidation whilst anaerobiosis caused a reduction. This unique redox response affords a distinction between metabolic activation and hypoxia. Both the techniques of positron emission transmission (PET) and magnetic resonance spectroscopy (MRS) signal glucose uptake and PCr decrease, respectively, and are ambiguous in their responses to these two transitions.

In the 1950s and 1960s, first absorption and then fluorescence methods were applied to the study of contracting muscle because of the intense interest, at that time, in the role of ATP, phosphocreatine, and ADP in muscle contraction (50). First, as I worked with C. M. Connelly (44, 45) and then Jobsis (30), Weber (41), and Mauriello & Aubert (33), we observed that mitochondria in muscle responded in the typical state 4-to-state 3 transition involving an oxidation of NADH within a fraction of a second, for example in gastrocnemius muscles of the toad, frog, turtle, and indeed in the heart of the turtle (115, 116). Thus, the optical method afforded crucial data on the formation of ADP, which could only arise from ATP breakdown at an early point in muscle contraction. Whilst ^{31}P NMR has now clarified the relationships between ADP formation, phosphocreatine breakdown, and the homeostasis of ATP in oxidative muscle fibers (Type I) (107), this demonstration by J. Park and M. Cohn came at a time when the analytical method for measuring ADP was inadequate, phosphocreatine was thought by some to be the primary energy donor, and changes of ATP commensurate with the need for muscle contraction were only obtained in the delicately balanced inhibition of creatine kinase by dinitrofluorodinitrolbenzene in a system that was by no means physiological (15). Here, the measurements of muscle with the spectroscopic method were soon superseded by the greater sensitivity of the NADH fluorescence, which not only showed essentially the same results as the dual-wavelength spectroscopic method, but also gave unambiguous information on the difference between metabolic activation under oxygen-sufficient and oxygen-limited conditions. These results presaged much of the subsequent work on distinguishing metabolic activation from oxygen limitation.

Intracellular Microspectrophotometry of Cytochromes and Microfluorometry

An interest that began at the Old Karoline Institute at Hantverkargatan was inspired by my first-hand observation of Caspersson's well-advanced quartz microspectrophotometry of DNA in tissues. This technique was at that time being extended to the visible region by a young scientist, Dr. Bo

Thorell, to study hemopoesis in reticulocytes. The need to localize optically the intracellular organelle responsible for the redox changes of cytochromes and NADH was manifest in the ongoing studies. This localization required approximately 15 years to effect (128, 130, 131). Two possibilities were presented: (a) that of the Caspersson-Thorell Laboratory (16–18), namely optical spectroscopy of single mitochondria in cells requiring extremely high sensitivity because of the low absorbance of cytochromes in single mitochondria, or (b) an alternative approach of fluorescence microscopy.

This need led us to embark upon the development of microfluorometer for NADH fluorescence that would measure the signals from a single mitochondrion in a living cell and thereby resolve in vivo the difficult question of how much NADH/NADPH in the cytosol contributed to the mitochondrial NADH signal.

In the first in vivo study of NADH fluorescence in a single cell, I chose the mitochondrial aggregate or Nebenkern meiotic telophase of the insect spermatid (33). Here the development led to a completely new track, namely the optimal fluorescence microscope technology for such studies. However, the work of Holtzer et al (66a) of the University of Pennsylvania, Department of Anatomy, on fluorochrome-stained muscle gave many clues as to how the experiments should be done. The use of the 1000-watt water-cooled mercury arc provided a very powerful excitation source; the cardioid dark-field condenser and the high-aperture oil immersion object solved the optical problem, whilst the Brown chopper converted to a vibrating diaphragm in the image plane allowed the phase-sensitive detection of two signals, one from the cytosol and one from the Nebenkern. In studies with Bo Thorell, the covered spermatid preparation became anaerobic in 30 to 40 minutes, based upon calculation from respiratory data, and a transition of increased fluorescence from the mitochondrial aggregate or Nebenkern was clearly observed whilst the cytosol did not change significantly under the conditions of the experiment. This study satisfied me that we were on the right track in our tissue studies and that mitochondrial fluorescence increase would be a sensitive indicator of mitochondrial hypoxia in tissues.

To better visualize the cells, in 1966 Eden & Akerman at the Karolinska suggested the use of dichroic filters for separation of fluorescence emission (blue-yellow) from red light used for cell and microinstrument visualization. Kohen & Hirschberg designed a family of multichannel microspectrofluorometers, first around the Leitz Ultropak and then around the Leitz Ploemopak (64–66). They developed a long-working-distance phase microscope. The development of controlled micro-injection in the laboratory of Kohen

& Kohen has opened the study of enzyme kinetics and metabolic control in single cells (77–80; see also 120). Barry Masters (96, 97) used optical methods of redox fluorometry to measure oxidative metabolism in the component layers of the cornea.

Subsequently, fluorescence microscopy has proliferated in many commercial forms as discussed below, generally using epi or remittance optics for one-sided study of thicker samples, but none has matched the sensitivity of the original method in which only the "autofluorescence" from a single mitochondrion was measured.

Microspectrophotometry

A happy collaboration with Bo Thorell was undertaken. He had one of the clearest visions of what is most relevant and essential in single-cell research, which in microspectrophotometry, was the instrument developed in collaboration with Lennart Ackerman (129, 130). A vibrating diaphragm in the image plane, or later a rotating disc, provided the necessary resolution in time and space. An over-voltaged tungsten light source and a $f = 3.5$ grating monochromator were also used. In Philadelphia, we extended the use of the microspectrophotometer at liquid nitrogen temperature to study the kidney cell. Arvanitaki (2) studied visual pigments of the retina and Thorell studied those of butterflies and flies, which resulted in the identification of three photosensitive (bleaching) and three screening pigments. Thorell collaborated with Langer on the eye pigments of the fly (87).

Fluorescence and Absorption Microscopy of Intracellular Signals with Intrinsic and Extrinsic Probes

Just as in the 1950s, when fluorescence and absorption vied for leadership in the study of mitochondria, they now vie in the study of extrinsic and intrinsic probes, especially because intracellular probes are available for pH, membrane potential, calcium, etc, particularly in thin preparations such as ganglion cells. At the same time, comparisons of intrinsic and extrinsic probes must be considered. The extrinsic probes of mitochondrial function such as rhodamine 123 should be appropriately compared with signals that could be obtained directly from NADH or cytochrome. Although the extrinsic probes are easier to use than the intrinsic probes, they are less safe because of problems of distribution among compartments (cytosol and mitochondrial matrix), confusion of plasma and intracellular membranes, and generalized damage to the membranes by light-activated free-radical generation from extrinsic probes. In all cases, minimization of excitation intensity is required for sample stability, and the dark-field cardioid condenser has so far appeared to be optimal in this respect. At the same time, significant developments in signal acquisition have been obtained, such as two-dimensional silicon diode detectors, microchannel plate detectors, etc. Also, confocal microscope optics have led to a better resolution in the third dimension than has previously been possible.

The development of appropriate extrinsic probes and their delivery to appropriate membrane systems by Waggoner (134, 135), Cohen (43, 144), B. M. Salzberg (personal communication), and others have enabled two-dimensional mapping of membrane potentials in many systems such as ganglion cells. Salama has applied these techniques of NADH fluorescence and membrane potential determination to the ischemic myocardium (117).

In sum, perturbation of cell function by electrical activity and controlled injection of substrates has led to the current research on localized spectroscopy of cell function.

Fiber-Optics Coupling

REDOX STATES AT HPO   The perfection of fiber-optics coupling of excitation and emission of optical signals to the surface of various organs in subcellular preparations has afforded reasonable localization and great mechanical convenience. Examples of this are provided by the fiber coupling of NADH fluorescence signals to remote tissues, for example in studies of the effect of high-pressure oxygen (HPO) upon the redox state of the rat brain. Here, the animal was enclosed in a pressure chamber and the fiber coupling conducted light to and from the brain of the animal inside the chamber through a pressure light coupling. The technique afforded the complete profile of redox states of NADH from zero pressure of oxygen to 5 to 10 atmospheres where convulsions occurred. Atmospheres of 0.02 to 1 were found to allow maintenance of the normal redox state whilst hypoxic and hyperoxic states occurred below and above this region. Again, NADH components of mitochondria provided an indicator not only of hypoxia but also hyperoxia.

INTRAOPERATIVE STUDIES   Other important applications of fiber optic–coupled tissue fluorometry have occurred in the development of intraoperative monitoring of relief of brain hypoxia in adult humans whose arterial oxygen supply was supplemented by anastomosis procedures. In such a case, a two-dimensional image of mitochondrial fluorescence from the brain surface was displayed. In order to ensure freedom from actinic damage to the brain, excitation at the 460-nm absorption band of flavoprotein generated emission at 560 nm. Relatively sophisticated data presentation was available to the surgeons, providing not only a two-dimensional picture of hypoxic regions, but also a histogram display of the frequency of the regions.

Such displays of tissue metabolism can be combined with many electrometric measures of oxygen, potassium, sodium, calcium, and more recently Doppler blood flow affording an optode of relatively small size (100). Lubbers (63) undertook similar approaches for measuring arterial blood chemistry in which the level of many blood constituents are converted into appropriate fluorescence signals by solid-state enzyme systems and the signals coupled to external detectors through fiber optics.

Freeze Trapping—Time Resolution and Localization

In many cases, the time resolution, the localization, and the selectivity of the analysis are insufficient, and the researcher resorts to freeze trapping, as pioneered by Von Herrevald (133). In general, the two-dimensional resolution of microscopy is retained, whilst that in the third dimension is greatly increased because, according to Gayesky et al (53, 54), the penetration in the frozen material may be only tens of microns.[3] However, confocal microscopy can also be called upon as well to determine the depth of penetration. Finally, the depth may be controlled by a technique introduced by Quistorff (27, 28, 35, 98, 112, 113), namely grinding the surface of the frozen tissue with a fine milling head under liquid nitrogen cooling, affording excellent results. Remarkably fast freezing of tissue slices directly from the animal is obtained by the contra-rotating saws of Quistorff (112, 113).

Most important to this method of low-temperature study are two factors: (a) the nonradiative transfers from the excited state are often diminished at low temperatures and the quantum yield of several fluorochromes is enhanced; and (b) the integration time of the method significantly increases because metabolism of substrates is stopped at liquid nitrogen temperatures. However, two limitations arise. First, photodecomposition of the fluorochromes may occur and damage the sample, and second, some reactions are not stopped at cryogenic temperatures, particularly those in hemoglobin that involve nuclear tunneling of ligands such as oxygen to rebind the active site of the heme iron or indeed to become photolyzed therefrom, although the latter is less likely. However, kinetic methods readily verify that the NADH and flavoprotein components at higher temperatures are in an effectively trapped state at liquid-nitrogen temperatures. Thus, the redox state of this portion of the respiratory chain can be preserved for long periods, and it may be assayed at any time without alteration. This technique, while available in only a few laboratories, is often called upon to provide the "gold standard" of the substrate and oxygen utilization in localized regions of tissues in three dimensions.

[3] A crucial test of this calculation with pulsed light is appropriate to actually determine this value directly (see below).

photometric technique in the 1930s occurred in the laboratory of Otto Warburg (138–140) as applied to the spectrophotometry of soluble substances, whilst Nikolai (105a) at the very same time took advantage of the lines of the Mercury arc and the absorption difference spectrum of hemoglobin in visible region (546–577 nm), which were selected with a rotating filter wheel (105a). He further applied this method to the measurement of the kinetics of hemoglobin deoxygenation in skin folds of the human hand using a gas-filled cesium detector, an A/C amplifier, and a rectifier (phase-insensitive) detector. Indeed, this devise was a precursor of Millikan's dual-wavelength detector, which employed the Weston phototronic cell cut into two parts appropriate to the two wavelengths of the Mercury arc. Closely following Millikan was the work of Matthes & Gross (97a) who made a hemoglobinometer that took advantage of the fact that the reduced-blood deoxyhemoglobin is more absorbing than oxyhemoglobin with red light, whilst with infrared light the deoxyhemoglobin is more transmitting than the oxyhemoglobin, setting forth the rationale for NIR hemoglobin in 1938. In 1939, I designed a very fast photoelectric colorimeter using three wavelengths, two to measure the peroxidase intermediates differentially, i.e. using wavelengths on each side of the isosbestic point in the region of the Soret band, and a third to measure the reaction product in the near-red region. This was the first spectrophotometer that employed a cathode ray tube for fast recording of enzyme substrate kinetics. This system has improved significantly since World War II technology in the post-war interval. In 1941, Millikan & Pappenheimer streamlined the Millikan hemoglobinometer to make an ear-oximeter, which again operated on the filter and split detector principle, although in this case they used a tungsten light source. I worked on the employment of monochromators time-shared into a sample containing biological material, initially cell suspensions and later perfused tissues, as well as the innovation of large-area detectors close to the sample to gather large solid angles of scattered light. Lubbers pioneered the way to the "complete" acquisition of spectral data by rapid scanning (92a,b).

The most complete study of spectroscopic responses of absorbers and scattering medium is that of Lubbers and coworkers, who constructed a mirror galvanometer scanner for a split-beam spectrophotometer. The split-beam spectral scan was accomplished in 10 ms, and with the dual-wavelength time-sharing instrument the scan was accomplished in 20 μs. Dynode feedback was used to obtain uniform sensitivity over the spectral region, affording logarithmic transformation to give absorbancy recording. The recording was serial—photography, magnetic tape, and finally on-line computers were used. Considerable attention was paid to the multicomponent analysis of the data, taking into account the inhomo-

This method has been used to produce a three-dimensional image of the progression of spreading depression in the gerbil brain, or of infarcts in a perfused heart caused by LAD occlusion (28, 61, 62, 114). It has been of further value in analyzing redox gradients in the acinus of animal liver. It has been used to record the progressive deoxygenation of the hemoglobin preceding the appearance of reduced absorption bands of cytochromes in a progressive transition from normoxia to hypoxia in gerbil brain. The absorption bands of cytochromes did not appear until the inspired oxygen was less than 5% (5–8). These observations of course could be localized to different portions of the brain, although they were not in that particular study. Finally, the results controverted previous ideas of the fuzziness of the border zone in LAD occlusion models and showed a close correlation of measures of NADH fluorescence and analytical biochemistry of the redox gradient from the ischemic tissue to the surrounding normoxic tissue in distances on the surface of the myocardium of approximately 100 μ.

Tissue Oxygen Gradients

Thus, the dimensions of tissue oxygen gradients and the present concept of localized hypoxic-ischemic tissue volumes emerged and were confirmed by spectroscopic studies of highly correlated or coherent deoxygenation of myoglobin and reduction of cytochrome oxidase in the crystalloid-perfused myocardium in a normoxic to anoxic transition (24).

The use of multidiode arrays as detectors of optical signals is now a popular technology and also affords a tomography of optical events (117). Because large signals are required by the silicon diode arrays usually employed, monitoring of signals from extrinsic probes such as voltage-sensitive or Ca^{2+}-sensitive dyes is usually employed.

TISSUE IMAGING IN VIVO

While freeze trapping was used in the above study of an organ in vivo, the imaging of localized regions of substrate or oxygen deficiency in a two- or three-dimensional display in vivo has been a goal of many laboratories, particularly in view of the need for identification of tissue heterogeneity, i.e. regions of the tissue that respond differently to these deficiencies because of their differing functional activities. A particularly striking success is that of Grinvald in imaging the columnar structures of the visual cortex (60, 91).

Spectroscopy of Hemoglobin in Tissues

The history of the development of tissue hemoglobinometry is an especially important aspect of the optical method. Early developments of the spectro-

geneous distribution of the pigments. The effective light scattering was quantitated by the pathlength distribution functions, which gave satisfactory results in several cases. Monte Carlo distributions and Kubelk-Munck (80a) theories were employed to derive an algorithm in which the information content of the spectrum of a single component in a mixture of spectra could be deconvoluted. This was applied in detail to the redox state of the respiratory chain (10a). Using the visible light (570–580) and a multifiber optical probe, Kessler (99) obtained a multichannel analysis of heterogeneity of hemoglobin oxygenation on the myocardium in both animal models and in humans intraoperatively. In this case, the multiple channels are time-shared outputs from a fiber probe several mm in diameter. The output is displayed as a histogram and illustrates significant heterogeneity of the surface of the myocardium under pathological conditions.

The dual-wavelength spectroscopy of hemoglobin and cytochrome in the animal brain has been most successful in recording the response to local stimulation using a single input-output fiber coupling of wavelengths in the 590- to 605-nm region (86). The response to stimulation corresponds to a decrease of absorption at 605 nm under normoxic conditions and an increase under hypoxic conditions and is thus regarded as an indicator of oxygen sufficiency in tissues. The signal is attributed to cytochrome oxidase, but as we see from Grinvald's (60, 91) data, a massive change of blood volume occurs upon stimulation of neurons and the optical path length is also varied. Thus, a careful deconvolution is necessary.

The Deep-Red or Near-Infrared Spectroscopy

The use of deep-red, near-infrared, and infrared light in tissue spectroscopy originated in the study of bacterial photosynthesis (48), was adapted to plant materials by Butler & Norris (13, 14), and showed a clear spectrum of the hemoglobin/myoglobin of the human hand. Jobsis (68, 69) pioneered the use of these wavelengths to study the absorption of the copper component of cytochrome oxidase in the region of 830 nm, in particular in animal models (cat) and in the heads of neonates in what he termed "transcranial spectroscopy." He further developed algorithms based upon fluorocarbon-perfused cat brain that gave optical path lengths that were believed to be transferable to the neonate brain and thus allow a deconvolution of hemoglobin volume and saturation changes from those of cytochrome oxidase signals using a four-wavelength algorithm. Delpy and coworkers (145) and others constructed similar instruments with related algorithms. However, the striking and indeed puzzling feature of the data has been the close correlation of the changes of hemoglobin and cytochrome copper in hypoxia, leading to the initial suggestions that brain

mitochondria contained a low-affinity cytochrome oxidase that responds to tissue pO_2 similar to that of hemoglobin. Indeed, Delpy has published cytochrome changes in response to variation of high pO_2s that also correlated with the hemoglobin changes. Isolation and prior study of brain mitochondria did not bear out this contention, and the freeze-trapped brain failed to show reduced cytochrome c in either normoxia or mild hypoxic stress. The absorption band of reduced cytochrome c was not observed until the doublet band of oxyhemoglobin was no longer detectable.

Time-Resolved Spectroscopy Techniques

A resolution of this apparently irresolvable discrepancy came, as might be expected, from a very different line of research. Pulse-time spectroscopy afforded two key technologies:

PULSE-TIME STUDIES   Pulse light technology is well known in biophysics for measuring very rapid reactions in gaseous ligand exchange, photobiology, and fluorescence life-time studies. Further developments of time-resolved spectroscopy (TRS) led to the use of liquid dye lasers capable of 100-MW tunable power generation, and detector developments led to the single-photon steak camera responsive in the picosecond (10^{-12} s) region.

PHASE MODULATION   At the same time, Weber's & Spencer's (125) phase modulation technology was extended to the gigahertz region by Lakowitz & Gratton (57, 58, 82–85), who used the microchannel plate photomultiplier as a detector. These ultra-fast technologies led to many kinetic studies of fast reactions and to life-time studies of multicomponent fluorochromes.

TRS OF TISSUES   These methods permitted a test in late 1987 (25, 34, 38) of the time-resolved spectroscopy or path length of photon migration in the animal brain, either perfused with crystalloid or containing hemoglobin. The input-output time delays greatly exceeded those corresponding to the linear distance between light input and light collection points. Furthermore, the time delay decreased when deoxyhemoglobin was present and absorbed light. The explanation of this result, and indeed of the results of Jobsis (68) and others, lay in the time course of photon arrival at the receiver. The received waveform rises to a peak with a time delay slightly greater than the input-output spacing and falls in an exponential decay; the overall response approximates that of a resistance capacitance network to an impulse function. What was remarkable was the effect of a specific absorber such as hemoglobin upon the decay constant; the intensity decay or the exponential decay rate was proportional to the absorber concentration. In fact, the simple relation

$$\frac{1}{L}\log I = \varepsilon C$$

appears to express the Beer-Lambert law for time resolved spectroscopy. Thus, the path length does decrease with absorber concentration. The values of path length from 10 to 20 cm are observed in dog and human brain, respectively, and these path lengths shorten with increased Hb absorption, for example, at 760 nm, or when the blood volume increases, for example, at 800 nm, an isosbestic point in the Hb/HbO_2 spectrum. Another important result was that the optical path length was greater when the brain was encased in the skull. These phenomena are consistent with theories of photon migration in highly scattering media by random walk or diffusion processes (108, 109). The absorption of migrating photons indeed shortens the path length and, in fact, the equations for photon migration show that at long times, the exponential decay predominates, whilst the delay at the peak of the pulse output is attributable mainly to the scattering factor, μ_s, and very little to μ_a, the absorption coefficient. Thus theory and experiment seem strongly correlated. Here, using imaging studies may be more meaningful because the path length is highly determined and the penetration depth appears to follow a simple banana-like figure between input and output as indicated by Monte Carlo computer modeling. To provide multipoint optical coupling for imaging studies, multi-input streak cameras or a 16-anode multichannel plate PMT have been employed.

Phase and Amplitude Modulation

The bulkiness and precision alignment of the optical pump for the liquid dye laser and the complexity of the single-photon counting system is not currently appropriate to critical care, especially under intraoperative conditions as has been possible with the continuous light spectrophotometers and fluorometers.

The photon migration in tissue not only increases the time delay between a pulse input and output but also shifts the phase and amplitude of the received signal, providing the oscillation frequency of the light input is in the correct range or is varied through an appropriate range of values according to the usual equations between phase shift and oscillator frequency (57, 84). By using 220-MHz modulation of 3-MW laser diodes in the appropriate region for measuring hemoglobin absorption (754 and 816 nm), a simple portable phasemeter has been constructed and employed in a series of studies of adults' and neonates' heads, arms, and legs (25).

The reference carrier is coupled to dynode No. 2 of the squirrel cage type of photomultiplier. This modulation is efficient at 220 MHz. The use of two or more laser diodes is made possible by oscillator frequencies that are 10–20 kHz offset from the reference frequency. These features, combined with amplitude-insensitive phase detection, afford a system that is reproducible to 1 mm of path length and has a drift of 0.5 mm/h. The path lengths measured in vivo are 15–30 cm (the mean value for seven adult human heads is 21 ± 3 mm) when the input-output fiber separation is 6 cm. Direct calculation of the deoxyhemoglobin content for the brain using a dual-wavelength phase modulation system gives 20 μM for several subjects. This instrument has most recently been applied to the study of optical path length increases in developing neonate brain (81), and the expected increase of photon migration path with increasing age was found. These results emphasize the need for direct determination of the optical path length in the particular brain under study; the transferability from animal models to human brain is probably invalid, and transferability among neonates of different head sizes has yet to be demonstrated (10).

At this point, the dual-wavelength method of TRS and PMS (phase modulation spectroscopy) provides a new and greatly extended usefulness of quantitative tissue spectroscopy.

Imaging

Several laboratories have considered the problem of obtaining images of objects within tissues such as the brain using photon migration. Two general solutions emerge: First, no image can be obtained from the scattered light; it should be eliminated and only coherent rays should be obtained by selecting those photons that make either the shortest trip or those that do not loose coherence from input to output. Thus a CT type of algorithm may be employed for image reconstruction. This idea has been pursued in several laboratories, particularly by Callis at Seattle (142), Alfano at New York (150), Yamashita et al at Hamamatsu (146), and Tamura et al at Sapporo (126, 127). Obviously, these solutions will require high-power light inputs and will operate most effectively over short distances, particularly in animal models such as the rat brain. H. Inaba (personal communication) has employed heterodyne mixing at the optical frequency to ensure that only those light rays of near-zero phase shift are measured. Again, the direct ray is detected.

The second method approaches the more difficult topic of imaging by means of the probability functions for photon migration between a variety of object points on, for example, the adult human brain. As shown early on, an absorbing object such as a tube containing deoxyhemoglobin placed within a bowl of highly scattering yeast would give not only shorter path lengths for photon migration proximal to the absorbing object but also absorbing object would give decays that suggested that the shorter path–length photons that passed through the object had a more rapid rate of decay than those that took longer paths that did not include the object to the same degree. This stimulated the study of imaging with phase modulation, initially at the University of Pennsylvania where edge resolution of approximately 1 cm was obtained for an absorbing object of several-cm dimension within a larger-diameter object (14 cm). An anomaly was observed in that the edge resolution, i.e. the steepness of the edge, seemed to be better at 97 MHz than at 220 MHz. Joint experiments done with Gratton, in which mechanical scanning of a fiber optic setup on each side of a large volume of intralipid, or indeed brain tissue, within which an absorbant object was placed, suggested that the spatial resolution at 100 MHz could be at least 0.5 cm (31). In addition, Gratton indicated that this high resolution results from advancing wavefronts of 100-MHz-amplitude modulated light of wavelengths of 2–6 cm as computed from a diffusion equation from photon migration.

Studies of photon migration using Monte Carlo methods (108, 109; B. Chance & J. S. Leigh, in preparation) simulated photon migration in a vessel containing an absorbing object. We observed: (a) that paths in a channel between the absorbing object and the periphery of the vessel are highly unfavored, i.e. photons can become absorbed in the object and can escape the system completely at the periphery of the object and (b) that photon migration paths "around/behind" the absorbing object are highly feasible (32).

Algorithms

The simplest algorithm for image formation is simply to subtract migration pathways before and after inserting the absorbing object. These give high contrast and a ready solution. Also, experimental and theoretical (Monte Carlo) simulations may be matched. It is not known at present how much needs to be assumed about the object to reconstruct the image of an object without a prior baseline. This topic is being actively pursued by several laboratories from the experimental and the theoretical standpoints. It is indeed satisfying to note that a new field of tissue optics is emerging.

Problem for the Future

The possibilities for localization of inhomogeneities of pigment distribution, for example hemoglobin in stroke and head injury, are pointed to by studies of model systems in which resolutions currently of half a cen-

timeter are obtainable at a frequency of 100 MHz. Presumably, the power-ful algorithms of data analysis employed to improve magnetic resonance imaging (MRI) images can also be applied here. Furthermore, microscopic imaging with frequencies in the GHz region seem possible.

An important application of optical imaging is the evoked activation of oxygen delivery to functional volumes of the exposed primate and feline brain in response to crossed-field stimulation of the visual cortex (60). In this case, the region of the columnar structure can be imaged in terms of measured blood-flow volume (91). Although this image can be identified through the dura, time-resolved technology may be required for non-invasive studies through skin and skull.

SUMMARY

I have traced the development of the optical method from Millikan's colorimetry of cat muscle myoglobin to today's high-frequency laser diode time-resolved phase modulation system study of hemoglobin and myoglobin in muscle and brain in adult humans. The path length as well as specific absorption information is obtained in terms of the rate of photon decay or by equivalent measurements using phase modulation. Localization of inhomogeneities of deoxyhemoglobin concentrations in stroke and head injury appears possible.

ACKNOWLEDGMENT

The rapid progress on image formation in several laboratories testified to the vigor and versatility of the optical method at the cutting edge of biophysical science. This development has required the collaboration of the many gifted colleagues mentioned in this text and to many others not mentioned. It has been most gratifying to have been able to play a role in the development of these frontiers of biophysics. This work is currently supported in part by NIH grants HL 44125 and NS 27346.

Literature Cited

1. Allen, J. P., Feher, G., Yeates, T. O., Komiya, H., Rees, D. C. 1987. *Proc. Natl. Acad. Sci. USA* 84: 5730
2. Arvanitaki, A., Chalazonitis, N. 1947. *Arch. Intern. Physiol.* 54: 406
3. Austin, R. H., Beeson, K. W., Eisenstein, L., Frauenfelder, H., Gunsalus, T. S., Marshall, V. 1975. *Biochemistry* 14: 5355
4. Ball, E. C., Chen, T. T. 1933. *J. Biol. Chem.* 107: 767
5. Barlow, C. H., Harden, W. R., Harken, A. H., Simson, M. B, Haselgrove, J. C., et al. 1979. *Crit. Care Med.* 7: 402
6. Barlow, C. H., Harken. A. H., Chance, B. 1977. *Ann. Surg.* 186: 737
7. Bashford, C. L., Barlow, C. H., Chance, B., Haselgrove, J. 1980. *FEBS Lett.* 113: 78
8. Bashford, C. L., Chance, B., Lloyd, D., Poole, R. K. 1980. *Biophys. J.* 29: 1
9. Bauman, N. 1939. *Cold Spring Harbor Symp. Quant. Biol.*
10. Benaron, D. A., Gwiazdowski, S,

10a. Kurth, C. D., Steven, J., Delivoria-Papadopoulos, M., Chance, B. 1990. *Ann. Int. Conf. IEEE Med. Biol.* 12: 1117
11. Bruley, D., Bicher, H. I., Reneau. D. 1984. In *Oxygen Transport to Tissue VI*, p. 555. New York: Plenum
12. Bücher, T. 1989. *Biochim. Biophys. Acta* 1000: 223
13. Bücher, T. 1947. *Biochim. Biophys. Acta* 1: 292
13. Butler, W. L. 1972. *Methods Enzymol.* 23: 3
14. Butler, W. L., Norris, K. H. 1960. *Arch. Biochem. Biophys.* 87: 31; See also 1977. In *The Science of Photobiology*, ed. K. C. Smith, p. 400. New York: Plenum
15. Cain, D. F., Davies, R. E. 1962. See Ref. 116a, p. 84
16. Caspersson. T. 1990. *J. R. Microsc. Soc.* 60: 8x
17. Caspersson, T. 1940. *Chromosoma* 1: 562
18. Caspersson, T. 1936. *Scand. Arch. Physiol.* 73(Suppl.): 81
19. Chance, B. 1940. *J. Franklin Inst.* 229: 455
20. Chance, B. 1943. *J. Biol. Chem.* 151: 553
21. Chance, B. 1951. *Rev. Sci. Instrum.* 22: 634
22. Chance, B. 1952. *2nd Int. Congr. Biochem. Paris*, p. 32 (Abstr.); Chance, B. 1954. See Ref. 100a, p. 399; Chance, B. 1955. *Harvey Lect.* 49: 145
23. Chance, B. 1983. *Curr. Cont.* 49: 20
24. Chance, B. 1989. *J. Appl. Cardiol.* 4: 207
25. Chance, B., ed. 1989. *Photon Migration in Tissues.* New York: Plenum
26. Chance, B., Baltscheffsky, H. 1958. *J. Biol. Chem.* 233: 736
27. Chance, B., Barlow, C. H. 1976. *Science* 193: 909
28. Chance, B., Barlow, C., Haselgrove, J., Nakase, Y., Quistorff, B., et al. 1978. In *Microenvironments and Metabolic Compartmentation*, ed. P. Srere, R. Estabrook, p. 131. New York: Academic
28a. Chance, B., Frank, K. H., Kessler, M., Lubbers, D. W., Mayevsky, A., Tamura, T., eds. 1990. *Scientific Committee, "Workshop on Quantitative Spectroscopy in Tissue."* Erlangen-Nurenberg: Univ. Erlangen-Nurenberg. In press
29. Chance, B., Hughes, B., MacNichol, E. F., Sayre, D., Williams, F. C., eds. 1949. *Waveforms.* Lexington: MIT Radiation Laboratory Series, Boston Technical
30. Chance, B., Jobsis, F. 1959. *Nature* 184: 195
31. Chance, B., Leigh, J., Miyake, H.,

32. Smith, D. S. Nioka, S., et al. 1988. *Proc. Natl. Acad. Sci. USA* 85: 4971
32. Chance, B., Maris, M., Sorge, J., Zhang, M. Z. 1990. In *Time Resolved Laser Spectroscopy in Biochemistry II*, ed. J. R. Lakowicz, 1204: 481. Proc. Soc. Photo Opt. Instrum. Eng.
33. Chance, B., Mauriello, G., Aubert, X. M. 1962. See Ref. 116a, p. 128
34. Chance, B., Nioka, S., Kent, J., McCully, K., Fountain, M., et al. 1988. *Anal. Biochem.* 174: 698
35. Chance, B., Quistorff, B. 1978. In *Oxygen Transport to Tissue—III*, ed. I. A. Silver, M. Erecinska, H. I. Bicher, p. 331. New York: Plenum
36. Chance, B., Schleyer, H. 1963. *6th Annu. Biophys. Soc. Meeting*, Washington (Abstr.)
37. Chance, B., Schoener, B., Yonetani, Y. 1965. In *Oxidases and Related Redox Systems*, ed. T. E. King, M. Morrison. p. 609. New York: Wiley
38. Chance, B., Smith, D. S., Nioka, S., Miyaka, H., Holtom, G., Maris, M. 1989. See Ref. 25, p. 121
39. Chance, B., Smith, L., Castor, L. 1989. *Biochim. Biophys. Acta* 398: 348
40. Chance, B., Thorell, B. 1959. *J. Biol. Chem.* 234: 3044
41. Chance, B., Weber, A. 1963. *J. Physiol.* 169: 263
42. Chance, B., Williams, G. R. 1955. *J. Biol. Chem.* 217: 383
43. Cohen, I. B., Lesher, S. 1986. *Soc. Gen. Physiol. Ses.* 40: 71
44. Connelly, C. M., Brink, F. 1953. *Rev. Sci. Instrum.*
45. Connelly, C. M., Chance, B. 1954. *Am. Phil. Soc.* 227: 710
46. DeVault, D., Chance, B. 1966. *Biophys. J.* 6: 825
47. DeVault, D. 1980. *Q. Rev. Biophys.* 13: 387
48. Duysens, L. M. N. 1951. PhD thesis. Utrecht: Univ. Utrecht; See also 1964. *Progress in Biophysics in Molecular Biology*. Oxford: Pergamon
49. Estabrook, R. W., Cooper, D. Y., Rosenthal, O. 1963. *Biochem. Z.* 338: 741
50. Fleckenstein, A., Janke, J., Davies, R. E., Krebs, H. A. 1954. *Nature* 174: 1081
51. Foggerty. 1990. International Center for Advanced Study in the Health Sciences, National Institutes of Health, June 25–27
52. Garfinkel, D. 1958. *Arch. Biochem. Biophys.* 77: 493
53. Gayesky, T. E. J., Connett, R. J., Honig, C. R. 1987. *Am. J. Physiol.* 252: H906

54. Gayesky, T. E. J., Honig, C. R. 1986. *Adv. Exp. Med. Biol.* 100: 487
55. Gibson, Q. H. 1966. *Annu. Rev. Biochem.* 35: 435
56. Gibson, Q. H., Greenwood. C., Wharton, D. C., Palmer, G. 1965. In *Oxidases and Related Redox Systems*, ed. T. E. King, H. S. Maston, M. Morrison, p. 591. New York: Wiley
57. Gratton, E., Jameson. D. M., Rosato. N., Weber, G. 1984. *Rev. Sci. Instrum.* 55: 486
58. Gratton, E., Lakowicz, J. R., Maliwal, B., Cherek, H., Laczko, G., Linkeman. M. 1984. *Biophys. J.* 46: 479
59. Green, D. E. 1954. See Ref. 100a
60. Grinvald. A. 1985. *Annu. Rev. Neurosci.* 8: 263
61. Haselgrove. J. C., Barlow, C. H. Chance, B. 1980. In *Cerebral Metabolism and Neural Function*, ed. J. V. Passoneau, R. A. Haskins, W. D. Lust. p. 72. Baltimore: William & Wilkins
62. Haselgrove. J. C., Barlow, C. H., Eleff, S., Chance, B., Lebordais, S. 1981. In *Oxygen Transport to Tissue: Advances in Physiological Sciences*, ed. A. G. B. Kovach, E. Dora, M. Kessler, I. A. Silver, p. 25. Budapest: Pergamon
63. Heinrich, U., Hoffmann, J., Lubbers, D. W. 1987. *Pflugers Arch.* 409: 152
64. Hirschberg, J. G., Kohen, E., Kohen, C. 1989. See Ref. 77a, p. 253
65. Hirschberg, J. G., Wouters, A. W., Kohen, Kohen, C., Thorell, B., et al. 1978. In *Multichannel Image Detectors*, ed. Y. Talmi, p. 235. Washington, DC: Am. Chem. Soc.
66. Hirschfeld, T. 1976. *App. Opt.* 15: 2965
66a. Holtzer, H., Marshall, J., Fink, H. 1957. *J. Biophys. Biochem. Cytol.* 3: 705
67. Huch, R., Huch, A., Lubbers, D. W., eds. 1981. *Transcutaneous PO₂*. New York: Thime-Stratton
68. Jobsis, F. F. 1977. *Science* 198: 1264
69. Jobsis, F. F., Mayevsky, A., Piiper, J., Hoper, J., Acker, H., et al. 1990. See Ref. 28a. In press
70. Kasten, F. H. 1983. In *History of Staining*, ed. G. Clark, F. H. Kasten, p. 147. Baltimore: Williams & Wilkins. 3rd ed.
71. Kasten, F. H. 1989. See Ref. 77a, p. 3
72. Keilin, D. 1925. *Proc. R. Soc. London Ser. B* 98: 313
73. Keilin, D. 1966. *The History of Cell Respiration and Cytochrome*. Cambridge: Cambridge Univ. Press
74. Keilin, D., Hartree, E. F. 1939. *Proc. R. Soc. London Ser. B* 127: 167
75. Keilin, D., Slater, E. C. 1953. *Brit. Med. Bull.* 9: 53

76. Klingenberg, M. 1958. *Arch. Biochem. Biophys.* 75: 376
77. Kohen. C., Kohen, E., Hirschberg, J. G., Prince, J. 1990. In *Foundations of Medical Cell Biology*, ed. E. E. Bittar. Greenwich, CT: JAI. In press
77a. Kohen, E., Hirschberg, J. G., eds. 1989. *Cell Structure and Function by Microspectrofluorometry*. San Diego/New York: Academic
78. Kohen, E., Kohen, C., Hirschberg, J. G., Fried, M., Prince, J. 1989. *Opt. Eng.* 28: 222
79. Kohen. E., Kohen, C., Hirschberg, J. G., Wouters, A. W., Thorell, B. et al. 1983. *Cell Biochem. Funct.* 1: 3
80. Kohen. E., Kohen. C., Prince, J., Schachtschabel, D. O. Hirschberg. J. G., et al. 1990. *J. Biotechnol.* 13: 1
80a. Kubelka. P. Munk, F. 1931. *Z. Tech. Physik.* 12: 593; See also Kubelka, P. 1948. *J. Opt. Soc. Am.* 38: 448; 1954. *J. Opt. Soc. Am.* 44: 330
81. Kurth. C. D. Steven, J. M. Nicholson, S. C., Norwood. W. I., Chance, B., Delivoria-Papadopoulos. M. 1989. *FASEB J.* 3: 241 (Abstr.)
82. Lakowicz, J. R., Cherek. H., Laczko, G., Gratton, E. 1984. *Biochim. Biophys. Acta* 777: 183
83. Lakowicz, J. R., Cherek, H., Maliwal, B., Gratton, E. 1985. *Biochemistry* 24: 376
84. Lakowicz, J. R., Gratton, E., Cherek, H., Maliwal, B. P., Laczko, G. 1984. *Biophys. J.* 46: 463
85. Lakowicz, J. R., Laczko, G., Gryczynski, I. 1986. *Rev. Sci. Instrum.* 57: 2499
86. LaManna. J. C., Light, A. I., Peretsman, S. J., Rosenthal, M. 1983. *Brain Res.* 293: 313
87. Langer, H., Thorell, B. 1965. *Exp. Cell Res.* 41: 673
88. Lardy, H. A., Copenhaver, H. Jr. 1954. *Nature* 174: 231
89. Lehninger, A. 1955. *The Harvey Lectures, 1953, 1954*, pp. 49, 176. New York: Academic
90. Lemke, R., Klaus, D., Lubbers, D. W., Oevermann, G. 1989. *Crit. Care Med.* 16: 353
91. Lieke, E. E., Frostig, R. D., Arieli, A., Ts'o, D. Y., Hildesheim, R., Grinvald. A. 1989. *Annu. Rev. Physiol.* 51: 543
92. Lipmann, F. 1946. In *Currents in Biochemical Research*, ed. D. E. Green, p. 137. New York/London: Interscience
92a. Lubbers, D., Niesel, W. 1957. *Naturwissenschaften* 44: 60
92b. Lubbers, D., Niesel, W. 1959. *Pflugers Arch.* 268: 2861
93. Lundegardh, H. 1964. *Biochim. Biophys. Acta* 88: 7

94. MacMunn, C. A. 1885. *Phil. Trans. R. Soc. London* 177: 267
95. Deleted in proof
96. Masters, B. M. 1986. *Curr. Top. Eye Res.* 4: 139
97. Masters, B. R. 1990. *Noninvasive Techniques in Ophthalmology.* New York/Berlin/Heidelberg: Springer-Verlag
97a. Mathes, K., Gross, F. 1939. *Arch. Exp. Pathol. Pharmakol.* 191: 831
98. Matschinsky, F. M., Hintz, C., Reichlmeier, K., Quistorff, B., Chance, B. 1978. In *Microheterogeneities and Metabolic Compartmentation,* ed. P. Srere, R. Estabrook. p. 149. New York: Academic
99. Mauch, E. D., Frank, K. H., Albrecht. H. P., Kessler, M. 1990. See Ref. 28a. In press
100. Mayevsky. A. 1990. See Ref. 28a. In press
100a. McElroy, W. D., Glass, B., eds. 1954. *The Mechanism of Enzyme Action.* Baltimore: The Johns Hopkins Press
101. Michel, H., Epp, O., Deisenhofer, J. 1986. *EMBO J.* 5: 2445
102. Millikan, G. A. 1937. *Proc. R. Soc. London Ser. B* 123: 218
103. Millikan, G. A. 1936. *Proc. R. Soc. London Ser. B* 120: 366
104. Millikan, G. A. 1941. *Rev. Sci. Instrum.* 13: 434
105. Ochoa, S. 1943. *J. Biol. Chem.* 151: 493
105a. Nicolai, L. 1932. *Arch. Ges. Physiol.* 229: 372, 389
106. Pappenheimer, J. R. 1941. *J. Physiol.* 99: 184
107. Park, J. H., Brown, R. L., Park, C. R., Cohn, M., Chance, B. 1988. *Proc. Natl. Acad. Sci. USA* 85: 8780
108. Patterson, M. S., Chance, B., Wilson, B. C. 1989. *J. Appl. Opt.* 28: 2331
109. Patterson, M. S., Moulton, J. D., Wilson, B. C., Chance, B. 1990. *Proc. Soc. Photo. Opt. Instrum. Eng.* 1203: 62
110. Perry, R., Thorell, B., Akerman, L., Chance, B. 1960. *Biochim. Biophys. Acta* 39: 24
111. Policard, A. 1925. *Bull. Histol. Appl.* 2: 167
112. Quistorff, B., Chance, B. 1980. *Anal. Biochem.* 108: 237
113. Quistorff, B., Chance, B. 1986. In *Regulation of Hepatic Metabolism, Inter- and Intracellular Compartmentation,* ed. T. Thurman, E. C. Kaufmann, K. Jungeman, p. 185. New York: Plenum
114. Quistorff, B., Haselgrove, J., Chance, B. 1985. *Anal. Biochem.* 148: 389
115. Ramirez, J. 1959. *J. Physiol.* 147: 14
116. Ramirez, J. 1964. *Biochim. Biophys. Acta* 88: 648
116a. Rodahl, K., Horvath, S. M., eds. 1962. *Muscle as a Tissue.* New York: McGraw-Hill
117. Salama, G., Lombardi, E., Elson. J. 1987. *Am. J. Physiol.* 25: H384
118. Deleted in proof
119. Shibata, K., Benson. A. A., Calvin. M. 1954. *Biochim. Biophys. Acta* 15: 461
120. Shires, T. K. 1969. *Cancer Res.* 29: 1277
121. Slater. E. C., Holton, F. A. 1953. *Biochem. J.* 55: 553
122. Slator, W. 1955. PhD thesis. Urbana: Univ. Illinois
123. Smith. L. 1953. *Fed. Proc.* 12: 270 (Abstr.)
124. Smith. L., Baltscheffsky, M. 1959. *J. Biol. Chem.* 234: 1575: See also 1956. *Fed. Proc.* 15: 357 (Abstr.)
125. Spencer, R. D., Weber, G. 1969. *Ann. NY Acad. Sci.* 158: 361
126. Tamura, M., Hazeki, O., Nioka, S., Chance, B. 1989. In *Chemoreceptors and Reflexes in Breathing,* ed. S. Lahiri, p. 159. New York: Oxford Univ. Press
127. Tamura, M., Oshino, N., Chance, B., Silver, I. A. 1978. *Arch. Biochem. Biophys.* 191: 8
128. Thorell, B. 1947. *Studies on the Formation of Cellular Substances during Blood Cell Production,* ed. King. Stockholm/Kimpton/London: Stockholm Boktryckeriet Norstedt Söner
129. Thorell, B., Akerman, L. 1957. *Exp. Cell Res. Suppl.* 4: 83
130. Thorell, B., Chance, B. 1960. *Exp. Cell Res.* 20: 43
131. Thorell, B., Chance, B., Legallais, V. 1965. *J. Cell Biol.* 26: 741
132. Tyndall, J. 1873. *Contributions to Molecular Physics in the Domain of Radiant Heat.* New York: Appleton
133. Von Herrevald
134. Waggoner, A. S. 1979. *Annu. Rev. Biophys. Bioeng.* 8: 47
135. Waggoner, A. S., Grinvald, A. 1977. *Ann. NY Acad. Sci.* 303: 217
136. Warburg, O. 1923. *Biochem. Z.* 142: 518
137. Warburg, O. 1924. *Biochem. Z.* 152: 479
138. Warburg, O., Christian, W. 1938. *Biochem. Z.* 303: 400
139. Warburg, O., Christian, W. 1942. *Biochem. Z.* 310: 384
140. Warburg, O., Christian, W. 1943. *Biochem. Z.* 314: 401
141. Warburg, O., Negelein, E. 1929. *Biochem. Z.* 214: 64
142. Warner, I. M., Christian, G. D., Davidson, E. R., Callis, J. B. 1977. *J. Anal. Chem.* 49: 565
143. Williams, A. T., Tarpley, W., Clark, C. 1948. *Trans. Am. Inst. Electr. Eng.* 67: 1
144. Wu, J.-Y., London, J. A., Zecevic. D., Loew, L. M., Orbach, H. S., et al. 1989. See Ref. 77a, p. 329
145. Wyatt, J. S., Cope, M., Delpy, D. T., Wray, S., Reynolds, E. O. R. 1986. *Lancet* 2: 1063
146. Yamashita, Y., Suzuki, S., Miyaki, S., Hayakawa, T. 1989. See Ref. 25, p. 50
147. Yang, C. C. 1952. *Proc. Inst. Radio Eng.* 49: 220
148. Yang, C. C. 1954. *Rev. Sci. Instrum.* 25: 807
149. Yang, C. C., Legallais, V. 1954. *Rev. Sci. Instrum.* 25: 801
150. Yoo, K. M., Alfano, R. R. 1989. *Phys. Rev. B* 39: 5806
151. Zhang, K., Chance, B., Reddy, K. S. 1988. *Am. Phys.* 33: 691 (Abstr.)

Reprinted from *Applied Optics,* Vol. 28(12), pp. 2210-2215 (June 15, 1989).
©1989 Optical Society of America.

Diffusion of light in turbid material

Akira Ishimaru

This paper discusses some of the present knowledge of the mathematical techniques used to describe light diffusion in turbid material such as tissues. Attention will be paid to the usefulness and limitations of various techniques. First, we review the transport theory, radiance, radiant energy fluence rate, phase functions, boundary conditions, and measurement techniques. We then discuss the first-order solution, multiple scattering, diffusion approximation, and their limitations. The plane wave, spherical wave, beam wave, and pulse wave excitations are discussed followed by a brief review of the surface scattering effects due to rough interfaces.

I. Introduction

The scattering of light by turbid media has been studied extensively in the past,[1] and its applications include atmospheric optics, optics in the ocean, optical scattering in biological media, and scattering by stellar and interstellar media. In spite of these studies, however, the existing theoretical models are still not satisfactory for explaining the experimental data in many important and practical applications. This paper attempts to show some of the existing theoretical models and indicate their limitations and usefulness.

In turbid material, light is scattered and absorbed due to the inhomogeneities and absorption characteristics of the medium. A mathematical description of the propagation and scattering characteristics of light can be made in two different manners: analytical theory and transport theory.[1] In analytical theory, we start with Maxwell's equations, take into account the statistical nature of the medium, and consider the statistical moments of the wave. In principle, this is the most fundamental approach, including all diffraction effects, and many investigations have been made using this approach.[1-4] However, its drawback is the mathematical complexities involved, and its usefulness is limited.

Transport theory,[1] on the other hand, does not start with Maxwell's equations. It deals directly with the transport of power through turbid media. The development of the theory is heuristic and lacks the rigor of the analytical theory. Since both the analytical and transport theories deal with the same physical problem, there should be some relation between them. In fact, many attempts have been made to derive the transport theory from Maxwell's equations with varying degrees of success. In spite of its heuristic development, however, the transport theory has been used extensively, and experimental evidence shows that the transport theory is applicable to a large number of practical problems.[1]

We first review the transport theory and the first-order and multiple scattering theories. We then devote most of our discussion to the diffusion theory with its limitations and usefulness.

II. Transport Theory

The fundamental quantity in transport theory is the radiance $I(\mathbf{r},\hat{s})$, which is also called the specific intensity in radiative transfer theory and the brightness in radiometry. Its unit is W m^{-2} sr^{-1} Hz^{-1} and is the average power flux density in a given direction $\hat{s}$ within a unit solid angle within a unit frequency band (see Ref. 1, p. 149 for details). Since we normally use a laser source with a narrow bandwidth and a detector with sufficient bandwidth, we integrate over the frequency and redefine the radiance with the unit W m^{-2} sr^{-1}.

The fundamental differential equation for the radiance is the transport equation

$$\frac{d}{ds} I(\mathbf{r},\hat{s}) = -\gamma_t I(\mathbf{r},\hat{s}) + \frac{\gamma_t}{4\pi} \int p(\hat{s},\hat{s}') I(\bar{r},\hat{s}') d\omega', \tag{1}$$

where $\gamma_t = \gamma_s + \gamma_a$ is the extinction coefficient in m^{-1}, γ_s is the scattering coefficient, γ_a is the absorption coefficient, $p(\hat{s},\hat{s}')$ is the phase function, and $d\omega'$ is the elementary solid angle about the direction $\hat{s}'$.

The quantity most useful in light diffusion in tissue is called the radiant energy fluence rate and is denoted

The author is with University of Washington, Department of Electrical Engineering, Seattle, Washington 98195.

Received 12 January 1989.
0003-6935/89/122210-06$02.00/0.
© 1989 Optical Society of America.

17

by $\psi(\mathbf{r})$.[5] It is the sum of the radiance over all angles at a point $\mathbf{r}$ and is measured by W m^{-2}:

$$\psi(\mathbf{r}) = \int_{4\pi} I(\mathbf{r},\hat{s})d\omega. \qquad (2)$$

The flow of the power per unit area is represented by the flux $\mathbf{F}(\mathbf{r})$, or the radiant flux density, defined by

$$\mathbf{F}(\mathbf{r}) = \int_{4\pi} I(\mathbf{r},\hat{s})\hat{s}d\omega, \qquad (3)$$

and is measured in W m^{-2}. Note that ψ and $\mathbf{F}$ have the same dimension, but ψ is a scalar while $\mathbf{F}$ is a vector.

From the transport Eq. (1), we can derive the following continuity equation:

$$\nabla \bullet \mathbf{F} + \gamma_a\psi = 0, \qquad (4)$$

where γ_a is the absorption coefficient (m^{-1}). Note that $\gamma_a\psi$ (W m^{-3}) is the amount of power absorbed by a unit volume of the medium and Eq. (4) means that the total power flux $-\nabla \bullet \mathbf{F}$ entering a unit volume is equal to the power absorbed within this volume.

Next let us consider the phase function $p(\hat{s},\hat{s}')$, which represents the scattering characteristics of the medium. If the scattering is symmetric about the direction of the incident wave, the phase function is a function of the scattering angle between $\hat{s}$ and $\hat{s}'$. In many practical cases, the following Henyey-Greenstein formula gives a good approximation for the phase function:

$$p(\theta) = \frac{W_0[1 - g^2]}{(1 + g^2 - 2g\cos\theta)^{3/2}}, \qquad (5)$$

where W_0 is the albedo (γ_s/γ_t) and g is the mean cosine of the scattering function:

$$W_0 = \frac{1}{4\pi}\int_{4\pi} p(\theta)d\omega, \qquad g = \frac{\int_{4\pi} p(\theta)\cos\theta d\omega}{\int_{4\pi} p(\theta)d\omega}. \qquad (6)$$

The mean cosine g (sometimes written as μ in the radiative transfer) ranges from zero for isotropic scattering where p is constant W_0 to one for the complete forward scattering when p is proportional to a delta function in the forward direction. The albedo W_0 ranges from zero for a completely absorbing medium to one for a completely scattering medium.

When a laser beam is incident on turbid material, the radiance inside the medium can be divided into the coherent intensity I_c and the diffuse intensity I_d:

$$I = I_c + I_d. \qquad (7)$$

The coherent intensity is the incident intensity reduced by the attenuation due to scattering and absorption and is called the reduced incident intensity. It is given by

$$I_c = F_0\delta(\hat{\omega} - \hat{\omega}_0) \exp(-\tau), \qquad (8)$$

where F_0 is the incident radiant flux density or irradiance (W m^{-2}) and $\delta(\hat{\omega} - \hat{\omega}_0)$ is a solid angle delta function pointed in the direction $\hat{\omega}_0$. The quantity τ is called the optical depth and is defined by

$$\tau = \int_0^s \gamma_t ds. \qquad (9)$$

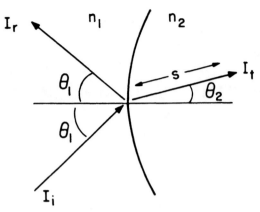

Fig. 1. Boundary conditions for the radiance at the interface between two homogeneous mediums.

The mean free path l_t is equal to γ_t^{-1} and is the distance over which the coherent intensity decreases to $\exp(-1)$ of the initial value.

Let us next consider the boundary conditions to be satisfied by the radiance at the interface between the homogeneous media with the refractive index n_1 and the refractive index n_2. First, Snell's law must be satisfied (Fig. 1):

$$n_1 \sin\theta_1 = n_2 \sin\theta_2. \qquad (10)$$

The reflected radiance I_r is given by

$$I_r = R_pI_i, \qquad (11)$$

where R_p is the power reflectivity and is given by

$$R_p = |R|^2. \qquad (12)$$

R is the Fresnel reflection coefficient and is equal to R_{11} or $R_\perp$ dependent on the polarization. If the wave is completely unpolarized, R_p is equal to $(\tfrac{1}{2})[|R_{11}|^2 + |R_\perp|^2]$. Similarly, the transmitted radiance I_t is given by

$$I_t = \frac{n_2^3 \cos\theta_2}{n_1^3 \cos\theta_1}|T|^2I_i, \qquad (13)$$

where T is the Fresnel transmission coefficient and is equal to T_{11} or $T_\perp$ depending on the polarization. For an unpolarized wave, $|T|^2$ is equal to $(\tfrac{1}{2})[|T_{11}|^2 + |T_\perp|^2]$ (see Ref. 1, p. 154 for the expression of R and T). Also note that if n_1 and n_2 are lossless and $n_1 > n_2$, the total reflection takes place if $\theta_1 > \theta_c$ where the critical angle θ_c is given by $\theta_c = \sin^{-1}(n_2/n_1)$.

If the medium with n_1 is homogeneous (air, for example) and the medium with n_2 is a turbid medium (tissue, for example), the above relationships (10)–(13) are applicable to the coherent intensity. The transmitted coherent intensity (13) is then reduced by the total attenuation:

$$I_t(s) = I_t(o) \exp(-\tau). \qquad (14)$$

The boundary condition for the diffuse intensity on the surface of the turbid medium is that no diffuse intensity enters the turbid medium:

$$I_d(\hat{s}) = 0 \qquad (15)$$

when $\hat{s}$ is pointed inward. The diffuse intensity incident on the boundary from the medium side also satisfies relationships (10)–(13).

Now, let us consider the measurement technique. If a detector has a certain receiving cross section $A(\hat{s})$, the received power output P_r is given by

$$P_r = \int_{4\pi} A(\hat{s})I(\hat{s})d\omega. \qquad (16)$$

If the detector is isotropic, $A(\hat{s}) = A_0$ is constant and independent of the direction, and we have

$$P_r = A_0 \int_{4\pi} I(\hat{s})d\omega = A_0\psi. \qquad (17)$$

Therefore, the output of an isotropic detector is proportional to the radiant energy fluence rate (Fig. 2).

If the detector is pointed in one direction and receives all the radiance equally from all directions on one side within the field of view, FOV $= 2\pi$, we have $A(\hat{s}) = A_0 \cos\theta$ and

$$P_r = A_0 \int_{2\pi} I(\hat{s})\cos\theta d\omega. \qquad (18)$$

If the field of view FOV $= \Delta\omega$ is very narrow, we have

$$P_r = A_0\Delta\omega I(\hat{s}). \qquad (19)$$

If the radiance consists of the coherent and the diffuse intensity as in Eq. (7), the received power is given by

$$P_r = A_0F_0 \exp(-\tau) + A_0\Delta\omega I_d. \qquad (20)$$

The first term is the coherent power when the coherent intensity is within $\Delta\omega$ of the detector. Note that the diffuse part of the received power is proportional to the field of view $\Delta\omega$.

In the above, we assumed that the radiance is scalar and the polarization effects are not included. In recent years, several extensive studies have been reported on the transport theory including all the polarization effects.[6] The radiance is then replaced by the 4×1 Stokes vector, the extinction coefficient is replaced by the 4×4 extinction matrix, and the phase function is replaced by the 4×4 Mueller matrix. The transport equation then becomes the matrix integro-differential equation and is called the vector transport equation or the vector radiative transfer equation.

III. First-Order Solution and Multiple Scattering

If the diffuse intensity is considerably smaller than the coherent intensity, the diffuse intensity is calculated by assuming that the total intensity $I_c + I_d$ illuminating the turbid medium is approximately equal to the coherent intensity I_c. This is called the first-order scattering, and the details are given in Ref. 1 (Chap. 8).

The first-order solution is simple and useful for many practical problems. However, it applies only to the cases where the diffuse intensity is much smaller than the coherent intensity. This happens when a plane wave is incident on a medium and the optical depth τ is smaller than one and the medium is absorbing (albedo $W_0 < 0.5$). If the incident beam is narrow, the first-order solution is applicable to a much greater

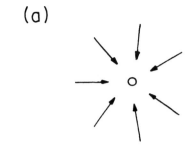

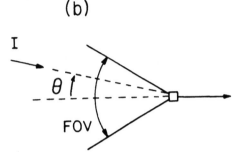

Fig. 2. (a) Isotropic detector; (b) detector with FOV.

optical depth than one when the medium is absorbing ($W_0 < 0.9$). In some tissues at some wavelengths, especially 600 nm to 1.3 μm, the albedo is close to unity, and, therefore, the first-order solution cannot be used unless the optical depth is much smaller than unity ($\tau \ll 1$).

Let us next consider a more general case where the first-order solution is not applicable. If the medium can be represented by a plane-parallel medium and the incident wave is a plane wave, the transport equation can be converted into a matrix differential equation by considering the radiance at many discrete angles (Fig. 3). This method is called the discrete ordinates method or the many flux theory (Ref. 1, Chap. 11).

$$\frac{d}{d\tau}\begin{bmatrix} I_1 \\ I_2 \\ \cdot \\ \cdot \\ \cdot \end{bmatrix} + \begin{bmatrix} S_{11} S_{12} \ldots \\ S_{21} S_{22} \\ \cdot \\ \cdot \\ \cdot \end{bmatrix}\begin{bmatrix} I_1 \\ I_2 \\ \cdot \\ \cdot \\ \cdot \end{bmatrix} = \begin{bmatrix} B_1 \\ B_2 \\ \cdot \\ \cdot \\ \cdot \end{bmatrix} \exp(-t) \qquad (21)$$

This matrix equation can be solved exactly by the eigenvalue–eigenvector method. By increasing the number of angles, the matrix solution should approach the exact solution. It is also possible to expand the radiance in a series of spherical harmonics and to separate the transport equation into spherical harmonics components. With a sufficient number of spherical harmonics, this should also approach the exact solution. These are useful and practical techniques, and even though it is limited to a plane-parallel medium illuminated by a plane wave, they can be used as a useful check of the other approximate solutions. There is a drawback to these methods, however. Usually the matrix is dense, and the matrix size cannot be too large even with the use of supercomputers. The

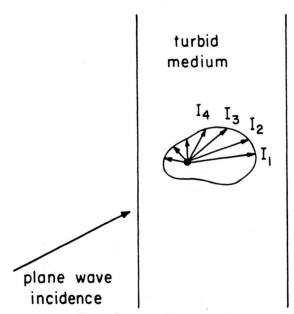

Fig. 3. Discrete ordinates method.

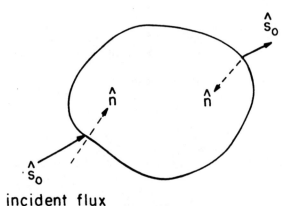

incident flux

Fig. 4. Boundary conditions for diffuse intensity.

solution is also unstable for a large matrix. In particular, if the phase function is peaked in the forward direction (g close to unity), the discrete ordinates method often does not yield good solutions.

There are several approximate solutions available. The simplest and most widely used method is the Kubelka-Munk two-flux theory and four-flux theory (Ref. 1, Chap. 10). For laser beam applications, the four-flux theory makes use of two diffuse fluxes and one forward and one backward coherent intensities. This is equivalent to representing many fluxes in the discrete ordinates method by only two fluxes. It is simple and convenient, but obviously it is too much of an approximation for the problem of optical diffusion in tissues. Therefore, the Kubelka-Munk theory can be used only if we need a very approximate estimate of the solution.

In the above, we discussed the first-order solution, the discrete ordinates method, and the Kubelka-Munk theory. For optical scattering in tissues where the albedo is close to one and the optical depth can become much greater than one, only the discrete ordinates method gives a useful exact solution. However, it is limited to the case of plane wave incidence on a plane-parallel medium, and it requires extensive computer calculations. A useful and practical approximate method of dealing with the problem of optical scattering in tissues is, therefore, the diffusion theory which is applicable when the medium is mostly scattering. In the next section, we describe the essence of the diffusion theory (Ref. 1, Chap. 9).

IV. Diffusion Theory

When a laser beam enters a medium, the radiance can be expressed as the coherent intensity and diffuse intensity. If the medium is mostly scattering, the diffuse intensity tends to be almost isotropic and the diffuse radiance has a broad angular spread. There-

fore, we can expand the diffuse intensity I_d in a series of spherical harmonics. The first two terms of the expansion constitute the diffusion theory:

$$I_d = \sum_{n=0}^{\infty} I_n = \frac{1}{4\pi}(\psi_d + 3\mathbf{F}_d \cdot \hat{s}) + \dots . \quad (22)$$

The diffuse radiant energy fluence rate ψ_d satisfies the following diffusion equation:

$$(\nabla^2 - \kappa^2)\psi_d = -Q, \quad (23)$$

where $Q \;\;= 3\gamma_s(\gamma_t + g\gamma_a)F_0\exp(-\tau)$,

$\kappa^2 = 3\gamma_a\gamma_{tr}$, and

$\gamma_{tr} = \gamma_s(1 - g) + \gamma_a$,

where the incident coherent beam is given in Eq. (8) and γ_{tr} is called the transport coefficient. Note that the transport coefficient is much smaller than the extinction coefficient, and, therefore, the transport mean free path $l_{tr} = \gamma_{tr}^{-1}$ is much greater than the mean free path $l_t = \gamma_t^{-1}$. Note also that the total radiant energy fluence rate is given by

$$\psi_t = \psi_c + \psi_d, \qquad \psi_c = F_0\exp(-\tau). \quad (24)$$

The boundary condition for ψ_d at the surface illuminated by the incident intensity (8) is

$$\psi_d + h\frac{\partial}{\partial n}\psi_d + 2(\hat{n}\cdot\hat{s}_0)Q_1 = 0, h = \frac{2}{3\gamma_{tr}}, \quad (25)$$

where $Q_1 = \gamma_s g F_0/\gamma_{tr}, \hat{s}_0$ is the unit vector pointed in the direction of the incident flux, and $\hat{n}$ is the normal unit vector toward the volume. In the exit surface, Q_1 is multiplied by $\exp(-\tau)$ (Fig. 4).

When an optical beam enters a turbid medium, the first-order scattering is dominant near the surface, and as the observation point moves into the medium, more and more second-order and higher-order scattering takes place. The diffusion solution is an approximation representing the limiting case where the multiple scattering is dominant. It is, therefore, clear that near the surface the diffusion solution may not be applicable.

The diffusion approximation for a beam wave incident on a turbid medium has been studied and compared with experimental data.[7] It is noted that if g is much smaller than unity ($g = 0.0895$) and the albedo is close to one, the diffusion solution is an excellent approximation within a fraction of decibels for all optical distances greater than one. Also if g is close to unity ($g = 0.925$), the difference between the diffusion solution and experimental data is 10–5 dB for $\tau = 1$–10 and 5–1 dB for $\tau = 10$–20. For tissues[5] the value of g is in the 0.6–0.98 range, and, therefore, it is expected that the difference between the diffusion and the true value may be much smaller for $g < 0.9$ than the above figures for $g = 0.925$.

Let us next consider the diffusion of a pulse in a turbid medium.[8] First, the coherent intensity pulse $\psi_c(t)$ propagates through the medium with the velocity v of light in that medium ($v = c/n$, n is the refractive index). This coherent pulse is scattered by the medium and generates the diffuse pulse $\psi_d(t)$. The diffuse pulse $\psi_d(t)$ satisfies the following equation:

$$\left[\nabla^2 - \frac{3}{v^2}\frac{\partial^2}{\partial t^2} - \frac{1}{D}\frac{\partial}{\partial t} + 3\gamma_a\gamma_{tr} \right]\psi_d(t) = 0, \qquad (26)$$

where D is the diffusion coefficient given by

$$D = \frac{v}{3(\gamma_a + \gamma_{tr})} .$$

Equation (26) shows that the wavefront of the diffuse pulse propagates with the velocity $v/\sqrt{3}$. It also shows that the pulse front is followed by a long tail.[8] A sketch of the general characteristics is shown in Fig. 5. At a given point in the medium, the coherent pulse ψ_c arrives with the velocity v followed by the diffuse pulse ψ_d, which is generated by ψ_c. Since ψ_d is generated at all points in the medium, the pulse has a broad peak in the neighborhood of $vt/\sqrt{3}$, but it is not a sharp peak. Figure 5 shows the pulse intensity inside the medium when a short pulse is incident. The figure in the middle shows the pulse intensity as a function of distance at two different times $t_1 < t_2$. Note that the leading edge propagates with the velocity v, but the broad peak appears in the neighborhood corresponding to the velocity $vt/\sqrt{3}$. It also indicates that there is a long tail contributed by the light diffusion through all points of the medium. The bottom figure shows the same phenomena as a function of time at a fixed point. A similar analysis was also given by Furutsu.[9]

Some experimental verification of this theory was reported.[10,11] In recent years, there has been increased interest in the coherent backscattering from diffuse media[12,13] as well as the temporal correlation of the scattered intensity.[13] These may prove to be useful tools in the determination of media characteristics.

Now let us consider the scattering due to a rough surface or a rough interface.[1] If the surface height is given by $z = f(x,y)$ and its variance is given by $\sigma^2 = \langle f^2 \rangle$, the surface is considered rough only if the standard deviation σ satisfies the following Rayleigh criterion:

$$\sigma > \lambda/(8 \cos\theta_i), \qquad (27)$$

where λ is the wavelength and θ_i is the incident angle (Fig. 6). In general, the rough surface is characterized

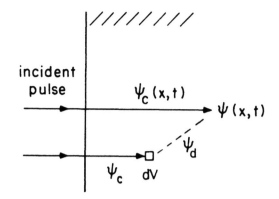

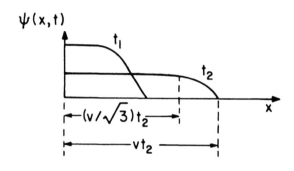

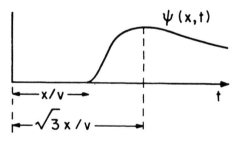

Fig. 5. Pulse propagation in a turbid medium.

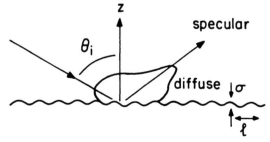

Fig. 6. Rough surface scattering.

by the height variance σ and the correlation distance l. If $\sigma \ll 1$ and $l \leq 1$, the perturbation technique is applicable. If the radius of curvature of the surface is much greater than a wavelength, the Kirchhoff approximation is applicable. In general, the specular reflection is reduced by the roughness, while the diffuse scattering increases as the roughness increases. Detailed studies of the problem and several new developments have been well documented.[1,14]

The rough surface effects become important when the light propagates across the rough interfaces between two media with different refractive indices. Then Snell's law and the boundary conditions stated in Eqs. (10)–(13) are not applicable and must be replaced by the appropriate solutions of the rough surface scattering problem in addition to the volume scattering discussed above.

V. Conclusion

We reviewed some of our present knowledge of optical diffusion in turbid media. We first reviewed transport theory including measurements. Then we discussed the first-order and multiple scattering theories. In discussing these, we attempted to indicate the usefulness and limitations of these methods. Then we concluded that the diffusion theory is the most useful approximate theory at the present time. We discussed the diffusion theory in some detail including beam wave, pulse wave, and rough surface scattering. The emphasis is on its limitations and usefulness in applying it to the problem of optical diffusion in tissues.

This work was supported by the National Science Foundation.

References

1. A. Ishimaru, *Wave Propagation and Scattering in Random Media* (Academic, New York, 1978).
2. J. A. Kong, *Electromagnetic Wave Theory* (Wiley, New York, 1986).
3. L. Tsang, J. A. Kong, and R. T. Shin, *Theory of Microwave Remote Sensing* (Wiley, New York, 1985).
4. V. V. Varadan and V. K. Varadan, Eds., *Multiple Scattering of Waves in Random Rough Surfaces* (Pennsylvania State U., University Park, 1987).
5. W. M. Star and J. P. A. Marijnissen, "New Trends in Photobiology (Invited Review) Light Dosimetry: Status and Prospects," J. Photochem. Photobiol. B Biol. 1, 149 (1987).
6. A. Ishimaru and C. Yeh, "Matrix Representations of the Vector Radiative-Transfer Theory for Randomly Distributed Nonspherical Particles," J. Opt. Soc. Am. A 1, 359–364 (1984).
7. A. Ishimaru, Y. Kuga, R. L.-T. Cheung, and K. Shimizu, "Scattering and Diffusion of a Beam Wave in Randomly Distributed Scatterers," J. Opt. Soc. Am. 73, 131–136 (1983).
8. A. Ishimaru, "Diffusion of a pulse in densely distributed scatterers," J. Opt. Soc. Am. 68, 1045–1050 (1978).
9. K. Furutsu, "Diffusion Equation Derived from a Space-Time Transport Equation," J. Opt. Soc. Am. 70, 360–366 (1980).
10. K. Shimizu and A. Ishimaru, "Experimental Test of the Reduced Velocity of Light in a Diffuse Medium," Opt. Lett 5, 205–207 (1980).
11. Y. Kuga, A. Ishimaru, and A. P. Bruckner, "Experiments on Picosecond Pulse Propagation in a Diffuse Medium," J. Opt. Soc. Am. 73, 1812–1815 (1983).
12. A. Ishimaru and L. Tsang, "Backscattering Enhancement of Random Discrete Scatterers of Moderate Sizes," J. Opt. Soc. Am. A 5, 228 (1988).
13. P. E. Wolf, G. Maret, E. Akkermans, and R. Maynard, "Optical Coherent Backscattering by Random Media," J. Phys. France 49, 63 (1988).
14. J. A. DeSanto and G. S. Brown, "Analytical Techniques for Multiple Scattering from Rough Surfaces," Prog. Opt. 23, 3–62 (1986).

Reprinted from *Clinical Applications of Modern Imaging Technologies,* Proc. SPIE
Vol. 1894, pp. 4-7 (1993).

New dermatological biomedical microscopes for early clinical diagnostics

Leon Goldman

Laser Consultant, Department of Dermatology
Naval Hospital, San Diego, California

ABSTRACT

With the current developments in optics, including laser optics, there should be more progress on the development of instrumentation for dermatological diagnostics, even clinical diagnostics. This report introduces new microscopy, much still under development, and research. A frank appeal for this program is made for multi-discipline help from optical physicists, biophysicists, biomedical engineers, even laser biomedical engineers, investigative dermatologists and pathologists. If one is allowed to say, the most current advanced clinical diagnostic microscope is the polarizing microscope under the stimulus of Rox Anderson, Lynn Drake, Steven Jacques and Peter Dorogi. The other microscopes for clinical dermatological research to be developed include the confocal scanning microscopy with the emphasis for living tissue, the ultrasonic biomedical microscope (UBM) for dermatology, and the holographic microscope, related to our studies on the biomedical aspects of optical phase conjugation. All these are introduced briefly for our studies and for definite pleas to help us.

2. INTRODUCTION

From colored drawings and paintings, then moulages and photographs to long years in developments of skin microscopy of living skin to the current studies of epiluminescence of Wolff and Kopf[1,2] to computer programmed patient pictures[3], imagery in dermatologic diagnostics continues to progress. These investigations stimulate challenges with modern technology, especially as concerns experiments with modern optics of the living skin. Imagery is now an important phase of laser optics.[4]

Years ago, stimulated by the prophetic words of Goethe, that "Man sees only what he knows," we started to develop special microscopes to look at the surface of the skin. For clinical diagnostics, we found these more valuable than the usual magnifiers.[5-10] An attempt was made to develop a simple portable stereo microscope and to design an examining and operating dermatological table for the dermatologist with an attached stereomicroscope for detailed examination of the skin from the scalp to the plantar surfaces of the feet. The recent developments of the skin microscope, as indicated above, show what progress has been made. Again, with new developments in current optics, there can be much progress in the future for dermatological clinical diagnostics. Actually, the real founder of skin surface microscopy is Hinselmann, a gynecologist. He suggested in 1933 that dermatologists should use the colposcopic microscope for dermatology lesions, especially about the vulva.[6a]

3. MATERIALS

The first approach is to attempt to use imagery for clinical diagnostics in a practical fashion beyond the previous studies of skin microscopy. The current instrument, at the suggestion of Kligman, is the coaxial polarizing microscope of Carl Zeiss Company.[11] The coaxial arrangement makes for better imagery. The 4% reduction in reflectance allows for some subsurface illumination.

In order to assay its practical value, this microscope is being used in the Dermatology Clinic of the Naval Hospital, San Diego. Photography with this polarizing microscope is of importance as a monitor for using illumination besides the usual illumination of light microscopy. The use of laser systems for illumination, especially as regards study of laser transillumination of the skin, means laser protective glasses, which would not be necessary for just the color photographic microscopy. As indicated previously, the stimulus for clinical research with the new coaxial polarizing microscope is due to Rox Anderson,[12] Lynn Drake,[13] Steven Jacques[14] and Peter Dorogi,[15] all now working with us. Vertical and oblique polarization will be compared. The polarizing microscope will be used also for capillaroscopy, such as HeNe and Kr will be studied for illumination. Dorogi will develop a supersensitive CCD color camera for this microscope.

We have used the old techniques of transillumination of the skin for current studies of laser transillumination.[16,17] Now, with many laser systems for energizing chromophores, endogenous or exogenous, some specific for certain tissues, all this may give rise to localized diagnostics by fluorescence. So we are now initiating laser transillumination with microscopes, besides the skin microscopes. We start with polarizing microscopy for clinical lesions. As indicated, the value of the different laser systems for clinical polarizing stereo microscopy has not been determined as yet. In an effort to improve reduction in reflectance for clinical polarizing microscopy, we are using on the surface such coverings as glass, quartz and synthetic sapphire coverings. Controls are being done with photography under all these different antireflectant materials.

The exogenous chromophores have been shown in the Photo Dynamic Therapy (PDT) for cancer diagnostics in tissue. Many new photosensitive chromophores have been developed in addition to our initial studies with hematoporphyrin derivative compounds.[19,20] Another group of chromophores widely used in the PDT program are the metallophthalocyanines. These are excellent for tumor treatment but do not offer much for the initial diagnostic fluorescence. Adding a photosensitive conjugate to these compounds would permit these compounds to be used for cancer diagnostics. D'Arreo is doing these studies for us with photosensitizing conjugates for the metallocyanines.[21]

At the suggestions of Dougherty and Kennedy,[22] 5-aminolevulinic (5-ALA) is being used for imagery of basal cancer in Mohs' fresh tissue technology. This is under study now by the Mohs Division of the Department of Dermatology of the Naval Hospital for recognition of basal cell cancer as contrasted with cellular differentiation between follicular basaloid proliferation.

The laser induced diagnostic fluorescence as the 5-ALA staining of basal cell cancer are examples of color induced for cancer diagnostics. For 5-ALA in Mohs' technology there is often absence of concern about transmission through the barrier of the stratum corneum.

For deep transmission of the exogenous tissue coloring chromophore or transmission of the laser for energizing specific chromophores previously brought, especially by the cancer tissue circulation, to the cancer mass, laser transmission through tissue fiber optics is necessary as the laser photons impact tissues everywhere; there is reflectance, scattering, absorption and even transmission through the cancer.

5-ALA is in use now by Anderson and Lui at the Wellman Laboratory as part of the PDT therapy for skin cancer.[23] 5-ALA is also under detailed study by Jacques at the M.D. Anderson Cancer Center of the University of Texas.[14]

Our studies, then, in the cooperative polarizing microscopy and chromophore energizing diagnostic induced fluorescence are a form of biomedical diagnostic consortium for the development and critical evaluation of new diagnostic instrumentation for the future. There are other types of diagnostic microscopy for clinical use still to be developed.

4. NEW DERMATOLOGICAL DIAGNOSTIC MICROSCOPY TECHNOLOGIES

We have to consider also what new technologies are now available besides the incoherent light skin microscopy and the laser transillumination microscopy. With J.H. Kerr, CAPT MC USN, Chairman of the Department of Dermatology of the Naval Hospital San Diego,[2,4] an effort is being made to try to use the military technologies of subsurface imagery diagnostics for the early diagnostics of solar induced lesions and cancer of sailor skin. This series will provide material to use some of the new optical technologies from optical tomography down deep into the dermis and below.

One of the important new technologies, especially for dermatopathology of the future, is the complex confocal microscopy. We are working with Gmitro of the Optical Sciences Center of the University of Arizona for the development with Gmitro for the use of confocal scanning microscopy in living subsurface tissues.[25] With the instrumentation developed at the Optical Sciences Center, this confocal microscopy instrumentation will be applied to the surface of the skin with skin biopsies. It is possible also that other laser systems will be used besides the argon laser for confocal microscopy. O'Grady, the dermatopathologist in the Department of Dermatology of the Naval Hospital in San Diego, will initiate the studies with the confocal scanning microscope with fresh tissue skin biopsies of animals.[29] The value of 3D imagery and diagnostic fluorescence here will be determined.

Another special investigative microscopy is the polarizing biomedical microscope of the ophthalmologists at the Humphrey Instrument Company of Carl Zeiss Company in San Leandro, California. This instrument is called UBM, Ultrasonic Biomedical Microscope. This was developed by Foster and Pavlin of the Ontario Cancer Institute/Princess Margaret Hospital in Ontario for ophthalmology. This is an important new instrument for studies of the superficial tissues of glaucoma. Alex Ilori of the Humphrey Instrument Company is developing this for dermatology.[30] It appears that this ultrasonic microscope can penetrate 4 mm under the skin surface. This will be of value in dermatology for early cancer detection, and for true imagery of the very early lesions of such disorders as psoriasis and lichen planus and other lesions. So this will give us detailed cellular and tissue imagery for early diagnostics, with controls with the dermatopathologists as indicated. Currently developments in ultrasonics in dermatology relate primarily to the evaluation of thickness of the skin. This will be of value in early and progressive lesions of morphoea, scleroderma and scleredema, especially when these studies are controlled with new tissue pressure transducers which we are attempting now to develop. Again, ultrasonics with better imagery, perhaps even by lasers, will offer considerable interest in investigative dermatology.

Another new biomedical microscopy is the holographic microscopy to be developed from our current studies in optical phase conjugation. We have established a biomedical laboratory for optical phase conjugation at Navy Oceans Service Center (NOSC). Optical phase conjugation, in brief, is an attempt to develop imagery in tissue where the reflected light, in phase, returns along its own incident ray.[26] A striking example of optical phase conjugation is the picture of a cat taken through frosted glass before and after the use of optical phase conjugation mirror. Without the optical phase conjugation mirror, there are no eyes or whiskers shown, evident clearly through the optical phase conjugation mirror. Our first experiments have been with attempts to recognize unstained different structures of the dermis and, as indicated previously, the recognition of coloring by 5-ALA, of basal cancer tissue in the fresh tissue of a Mohs' fresh tissue sections. These studies have just started by the Director of the Biomedical Optical Phase Conjugation Laboratory, Bendell.[27]

The studies of Castro and his associates in MRI tumor diagnostics[28] also present challenges for continued interest of dermatologists in MRI diagnostics.

5. CONCLUSIONS

This brief superficial introduction to new optical technology relates primarily to efforts for early dermatologic diagnostics, even for clinical dermatology. This preliminary report is to show the paths of the developments of modern imagery with optics and in some instances with lasers. Imagery, as indicated, is one of the important phases of modern laser technology and the biomedical applications of optical technology including optical tomography should continue to be of interest to dermatologists as regards clinical polarizing microscopy, the many facets of laser skin transillumination, both superficial and deep, and now with new special microscopes now under development. There is ultrasonic microscopy of tissue at high magnification. As yet, we have not initiated clinical studies in this new field. There are also now attempts at fresh tissue biopsies with confocal scanning microscopy for dermatology, ultrasonic biomedical microscopy and holographic microscopy from optical phase conjugation. All this is but a complex introduction to what we are just starting after long studies for instrumentation for surface skin microscopy and many phases of diagnostic transmission, both with and without lasers. These scattered pieces are offered to investigators especially in opto-electronics and dermatology as new challenges. Again, all this, with our dermatological dermatopathologist, will make for considerable progress in dermatologic diagnostic technologies of the future.

6. REFERENCES

1. Wolff, Klaus, personal communication.

2. Kopf, Alfred, personal communication.

3. Bath, James, DoDoCam Vision Sciences Inc., Natick, MA 01760, USA.

4. Biometrics Optical Society of Society Photoptic Instrument Engineering of USA (SPIE)

5. Goldman, Leon and Younker, W. "Studies in microscopy of surface of skin. Preliminary report of techniques." J Invest Derm, 9:11-16, 1947

6. Goldman, L. "Some investigative studies of pigmented nevi with cutaneous microscopy." J Invest Derm 16:407-427, 1951

6A. Hinselmann, Hans, Die Beuting der Kolposkopie fur den Dermatologen. Derm.Wschr 96 Nov 16:38-534-543; 1933

7. Goldman, Leon. "Clinical studies in microscopy of the skin at moderate magnification. Summary of ten years of experience." Arch Derm 75:345-360, 1957

8. Goldman, Leon. "A Simple portable skin microscope for surface microscopy." Arch Derm 78:246-247, 1958

9. Goldman, L., Vahl, J. and Rockwell, R. Jr., "Replica microscopy on scanning electron microscopy or laser impacts on the skin." J Invest Derm 52:18-24, 1969

10. Goldman, L. "Direct skin microscopy of the skin in vivo as a diagnostic and as a research tool (in color)." <u>J Dermatol Surg Oncol</u> 6:9, 1980

11. Kligman, A, personal communication

12. Anderson, R. Rox. "Polarized light examination and photography of the skin." <u>Arch Dermatol</u> 127:106-1991

13. Drake, Lynn, personal communication

14. Jacques, Steven, personal communication

15. Dorogi, P, personal communication

16. Goldman, L. and Kerr, J.H., "Biomedical subsurface imagery." <u>Journal Laser Applications</u>, vol 3, Fall 1991

17,18. Goldman, Leon and Kerr, JH, "Laser medicine subsurface imagery."
B. Transillumination with fiber optics, SPIE, 1641:2-4, 1992

19. Goldman, L. "Exogenous chromophores for laser Photosurgery, Laser Systems for Photobiology and Photomedicine, Edited by A.N. Chester et al., Plenum Press, New York 143-147, 1991

20. Goldman, L. "Exogenous chromophores for Laser Non-Surgical Photomedicine. Laser Systems for Photobiology and Photomedicine." Edited by A.N. Chester et al., Plenum Press, New York, 1991, 7-12

19. D'Arreo, A. CDR MS USN, personal communication

22. Dougherty, T., personal communication

23. Lui, Harvey, "Photodynamic Therpapy." 18th International Congress of Dermatology, New York, June 13, 1992

24. Kerr, JH, CAPT MC USN, personal communication

25. Gmitro, A., personal communication

26. Gross, Graham, L., personal communication

27. Bendell, I., personal communication

28. Castro, D., personal communication

29. O'Grady, TC, personal communication

30. Ilori, Alex, personal communication

Section Two
Optics of Tissues
with Strong Scattering

Reprinted with permission from *Journal of Investigative Dermatology*, Vol. 77(1), pp. 13-19 (1981). ©1981 Williams & Wilkins.

The Optics of Human Skin

R. Rox Anderson, B.S. and John A. Parrish M.D.

Department of Dermatology, Harvard Medical School, Massachusetts General Hospital, Boston, Massachusetts, U.S.A.

An integrated review of the transfer of optical radiation into human skin is presented, aimed at developing useful models for photomedicine. The component chromophores of epidermis and stratum corneum in general determine the attenuation of radiation in these layers, moreso than does optical scattering. Epidermal thickness and melanization are important factors for UV wavelengths less than 300 nm, whereas the attenuation of UVA (320–400 nm) and visible radiation is primarily via melanin. The selective penetration of all optical wavelengths into psoriatic skin can be maximized by application of clear lipophilic liquids, which decrease regular reflectance by a refractive-index matching mechanism. Sensitivity to wavelengths less than 320 nm can be enhanced by prolonged aqueous bathing, which extracts urocanic acid and other diffusible epidermal chromophores. Optical properties of the dermis are modelled using the Kubelka-Munk approach, and calculations of scattering and absorption coefficients are presented. This simple approach allows estimates of the penetration of radiation *in vivo* using noninvasive measurements of cutaneous spectral remittance (diffuse reflectance). Although the blood chromophores Hb, HbO_2, and bilirubin determine dermal absorption of wavelengths longer than 320 nm, scattering by collagen fibers largely determines the depths to which these wavelengths penetrate the dermis, and profoundly modifies skin colors. An optical "window" exists between 600 and 1300 nm, which offers the possibility of treating large tissue volumes with certain long-wavelength photosensitizers. Moreover, whenever photosensitized action spectra extend across the near UV and/or visible spectrum, judicious choice of wavelength allows some selection of the tissue layers directly affected.

Whenever the skin is involved as the site for photobiologic reactions, its optical properties play some role, and very often a major role, in affecting the response. Radiation must pass through the stratum corneum before reaching viable tissues, and hence the thickness, composition, and morphology of the stratum corneum is always a modifying factor. Having reached viable tissue, the radiation is scattered and absorbed by structures and chromophores which vary dynamically and between individuals. Ultimately, our quantitative understanding of all cutaneous and many systemic photobiologic responses, whether photochemically or photothermally induced, depends in part upon being able to quantitatively model and understand the transfer of optical radiation within skin.

New knowledge of cutaneous optics enters into the design of new therapies involving either photochemical reactions with known action spectra and metabolic consequences (phototherapies, photochemotherapies) or selective thermal destruction of pigmented target tissues. Different wavelengths across the optical spectrum, defined here as approximately 250 nm in the

ultraviolet to approximately 3000 nm in the infrared, reach vastly different depths within tissue, and essentially all photobiologic effects are both wavelength and dose-dependent. If an action spectrum is broad, one therefore has some control, by choice of wavelength, over the depth to which tissues are directly affected by the radiation. Our rapidly increasing knowledge of cellular and molecular photobiology gained from *in vitro* bacterial and tissue culture studies can, in theory, be related to observed responses of cells *in situ* by comparing the dose-related effects of optical radiation *in vitro* to those *in vivo*. Conversely, on the basis of knowing the practical upper limits of spectral radiant exposure doses experienced by cell layers, blood, or other structures *in vivo*, one can then concentrate on basic studies of repair, mutation, and metabolic changes induced by equivalent doses *in vitro*. Optics of skin modify spectra for photobiologic responses, and the transmittance of radiation to a given tissue layer should be considered when analyzing such spectra. Unfortunately, the "target" tissue layer is often poorly defined, and other factors, such as competing photochemical pathways, can modify action spectra as well.

Another broad potential application involving the optics of skin is that of noninvasive *in vivo* optical spectroscopic measurements which can be used to monitor major cutaneous chromophores of interest. These include melanin, oxygenated and reduced hemoglobin, and bilirubin, all of which have been monitored with varying degrees of success by analysis of skin remittance (diffuse reflectance) spectra [1–12]. Although clinicians have used grossly visible cutaneous autofluorescence excited by UVA wavelengths as a diagnostic tool for decades, there has been no successful quantitative analysis of *in vivo* cutaneous fluorescence spectra. Such an endeavor would probably yield useful information.

Central to the basic understanding or application of the optics of skin is the development of a quantitative, general model for radiation transfer in this complex, dynamic, variable, and multilayered optical medium. This has yet to be accomplished in anything but an approximate fashion, because the microscopically complex structure of the skin makes an entirely rigorous analysis of its optics virtually impossible. However, on the macroscopic scale, phenomenological theories of radiation transfer in turbid media can be applied to model the optics for each skin layer. Fortunately, many of the major chromophores are normally confined to a single layer. Melanin is confined to the epidermis and stratum corneum, whereas the various forms of hemoglobin are confined to vessels of the dermis, and only indirectly exert any influence on optical radiation densities within the overlying epidermis. Considering the absorption spectra and localization of the major cutaneous pigments, and optical scattering for each layer, it is in theory possible to arrive at mathematical descriptions of cutaneous optics which include many of the major variables *in vivo*, and which can be used to analyze the skin and its photobiologic responses and to approximate actual optics of human skin.

AN OVERVIEW

Initially it is helpful to schematize the optics of normal skin as shown in Fig 1. At near-normal (nearly perpendicular) incidence, a small fraction of an incident radiation is reflected due to the change in refractive index between air ($n_D = 1.0$) and stratum corneum ($n_D \cong 1.55$) (13). For normally incident radiation, this *regular reflectance* of an incident beam from normal

This work was supported by NIH grant AM25395-02, and funds from the Wellman Labs.

Reprint requests to: John A. Parrish, Department of Dermatology, Harvard Medical School, Massachusetts General Hospital, Boston, MA 02114.

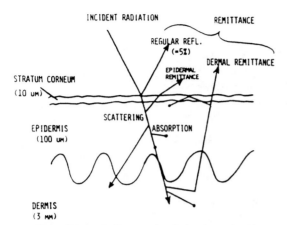

FIG 1. Schematic diagram of optical pathways in skin.

skin is always between 4% and 7% over the entire spectrum from 250–3000 nm, for both white and black skin [14,15]. This same air-tissue optical interface also causes internal reflection of diffuse, back-scattered radiation, which is an important consideration when analyzing remittance spectra of skin. Because the surface of the stratum corneum is not smooth and planar: (1) the regular reflectance from skin is not specular, i.e., skin reflectance does not maintain an image and (2) a beam of collimated incident radiation, upon passing through this surface and into the skin, is refracted and therefore made somewhat more diffuse by this rough surface. These effects are similar to those which make ground glass translucent, compared with the transparency of polished glass.

Regular reflectances occurring at the skin surface can be clinically important. Whereas normal skin has a single continuous air-tissue interface, the surface of psoriatic plaques is generally torturous and consists of stacked flakes of abnormal corneocytes, with some air spaces between them. These present multiple optical interfaces, and hence the regular reflectance occurring at the surface of psoriasis vulgaris plaques is greater than that for normal skin, giving the plaques a white, scaly appearance. When lipophilic compounds capable of spreading to and filling the spaces are applied, the regular reflectance of the plaque immediately decreases to values within the range for normal skin [16]. The broad spectral character, magnitude, and rapidity of the decreases in reflectance indicate that the mechanism involved is the closer matching of the refractive index between the applied compound and the skin, as compared to air and skin. As would be expected, similar application to normal skin does not affect its regular reflectance, because it possesses only a single interface. Because the observed decrease in psoriatic skin reflectance is unrelated to optical absorption by the applied compounds, a greater fraction of the incident radiation must penetrate the plaque, but not normal skin sites, after application of oils. These observations explain in part why nonphotosensitizing oily lubricants when applied prior to phototherapy treatments significantly enhance therapeutic effectiveness [16].

Within any of the layers of skin, the 93% to 96% of the incident radiation not returned by regular reflectance may be absorbed or scattered. These two processes taken together essentially determine the penetration of radiation into skin, as well as the remittance of scattered radiation from the skin. Scattering results from inhomogeneities in a medium's refractive index, corresponding to physical inhomogeneities. The spatial distribution and intensity of scattered light depends upon the size and shape of the inhomogeneities relative to the wavelength, and upon the difference in refractive index between the medium and the inhomogeneities. For molecules or small particles with dimensions less than roughly one-tenth of the wavelength, scattering is generally weak, nearly isotropic

(equally distributed spatially), polarized, and varies inversely with the 4th power of wavelength (Rayleigh scattering). For particles with dimensions on the same order as the wavelength, scattering is much stronger, more forward-directed, and, while varying inversely with wavelength, is not such a strong inverse function. When the particle size greatly exceeds the wavelength (so-called Mie scattering), scattering is again diminished and becomes highly forward-directed. Within the skin all of these general types of scattering occur, but quantitatively, scattering by stuctures with dimensions on the order of optical wavelengths or somewhat larger must dominate over Rayleigh scattering. In particular, scattering by collagen fibers appears to be of major importance in determining the penetration of optical radiation within the dermis [15].

If scattering is marked, most photons experience multiple scattering before being absorbed or back-scattered from the sample. In this case, the spatial distribution of the radiation as it passes through the sample quickly becomes isotropic (i.e., diffuse), regardless of spatial distribution obtained for single scattering. If the radiation is isotropic, one can show that the average pathlength of photons through an infintesimal pathlength dx in any one direction is simply 2 dx [17]. For perfectly diffuse (isotropic) radiation, the situation therefore becomes somewhat simplified, and one can derive absorption and scattering coefficients for diffuse radiation, equal to twice those for collimated radiation because of the pathlength argument given above, in terms of measurements of transmittance and remittance. One popular model for this analysis is that derived by Kubelka and Munk [18–20]. The differential (continuous) model proposed by Kubelka and Munk is neither an elegant nor thorough model of optical radiation transfer, but it is simple and can be most readily applied to skin. In general, the more physically rigorous theories of radiation transfer require a knowledge of structure and optical parameters which is difficult to obtain for skin [21].

The Kubelka-Munk theory assumes that the sample possesses inhomogeneities which are small compared with the sample thickness; that the incident radiation is diffuse; and that regular reflection occurring at the boundaries of a sample can be neglected. Although not all of these assumptions are easily met, especially the latter two, the theory nonetheless offers a means for a simple quantitative treatment of skin optics. Radiation within the sample is divided into 2 opposing diffuse fluxes, I and J (Fig 2). The sample's back-scattering (S) and absorption (K) coefficients for diffuse radiation are defined in two differential equations as the fraction of diffuse radiation either back-scattered or absorbed per unit differential pathlength of the sample. These differential equations are:

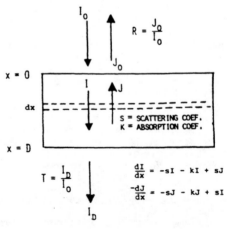

FIG 2. The Kubelka-Munk model for radiation transfer in a turbid, absorbing medium.

$$dI = (-KI - SI + SJ) \, dx \qquad (1)$$

$$-dJ = (-KJ - SJ + SI) \, dx \qquad (2)$$

which simply state that the change, dI, in flux I over some layer of thickness dx is equal to that fraction of I removed by absorption and back-scattering plus some fraction contributed to I by back-scattering from J. The 2nd differentiation equation is an analogous statement for J. Integration and substitution of boundary conditions gives a particular solution, which can then be rearranged to express S and K (the 2 unknowns) in terms of R and T (the measurable quantities). Written in the forms derived by Kubelka and Munk, these are:

$$K/S = [(1 + R^2 - T^2)/2R] - 1 \qquad (3)$$

$$S = \frac{1}{d} [K/S(K/S + 2)]^{-1/2} \coth^{-1} \left[\frac{1 - R(K/S + 1)}{R[K/S(K/S + 2)]^{1/2}} \right] \qquad (4)$$

Because a minimum of two different measurements are always necessary to determine the 2 unknowns S and K, measurements of both remittance and transmittance, or remittance with two different reflective "backgrounds," are required. In order to use this model practically, one must also account for regular reflection occurring at both sample boundaries, and adhere to the use of diffuse incident radiation. This has been accomplished for thin samples of human dermis in vitro [15]. Once S and K are known, the two fluxes I and J can be reconstructed, and the radiation density at a given depth can be estimated by summing I and J at that depth. Near the front surface of a scattering sample, the sum of I and J can easily exceed I_0, the incident density of optical radiation. In the extreme case, I plus J just inside the surface of a sample with 100% remittance is twice I_0. Such "concentration" of radiation density due to scattering occurs in fair-skinned individuals for most visible wavelengths, where remittance is high. If a sample is infinitely thick, or simply thick enough that T approaches zero, one can rewrite equation 3 as:

$$\frac{K}{S} = \frac{(R - 1)^2}{2R} \qquad (5)$$

Here, the remittance of a thick sample depends solely upon the ratio of its absorption and scattering coefficients. The dermis is sufficiently thick that for wavelengths less than 600 nm, its transmittance approaches zero, which potentially simplifies analysis of remittance spectra. If one treats S as a known constant, K can be estimated directly from R.

Fortunately, the structures of skin which lead to strong scattering, and hence determines S, appear to be different than those chromophores present which determine K. For any given layer of skin, K is compositely determined by the concentration and distribution of those chromophores present. This is convenient because in normal skin certain chromophores such as hemoglobins, bilirubin, and melanin change rapidly, causing changes in absorption coefficients, whereas scattering coefficients should not change significantly until some gross alteration of structure occurs.

Finally, it is apparent that as the thickness of any particular sample decreases, R always decreases and T always increases. In the case of the stratum corneum, and to a large extent the entire normal human epidermis, the layer is thin enough that its contribution to remittance (other than the regular reflectance discussed above) is minimal over the entire visible and near infrared spectral regions [15].

OPTICS OF THE STRATUM CORNEUM AND EPIDERMIS

Many studies of the transmission of ultraviolet radiation through excised human epidermis and stratum corneum have been reported since the original work of Hasselbalch [22]. Much of the early work failed to account accurately for the diffuse nature of transmission through skin samples. Since the advent of commercially-available spectrophotometers with integrating spheres, several groups have measured and published total transmission spectra of human epidermis [23,24]. The ultraviolet-visible transmission of fair-skinned Caucasian stratum corneum or epidermis qualitatively resembles that of protein containing the aromatic amino acids tryptophan and tyrosine, with a minimum in transmittance near 275 nm due to absorption by these and other aromatic chromophores. Nucleic acids, with an absorption maximum near 260 nm, and numerous small aromatic molecules, especially urocanic acid, with an absorption maximum at 277 nm at pH 7.4, also contribute to the broad 275 nm absorption band seen in epidermis and stratum corneum. Melanin content and distribution usually plays a major but highly variable role in determining the transmission of optical radiation through the statum corneum and epidermis, depending upon the genetically determined capacity of an individual for constitutive and facultative pigmentation. The high absorbance of epidermis and stratum corneum for wavelengths less than 240 nm is largely due to peptide bonds.

The measurement of epidermal transmittance is complicated by a broad fluorescence excitation band centered near 280 nm, associated with an emission band between 330 and 360 nm, consistent with tryptophan or tyrosine fluorescence [25]. This emission band is of sufficient intensity to cause suspicion of epidermal transmission spectra in the region less than 300 nm, when taken with integrating spheres equipped with broadband (UV-visible sensitive) photomultipliers, as in essentially all standard spectrophotometer systems. A second problem arises if the epidermal sheet is suspended in air or placed against a quartz slide, typically at the entrance port of an integrating sphere. Some total internal reflection of forward-scattered and refracted off-axis rays occurs, which are then lost for measurement purposes.

The autofluorescence error can be overcome by using a "solar-blind" detector, which is insensitive to wavelengths longer than 320 nm, and the problem of total internal reflection can be overcome by using normal saline as the optical medium on the dermal side of epidermal samples. This also maintains the samples in a physical environment similar to that in vivo. Representative fair-skinned Caucasian epidermal and stratum corneum transmission (T) spectra taken with such a system, and expressed in apparent optical density (O.D. = log T) units, are presented in Fig 3a and 3b and compared with conventional spectra not corrected for autofluorescence [25].

Absorption spectra of major epidermal pigments are given in Fig 4. It can be seen that epidermal or corneal transmittance spectra are compositely determined by absorption by these (and certainly other) substances. Variations in the concentrations, distributions, or amounts of these chromophores, and in epidermal thickness, largely determine individual and anatomic variations in epidermal spectral transmission. One would expect the protein- and nucleic-acid-bound chromophores to be of rather constant concentration and distribution in normal skin, since these chromophores are inherent necessities of the cellular tissue. Both melanin and urocanic acid, however, have variable concentrations and distributions and unlike protein or nucleic acid, ultraviolet optical absorption may be their major functional role in human skin.

There are conflicting reports on the possible photoinduction of urocanic acid synthesis in the epidermis [26,27] but melanin is certainly photoinducible. In the visible portion of the spectrum, melanin is essentially the only pigment affecting the transmittance of normal human epidermis, giving rise to the wide range of discernable skin colors from "black" to "white." The 300 nm transmittance of full-thickness suction-separated epidermis including the basal cell layer varies by 2 to 3 orders of magnitude from very fair-skinned Caucasian to darkly pigmented Negro individuals.

Melanin is not a "neutral density" filter of the skin; its absorption increases steadily toward shorter wavelengths over the broad spectrum of 250 to 1,200 nm. In the near infrared,

31

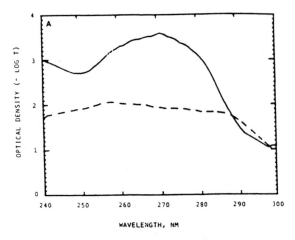

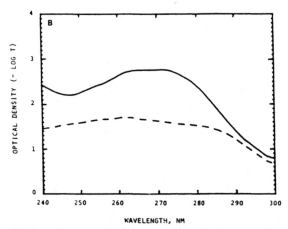

FIG. 3. *a*, Apparent optical density of Caucasian human epidermis sample taken with (——) and without (- - - - -) correction for tissue autofluoresence. Overestimation of transmittance occurs due to auto-fluorescence. Sample was obtained from amputated thigh skin, was separated by immersion in 60°C water for 30 sec, and consisted of the entire epidermis minus the basal cell layer. *b*, Apparent optical density of stratum corneum from skin adjacent to that shown in Fig 3*a*. Sample was separated by 8-h incubation at 37°C in the presence of 10 mg/ml staphylococcal scalded skin syndrome epidermolytic toxin [45] in Hepe's buffer with 20% FCS, and consisted of stratum corneum plus stratum granulosum.

beyond about 1100 nm, absorption by melanin is essentially negligible. For wavelengths longer than 1100 nm, both skin transmittance [28] and remittance [29,30] (Fig 5) are unaffected by melanin pigmentation.

In addition to increasing melanogenesis, UV exposures of skin cause epidermal hyperplasia [31,32]. The relative degree of UV-induced photoprotection offered by melanogenesis versus epidermal hyperplasia depends upon the wavelengths in question, and individual factors. For wavelengths less than 300 nm, and certainly at 275 nm, hyperplasia can offer effective photoprotection, but at longer wavelengths, melanin is the only major epidermal chromophore in normal skin. The capacity for inducing various degrees of hyperpigmentation (tanning) is variable and complexly genetically determined. Precíse dose-response, action spectrum, or photoprotective-effect studies for single exposures or for multiple exposures leading to steady-state equilibria of this interesting photoinducible, photoprotective system are lacking. The action spectrum for induction of melanogenesis grossly resembles that for induction of delayed erythema, but at longer wavelengths in the near UV or visible

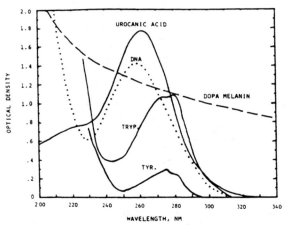

FIG. 4. UV absorption spectra of major epidermal chromophores. DOPA-melanin, 1.5 mg% in H_2O; urocanic acid, 10^{-4} M in H_2O; calf thymus DNA, 10 mg% in H_2O (pH 4.5); tryptophane, 2×10^{-4} M (pH 7); tyrosine, 2×10^{-4} M (pH 7). The broad epidermal absorption band near 275 nm is the result of absorption by protein, urocanic acid, nucleic acids, and other aromatic chromphores.

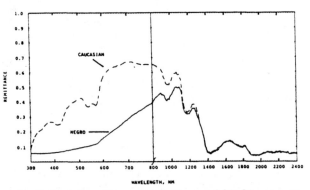

FIG 5. Spectral remittance of dark Negro and fair Caucasian skin (flexor surface of forearm in each case). The lack of significant absorption by melanin for wavelengths longer than approximately 1,100 nm, and increased absorption at shorter wavelengths, is apparent. Note also that, because of regular reflectance at the skin surface, remittance is never less than 5% in either case.

spectral regions, melanogenesis can be induced by suberythemogenic exposure doses [33,34]. UVA (320–400 nm)-induced tanning may be less protective against UVB (290–320 nm) radiation than UVB-induced tanning [35]. The mechanism for this difference is unknown.

Melanin is a remarkably stable protein-polymer complex, the chromophoric backbone of which survives attack by proteases, acids and bases. Caucasian melanosomes typically contain a greater number of melanin granules, but less total melanin, than Negroid or Mongolian melanosomes, and also appear to suffer greater degradation within keratinocytes. The optical effects associated with dispersed "melanin dust" in Caucasians versus intact melanosomes have not been quantitated, but it is likely that, unless the chromophoric backbone is degraded, dispersal of melanin pigment in Caucasian stratum corneum affords somewhat greater protection than would the same quantity of melanin sequestered in intact melanosomes. An interracial study of epidermal transmittance by Kaidbey, et al [36] suggests that the large racial differences in sensitivity to UV of 10- to 30-fold [37,38] correlate poorly with the small racial differences of approximately 3-fold noted in stratum corneum transmission. However, the minimal erythema dose of black and white subjects has never been directly compared with accurate stratum corneum or epidermal transmittance measurements of samples from the same subjects, split at various levels in the tissue.

Urocanic acid is thought to play some role as an "endogenous sunscreen" of the epidermis and stratum corneum [39,40]. Recent observations [41] show that extraction of water soluble, diffusible, UV-absorbing compounds from skin into topically applied water accounts for the up to 50% increased sensitivity of skin to UVB radiation after hydrating the skin for prolonged periods. While most of the material extracted is lipid or protein, a small fraction (about 0.2%) of the material is urocanic acid. Because of its high extinction coefficient (18,800 lM^{-1} cm^{-1} at 277 nm, pH 7.4), however, urocanic acid accounted for approximately 75% of the optical absorbance of the extracted materials. Because extensive exposure to sunlight is often associated with sweating, which deposits urocanic acid on the skin surface [39], it is possible that sweating may serve to some extent as a thermally-induced photoprotective mechanism.

In those studies that have compared diffuse versus direct (total transmittance versus transmittance along an optical path in line with the incident beam) transmittance of epidermis or stratum corneum, the ratio of diffuse/direct transmission does not appear to be wavelength dependent [23,42] for either UV or visible wavelengths. This broadband independence of wavelength suggests that the diffuse nature of epidermal transmission of ultraviolet wavelengths is due more to the irregular refractive surface of skin than to particle scattering within the epidermis. Furthermore, other than regular reflectance, only about 5% of collimated incident radiation in the 350-3000 nm region is remitted by scattering within Caucasian epidermis [15]. This observation is consistent with a thin sample in which the back-scattering coefficient (S), is small compared with the reciprocal of the sample thickness (<100 cm^{-1}) and/or absorption relative to scattering is large. Epidermal transmittance spectra of fair Caucasians indicate that most of incident near UV, visible, and near infrared radiation is transmitted through epidermis; one must conclude from the above that whatever back-scattering occurs in normal epidermis over this spectral region is for practical purposes weak, and that any strong scattering within epidermis that does occur must be forward-directed, i.e., off-axis refraction occurring at the skin surface, and large-particle scattering within the tissue. It must be pointed out, however, that despite the central role of the epidermis in providing optical protection for humans, a thorough attempt to model epidermal optics is still lacking.

OPTICS OF THE DERMIS

The dermis has distinctly different optical properties than the epidermis, reflecting differences in structure and composition. Perhaps because the epidermis is easily isolated and forms the first "optical element" of skin, relatively few studies have concentrated upon dermal optics. Hardy, Hammell, and Murgatroyd [28] goniometrically measured visible and near infrared transmittance of skin sections in vitro, which included various fractions of dermis. The data indicates that the Beer-Lambert relation is invalid for dermis, and that transmittance is both higher and more forward-directed for longer wavelengths over the region between 0.5 and 1.23 μm. These observations suggest that scattering is of major importance in the dermis. Findlay [43] measured transmittance and remittance spectra of dura mater and pig dermis and found that thin sections, which appeared blue when placed on a black background, showed greater transmittance of longer wavelengths, similar to Hardy et al.'s findings, but exhibited greater remittance of shorter wavelengths. Summing Findlay's transmittance and remittance spectra gives values close to 1.0 (100%) across the entire visible spectrum, indicating that very little visible light was actually absorbed. The best explanation for his data is that scattering in the dermis must vary inversely with wavelength. Anderson, et al. [15] have presented calculations of spectral scattering (S)

and absorption (K) coefficients for human dermis in vitro by application of a modified Kubelka-Munk theory to measurements of transmittance and remittance of thin dermal sections. Measurements were made under conditions appropriate to the assumptions inherent in this model. The spectral transmittance and remittance of a typical 200 μm thick human papillary dermis section, analogous to those of Findlay, are shown in Fig 6. Calculated values for S and K are shown in Fig 7. Dermal scattering is markedly increased at shorter wavelengths. The absorption coefficient, D, for bloodless dermis is smaller than S except at the prominent absorption bands of water in the infrared region. Dermal scattering therefore plays a major role in determining the depth to which radiation of various wavelengths penetrates the dermis, and largely accounts for observations [28, 44] that, in general, longer wavelengths across the UV-visible-near infrared spectrum penetrate the dermis to a greater extent than do shorter wavelengths.

The appearance of blue skin nevi can be explained based upon this fact. The average dermal pathlength and depth of penetration of remitted shorter wavelengths (blue) light is much less than that of longer wavelengths (red) light. This is because of increased scattering at shorter wavelengths. In blue nevi, melanin is pathologically deposited in the dermis. Blue light encounters less of the dermally deposited melanin than red light, and may therefore suffer less absorption. Such scattering is the only means by which a pigment, such as melanin, which absorbs shorter wavelengths more strongly than longer wavelengths, can produce blue colors.

In vivo, the blood-borne pigments hemoglobin, oxy-hemoglobin, beta-carotene, and bilirubin are the major absorbers of

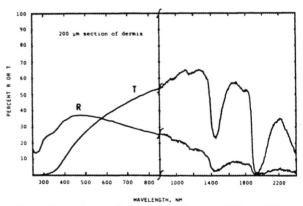

FIG 6. Spectral transmittance and remittance of 200 μm thickness section of human dermis.

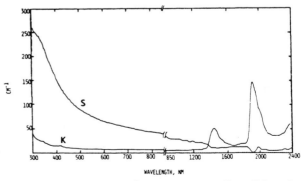

FIG 7. Diffuse scattering (S) and absorption (K) coefficients for human dermis in vitro, calculated from measurements of spectral remittance and transmittance of thin dermal sections under conditions appropriate to application of the Kubelka-Munk theory of radiation transfer [15].

33

visible radiation in the dermis. Absorption spectra for these dermal chromophores, and for dopa-melanin, are shown in Fig 8. In addition, typically less than 1% of the total hemoglobin in blood is methemoglobin, which has an absorption band in the red visible region. The effect of these substances on K is not seen in the *in vitro* dermal spectra presented above but can be estimated or inferred from *in vivo* remittance spectra. This is done in the near UV and visible spectrum by assuming S to be the same *in vivo* as measured *in vitro*, and using the *in vivo* remittance of very fair or vitiliginous skin as an approximation of R for an infinitely thick sample, with no melanin pigmentation. K can therefore be determined from eq. 5 above. The 2 fluxes I and J can then be reconstructed, and summed to find the total flux density at a depth x. It can be shown that this sum is $I_o e^{-1}$ when

$$x = \beta/K\left[1 + \ln\left(\frac{2}{1 + \beta}\right)\right]$$

where β is given by

$$\beta = \left[\frac{K}{K + 2S}\right]^{1/2}.$$

For shorter wavelengths, the 1/e values can be estimated from epidermal transmittance spectra. The Table gives estimated depths for which radiation is attenuated to 1/e of the incident radiation density, for fair Caucasian skin *in vitro*. It must be realized that the values given in the Table are only estimations of the depths of penetration of various wavelengths, based on a highly simplified model, and for vitiliginous skin. The epider-

mis of pigmented individuals can greatly reduce these values, especially at shorter wavelengths, as discussed above.

Since the penetration of optical radiation in the tissue is wavelength-dependent, stratification of pigments at different depths influences the spectral distribution of the radiation reaching a given stratum. For example, only the superficial vessels—capillaries and the venular plexus—will be exposed to significant blue or UV radiation. Conversely, an optical "window" exists in skin and most other soft tissue in the region 600–1300 nm. Whenever it is possible to use some portion of the penetrating 600–1300 nm wavelength region to cause phototoxicity, the volume and depth of tissue affected will be large. Preliminary measurements show that up to 1% of the 605 to 850 nm wavelength region penetrates the entire human chest wall, post mortem. The transmittance of wavelengths less than 550 nm is less than 10^{-5}, however [25].

SUMMARY

The stratum corneum and epidermis provide an optical barrier primarily by absorption of radiation, and to a lesser degree, by optical scattering. In the ultraviolet region less than 300 nm, aromatic amino acids, nucleic acids, urocanic acid, and melanin can be defined as major epidermal absorbers. Hyperplasia, melanogenesis, and perhaps urocanic acid synthesis, form an inducible photoprotective system. The relative importance of these variable protective factors is wavelength-dependent and varies between skin sites and individuals. In the wavelength region 350–1200 nm, melanin is the major absorber of radiation in the epidermis, especially at shorter wavelengths. One can manipulate the optics of the epidermis by various stimuli including UV radiation, by extraction *in vivo* of UV-absorbing compounds, most notably urocanic acid, and in the case of psoriasis by a superficial refractive index matching mechanism when oil is applied. A rigorous model, with data, for epidermal optics is lacking.

The dermis may be considered a turbid tissue matrix with which optical scattering is an inverse function of wavelength and largely defines the depth of optical penetration. Absorption bands of blood-borne chromophores, especially bilirubin and oxyhemoglobin, are apparent in remittance spectra of skin, and such spectra can be used to monitor or analyze serum bilirubin, vascular, or pigmentation responses. Despite many complicating factors, it is possible to approximate the optics of the dermis using radiation-transfer theories, and a simple model is presented.

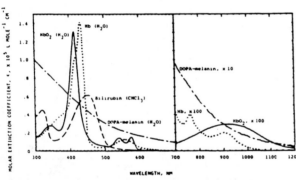

FIG 8. Absorption spectra of major visible-absorbing pigments of human skin, HbO$_2$ (——), Hb (. . . . .), bilirubin (- - - - -), and DOPA-melanin (— · —). Parentheses indicate solvent. The spectrum shown for DOPA-melanin is the absorbance on a scale of 0 to 1.5 of 1.5 mg% aqueous solution. Not shown is β-carotene, which has a broad absorption band qualitatively similar to that for bilirubin in the 400–500 nm region, with maxima at 466 and 497 nm in CHCl$_3$. Note scale changes in the near infrared.

Approximate depth for penetration of optical radiation in fair Caucasian skin to a value of 1/e (37%) of the incident energy density

Wavelength (nm)	Depth (μm)
250	2
280	1.5
300	6
350	60
400	90
450	150
500	230
600	550
700	750
800	1200
1000	1600
1200	2200

REFERENCES

1. Edwards EA, Duntley SQ: The pigments and color of human skin. Am J Anat 65:1–33, 1939
2. Goldzieher JW, Roberts IS, Rawls WB, Goldzieher MA: "Chemical analysis of the intact skin by reflectance spectrophotometry. Arch Dermatol Syphilol 64:533–548, 1951
3. Edwards EA, Finkelstein NA, Duntley SQ: Spectrophotometery of living human skin in ultraviolet range. J Invest Dermatol 16:311–321, 1951
4. Sheard C, Brown E: The spectrophotometric analysis of the color of the skin. Arch Int Med 38:816–831, 1926
5. Daniels F, Imbrie JD: Comparison between visual grading and reflectance measurements of erythema produced by sunlight. J Invest Dermatol 30:295–301, 1958
6. Breit R, Kligman AM: Measurement of erythemal and pigmentary responses to ultraviolet radiation of different spectral qualities, The Biologic Effects of Ultraviolet Radiation (with Emphasis on the Skin). Edited by F. Urbach. Oxford, Pergamon Press, 1969, pp 267–275
7. Frank L, Rapp Y, Bergman LV: An instrument for the objective measurement of erythema. J Invest Dermatol 38:21–24, 1962
8. Tronnier H: Evaluation and measurement of ultraviolet erythema, The Biologic Effects of Ultraviolet Radiation (with Emphasis on the Skin). Edited by F. Urbach. Oxford, Pergamon Press, 1969, pp 255–265
9. Feather JW, Dawson JB, Barker DJ, Cotterill JA: A theoretical and experimental study of the optical properties of skin *in vivo*, Proceedings of the Symposium on Bioengineering and the Skin. Cardiff, MTP Press, Ltd., International Medical Publishers, 1980, in press

10. Ballowitz L, Avery ME: Spectral reflectance of the skin. Biology of the Neonate 15:348–360, 1970
11. Bruce RA: Noninvasive estimation of bilirubin and hemoglobin oxygen saturation in the skin by reflection spectrophotometry. Ph.D. Thesis, Duke University, Durham, North Carolina, 1978
12. Haunemann RE, DeWitt DP, Weichel JF: Neonatal serum bilirubin from skin reflectance. Pediat Res 12:207–210, 1978
13. Scheuplein RJ: A survey of some fundamental aspects of the absorption and reflection of light by tissue. J Soc Cosmet Chem 15:111–122, 1964
14. Parrish JA, Anderson RR, Urbach F, Pitts D: UV-A: Biologic Effects of Ultraviolet Radiation with Emphasis on Human Responses to Longwave Ultraviolet. New York, Plenum Press, 1978
15. Anderson RR, Hu J, Parrish JA: Optical radiation transfer in the human skin and application in in vivo remittance spectroscopy, Proceedings of the Symposium on Bioengineering and the Skin, Cardiff, Wales, July 19–21, 1979. MTP Press, Ltd., London, 1980, in press
16. Anderson RR, LeVine MJ, Parrish JA: Selective modification of the optical properties of psoriatic vs. normal skin. Book of Abstracts, 8th International Photobiology Congress, Strasbourg, France, July 1980, p 152
17. Kortum G: Reflectance Spectroscopy. New York, Springer-Verlag, 1969
18. Kubelka P, Munk F: Ein Beitrag zür Optik der Farbanstriche. Z Technichse Physik 12:593–601, 1931
19. Kubelka P: New contributions to the optics of intensely light-scattering materials. Part I. J Opt Soc Am 38:448–457, 1948
20. Kubelka P: New contributions to the optics of intensely light-scattering materials. Part II: nonhomogeneous layers. J Opts Soc Am 44:330–335, 1954
21. Atkins JT: Optical properties of turbid materials, The Biological Effects of Ultraviolet Radiation (with Emphasis on the Skin). Edited by F Urbach. Oxford, Pergamon Press, 1969, pp 141–150
22. Hasselbalch KA: Quantitative Untersuchungen uber die Absorption der menschlichen Haut von ultravioletten Strahlen. Skand Arch Physiol 25:5–68, 1911
23. Everett MA, Yeargers E, Sayre RM, Olson RL: Penetration of epidermis by ultraviolet rays. Photochem Photobiol 5:533–542, 1966
24. Pathak MA: Photobiology of melanogenesis: biophysical aspects, Advances in Biology of the Skin, Vol. VIII, The Pigmentary System. Edited by W. Montagna, F. Hu. Oxford, Pergamon Press, 1967, pp 397–420
25. Anderson RR, Parrish JA: Unpublished observations.
26. Hais IM, Strych A: Increase in urocanic acid concentration in human epidermis following insolation. Coll Czech Chem Comm 34:649–655, 1969
27. Baden HP, Pathak MA: The metabolism and function of urocanic acid in skin. J Invest Dermatol 48:11–17, 1967
28. Hardy JD, Hammell HT, Murgatroyd D: Spectral transmittance and reflectance of excised human skin. J Appl Physiol 9:257–264, 1956
29. Jacquez JA, Huss J, McKeehan W, Dimitroff JM, Kuppenheim HF: Spectral reflectance of human skin in the region 0.7–2.6 μ. J Appl Physiol 8:297–299, 1956
30. Kuppenheim H, Heer RR, Jr.: Spectral reflectance of white and Negro skin between 400 and 1000 mμ. J Appl Physiol 4:800–806, 1952
31. Baden HP, Pearlman C: The effects of ultraviolet light on protein and nucleic acid synthesis in the epidermis. J Invest Dermatol 48:71–75, 1964
32. Epstein JH, Fukuyama K, Fye K: Effects of ultraviolet radiation on the mitotic cycle and DNA, RNA and protein synthesis in mammalian epidermis in vivo. Photochem Photobiol 12:57–65, 1970
33. Parrish JA, Zaynoun S, Anderson RR: Cumulative effects of repeated subthreshold doses of ultraviolet radiation. J Invest Dermatol, May, 1981
34. Langner A, Kligman A: Tanning without sunburn with aminobenzoic acid type sunscreen. Arch Dermatol 106:338–343, 1972
35. Kaidbey KH, Kligman AM: Sunburn protection by longwave ultraviolet radiation-induced pigmentation. Arch Dermatol 114:46–48, 1978
36. Kaidbey KH, Poh-Agin P, Sayre RR, Kligman AM: Photoprotection by melanin—A comparison of black and Caucasian skin. J Am Acad Dermatol 1:249–260, 1979
37. Olson RL, Gaylor J, Everett MA: Skin color, malanin, and erythema. Arch Dermatol 108:541–544, 1973
38. Hausser KW, Vahle W: Sunburn and suntanning, The Biologic Effects of Ultraviolet Radiation (with Emphasis on the Skin). Edited by F Urbach. Oxford, Pergamon Press, 1969, pp 3–21
39. Zeniske A, Krahl JA: The occurrence of urocanic acid in sweat. Biochim Biophys Acta 12:479–484, 1953
40. Everett MA, Anglin JH, Bever AT: Ultraviolet-induced biochemical alterations in skin. Arch Dermatol 84:717–724, 1961
41. Anderson RR, Blank IH, Parrish JA: Mechanisms of increased ultraviolet transmittance through human skin after topical applications (abstract), Program and Abstracts, 7th Annual Meeting of the American Society for Photobiology, Pacific Grove, California, June 1979, p 141
42. Lucas NS: The permeability of human epidermis to ultraviolet radiation. Biochem J 25:57–70, 1930
43. Findlay GH: Blue skin. Br J Dermatol 83:127–134, 1970
44. Bachem A, Reed CI: The transparency of live and dead animal tissue to ultraviolet light. Am J Physiol 90:600–606, 1929
45. Elias PM, Fritsch P, Dahl MV, Wolff K: Staphylococcal toxic epidermal necrolysis: Pathogenesis and studies on the subcellular site of action of exfoliation. J Invest Dermatol 65:501–512, 1975

Reprinted with permission from *Applied Optics,* Vol. 22(16), pp. 2456-2462
(August 15, 1983). ©1983 Optical Society of America.

Scattering and absorption of turbid materials determined from reflection measurements.   1:   Theory

R. A. J. Groenhuis, H. A. Ferwerda, and J. J. Ten Bosch

To allow the determination of scattering and absorption parameters of a turbid material from reflection measurements the relation of these parameters to the reflection has been described by two theoretical approaches. One approach is based on the diffusion theory which has been extended to include anisotropic scattering. This results in a reflection formula in which the scattering and absorption are described by one parameter each. As a second more general approach a Monte Carlo model is applied. Comparison of the results indicates the range of values of the scattering and absorption parameters where the computationally fast diffusion approach is applicable.

I.   Introduction

Up to now experimental methods to determine the scattering and absorption characteristics of turbid materials mostly are based on measurements of the reflection and transmission of slabs of the material. This may pose a problem if only the reflection can be measured, i.e., in bulk material. Therefore, a method was developed to determine the scattering and absorption characteristics of turbid materials from reflection measurements only. A related approach was recently proposed by Langerholc.[1]

Figure 1 shows schematically the measuring arrangement. Light normally incident upon a sample is scattered and possibly also partly absorbed. The reflected light is measured as a function of the distance between the center of the incident beam and the measuring spot. The detector measures mainly multiply scattered light.

Multiple-scattering theory has to be used to describe the reflection properly. Three approaches in dealing with 3-D multiple-scattering problems have been developed: analytical theories; transport theory; and a Monte Carlo method.[2,3]

(1) Analytical theory is based on the fundamental equations governing field quantities: the Maxwell equations in particular. The scattering and absorption characteristics of the scattering particles are introduced via the material equation, and so differential or integral equations for statistical quantities such as correlation functions are obtained. Although in principle mathematically rigorous, in practice approximations have to be made to get useful results.[2,3] Twersky's theory is an example of these analytical theories.[4]

(2) Transport theory[5,6] deals directly with transport of photon energy through a medium containing scattering particles. This theory has been developed independently of the analytical theory. Its foundation on the Maxwell equations has not been clarified completely. Wolf[7] has developed a new theory of radiative transfer related to Maxwell's equations. Only recently Fante[8] has extended Wolf's theory to material media. For the case of isotropic nondispersive media he has derived the conditions under which the radiative transport theory is consistent with Maxwell's equations. The basic equation in transport theory is the equation of transfer, which is also used in neutron transport theory.[9] The transport theory is often used in the diffusion approximation, i.e., at every point (outside the incident beam) radiative transfer is described only by the photon number density and the net photon flux. This is allowed if the light is scattered many times and as a result has an almost uniform angular distribution. The transport theory in the diffusion approximation or, briefly, diffusion theory was used by Reynolds *et al.*[10] to determine the relative reflectance by a whole blood

H. A. Ferwerda is with State University Groningen, Department of Applied Physics, Nijenborgh 18, 9717 AG Groningen, The Netherlands. J. J. Ten Bosch is with State University Groningen, Laboratory for Materia Technica, A. Deusinglaan 1, 9716 AV Groningen, The Netherlands, as was R. A. J. Groenhuis, when this work was done; he is now with U.S. National Institutes of Health, National Institute of Dental Research, Bethesda, Maryland 20205.

Received 10 September 1982.
0003-6935/83/162456-07$01.00/0.

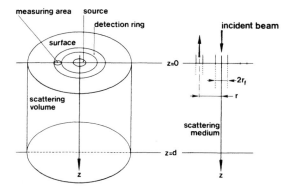

Fig. 1. Geometry to measure the reflected light as a function of the distance to a small incident beam: 3-D representation and cross section through the z axis.

medium. The geometry used in their treatment strongly resembles ours.

(3) In a Monte Carlo simulation of radiative transfer[11-13] photons generated to represent a light source are followed on their pathways in the material until detection, escape, or absorption occurs. The pathways are calculated on the basis of the scattering and absorption characteristics of the material and random distribution of scattering events. Usually much computer time is required for Monte Carlo calculations. In every geometry a Monte Carlo simulation can be used.

This paper discusses two approaches: the diffusion theory and the Monte Carlo method. The methods are applied to materials with various scattering and absorption characteristics. The results are compared yielding the ranges of the scattering and absorption parameters where the diffusion theory may be applied.

The scattering in the material is described by the number density ρ of the scattering particles, the scattering cross section σ_s, and the scattering phase function and the absorption by the number density and the absorption cross section σ_a.

One application of the measuring method shown in Fig. 1—an application we are interested in—refers to human dental enamel, the tissue ~2 mm thick which covers the crowns of the teeth. Sound enamel is rather translucent. Incipient caries results in structural changes inside the enamel appearing as opaque spots in the enamel, the white spots. Measurements of the optical parameters of teeth may indicate the stage of the caries process.[14] Other applications of the method seem to be obvious in biological as well as other fields.

II. Diffusion Theory

A. Derivation of the Diffusion Theory

The derivation of the diffusion theory described here closely follows the treatment given by Ishimaru.[2,3] However, scattering by anisotropic scatterers is introduced in a different way in the derivation of the diffusion equation as will be shown.

Transport theory is based on the equation of transfer[3]:

$$(\mathbf{s} \cdot \nabla_r)L(\mathbf{r,s}) = -\rho\sigma_t L(\mathbf{r,s}) + \frac{\rho\sigma_t}{4\pi} \int_{4\pi} p(\mathbf{s,s'})L(\mathbf{r,s'})d\omega', \quad (1)$$

where $L(\mathbf{r,s})$ = radiance in point $\mathbf{r}$ in the direction defined by unit vector $\mathbf{s}$ (W m^{-2} sr^{-1}Hz^{-1});

ρ = number of scattering particles per unit volume (m^{-3});

σ_s = single-particle scattering cross section (m^2);

σ_a = single-particle absorption cross section (m^2);

$\sigma_t = \sigma_s + \sigma_a$ = total cross section (m^2);

$\omega_0 = \sigma_s/\sigma_t$ = single-particle albedo;

$p(\mathbf{s,s'})$ = phase function describing the part of the photon flux scattered from the direction $\mathbf{s'}$ into the direction $\mathbf{s}$(sr^{-1}). The normalization is such that

$$\frac{1}{4\pi} \int_{4\pi} p(\mathbf{s,s'})d\omega' = \omega_0;$$

$d\omega'$ = element of solid angle (sr); and

$\mu = \mathbf{s} \cdot \mathbf{s'}$ = cosine of the scattering angle, the angle between the unit vectors $\mathbf{s}$ and $\mathbf{s'}$.

We assume that the phase function is only a function of μ and ω_0. Physically this means that the scattering particles are randomly oriented. Often in this case the Henyey-Greenstein phase function[15] is used:

$$p(\mu) = \omega_0(1 - g^2)(1 + g^2 - 2g\mu)^{-3/2}, \quad (2)$$

where $g = \bar{\mu}$, the mean cosine of the scattering angle.

The anisotropy of the scattering is described by g: the scattering varies continuously from backwardly peaked ($g = -1$) via isotropical ($g = 0$) to forwardly peaked ($g = 1$). The phase function is a useful model for scattering processes occurring, e.g., in blood,[10] in the sky.[15]

We will adopt a simpler phase function:

$$p(\mu) = \omega_0[(1 - g) + 4g\delta(\mu - 1)]. \quad (3)$$

The first term describes isotropic scattering, the second term strongly forwardly peaked scattering as indicated by the delta function $\delta(\mu - 1)$. This phase function permits separation of the radiance of the scattered light into a nearly diffuse part and a part parallel to the incident beam [see Eq. (6)]. The constants in Eq. (3) have been chosen so that the first two moments in Eqs. (2) and (3) are the same.

Substitution of Eq. (3) into Eq. (1) yields

$$(\mathbf{s} \cdot \nabla_r)L(\mathbf{r,s}) = -\rho\sigma_{tr}L(\mathbf{r,s}) + \frac{\rho\sigma_s'}{4\pi} \int_{4\pi} L(\mathbf{r,s'})d\omega', \quad (4)$$

where $\sigma_s' = \sigma_s(1 - g)$ = effective scattering cross section; $\sigma_{tr} = \sigma_s' + \sigma_a$ = transport cross section.

The scattering medium is supposed to be bound by two parallel planes. The z axis is chosen perpendicular to these planes. One of the planes ($z = 0$) is illuminated by a cylindrical beam of light parallel to the z axis. The radiance of this beam is given by

$$L_{inc}(\mathbf{r},\mathbf{s}) = E_0 u(r - r_f) \cdot \delta(\mu' - 1), \tag{5}$$

where E_0 = constant irradiance (W m^{-2} Hz^{-1});
    r_f = radius of the incident beam (m);
    r = distance to the z axis, the axis of the incident beam (m);
    $u(r - r_f)$ = unit step function = 1 if $r < r_f$, = 0 if $r > r_f$, and
    μ' = cosine of the angle with the z axis.

It is convenient to divide the radiance in the medium into two parts:

$$L(\mathbf{r},\mathbf{s}) = L_{ri}(r,z) + L_d(\mathbf{r},\mathbf{s}), \tag{6}$$

where $L_{ri}(r,z)$ = reduced incident radiance (W m^{-2} sr^{-1}Hz^{-1}), and $L_d(\mathbf{r},\mathbf{s})$ = (nearly) diffuse radiance (W m^{-2}sr^{-1}Hz^{-1}). The reduced incident radiance includes the unscattered and the forward-scattered incident radiance. This indicates that $L_{ri}(r,z)$ satisfies the following equation [see also Eq. (4)]:

$$\frac{d}{dz}L_{ri}(r,z) = -\rho\sigma_{tr}L_{ri}(r,z). \tag{7}$$

This means that $L_{ri}(r,z)$ is reduced by losses due to absorption and nonforward scattering. Temporarily surface reflection is left aside (see Sec. II.C). Then Eq. (5) gives the boundary condition at the surface ($z = 0$): $L_{ri}(r,z)|_{z=0} = L_{inc}$. The solution of Eq. (7) becomes

$$L_{ri}(r,z) = E_0 u(r - r_f)\delta(\mu' - 1)\exp(-\rho\sigma_{tr}z). \tag{8}$$

Substitution of Eqs. (6) and (8) into Eq. (4) yields

$$(s \cdot \nabla_r)L_d(\mathbf{r},\mathbf{s}) = -\rho\sigma_{tr}L_d(\mathbf{r},\mathbf{s}) + \frac{1}{4}\rho\sigma'_s E_0 u(r - r_f)\exp(-\rho\sigma_{tr}z)$$
$$+ \frac{1}{4\pi}\rho\sigma'_s \int_{4\pi} L_d(\mathbf{r},\mathbf{s}')d\omega'. \tag{9}$$

Since $L_d(\mathbf{r},\mathbf{s})$ describes nearly diffuse radiation (which is almost isotropic) it may be approximated by the first two terms of its Taylor series expansion[3]:

$$L_d(\mathbf{r},\mathbf{s}) = U_d(\mathbf{r}) + \frac{3}{4\pi}\mathbf{F}_d(\mathbf{r}) \cdot \mathbf{s}, \tag{10}$$

where $U_d(\mathbf{r})$ = average diffuse radiance (W m^{-2} sr^{-1}Hz^{-1}) and $\mathbf{F}_d(\mathbf{r})$ = net diffuse photon flux (W m^{-2} sr^{-1}Hz^{-1}). From Eqs. (9) and (10) we may derive the diffusion equation. Substitution of Eq. (10) into Eq. (9) yields

$$\mathbf{s} \cdot \nabla_r U_d(\mathbf{r}) + \frac{3}{4\pi}(\mathbf{s} \cdot \nabla_r)[\mathbf{s} \cdot \mathbf{F}_d(\mathbf{r})]$$
$$= -\rho\sigma_a U_d(\mathbf{r}) - \frac{3}{4\pi}\rho\sigma_{tr}[\mathbf{F}_d(\mathbf{r}) \cdot \mathbf{s}]$$
$$+ \tfrac{1}{4}\rho\sigma'_s E_0 u(r - r_f)\exp(-\rho\sigma_{tr}z). \tag{11}$$

Integration of Eq. (11) over all directions yields

$$\nabla_r \cdot \mathbf{F}_d(\mathbf{r}) = -4\pi\rho\sigma_a U_d(\mathbf{r}) + \pi\rho\sigma'_s E_0 u(r - r_f)\exp(-\rho\sigma_{tr}z). \tag{12}$$

Integration of Eq. (11) over all directions after multiplication by $\mathbf{s}$ gives

$$\nabla_r U_d(\mathbf{r}) = -\frac{3}{4\pi}\rho\sigma_{tr}\mathbf{F}_d(\mathbf{r}). \tag{13}$$

Elimination of $\mathbf{F}_d(\mathbf{r})$ from Eqs. (12) and (13) yields the time-independent diffusion equation for the average diffuse intensity $U_d(\mathbf{r})$:

$$(\nabla_r^2 - \rho\sigma_a D^{-1})U_d(\mathbf{r}) = -\frac{1}{4}\rho\sigma'_s D^{-1}E_0 u(r - r_f)\exp(-\rho\sigma_{tr}z). \tag{14}$$

where $D = (3\rho\sigma_{tr})^{-1}$ = diffusion coefficient (m).

B. Boundary Conditions

In the most simple case no diffuse surface reflection occurs. As Fig. 1 shows boundary conditions occur at $z = 0$ and $z = d$, where d is the thickness of the material. We confine ourselves to the surface $z = 0$. The exact boundary condition for the diffuse radiance cannot be satisfied.[3] A generally used boundary condition is that at the surface the total diffuse flux directed inward is zero[9]:

$$\int_{2\pi,\mu'>0} L_d(\mathbf{r},\mathbf{s})(\mathbf{s} \cdot \mathbf{z})d\omega = 0 \quad \text{at } z = 0. \tag{15}$$

Outside the incident beam this boundary condition can be expressed in $U_d(\mathbf{r})$ using Eqs. (10) and (13)[3]:

$$U_d(\mathbf{r}) - h\frac{\partial}{\partial z}U_d(\mathbf{r}) = 0 \quad \text{at } z = 0, \tag{16}$$

where $h = 2D = 2(3\rho\sigma_{tr})^{-1}$. (This holds only in case no diffuse surface reflection occurs.)

Here we consider the more realistic case that diffuse surface reflection occurs. The boundary condition in Eq. (15) can be extended to this case. The boundary condition is that the total diffuse flux directed inward is equal to the reflected part of the total flux directed outward:

$$\int_{2\pi,\mu>0} L_d(\mathbf{r},\mathbf{s})(\mathbf{s} \cdot \mathbf{z})d\omega = r_d \int_{2\pi,\mu<0} L_d(\mathbf{r},\mathbf{s})(\mathbf{s} \cdot \mathbf{z})d\omega. \tag{17}$$

The internal reflection r_d of uniformly diffuse radiation can be calculated using a curve fit by Egan and Hilgeman[16]:

$$r_d \simeq -1.4399n^{-2} + 0.7099n^{-1} + 0.6681 + 0.0636n, \tag{18}$$

where n is the index of refraction of the medium.

Outside the incident beam Eq. (17) can be expressed in $U_d(\mathbf{r})$ using Eqs. (10) and (13):

$$U_d(\mathbf{r}) - 2D\frac{\partial}{\partial z}U_d(\mathbf{r}) = r_d\left[U_d(\mathbf{r}) + 2D\frac{\partial}{\partial z}U_d(\mathbf{r})\right]$$

or

$$U_d(\mathbf{r}) - h\frac{\partial}{\partial z}U_d(\mathbf{r}) = 0 \quad \text{at } z = 0. \tag{19}$$

Analogously,

$$U_d(\mathbf{r}) + h\frac{\partial}{\partial z}U_d(\mathbf{r}) = 0 \quad \text{at } z = d,$$

where $h = 2D(1 + r_d)(1 - r_d)^{-1}$. (This holds in case diffuse surface reflection occurs.)

C. Solution of the Diffusion Equation

We want to determine the relative radiance, defined as the ratio of the detected radiance and the incident radiant flux. The geometry is shown in Fig. 1. A cylindrical beam of radius r_f is normally incident on a slab medium of thickness d. A detector measures the light flux emitted from an area A into an aperture A_1.

Reynolds et al.[10] applied the diffusion equation to light scattering in a whole blood medium. They used almost the same geometry as we do here. They have derived a formula to describe the relative radiance at an arbitrary location in the plane $z = 0$.

Although in general our approach is the same as theirs, many details differ:

(1) We use other boundary conditions [Eq. (19)] because of the diffuse surface reflection.

(2) We use another diffusion equation [Eq. (14)].

(3) We take into account the specular reflection of the incident and emitted beams.

The consequences of these differences are as follows:

(1) Their boundary condition satisfied the same formula as ours [Eq. (19)]. The form of the solution is the same; only the meaning of the parameter h is different.

(2) The diffusion equation that they have used differs from ours [Eq. (14)] in the last term in two respects. First, instead of $\rho\sigma_s$ they have used $\rho\sigma_s(1 + 3g\sigma_t D)$. This difference returns in the final solutions. Second, instead of $\exp(-\rho\sigma_{tr}z)$ they have used $\exp(-\rho\sigma_t z)$. As a consequence the parameter z_i which occurs in the solution has to be solved from the equation

$$\int_0^d \exp(-\rho\sigma_{tr}z')\sin(k_i z' + \gamma_i)dz' = z_i[k_i^2 + (\rho\sigma_{tr})^2]^{-1},$$

where $\gamma_i = \tan^{-1}(hk_i)$,
k_i = solutions of the equation $\tan k_i d = 2hk_i(h^2k_i^2 - 1)^{-1}$,
d = thickness of the slab medium, and
$h = 2D(1 + r_d)(1 - r_d)^{-1}$ [see Eq. (19)].
The result is

$$z_i = \sin\gamma_i[\rho\sigma_{tr} + \exp(-\rho\sigma_{tr}d)(k_i \sin k_i d - \rho\sigma_{tr} \cos k_i d)]$$
$$+ \cos\gamma_i[k_i - \exp(-\rho\sigma_{tr}d)(\rho\sigma_{tr} \sin k_i d + k_i \cos k_i d)]. \quad (20)$$

(3) The coefficient of specular reflection r_s of the incident and emitted beam which both are (almost) perpendicular to the surface is taken into account by multiplying the solution by $(1 - r_s)^2$.

After inserting the modifications mentioned above into the solution obtained by Reynolds et al.[10] the relative radiance $R(r)$ is obtained:

$$R(r) = \frac{1}{2\pi} \frac{(1 - r_s)^2}{\pi r} \frac{dR_d(r)}{dr} \quad (m^{-2}sr^{-1}), \quad (21)$$

where $R_d(r) = \frac{8\rho\sigma_s'}{Dr_f^2} \sum_{i=1}^{\infty} \frac{\Gamma_i z_i R_i(r)}{(k_i^2 + \rho^2\sigma_{tr}^2)\lambda_i^2}$,

$R_i(r) = r_f^2/2 - rr_f I_1(\lambda_i r_f)K_1(\lambda_i r) \quad r \geq r_f$,

$\Gamma_i = \dfrac{k_i[(\sin\gamma_i)/2 + k_i D \cos\gamma_i]}{2k_i d + \sin(2\gamma_i) - \sin[2(k_i d + \gamma_i)]}$,

$\lambda_i = (k_i^2 + \rho\sigma_a D^{-1})^{1/2}$,

I_1, K_1 are modified Bessel functions,
r_s = specular reflectance at normal incidence = $(n - 1)^2(n + 1)^{-2}$,
n = index of refraction of the medium.

D. Validity of the Solution

By comparing rigorous results for the Milne problem and some other problems with results obtained using the diffusion equation Case and Zweifel[9] concluded that the diffusion equation is valid if the albedo is near 1 and the characteristic dimensions of the medium are larger than the mean free path. Recently, the conditions under which the diffusion equation is valid were derived more rigorously by Furutsu[17] and Ishimaru.[18] They found that the absorption coefficient should be much smaller than the scattering coefficient and that the average distance light travels in the medium should be larger than the effective mean free path $(\rho\sigma_{tr})^{-1}$.

In the geometry we are dealing with the second condition has the following consequences. The slab thickness must be larger than the effective mean free path. Due to the normal incidence of the source beam, light has been scattered several times, usually before being detected at the surface. So except within and near the area where the incident beam enters the medium the results obtained with the diffusion equation will be accurate if the other conditions are fulfilled.

The validity of the diffusion equation has been determined quantitatively by comparison with results obtained by Monte Carlo calculations.

III. Monte Carlo Method

A. Simulation Model

Monte Carlo calculations were done using a modification of the computer program described by Meier et al.[12] The basic simulation steps are:

(1) Source photon generation. The photons are generated at the surface of the sample. Their spatial and angular distributions correspond to those of the light source used in the experiments. For our comparison of the results of the Monte Carlo calculations to the diffusion results a normally incident beam [Eq. (5)] has been simulated too (see Sec. III.B).

(2) Pathway generation. After generating a photon, the average distance to the first collision is determined. The scattering particles are supposed to be randomly distributed. The mean free path is $(\rho\sigma_s)^{-1}$. We may use then[13]

$$\tau = -\ln RN/\rho\sigma_s, \quad (22)$$

where RN is a random number from a sequence of independent uniformly distributed random numbers between 0 and 1.

Thus a scattering point has been determined. Then some checks and calculations described in steps 3, 4, and 5 are performed. If the photon has not been eliminated (see steps 3 and 4) a new direction is determined. The azimuth angle ϕ and the cosine μ of the scattering angle with respect to the old direction are simulated by

$$\phi = 2\pi RN,$$

$$\mu = [(1 + g^2) - (1 - g^2)^2(1 - g + 2gRN)^{-2}][2g]^{-1}. \quad (23)$$

The last formula is derived from the Henyey-Greenstein phase function [Eq. (2)].[19] A new pathway is generated

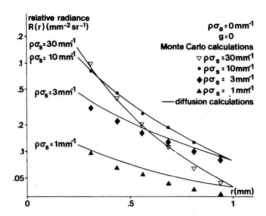

Fig. 2. Relative radiance R is calculated as a function of the distance r (Fig. 1) between source and detector using the diffusion theory (full lines) and the Monte Carlo method (symbols). Several values of $\rho\sigma_s$, the linear scattering coefficient, are used. For clarity, symbols and full lines are used instead of histograms.

using Eq. (22). Then a new scattering point is determined. This procedure is continued until the photon is eliminated.

(3) Reflection and absorption. For calculational reasons a weight is attributed to the photon. At the moment the photons leave the light source their weight is 1. Due to reflection and absorption the weight is reduced. If the calculated position of the photon is above the surface, specular reflection occurs. The weight of the photon is multiplied by the reflection coefficient calculated using Fresnel's law and the position of the photon is determined by reflection of the calculated position: z becomes $-z$. In the Monte Carlo calculations we suppose that absorption occurs between the scatterers, not inside the scatterers as supposed in the diffusion theory. The absorption is taken into account by multiplying the weight of the photon by $\exp(-a\tau)$, where a is the linear absorption coefficient. The relation of a to σ_a is explained in Sec. III.B.

(4) Elimination. Before a new scattering point is simulated the weight is compared with a critical weight. Photons whose weight is lower than the critical weight are eliminated. For computational efficiency the scattering volume is confined to a cylinder (see Fig. 1 and Sec. III.B). If the calculated position of the photon is beside or under this cylinder, the photon is eliminated too.

(5) Detection. For each scattering point the probability P that the photon is detected is computed and stored. We suppose that the photon is detected only by the detection ring positioned vertically over the scattering point (see Fig. 1). This is acceptable because the viewing angle of the detector is small. The probability P is given by

$$P = wp(\mu_0)d\omega_0 \exp[-(\rho\sigma_s + a)z_0], \qquad (24)$$

where w = photon weight,
$p(\mu_0)$ = phase function [Eq. (2)],
μ_0 = cosine of the angle between the photon's direction before scattering and a normal on the surface $z = 0$ pointed outward,

$d\omega_0$ = solid angle of detection in the sample, and
z_0 = depth of the scattering position.

The function $\exp[-(\rho\sigma_s + a)z_0]$ is the probability that a photon will reach the detector from its present position without being scattered or absorbed. We assume that the summation of the probabilities yields the detected radiance for the detection rings.

B.   Remarks

(1) In the Monte Carlo method it is supposed that the scattering events are independent.

(2) In the diffusion theory the absorption is described by the absorption cross section σ_a of the scatterers and the number of scattering particles ρ, in the Monte Carlo method by the linear absorption coefficient a, which accounts for the absorption between the scattering particles. According to Meier et al.[12] a is equal to $\rho\sigma_a$. So we may replace a by $\rho\sigma_a$.

(3) Numerical experience has shown that 10^4 photons are necessary to obtain results with the statistical error in the results of <5%. The statistical error occurs because only a finite amount of photons is used in the calculations.

(4) Numerical results were computed with a simulation of a normally incident beam as a photon source and also with a simulation of the fiber used in the experiments. Comparison showed that the differences are far below the statistical error of 5%. Thus incident light from the fiber may be approximated by a normally incident beam.

(5) Termination of the computing process due to elimination of the photons because their weight is below the critical weight yields negligible errors. Termination of the computing process due to elimination of the photons because the scattering point is beside or under the scattering volume causes considerable errors, especially if no absorption occurs. This error can be reduced by enlarging the scattering volume, which on the other hand increases the required computer time. Usually this error was reduced to ~5%.

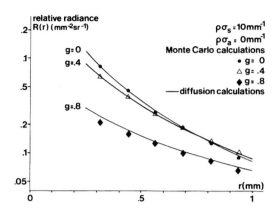

Fig. 3. Relative radiance R for several values of g, the average cosine of the scattering angle (see Fig. 2).

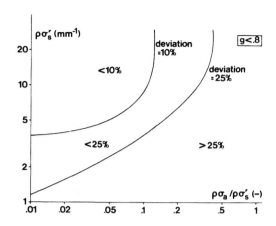

Fig. 5. Average proportional deviation of the relative radiance values calculated with the diffusion theory and those calculated with the Monte Carlo method mapped as a function of $\rho\sigma_s' = \rho\sigma_s(1-g)$ and $\rho\sigma_a/\rho\sigma_s'$. Three areas are indicated: deviation $< 10\%$; $10\% <$ deviation $< 25\%$; and deviation $> 25\%$.

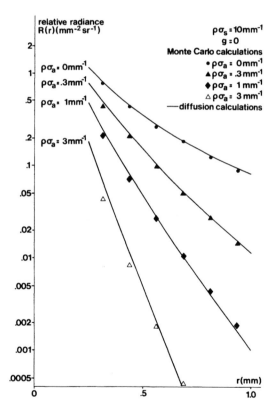

Fig. 4. Relative radiance R for several values of $\rho\sigma_a$, the linear absorption coefficient (see Fig. 2).

We would like to thank R. R. Meier for providing us with a Monte Carlo computer program which we used for our calculations in a modified version.

IV. Results

The diffusion and Monte Carlo calculations were performed with parameter values that were taken from the experimental situation. The light source diameter is 0.20 mm; its numerical aperture is 0.38. The detector area is 0.05×0.20 mm²; its viewing angle in air is 0.07 rad. The detection was simulated by six detection rings, of 0.125-mm width, between 0.25 and 1.00 mm. The material is supposed to have an index of refraction of 1.62.

The relative radiance values obtained with both methods were compared. In Fig. 2 various values of the scattering cross section σ_s were used: At $\rho\sigma_s = 30$ and 10 mm⁻¹ the fit is excellent; at lower values of $\rho\sigma_s$ a deviation occurs. In Fig. 3 various values of the average cosine g of the scattering angle were used. At $g = 0$ and $g = 0.4$ an excellent fit is observed; some deviation occurs at $g = 0.8$. The reason for the deviations in Figs. 2 and 3 may be the same: the effective mean free path $[\rho\sigma'_{tr}]^{-1}$ is about as long as the distance from the source to the detection spots. In that case the diffusion theory is not totally valid (see Sec. II.D). In Fig. 4 various values of the absorption cross section were used. If $\rho\sigma_a$ increases, the deviation increases too. This is due to the validity of the diffusion equation, which is confined to the case that $\rho\sigma_a/\rho\sigma_s \ll 1$ (see Sec. II.D).

The average proportional deviation of the value of the relative radiance calculated with the diffusion theory with respect to those calculated with the Monte Carlo method has been determined. Results are shown in Fig. 5 in a plot of $\rho\sigma'_s = \rho\sigma_s(1-g)$ and $\rho\sigma_a/\rho\sigma'_s$. It is indicated where the average proportional deviation is <10%, between 10 and 25% and more than 25%. If $\rho\sigma'_s > 5$ mm⁻¹ and $\rho\sigma_a/\rho\sigma'_s < 0.1$, an excellent fit occurs (deviation of <10%); if $\rho\sigma'_s > 2$ mm⁻¹ and $\rho\sigma_a/\rho\sigma'_s < 0.3$, usually a reasonable fit occurs (deviation of <25%).

On the Cyber 170/760 computer it takes ~0.5 sec to calculate the relative radiance at the six detection locations using the diffusion theory and 50–4000 sec using the Monte Carlo method: ~50 sec for strongly absorbing to 4000 sec for nonabsorbing media.

V. Conclusions

Two theoretical approaches are provided in this paper. They relate values of relative radiance measured with an experimental arrangement shown schematically in Fig. 1 to parameters describing the scattering and absorption characteristics of a sample, which are to be determined.

The first approach is the diffusion theory, which is only valid for multiply scattered light. It has been derived here that in the equation for the relative radiance [Eq. (21)], the scattering cross section σ_s always appears in the combination $\rho\sigma'_s = \rho\sigma_s(1-g)$. Samples with anisotropic scatterers described by $\rho\sigma_s$ and g have the same relative radiance as samples with isotropic scatterers described by $\rho\sigma'_s = \rho\sigma_s(1-g)$. Thus the scattering and absorption in turbid materials are determined completely by two parameters $\rho\sigma_a$ and $\rho\sigma_s(1-g)$ when the diffusion theory is valid.

The parameter $\rho\sigma_a$ can be identified with the linear absorption coefficient a, $\rho\sigma_s$ with the linear scattering coefficient s. As Meador and Weaver[20] show, the widely used Kubelka-Munk method yields the parameters a and $s(1-g)$ by measuring the reflectance and transmittance of a slab medium. By measuring the relative radiance curve the same parameters may be determined for a bulk material.[21]

The second approach is the Monte Carlo method, which is more generally applicable than the diffusion theory but requires much more computer time.

A comparison of the results obtained with the diffusion theory with those obtained with the Monte Carlo method shows a good fit when only multiply scattered light is measured. Then the computationally fast diffusion theory should be used; otherwise Monte Carlo calculations should provide the relative radiance curves.

Although the calculations were performed for given dimensions of the experimental setup an extension to other dimensions is possible.[21]

References

1. J. Langerholc, Appl. Opt. **21**, 1593 (1982).
2. A. Ishimaru, Proc. IEEE **65**, 1030 (1977).
3. A. Ishimaru, *Wave Propagation and Scattering in Random Media, Vol. 1* (Academic, New York, 1978).
4. V. Twersky, J. Opt. Soc. Am. **69**, 1567 (1979).
5. S. Chandrasekhar, *Radiative Transfer* (Oxford U. P., New York, 1960).
6. V. V. Sobolev, *A Treatise on Radiative Transfer* (Van Nostrand-Reinhold, Princeton, N.J., 1963).
7. E. Wolf, Phys. Rev. D **13**, 869 (1976).
8. R. L. Fante, J. Opt. Soc. Am. **71**, 460 (1981).
9. K. M. Case and P. F. Zweifel, *Linear Transport Theory* (Addison-Wesley, Reading, Mass., 1967).
10. L. Reynolds, C. Johnson, and A. Ishimaru, Appl. Opt. **15**, 2059 (1976).
11. L. L. Carter, H. G. Horak, and M. T. Sandford, J. Comput. Phys. **26**, 119 (1978).
12. R. R. Meier, J.-S. Lee, and D. E. Anderson, Jr., Appl. Opt. **17**, 3216 (1978).
13. E. D. Cashwell and C. J. Everett, *Monte Carlo Method for Random Walk Problems* (Pergamon, London, 1959).
14. R. A. J. Groenhuis, in *Technical Digest, Topical Meeting on Optical Phenomena Peculiar to Matter of Small Dimensions* (Optical Society of America, Washington, D.C., 1980), paper WB-6.
15. H. C. van de Hulst, *Multiple Light Scattering, Vol. 2* (Academic, New York, 1980).
16. W. G. Egan and T. W. Hilgeman, *Optical Properties of Inhomogeneous Materials* (Academic, New York, 1979).
17. K. Furutsu, J. Opt. Soc. Am. **70**, 360 (1980).
18. A. Ishimaru, J. Opt. Soc. Am. **68**, 1045 (1978).
19. A. N. Witt, Astrophys. J. Suppl. **35**, 1 (1977).
20. W. E. Meador and W. R. Weaver, Appl. Opt. **18**, 1204 (1979).
21. R. A. J. Groenhuis, J. J. Ten Bosch, and H. A. Ferwerda, Appl. Opt. **22**, 2463 (1983).

Reprinted with permission from *Applied Optics*, Vol. 22(16), pp. 2463-2467
(August 15, 1983). ©1983 Optical Society of America.

Scattering and absorption of turbid materials determined from reflection measurements. 2: Measuring method and calibration

R. A. J. Groenhuis, J. J. Ten Bosch, and H. A. Ferwerda

A new experimental method has been developed to determine the scattering and absorption characteristics of a turbid material. Existing methods usually require transmission and reflection measurements carried out on a thin slab of the material under study; this method is based on reflection measurements carried out on bulk material. This will be of great advantage in many applications. This paper describes the measuring system and indicates the area of application of the method. Calibration measurements have been carried out to substantiate the approach.

I. Introduction

The scattering and absorption characteristics of turbid materials usually are determined from reflection and transmission measurements on a thin slab of the material.[1] We present a method to determine these characteristics from reflection measurements on bulk material.

Figure 1 shows the measuring geometry. Light incident about normally onto a sample is scattered in that sample and possibly also partly absorbed. Some light is scattered back into the detector. The backscattered light is measured as a function of the distance r between the axis of the incident beam and the detection spot. From this curve the relative radiance $R(r)$ is derived as a function of the distance r. The relative radiance $R(r)$ is defined as the ratio of the detected radiance to the incident radiant flux.

Scattering is described by the linear scattering coefficient s, the average cosine g of the scattering angle, and absorption by the linear absorption coefficient a. From slab measurements the parameters $s(1 - g)$ and a of the

material under study can be determined. This paper describes how they can be determined from the relative radiance curve $R(r)$. Two theoretical approaches have been used to relate the relative radiance curve $R(r)$ to $s(1 - g)$ and a: the photon transport theory in the diffusion approximation (diffusion theory) and the Monte Carlo method.[2]

In this paper the measuring arrangement and its properties are described. A relatively simple procedure to derive $s(1 - g)$ and a from the relative radiance curve is pointed out. To check the measuring method calibration measurements have been carried out.

We will use the method in future to determine the scattering and absorption characteristics of dental enamel, a tissue ~2 mm thick which covers the crowns of the teeth. This may indicate the stage of the caries process.[3] The method is nondestructive, which is an advantage over the methods which are being used.

II. Measuring Method

A. Principle

In Fig. 1 the measuring geometry is shown schematically. A small area of the upper surface of a sample is illuminated by a beam of monochromatic light. The relative radiance $R(r)$, defined as the ratio of the detected radiance and the incident radiant flux, is determined as a function of the distance from the center of the spot of illumination to the detection spot.

The relative radiance depends on the scattering and absorption properties of the sample.[2] The photon transport is determined by the effective mean free path

H. A. Ferwerda is with State University Groningen, Department of Applied Physics, Nijenborgh 18, 9717 AG Groningen, The Netherlands. J. J. Ten Bosch is with State University Groningen, Laboratory for Materia Technica, A. Deusinglaan 1, 9716 AV Groningen, as was R. A. J. Groenhuis, when this work was done; he is now with National Institute of Dental Research, Bethesda, Maryland 20205.

Received 10 September 1982.

0003-6935/83/162463-05$01.00/0.

© 1983 Optical Society of America.

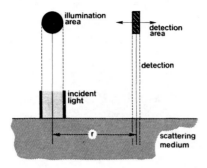

Fig. 1. Geometry to measure backscattered light as a function of the distance r from the axis of the incident beam to the center of the detection area: top, top view; below, cross section.

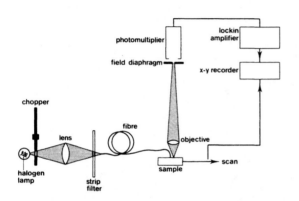

Fig. 2. Experimental arrangement: the relative radiance of the sample is measured as a function of r (see Fig. 1).

between the scatterers: $[s(1 - g)]^{-1}$. We may say that at low values of $s(1 - g)$ the photons are distributed over a larger volume than at high values of $s(1 - g)$, and consequently the relative radiance curve is less steep. When absorption occurs larger distances are relatively more affected than short distances. The curve becomes steeper and lower. The relative radiance curve depends also on the surface reflection, which is determined by the index of refraction of the material.[2] Due to surface reflection the relative radiance curve becomes less steep.

To facilitate the practical use of the method a measured relative radiance curve can be fitted to a function $C_1 r^{-1/2} \exp(-C_2 r)$. This yields values of C_1 and C_2 for the measured curve. On the basis of theoretical calculations[2] the relation of C_1 and C_2 to a and $s(1 - g)$ has been derived. The curve fitting thus acts as an intermediate step to find a and $s(1 - g)$ from the experimental curve.

B. Measuring Arrangement

In Fig. 2 the measuring equipment is shown. Light emitted by a halogen lamp (12 V, 50 W) is interrupted by a chopper at $\sim$500 Hz and then focused by a microscope objective (25× magnification) on the end of a plastic coated silica fiber (trademark, Fibrox; 0.20-mm effective diam; 0.38 N.A.). The wavelength of the light is adjusted by a strip filter between 400 and 700 nm

(20-nm bandwidth). The other end of the fiber was bent by local heating (12-mm minimum curve radius). This end is positioned normally to the sample surface, which is touched. Light emerging from a measuring area of $\sim$0.05 × 0.20 mm^2 is detected by a microscope densitometer (Leitz MPV, 3.2× objective, 0.07 N.A., photomultiplier EMI 9558 S20). Sample and fiber together can be displaced with respect to the measuring area, perpendicularly to the length of this area, at a rate of $\sim$0.1 mm sec^{-1} (Fig. 1). The output signal is amplified by a lock-in amplifier (Ortec Brookdeal 9501E) and then recorded as a function of the distance between the measuring area and the spot of illumination.

C. Parameter Determination

It is cumbersome to fit a complicated theoretical curve to an experimental one. Therefore, the experimental curve of the relative radiance is adapted to a function $C_1 r^{-1/2} \exp(-C_2 r)$, in which C_1 and C_2 are parameters and r is the distance from the center of the illumination spot to the measuring spot. This is an approximation for large values of $C_2 r$ of the formula for the relative radiance derived with the diffusion theory (see Appendix). For this adaptation linear regression analysis was applied in the $0.25 < r < 1.00$-mm range to the function $\ln[R(r) r^{1/2}]$, which ideally should equal $\ln(C_1) - C_2 r$.

Furthermore, C_1 and C_2 have to be related to $s(1 - g)$ and a of the material. To this end functions $C_1 r^{-1/2} \exp(-C_2 r)$ were fitted to theoretical curves of $R(r)$, calculated for the experimental geometry used and for the index of refraction of the material under study.[2] Diffusion theory was used when permittable, Monte Carlo calculations when necessary. Figure 3 shows an example of the relation of C_1 and C_2 to $s(1 - g)$ and a for our geometry and for an index of refraction $n = 1.62$. In this way a measured curve yields C_1 and C_2, which in turn provide values of $s(1 - g)$ and a of the material under study.

D. Measuring Procedure

Using the experimental setup described in Sec. III.B a signal is recorded as a function of the distance r between the illumination spot and the measuring spot. This curve is digitized with a CETEC-Ferranti digitizing table connected to a PDP 11/05 computer.

In addition to light scattered in the sample also some light directly radiated from the fiber to the detector is collected. The small amount of this light is determined separately, digitized, and subtracted from the signal measured on the sample.

To calculate the relative radiance (the ratio of the radiance of the detected signal to the radiant flux of the incident light), the radiant flux of the fiber should be known. The angular distribution of the fiber output is measured by a detector rotating around the fiber end. Then the output of the fiber is determined from a measurement with the measuring arrangement described before. The fiber is placed upside down under the microscope, the photomultiplier amplification is

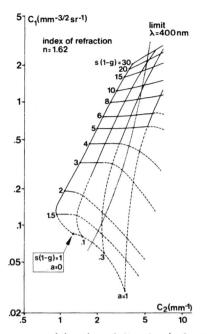

Fig. 3. Diagram to read the values of $s(1-g)$ and a from the values of C_1 and C_2, which fit the calculated relative radiance curves (full line, diffusion theory; dashed line, Monte Carlo method[2]). The applicability area at a wavelength of 400 nm is the area on the left of the indicated limit (dotted line); at wavelengths between 500 and 700 nm the whole area may be used. The diagram is valid for the geometry used and for an index of refraction of 1.62.

reduced by a factor of 1000, and the fiber output is determined.

The relative radiance is calculated by the PDP 11/05 computer. It carries out the correction for direct radiation and the adaptation to the function $C_1 r^{-1/2} \exp(-C_2 r)$, which yields the values of C_1 and C_2. Using maps such as the one shown in Fig. 3 the values of $s(1 - g)$ and a are determined by hand.

III. Calibration

A. Calibration Method

To check the newly developed method, measurements were carried out on calibration samples of turbid plastic. With the new method the values of a and $s(1 - g)$ were determined. Then a thin slab was cut from these samples and the diffuse transmission and reflection were measured with an integrating sphere built in a spectrophotometer (Perkin-Elmer 124). From these values the Kubelka-Munk coefficients S and K for scattering and absorption, respectively, were calculated using formulas given by Spitzer and Ten Bosch.[4] The approximate relations of $s(1 - g)$ and a to S and K have been derived by Mudgett and Richards[5,6] and Meador and Weaver[7]:

$$s(1 - g) = \tfrac{4}{3}S + \tfrac{1}{6}K,$$
$$a = \tfrac{1}{2}K. \qquad (1)$$

With these equations we determined $s(1 - g)$ and a from S and K. The estimated error in $s(1 - g)$ and a is $\sim$30%.

B. Calibration Samples

As calibration samples we used acrylonitrile–butadiene–styrene (ABS) copolymer blocks with 0, 0.1, and 1 wt. % TiO_2 grains (Borg Warner, Amsterdam, The Netherlands). Other calibration samples were prepared from distilled styrene (Merck, F.R.G.) with 10 wt. % quartz (nearly spherical particles, 40-nm average diam, Aerosil, Degussa, F.R.G.) and 0, 0.01, 0.03, and 0.1 wt. % of a red dye (Fett Rot RR, Hoechst, F.R.G.). After adding 1 wt. % α,α'-azo-iso-butyronitrile (Merck, F.R.G.) the mixture of distilled styrene, quartz, and red dye was polymerized (free radical polymerization) at 50°C during one day.

IV. Results

Factors which determine the total accuracy of the measuring method are the error in the determination of the incident radiant flux, appearing in the level of the relative radiance, 5%, and the error in the theoretical curve[2]: 5–25%. This results in an estimated error in the absolute values of $s(1 - g)$ and a of $\sim$30%.

The accuracy of the measuring method is only slightly influenced by the adaptation process. Figure 4 shows three experimental curves from which C_1 and C_2 were determined and from these subsequently $s(1 - g)$ and a. With these values theoretical points were calculated which are shown together with the experimental curves in Fig. 4. Agreement appears to be very good: the average deviation between the theoretical points and the adaptation curve is <3% for the range of values covered by Fig. 3.

The range of the method appeared to be limited by digitizing accuracy, noise, and sensitivity of the method to parameter changes.

As the full $R(r)$ curve is plotted on a single sheet of graph paper, the maximum ratio of the relative radiance

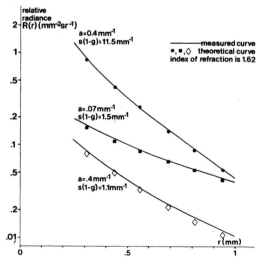

Fig. 4. Experimental relative radiance of three samples shown as a function of r (full lines). These curves were each fitted to six theoretical points calculated for definite values of $s(1 - g)$ and a. These values are attributed to the respective measured curve.

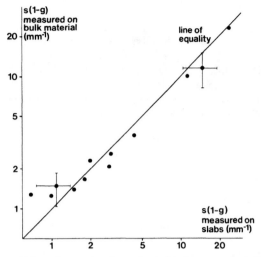

Fig. 5. Values of $s(1 - g)$ as determined with the new method plotted vs those determined with the calibration method. The line shows the desired equality.

values in the measuring range, i.e., at $r = 0.25$ mm and $r = 1$ mm, is 100 due to the limited accuracy in digitizing. This limits the maximum value of C_2 to 7 mm^{-1}.

The noise of the measuring system corresponds to a relative radiance level of $\sim 1 \times 10^{-8}$ m^{-2} sr^{-1} at wavelengths between 500 and 700 nm increasing to 3×10^{-7} m^{-2} sr^{-1} at 400 nm. The latter value is caused by high absorption in the fiber and low sensitivity of the photomultiplier system at 400 nm. High noise levels decrease the maximum value of C_2 that can be determined.

Theoretical calculations[2] show that if $s(1 - g) > 30$ mm^{-1} or $s(1 - g) < 1$ mm^{-1} the relative radiance curves and thus C_1 and C_2 are not sensitive to changes in the values of $s(1 - g)$ and a.

The applicability limits for the measuring system as described in this paper are indicated in Fig. 3.

The results of the calibration experiments are shown in Figs. 5 and 6. Figure 5 shows the values of $s(1 - g)$ for the three ABS blocks and the polystyrene block without dye measured at three wavelengths: 500, 600, and 700 nm. Figure 6 shows the values of a for the four polystyrene blocks measured at 600 and 700 nm. At 500 nm the absorption was too high to apply any of the measuring methods. The deviation of the measuring points in both figures from the line of equality is almost always within the estimated measuring error for both methods, 30%.

V. Conclusions

The method in this paper determines $s(1 - g)$ and a of bulk material from reflection measurements. For the equipment used by us the method has an accuracy for absolute measurements of 30% in the ranges of 1 mm^{-1} $< s(1 - g) < 30$ mm^{-1}, $a < 1$ mm^{-1} (500 nm $< \lambda < 700$ nm), or $a < 0.3$ mm^{-1} ($\lambda = 400$ nm).

The range of $s(1 - g)$ is determined by the fiber diameter. If lower values of $s(1 - g)$ are to be determined, the fiber diameter should be enlarged. However, this reduces the maximum value of $s(1 - g)$ that can be determined. If, for example, values of $s(1 - g)$ between 0.5 and 15 mm^{-1} are to be determined instead of values between 1 and 30 mm^{-1}, the fiber diameter should be 0.4 mm instead of 0.2 mm; the range of r should be 0.5 $< r < 2$ mm instead of $0.25 < r < 1$ mm. Figure 3 still may be used, but the scale factors should be changed: $C_1, C_2, s(1 - g)$, and a should be replaced by $2^{3/2}C_1, 2C_2,$ $2s(1 - g)$, and $2a$, respectively.

Higher values of a may be measured if the noise level is reduced ($\lambda \simeq 400$ nm) or the digitizing accuracy is enlarged (500 nm $< \lambda < 700$ nm).

We developed the method to carry out measurements on dental enamel. The values of $s(1 - g)$ and a of dental enamel are usually within the applicability range of the method, although sometimes the values of $s(1 - g)$ may be too low.[4] The present experimental arrangement is not suitable in clinical practice; replacement of the microscope by fibers to transport the reflection signal to a detector may solve the problem.

The method seems to be applicable to other bulk materials such as biological ones (e.g., the white of the eye) and others (e.g., plastics, fluids with scattering particles like milk). An advantage is that no thin slabs have to be made as the often used Kubelka-Munk method requires.

Summarizing, we have developed a method to measure $s(1 - g)$ and a of a bulk material. It is suitable to dental enamel as we required, and it may be applicable to other materials.

The authors like to thank T. Bartels for his advice in preparing polystyrene samples, L. Dijkema for providing the red dye, P. G. Koops for his experimental work, and Borg Warner (Amsterdam) for providing the ABS blocks.

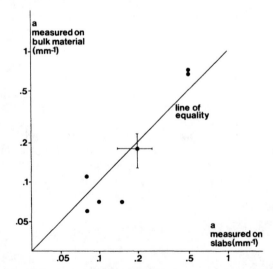

Fig. 6. Values of a as determined with the new method plotted vs those determined with the calibration method. The line shows the desired equality.

Appendix A: Approximation of the Relative Radiance

A formula for the relative radiance $R(r)$ has been derived [Eq. (21) of Ref. 2]. Now we are interested in the r dependence only:

$$R(r) = \sum_{i=1}^{\infty} C_i' \frac{1}{r} \frac{\partial}{\partial r} K_1(\lambda_i r), \qquad (A1)$$

where C_i' and λ_i are constant [Eq. (21) of Ref. 2], r is the distance to the axis of the incident beam, and K_1, K_0 are modified Bessel functions.

Using the formula[8]

$$\frac{1}{x} \frac{\partial}{\partial x} [x K_1(x)] = K_0(x), \qquad (A2)$$

we replace Eq. (A1) by

$$R(r) = \sum_{i=1}^{\infty} C_i' \lambda_i^2 K_0(\lambda_i r). \qquad (A3)$$

We assume that $\lambda_i r \gg 1$ for the dominating terms. Since for $x \gg 1, K_0(x) \rightarrow 1.253 x^{-1/2} \exp(-x)$,[8] we may approximate $R(r)$ by

$$R(r) \simeq \sum_{i=1}^{\infty} 1.253 C_i' \lambda_i^{3/2} r^{-1/2} \exp(-\lambda_i r). \qquad (A4)$$

Calculations indicate that a few terms dominate in the sum. Those terms have almost identical values of λ_i. So we approximate Eq. (A4) by

$$R(r) \simeq C_1 r^{-1/2} \exp(-C_2 r), \qquad (A5)$$

where C_1 and C_2 are constants. This formula is used as an approximation of the relative reflectance. Results show that the assumptions used are permitted.

References

1. W. G. Egan and T. W. Hilgeman, *Optical Properties of Inhomogeneous Materials* (Academic, New York, 1979).
2. R. A. J. Groenhuis, H. A. Ferwerda, and J. J. Ten Bosch, Appl. Opt. **22**, 2456 (1983).
3. R. A. J. Groenhuis, in *Technical Digest*, *Topical Meeting on Optical Phenomena Peculiar to Matter of Small Dimensions* (Optical Society of America, Washington, D.C., 1980), paper WB-6.
4. D. Spitzer and J. J. Ten Bosch, Calcif. Tissue Res. **17**, 129 (1975).
5. P. S. Mudgett and L. W. Richards, Appl. Opt. **10**, 1485 (1971).
6. P. S. Mudgett and L. W. Richards, J. Colloid Interface Sci. **39**, 551 (1972).
7. W. E. Meador and W. R. Weaver, Appl. Opt. **18**, 1204 (1979).
8. M. Abramowitz and I. A. Stegun, Eds. *Handbook of Mathematical Functions* (Dover, New York, 1965).

Reprinted with permission from *Medical Physics,* Vol. 10(6), pp. 824-830 (1983).
©1983 American Institute of Physics.

A Monte Carlo model for the absorption and flux distributions of light in tissue

B. C. Wilson

*Department of Physics, Ontario Cancer Treatment and Research Foundation, 711 Concession Street,
Hamilton, Ontario, Canada L8V 1C3*

G. Adam

Department of Radiobiology, Nuclear Research Centre, Negev, Beersheva, Israel

A Monte Carlo computer model has been developed to study the propagation of light in tissues. Light attenuation is assumed to result from absorption and isotropic scattering. The model has been used to predict the distribution of absorbed dose in homogeneous tissues of different absorption/scattering ratios, for illumination both by external light beams and via implanted optical fibers. The photon flux into optical fibers placed in the tissue as detectors has also been investigated. The results are interpreted in relation to the use of visible light irradiation for photo radiation therapy.

I. INTRODUCTION

Recent clinical and laboratory studies[1-5] have reawakened interest in photo radiation therapy (PRT) and have indicated that the technique may represent a highly significant advance in our ability to provide local control of a variety of malignant tumors. Localized visible light irradiation is applied to the tumor some time after administration of a photosensitizing drug. Cytotoxicity is believed to result from the production of singlet oxygen generated by the absorption of visible light by the photosensitizer.[6,7] The therapeutic efficacy is determined by three main factors: (1) the differential concentration of photosensitizer between the tumor and surrounding normal tissue,[8] (2) the light energy absorbed by the cells, and (3) the inherent cell sensitivity. Thus, as discussed by several authors,[1,9-12] the establishment of a system to quantitate the light delivered to the treated tissue is an important factor for improving clinical results.

There are very few data on the optical properties of tissues in the visible wavelength range. Ideally one would like to have information on the reflectance, absorption, and scattering properties as a function of wavelength for the tissues of interest. There have been no systematic *in vivo* measurements, even for animal tissues. Most of the *in vitro* work to date has been on the transmission of skin, carried out using excised specimens. Hardy *et al.*,[13] using a spectrophotometer, observed that, at infrared wavelengths, the attenuation due to photon scattering and that due to absorption in various components of skin could be combined, and the transmittance described by a simple exponential form (Beer's law). However, in the visible light range, a single exponential did not adequately fit the data. This was attributed to the heterogeneity in the attenuating properties of skin with increasing depth (for example, the distribution of melanin). Wan *et al.*[14] modeled the diffuse transmittance and reflectance of multilayer structures, and applied the model to determine the absorption and scattering coefficients for a number of differently pigmented human skin samples, in the

wavelength range 250–800 nm. Parrish[15] has recently reported on the penetration depth (depth at which the incident intensity is reduced to 37%) in the range 350–800 nm for fair and black skin measured *in vitro,* and observed a significant increase in the penetration at longer wavelengths.

For tissues other than skin, the data are sparse, both for animals and humans. Eichler *et al.*[16] in 1977 measured the penetration through excised specimens of human and pig liver and kidney. Using a narrow beam in the wavelength range 350–1000 nm, it was found that the transmitted intensity, including diffuse scattering in the forward direction, decreased exponentially with increasing tissue thickness. The penetration depth was strongly dependent on wavelength. No attempt was made to separate the absorption and scattering contributions to the total attenuation.

Wan *et al.*[17] have reported measurements of the gross transmission of light in the range 400–865 nm through *post-mortem* specimens of various human tissues (skull bone, chest wall, abdominal wall, scrotal sac). They observed a strong wavelength dependence and noted the influence of both absorption and scattering in the attenuation of the light.

The most recent and extensive work has been done by Svaasand *et al.*,[10-12] who used inserted optical fibers coupled to a photodetector to estimate the space irradiance ϕ, in a number of animal and human tissues exposed to light at selected wavelengths. ($\phi = \int_\Omega L d\Omega$, where the radiance L = flux of optical energy in a particular direction per unit solid angle Ω, and per unit area normal to the direction of propagation.) By varying the position and orientation of the detector fiber, they were able to measure the radiance in the forward, sideways, and backward directions at different depths along the central axis of the incident light beam. This allowed a qualitative separation of the absorption and scattering components of the attenuation. The penetration depth was found to be strongly dependent on the tissue type and on the wavelength. For example, at 633 nm the penetration depth for pig liver *in vitro* was 0.8 mm, while that of cow brain was 4.0 mm. In rabbit thigh muscle *in vivo* at 633 nm, the values ranged between 4.4 and 6.1 mm, and at 514 nm between 1.3 and 2.1 mm. The corresponding values *in vitro* were 6.6–8.8 and 4.0–5.1 mm. In *postmortem* adult human brain specimens, the penetration depth ranged from 0.4 mm at 488 nm to 3.2 mm at 1060 nm. The corresponding values for fetal specimens were 1.7 and 8.8 mm, respectively.[18] In addition, the tissues were found to differ substantially in the relative importance of scattering and absorption to the total attenuation. Brain was highly scattering and the distribution of light could be described adequately by diffusion theory, whereas, in heavily pigmented tissues such as liver, absorption appeared to be the dominant process. In these studies, the tissues were illuminated both by an external beam incident normally on the tissue surface, and by inserting an optical fiber coupled to the light source into the tissue substance. The space irradiance decreased exponentially along the central axis of the beam for plane beam irradiation, but was of a more complex form with an implanted fiber source.

To date, there has been no full analytic description of the propagation of light in tissues, and only a few simple cases have been examined theoretically. Kubelka[19,20] and, more recently, Wan *et al.*[14] have developed models for the diffuse transmittance and reflectance in plane tissue layers illuminated by broad-beam light. For a homogeneous layer, infinite in extent perpendicular to the beam direction, the transmission of optical power is exponential with depth. At sufficient depth in turbid media such as tissue, where scattering is important, the effective attenuation coefficient, μ_{eff}, may be expressed in terms of the absorption and scattering coefficients, μ_a and μ_s, by

$$\mu_{\text{eff}}^2 = \mu_a^2 + 2\mu_a\mu_s. \tag{1}$$

Svaasand *et al.*[10] have investigated the extreme cases of strong absorption and strong scattering. Two forms of illumination were considered: (i) a parallel collimated light beam incident normally on the tissue surface and, (ii) an implanted optical fiber light source. The tissue is assumed to be of infinite (or semi-infinite) extent, both along beam direction and perpendicular to it. For high scattering, it is possible to apply diffusion theory to calculate the dependence of the space irradiance as a function of distance from the source. For case (i), the space irradiance falls off exponentially with depth in the tissue. The effective attenuation coefficient μ_{eff} equals μ_a for pure absorption. For high scattering, $\mu_{\text{eff}}^2 = \mu_a/\zeta$, where ζ is the space irradiance diffusion constant. For a point source within the tissue [case (ii)], the space irradiance ϕ, at distance ρ is given by

$$\phi = \phi_0 \left(\frac{c}{\rho} \right)^n \cdot e^{-\mu_t(\rho - c)}, \tag{2}$$

where μ_t is the total attenuation coefficient, ϕ_0 and c are constants, $n = 1$ for high scattering, and $n = 2$ for high absorption.

The main limitation of this formulism is that it does not allow one to deal with the case where both absorption and scattering processes are significant. Incorporating the effect of real source geometries will also be difficult; for example, where an implanted optical fiber of limited numerical aper-

ture, or an external beam of limited dimension are used to illuminate the tissue.

In order to study the general case of mixed absorption and scattering for more realistic geometries, we have used a Monte Carlo approach. This permits the calculation of both the distribution of absorbed "dose" in the tissue and the response of implanted optical fibers used as detectors of the photon flux. In the following section, we shall describe the basis and assumptions of the model, and will then present the results of a series of computer simulations which have been carried out using it.

II. METHOD

Monte Carlo techniques have been widely applied in radiation transport studies (see, for example, Ref. 21). The technique is based on the stochastic nature of radiation interactions. Thus, in the present study, the attenuation of light photons in tissue can be described by computer simulation of appropriately weighted random absorption and scattering interactions.

The parameters of the model are as follows. A beam of light is introduced into a volume of tissue having absorption and scattering coefficients μ_a and μ_s, respectively. The two geometries that we have examined are illustrated in Fig. 1. In the first, illumination is by an external parallel beam of given diameter B, and in the second the light is introduced *via* an implanted optical fiber with a given numerical aperture NA_s. For each, in the absence of attenuating medium, the light intensity within the geometric edge of the field is uniform across a plane perpendicular to the central x axis of the beam.

Each incident photon was generated via a random number algorithm so as to produce this initial intensity distribution, and the ray was then "traced" through the tissue volume. The path length between successive interactions was calculated as

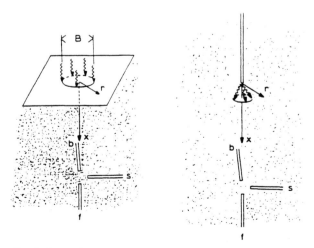

FIG. 1. Geometries for the Monte Carlo model with external beam and implanted fiber illumination. Tissue is represented by stippling. The detector fiber orientations for measuring the forward, sideways, and backward flux on the central axis ($r = 0$) are indicated.

$$L = -\ln(R)/\mu_t, \qquad (3)$$

where $0 < R < 1$ is a uniformly distributed pseudorandom number, and $\mu_t = \mu_a + \mu_s$ is the total attenuation coefficient. This formulism generates an exponential distribution of interaction path lengths.

At the interaction point, the photon was assumed to deposit a fraction, μ_a/μ_t, of its current weight, WT_i (set initially equally to 1), as absorbed energy, and to emerge from the interaction with weighting factor

$$WT_{i+1} = (\mu_s/\mu_t) \cdot WT_i.$$

The direction of the scattered photon was selected from a random distribution such that the probability per unit solid angle was the same in all directions. A new path length was calculated as before and the ray tracing continued. Figure 2 illustrates the photon history. Weighting the rays in this way results in better statistical precision for a given number of input photons. Also, it is computationally more efficient than increasing the number of incident photons but terminating ray tracing upon the first absorption.[21]

It should be noted that, in this model, the scattered photons are assumed to have the same absorption and scattering coefficients as the incident photons. That is, the energy (and polarization) is unchanged by the scatter interaction. Other effects such as fluorescence have also been ignored.

The number of interactions per photon was selected so that, for any combination of μ_a and μ_s, at least 85% of the integrated weighting factor was absorbed in the tissue volume (typically four interactions for $\mu_a/\mu_s = 4/1$, eight interactions for $\mu_a/\mu_s = 1/4$).

For an implanted fiber source, an infinite tissue volume was assumed in all directions. For an external beam with the tissue surface at $x = 0$, the tissue occupied the semi-infinite space defined by $x > 0$; rays exiting back through the surface were assumed lost and ray tracing terminated. In both cases, reflection from surfaces (fiber–tissue, air–tissue) was ignored, and the tissue volume was assumed homogeneous.

Where possible, cylindrical symmetry was invoked to minimize computation.

Two separate FORTRAN computer programs were written and run on a D.E.C. PDP 11/34 computer. In the first, the distribution of absorbed dose (i.e., photons absorbed per unit volume) was calculated as a matrix in x (depth along central axis) and r (radial distance from central axis). The matrix element, i.e., voxel size, was chosen as a compromise between statistics and spatial resolution. The program was run firstly for an external beam of diameter B incident normally on the tissue surface and centered on $x = 0$, $r = 0$; secondly, for an implanted source fiber, of numerical aperture NA_s, aligned along the $+x$ direction with the tip at $x = 0$, $r = 0$. For each, the two cases of $\mu_a/\mu_s = 4/1$ and $1/4$ were examined in detail. Runs were carried out for $B = 0, 5, 10$ (in units of δ—see below), and for $NA_s = 0.2, 0.8$ radians. For most runs 10 000 input photons were generated.

The second calculation was for the photon flux into a "detector fiber" positioned within the tissue volume, as illustrated in Fig. 1. For each ray segment, the program checked whether the photon crossed the detector fiber tip at an angle smaller than its numerical aperture; if so, then the detected flux was incremented by the current ray weight WT_i. However, the ray tracing was continued, assuming that the presence of detector fiber does not affect the distribution of light in the tissue. This flux program was also run for a variety of input parameters: external beam, $B = 0, 5\delta$; implanted fiber source, $NA_s = 0.2, 0.8$; $\mu_a/\mu_s = 4/1, 1/4$. For each, the detected flux was determined for both narrow and wide acceptance detector fibers (numerical apertures, $NA_D = 0.2, 0.8$), positioned along the central beam axis at depths of 2.5δ and 5δ from the tissue surface or source fiber tip. At these positions, the angle of the detector fiber was selected as 180°, 90°, or 0° to the beam. This allowed calculation of "forward," "sideways," and "backward" detected flux, respectively (see Fig. 1). Typically 100 000 input photons were used, which required around 75 or 125 min of computer time for 4 or 8 scatters per photon trace, respectively.

A. Distance scaling and normalization

All results presented below have distances measured in units of the mean free path, $\delta = 1/\mu_t$, in order that they may be scaled for use with any tissue once the total attenuation coefficient μ_t is known.

The absorbed dose D has been normalized so as to represent the number of photons absorbed per unit volume of tissue (δ^3) per input beam photon. The detected flux F is given as the number of photons entering a detector fiber of unit area (δ^2) per input beam photon. Since reflecting interfaces have been ignored, all input photons generated were assumed to enter the tissue, and, within the area and numerical aperture of the detector fiber, all photons contributed to the detected flux.

III. RESULTS

A. Absorbed dose

Figure 3 shows the "isodose distributions" with both external beam and inserted fiber irradiation, for high absorp-

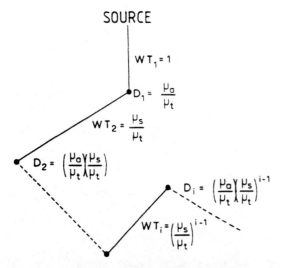

FIG. 2. Schematic of photon history showing the weighting factors WT_i, for each ray, and the absorbed dose D_i, at each interaction vertex. μ_a, μ_s, and μ_t are the attenuation coefficients as defined in the text.

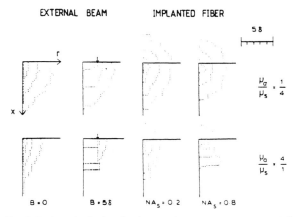

EXTERNAL BEAM   IMPLANTED FIBER

FIG. 3. Isodose distributions for the two illumination geometries and the two tissue types. Moving inwards, the contour lines on each plot represent $D = 10^{-4}, 10^{-3}, \ldots$. The size scale is shown in the upper right-hand corner. For $B = 5\delta$, the arrow indicates the geometric edge of the incident light beam.

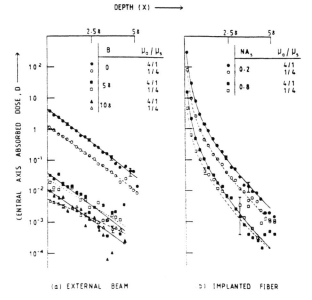

FIG. 4. Absorbed dose as a function of depth along the central beam axis. For the external beams, the straight lines are the linear regression fits. For the implanted fiber source, the curves are the best chi-square fits to the data points. The typical errors shown are 1 standard deviation from the photon statistics.

tion ($\mu_a/\mu_s = 4/1$) and high scattering ($\mu_a/\mu_s = 1/4$) tissues. Each contour line represents a tenfold change in the absorbed dose.

The dimension scale on the distributions is shown in units of the value of the mean free path δ. It is known,[10-12] that, for visible light in mammalian tissues, δ is likely to be in the order of a few millimeters. Thus, to treat a tumor a few centimeters in diameter, tumoricidal doses may be required at distances of say, 5δ–10δ.

In the low-dose regions, the number of photons contributing to the calculated absorbed dose is small, since most of the distributions of Fig. 3 are for only 10 000 input photons. For example, for $D = 10^{-3}$ the weighted photon number at each point is typically 10–20 ($= \Sigma_i n_i WT_i$, where n_i is the number of absorbed photons of weight WT_i). Thus, the statistical precision is rather poor. Nevertheless, the overall shape and position of the isodose levels is well demonstrated.

The distribution of absorbed dose along the central beam axis (D versus x) is shown in Fig. 4 for the different illumination geometries and the two tissue types. These data have been plotted on a logarithmic dose scale to test the exponential behavior of the curves. The statistical errors are indicated at selected points.

The dose profiles (D versus r) are shown in Fig. 5 at depths of 0.5δ, 2.5δ, and 5δ. Each set of curves has been normalized to the value of D at $x = 0.5\delta$, $r = 0$. Again, a logarithmic scale has been used for the dose axis.

B. Detected flux

Figure 6 shows the detected flux F into narrow and wide aperture fibers ($NA_D = 0.2, 0.8$) in both absorbing and scattering tissue illuminated either via an implanted source fiber or by an external beam. The flux detected in the forward, sideways, and backward directions is given for the detector fiber positioned along the beam axis at a distance of 2.5δ from the implanted source fiber tip or tissue surface ($x = 2.5\delta$, $r = 0$). The forward detected flux at $x = 5\delta$ is also shown; the sideways and backward results at this depth have been omitted because of poor statistics.

The representative errors shown in Fig. 6 are the standard deviations on the number of photons detected, taking the ray weighting factors into account.

Since detector fibers would be used in patients or animal tissues to measure the local absorbed dose, we have examined the relationship between the detected flux F and the absorbed dose D along the central axis. The results are illustrated in Fig. 7, where the values of F/D are plotted for the same set of parameters as in Fig. 6.

IV. DISCUSSION

A. Isodose distributions

Referring to Fig. 3, we see the following.

1. External beam

With high absorption and a finite beam width ($B = 5\delta$), the isodose distribution is nearly cylindrical except at the

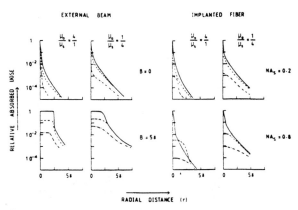

FIG. 5. Absorbed dose profiles perpendicular to the central beam axis. In each plot the three lines correspond to $x = 0.5\delta$(—), $x = 2.5\delta$(----), and $x = 5\delta$(·····).

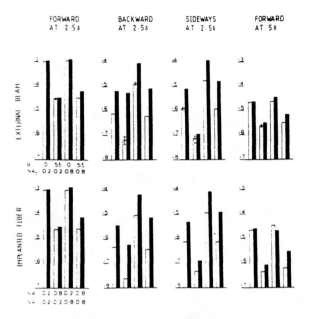

FORWARD AT 2·5δ BACKWARD AT 2·5δ SIDEWAYS AT 2·5δ FORWARD AT 5δ

FIG. 6. Detected photon flux, plotted as histograms for the two illumination geometries and the two tissue types: ☐ $\mu_a/\mu_s = 4/1$, ■ $\mu_a/\mu_s = 1/4$. The value of $\log_{10}(F)$ is given for the three detector fiber orientations at $x = 2.5\delta$. $r = 0$, and for the forward direction at $x = 5\delta$, $r = 0$. The parameters for the source geometry (B,NA_s) and for the detector numerical aperture (NA_D) are as defined in the text.

lowest dose level. Even for a pencil beam $(B = 0)$, a significant volume of tissue is irradiated at the 10^{-4} dose level, this isodose line extending to a radius, $r \sim 3\delta$ at the surface.

As expected, the distributions become more isotropic as the absorption scatter ratio decreases. For high scattering, the "treated" volume extends considerably beyond the geometric edge of the beam.

2. Implanted fiber

For high absorption, the shape of the isodose distributions depends strongly on the numerical aperture of the source

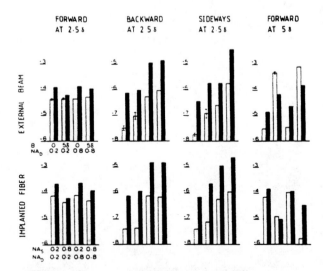

FORWARD AT 2·5δ BACKWARD AT 2·5δ SIDEWAYS AT 2·5δ FORWARD AT 5δ

FIG. 7. Ratio of detected flux to absorbed dose F/D for the different geometries and tissues. All symbols are as for Fig. 6.

fiber. Higher scattering removes this dependence, except for the high doses near the fiber tip.

B. Central axis depth doses

1. External beam

We have fitted each data set in Fig. 4(a) by linear regression to the exponential form

$$D = D_0 e^{-\mu_{eff}x}, \tag{4}$$

where μ_{eff} is interpreted as the effective attenuation coefficient. Table I shows the results of these fits; μ_{eff} has been expressed here in units of $1/\delta$ where $\delta = 1/\mu_t$ is the mean free path used as input to the Monte Carlo program.

For no scatter, i.e., $\mu_s = 0$, we expect $\mu_{eff} = \mu_t = 1.0/\delta$. This is close to the results found for $\mu_a/\mu_s = 4/1$, both for a narrow and wide external beam. With significant scattering, i.e., $\mu_a/\mu_s = 1/4$, the slope of the depth dose curves is less. With increasing beam diameter B, the value of μ_{eff} should tend to the value given in Eq. (1) above,[19,20] which predicts $\mu_{eff} = 0.6/\delta$ for $\mu_a/\mu_s = 1/4$. This is an excellent agreement with our result of $0.57/\delta$ for a beam diameter of 10δ.

2. Implanted fiber

With a fiber inserted into the tissue to deliver the light, we expect that the falloff in absorbed dose along the central axis will be due to both the beam divergence and to the attenuation by the tissue. For the pure absorption case, the behavior should be

$$D \propto \frac{1}{x^2} e^{-x/\delta}, \tag{5}$$

where the divergence factor $1/x^2$ is simply the inverse square law. According to Eq. (2), in the highly scattering situation, this term should be $1/x$ rather than $1/x^2$. In this case, however, the exponent is no longer expressible simply in terms of μ_a and μ_s, and one requires a knowledge also of the diffusion constant ζ.

To determine the behavior of the distributions shown in Fig. 4(b), we have carried out chi-square (χ^2) fits to the form

$$D = \frac{D_0 e^{-\mu_{eff}x}}{x^n}, \tag{6}$$

where D_0, μ_{eff}, and n were variables in the fit. The results are summarized in Table II. For the high-absorption case $(\mu_a/\mu_s = 4/1)$, the best fits were $\mu_{eff} \sim 1.0/\delta$, $n \sim 1.9$–2.0. This is in good agreement with the predictions of Eq. (2). With higher scattering $(\mu_a/\mu_s = 1/4)$, however, the results

TABLE I. Effective attenuation coefficient, in units of $1/\delta$, for external beam irradiation. The correlation coefficient of each linear regression fit is given in brackets.

μ_a/μ_s	Beam diameter (B)		
	0	5δ	10δ
4/1	1.01 (0.998)	0.95 (0.882)	0.94 (0.946)
1/4	0.97 (0.967)	0.78 (0.941)	0.57 (0.966)

TABLE II. Effective attenuation coefficient, in units of $1/\delta$, and divergence exponent for implanted fiber irradiation. The reduced χ^2 $(\chi^2/\text{degrees of freedom})$ of each fit is given in brackets.

| μ_a/μ_s | Source fiber aperture (NA_s) | | Variable |
	0.2	0.8	
4/1	0.99	0.98	μ_{eff}
	1.92	2.0	n
	(2.3)	(1.6)	
1/4	0.87	0.82	μ_{eff}
	1.94	1.77	n
	(1.3)	(0.8)	

are less clear cut. The data do not fit well to Eq. (6) if n is fixed at 1.0 (reduced $\chi^2 > 10$, $\mu_{\text{eff}} > 2.5/\delta$); i.e., the simple diffusion model does not hold. Statistically good fits were, however, obtained with $\mu_{\text{eff}} \sim 0.8\text{--}0.9/\delta$, $n \sim 1.75\text{--}1.95$. Thus, both μ_{eff} and n are certainly decreased by scattering, but not to the degree which might be expected.

In examining Fig. 4(b), and in particular that for $\mu_a/\mu_s = 1/4$ and $NA_s = 0.8$, it is observed that the data for larger depths $(x \gtrsim 4\delta)$ lie systematically above the fitted values. This suggests that a two-component curve may be more appropriate. However, at this stage we do not have adequate statistics on the Monte Carlo data to test this hypothesis.

C. Dose profiles

The plots of D versus r, shown in Fig. 5, simply reflect in more detail the shape of the isodose distributions of Fig. 3. They do, however, demonstrate more clearly the changing form of the beam cross section as the light propagates to greater depths in the tissue. There is evidence in these profiles also for a two-component description, but again more detailed and precise modeling will be required to test this.

The apparently anomalous behavior for the implanted fiber profiles, for example the crossover in the curves for $\mu_a/\mu_s = 4/1$, $nA_s = 0.8$, is associated with the location of the geometric edge of the incident beam.

D. Detected flux

From the results in Fig. 6 for the photon flux detected by a fiber placed along the central axis and angled at 180°, 90°, and 0° to the incident beam direction, we observe the following.

The forward detected flux F_f is rather insensitive to the absorption/scatter ratio, both for narrow $(NA_s = 0.2$ or $B = 0)$ and wide $(NA_s = 0.8$ or $B = 5\delta)$ incident light beam geometries. Only at larger depths $(x = 5\delta)$ and with a wide incident beam and a large aperture detector fiber $(NA_D = 0.8)$, does F_f show significant dependence on μ_a/μ_s (where, by "significant," we mean a factor of 5 or more).

At $x = 5\delta$, there are large differences in the behavior of F_f between the external beam and the implanted fiber illumination techniques. These differences can be attributed mainly to the beam divergence with the implanted source fiber.

Unlike F_f, the sideways and backward detected fluxes are significantly affected by the absorption/scatter ratio, and also depend strongly on the source geometry and detector fiber aperture. This is to be expected, since a detector fiber in

either of these orientations along the central axis will detect only scattered photons. At a depth of $x = 2.5\delta$, F_s and F_b are less by one to three orders of magnitude compared with F_f. Note also that F_s can be less than F_b due to the different solid angle covered by the detector fiber in the two orientations, as discussed in detail by Svaasand et al.[10]

It is of interest to compare the results of the Monte Carlo model with available experimental data. The only directly comparable results in the literature are again those of Svaasand et al.,[10] whose experimental value of the penetration depth in cow muscle at 633 nm is 1.8 mm, measured using an implanted fiber source and a fiber detector of numerical aperture around 0.35. In Table III, we have calculated from Svaasand's data the experimental values of the ratio of F_b to F_f at depth 2.5δ, and the ratio of F_f at 2.5δ to F_f at 5δ (assuming $\delta = 1.8$ mm). The comparison with the predictions of the Monte Carlo model indicates that for this tissue at least, the scattering is greater than that corresponding to $\mu_a/\mu_s = 1/4$. Alternately, the scattering in muscle may be nonisotropic. By increasing the scattering to $\mu_a/\mu_s = 1/20$ in the Monte Carlo program, we have found that the predicted ratios are roughly double those of Table III, thus overlapping with the experimental values.

E. Ratio of detected flux to absorbed dose

The main interest in the F/D ratio is whether the response of a detector fiber can be used to measure the local absorbed dose, and how much knowledge of the illumination and detector geometries, and of the tissue characteristics is needed to achieve this. Ideally, one would like F/D to be insensitive to these factors. We shall consider the behavior of F/D for the forward, sideways, and backward detected flux, referring to Fig. 7.

At $x = 2.5\delta$, for all source and detector geometries, and in the three detector fiber orientations, the value of F/D is higher in the higher scattering tissue. The dependence on the absorption/scatter ratio is least in the forward direction, where there is also little variation with the source and detector parameters.

However, at greater depth, the dependence of F/D on the various factors becomes very complex, even in the forward direction. No longer does the higher scattering tissue necessarily result in a higher F/D value, and there is no clear pattern as the source and detector characteristics change.

The two ratios F_s/D and F_b/D show the same overall behavior at depth $x = 2.5\delta$. The values increase, both for scattering and absorbing tissues, as the beam size increases, and as the detector fiber aperture increases. The first effect is

TABLE III. Comparison of detected flux measurements in cow muscle with predictions of Monte Carlo model.

| | Measured (Ref. 10) | Monte Carlo $(\mu_a/\mu_s = 1/4)$ | |
		$NA_{s,D}$: 0.2	0.8
$\dfrac{F_b \text{ at } x = 2.5\delta}{F_f \text{ at } x = 2.5\delta}$	0.2	4.10^{-3}	0.1
$\dfrac{F_f \text{ at } x = 5.0\delta}{F_f \text{ at } x = 2.5\delta}$	0.06	0.03	0.05

due to reduction in dose more than compensating for the decreased detected flux. The increase with larger NA_D is due simply to a greater fraction of the total photon flux being within the detector fiber aperture, and so contributing to the detected flux.

V. CONCLUSIONS

Although Monte Carlo modeling has been used widely in the study of ionizing radiations in medicine, we are unaware of any work on applying the technique to light dosimetry in tissues. The results presented here are, of course, very preliminary, and we have examined only a limited range of illumination conditions and model tissue types. Other studies are underway, and a number of important refinements and extensions can be identified, namely; (1) improved statistical precision through increasing the number of photon histories, (2) allowing nonisotropic scattering, (3) allowing nonhomogeneous model tissue, (4) accounting for interfaces and tissue boundaries, (5) increasing the range of illumination geometries and tissue parameters, and (6) more detailed study of the spatial and directional distributions of photon flux.

More importantly, it will be essential to test the predictions of the model against experimental data. A number of groups, including our own, are presently carrying our measurements on different animal and human tissues in various wavelength ranges. However, as we have demonstrated above, it may be difficult to separate out the tissue-dependent parameters in these experiments from the effects of illumination geometry and detector fiber characteristics. It will therefore be desirable to test the Monte Carlo approach by making measurements in suitable tissue-simulating phantoms, where the absorption and scattering characteristics can be varied at will and independently measured. This work is in progress, and preliminary experiments using agar doped with charcoal (for absorption) and glass microspheres (for scatter) show promise.

If the model stands up to these tests, then it can be used for several purposes: (1) to analyze and interpret experimental measurements in real tissues, particularly in determining the absorption and scattering coefficients (and the angular dependence of scatter), (2) to study the effects on the absorbed dose distributions of changing the illumination conditions, once the absorption/scattering properties of the tissue are known, and (3) thus, to optimize techniques of light exposure in the treatment of patients by photo radiation therapy.

ACKNOWLEDGMENTS

The authors would like to thank Diane Lowe and James Stang for technical assistance, and Anne Devries for preparing the manuscript. This work was supported by the National Cancer Institute of Canada and the Ontario Cancer Treatment and Research Foundation.

[1]T. J. Dougherty, K. R. Weishaupt, and D. G. Doyle (review article) in *Cancer: Principles and Practice of Oncology*, edited by Vincent T. De Vita, Samuel Hellman, and Steven A. Rosenberg (Lippincott, Philadelphia, 1982), p. 1836.

[2]T. J. Dougherty, J. Invest. Dermatol. **77**, 122 (1981).

[3]Y. Hayata, H. Kato, C. Konaka, J. Ono, and N. Takizawa, Chest **81**, 269 (1982).

[4]M. C. Berenbaum, R. Bonnett, and P. A. Scourides, Br. J. Cancer **45**, 571 (1982).

[5]J. H. Kinsey, D. A. Cortese, H. L. Moses, R. J. Ryan, and E. L. Branum, Cancer Res. **41**, 5020 (1981).

[6]T. J. Dougherty, C. J. Gomer, and K. R. Weishaupt, Cancer Res. **36**, 2330 (1976).

[7]J. P. Pooler and D. P. Valenzo, Med. Phys. **8**, 614 (1981).

[8]C. J. Gomer and T. J. Dougherty, Cancer Res. **39**, 146 (1979).

[9]A. E. Profio and D. R. Doiron, Med. Phys. **8**, 190 (1981).

[10]L. O. Svaasand, D. R. Doiron, and A. E. Profio, University of Southern California, Institute for Physics and Imaging Science, Report MISG 900-02, 1981.

[11]L. O. Svaasand and D. R. Doiron, University of Southern California, Institute for Physics and Imaging Science, Report MISG 900-05, 1982.

[12]D. R. Doiron, L. O. Svaasand, and A. E. Profio, in *Porphyrin Photosensitization*, edited by D. Kessel and T. J. Dougherty (Plenum, New York, 1983), pp. 63–76.

[13]J. D. Hardy, H. T. Hammel, and D. Murgatroyd, J. Appl. Physiol. **9**, 257 (1956).

[14]S. Wan, R. R. Anderson, and J. A. Parrish, Photochem. Photobiol. **34**, 493 (1981).

[15]J. A. Parrish, J. Natl. Cancer Inst. **69**, 273 (1982).

[16]J. Eichler, J. Knof, and H. Lenz, Radiat. Environ. Biophys. **14**, 239 (1977).

[17]S. Wan, J. A. Parrish, R. R. Anderson, and M. Madden, Photochem. Photobiol. **34**, 679 (1981).

[18]L. O. Svaasand (private communication, 1982).

[19]P. Kubelka, J. Opt. Soc. Am. **38**, 448 (1948).

[20]P. Kubelka, J. Opt. Soc. Am. **44**, 330 (1954).

[21]A. E. Profio, in *Radiation Shielding and Dosimetry* (Wiley, New York, 1979), pp. 168–199.

Reprinted with permission from *IEEE Journal of Quantum Electronics,*
Vol. QE-23(10), pp. 1721-1733 (October 1987). ©1987 IEEE.

Development and Application of Three-Dimensional Light Distribution Model for Laser Irradiated Tissue

GILWON YOON, ASHLEY J. WELCH, SENIOR MEMBER, IEEE, MASSOUD MOTAMEDI,
AND MARTINUS C. J. VAN GEMERT

Abstract—A three-dimensional model for estimating light distribution in laser irradiated tissue is presented. Multiple scattering and absorption of the laser beam are modeled using seven fluxes. One-, two-, and three-dimensional solutions are discussed and light distributions computed from the seven flux model are compared to those computed with the diffusion approximation. Methods for obtaining the phase function, absorption coefficient, and scattering coefficient for tissue are discussed and illustrated with measurements for human aortic vessel wall at the wavelength of 632.8 nm. Measured values are used in the seven flux model to estimate the rate of heat generation in the vessel wall.

Introduction

THIS paper presents a theoretical investigation of light absorption and scattering in biological media irradiated by lasers. Methods are presented for estimating the light energy distribution in the tissue, which is essential for dosimetry for either photodynamic or for thermal coagulation therapy. Also, the models provide a technique for analyzing reflected or transmitted light as a diagnostic tool, or for evaluation of the progress of laser treatment.

In the first two sections we briefly review "optical interaction of lasers with tissue" and "methods for determining optical properties." In addition, new methods are presented for measuring the optical properties for tissue that scatters light anisotropically. These methods are used to measure the absorption coefficient, the scattering coefficient, and the phase function for healthy vessel wall *in vitro* samples at a wavelength of 632.8 nm.

Following these sections, we examine a technique for approximating multiple scattering and absorption which represents scattered light with six directional fluxes and solutions for one-, two-, and three-dimensional cases are presented. Light distributions computed with the flux model are compared to distributions computed with the diffusion approximation of the radiative transfer equation and appropriate conditions for applying the flux model are suggested. Measured optical properties are used with the model to predict the rate of heat generation in tissue due to the absorption of the laser light.

Manuscript received February 19, 1987; revised May 5, 1987. This work was supported in part by the Free Electron Laser Biomedical/Materials Program under ONR Contract N00014-86-K-0875.

G. Yoon, A. J. Welch, and M. Motamedi are with the Department of Electrical and Computer Engineering, Biomedical Engineering Program, the University of Texas at Austin, Austin, TX 78712.

M. C. J. van Gemert is with the Experimental Laser Unit, Academic Medical Centre, University of Amsterdam, Amsterdam, The Netherlands.

IEEE Log Number 8716268.

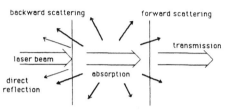

Fig. 1. Laser beam interaction with tissue.

I. Optical Interaction of Lasers with Tissue

Possible interactions of light and tissue are illustrated in Fig. 1. A small percentage, usually about 5 percent of a normally incident laser beam is reflected (Fresnel reflection) from the surface due a mismatch in refractive index. The rest of the beam is transmitted into the tissue and encounters the process of multiple scattering and absorption. Absorbed light energy is converted to heat which increases the temperature of the tissue.

The degree of scattering depends upon the wavelength of the laser beam and the optical properties of the tissue. For example, the 193, 248, and 308 nm ultraviolet wavelengths of the ArK, KrF, and XeCl excimer lasers and the 2.94 and 10.6 μm infrared wavelengths of the Er:YAG and CO_2 laser, respectively, are highly absorbed in vascular tissue; penetration depth (i.e., the depth at which the magnitude of the light intensity is reduced by a factor of e^{-1} due to absorption and scattering) of these wavelengths is approximately 1 to 20 μm. At these wavelengths, scattering is not significant compared to absorption, as illustrated in Fig. 2(a).

However, for wavelengths between 450 and 590 nm, which include the argon laser wavelengths, the penetration depth of the laser beam is approximately 0.5 to 2.5 mm. Both absorption and scattering are substantial, and light in the tissue has a strongly collimated component surrounded by a region where light is multiply scattered [see Fig. 2(b)]. The back scattered component of light is a major component of the total measured reflectance; measurements of 15 to 40 percent of the incident beam are typical for these wavelengths. Between 590 nm and 1.5 μm, which includes the 1.06 and 1.32 μm wavelengths of the Nd:YAG laser, scattering dominates absorption and the penetration depth varies from 2.0 to 8.0 mm. As the light passes through the tissue, the collimated structure of the beam is replaced by completely diffuse

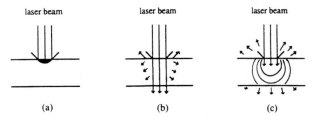

Fig. 2. Scattering and absorption of laser light. (a) Absorption dominant. (b) Equal scattering and absorption. (c) Scattering dominant.

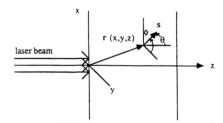

Fig. 3. Normal incidence of laser beam on the slab geometry. $L(r, s)$ is the radiance in $s(\theta, \phi)$ direction at $r(x, y, z)$ position.

light, as depicted in Fig. 2(c). Backscattering is markedly increased and the range of total measured reflected light is as high as 35–70 percent of the incident light. For a normally incident beam, total reflectance is primarily due to backscattering except when absorption is much larger than scattering, in which case mainly Fresnel reflection occurs. The degree of backscattering is a function of the wavelength-dependent optical properties of the tissue.

Laser Light Distribution in Tissue

Electromagnetic wave interaction with biological media varies depending upon wavelength and the optical properties of the tissue. For wavelengths that are much longer than cell diameters (frequencies lower than 300 GHz) where there is little scattering from the cellular structures, and therefore reflection, absorption, and transmission are described best using electromagnetic theory [1], [2]. However, the electromagnetic spectrum of lasers lies in the infrared to ultraviolet wavelength band; substantial multiple scattering in tissue occurs in this band due to the comparable size of cells with respect to the irradiation wavelength. For laser wavelengths, the radiative transfer theory provides a practical description for the optical propagation of light in tissue [3].

By assuming that scattering and absorbing centers are uniformly distributed in tissue and neglecting internal light generation by fluorescence, a mathematical description for laser beam normally incident on a slab (Fig. 3) is given in (1) and (2). The radiance of the collimated light is attenuated by direct absorption and scattering (1).

$$dL_c(r, z)/dz = -\gamma L_c(r, z) \qquad (1)$$

where $L_c(r, z)$ is the collimated radiance [watt/unit area-steradian] at position r in the z incident direction, r is a position vector, γ is the attenuation coefficient defined as the sum of the absorption coefficient κ and the scattering coefficient σ. The radial profile of the collimated beam within the tissue has the same shape as the incident beam. Scattered collimated light goes through multiple scattering. The distribution of light scattered from the laser beam can be described by the radiative transfer equation [4].

$$s \cdot \nabla L_s(r, s) + \gamma L_s(r, s)$$

$$= \frac{\gamma}{4\pi} \int_{4\pi} p(s, s') L_s(r, s') \, d\omega'$$

$$+ \frac{\gamma}{4\pi} p(s, z) L_c(r, z) \qquad (2)$$

where $L_S(r, s)$ is the scattered radiance [watt/unit area-steradian] at position r in the s direction (s is the directional unit vector). The phase function, $p(s, s')$, represents scattering contribution from s' to the s direction; ω denotes the solid angle. The solid angle integration of this phase function is defined as

$$(1/4\pi) \int_{4\pi} p(s, s') \, d\omega' = \sigma/\gamma. \qquad (3)$$

The second term in (2) is the decrease in intensity of scattered light by absorption and scattering. The first term of the right-hand side is the gain in intensity in the s direction due to scattering from all over directions and the second term of the right-hand side is the gain due to scattering from the collimated beam. The scattered light L_S, must be added to the collimated beam L_c, when determining the radiance distribution in tissue:

$$L(r, s) = L_c(r, s) + L_s(r, s). \qquad (4)$$

This flexible theory has been applied to different areas such as light scattering in stellar atmosphere and neutron transfer in nuclear engineering [5], [6]. Even though the radiative transfer theory gives an adequate description of light absorption and scattering, a general solution of the resulting "radiative transfer equation" is not known. Solutions are available only for simple cases such as isotropic scattering and infinitely extended geometry [4]. Numerical solutions for two- and three-dimensional problems using the general transport equation require extensive computer time and memory. In the majority of practical cases, it is desirable to obtain approximate solutions.

II. METHODS FOR DETERMINING OPTICAL PROPERTIES

Calculation or computer modeling of the distribution of laser light in tissue requires 1) measurement of the optical properties of the media of interest and 2) a theory or model for computing the light distribution. Unfortunately these are not independent steps. In practice, it is convenient to measure the optical properties in a manner that is consistent with the model for light distribution. Methods for dominant absorption, isotropic scattering, and anisotropic scattering cases are described as follows.

Dominant Absorption Case

When absorption is much larger than scattering, light is attenuated exponentially mainly by absorption (Beer's law); that is, the radiance at depth z is

$$L(z) = L_{inc} \exp(-\kappa z) \qquad (5)$$

where L_{inc} is the incident radiance (neglecting surface reflection). In this case the tissue is characterized by the absorption coefficient κ. This coefficient can be determined experimentally by measuring the attenuation of the laser beam through a tissue sample of thickness d. By solving (5) for κ

$$\kappa = \left[\ln\left(L_{inc}/L(d)\right)\right]/d. \qquad (6)$$

Unfortunately, if κ is larger than a few hundred per centimeter, it is difficult to obtain tissue samples thin enough for accurate measurements.

As previously mentioned, wavelengths in the ultraviolet and far-infrared bands are highly absorbed by tissue and scattering is insignificant compared to absorption. For example, penetration depths for the wavelengths of the ArF, KrF, and XeCl excimer lasers (193, 248, 308 nm), Er:YAG (2.94 μm), and CO_2 (10.6 μm) lasers are approximately 1 μm, 10 μm, 50 μm, 1 μm, and 20 μm, respectively. Values for 193 μm are based on the data of Srinivasan [7]. The numbers for 248 and 308 μm are derived from epidermal data by Wan *et al.* [8] and dermal data by Anderson and Parrish [9], respectively. Since water content affects sample thickness, penetration depths for ultraviolet wavelengths are dependent upon the percentage of nonabsorbing water in the tissue. Infrared wavelengths beyond 1.5 μm are highly absorbed by water and typically, the percentage of water content in tissue determines the absorption coefficient. Often water absorption data [10] such as Fig. 4 are cited as being equivalent to tissue absorption in the infrared spectrum. However, Berry has noted that there is a difference in the absorption properties of "free" and "bound" water in tissue [11]. Free water has an absorption peak at 2.94 μm whereas Berry has measured the peak of bound water at 3.05 μm. In the ultraviolet spectrum, absorption depends upon the protein content in tissue.

Isotropic Scattering Case

In contrast, if scattering is substantial, the distribution of the laser light in tissue cannot be predicted by Beer's law and neither absorption nor scattering can be individually estimated from attenuation measurements of the laser beam.

For isotropic scattering, absorption and scattering coefficients can be determined by measuring diffuse reflection and diffuse transmission for a thin sample of tissue. From these measurements, the Kubelka–Munk absorption and scattering coefficients, K and S, respectively, can be calculated using the simple relations of transmission and reflection to K and S [12]. This method typically makes use of an integrating sphere to measure reflection and transmission; values for K and S have been reported for skin [8] and for blood [13]. Typically these measurements have been made without index matching of the tissue to the environment and using collimated light rather than diffuse light as required by the theory. Techniques to compensate

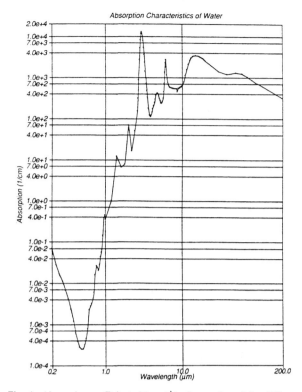

Fig. 4. Absorption coefficients [1 cm^{-1}] of water from 0.2 to 200 μm.

for index mismatching have been developed. For example, Egan *et al.* [14] obtained K and S graphically from a chart which relates reflection and transmission with K and S for given thickness and index of refraction of a sample. Kottler [15] computed volumetric reflection and transmission with an additional reflection measurement for a sample with black-backing, then K and S were obtained.

Kubelka–Munk coefficients K and S computed from measurements of diffuse reflection and diffuse transmission can be used to calculate the absorption and scattering coefficients of the radiative transfer equation, κ and σ. These relations between the Kubelka–Munk theory and the radiative transfer theory have been studied for isotropic scattering by Klier [16]. Another method for determining κ and σ using only diffuse transmission measurements has been described by Yoon *et al.* [17]. This approach requires transmission measurement from samples of various thickness.

Anisotropic Scattering Case

For many cases, isotropic scattering in tissue has been assumed for convenience. However, an analysis of light interaction with tissue requires complete determination of absorption coefficient, scattering coefficient, and phase function, which are functions of wavelength. Estimation of these optical properties for anisotropic scattering is much more complicated since there are no simple inverse relations between reflection/transmission measurement and the radiative transfer equation.

Thus, it has been necessary to develop techniques based on somewhat limited conditions. For instance, techniques based upon diffusion approximation have been developed for determining κ, σ, and the average cosine angle of the phase function, g by Jacques et al. [18] and by Marynisses et al. [19]. Based upon these recent measurements, phase functions for some tissues are highly forward scattering and the isotropic scattering assumption is not adequate. Another method using relations of the Kubelka–Munk theory and the one-dimensional diffusion approximation has been reported by van Gemert et al. [20]. This technique evaluates κ, σ, and g from K and S with an additional measurement of the on-axis transmission of the collimated beam.

However, estimation of optical properties require direct measurement of the phase function and related experiments to evaluate κ and σ. It is not possible to isolate absorbing/scattering particles in the tissue structure, however the phase function can be estimated by measuring the angular light distribution of a small diameter beam through a thin sample (ideally, the tissue samples should be thin enough to ensure single scattering events). Spatial variations can be expected in any tissue sample due to the non-homogeneous nature and complex structure of tissue.

III. Optical Properties of Vessel Wall at 632.8 nm

A method for determination of the absorption coefficient and scattering coefficient and phase function using measurements of phase function, collimated attenuation, and diffuse transmission is discussed in this section. This method is applied to *in vitro* samples of human vessel wall; optical properties measured at 632.8 nm are used to compute the rate of heat generation in a later section.

Phase Function Measurement

Experimental Setup: The setup for measuring angular distributions of light scattered from a laser beam passing through a thin tissue sample is illustrated in Fig. 5. Samples placed in the center of a water-filled tank were irradiated by a 1 mm diameter beam from a He–Ne laser. Scattered light was measured with a photodiode detector (1 mm aperture) that was rotated through 360°, with the midpoint of tissue as the center point of the circle. The sample and the detector were submerged in the water tank to minimize the difference of indexes of refraction and the inside-walls of the tank were painted black. The radius of the circle was 24 cm and the angular step size was 0.6°, except for the use of a 0.3° step for alignment of the detector precisely with the collimated beam, and for measurements of light intensities in regions of highly-peaked forward scattering. An IBM XT personal computer was used to control angular steping of the detector and to acquire data.

Light detected using the system illustrated in Fig. 5 is proportional to "radiance/cos θ" because of the angular difference between the sample surface and the detector. In addition, measured radiance around $\theta = 90°$ (at right angle to the laser beam) do not represent the real scattering pattern because of the increased path length of the scattered light in the slab geometry of the tissue sample.

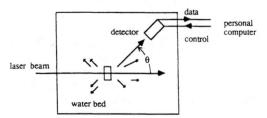

Fig. 5. Experimental setup of phase function measurement.

Measured angular distributions of scattered light for an 80 μm thick sample of cadaveric aorta are shown by dots in Fig. 6(a).

Analysis of Measured Phase Function: Calculation of light distribution can be simplified if the measured angular distribution can be expressed in a closed mathematical form. The Henyey–Greenstein function has been used to represent highly-peaked forward scattering by Danielson et al. [21] to describe scattering in clouds. Reynolds et al. [22] have described a two-parameter phase function for blood which provides a better correlation with experimental data. Also, the Henyey–Greenstein term has been combined with an isotropic term to create a composite phase function to characterize the angular scattering pattern for human dermis by Jacques et al. [23]. In a like manner, the measured data of Fig. 6(a) can be fit by a composite phase function consisting of an isotropic term and the Henyey–Greenstein term as follows:

$$p(\cos \theta) = (\sigma/\gamma) \left[u + (1 - u)(1 - g_H^2) \right.$$
$$\left. \cdot (1 + g_H^2 - 2g_H \cos \theta)^{-1.5} \right] \quad (7)$$

where the first term u represents the isotropic scattering and the second term is the Henyey–Greenstein formula. The average cosine angle of this phase function g, is $(1 - u) g_H$ where $g = \int_{4\pi} p(\cos \theta) \cos \theta \, d\omega / \int_{4\pi} p(\cos \theta) \, d\omega$. g_H is g for the Henyey–Greenstein term only.

The phase function in (7) was fit to the measured data of Fig. 6(a) using the least squares method. Values of $g_H = 0.945$ and $u = 0.071$ for 80 μm thick sample were obtained. The composite phase function computed with these values is presented in Fig. 6(a) (in solid line). Several measurements for samples whose thickness was less than 130 μm were made and computed values of u and g_H for these phase functions were plotted in Fig. 6(b). The 127 μm thick sample was fresh tissue and other samples such as 10, 30, and 80 μm thick were obtained by using a microtome to slice a frozen section. In reality, it is not possible to ensure single scattering events in the samples. As the thickness of the sample is decreased the number of scattering events are decreased and the measured distribution approaches a real phase function. From the linear regressions for g_H and u in Fig. 6(b), the obtained asymptotic values were 0.976 for g_H and 0.094 for u. Thus the average cosine angle of the phase function g, was 0.882.

Attenuation Coefficient Measurement

The attenuation coefficient $\gamma = \kappa + \sigma$ was measured from the attenuation of the collimated beam. The same

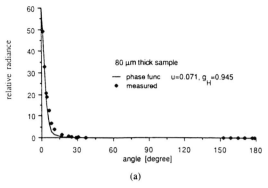

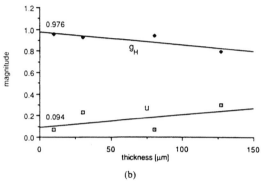

Fig. 6. (a) Angular distributions of measured light intensities (in dots) and the phase function described by (7) fit by the least squares method (in solid line) for an 80 μm thick sample of aortic wall. (b) Measured values of g_H and u for thin tissue samples. The linear regressions (in solid lines) give 0.976 and 0.094 as the asymptotic values for g_H and u, respectively.

system described in Fig. 5 was used with the detector placed on the beam axis. The solid angle of the detector was 1.36×10^{-5} steradian which minimized detection of scattered light. Thin samples of various thickness, whose thickness did not exceed more than 310 μm, were used for this measurement. Under these conditions, collimated attenuation is $\exp(-\gamma d)$ where d is the sample thickness. The attenuation coefficient was obtained graphically; the logarithm of the measured collimated attenuation versus thickness was plotted and the slope was obtained by the linear regression, which gave 316 cm^{-1} for the attenuation coefficient with 0.98 as the sample correlation coefficient.

Diffuse Transmission Measurement

An additional measurement is required to separate absorption and scattering coefficients from the attenuation coefficient. For this purpose, we used diffuse transmission measurement; if the equation for Kubelka–Munk transmission T, is modified to include the external diffuse surface reflection coefficient r_{de}, and the internal diffuse surface reflection coefficient r_{di}, that is

$$T = \frac{(1 - r_{de})(1 - r_{di})b}{(r_{di}^2 - 2r_{di} + a)\sinh(bSd) + (1 - r_{di}^2)b\cosh(bSd)} \quad (8)$$

where a and b satisfy $b^2 = a^2 - 1 = K(K + 2S)/S^2$. The asymptotic solution for $\ln(T)$ is given by a linear equation.

$$\ln(T) \cong -\sqrt{K(K + 2S)}\, d + \text{constant.} \quad (9)$$

The slope of (9), $-\sqrt{K(K + 2S)}$, is no longer a function of r_{de} and r_{di}, which may not be known. This slope can be obtained from measurements of diffuse transmission through tissue samples of various thickness. In order to separate κ and σ, the following relations reported in [20] are applied.

$$K = 2\kappa \quad (10)$$

$$S = (3/4)(1 - g)\sigma - (1/4)\kappa. \quad (11)$$

Along with g obtained from the phase function measurement, the absorption coefficient is given by

$$\kappa = -(1 - g)\gamma/2g$$
$$+ \sqrt{[(1 - g)\gamma/2g]^2 + K(K + 2S)/3g}. \quad (12)$$

Experimental Setup: The system for measuring diffuse transmission is illustrated in Fig. 7. A He–Ne laser beam passed through a photoacoustic chopper. This modulated beam was expanded and was passed through a diffusing plate. The amount of transmission was detected using an integrating sphere. A photoacoustic chopper/lock-in amplifier system was used to minimize noise problems. The laser beam was expanded so that the relative size of beam to sample thickness was large enough to ensure proper conditions for a one-dimensional slab geometry required by (8). Transmission as a function of tissue thickness for human vessel wall is shown in Fig. 8. The slope in Fig. 8 calculated by the linear regression technique was -7.89 cm^{-1}.

The above three experimental results are summarized as follows:

$$g_H = 0.976, \quad u = 0.094, \quad g = 0.882, \quad \gamma = 316 \text{ cm}^{-1}$$
$$-\sqrt{K(K + 2S)} = -7.89 \text{ cm}^{-1}, \quad \kappa = 0.55 \text{ cm}^{-1},$$
$$\sigma = 315.45 \text{ cm}^{-1}.$$

IV. THREE-DIMENSIONAL LIGHT DISTRIBUTION MODEL

Because of the difficulties in obtaining the general solution of (2), approximate solutions have been employed. For instance, single scattering theory provides reasonable results when scattering centers are sparsely distributed and the diffusion approximation is a reasonable assumption when scattering is much more dominant than absorption. Halldorsson *et al.* [24] assumed single scattering to predict the temperature rise in a slab of human bladder irradiated by the Nd:YAG laser. However, single scattering is not a good approximation for most tissues because of their dense structure.

The diffusion approximation has been successfully used

by Reynolds *et al.* to model diffuse reflectance from blood [25] and by Groenhuis *et al.* [26] to compare computed

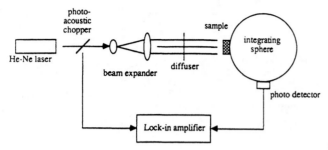

Fig. 7. Experimental setup for diffuse transmission measurement.

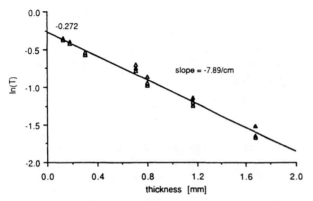

Fig. 8. Measured diffuse transmission through aortic wall at 632.8 nm. Thickness versus the logarithm of transmission. The straight line represents the linear regression for the measured data.

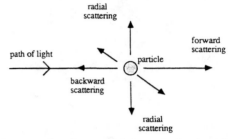

Fig. 9. Representation of scattered light by six directional fluxes in the seven flux model.

and measured reflected distributions of radiance from dental enamel. Jacques and Prahl [18] have also used measured optical properties in the one-dimensional diffusion approximation to compute light distribution in the mouse dermis. Special care must be exercised when the diffusion approximation is used for predicting light distribution and rate of heat generation inside tissue irradiated by a laser. Since the diffusion approximation assumes that the light is almost uniformly scattered in all directions, with more amplitude in the direction of the flux flow, the best results are obtained when scattering is much larger than absorption. The approximation becomes less appropriate when absorption is as substantial as scattering or when scattering is highly anisotropic. In addition, in regions within a few of optical depths of the surface or near the collimated laser beam, the scattered light has not yet reached the diffusion mode and should be characterized as a multiple scattering process. It is these regions which are our primary concern.

Seven-Flux Model

An approximation of laser light scattering in tissue is achieved by creating a simple pattern of weighted directional fluxes. As illustrated in Fig. 9, the scattering pattern is represented by six fluxes. This formation is obviously an approximation and not exact from a mathematical point of view. Nevertheless, the concept of discrete fluxes provides a practical model. The directions of the fluxes are selected in such a way to optimize the

geometrical relation between the incident beam and the medium. The x-y-z coordinate system presented in Fig. 3 is used to represent the laser-tissue geometry on a slab and x, $-x$, y, $-y$, z, and $-z$ are the components for the scattered light. A seventh flux in the $+z$ direction F_c, is introduced to represent the collimated light. Seven first-order coupled linear differential equations for these fluxes can be written as follows.

$$\partial F_c(x, y, z)/\partial z = -\gamma F_c(x, y, z) \qquad (13)$$

$$\partial F_{+z}(x, y, z)/\partial z + \gamma F_{+z}$$
$$= \gamma[\{p_{z,x}F_{+x} + p_{z,-x}F_{-x} + p_{z,y}F_{+y} + p_{z,-y}F_{-y}$$
$$+ p_{z,z}F_{+z} + p_{z,-z}F_{-z}\} + p_{z,z}F_c(x, y, z)] \qquad (14)$$

$$-\partial F_{-z}(x, y, z)/\partial z + \gamma F_{-z}$$
$$= \gamma[\{p_{-z,x}F_{+x} + p_{-z,-x}F_{-x}$$
$$+ p_{-z,y}F_{+y} + p_{-z,-y}F_{-y}$$
$$+ p_{-z,z}F_{+z} + p_{-z,-z}F_{-z}\} + p_{-z,z}F_c(x, y, z)] \qquad (15)$$

$$\partial F_{+x}(x, y, z)/\partial x + \gamma F_{+x}$$
$$= \gamma[\{p_{x,x}F_{+x} + p_{x,-x}F_{-x} + p_{x,y}F_{+y} + p_{x,-y}F_{-y}$$
$$+ p_{x,z}F_{+z} + p_{x,-z}F_{-z}\} + p_{x,z}F_c(x, y, z)] \qquad (16)$$

$$-\partial F_{-x}(x, y, z)/\partial x + \gamma F_{-x}$$
$$= \gamma[\{p_{-x,x}F_{+x} + p_{-x,-x}F_{-x} + p_{-x,y}F_{+y}$$
$$+ p_{-x,-y}F_{-y} + p_{-x,z}F_{+z} + p_{-x,-z}F_{-z}\}$$
$$+ p_{-x,z}F_c(x, y, z)] \qquad (17)$$

$$\partial F_{+y}(x, y, z)/\partial y + \gamma F_{+y}$$
$$= \gamma[\{p_{y,x}F_{+x} + p_{y,-x}F_{-x} + p_{y,y}F_{+y} + p_{y,-y}F_{-y}$$
$$+ p_{y,z}F_{+z} + p_{y,-z}F_{-z}\} + p_{y,z}F_c(x, y, z)] \qquad (18)$$

$$-\partial F_{-y}(x, y, z)/\partial y + \gamma F_{-y}$$
$$= \gamma \big[\{ p_{-y,x} F_{+x} + p_{-y,-x} F_{-x} + p_{-y,y} F_{+y}$$
$$+ p_{-y,-y} F_{-y} + p_{-y,z} F_{+z} + p_{-y,-z} F_{-z} \}$$
$$+ p_{-y,z} F_c(x, y, z) \big]. \qquad (19)$$

The exponential decrease of the collimated flux $F_c(x, y, z)$, by absorption and scattering is described in (13). The remaining six equations all have similar forms. Consider F_{+z}, which is the flux in the $+z$ direction from (14). The phase function $p(s, s')$ of (3) is represented by weights $p_{i,j}$. $p_{z,x}$ is the portion of flux from the x direction scattered into the z direction, $p_{z,-x}$ is the portion of flux from the $-x$ direction scattered into the z direction, etc. Flux in F_{+z} [the first term of the left-hand side in (14)] is decreased by absorption and scattering of F_{+z} (the second term of the left-hand side) and increased by scattering contributions from all other scattered fluxes as well as the collimated flux [the right-hand side of (14)]. In similar manner, the remaining equations are explained.

There have been similar approaches for representing scattering of electromagnetic waves. Chu et al. [27] introduced the representation of six fluxes for diffuse light, but their model was limited to uniform, diffuse incident irradiation. In order to describe the scattered light, Cummins et al. [28] used four light components: one in the direction of the beam propagation, one in the opposite direction, and two radial components. This approximation resulted in a two-dimensional geometry since all four light components were in the same plane. In addition, isotropic scattering was assumed by Cummins et al.

Typically, measured phase functions are axially symmetric. By assuming axial symmetry, a simpler expression can be obtained for (13)-(19). Using the representations; forward scattering (p_f), backward scattering (p_b), and four radial scatterings with the same magnitude (p_r) and defining $p_{i,j}$ as the portion of flux from the j direction scattered into the i direction, the following is easily understood; $p_f = p_{z,z} = p_{-z,-z} = p_{x,x} = p_{-x,-x} = p_{y,y} = p_{-y,-y}$, and $p_b = p_{z,-z} = p_{-z,z} = p_{x,-x} = p_{-x,x} = p_{y,-y} = p_{-y,y}$ and the rest are p_r. $p_{i,j} = p_{j,i}$ also holds. These $p_{i,j}$'s represent components of a weighted-discrete phase function.

Accuracy is dependent on how well the phase function can be represented by the scattering pattern illustrated in Fig. 9. A flux to a given reference direction s is the projected radiance into s direction over the half hemisphere. Therefore the probability of light being scattered into each direction is computed in terms of vectorial momentum or pressure into a given direction rather than integration of the scattering probabilities for the region represented by a flux. This pressure can be explained as the rate of transfer of the momentum component normal to a unit surface. Using this concept, the magnitudes of the components of the weighted-discrete phase function are obtained in the same manner as Chu et al. [27].

$$p_f = (1/4\pi) \int_{2\pi, z} p(s, s')(z \cdot s')^2 \, d\omega' \qquad (20)$$

$$p_b = (1/4\pi) \int_{2\pi, -z} p(s, s')(-z \cdot s')^2 \, d\omega' \qquad (21)$$

$$p_r = (1/4\pi) \int_{2\pi, v} p(s, s')(v \cdot s')^2 \, d\omega'$$
$$\text{where } v \text{ is one of } x, -x, y, -y. \qquad (22)$$

Solid angle integration over 2π is evaluated with its reference direction as the center of 2π hemisphere. $p_f + p_b + 4p_r = \sigma/\gamma$ holds and, for isotropic scattering, p_f, p_b, and p_r each equal $\sigma/6\gamma$. The solutions of (13)-(19) are obtained with appropriate boundary conditions. An analytic solution is available for an uniform incident beam, where there are no light intensity variations in the x and y directions. However for two- and three-dimensional cases, where it is difficult to solve these equations analytically, a finite difference code has been implemented. Analytical and numerical solutions as well as applied boundary conditions are discussed in Appendix I.

Radiance

The light component of the collimated flux, $F_c(x, y, z)$, is only in the z direction whereas scattered fluxes have light components in all directions. Once the values of the discrete fluxes (W/cm^2) are determined, radiance (W/cm^2-sr) can be reconstructed. This is accomplished by expressing the radiance as the terms of the associate Legendre polynomials. Reconstruction of the radiance in this manner allows us to use only six terms for our case, which are selected subjectively in order to give probable scattering patterns. The radiance at position $r(x, y, z)$ into $s(\cos\theta, \phi)$ direction of the spherical coordinate (Fig. 3) is

$$L_c(\cos\theta, \phi) = F_c \delta(\cos\theta - 1)\delta(\phi) \quad \text{at a given } r$$
$$(23)$$

$$L_S(\cos\theta, \phi) = m_0 \psi_0^0(\cos\theta) + m_1 \psi_1^0(\cos\theta)$$
$$+ m_2 \psi_1^1(\cos\theta)\sin\phi + m_3 \psi_1^1(\cos\theta)$$
$$\cdot \cos\phi + m_4 \psi_2^0(\cos\theta)$$
$$+ m_5 \psi_2^2(\cos\theta)\cos 2\phi \quad \text{at a given } r$$
$$(24)$$

where ψ's are the associate Legendre polynomials. Since fluxes can be represented as in (25),

$$F_S = \int_{2\pi, s} L_S(r, s')(s \cdot s') \, d\omega'$$
$$\text{where } s = \pm z, \pm x, \pm y \qquad (25)$$

coefficients, $m_0 - m_5$, are computed by applying L_S of (24) into (25) and calculated $m_0 - m_5$ are

$$m_0 = (1/6\pi)(F_{+z} + F_{-z} + F_{+x} + F_{-x} + F_{+y} + F_{-y})$$
$$(26)$$

$$m_1 = (3/4\pi)(F_{+z} - F_{-z}) \qquad (27)$$

$$m_2 = (3/4\pi)(F_{+y} - F_{-y}) \qquad (28)$$

$$m_3 = (3/4\pi)(F_{+x} - F_{-x}) \qquad (29)$$

$$m_4 = (4/3\pi)(F_{+z} + F_{-z})$$
$$- (2/3\pi)(F_{+x} + F_{-x} + F_{+y} + F_{-y}) \qquad (30)$$

$$m_5 = (1/3\pi)(F_{+x} + F_{-x} - F_{+y} - F_{-y}). \qquad (31)$$

Fluence Rate and Rate of Heat Generation: The fluence rate, Φ, is defined as the solid angle integration of radiance.

$$\Phi(r) = \int_{4\pi} [L_c(r, s) + L_s(r, s)] \, d\omega$$
$$= F_c(r) + 4\pi m_0(r). \qquad (32)$$

Integration of $L_s(r, s)$ over 4π solid angle cancels out all the associated Legendre polynomial terms except the m_0 term. The m_0 term represents the average radiance. The rate of heat generation $H\,[\mathrm{W/cm^3}]$ due to the absorption of light in tissue is proportional to the fluence rate and the absorption coefficient according to the relation

$$H(r) = \kappa \Phi(r). \qquad (33)$$

Comparison with Diffusion Approximation

A quantitative comparison of light distributions computed with the seven flux model and the diffusion approximation (Appendix II) was made for a laser beam with a Gaussian profile that had a 1.0 mm e^{-2} radius and a peak irradiance at the beam center of 100 W/cm² (i.e., 1.57 W laser power) for convenience. The thickness of the medium was 2.0 mm. Absorption and scattering coefficients were selected to represent equal absorption and scattering ($\kappa = 10$, $\sigma = 10\ \mathrm{cm^{-1}}$), scattering larger than absorption ($\kappa = 1$, $\sigma = 10\ \mathrm{cm^{-1}}$), and dominant scattering ($\kappa = 1$, $\sigma = 100\ \mathrm{cm^{-1}}$). To reduce the complexity of the problem, isotropic scattering and index matching between tissue and environment were assumed. Fluence rate as a function of depth was computed for three sets of absorption and scattering coefficients.

The results are compared in Figs. 10 and 11. The fluence rates at the beam center (Fig. 10) and at the e^{-2} radius (Fig. 11) are illustrated as a function of depth. The e^{-2} radius is defined as the radial distance where the fluence rate drops to e^{-2} of the fluence rate of the beam center. The light intensity at the surface is higher than the intensity of the incident beam due to volumetric back scattering. There are a few differences between the seven flux model and the diffusion approximation. Fluence rate at the front surface computed with the seven flux model is higher than that computed from the diffusion approximation. However, fluence rate computed with the former drops intensity more rapidly deeper in the tissue. The computed radial spread can be seen in Fig. 12 in terms of the e^{-2} radius relative to the center fluence rate at the

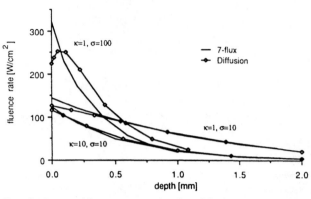

Fig. 10. Computed fluence rate as a function of depth at the beam center.

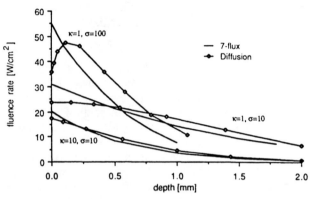

Fig. 11. Computed fluence rate as a function of depth at the radius of 1.0 mm.

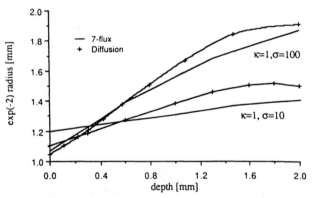

Fig. 12. Beam broadening in tissue due to scattering. Radial distances where the fluence rate drops to e^{-2} of that of the beam center were plotted as function of depth.

depth z. The e^{-2} radius of the diffusion approximation at the surface is smaller than that of the seven flux model even though broadening of the e^{-2} radius is more distinct in the diffusion approximation. It is interesting to note that in Fig. 12 the image sizes expands somewhat linearly as a function of depth in the tissue. A similar linear expansion has been noted by Sinofsky and Dumont [29] in the measurements of transmitted intensity profiles in arterial vessel irradiated with an argon laser.

V. Prediction of the Rate of Heat Generation on Vessel Wall

For an application of the seven flux model for predicting the rate of heat generation, we choose the case of normal aortic wall irradiated by a laser wavelength of 632.8 nm. Measured optical properties from Section III are used. A Gaussian beam with 2.0 mm spot size and 100 W/cm² irradiance at the beam center (1.57 W) are selected.

Values of p_f, p_b, and p_r are computed from the estimated phase function using (20)-(22). As an example these values are plotted in Fig. 13 for the Henyey-Greenstein phase function. For $g = 0$, $p_f = p_b = p_r = p_{iso}$ where p_{iso} is the value for an isotropic scattering and equal to $\sigma/6\gamma$. As the phase function becomes more forward scattering, the value of p_f increases and the values of p_b and p_r decrease until $p_f = 6p_{iso}$, $p_b = p_r = 0$ for $g = 1$ (Fig. 13). For backward scattering, the value of p_b increases until $p_b = 6p_{iso}$, $p_f = p_r = 0$ for $g = -1$. Based on the measurements in the Section III where the phase function in (7) was represented by $u = 0.094$ and $g_H = 0.976$, values of $p_f = 5.23\ p_{iso}$, $p_b = 0.09\ p_{iso}$, $p_r = 0.17\ p_{iso}$ were calculated.

Using $\kappa = 0.55$ and $\sigma = 315.45$ cm^{-1}, the estimated rate of heat generation is illustrated in Figs. 14 and 15. The reflection coefficient for the collimated beam, r_{ce}, at the front surface was set to 2 percent and the internal diffuse surface reflection coefficient r_{di}, 47 percent (these values were computed from (A-6) for the index of refraction of 1.33). Axial profiles along the beam center are illustrated in Fig. 14. Rate of heat generation due to collimated light is very small because of high scattering; the profile is dominated by noncollimated scattered light (Fig. 14). Although the optical penetration depth is approximately 30 μm, the axial profile indicates much deeper penetration of the light in tissue. These distributions are a result of high forward scattering of vessel wall ($g = 0.882$) and very little absorption inside the tissue. Radial profiles at different depths are shown in Fig. 15. Deep and radial spread of the rate of heat generation patterns are observed.

VI. Summary

For most laser wavelengths except in the ultraviolet and infrared bands scattering is an important parameter in determining the light distribution in tissue irradiated by laser light. Methods have been described for measuring phase function, absorption, and scattering coefficients. Using these methods, the optical properties of aortic vessel wall have been measured at 632.8 nm wavelength. Measurements confirm the anisotropic scattering noted in other tissues and prove that the isotropic scattering assumption, which has often been used, is not appropriate. The measured phase function appears to fit well a phase function composed of an isotropic term and a Henyey-Greenstein term. For estimation of light distribution and rate of heat generation, the seven flux model has been introduced.

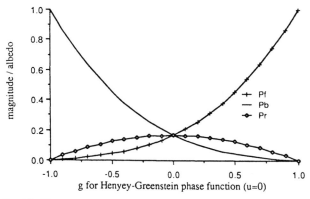

Fig. 13. The magnitudes of computed p_f, p_b, and p_r for the Henyey-Greenstein phase function (i.e., $u = 0$). These values are shown with respect to the average cosine angle g.

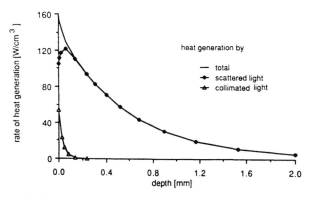

Fig. 14. Rate of heat generation in aortic wall as a function of depth at the beam center. 1.57 W power and 2 mm spot size are assumed. The $\triangle$ curve would represent the lower bound estimate of rate of heat generation due to the collimated beam.

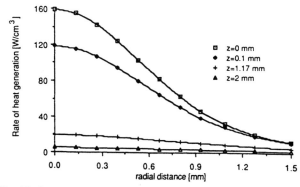

Fig. 15. Rate of heat generation in aortic wall as a funciton of radial distance at different depths. 1.57 W power and 2 mm spot size are assumed.

Multiple scattering assumed in the model is considered more appropriate than single scattering or the diffusion process. In addition, the model can be extended to other geometries with its flexibility. Accuracy depends on how well the scattering pattern represented by six directional fluxes can describe a real phase function. The model is expected to give reasonable results for the phase functions observed in the tissues which show very highly forward peak. However, the model is less accurate when the distribution pattern of the phase function becomes complex.

APPENDIX I
SOLUTIONS OF SEVEN-FLUX MODEL

A. Uniform Incidence Upon a Slab Geometry

For a uniform incidence upon a slab geometry (Fig. 3), fluxes do not vary with respect to x, $-x$, y, and $-y$. Under these conditions, (13)–(19) can be rewritten as

$$\partial F_c(z)/\partial z = -\gamma F_c(z) \tag{A-1}$$

$$\partial F_{+z}(z)/\partial z = C_1 F_{+z}(z) + C_2 F_{-z}(z) + D_1 F_c(z) \tag{A-2}$$

$$-\partial F_{-z}(z)/\partial z = C_1 F_{-z}(z) + C_2 F_{+z}(z) + D_2 F_c(z) \tag{A-3}$$

$$
\begin{aligned}
F_{+x}(z) &= F_{-x}(z) = F_{+y}(z) = F_{-y}(z) \\
&= p_r \frac{F_{+z}(z) + F_{-z}(z) + F_c(z)}{1 - (p_f + p_b) - 2p_r}
\end{aligned} \tag{A-4}
$$

where

$$C_1 = \gamma p_f - \gamma + 4\gamma p_r^2 / \left\{ 1 - (p_f + p_b) - 2p_r \right\}$$

$$C_2 = \gamma p_b + 4\gamma p_r^2 / \left\{ 1 - (p_f + p_b) - 2p_r \right\}$$

$$D_1 = \gamma p_f + 4\gamma p_r^2 / \left\{ 1 - (p_f + p_b) - 2p_r \right\}$$

$$D_2 = C_2.$$

Three boundary conditions for a slab of finite thickness have been applied as follows. 1) $F_c(0) = (1 - r_{ce}) F_{inc}$; r_{ce} is the external reflectance of the collimated light, F_{inc} is the incident collimated flux. 2) $F_{+z}(0) = r_{di} F_{-z}(0)$; r_{di} is the internal reflectance of scattered light. 3) At the rear surface, $F_{-z}(d) = r_{di} F_{+z}(d)$; d is the slab thickness. No boundary conditions for the rest fluxes are imposed since these fluxes are assumed to propagate along the boundaries without traveling across the discontinuity. The collimated irradiation, F_{inc}, has spatial light only in the z direction, a portion of which is reflected at the front surface by the Fresnel reflection. r_{ce} is given by

$$r_{ce} = \left[(n_r - 1)/(n_r + 1) \right]^2 \tag{A-5}$$

where n_r is the relative index of refraction between the medium and the surroundings. On the other hand, the fluxes representing scattered light have light components in all directions. Values for r_{di} should be determined by experiment especially for anisotropic scattering or for thin tissues. For diffused light the following relation can be used [14]:

$$r_{di} = -1.4399/n_r^2 + 0.7099/n_r + 0.6681 + 0.0636\, n_r. \tag{A-6}$$

The value of r_{di} at the front surface is usually closer to that in (A-6) than r_{di} at the rear surface [23]. Therefore, if the experimental data are not available for *in vivo* treatment where the tissue thickness is much larger than the optical depth, the above equation may be used. The solution for (A-1)–(A-4) is

$$F_c(z) = (1 - r_{ce}) F_{inc}\, e^{-\gamma z} \tag{A-7}$$

$$F_{+z}(z) = A_1 e^{vz} + A_2 e^{-vz} + A_3 e^{-\gamma z} \tag{A-8}$$

$$F_{-z}(z) = A_4 e^{vz} + A_5 e^{-vz} + A_6 e^{-\gamma z} \tag{A-9}$$

where

$$v = \sqrt{C_1^2 - C_2^2}$$

$$
\begin{aligned}
A_1 = F_c(0) \Big[& (r_{di}\Psi_1 - \Psi_2) \left\{ r_{di} + (v + C_1)/C_2 \right\} e^{-vd} \\
& - (\Psi_1 - r_{di}\Psi_2) \left\{ 1 + r_{di}(v + C_1)/C_2 \right\} \\
& \cdot e^{-\gamma d} \Big] / \left\{ \Delta(v^2 - \gamma^2) \right\}
\end{aligned}
$$

$$\Psi_1 = D_1 C_2 - D_2(C_1 + \gamma)$$

$$\Psi_2 = D_2 C_2 - D_1(C_1 + \gamma)$$

$$
\begin{aligned}
\Delta = & \left\{ 1 - r_{di}(v - C_1)/C_2 \right\} \\
& \cdot \left\{ r_{di} + (v + C_1)/C_2 \right\} e^{-vd} \\
& - \left\{ 1 + r_{di}(v + C_1)/C_2 \right\} \\
& \cdot \left\{ r_{di} - (v - C_1)/C_2 \right\} e^{vd}
\end{aligned}
$$

$$
\begin{aligned}
A_2 = F_c(0) \Big[& (\Psi_1 - r_{di}\Psi_2) \\
& \cdot \left\{ 1 - r_{di}(v - C_1)/C_2 \right\} e^{-\gamma d} \\
& - (r_{di}\Psi_1 - \Psi_2) \left\{ r_{di} - (v - C_1)/C_2 \right\} \\
& \cdot e^{vd} \Big] / \left\{ \Delta(v^2 - \gamma^2) \right\}
\end{aligned}
$$

$$A_3 = \Psi_2 F_c(0)/(v^2 - \gamma^2)$$

$$A_4 = A_1(v - C_1)/C_2$$

$$A_5 = -A_2(v + C_1)/C_2$$

$$A_6 = \Psi_1 F_c(0)/(v^2 - \gamma^2).$$

B. Numerical Computation of Two- and Three-Dimensional Problems

A finite difference method has been implemented for two- and three-dimensional problems. Since the same algorithm is used for both 2-D and 3-D cases, the 2-D case will be examined first. Then, unique features of the 3-D geometry will follow. No variation in the y axis is assumed for the 2-D case.

The notation for the finite difference algorithm uses z_i and x_j to represent discrete points of z and y. The indexes of grid points of z and x axis are i and j, respectively. The midpoint between z_{i+1} and z_i is $z_{i+1/2}$, i.e., $z_{i+1/2} = (z_{i+1} + z_i)/2$ and the flux at the midpoint is represented by the average flux of two adjacent points. For example, the finite difference representation of (14) of the seven flux model (the independent variable y is omitted in the expression) is

$$F_{+z}(z_{i+1}, x_j) = \frac{2 - \gamma(z_{i+1} - z_i)}{2 + \gamma(z_{i+1} - z_i)} F_{+z}(z_i, x_j)$$

$$+ \frac{z_{i+1} - z_i}{2 + \gamma(z_{i+1} - z_i)} \left[S_{+z}(z_{i+1}, x_j) \right.$$

$$\left. + S_{+z}(z_i, x_j) \right] \qquad \text{(A-10)}$$

where

$$S_{+z}(z_i, x_j) = (\gamma/6) \left[p_{z,x} F_{+x}(z_i, x_j) + p_{z,-x} F_{-x}(z_i, x_j) \right.$$

$$+ p_{z,y} F_{+y}(z_i, x_j) + p_{z,-y} F_{-y}(z_i, x_j)$$

$$+ p_{z,z} F_{+z}(z_i, x_j) + p_{z,-z} F_{-z}(z_i, x_j)$$

$$\left. + p_{z,z} F_c(z_i, x_j) \right].$$

Other equations (15)–(19) are implemented in the same manner. Boundary conditions are applied as follows:

$$F_c(0, x) = (1 - r_{ce}) F_{\text{inc}}(x)$$

$$F_{+z}(0, x) = r_{di} F_{-z}(0, x)$$

$$F_{-z}(d, x) = r_{di} F_{+z}(d, x)$$

$$F_{+x}(z, -X) = 0$$

$$F_{-x}(z, X) = 0 \qquad \text{(A-11)}$$

where d is the tissue thickness and X is an arbitrarily far distance where the F_{-x} component can be assumed to be zero. A symmetric boundary condition, i.e., $F_{+x}(z, 0) = F_{-x}(z, 0)$, should be used in order to reduce memory size and computation time if the profile of the incident beam is symmetric with respect to $x = 0$ axis. In order to minimize the accumulation of numerical error and to ensure stable convergence, iteration procedures follow the direction of each flux. This is from z_i to z_{i+1} for F_{+z} flux whereas F_{-z} follows in the direction from z_{i+1} to z_i. In the same manner, iteration of F_{+x} is along the direction from x_j to x_{j+1} and that of F_{-x} from x_{j+1} to x_j. This algorithm converges faster and is less dependent on the grid size than other forms of the partial differential equation. However, the grid size is larger than $2/\gamma$, the coefficient of F_{+z} on the right-hand side of (A-10) becomes negative and the solution does not converge. If the grid size is too large with respect to gradients of the flux, the accuracy is decreased.

Three-dimensional implementation is a natural extension of the two-dimensional algorithm. A geometry is expanded into an x, y, z volume and all six fluxes are implemented in finite difference code as described in (A-10). The boundary conditions in (A-11) are expanded as follows:

$$F_c(0, x, y) = (1 - r_{ce}) F_{\text{inc}}(x, y);$$

$$F_{+z}(0, x, y) = r_{di} F_{-z}(0, x, y)$$

$$F_{-z}(d, x, y) = r_{di} F_{+z}(d, x, y); \quad F_{+x}(z, -X, y) = 0$$

$$F_{-x}(z, X, y) = 0$$

$$F_{+y}(z, x, -Y) = 0; \quad F_{-y}(z, x, Y) = 0. \qquad \text{(A-12)}$$

Except for complicated geometries, the volume required for numerical computation can be reduced if the profile of the incident beam has certain symmetry. For example, only one-eighth volume of the whole geometry needs to be computed when the incident beam is axially symmetric and the optical properties do not vary in the tissue.

APPENDIX II

DIFFUSION APPROXIMATION

The diffusion approximation is a well-established theory (Ishimaru [30], an excellent reference). Light is scattered almost uniformly with more amplitude in the direction of the flux flow after encountering numerous scattering events. $L_s(r, s)$ in (2) is represented by the summation of a constant radiance term for any s direction and a term to compensate for forward peaking, thus

$$L_S(r, s) = U(r) + \int_{4\pi} L_S(r, s) \, s \cdot z \, d\omega (3/4\pi)$$

$$\text{(A-13)}$$

where $U(r)$ is defined as $\int_{4\pi} L_S(r, s) \, d\omega / 4\pi$. The above two terms correspond to the first two terms of Taylor's series expansion of $L_S(r, s)$. Boundary conditions are applied for the forward and backward fluxes; at the front surface, the forward flux equals the internally reflected portion of the backward flux and, at the rear surface, the backward flux equals the internally reflected portion of the forward flux, i.e.,

$$\int_{2\pi, +z} L_S(r, s) \, s \cdot z \, d\omega = r_{di} \int_{2\pi, -z} L_S(r, s) \, s \cdot z \, d\omega$$

$$\text{at } z = 0 \qquad \text{(A-14)}$$

$$\int_{2\pi, -z} L_S(r, s) \, s \cdot z \, d\omega = r_{di} \int_{2\pi, +z} L_S(r, s) \, s \cdot z \, d\omega$$

$$\text{at } z = d. \qquad \text{(A-15)}$$

Applying (A-13) and (A-15) into (2), we can obtain an equation in terms of $U(r)$.

$$\nabla^2 U(r) - 3\kappa\gamma_e U(r)$$

$$= -[3\sigma\gamma_e + 3\sigma\gamma g] F_c(r)/4\pi \qquad \text{(A-16)}$$

with two boundary conditions at the front and rear surfaces

$$U(r)(1 - r_{di})/(1 + r_{di}) - (2/3\gamma_e) \partial U(r)/\partial z$$

$$= -(g\sigma/2\pi\gamma_e) F_c(r) \quad \text{at } z = 0$$

$$U(r)(1 - r_{di})/(1 + r_{di}) + (2/3\gamma_e) \partial U(r)/\partial z$$

$$= (g\sigma/2\pi\gamma_e) F_c(r) \quad \text{at } z = d.$$

where

$$\gamma_e = \kappa + \sigma(1 - g) \quad \text{and}$$

$$F_c(r) = F_{\text{inc}}(x, y) \exp(-\gamma z).$$

Analytic solutions for the axially symmetric geometry for the diffusion approximation have been discussed in [26] and [30]. In addition, a numerical technique using the finite difference code for the same geometry has been implemented in our work.

ACKNOWLEDGMENT

The authors would like to thank S. A. Prahl for valuable discussions on applying the phase function described in (7).

REFERENCES

[1] C. C. Johnson and A. W. Guy, "Nonionizing electromagnetic wave effects in biological materials and systems," *Proc. IEEE*, vol. 60, pp. 692–718, June 1972.

[2] H. P. Schwan, "Interaction of microwave and radio frequency radiation with biological systems," *IEEE Trans. Microwave Theory Tech.*, vol. MTT-19, pp. 146–152, Feb. 1971.

[3] A. J. Welch, "The thermal response of laser irradiated tissue," *IEEE J. Quantum Electron.*, vol. QE-20, pp. 1471–1481, Dec. 1984.

[4] S. Chandrasekar, *Radiative Transfer*. London, England: Oxford University Press, 1960.

[5] E. Novotny, *Introduction to Stellar Atmospheres and Interiors*. London, England: Oxford University Press, 1973.

[6] G. Bell and S. Glasstone, *Nuclear Reactor Theory*. Malabar, Florida: Robert E. Krieger, 1970.

[7] R. Srinivasan, "Ablation of polymers and biological tissue by ultraviolet lasers," *Science*, vol. 234, pp. 559–565, 1986.

[8] S. Wan, R. R. Anderson, and J. A. Parrish, "Analytical modeling for the optical properties for the skin with in vitro and in vivo applications," *Photochem. Photobiol.*, vol. 34, pp. 493–499, 1981.

[9] R. R. Anderson and J. A. Parrish, *The Science of Photomedicine*. New York: Plenum, 1982, pp. 147–194.

[10] G. M. Hale and M. R. Querry, "Optical constants of water in 200 nm to 200 μm wavelength region," *Appl. Opt.*, vol. 12, no. 3, pp. 555–563, Mar. 1973.

[11] M. J. Berry, personal communication, Rice University, Houston, TX, 1987.

[12] P. Kubelka, "New contributions to the optics of intensely light-scattering materials," *J. Opt. Soc. Amer.*, vol. 38, no. 5, pp. 448–457, May 1948.

[13] M. C. J. van Gemert and J. P. H. Henning, "Model approach to laser coagulation of dermal vascular lesions," *Arch. Dermatol. Res. 270*, pp. 429–439, 1981.

[14] W. G. Egan and T. W. Hilgeman, *Optical Properties of Inhomogeneous Materials*. New York: Academic, 1979.

[15] F. Kottler, "Turbid media with plane-parallel surfaces," *J. Opt. Soc. Amer.*, vol. 50, no. 5, pp. 483–490, May 1960.

[16] K. Klier, "Absorption and scattering in plane parallel turbid media," *J. Opt. Soc. Amer.*, vol. 62, no. 7, pp. 882–885, July 1972.

[17] G. Yoon, W. F. Cheong, and A. J. Welch, "Determination of absorption and scattering coefficients from diffuse transmission measurement," *Lasers in Surg. Med.*, vol. 7, no. 1, p. 71, 1987.

[18] S. L. Jacques and S. A. Prahl, "Modeling optical and thermal distribution in tissue during laser irradiation," *Lasers in Surg. Med.*, vol. 6, no. 6, pp. 494–503, 1987.

[19] J. P. A. Marynisses and W. M. Star. *Porphyrin Localization and Treatment of Tumors*, D. R. Doiron and C. J. Gomer, Eds. New York: Alan Liss, 1981, pp. 133–148.

[20] M. C. J. van Gemert, A. J. Welch, W. M. Star, M. Motamedi, and W. F. Cheong, "Tissue optics for a slab geometry in the diffusion approximation," *Lasers in Med. Sci.*, in press.

[21] R. E. Danielson, D. R. Moore, and H. C. van de Hulst, "The transfer of visible radiation through clouds," *J. Atmos. Sci.*, vol. 26, pp. 1078–1087, 1969.

[22] L. O. Reynolds and N. J. McCormick, "Approximate two-parameter phase function for light scattering," *J. Opt. Sci. Amer.*, vol. 70, no. 10, pp. 1206–1212, Oct. 1980.

[23] S. L. Jacques, C. A. Alter, and S. A. Prahl, "Angular dependence of He–Ne laser light scattering by human dermis," *Lasers in Life Sci.*, vol. 1, no. 4, 1987.

[24] T. Halldorsson and J. Langerholc, "Thermodynamic analysis of laser irradiation of biological tissue," *Appl. Opt.*, vol. 17, no. 24, pp. 3948–3958, Dec. 15, 1978.

[25] L. O. Reynolds, C. Johnson, and A. Ishimaru, "Diffuse reflectance from a finite blood medium: Applications to the modeling of fiber optic catheters," *Appl. Opt.*, vol. 15, no. 9, pp. 2059–2067, Sept. 1976.

[26] R. A. J. Groenhuis, H. A. Ferwerda, and J. J. T. Bosch, "Scattering and absorption of turbid materials determined from reflection measurements," *Appl. Opt.*, vol. 22, no. 16, pp. 2456–2467, Aug. 15, 1983.

[27] C. Chu and S. W. Churchill, "Numerical solutions of problems in multiple scattering of electromagnetic radiation," *J. Phys. Chem.*, vol. 59, pp. 855–863, Sept. 1955.

[28] L. Cummins and M. Nauenberg, "Thermal effects of laser radiation in biological tissue," *Biophys. J.*, vol. 42, pp. 99–102, Apr. 1983.

[29] E. Sinofsky and M. Dumont, "Measurement of argon laser beam spreading through arterial plaque," *Lasers Life Sci.*, vol. 2, pp. 143–150, Oct. 1987.

[30] A. Ishimaru, *Wave Propagation and Scattering in Random Media*. New York: Academic, 1978, vol. 1.

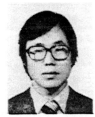

Gilwon Yoon was born in Jinjoo, Korea, on April 27, 1955. He received the B. S. degree from Seoul National University, Korea, in 1977, and the M.S. degree from the University of Texas at Austin in 1984, both in electrical engineering.

He is currently a Ph.D. candidate at the University of Texas at Austin. From 1977 to 1982, he was a research engineer at the Agency for Defense Development in Daejeon, Korea. From 1984 to 1985, he worked as a teaching assistant, and from 1983 to present he is working as a research assistant, both with the Department of Electrical and Computer Engineering. His research interest is optical and thermal interaction of laser light with tissue.

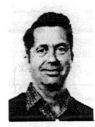

Ashley J. Welch (M'66–SM'79) was born in Ft. Worth, TX, on May 3, 1933. He received the B.S.E.E. degree from Texas Technological College, Lubbock, in 1955, the M.S.E.E. degree from Southern Methodist University, Dallas, TX, in 1959, and the Ph.D. degree from Rice University, Houston, TX, in 1964.

He joined the Faculty of the University of Texas at Austin, in 1964, as an Assistant Professor with the Department of Electrical Engineering. Administrative duties at the University of Texas have included: Director of the College of Engineering Hybrid Computing Facility from 1970 to 1971, and Director of the Biomedical Engineering Program from 1971 to 1976. He is currently the Marion E. Forsman Centennial Professor of Electrical and Computer Engineering and Biomedical Engineering at the University of Texas at Austin. His research interests include analysis of laser-tissue interactions and computer-aided analysis of electrophysiological data. He was Co-Chairman of the 1982 Gordon Conference on Lasers in Medicine and Biology and is currently Editor-in-Chief of the journal *Lasers in the Life Sciences*.

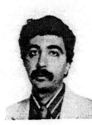

Massoud Motamedi was born in Esfahan, Iran, on May 22, 1957. He received the B.S. and M.S. degrees from the University of Texas at Austin in 1980 and 1982, respectively, both in electrical engineering. For his M.S. thesis, he conducted experimental and theoretical studies on thermal response of tissue irradiated by the Nd:YAG laser.

Since 1983, he has been working towards the Ph.D. degree in the area of experimental and theoretical studies of laser beam propagation in biological media. He is expected to receive the Ph.D.

degree from the University of Texas at Austin, in 1987. He is currently conducting research in laser angioplasty at the Department of Cardiology at Harper Hospital, Detroit, MI.

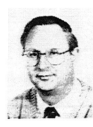

Martinus C. J. van Gemert was born in Delft, The Netherlands, on March 25, 1944. He received the M.Sc. degree from Delft University in 1969, and the Ph.D. degree from Leiden University, The Netherlands, in 1972, both in physics.

He was with Philips Research Laboratories, Eindhoven, The Netherlands, as a member of the Gaseous Electronics Group from 1972 to 1978. From 1978 to 1987, he worked as a clinical physicist at St. Joseph Hospital, Eindhoven. He was on leave during 1984–1985 and joined A. J. Welch's research group at the University of Texas at Austin supervising various projects on laser applications in medicine. Since July 1987, he has been working as director of the Experimental Laser Unit of the Academic Medical Centre, University of Amsterdam, The Netherlands.

Reprinted with permission from *Applied Optics,* Vol. 27(16), pp. 3382-3391
(August 15, 1988).

Photon migration in layered media

Ralph Nossal, J. Kiefer, G. H. Weiss, R. Bonner, H. Taitelbaum, and S. Havlin

Surface emission profiles and related functions are computed for particles (photons) migrating within a semi-infinite medium containing a surface layer whose absorbance differs from that of the underlying layer. Photons are assumed to be inserted at a single point on the surface. In certain cases distinct features appear in the emission profiles which enable determination of the thickness of the top layer and of the absorption coefficients of both layers. Computations are performed to provide estimates of parameter ranges for which the presence of one layer distorts photon emission profiles from the other. Several ancillary functions are calculated, including the absorbance profile as a function of depth, the expected path length of photons that are reemitted at a distance ρ from the point of insertion, and the average depth probed by those reemitted photons.

I. Introduction

Many therapeutic and diagnostic techniques in medicine depend on specific local interactions of light with tissue and other biological media. In several applications radiation is incident at the surface of a tissue, and the reemission of photons from that surface provides information about the medium. We, therefore, recently developed a mathematical model to describe photon migration in turbid media.[1] Formulas were obtained for the spatial intensity distribution of diffuse emission at the surface and for the mean total path length traveled by a photon between the point of incidence and the point of reemission. We also were able to find the probability density for photon absorption as a function of depth in the tissue and the average depth at which a photon travels before reemission. These all are useful for interpreting data acquired by remote optical sensing of biological tissue, an example of which is laser Doppler velocimetry to measure microvascular blood flow.[2,3]

As light penetrates biological tissue, it is scattered by many refractive-index variations, which, over distances of the order of 1 mm, lead to the randomization of the direction of propagation. The great variability in microscopic refractive index within the medium makes it almost impossible to analyze scattering in detail for living tissues. However, the specifics of the short range behavior by which light is partially scattered from its initial direction do not need to be understood to describe light propagation over distances substantially greater than that required for the randomization of the direction of propagation. Thus we previously adapted a discrete lattice model as a convenience in carrying out both analytic and numerical calculations. The use of such a lattice random walk should be regarded as a phenomenological approach, justified by comparison to calculations for more physically realistic models, such as in Ref. 1 for a semi-infinite continuum model having random scattering lengths. The continuum model corresponds to a lattice with vanishingly small lattice spacing where randomization of direction occurs over distances which are exponentially distributed about a constant mean value. Such lattice models underly the development of many theories of diffusive motion.[4]

In our earlier work,[1] the homogeneous tissue was assumed to be so thick that only a single surface—the interface between the tissue and the exterior medium—needs be taken into account. In the present work we use the lattice model to examine the effects of tissue heterogeneity by including an additional superficial tissue layer whose absorptive properties differ from those in the underlying bulk medium. Examples of layered biological tissues are skin (epidermis, dermis, subcutaneous fat) and the walls of arteries (intima, muscle, adventitia), stomach, bladder, intestine, and esophagus. Also, different tissues in contact, or tumors within a single tissue, in certain cases might be modeled as being such layers. Two potential clinical applications involve tumor detection and therapy: (1) to detect a deep-lying tumor by examining diffuse

H. Taitelbaum and S. Havlin are with Bar-Ilan University, Physics Department, Ramat-Gan, Israel; the other authors are with National Institute of Health, Bethesda, Maryland 20892; R. Bonner is in the Biomedical Engineering Branch, Division of Research Services, and the other authors are in the Physical Sciences Laboratory, Division of Computer Research & Technology.

Received 14 September 1987.

surface emissions,[5] it is necessary to know how the emitted image is distorted by the intervening tissue, e.g., how thin the upper layer has to be to detect the underlying abnormality; (2) when irradiating pigmented epithelia of finite thickness, such as a region of malignant melanoma tissue in which one is trying to apply phototherapy,[6] one needs to know the depth distribution of light absorption and how the underlying tissue layer affects the absorption profile. A third example derives from attempts to destroy atherosclerotic plaque using laser angioplasty[7]: A scheme by which plaque can be identified optically, and its thickness quantified by remote sensing, might be used to control therapeutic laser ablation. Because in these cases one cannot readily make measurements within the tissues, information may only be available from photons that penetrate and subsequently are reemitted from the surface.

Although Monte Carlo calculations can be carried out for heterogeneous tissue geometries, such simulations are almost useless for examining the characteristics of photon reemission at distances far from the point of insertion because long migration paths occur with low probability. Hence we devised an iterative computational scheme for the lattice occupancy probabilities of migrating particles. This methodology is described in the next section (Sec. II). It is particularly useful when the scattering cross sections (i.e., the scattering lengths) of the various regions of the composite material are similar but when the regions have different average absorptions. For illustration, we specifically consider a two-region composite with a surface layer lying on top of a semi-infinite substrate.

Results from these calculations are presented in Sec. III. First we consider a case where the absorbances of the two layers differ by a factor of 20. Because of this disparity, the effects of the more highly absorbing layer are distinct, and results are easily interpretable (see Figs. 2–9). Insights gained from these studies then facilitate an understanding of the results of corresponding computations performed for layered media in which the absorptive properties are similar (e.g., Figs. 10 and 11).

At this stage of the investigation our principal goal is to provide general qualitative insights into the behavior of photons migrating in layered media rather than to obtain precise numerical results. In Sec. IV we briefly discuss other calculations that are possible using the present methods. The present numerical investigations suggest that it is feasible to estimate useful physical parameters for a two-layered medium from experimental data, especially if the absorbances are dissimilar.

II. Computational Methodology

We wish to simulate the history of a photon after it is injected into a semi-infinite two-layered medium. The kinetics of photon migration are modeled in terms of a random walk on a discrete lattice. However, instead of simulating many random walks and calculating averaged quantities from them, we are able to

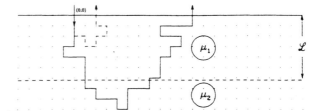

Fig. 1. Two-dimensional projection of semi-infinite layered medium, approximated by a lattice of discrete scattering loci surrounded by continuously absorbing material. The scattering length here is understood to be identical in the two regions, and the absorption coefficients in the top and the bottom layers are μ_1 and μ_2.

calculate exact probabilities. The scheme for doing this has been used recently in a number of physical applications.[8,9] Specifically, we assume that a walker starts at radius $r = 0$ and depth $z = 1$ (see Fig. 1). After n steps each site contains a fractional number of walkers corresponding to the probability that a single walker, starting from (0,0,1), will be at that site. Any random walker reaching the surface is considered to be absorbed there and is so recorded.

In the present work the scattering is presumed to be angularly isotropic. Thus, if we were to use ordinary rectangular coordinates, the probability of moving would be equal to one-sixth in each of the six possible directions. To simplify the computations, we utilize the circular symmetry and divide the migration space into concentric annuli, or rings, whose inner and outer radii are given by $j \pm \frac{1}{2}$ ($j = 1,2,...$). In this case the probability of moving in either direction along the z axis still is one-sixth, but different probabilities are used to describe lateral movements. For a walker in the central core (inner radius = 0, outer radius = $\frac{1}{2}$), the probability of a move outward to the annulus whose ring index is $r = 1$ is two-thirds. However, for a walker in a ring of index $r > 0$, the probability of moving inward is $(\frac{1}{6})[1 - 1/(2r)]$, while the probability of moving outward is $(\frac{1}{6})[1 + 1/(2r)]$. Furthermore, in all cases except the central core, the probability of staying in the same annulus and moving around it one step clockwise or counterclockwise, without changing depth or radius, is one-third. We verify these formulas by the following observations: (1) If the circular shells are replaced by nested squares or hexagons, the probabilities of migration, within a given shell or to its neighbors, also are given by these formulas. (2) If infinite space is uniformly populated by photons, migration according to these formulas keeps the distribution uniform.

One complication is that at each step some of the walkers are absorbed. Absorption is assumed to be described by Beer's law, i.e., $\exp(-\mu)$ is the survival probability per unit step, where μ is the absorption coefficient per unit scattering length.[1] By convention, we assume that, at the interface between the two tissue phases, the material of the upper layer extends to a depth of $\mathcal{L} + \epsilon$, where ϵ is a vanishingly small quantity.

Thus, when scattering occurs toward the surface or in the plane defined by $z = \mathcal{L}$, the subpopulation of random walkers is decreased by a term depending on the absorption of the upper region; when scattering at the $\mathcal{L}$th layer is directed downward into the material, the absorbed fraction is given by the properties of the lower region.

In our numerical work, the lattice typically contains $z_m = 130$ total depth levels and $r_m = 130$ concentric rings. To obtain the number of walkers that decay at each of the i levels, we count the total number of walkers at depth i and multiply by the fraction $[1 - \exp(-\mu_i)]$, where μ_i is the absorption coefficient per unit scattering length at the ith level. {In accordance with our convention, at the interface $z = \mathcal{L}$ we multiply by $[1 - (5/6) \exp(-\mu_{upper}) - (1/6) \exp(-\mu_{lower})]$.} Then, beginning at the center, we process each ring successively. The use of two grids, old walker and new walker, facilitates the procedure of dividing and allocating probability densities. We count and remove the walkers that reach the remote surfaces of our large but finite array, asserting that only a fraction of the walkers impinging on the fictitious boundary is absorbed. (We arbitrarily take that fraction to be one-half but find that the particular choice does not significantly affect results.) Next, for each ring, we compute the cumulative number of walkers that have surfaced, both unweighted and weighted by step number. At the end of the simulation the unweighted number is used to determine the photon emission profile. The step-weighted quantity is used to calculate the average path length (step number) of those photons that surface within any given ring. All calculations are repeated until the number of active walkers (those which neither leaked at the boundaries nor were absorbed within the medium) falls below a preset value (typically 10^{-10}, which corresponds to ~1000–2000 iterative steps).

An additional parameter of physical interest is the average depth of a photon that emerges at a distance ρ from the injection point. An adaptation of the exact enumeration method, utilizing two registers at each site, is used to calculate this quantity.

III. Results

A. Disparate Absorption

We begin by examining cases in which the absorption coefficients of the two layers are very different. Insights gained from this part of the investigation facilitate later interpretation of calculations for photon migration in layered media having similar absorption coefficients.

Measurable quantities in the anticipated applications consist of surface emission data obtained at various distances ρ from the entrance point of the laser beam. However, because the numerical simulations are performed for a lattice model, results will be given in terms of the function G_r, defined to be the fraction of photons reemitted within the rth annulus on the surface. These data can be related to the function $\gamma(\rho)$,

defined as the probability density that a photon exits the medium at distance ρ; i.e., $\gamma(\rho)d\rho$ is the reemitted radiation at a distance lying between ρ and $\rho + d\rho$ [see Eq. (11) of Ref. 1].

1. Form of the Surface Emission Profile

First we consider the case where absorption within the surface layer is very much greater than that within the lower region ($\mu_1 \gg \mu_2$). In Fig. 2(a) we show surface profiles G_r for $\mu_1 = 0.2$, $\mu_2 = 0.01$, computed for differing values of the thickness $\mathcal{L}$ (in lattice units) of the upper layer, where the quantities μ_1 and μ_2 are the absorption coefficients of the upper and lower layers, respectively. It has been shown in Ref. 1 [from Eqs. (12) and (14)] that the function $\gamma(\rho)$ for a homogeneous medium is

$$\gamma(\rho) \sim \rho^{-1} \exp[-\rho(6\mu)^{1/2}], \tag{1}$$

for sufficiently large ρ. Thus, when the bottom layer has the same absorption coefficient as does the top, we expect the quantity $\log(rG_r)$ to vary as a straight line with the slope given as $-(6\mu_1)^{1/2}$. This is demonstrated in Fig. 2(b), where the results shown in Fig. 2(a) are replotted as rG_r on semilogarithmic axes. The slope of the line marked ∞, which corresponds to a homogeneous material, indeed has the expected behavior. More interesting, however, is the fact that for large r the slopes of the other lines on the graph are given as $d[\log(rG_r)]/dr = -(6\mu_2)^{1/2}$. Thus, in principle, the absorption coefficients of both layers can be determined from the surface emission, the absorption of the bottom layer being obtained from the emission profile at large r, and that of the top layer being obtained from the emission profile close to the point where photons are injected.

A simple heuristic interpretation of these results is that photons reemitted close to their insertion point mostly travel in the upper layer, whereas those reemitted far from the insertion point mostly move within the bottom layer. Indeed, the large absorption coefficient of the top layer makes it very unlikely that any photons that travel for significant distances in that region will survive. The fact that the initial slope persists to ever greater r when the upper layer becomes increasingly thick is consistent with this interpretation. In Fig. 2(c) we plot the function $[\log(rG_r) + r(6\mu_2)^{1/2}]$ vs r. The line marked ∞ now has as its slope $(6\mu_2)^{1/2} - (6\mu_1)^{1/2}$. The regular spacing noted between the horizontal lines suggests that with proper calibration it may be possible to infer the thickness of the upper layer from the surface emission data.

2. Absorption as a Function of Depth

Similar features are seen in the curves for $A(z)$, which we designate here as the absorption at depth z. In Fig. 3(a) we show the absorption as a function of depth, and in Fig. 3(b) we plot the quantity {$\log[A(z)] + z(6\mu_2)^{1/2}$}. In accordance with analytical predictions[1] the diffential absorption in each region, far from the interface, is proportional to $\exp[-z(6\mu_i)^{1/2}]$, where μ_i is the absorption coefficient at the ith level. Figure 3(b)

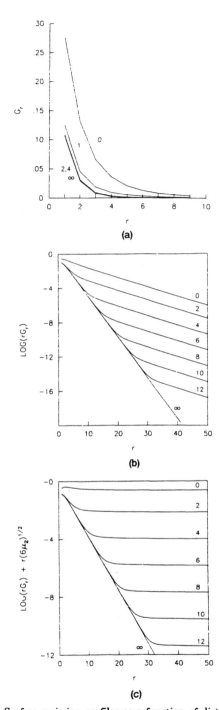

(a)

(b)

(c)

Fig. 2. Surface emission profiles as a function of distance from point of photon insertion for various values of top layer thickness $\mathcal{L}$. The absorption coefficient of the top layer is much greater than that of the bottom, namely, $\mu_1 = 0.2$, $\mu_2 = 0.01$: (a) the intensity in the rth ring G_r vs r; (b) $\log r G_r$ vs r; (c) $[\log r G_r + r(6\mu_2)^{1/2}]$ vs r (skewed values, see text). Note that distinguishing features appear only in the tails of the emission profiles, where the intensity has fallen off by several decades.

shows that the flux which enters the lower layer has been depleted exponentially by a factor that depends on the thickness of the upper layer.

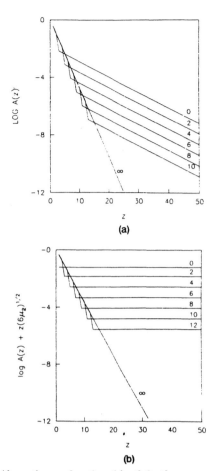

(a)

(b)

Fig. 3. Absorption as a function of depth for the same conditions as in Fig. 2: (a) $\log A(z)$ vs z; (b) $[\log A(z) + z(6\mu_2)^{1/2}]$ (skewed values).

3. Average Path Length in the Medium

We also have calculated the average total path length traversed by a photon that emerges within the rth ring. This quantity is of general interest when interpreting optical signals obtained from remote sensing measurements. In such cases the probability of photon interaction depends on the total path length over which photon migration occurs within the tissue. For example, knowledge of the mean path length is required for absolute measurement of microvascular blood flow and blood volume by laser Doppler techniques.[2]

When the medium through which the photons migrate is homogeneous, the average total path length, given that a photon is emitted at distance ρ from the point of injection, varies linearly with ρ as[1] $\langle n|\rho \rangle = 2 + 3\rho/(6\mu)^{1/2}$. Such behavior is indicated in Fig. 4(a) by the line designated as ∞, where we show results of calculations of $\langle n|r \rangle$ for a uniform medium having the absorption of the upper layer (approximating thereby a homogeneous semi-infinite medium). The other curves in that figure correspond to photons moving in a medium containing an upper region of finite thickness layered on top of a semi-infinite medium of lower absorption. Again, the interpretation of the figure is that photons emerging close to the point of insertion mostly travel in the upper region. To be detected at a surface point far from the point of insertion, a photon has to travel within the lower region, as otherwise it tends to be absorbed. Indeed, for very large values of r, the average cumulative path length closely approximates that for photons which travel entirely in a medium having the properties of the bottom layer. This is indicated by the fact that the slope of the asymptotic curve marked 0 in Fig. 4(a) is given as $3/(6\mu_2)^{1/2}$.

An interesting representation of these data is achieved by dividing the curves $\langle n|r\rangle$, pertaining to different $\mathcal{L}$, by the corresponding values of the curve $\langle n|r\rangle_\infty$ for a homogeneous semi-infinite medium having the absorptive properties of the upper layer. In Fig. 4(b) we show the data of Fig. 4(a) plotted in this way. The curves seem to be evenly spread along the r axis for $\mathcal{L} \geq 2$ and spaced in proportion to $\mathcal{L}$. If the curves are shifted along the r axis, they overlap. Accordingly, if the curves of Fig. 4(b) are scaled along the abscissa by the factor $r/\mathcal{L}$, the midpoints coincide, although the curves do not otherwise superimpose.

4. Average Depth of an Emitted Photon

Another quantity that we are interested in—needed to determine which region of tissue is probed in remote sensing applications—is the average depth $\langle z|r\rangle$ at which a photon travels before surfacing within ring r. Results (still for the situation $\mu_1 = 0.2$, $\mu_2 = 0.01$) are shown in Fig. 5. Again, for photons emitted at small values of r, the average depth of penetration is almost identical to that of a lattice of infinite thickness. The transition noted in the curve at larger r indicates that photon migration occurs within the lower layer. As shown in Fig. 5, photons reemitted at larger r probe ever deeper regions of the tissue as the surface layer is thickened. The even spacing between the curves marked $\mathcal{L} = 2$, $\mathcal{L} = 4$, $\mathcal{L} = 6$, etc., indicates that, whatever the thickness of the upper layer, the lower layer is probed to nearly the same depth below its boundary with the upper layer. Due to the high absorption coefficient of the upper layer, the photons that surface are predominantly those which pass directly through the upper layer to the lower layer, where migration without absorption is more likely.

An ancillary point which now can be established is that, in a homogeneous medium, $\langle z|r\rangle$ seems to vary as r^α for sufficiently large r. The coefficient α is given approximately as $\alpha \doteq 0.5$. (Actually, present calculations indicate $\alpha = 0.54$ for $\mu = 0.01$, $\alpha = 0.50$ for $\mu = 0.2$, and $0.50 < \alpha < 0.54$ for $0.01 < \mu < 0.2$ with a tendency toward $\alpha = \frac{1}{2}$ as μ increases.) We recently found that, in a single-layer medium, the correct value of α indeed is 0.5.[10]

5. Case $\mu_1 \ll \mu_2$

We now examine what happens when the absorption of the top layer is much weaker than that of the bottom ($\mu_1 \ll \mu_2$). Let us consider as an example the inverse of the situation examined above, i.e., now assume $\mu_1 =$

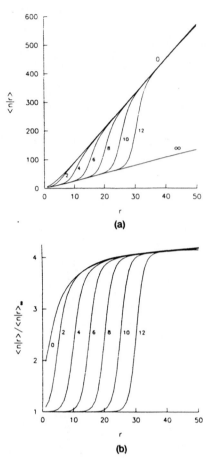

(a)

(b)

Fig. 4. Expected path length $\langle n|r\rangle$, given that a photon emerges at a point separated by r scattering lengths from the point of incidence: (a) $\langle n|r\rangle$ vs r; (b) normalized values, $\langle n|r\rangle/\langle n|r\rangle_\infty$ vs r, where $\langle n|r\rangle_\infty$ are values expected when $\mathcal{L} \to \infty$ (a homogeneous semi-infinite medium with the absorptive properties of the top layer). Conditions are identical to those stated in the caption of Fig. 2.

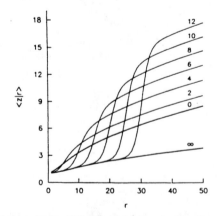

Fig. 5. Expected value of the depth $\langle z|r\rangle$ probed by photons emerging at r. Conditions are as described in Fig. 2 caption.

0.01, $\mu_2 = 0.20$. Surface emission profiles for this case are shown in Fig. 6. In accordance with our intuition, the profiles corresponding to a surface layer of vanishing thickness decay more rapidly, as a function of r, than those for a medium with an overlaying region of

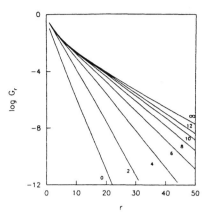

Fig. 6. $\log G_r$ vs r. The top layer absorption coefficient here is much smaller than that of the lower region ($\mu_1 = 0.01$, $\mu_2 = 0.2$).

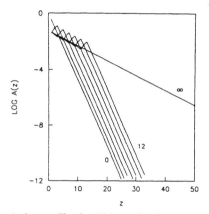

Fig. 7. Absorption profiles, $\log A(z)$, vs z for the same conditions as shown in Fig. 6.

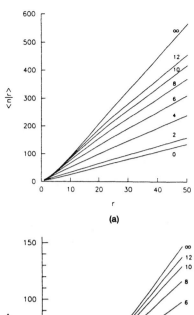

Fig. 8. (a) Expected path length, $\langle n|r \rangle$ vs r. Conditions identical to those of Fig. 6. (b) Same as (a), except the abscissa is expanded.

low absorption. However, it is somewhat surprising that, in contrast with the results in Fig. 2, the slope associated with the large r decay seems to change continuously with layer thickness $\mathcal{L}$. Thus it would be difficult to extract information about the two regions unless, perhaps, the absorbance of one of the regions were known. Additionally, we note the absence of any sharply delineated breakpoints in $\log G_r$ from which the thickness of the top layer can be ascertained. If properly calibrated, however, the slope of the large r decay might provide such information.

The absorption profiles, determined as a function of depth, also lack surprising features. In Fig. 7 we show $\log A(z)$ vs z and note that the curves corresponding to different $\mathcal{L}$ are parallel, being displaced from one another by a factor proportional to the thickness of the upper, low absorbance, layer. The only unusual feature occurs at the boundary between the two layers, where a discontinuity in the number of absorbed photons is observed. This attribute reflects the fact that the number of absorbed photons is proportional to both the absorption coefficient and the flux; although the flux at the boundary is continuous, the absorption coefficients are discontinuous and cause a jump in an absorption profile. However, other than this, the

curves shown in Fig. 7 have a simple interpretation, namely, that the top layer acts as a low absorption screen that decreases the flux arriving at the top of the lower layer, whence normal absorption subsequently occurs. In other words, the absorption in the lower layer can be estimated simply by decreasing the flux by an exponential factor whose argument is proportional to the product of the absorbance and the thickness of the upper layer.

The expected number of steps in a migration path $\langle n|r \rangle$ given that a photon is reemitted at r and the average depth probed by those photons $\langle z|r \rangle$ similarly lack any dramatic characteristics. In Fig. 8(a) we show $\langle n|r \rangle$. Note that the slopes of the curves at large r lie between the limiting values given by results for uniform media of either high or low absorbance, the value for the layered media changing continuously with layer thickness. However, the behavior for small r [Fig. 8(b)] indicates that, if the top layer is sufficiently thick, the average number of lattice collisions experienced by reemitted photons is approximately that of photons moving in material of uniform low absorbance, provided that $r \lesssim 0.6\mathcal{L}$. In Fig. 9 we show $\langle z|r \rangle$. The seemingly anomalous position of the curve for $\mathcal{L} = 0$ (corresponding to a homogeneous medium with $\mu = \mu_2$) reflects the fact that reemitted photons mostly

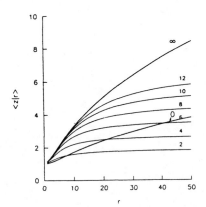

Fig. 9. Expected depth, $\langle z|r \rangle$ vs r. Conditions identical to those of Fig. 6.

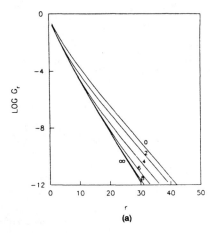

(a)

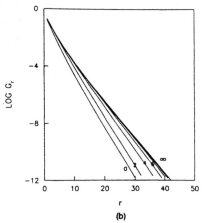

(b)

Fig. 10. Surface emission profiles, $\log G_r$ vs r, for media with layers having similar absorbance: (a) $\mu_1 = 0.1$, $\mu_2 = 0.05$; (b) $\mu_1 = 0.05$, $\mu_2 = 0.1$.

move in the upper layer if the absorbance of that layer is much lower than that of the base. Although photons seemingly probe deeper into a uniform medium of high absorbance, fewer will escape from the surface.

Before concluding this section we remark that, by setting the absorbance of the bottom layer to a very large value, it is possible to mimic a thin tissue where the photons that pass through the upper layer are lost forever. This condition is approached, for example, in photoradiation treatment of metastatic ovarian cancer cells lying on top of highly absorbing spleen or liver tissue. An analogous situation arises when the underlying layer has a very long characteristic scattering length (as in free space). In this case, even if absorption is negligible, the lower layer cannot efficiently reflect photons back into the upper layer. Illumination of the wall of an inflated bladder within the peritoneal cavity might be modeled in this manner.

B. Layers of Similar Absorbance

1. Surface Emission Profiles

In almost all biological tissues, differences in absorption of different layers are due to small variations in the concentrations of ubiquitous chromophores. Thus the absorptions of different layers usually are similar, even if the tissue shows visible heterogeneity. For example, the marked yellow color of fatty atheroma, compared to a normal artery, results from only an approximately twofold difference in blue light absorption coefficients.[11] Another example where adjacent tissues might have slight, but discernible, differences in absorption is one in which tumors are present. Indeed, the detection of underlying tumors might be possible because of an increase in absorption arising from the hemoglobin in blood within such highly vascularized and hemorrhagic tissues.

In Fig. 10 we show the emission profiles $\log G_r$ for the cases (a) $\mu_1 = 0.1$, $\mu_2 = 0.05$ and (b) $\mu_1 = 0.05$, $\mu_2 = 0.1$. These values are typical of those for real biological tissues.[11-13] We infer from the computed data that it may be very difficult to discern the presence of a heterogeneous structure by cursory examination of the

gross features of the emission profile. Yet some success might be realized in this regard if the absorbance of the top layer is greater than that of the bottom. In such cases [see Fig. 19(a)], sharp changes in slope should be observable in the curves of $\log G_r$ if data can be acquired at sufficiently large r. The presence of such sharp breaks will be a general characteristic of overlying layers of higher absorbance, provided that the data are free of noise. Similar features are seen in Fig. 2(a) ($\mu_1 = 0.2$, $\mu_2 = 0.01$), but, in that case of disparate absorptions, they are much more prominent. Also, as noted before in Fig. 6, when the top layer is less absorbing, the surface emission profiles seem to be smoother [see Fig. 10(b)]. The absorption profiles $A(z)$ and the curves of average migration (path) length $\langle n|r \rangle$ also have the same general appearance as those for the disparate layers case, except that the distinguishing features are less evident.

2. Average Depth of an Emitted Photon

In Fig. 11 we present results of calculations of the average depth $\langle z|r \rangle$, conditional on photon reemission within the rth ring. We again observe that the presence of a more highly absorbing layer strongly affects the depth probed by the photons that are reemitted at

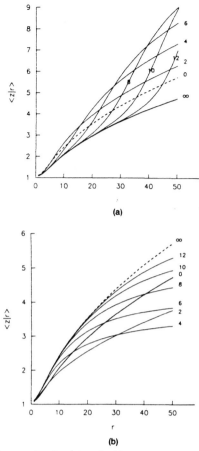

(a)

(b)

Fig. 11. Average depth $\langle z|r \rangle$ probed by emergent photons. Conditions are the same as in Figs. 10(a) and (b). The thick solid lines correspond to the situation where the entire medium has absorption $\mu = 0.1$; dotted lines correspond to the situation where the entire medium has absorption $\mu = 0.05$.

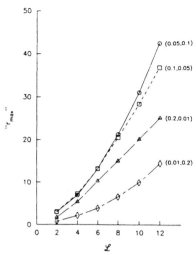

Fig. 12. Maximum distance along the surface for which emergent photons primarily probe the upper layer r_{max} as a function of $\mathcal{L}$. Numbers in parentheses are the values (μ_1, μ_2) corresponding to each curve. Data are determined by extrapolations of curves of $\langle z|r \rangle$, such as given in Fig. 11, to the point where $\langle z|r \rangle = (1 \pm 0.05)\langle z|r \rangle_\infty$.

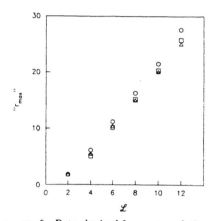

Fig. 13. r_{max} vs $\mathcal{L}$. Data obtained from extrapolations of surface emission curves, $\log G_r$, ●, and curves of $[\langle n|r \rangle / \langle n|r \rangle_\infty - 1]$, ■, compared with data for $\langle z|r \rangle$ shown in Fig. 12, ▲.

larger r (see Figs. 5 and 9). The thick solid lines in Figs. 11 correspond to a situation where the entire medium is composed of the more highly absorbing material, and the dotted lines correspond to a uniform medium of lower absorbance. By comparing the results shown in Fig. 11(a) with those in Fig. 11(b), we note that if the higher absorbance material underlies the lower ($\mu_1 < \mu_2$), the average depth probed by reemitted photons is less than that which would occur in a homogeneous medium consisting of the material of the top layer. In contrast, if the higher absorbance material constitutes the surface layer ($\mu_1 > \mu_2$), the depth that is probed increases by an amount proportional to the thickness of the upper layer. For photons detected at sufficiently large r, the additional depth is approximately equal to a fraction of the surface layer, where the fraction varies from 0 to 1 as μ_1/μ_2 varies from 1 to a large value.

Of course, essentially only the properties of the top layer are probed if the reemitted photons are detected close to the point of insertion. A rough estimate of the maximum value of r at which the reemitted photons primarily probe the surface can be obtained from Fig.

11 by extrapolating to the points where the curves for finite layer thickness superimpose on the curve for infinite thickness. Results are shown in Fig. 12, not only for the cases considered above but also for several other combinations of absorption coefficients. These estimates of r_{max} are consistent with estimates obtained from other quantities that we have calculated. For example, in Fig. 13 we show (for $\mu_1 = 0.2$, $\mu_2 = 0.01$) the values of r_{max} obtained by determining where the surface emission profiles differ by 5% (i.e., $\log G(r|\mathcal{L})/G(r|\mathcal{L} = \infty) = \log 1.05 = 0.0212$). The values are close to those given in Fig. 12 and agree also with estimates of r_{max} obtained by setting $|\langle n|r \rangle / \langle n|r \rangle_\infty - 1| = 0.05$ [see Figs. 2(b) and 4(b)].

IV. Remarks

The methodology of exact enumeration provides a means to test accurately, with greater precision than

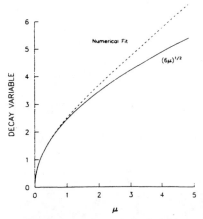

Fig. 14. Comparison between theoretical value of decay rate of $A(z)$ in homogeneous media $(6\mu m)^{1/2}$, as given by the theory developed in Ref. 1, and the rate obtained from direct enumeration of probability densities, as described in Sec. II. Solid line, theoretical value; dotted line, numerical computation.

by our earlier Monte Carlo simulations,[1] several of the mathematical expressions that we previously derived. For the most part, our earlier analytical work has been substantiated. However, an interesting point that now seems to be established by these calculations, particularly results shown in Figs. 5, 9, and 11, is that the power law dependence of $\langle z|r \rangle$ on r is given as $\langle z|r \rangle \sim r^{1/2}$.[10] Another mathematical point that can be clarified is whether the depth profile for homogeneous absorption $A(z)$ truly is given by the expression $A(z) \sim \exp[-z(6\mu)^{1/2}]$, even if the absorption coefficient μ is very large. In the latter case the flux would decrease rapidly near the surface, and the mixing of lattice and continuum models, as done in Ref. 1, might not be appropriate. Indeed, as shown in Fig. 14, when μ exceeds a value of ~ 3, the errors in the decay rate exceed 10%.

As pointed out in Sec. I, we have ignored anisotropic scattering. We previously argued[1] that the artifice of isotropic scattering, such as is used here, is equivalent to redefining the mean scattering length. By asserting that the scattering angle distribution is uniform, we implicitly set the scattering length to be the rms distance (number of steps) that a photon travels before it turns on average through an angle of 90° with respect to its incident direction. We have performed a limited number of Monte Carlo simulations for homogeneous media whose scattering is spatially anisotropic and indeed have found that the results can be scaled to mimic those of isotropic media.[10] If necessary, the computational scheme used here could be extended to account for unequal scattering angle probabilities by increasing the size of probability density matrices to provide a memory of preceding steps. Another factor not accounted for is the possible difference in scattering length in the different layers. This too presumably could be taken into account by modifying the transition matrices for probability densities.

Our present results indicate that, when an underlying tissue layer has a lower absorption than the upper

layer, photons reemitted sufficiently far from the point of insertion most likely will have moved primarily within the underlying layer. Thus the optical characteristics of the lower tissue layer can be evaluated by examining surface emission at values of ρ greater than $\mathcal{L}$, where $\mathcal{L}$ is the thickness of the superficial layer. Unless obscured by noise, a discontinuity in the diffuse surface emission will be observed, and the optical properties of the lower layer can be ascertained with good precision. In contrast, when the lower layer is more highly absorbing than the superficial layer, the uncovering of detailed information about the lower layer is more problematic. In this case the discontinuity in tissue properties causes an increased loss of deeper photon trajectories, and photons that emerge at larger ρ predominantly sample the interface between the two layers. Consequently, the reemission profile at large ρ depends in a complicated way on optical characteristics of both homogeneous layers, with the consequence that the optical identity of the lower layer may remain ambiguous.

In both cases, one might have to measure emission profiles in a region of ρ where the intensities are very weak compared with those near the point of photon insertion. Alternatively, by using multiple wavelengths for which the absorption coefficients vary in different fashions, it might be possible to discern differences in the emission profiles at smaller ρ that contain significant information. In either case it might be necessary to design special instrumentation to achieve the necessary range and sensitivity, but, as suggested by these calculations, such an effort could be very rewarding. Concomitant theoretical analysis is required, however, whenever remote sensing of biological tissue is undertaken in which the mean depth sampled is greater than the thickness of a homogeneous layer.

S. Havlin gratefully acknowledges support from the USA-Israel Binational Science Foundation.

References

1. R. Bonner, R. Nossal, S. Havlin, and G. H. Weiss, "Model for Photon Migration in Turbid Biological Media," J. Opt. Soc. Am. A **4**, 423 (1987).
2. R. Bonner and R. Nossal, "Model for Laser Doppler Measurements of Blood Flow in Tissue," Appl. Opt. **20**, 2097 (1981).
3. R. F. Bonner, T. R. Clem, P. D. Bowen, and R. L. Bowman, "Laser Doppler Real-Time Monitor of Pulsatile and Mean Blood Flow in Tissue Microcirculation," in *Scattering Techniques Applied to Supramolecular and Nonequilibrium Systems*, S-H. Chen, B. Chu, and R. Nossal, Eds. (Plenum, New York, 1981).
4. G. H. Weiss and R. J. Rubin, "Random Walks, Theory, and Selected Applications," Adv. Chem. Phys. **52**, 363 (1983).
5. W. E. Blumberg, "Light Propagation in Human Tissues," Biophys. J. **51**, No. 2, Part 2), 288a (1987).
6. D. R. Dorion, L. O. Svaasand, and A. E. Profio, "Light Dosimetry in Tissue, Application to Photoradiation Therapy," in *Porphyrin Photosensitization*, D. Kessel and T. J. Dougherty, Eds. (Plenum, New York, 1983).
7. C. Kittrell, R. L. Willett, C. Santos-Pacheo, N. B. Ratliff, J. R. Kramer, E. G. Malk, and M. S. Feld, "Diagnosis of Fibrous

Arterial Atherosclerosis Using Fluorescence," Appl. Opt. **24,** 2280 (1985).

8. D. Ben-Avraham and S. Havlin, "Diffusion of Percolation Clusters at Criticality," J. Phys. A **15,** L691 (1982); S. Havlin and D. Ben-Avraham, "Diffusion in Disordered Media," Adv. Phys. **36,** 695 (1987).

9. S. Havlin, G. H. Weiss, J. E. Kiefer, and M. Dishon, "Exact Enumeration of Random Walks with Traps," J. Phys. A **17,** L347 (1984).

10. G. H. Weiss, R. Nossal, and R. J. Bonner, "Statistics of Penetration Depth of Photons Re-Emitted from Irradiated Tissue," Mod. Optics (in press).

11. M. R. Prince, T. F. Deutsch, M. M. Mathews-Roth, R. Margolis, J. A. Parrish, and A. R. Oseroff, "Preferential Light Absorption in Atheromas *in vitro*," J. Clin Invest. **78,** 295 (1986).

12. P. J. Kolari, "Penetration of Unfocused Laser Light into the Skin," Arch. Dermatol. Res. **277,** 342 (1985).

13. B. C. Wilson and M. S. Patterson, "The Physics of Photodynamic Therapy," Phys. Med. Biol. **31,** 327 (1986).

Reprinted with permission from *Applied Optics,* Vol. 28(12), pp. 2216-2222
(June 15, 1989). ©1989 Optical Society of America.

Light transport in tissue

A. Edward Profio

The propagation of light in tissue may be calculated by exact transport theory, or the approximate diffusion theory, provided the optical properties are known at the source wavelength. Optical properties for the exact methods are the absorption coefficient, scattering coefficient, and angular distribution of scattering. Appropriate properties for diffusion theory are the diffusion length and diffusion coefficient (corrected for anisotropic scattering). Computer programs and analytical solutions (for some simple geometries) exist, but the optical properties have to be determined experimentally and are not well defined as yet. The radiant energy fluence rate and the diffuse transmittance and reflectance have been measured in several tissues and in a few geometries, but there are gaps in the data as a function of wavelength. Calculations and measurements reveal that very large errors can result if the optical properties (for example, the diffusion length) are inaccurate, if anisotropic scattering is neglected, or if the finite size of the irradiating light beam is not taken into account. Furthermore, the radiant energy fluence and transmittance are perturbed by local regions of lesser or greater absorption, although recovery of the fluence and transmittance occurs beyond some three diffusion lengths.

I. Introduction

The transport of light in mammalian tissue is important in photochemotherapy and photothermotherapy as well as in diagnosis by fluorescence, diaphanography, and photography. Photochemotherapy is exemplified by photodynamic therapy (PDT), where light is absorbed in a previously administered chemical (e.g., a porphyrin), generating cytotoxic singlet oxygen in the presence of ordinary molecular oxygen. Photothermotherapy refers to denaturation, vaporization, or carbonization of tissue because of the temperature rise associated with absorption of light in a chromophore. This is the usual mode of laser surgery. Fluorescence diagnosis may be achieved by detection of fluorescence emission from either a previously administered fluorescent chemical that concentrates in a lesion or perhaps from an endogenous fluor.

Diaphanography, or transillumination, is detection of a lesion by differences in diffuse transmittance. Photography depends on differences in diffuse (or perhaps specular) reflectance. Thus the quantities of interest are the absorbance as a function of position in the irradiated volume, the diffuse transmittance from the surface opposite the source, and the diffuse reflectance from the surface on which the light is incident.

One may choose either a computational or experimental approach to obtaining these quantities. The former requires an algorithm or computer program to solve the transport equation together with a set of material optical properties as a function of wavelength: absorption coefficient; scattering coefficient; and angular distribution of scattering (phase function). Approximate results, often adequate for the purpose, may be obtained from a diffusion theory approach using the diffusion coefficient (which includes the mean cosine of scattering) and diffusion length. The diffusion coefficient and diffusion length involve differing combinations of the absorption and scattering coefficients and may be measured directly.

The experimental approach requires instruments to measure energy absorption rate (dose rate) or the radiant energy fluence rate (from which the absorption rate can be calculated knowing the absorption coefficient) or the transmitted or reflected radiance.

Computational and experimental techniques and some results are presented and discussed.

II. Theory

The propagation of visible or IR photons in a turbid medium such as tissue is described by the Boltzmann transport equation (1) without change in energy (neglecting Raman scattering and fluorescence). The steady state equation for a monochromatic source is

The author is with University of California, Santa Barbara, Department of Chemical & Nuclear Engineering, Santa Barbara, California 93106.

Received 10 December 1988.

0003-6935/89/122216-07$02.00/0.

© 1989 Optical Society of America.

$$\nabla \cdot \Psi(r,\Omega) + \mu_t(r)\Psi(r,\Omega) = \int \mu_s S(\theta)\Psi(r,\Omega')d\Omega' + Q(r,\Omega'), \quad (1)$$

where $\Psi(r,\Omega)$ = radiance at position r in direction Ω (after scattering), Ω' refers to direction before scattering;

μ_t = total interaction coefficient ($\mu_a + \mu_s$);

μ_a = absorption coefficient;

μ_s = scattering coefficient;

$S(\theta)$ = phase function, normalized angular distribution of scattering, and

$Q(r,\Omega)$ = source density.

The transport equation is solved subject to boundary conditions (e.g., no return of photons emitted at a surface or a surface source).

The radiant energy fluence rate is found by integrating the radiance over 4π solid angle

$$\Phi(r) = \int_{4\pi} \Psi(r,\Omega)d\Omega. \quad (2)$$

The angle integrated transmittance or reflectance is obtained by an appropriate integration of the outward directed radiance at the surface.

Analytical solutions may be obtained but only for a few simple geometries. Thus the Boltzmann transport equation is usually solved numerically on a computer. Programs developed for neutron and gamma ray transport calculations may also be used for visible and IR photons. The principal methods used are discrete ordinates[1,2] or the equivalent solution obtained by a Monte Carlo technique.

The discrete ordinates method is a numerical technique, in which the angular distribution as well as the spatial distribution is defined by a finite number of coordinates (cosines of the angle or dimensions of volume cells) rather than continuously. The absorption and scattering coefficients are represented as the average or group values, and the angular distribution of scattering is input as coefficients of the Legendre polynomial expansion of the phase function. The program calculates the radiance at each spatial cell and angle and iterates until the solution converges to a distribution that is consistent with the boundary conditions and sources. There are programs that solve 1-D problems (infinite slab, sphere, or infinitely long cylinder), 2-D problems (infinitely long bars or wedges or finite cylinders), or 3-D problems. Laminated slabs, nested spheres, cylinders, etc. can be handled. In practice, most geometries of interest for light transport in the body can be handled with a 2-D program including a finite beam radius. However, the program is large and computation intensive, so rather large and fast mainframe or superminicomputers are required.

Wilson and Adam[3] have developed a simplified Monte Carlo program for light transport, emphasizing calculation of the dose. It was run on a minicomputer. We are developing a Monte Carlo program to run on a microcomputer. The Monte Carlo method essentially runs a computer simulation of the random walk of the photon. The distance from the source or last collision is selected from an exponential distribution (characterized by the mean free path or inverse of μ_t) using a pseudorandom number generated by the computer.

The new coordinates are then calculated by trigonometry. The weight of the photon is multiplied by the ratio of the scattering to total coefficient. At the end of the random walk tracking, the loss in weight at each collision is tallied to compute the absorption. The angle of scattering is selected from the phase function, again using a pseudorandom number. The new direction in the fixed coordinate system is then computed, and the process continues until the weighted photon escapes or its weight reaches a cutoff. Then a new source photon is launched.

When absorption is small compared to scattering, scattering is not very anisotropic, and the radiant energy fluence rate is not needed close to the source or a strong absorber or boundary; then diffusion theory[4] may be used. The diffusion equation is

$$D\nabla^2\Phi(r) - \mu_a\Phi(r) + Q(r) = 0 \quad (3)$$

and is solved subject to boundary and surface source conditions. The diffusion coefficient D (centimeters) is given by

$$D = \frac{1}{3[\mu_a + \mu_s(1-w)]}, \quad (4)$$

where w (also called g in some papers) is the mean cosine of the angle of scattering,

$$w = \int S(\theta) \cos\theta d(\cos\theta). \quad (5)$$

The diffusion length

$$L = \sqrt{D/\mu_a}. \quad (6)$$

Diffusion theory solutions can be obtained analytically for 1-D geometries, but for 2- or 3-D geometries a computer program is needed.

Wilson and Patterson[5] have compared diffusion theory, discrete ordinates theory, and Monte Carlo theory calculations of the radiant energy fluence rate in a fictitious medium with isotropic scattering for plane geometry with a perpendicularly incident source. The albedo c, or ratio of scattering coefficient to total interaction coefficient, was either 0.90 or 0.99. Good agreement was obtained between the three methods in this problem. On the other hand, the error using a modified Kubelka-Munk approximation was significantly larger, and K-M is only applicable to 1-D geometries.

Svaasand[6] has compared diffusion theory calculations with measured radiant energy fluence distributions in plane and spherical geometry and found good agreement. Hence in many cases the simpler although approximate diffusion theory may be applied in lieu of the more complex discrete ordinates or Monte Carlo theories.

III. Computational Results

The effect of anisotropic scattering on the propagation of the light can be seen in Fig. 1, computed by the discrete ordinates method. The relative energy fluence rate is plotted as a function of the distance in mean free paths (μ_t^{-1}) for various values of the anisotropy parameter w for albedo $c = \mu_s/\mu_t = 0.90$ in spherical geometry. Although this does not account for the actual phase function $S(\theta)$, it does include the first

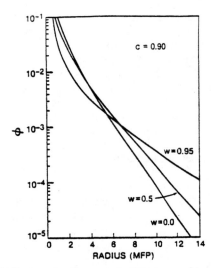

Fig. 1. Radiant energy fluence vs radius measured in units of the mean free path for anisotropic scattering compared to isotropic scattering by the discrete ordinates method.[1] By permission of Pergamon Press.

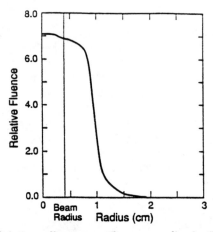

Fig. 2. Relative radiant energy fluence vs radius for finite beam irradiation of the surface (arbitrary source normalization). The diffusion length was 0.4 cm, and isotropic scattering ($w = 0$) was assumed.

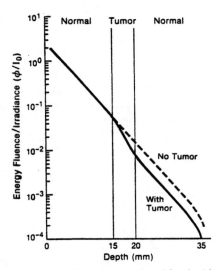

Fig. 3. Radiant energy fluence as function of depth with an absorbing lesion in 1-D slab geometry illustrating the depression of the fluence in and near the absorber.

term of the expansion of $S(\theta)$ in Legendre polynomials. The very different values of Φ for a highly forward peaked distribution ($w = 0.95$) compared to isotropic scattering ($w = 0$) are obvious.

The effect of finite beam radius may be seen in Fig. 2, where $w = 0$, $L = 0.4$ cm, and the radiant energy fluence is plotted as a function of radius for a perpendicular source beam of 0.4-cm radius. For a beam radius of the order of or smaller than the diffusion length (as in this example), the radiant energy fluence decreases with increasing radius. Although not plotted here, the calculations show that the radiant energy fluence decreases more rapidly with increasing depth, even on the beam axis. These effects should be taken into account in photodynamic therapy by making the beam radius a few diffusion lengths greater than the maximum extent of the tumor and by increasing the irradiance to compensate for the faster decrease with depth.

The effect of a localized absorber (e.g., a tumor region with increased blood concentration compared to surrounding tissue) is shown in Fig. 3 for laminated slab geometry (1-D). Note that $\phi/I_0 = 2.5$ at the surface because of backscattering. The radiant energy fluence is depressed within the absorbing region and after the absorber. It is also depressed near the exit surface because of escape of the photons. The radiant energy fluence is not noticeably decreased near the entrance surface (left-hand side) in this plot, because the discrete ordinates program used did not permit exact perpendicular incidence, but only a range of incident angles. But the 1-D geometry is not appropriate anyway for a small localized region (such as a tumor) in tissue with different scattering and absorbing properties.

Figure 4 shows a 2-D discrete ordinates calculation. A tumor was simulated by a cylindrical volume of height and diameter equal to 0.53 cm embedded in a matrix of 4-cm height and diameter. The optical properties of the simulated tumor material are $\mu_a = 1.2$ cm^{-1} and $\mu_s(1 - w) = 3.0$ cm^{-1}. The properties of the matrix simulating normal tissue are $\mu_a = 0.67$ cm^{-1} and $\mu_s(1 - w) = 2.6$ cm^{-1}. The light was incident on the left as in Fig. 3, but the depth is measured from the exit surface because the possibility of recovery before the exit surface is of interest. The radiant energy fluence is depressed before, within, and after the absorbing lesion but then recovers because of scattering around the lesion (possible in 2-D geometry but not in 1-D geometry). The fluence near the exit surface is essentially unaffected by the presence of the tumor.

IV. Experiment

A. Tissue Properties

To calculate the propagation of light in tissue, one needs to measure the scattering coefficient, phase

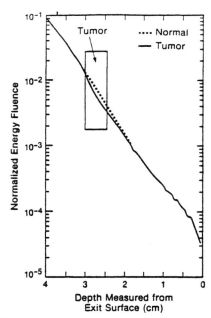

Fig. 4. Radiant energy fluence as function of depth with 0.53- × 0.53-cm absorbing lesion in 2-D nested cylinder geometry. Optical properties are given in the text. Light is incident from the left.

function (angular distribution of scattering), and absorption coefficient at the wavelengths of the source. The scattering coefficient of most tissues is large compared with the absorption coefficient. This makes it easier to measure the scattering than the absorption. A method of deriving the coefficients is to obtain the total interaction coefficient μ_t by measuring the transmittance of a thin specimen in a collimated beam with a collimated photodetector,

$$\mu_t = -(1/d) \ln I/I_0, \tag{7}$$

where d is the thickness of the specimen, I is the photodetector signal with the specimen in the beam, and I_0 is the signal with the specimen out of the beam.[7] Typical tissue specimens have interaction coefficients of 320–700 cm^{-1}, corresponding to mean free paths of 31–14 μm at 630 or 633 nm. The transmittance of the uncollided photons is only some 10^{-14} in 1 mm. The specimen has to be thin enough that multiple scattering is negligible, say 100 μm or less. The collimation has to be within a degree or so because scattering in tissue is very anisotropic. The scattering coefficient μ_s is obtained then by subtracting the absorption coefficient from μ_t. Often μ_s is essentially equal to μ_t.

The phase function is measured by irradiating the thin tissue specimen with a narrow collimated beam of the appropriate wavelength and rotating the collimated photodetector in a near 180° arc around the specimen.[7] Except near 0°, the scattered intensity from the thin specimen is low. A thick specimen would scatter more intensely, but the measurement would be compromised by multiple scattering. It has been found[7,8] that the angular distribution is highly forward peaked (clustered near 0° along the beam axis). Typical tissues have $w = 0.64$–0.97, correspond-

ing to angles of 50–14° at a wavelength of 633 nm. It should be noted that $w = 0.97$ results in an effective scattering cross section $(1 - w)\mu_s$. Anisotropy must be taken into account in calculations of the propagation of light either by explicit angular scattering cross sections in Monte Carlo and other exact transport theory methods or implicitly by a modified diffusion coefficient in diffusion theory.

One method of measuring the absorption coefficient is to measure the change in light intensity in an integrating sphere when the absorbing specimen is introduced compared to a standard.[8] One might also consider measuring the extinction coefficient in a spectrophotometer after cell lysis or separation of the absorber from the scatterer, if this can be done. Another method is to derive the absorption and modified scattering coefficient $\mu_s(1 - w)$ from measurements of the spatial attenuation of light in a large specimen as a function of added absorber of known absorption coefficient.[9] The diffusion length can be obtained with no added absorber, and the diffusion coefficient can be obtained from the slope of L^2 vs $\Delta\mu_a$ [Eq. (6)]. When diffusion theory is not sufficiently accurate, one could fit discrete ordinates or Monte Carlo solutions to the measurements of the spatial distribution of the radiant energy fluence rate. Theoretically, one might also integrate over the scattered light as a function of angle to obtain μ_s and subtract it from μ_t, but this is bound to be inaccurate.

A measured value of $\mu_a = 0.49$ cm^{-1} at 633 nm was obtained for a thin tumor tissue specimen[8] by the integrating sphere technique, but this may be too low because little blood was in the thin specimen. Generally, $\mu_a \approx 1$ cm^{-1}.

B. Radiant Energy Fluence Rate

The radiance Ψ may be measured at several angles and the radiant energy fluence rate Φ obtained by integration over the 4π solid angle.[8,10] It is even better to measure the radiant energy fluence rate (space irradiance) directly using a calibrated isotropic detector.[1,11] The detector consists of a diffusely scattering coating or scattering sphere on a fiber optic lightguide (single filament), which is coupled to a photodetector such as a photodiode. The composition and thickness of the scatterer are selected to achieve an isotropic response without a large decrease in sensitivity. The detection system is calibrated by measuring the response in a collimated beam of known irradiance, because the radiant energy fluence rate is equal to the irradiance in such a configuration. The response is affected by the index of refraction of the medium; hence the calibration should be performed in a transparent fluid with index matching that of tissue.

Results of some radiant energy fluence rate measurements are given in the references.[1,8,11] For plane (large slab) geometry, homogeneous tissue, and a large diameter, perpendicularly incident light beam, the radiant energy fluence rate as a function of depth below the surface $\Phi(x)$ is up to 4 times the irradiance at $x = 0$ because of scattering. Then $\Phi(x)$ decreases rapidly with increasing x in a transient region before reaching an asymptotic region with an exponential dependence

$$\Phi(x) = \text{const. } \exp(-\alpha x). \qquad (8)$$

In infinite plane geometry, $\alpha = L^{-1}$, where L is the diffusion length in diffusion theory. When either the beam or the tissue is finite, even on-axis $\Phi(x)$ decreases more rapidly than L^{-1} because of lateral leakage of photons. The decrease of Φ with cylinder radius (in cylindrical geometry with a line source of light on-axis) is more rapid than the decrease with x in plane geometry because of the geometrical spreading. The decrease with radius in spherical geometry with a point isotropic source at the center is even more rapid than for cylindrical or plane geometry, going as

$$\Phi(r) = \text{const. } \frac{\exp(-\alpha r)}{r}. \qquad (9)$$

Typical values of α at 630–633 nm are 2.5–5 cm^{-1}.[5] At shorter wavelengths, e.g., in the blue, and in colored tissue such as liver, α may be 20 cm^{-1} or even larger.[12]

Figure 5 plots measurements of the radiant energy fluence rate in a subcutaneous mouse tumor 3 mm thick using the isotropic fiber optic probe. The argon-dye laser beam (630 nm) was perpendicularly incident and expanded to ~1-cm diameter with an irradiance of 100 mW/cm^2. Depths were difficult to measure or control in practice. The distribution is not a simple exponential. It may be that the fiber optic probe was not located precisely where planned or because the tissue was inhomogeneous (e.g., measurements were made through skin).

A problem with the isotropic fiber optic probe is its relatively large size (order of 1 mm diameter) and the even larger hollow needle needed to make the hole for insertion of the probe (e.g., a fifteen gauge hypodermic needle). Bleeding may result, and it is not easy to position the needle and probe at the desired point. It may be preferable to use a thinner probe, even though isotropy is compromised. The radiance is nearly isotropic anyway at depth in tissue because of multiple scattering, even with anisotropic scattering. Of course, the magnitude at depth is affected by the anisotropic scattering and directionality of the source. It might be possible to dispense with the hollow needle if the fiber is supported so that it can be inserted by itself, as is done with an implanted irradiating fiber. Another problem is calibration. With an isotropic probe, calibration can be done in a collimated beam. With an anistropic probe, calibration depends on the angular distribution of incident light. More work needs to be done to facilitate measurements of the radiant energy fluence rate.

If the technique for making *in situ* measurements is improved, it would be desirable to monitor the radiant energy fluence or fluence rate during the treatment. The probe should be located at the base of the tumor (where the absorbed dose will be a minimum) to assure that the effective absorbed dose is sufficient to eradicate the tumor. It may also be desirable to locate a probe at the most irradiated point in normal tissue to assure damage to normal tissue is acceptable. Such

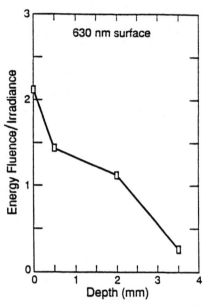

Fig. 5. Measured radiant energy fluence rate per unit irradiance vs depth in a 3-mm thick subcutaneous mouse tumor for perpendicular incidence of a 1-cm diam beam of 630-nm light.

measurements would automatically take into account variations in optical properties of the tissues during irradiation.

Inasmuch as the ratio of the concentration of photosensitizer in a tumor to the concentration in normal tissue is <10 in photodynamic therapy, it would be advisable to make the attenuation factor $\Phi/\Phi_0 < 0.1$, or some of the surrounding normal tissue may receive as large a dose as the least irradiated part of the tumor.

C. Diffuse Transmittance

Measurements of the diffuse transmittance are of interest in diaphanography and have been applied to derivation of the optical properties of tissues as well. The diffuse transmittance is measured by installing an integrating sphere on the exit surface with a small hole for admission of the transmitted light into the sphere. The photodetector of the sphere is calibrated against a standard of known diffuse transmittance or by ratioing the signal obtained with and without the specimen in place.

Measurements of the diffuse transmittance of 1-cm thick (breast) tissue specimens have been made as a function of wavelength from 600 to 1000 nm.[13] Typical transmittances vary from 9×10^{-3} to 2×10^{-4} depending on tissue and wavelength. *In vivo* measurements in a 4-cm thick compressed breast gave a diffuse transmittance of ~10^{-4} in the red and near IR. The principal absorber is hemoglobin, and transmittance is lower at shorter wavelengths and in well perfused peritumor regions. Measurements in other tissues have been made as well.[14]

Two-dimensional calculations of the radiant energy fluence rate and diffuse transmittance were performed by the discrete ordinates method[15] using optical properties derived from the specimen measurements. Attenuation was $\sim 10^{-4}$ for a 4-cm thickness.

D. Diffuse Reflectance

The diffuse reflectance can be calculated if the optical properties of the tissue are known. In diffusion theory, the diffuse reflectance

$$\gamma = (1 - 2D\alpha)/(1 + 2D\alpha) \tag{10}$$

in infinite plane geometry. The diffuse reflectance can be calculated directly in discrete ordinates or Monte Carlo theory.

The diffuse reflectance can be measured by placing an integrating sphere with photodetector on the incident surface with a through hole to admit the beam. Some measurements have been made instead with a bifurcated fiber optic cable, in which irradiating and receiving fibers are intermixed randomly in the common leg. Then one set of fibers is coupled to the light source, and the remaining set of fibers is coupled to the photodetector. Measurements in animal tissue specimens gave values of γ from 0.18 for brain to 0.60 for liver at 633 nm.[10] If γ and α are measured, D can be derived (or, in general, any one of the parameters if the other two are known). The value of D varies from ~ 0.05 to 0.06 cm^{-1} for brain, kidney, or muscle to 0.03 cm^{-1} for liver.

V. Discussion

Measurements are recommended for dosimetry, although calculations are useful in defining the protocol for treatment, consistent with the capabilities of the equipment, the desired duration of irradiation of the patient, and one's knowledge of the optical properties of the tissues.

Anisotropic scattering has to be included in calculations of the transport of light in tissue. Anisotropy is, of course, included in measurements of the diffusion coefficient and diffusion length. It is important to recognize that the absolute magnitude, as well as the shape, of the spatial distribution of the radiant energy fluence is affected by the anisotropic scattering.

Usually the tissue will extend several diffusion lengths beyond a tumor, so that lateral leakage may be neglected. However, the beam radius in surface irradiation for photodynamic therapy should exceed the radius of a tumor by at least three diffusion lengths (typically 6–12 mm, depending on the tissue properties) so that the decrease in radiant energy fluence near the edge of the beam does not extend into the tumor.

In transillumination or diaphanography, the radiant energy fluence and transmitted radiance are decreased only within about three diffusion lengths of the absorbing lesion. Thus, if the lesion is more than a few millimeters below the skin surface on the side opposite the light source, contrast will be very low, and the lesion may be undetectable by the transillumination method.

Theoretical methods seem to be satisfactory, except that programs suitable for small computers should be developed (2- and 3-D diffusion theory, Monte Carlo, discrete ordinates if feasible). But additional measurements are needed of the optical properties of vari-

ous human tissues (absorption and scattering coefficients, phase function) as a function of wavelength over a broad spectrum (UV through near IR). The methods of measuring the absorption coefficient probably need the most attention, as it is difficult to measure the small absorption in the presence of a large amount of scattering. Measurements of the phase function are also difficult and could be improved.

Experimental methods have been developed for measurements of the radiant energy fluence, in particular, the implantable isotropic fiber optic probe. If such a probe could be inserted at the base of a tumor, the irradiation could proceed until the energy fluence was sufficient to kill nearly all the malignant cells. This would be more reliable than irradiating to a certain irradiance at the surface or a certain flux (energy) from an interstitial fiber. Instruments for measuring the transmitted or reflected diffuse radiance (or emergent flux) are reasonably satisfactory, at least for relative values.

One other concern is that measurements of optical properties are nearly always made in specimens. There may be some changes in optical properties compared to the *in vivo* situation. In particular, the loss of blood flow and oxygenation may affect the properties, and this is important in transillumination and may be significant in photodynamic therapy. Additional experiments and comparisons of specimen and *in vivo* results are suggested.

The calculations were performed in part by G. A. Navarro. The research was supported by National Cancer Institute grants CA-31865 and CA-34483, NIH, PHS, Department of HHS.

References

1. A. E. Profio and D. R. Doiron, "Transport of Light in Tissue in Photodynamic Therapy," Photochem. Photobiol. 46, 591–599 (1987).
2. A. E. Profio, *Radiation Shielding and Dosimetry* (Wiley, New York, 1979), pp. 167–218.
3. B. C. Wilson and G. Adam, "A Monte Carlo Model for the Absorption and Flux Distributions of Light in Tissue," Med. Phys. 10, 824–830 (1983).
4. J. J. Duderstadt and L. J. Hamilton, *Nuclear Reactor Analysis* (Wiley, New York, 1979).
5. B. C. Wilson and M. S. Patterson, "The Physics of Photodynamic Therapy," Phys. Med. Biol. 31, 327–360 (1986).
6. L. O. Svaasand; unpublished. Quoted in A. E. Profio and D. R. Doiron.[1]
7. S. T. Flock, B. C. Wilson, and M. S. Patterson, "Total Attenuation Coefficients and Scattering Phase Functions of Tissues and Phantom Materials at 633 nm," Med. Phys. 14, 835–841 (1987).
8. M. R. Arnfield, J. Tulip, and M. S. McPhee, "Optical Propagation in Tissue with Anisotropic Scattering," IEEE Trans. Biomed. Eng. BME-35, 372–381 (1988).
9. A. E. Profio, "Dose Measurements in Photodynamic Therapy of Cancer," Lasers Surg. Med. 7, 1–5 (1987).
10. D. R. Doiron, L. O. Svaasand, and A. E. Profio, "Light Dosimetry in Tissue: Application to Photoradiation Therapy," in *Porphyrin Photosensitization*, D. Kessel and T. J. Dougherty, Eds. (Plenum, New York, 1983), pp. 63–76.
11. J. P. A. Marijnissen and W. M. Marijnissen, "Star Quantitative Light Dosimetry in Vitro and in Vivo," Lasers Med. Sci. 2, 235–242 (1987).

12. B. C. Wilson, W. P. Jeeves, and D. M. Lowe, "*In Vivo* and *Postmortem* Measurements of the Attenuation Spectra of Light in Mammalian Tissue," Photochem. Photobiol. 42, 153–162 (1985).

13. S. Ertefai and A. E. Profio, "Spectral Transmittance and Contrast in Breast Diaphanography," Med. Phys. 12, 393–400 (1985).

14. F. P. Bolin, L. E. Preuss, and B. W. Cain, "A Comparison of Spectral Transmittance for Several Wavelengths; Effects at PRT Frequencies," in *Porphyrin Localization and Treatment of Tumors*, D. R. Doiron and C. J. Gomer, Eds. (Liss, New York, 1984), pp. 221–225.

15. G. A. Navarro and A. E. Profio, "Contrast in Diaphanography of the Breast," Med. Phys. 15, 181–187 (1988).

Reprinted with permission from *IEEE Transactions on Biomedical Engineering*,
Vol. 36(12), pp. 1146-1154 (December 1989). ©1989 IEEE.

Skin Optics

M. J. C. VAN GEMERT, STEVEN L. JACQUES, H. J. C. M. STERENBORG, AND W. M. STAR

Abstract—Quantitative dosimetry in the treatment of skin disorders with (laser) light requires information on propagation of light in the skin related to the optical properties of the individual skin layers. This involves the solution of the integro-differential equation of radiative transfer in a model representing skin geometry, as well as experimental methods to determine the optical properties of each skin layer. These activities are unified under the name skin optics. This paper first reviews the current status of tissue optics, distinguishing between the cases of: dominant absorption, dominant scattering, and scattering about equal to absorption. Then, previously published data as well as some current unpublished data on (human) stratum corneum, epidermis and dermis, have been collected and/or (re)analyzed in terms of absorption coefficient, scattering coefficient, and anisotropy factor of scattering. The results are that the individual skin layers show strongly forward scattering (anisotropy factors between 0.7 and 0.9). The absorption and scattering data show that for all wavelengths considered scattering is much more important than absorption. Under such circumstances, solutions to the transport equation for a multilayer skin model and finite beam laser irradiation are currently not yet available. Hence, any quantitative dosimetry for skin treated with (laser) light is currently lacking.

INTRODUCTION

TREATMENT of skin disorders with light makes use of absorption of photons by chromophores present in viable cells of either the epidermis or the dermis. Optimizing such treatments requires quantitative knowledge of the fraction of incident light that reaches the target chromophore, its ability to absorb that light, and the short and long term biological response of the (host) tissue.

The present analysis of skin optics will concentrate upon relations for the fluence rate distribution of light within the skin, related to the absorbing and scattering properties of the various skin components, in response to incident irradiance. If successful, quantitative light dosimetry can be introduced in, e.g., PUVA for psoriasis, photodynamic therapy of cancer, portwine stain coagulation, and photodynamic therapy for jaundice in newborns.

At present, a rigorous theory is far from being available, partly because skin is irregularly shaped, has hair follicles and glands, is inhomogeneous, multilayered, and has anisotropic physical properties. So any fruitful attempt to understand skin optics requires a considerably

Manuscript received December 5, 1988; revised May 1, 1989.

M. J. C. van Gemert and H. J. C. M. Sterenborg are with the Laser Centre, Academic Medical Centre, Amsterdam, The Netherlands.

S. L. Jacques is with Laser Biology Research Laboratory, The University of Texas/M. D. Anderson Cancer Center, Houston, TX 77030.

W. M. Star is with the Department of Clinical Physics, Dr. Daniel den Hoed Cancer Center, Rotterdam, The Netherlands.

IEEE Log Number 8931098.

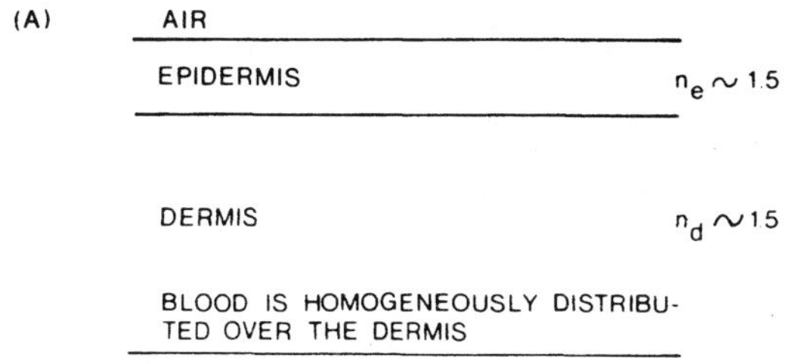

Fig. 1. Schematic model of skin with plane parallel epidermal and dermal layers. Each layer is homogeneous and has isotropic physical properties. Absorption and scattering are introduced by assuming a random but homogeneous distribution of absorbers and scatterers over the volume. Local scattering can be anisotropic. For convenience, blood is assumed here to be homogeneously distributed over the dermal volume. The refractive indexes of epidermis and dermis are considered identical. A number of 1.5 is mentioned for convenience.

simplified model for the skin. A diagram of the skin and a simplified model consisting of epidermis and dermis as two plane parallel layers with isotropic physical properties is shown in Fig. 1. The layers are assumed to have the same refractive index ($n \sim 1.37$–1.5 [1]) but a different number density of absorbers and scatterers that are randomly distributed over the volume. As a consequence, wavelength dependent absorption and scattering coefficients (mm^{-1}) can be assigned to both the epidermis and dermis. Blood may either be explicitly taken into account (see Fig. 4 below) or it may be assumed to be homogeneously distributed in the dermis (Fig. 1); this latter assumption will influence the dermal absorption coefficient at certain wavelengths but (presumably) hardly the scattering coefficient. An additional optical parameter is the scattering phase function, expressing the probability density function that a photon moving in direction s is scattered into another direction s'. Within the concepts of such a model, propagation of light can be described by radiative transfer theory which originates from astrophysics [2]. This theory requires that the scatterers are far enough apart to scatter independently from each other. An additional simplification used here is that polarization effects are neglected. Despite the simple model described in Fig. 1, two complicating factors remain. First, a general (analytical) solution of the integro-differential equation of radiative transfer is not available under all conditions relevant for skin treatments. Solutions are available under restricted conditions only such as, e.g., uniform irradiation or when either absorption or scattering strongly dominates. Second, determination of the optical parameters (absorption, scattering, and phase function) requires not only the solution to the transport equation (or a suitable approximation) for an experimental geometry (e.g., a thin slab of tissue) but also an inverse solution that relates measurements such as reflection and transmission to the optical properties. Such methods have only been developed recently, usually under conditions that scattering dominates over absorption (so-called diffusion approximation).

The purpose of this paper is to review the status of tissue optics (solutions to the transport equation as well as experimental methods to measure the optical properties involved), and collect previously published as well as currently unpublished information on skin optical parameters, rearranged if necessary according to present day knowledge.

General Aspects of Transport of Light in Tissue

Assume collimated light normally incident upon a slab of turbid material with refractive index $n > 1$. Due to the mismatch in refractive index a small portion of the incident beam is specularly reflected, also called Fresnel reflection (4 percent for $n = 1.5$). The remaining 96 percent enters the tissue where it is attenuated due to absorption and scattering. Photons scattered out of the collimated beam initially propagate in (random) directions described by the phase function. These scattered photons contribute to a diffuse distribution of light in the tissue that extends beyond the boundaries of the collimated incident beam. A back scattered photon from the diffuse part of the light distribution that reaches the tissue–air boundary at an angle with the inward normal larger than the so-called critical angle for total reflection, is reflected back into the tissue. The critical angle is defined as the arcsine of $1/n$, so arcsin $(1/1.5) = 41.8°$ for $n = 1.5$. This process of total internal back-reflection against the tissue–air boundary for perfectly diffuse light leads to a 55 percent theoretical diffuse back-reflectance for $n = 1.5$ [1]. However, a much smaller diffuse back-reflectance coefficient may be more appropriate for laser irradiated skin because light close to boundaries may not be perfectly diffuse, but more forward directed.

The phase function for scattering $p(s, s')$ representing the albedo times the probability density function that a photon is scattered from direction s into direction s' depends only on the angle θ between s and s' due to the assumption that the scatterers are randomly distributed over the tissue volume, expressing that the tissue lacks spatially correlated structures. Thus,

$$p(s, s') = p(\theta). \tag{1}$$

Various theoretical phase functions considered for tissue are illustrated in Fig. 2. Isotropic scattering shown in Fig. 2(a) is represented as a constant

$$p(s, s') = \text{constant}. \tag{2a}$$

Slightly forward scattering can be represented by the first

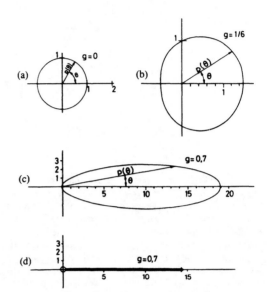

Fig. 2. Examples of phase functions $p(\theta)$. (a) Isotropic scattering, equation (2a). (b) Forward scattering, equation (2b) using an example of the first two moments of the phase function expansion in Legendre polynomials with $g = 1/6$. (c) The Henyey–Greenstein phase function, equation (2c), for $g = 0.7$. (d) An approximation to the Henyey–Greenstein phase function, identical in the first two moments, equations (2d) and (3).

two moments of the phase function (see, e.g., Ishimaru [3], p. 177).

$$p(\theta) = \text{constant } [1 + 3g \cos \theta] \tag{2b}$$

where g is the mean cosine of the scattering angle (called anisotropy factor), arbitrarily chosen as $g = 1/6$ for depiction in Fig. 2(b). Isotropic scattering has $g = 0$; purely forward scattering $g = 1$, and purely backward scattering $g = -1$. Forward scattering according to the so-called Henyey–Greenstein phase function [4], [5, p. 307] is presented in Fig. 2(c)

$$p(\theta) = \left(\frac{\sigma_s}{\sigma_s + \sigma_a}\right) \frac{(1 - g^2)}{(1 + g^2 - 2g \cos \theta)^{3/2}} \tag{2c}$$

where σ_a, σ_s are the absorption and scattering coefficients (mm^{-1}). An approximation to (2c) shown in Fig. 2(d) is

$$p(\theta) = \left(\frac{\sigma_s}{\sigma_s + \sigma_a}\right) [2g\delta(1 - \cos \theta) + (1 - g)]. \tag{2d}$$

The first term indicates strongly forward peaked scattering and the second term isotropic scattering. Equations (2c) and (2d) are identical in their first two moments, that is

$$\frac{1}{2} \int_{-1}^{1} p(\cos \theta) \, d(\cos \theta) = \frac{\sigma_s}{\sigma_s + \sigma_a} \tag{3a}$$

$$\frac{1}{2} \int_{-1}^{1} \cos \theta \, p(\cos \theta) \, d(\cos \theta) = g\left(\frac{\sigma_s}{\sigma_s + \sigma_a}\right). \tag{3b}$$

Equation (3a) is the normalization condition imposed on the phase function. Both phase functions (2c) and (2d) have been used to characterize scattering of tissue (see below). The ratio $[\sigma_s/(\sigma_s + \sigma_a)]$ is called the albedo for single particle scattering.

STRONG ABSORPTION

For some (laser) wavelengths in the UV (e.g., at the ArF excimer laser wavelength at 193 nm) and the IR (Er-YAG laser at 2.94 μm; the CO_2 laser at 10.6 μm) tissue absorption may be substantially larger than scattering. Transport theory is then simple. The fluence rate in the tissue decreases exponentially with increasing depth according to

$$I_c(z, r) = I_L(r)(1 - r_{sp})e^{-\sigma_a z} \qquad (4)$$

where $I_L(r)$ (watt m^{-2}) is the radial profile of the incident laser beam, $I_c(z, r)$ (watt m^{-2}) is the fluence rate in the tissue at coordinates z, r, and r_{sp} is the specular reflection coefficient (Fresnel reflection). Equation (4) is called Beer's law.

Experimentally, σ_a can be determined by measuring the transmittance (T) through a slab of material, with thickness t. From (4) this yields

$$\sigma_a = \frac{1}{t}\ln\left(\frac{1}{T}\right) \qquad (5)$$

and T defined as

$$T = \frac{I_c(t)}{I_L(1 - r_{sp})}. \qquad (6)$$

An experimental problem can be that thickness t should be extremely small when σ_a is large. For example, soft tissue has at the 10.6 μm wavelength of a CO_2 laser an absorption coefficient of approximately 60 mm^{-1}. In this case a thickness of $t = 38$ μm yields a 10 percent transmittance.

STRONG SCATTERING

Between about 300 and 1000 nm nonpigmented tissues have scattering dominating over absorption. Under these circumstances the transport equation can be approximated by a diffusion equation in the diffuse light fluence rate $\phi_d(z, r)$ (watt m^{-2}), defined as the total amount of diffuse light power that passes through a small sphere located at (z, r) divided by the cross sectional area of that sphere. Under conditions of cylindrical symmetry the diffusion equation reads

$$\left[\frac{d^2\phi_d(z, r)}{dz^2} + \frac{d^2\phi_d(z, r)}{dr^2} + \frac{1}{r}\frac{d\phi_d(z, r)}{dr}\right]$$
$$- 3\sigma_a[\sigma_a + \sigma_s(1 - g)]\phi_d(z, r)$$
$$= -3\sigma_s[\sigma_s + (1 + g)\sigma_a]I_c(z, r) \qquad (7)$$

where the first term on the left-hand side represents diffusion losses in the z and r directions (for cylindrical symmetry) which gives the name: diffusion equation. The right-hand side term involves the collimated laser beam

attenuated by absorption and scattering $I_c(z, r)$ which is the source for the diffuse light distribution. Note that the phase function for scattering is here represented by the anisotropy factor g, the first moment of the phase function, (3b). Equation (7) can be solved analytically or numerically with appropriate boundary value conditions such as the specular reflectance of the collimated source and internal reflection of diffuse light at tissue–air interfaces; see, e.g., Groenhuis et al. [6] and Keijzer et al. [7]. The total fluence rate, $\phi(z, r)$, is the sum of the collimated and the diffuse components

$$\phi(z, r) = \phi_c(z, r) + \phi_d(z, r) \qquad (8)$$

where $\phi_c(z, r) = I_c(z, r)$. Details of the derivation can be found in Ishimaru [3] and Groenhuis et al. [6]. For an infinite laser beam diameter (uniform irradiation of a semi-infinite slab), (7) can be rewritten as a set of first order differential equations in the diffuse forward and backward fluxes. This set can be solved analytically [8]–[10].

Solutions of (7) and (8) for $\sigma_a = 0.2$ mm^{-1}, $\sigma_s = 18.8$ mm^{-1}, and $g = 0.8$, which is a set of values that approximates in vitro dermal tissue at 633 nm wavelength [11] are shown in Fig. 3. A radially uniform intensity beam, radius w_L, was used. These results show that if w_L is large, $\phi(z = 0, r = 0)$ can be 3.3 times larger than the incident irradiance due to back scattering. This factor of 3.3 drops to 1 when w_L tends to zero. In other words, the viable light intensity distribution inside the tissue that is available for therapeutic benefits is a complicated function of σ_a, σ_s, g, and w_L. This makes any quantitative dosimetry extremely hard, especially because the relationships are not obvious.

In addition, for a multilayer (skin) model (7) has only been solved for uniform irradiation of a semi-infinite slab [3, pp. 216–219], [12]. A result of a four-layer skin model (from [12]) is shown in Fig. 4. The optical data used are from the present paper (Fig. 8 below). This four-layer skin model has been used to analyze portwine stain laser treatment [13], explicitly requiring a blood layer plexus. It therefore differs from the more general skin model of Fig. 1. For a finite laser beam a multilayer solution has not been published, but progress is being made with finite element and Monte Carlo models. The problem is that the second layer not only has an incident attenuated collimated beam, but also an incident diffuse beam from the first layer. In turn, the first layer, at the interface with the second, now has the back-reflected diffuse beam incident as well. As curves similar to Fig. 3 are not yet available for the skin model of Fig. 1 irradiated with a finite laser beam, any quantitative multiple layer dosimetry for skin treated with laser light is only possible when the laser spot is much larger than the penetration depth. In this case, the one-dimensional optical analysis provides an accurate estimate of fluence rate as a function of depth at the center of the beam. Fluence rate can be used to calculate the rate of heat generation in the tissue and then temperature can be calculated using the heat conduction equation.

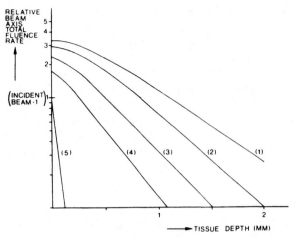

Fig. 3. Total fluence rate as a function of tissue depth z at $r = 0$ according to the diffusion model, equations (7) and (8), and optical parameters $\sigma_a = 0.2$ mm^{-1}, $\sigma_s = 18.8$ mm^{-1}, and $g = 0.8$ representing dermal tissue at 633 nm [11]. Beam diameters ($2w_L$) are: 1) infinite, 2) 2 mm, 3) 1 mm, and 4) 0.5 mm: curve 5) represents the collimated beam, attenuated according to exp $[-(\sigma_a + \sigma_s)z]$. The laser beam has uniform irradiance: $I_c(z = 0, r) = 1$ for $r \leq w_L$ and $I_c(z = 0, r) = 0$ for $r > w_L$. Index mismatching has been used.

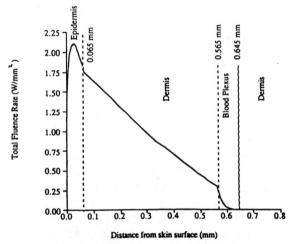

Fig. 4. Total fluence rate (watt/cm^2) versus depth from skin surface (mm) for a four-layer skin model. Refractive index matching with $n = 1.33$ is assumed for all layers. A collimated beam, of infinite dimension is assumed with 1 watt/mm^2 irradiance at 577 nm wavelength. Input data were as follows (Fig. 8). Epidermis: thickness 0.065 mm, $\sigma_{ae} = 3.8$ mm^{-1}, $\sigma_{se} = 50$ mm^{-1}, $g_e = 0.786$. Dermis: thickness 0.5 mm (upper dermis) and 0.3 mm (lower dermis), $\sigma_{ad} = 0.3$ mm^{-1}, $\sigma_{sd} = 21.7$ mm^{-1} (Jacques' value, Fig. 8), $g_d = 0.81$. Blood: thickness 0.08 mm, $\sigma_{ab} = 37.6$ mm^{-1}, $\sigma_{sb} = 0.96$ mm^{-1}, $g_b = 0$.

In calculating the curves of Figs. 3 and 4, we have assumed numbers for σ_a, σ_s, and g are available. Actually, reliable methods to measure these parameters for strongly scattering materials are only currently being developed. Determination of the three independent parameters σ_a, σ_s, and g requires three independent measurements. Usually, one measurement is σ_t, the collimated attenuation coefficient for a thin slab of tissue [14]. The other two measurements refer to properties measured with the diffuse part of the light. One possibility is to measure the diffuse

reflectance (R_d) and transmittance (T_d) of a slab of tissue with thickness t (e.g., in an integrating sphere geometry). First, these measurement yields parameters K, S via

$$S = \frac{1}{bt} \ln \left[\frac{1 - R_d(a - b)}{T_d} \right] \qquad K = S(a - 1) \quad (9a)$$

$$a = \frac{1 - T_d^2 + R_d^2}{2R_d} \qquad\qquad b = \sqrt{a^2 - 1} \quad (9b)$$

where K, S are absorption and scattering parameters of the Kubelka–Munk formalism [10]. Second, S and K have been related to the optical parameters by [15]

$$S = \tfrac{3}{4}\sigma_s(1 - g) - \tfrac{1}{4}\sigma_a \quad (10a)$$

$$K = 2\sigma_a. \quad (10b)$$

Adding the measured collimated attenuation coefficient σ_t

$$\sigma_t = \sigma_a + \sigma_s \quad (10c)$$

yields in a straightforward way to values of σ_a, σ_s, and g. Similar methods have been worked out by Marijnissen et al. [8], [9] and by Jacques and Prahl [16]. We recall, however, that scattering has to dominate over absorption $[\sigma_s(1 - g) >> \sigma_a]$. Below, [see (12)] relations between S, K and σ_a, σ_s, and g are presented that are more accurate than those of (10). In fact, (10) represent (12) in the limit that $\sigma_a/[\sigma_s(1 - g)]$ tends to zero.

SCATTERING ABOUT EQUAL TO ABSORPTION

In this situation no simplified solution to the transport equation [(11) below] is currently available and in order to find fluence rate distributions in tissue this equation needs to be completely solved. The transport equation reads [2], [3]

$$\frac{dL(r, s)}{ds} = -(\sigma_a + \sigma_s) L(r, s) + \frac{\sigma_a + \sigma_s}{4\pi} \int_{4\pi} p(s, s')$$
$$\cdot L(r, s') \, dw' \quad (11)$$

where $L(r, s)$ is the radiance (watt m^{-2} sr^{-1}) at tissue location r (z, r), expressing that $L(r, s) \, dw$ is the amount of light power confined within solid angle dw, moving in the direction s, which crosses a unit area located at r. The first term of the r.h.s. of (11) denotes the losses in $L(r, s)$ per unit of length in direction s due to absorption and scattering. The second term denotes the gain in $L(r, s)$ per unit length in direction s due to scattering from all other directions s'. The light power per unit area confined within solid angle dw' coming from direction s' is $L(r, s') \, dw'$ with scattering probability density function $p(s, s')$ for scattering from direction s' to direction s. Note that the transport equation is a *local* equation that considers the spatial balance of light power at coordinate r.

To our knowledge, no analytical solution or reasonable approximation is available to (11) for $\sigma_a \sim \sigma_s$ for an incident finite laser beam. Such solutions are now available, however, from Monte Carlo numerical techniques; see, e.g., Wilson and Adam [17] and Keijzer et al. [18].

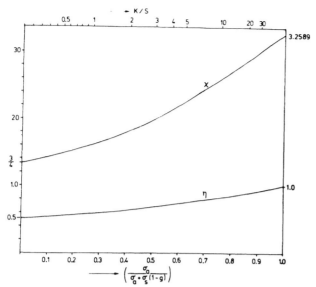

Fig. 5. Parameters η and χ, according to $\sigma_a = \eta K$ and $\sigma_s(1 - g) = \chi S$, as a function of $\sigma_a/[\sigma_a + \sigma_s(1 - g)]$ (lower scale) and K/S (upper scale). The phase function used in the derivation is according to (2d).

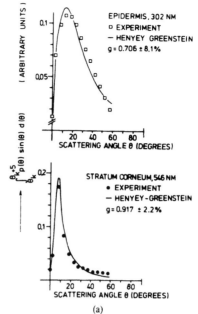

(a)

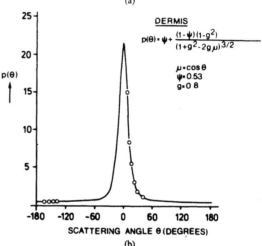

(b)

Fig. 6. The Henyey–Greenstein phase function, (2c), fit to the goniometer measurements of Bruls [20] on stratum corneum and epidermis and of Jacques *et al.* [11] and Prahl (S. A. Prahl: three-dimensional calculations of light distributions in tissue, The University of Texas at Austin, 1986, unpublished) on dermis. The measurements by Bruls [20, Fig. 7 and Table I] refer to $\int_{\theta_k}^{\theta_k + 5°} p(\theta) \sin \theta d\theta$, with θ_k varying between $\theta_1 = 0$, $\theta_2 = 5°$, $\theta_3 = 10°$, etc.

Methods to determine σ_a, σ_s, and $p(s, s')$ or g when $\sigma_a \sim \sigma_s$ have not received the attention that has been given to the conditions $\sigma_a \gg \sigma_s$. Chandrasekhar [2, p. 19] has solved (11) under the constraint of no collimated or diffuse source (or, if there is such a source, it is expected to be so far away that attenuation of the source has virtually been complete). He has assumed isotropic scattering or $p(s, s') = $ constant, (2a) and Fig. 2(a). It is also easy to show that this solution for isotropic scattering can be extended when the phase function involving strongly forward and isotropic scattering can be represented by the phase function of (2d). In this case, σ_s in Chandrasekhar's solution is replaced by $\sigma_s(1 - g)$ [15]. Once again, parameters K and S can be determined by similar integrating sphere methods using the relations in (9). Here, K and S are related to σ_a and $\sigma_s(1 - g)$ by

$$\sigma_a = \eta K \qquad (12a)$$

$$\sigma_s(1 - g) = \chi S \qquad (12b)$$

where curves for η and χ are shown in Fig. 5 as a function of $\sigma_a/[\sigma_a + \sigma_s(1 - g)]$ and of K/S. Equations (12) have originally been proposed by Klier [19] for isotropic scattering ($g = 0$). Klier's analysis used the observation that Chandrasekhar's and Kubelka–Munk's formulas for transmission and reflection coefficients were formally identical functions of the optical parameters involved. Equating these coefficients resulted in (12) and Fig. 5. Again, measurement of the collimated attenuation coefficient σ_t yields

$$\sigma_t = \sigma_a + \sigma_s \qquad (12c)$$

indicating that σ_a, σ_s, and g can be determined albeit under the constraint that the phase function of (2d) applies.

The authors are not aware that such measurements under these conditions of $\sigma_a \sim \sigma_s$ have been published. These measurements would also require special boundary conditions that may not be easy to realize in practice. Nevertheless, this method is used below to analyze published transmission and reflection data of skin layers in terms of transport equation parameters.

COMPILATION OF EXPERIMENTAL SKIN DATA

The following paragraphs describe optical properties of skin layers, from measurements performed in a number of different laboratories. No attempt has been made to incorporate the effect of tissue preparations and tissue con-

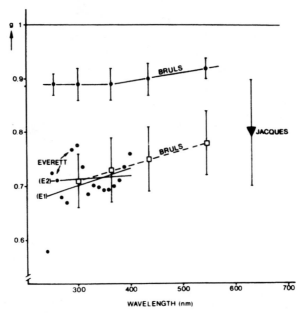

Fig. 7. Compiled experimental g values for: stratum corneum (●) from experimental data by Bruls [20]; and Everett *et al.* [21]; epidermis (▢), from data by Bruls [20], and dermis (▼), from Jacques *et al.* [11]. The analyzed data from Everett *et al.* show considerable scatter. A least squares analysis of that data, according to $g = A + B\lambda$ (wavelength λ in nanometers) shows: $A = 0.603$; $B = 3.23 \times 10^{-4}$, see line ($E1$). Neglecting, as Diffey [1] did the point at 240 nm yields: $A = 0.692$; $B = 6.7 \times 10^{-5}$, see line ($E2$), or an almost wavelength independent g value of about 0.715 (250–400 nm), in reasonable correlation with $g = 0.68$ deduced from Diffey's $\beta = 0.84$.

ditions (e.g., the amount of blood in the tissue), upon the reported values.

Stratum Corneum

Bruls [20] published goniometer measurements of *in vitro* stratum corneum. We used a least squares fit to analyze his data according to the Henyey–Greenstein phase function, (2c), extracting values of g (see Fig. 6). The results of g as a function of wavelength shown in Fig. 7 indicate that g is approximately 0.9 with a tendency to increase with increasing wavelength. Stratum corneum is a highly forward scattering layer but, more importantly, the Henyey–Greenstein phase function seems a good description for stratum corneum scattering behavior, see Fig. 6.

Everett *et al.* [21] measured collimated and diffuse transmission, and diffuse reflection from a 10 μm thick sample of "90 percent pure" stratum corneum, in the UV. Figs. 7 and 8 show the analyzed data for g and σ_a, σ_s, respectively, obtained using (12). Values of g found in this way are between 0.58 and 0.78 for wavelengths between 240 and 400 nm, so substantially lower than those derived from Bruls' data. A clear explanation of this discrepancy is not easy to give. However, as it is unknown whether Everett *et al.* used diffuse incidence or collimated incidence in their experiments, it seems at present that Bruls' data are more reliable. Recently, Diffey [1] also used these data by Everett to analyze the optical proper-

ties of stratum corneum using a strictly one-dimensional form of (11). The parameter β occurring in Diffey's analysis, describing the fraction of scattered light that is scattered in the forward direction [22], is then related to g by $g = 2\beta - 1$. Diffey's results of σ_a and σ_s, assuming $\beta = 0.84$ (or $g = 0.68$), are consistent with the results given in Figs. 7 and 8.

Epidermis

Goniometer measurements by Bruls [20] on epidermis were again analyzed according to the Henyey–Greenstein phase function (Fig. 6) yielding g values as a function of wavelength (Fig. 7). Again, the Henyey–Greenstein phase function fits well for epidermis, with values between 0.71 at 300 nm and 0.78 at 540 nm, varying linearly with wavelength.

Wan *et al.* [24] published epidermal diffuse integrating sphere measurements of K and S, see (9). Again using these values in conjunction with (12) and Fig. 5 leads to values of σ_a and $\sigma_s(1 - g)$. Assuming that the g values deduced from Bruls' experiments (assuming Henyey–Greenstein phase function behavior) also fit the analysis of (12) and assuming (2d) as the phase function, gives values for σ_s as well. The results are shown in Fig. 8. The epidermis is thus a strongly forward scattering layer with reasonable absorption in the visible but with substantial absorption in the UV. At all wavelengths considered, scattering coefficients appear larger than the corresponding absorption coefficients.

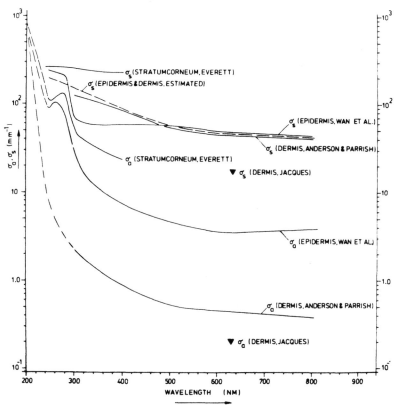

Fig. 8. Experimental absorption (σ_a) and scattering (σ_s) coefficients for stratum corneum (from data by Everett *et al.* [21]); epidermis (from data by Wan *et al.* [23]); and dermis (from data by Anderson and Parrish [25]; and from Jacques *et al.* [11]). For shorter UV wavelengths (<200 nm) absorption coefficients indicated by (— — —) are likely to reach values of $\sigma_a \sim 1000$ mm^{-1}. The dashed line (------------) shows the estimated epidermal and dermal scattering coefficient, assumed equal to each other.

Dermis

Values for K and S of dermal tissue, obtained from integrating sphere measurements were published by Anderson and Parrish [25]. Conversion of Kubelka–Munk coefficients to transport parameters using (12a) and (12b) yields values for σ_a and $\sigma_s(1 - g)$. Assuming g values vary with wavelength according to Fig. 7 it is possible to compute σ_s with (12b). These values for σ_s as a function of wavelength are illustrated in Fig. 8.

DISCUSSION

Experimental Data

The experimental g value presented in Fig. 7 suggest that skin layers are strongly forward scattering media for wavelengths between 240 and 633 nm. The g values of stratum corneum, analyzed from Everett's reflection and transmission data, show values that are more than 20 percent lower than those from Bruls' data. However, the trend as a function of wavelength is similar within measurement accuracy. The low g value at 240 nm may be an experimental artefact caused by the combined influence of the strong increase in stratum corneum absorption at 240 nm,

and experimental difficulties associated with these short UV wavelengths.

Interestingly, the dermal g values at 633 nm, from Jacques, is virtually identical to the extrapolated epidermal g factors from Bruls. In addition, these two goniometer experiments show a good fit to the Henyey–Greenstein phase function, (3c) and Fig. 6. As a result, epidermal and dermal g factors may be considered identical according to (wavelength λ in nanometer)

$$g_e \sim g_d \sim 0.62 + \lambda 0.29 \times 10^{-3} \, (\lambda \text{ in nm}). \quad (13)$$

Equation (13) may be used in practice until more goniometer data become available, preferably for skin layers from the same human skin samples. Equation (13) has also been used to analyze dermal σ_s values as a function of wavelength, shown in Fig. 8.

The absorption (σ_a) and scattering (σ_s) coefficients of Fig. 8 show that σ_s is always larger than σ_a for the wavelengths considered (full lines in Fig. 8). The epidermal (and stratum corneum) absorption coefficients show a strong maximum around 260 to 280 nm. This strong increase in σ_a in conjunction with the corresponding increased experimental inaccuracies in the diffuse transmittance and reflectance measurements is probably the reason

TABLE I
WAVELENGTH BANDS (IN NANOMETERS) FOR WHICH BEER'S LAW, (4), AND THE DIFFUSION MODEL, (7), ARE "REASONABLE" OR "GOOD" APPROXIMATIONS TO THE TRANSPORT EQUATION (11). CRITERIA FOR "REASONABLE" AND "GOOD" ARE GIVEN IN THE TEXT. WAVELENGTH BANDS FOR WHICH THE EXACT SOLUTION TO (11) IS *REQUIRED* ARE INDICATED IN THE LAST COLUMN

Skin-Layer	Beer's Law		Diffusion Model		Exact Solution Required
	"Reasonable"	"Good"	"Reasonable"	"Good"	
Epidermis	200–220 nm				220–2000 nm
Dermis	200–220 nm		220–300 nm	300–2000 nm	

that also the measured epidermal scattering coefficient increases strongly at 300 nm. This interpretation, and the observation in Fig. 8 that epidermal and dermal σ_s values virtually coincide between 500 and 633 nm, suggests the dashed curve in Fig. 8 may be a reasonable estimate for both epidermal and dermal scattering coefficients until more data become available. The dermal value of σ_s at 633 nm, from recent work by Jacques, may be the first of such additional data. The discrepancy by a factor of 2.4 is not alarming. Dermal absorption coefficients are about ten times smaller than those for epidermis. Again, Jacques' recent value at 633 nm is lower by a factor of 2.3. The σ_a, σ_s values for stratum corneum, from Everett et al., deviate somewhat from the other (epidermal and dermal) results except for the UV wavelengths around 250 nm. The reason is not clear although it may reflect experimental uncertainties. Fig. 8 incorporates (expected) increase in tissue absorption coefficients towards (an estimated) ~ 1000 mm^{-1} for wavelengths < 200 nm (dashed lines).

An interesting question is for what wavelength bands the approximate solutions to the transport equation (11) can be used. First, $\sigma_a \gg \sigma_s$ yields Beer's law, (4). We assume $\sigma_a > 10\sigma_s$ yields a good approximation and $\sigma_a > 5\sigma_s$ yields a reasonable approximation to (11). Similarly, the diffusion model (7) yields a good, respectively reasonable approximation to (11) when $\sigma_s(1 - g) > 10\sigma_a$ or $\sigma_s(1 - g) > 5\sigma_a$. Table I has been tabulated from Fig. 8 according to these criteria. Surprisingly, Table I suggests that a better approximation of the transport equation is required for epidermal tissue optics for almost all wavelengths of interest. For the short UV wavelengths (< 200 nm) one would intuitively expect Beer's law to apply. However, our analysis shows that Beer's law is only a "reasonable" model. For dermal tissue optics, the diffusion model seems adequate for $\lambda > 220$ nm, and Beer's law "reasonable" for the 200–220 nm band. Attempts to evaluate the accuracy of the diffusion approximation for computed fluxes, radiances, and fluence rates as a function of optical parameters has been recently described [26], [27].

Theoretical Methods

The method [see (12)], employed in this paper to determine transport equation absorption (σ_a) and scattering (σ_s, g) parameters from published data on collimated transmission and diffuse transmission and reflection of a slab of tissue, is exact in principle. However, a condition is that the theoretical boundary conditions can be satisfied experimentally. Another condition is that the phase function of the tissue can be represented by the sum of an isotropic and a strongly forward peaked component, (2d) and Fig. 2(d). Although certain tissues and tissue phantoms indeed show this behavior; see, e.g., the paper by Flock et al. [14], available goniometer data of skin layers show their phase functions to be represented quite reasonably by the Henyey–Greenstein phase function, (3c) and Figs. 2(c) and 6. These two phase functions have only their first two moments in common, (3), and Fig. 2(c) and (d) show the substantial difference between them for $g = 0.7$. This strongly suggests the need of theoretical relations, comparable to those of (12), for a Henyey–Greenstein phase function. Most likely, Chandrasekhar's approach [2, p. 19] will work here, transforming the transport integro-differential equation into an easier solvable integral-equation [23, (43)–(47)]. Again, as with (12), this method yields better results only if the theoretical boundary conditions can be satisfied experimentally, which may be difficult.

Summarizing therefore, the optical properties of the skin layers, compiled from different sources and shown in Figs. 7 and 8, can only be considered as approximations, although, most likely, the best values available today. In any case, these results stress both the need for theoretically sound methods and corresponding adequate measurements, as well as the dearth of current reliable optical data of skin layers.

REFERENCES

[1] B. L. Diffey, "A mathematical model for ultraviolet optics in skin," *Phys. Med. Biol.*, vol. 28, pp. 647–657, 1983.
[2] S. Chandrasekhar, *Radiative Transfer.* New York: Dover, 1960.
[3] A. Ishimaru, *Wave Propagation and Scattering in Random Media, Vol. 1.* New York: Academic, 1978.
[4] L. G. Henyey and J. L. Greenstein, "Diffuse radiation in the galaxy," *Astrophys. J.*, vol. 93, pp. 70–83, 1941.
[5] H. C. van de Hulst, *Multiple Light Scattering: Tables, Formulas and Applications, Vol. 2.* New York: Academic, 1980.
[6] R. A. J. Groenhuis, H. A. Ferwerda, and J. J. Ten Bosch, "Scattering and absorption of turbid materials determined from reflection measurements. I: Theory," *Appl. Optics*, vol. 22, pp. 2456–2467, 1983.
[7] M. Keijzer, W. M. Star, and P. R. M. Storchi, "Optical diffusion in layered media," *Appl. Optics*, vol. 27, pp. 1820–1824, 1988.
[8] J. P. A. Marijnissen and W. M. Star, "Phantom measurements for light dosimetry using isotropic and small aperture detectors," in *Por-*

phyrin Localization and Treatment of Tumors, D. R. Doiron and C. J. Gomer, Eds. New York: Alan Liss, 1984, pp. 133–148.

[9] J. P. A. Marijnissen, W. M. Star, J. L. van Delft, and N. A. P. Franken, "Light intensity measurements in optical phantoms and *in vivo* during HPD-photoradiation treatment using a miniature light detector with isotropic response," in *Photodynamic Therapy of Tumors and Other Diseases*, G. Jori and C. Perria, Eds. Padova: Libreria Progetto, 1985, pp. 387–390.

[10] M. J. C. van Gemert, A. J. Welch, W. M. Star, M. Motamedi, and W. F. Cheong, "Tissue optics for a slab geometry in the diffusion approximation," *Lasers Med. Sci.*, vol. 2, pp. 295–302, 1987.

[11] S. L. Jacques, C. A. Alter, and S. A. Prahl, "Angular dependence of He–Ne laser light scattering by human dermis," *Lasers Life Sci.*, vol. 1, pp. 309–333, 1987.

[12] M. J. C. van Gemert, G. A. C. M. Schets, M. Bishop, W. F. Cheong, and A. J. Welch, "Optics of tissue in a multi-slab geometry," *Lasers Life Sci.*, vol. 2, pp. 1–18, 1988.

[13] M. J. C. van Gemert, W. J. de Kleijn, and J. P. Hulsbergen Henning, "Temperature behavior of a model portwine stain during argon laser coagulation," *Phys. Med. Biol.*, vol. 27, pp. 1089–1104, 1982.

[14] S. T. Flock, B. C. Wilson, and M. S. Patterson, "Total attenuation coefficients and scattering phase functions of tissues and phantom materials at 633 nm," *Med. Phys.*, vol. 14, pp. 835–841, 1987.

[15] M. J. C. van Gemert and W. M. Star, "Relations between the Kubelka–Munk and the transport equation models for anisotropic scattering," *Lasers Life Sci.*, vol. 1, pp. 287–298, 1987.

[16] S. L. Jacques and S. A. Prahl, "Modeling optical and thermal distributions in tissue during laser irradiation," *Lasers Surg. Med.*, vol. 6, pp. 494–503, 1987.

[17] B. C. Wilson and G. A. Adam, "A Monte Carlo model for the absorption and flux distributions of light in tissue," *Med. Phys.*, vol. 10, pp. 824–830, 1983.

[18] M. Keijzer, S. L. Jacques, S. A. Prahl, and A. J. Welch, "Light distributions in artery tissue: Monte Carlo simulations for finite diameter laser beams," *Lasers Surg. Med.*, vol. 9, pp. 148–154, 1989.

[19] K. Klier, "Absorption and scattering in plane parallel turbid media," *J. Opt. Soc. Amer.*, vol. 62, pp. 882–885, 1972.

[20] W. A. G. Bruls and J. C. van der Leun, "Forward scattering properties of human epidermal layers," *Photochem. Photobiol.*, vol. 40, pp. 231–242, 1984.

[21] M. A. Everett, E. Yeargers, R. M. Sayre, and R. L. Olsen, "Penetration of epidermis by ultraviolet rays," *Photochem. Photobiol.*, vol. 5, pp. 533–542, 1966.

[22] J. T. Atkins, "Absorption and scattering of light in turbid media," Ph.D. dissertation, Univ. Delaware, June 1965.

[23] W. M. Star, J. P. A. Marijnissen, and M. J. C. van Gemert, "Light dosimetry in optical phantoms and in tissues. I. Multiple flux and transport theory," *Phys. Med. Biol.*, vol. 33, pp. 437–454, 1988.

[24] S. Wan, R. R. Anderson, and J. A. Parrish, "Analytical modeling for the optical properties of the skin with *in vitro* and *in vivo* applications," *Photochem. Photobiol.*, vol. 34, pp. 493–499, 1981.

[25] R. R. Anderson and J. A. Parrish, "Optical properties of human skin," in *The Science of Photomedicine*, J. D. Regan and J. A. Parrish, Eds. New York: Plenum, 1982, pp. 147–194.

[26] G. Yoon, S. A. Prahl, and A. J. Welch, "Accuracies of the diffusion approximation and its similarity relations for laser irradiated biological media," *Appl. Optics*, vol. 28, pp. 2250–2255, 1989.

[27] S. A. Prahl, "Light transport in tissue," Ph.D. dissertation, Univ. Texas, Austin, TX, Dec. 1988.

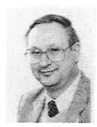

M. J. C. van Gemert was born in Delft, The Netherlands, on March 25, 1944. He received the M.Sc. degree from Delft University in 1969, and the Ph.D. degree from Leiden University, The Netherlands, in 1972, both in physics.

He was with Philips Research Laboratories, Eindhoven, The Netherlands, as a member of the Gaseous Electronics Group from 1972 to 1978. From 1978 to 1987, he worked as a clinical physicist at St. Joseph Hospital, Eindhoven. He was on leave during 1984–1985 and joined A. J. Welch's research group at The University of Texas at Austin supervising various projects on laser applications in medicine. Since July 1987, he has been working as director of the Experimental Laser Unit of the Academic Medical Centre, University of Amsterdam, The Netherlands.

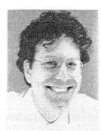

Steven L. Jacques was born in Spokane, WA, in 1950. He received the B.S. degree in biochemistry from Massachusetts Institute of Technology, Cambridge, the M.S. degree in electrical engineering, and the Ph.D. degree in biophysics, both from the University of California, Berkeley.

He worked for five years at the Wellman Laboratory for Photomedicine, Massachusetts General Hospital, Boston, MA, and attained the rank of Instructor in Dermatology (Biomedical Engineering) at Harvard Medical School. He now is Director of the Laser Biology Research Laboratory and Assistant Professor of Urology at the University of Texas M.D. Anderson Cancer Center, Houston.

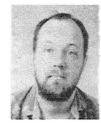

H. J. C. M. Sterenborg received the M. S. degree in physics at the Eindhoven University of Technology in 1982 and the Ph.D. degree from the Rijks Universiteit Utrecht in 1987. His Ph.D. work concerned the action spectrum of UV-carcinogenesis.

Currently he is working at the Laser Centre of the Academic Hospital of the University of Amsterdam. His present research interests are tissue optics, laser diagnostics, lithotripsy, and photodynamic therapy.

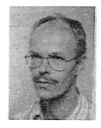

W. M. Star received the Ph.D. degree in low temperature solid state physics in 1971 from the University of Leiden. He did postdoctoral research at the Francis Bitter National Magnet Laboratory of MIT, Cambridge, MA.

Since 1974 he has been a clinical physicist in radiotherapy at the Dr. Daniel den Hoed Cancer Center in Rotterdam, The Netherlands. Since 1979 he has become increasingly involved in research on Photodynamic Therapy and tumor imaging with exogeneous photosensitizers. This includes animal studies, light delivery, and light dosimetry and clinical applications.

Reprinted with permission from *Applied Optics,* Vol. 28(12), pp. 2318-2324
(June 15, 1989). ©1989 Optical Society of America.

Extinction and absorption coefficients and scattering phase functions of human tissues *in vitro*

Renato Marchesini, A. Bertoni, S. Andreola, E. Melloni, and A. E. Sichirollo

Optical properties of different human tissues *in vitro* have been evaluated by measuring extinction and absorption coefficients at 635- and 515-nm wavelengths and a scattering angular dependence at 635 nm. Extinction was determined by the on-axis attenuation of light transmitted through sliced specimens of various thicknesses. The absorption coefficient was determined by placing samples into an integrating sphere. The Henyey-Greenstein function was used for fitting experimental data of the scattering pattern. The purpose of this work was to contribute to the study of light propagation in mammalian tissues. The results show that, for the investigated tissues, extinction coefficients range from ~200 to 500 cm^{-1} whereas absorption coefficients, depending on wavelength, vary from 0.2 to 25 cm^{-1}. Scattering is forward peaked with an average cosine of ~0.7.

I. Introduction

Much effort is being made in the study of light propagation in tissue due to the development and wide use of lasers for surgical and therapeutic applications. In particular, in photodynamic therapy (PDT)[1,2] treatment effectiveness is greatly influenced by photosensitizer content and light distribution in the irradiated tissue, and an accurate evaluation of energy fluence in depth should allow an estimate of whether the whole tumor mass will be properly irradiated.

To evaluate light flux in depth within a medium, two different approaches could be assayed: (1) direct measurements with a suitable probe[3] or (2) external description by means of theoretical models.[2,4,5] Unfortunately both methods could give unreliable results. The direct *in situ* measurement needs light detectors whose insertion into tissue does not alter flux distribution and whose response does not depend on the direction of incoming light. Optical probes fulfilling those requirements have not yet been fully developed. At present, an optical fiber embedded in a bulb of light-diffusing material is being used as an isotropic probe.[3,6]

Different approaches to solve the theoretical models have been proposed. Some of them are refined versions of the widely used Kubelka-Munk two-flux mod-

el,[7] others derive from transfer theory where the transport equation[8] is solved in particular boundary conditions. Finally, a different way to face the problem is the use of Monte Carlo methods to trace the fate of individual photons.[9]

In any case, for the evaluation of energy fluence rate inside a medium, optical characteristics of the irradiated material have to be known, namely, absorption and scattering coefficients and single scattering angular distribution (i.e., the phase function). In recent years, efforts to determine the optical properties of various human and animal tissues have produced much experimental data.[2] Nevertheless, agreement between the results is rarely found, since in most cases the optical parameters were not measured in a direct way but evaluated from measurements of transmittance and reflectance and following different light propagation models. The great issue related to the latter approach is the accuracy of the results obtained by the chosen model, which could be strongly dependent on the geometry of irradiation, the phase function of the medium, and the uniqueness of light propagation equation solutions. For example, scattering by mammalian tissue has been considered to be isotropic, whereas recently reported data suggest that a strongly forward component is present.[10,11]

The aim of this work was to contribute to the knowledge of optical characteristics of human tissues. To overcome the previous mentioned drawbacks, we used experimental methods which allowed direct determination of the tissues' optical properties, namely, the extinction coefficient, the absorption coefficient, and single scattering angular distribution. Measurements were performed in part at 635-nm and in part at 515-

The authors are with National Institute of Tumors, 1 via Venezian, 20133 Milan, Italy.

Received 4 November 1988.

0003-6935/89/122318-07$02.00/0.

nm wavelengths by using an argon and an argon-dye laser.

II. Materials and Methods

A. Tissue Preparation

Nontumoral human tissues obtained from breast (skin and underlying layers), lung (parenchymatous tissue), liver, uterus (smooth muscle of the inner wall), dermis (from the leg), and muscle (striated) were cut with a microtome from different frozen samples. Skin of the breast and dermis was cut parallel to the surface, and striated muscle was cut perpendicularly to the fibers. The sliced samples, with thicknesses from 20 to 100 μm and an area of $\sim$1 cm^2, were hydrated with saline to prevent loss of moisture and sealed between two optical grade glasses. Optical properties of samples thus prepared have been observed to remain unaffected for at least 24 h. A dummy sample made by sealing a drop of saline between two glasses was used for background correction.

B. Extinction Measurement

Figure 1 shows a scheme of the optical system for measuring extinction. The correctness of Beer's law was assumed for very thin sections of material, i.e., the strict proportionality between $\ln(I/I_0)$ and the extinction defined as the sum of scattering and absorption. An argon or argon-pumped dye laser was used. The light beam was delivered through an optical fiber, collimated, and split to monitor continuously the power of the incident beam. The beam size was kept much smaller than the sample area to prevent side effects but large enough to avoid that microstructures or small holes in the tissue would affect light transmission measurement. The photodiode viewing angle was 8×10^{-5} sr.

C. Absorption Measurement

Figure 2 shows the arrangement to measure absorption. The laser beam was delivered in an identical way as that used for extinction measurement. The sample and light-diffuser disk used as a standard were properly positioned into an integrating sphere, 125 mm in diameter. With this 4π geometry arrangement, only one measurement is made to determine the amount R_0, thereafter called the true reflectance, which represents the sum of the transmittance T and reflectance R.[12]

The integrating sphere was operated in a comparison mode. According to theories of the integrating sphere formulated by Jacquez and Kuppenheim[13] and Goebel,[14] the ratio F_s/F_{st} of the signals being measured when the primary beam is incident on the sample F_s or switched to the standard F_{st} can be related to the absorbance A. The flux $F_t(i)$ incident on a generical area a_i (e.g., the exit port) with reflectance r_i is defined as

$$F_t(i) = P_0 f_i r_t \bigg/ \left[1 - r_w\left(1 - \sum_0^m f_1\right) - \sum_0^m r_i f_i \right], \qquad (1)$$

where P_0 is the flux initially incident on the target, f_i is

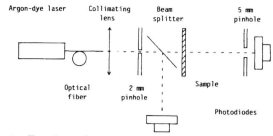

Fig. 1. Experimental arrangement for measuring on-axis light attenuation. The distance from the sample to the 5-mm diam pinhole is 1 m. The photodiode at 90° with respect to the light beam was used for normalizing attenuation readings.

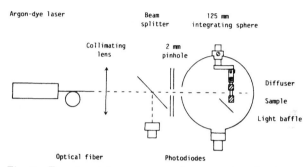

Fig. 2. Experimental arrangement for measuring absorbance. Sample and diffuser can simultaneously slide orthogonally to the laser beam.

the ratio between the generical area a_i and the sphere total area, r_t is the fraction of the unabsorbed flux in the sphere after primary beam interaction with a target having area f_0, and r_w is the coating reflectance of the sphere wall.

The term

$$r_w\left(1 - \sum_0^m f_i\right) + \sum_0^m r_i f_i$$

is the average reflectance $\bar{r}_w$ of the sphere. Since $\bar{r}_w$ remains practically unchanged when the sample or the standard is directly irradiated, it follows that[13]

$$F_s(i)/F_{st}(i) = r_s/r_{st}, \qquad (2)$$

when the sample (with reflectance r_s) and the standard (with reflectance r_{st}) reflected in a perfectly diffuse manner, and

$$F_s(i)/F_{st}(i) = \bar{r}_w r_s/r_{st}, \qquad (3)$$

when the sample has specular components. Since our specimens are neither perfectly diffusing nor specular, the maximum relative error in determining r_s is given by $1 - \bar{r}_w$.

The integrating sphere, formed by two half hemispheres, was provided with four ports located on the horizontal equator at 0, 90, 180, and 270°. The 0° entrance port has a diameter of 0.3 cm, (0.125 in.), and the others are 1.27 cm (0.5 in.) in diameter. The 180° port was closed with a port-plug coated with the same coating (i.e., barium sulfate) applied to the sphere

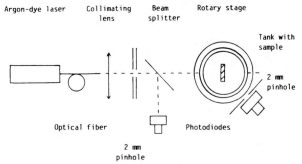

Argon-dye laser   Collimating   Beam   Rotary stage
lens   splitter

Tank with
sample

2 mm
pinhole

Optical fiber   Photodiodes

2 mm
pinhole

Fig. 3.   Experimental arrangement for measuring scattering angular dependence.

surface. The remaining ports were used for locating a photodiode (4-mm diam active area) and the holder for supporting the standard and sample. The holder consisted of Perspex rods which were assembled so as to obtain 3 degrees of freedom for properly positioning the targets. The baffle assured that the radiation did not reach the detector without undergoing multiple reflections. Measurement of the flux passing through the photocell aperture determined with the aid of Eq. (1) a wall reflectance of 0.92 at the employed wavelengths. Introduction of the target holder reduced the sphere average reflectance to 0.89. The additional insertion of the light diffuser did not further alter flux reading; thus a reflectance value close to 1 was assumed for the diffuser standard.

Since in the 4π geometry both the transmitted and reflected fractions of light flux from the sample contribute to diffuse illumination, we may identify reflectance r_s with the true reflectance R_0, and from the conservation of energy it follows that the absorbance A_s can be expressed as

$$A_s = 1 - r_s = 1 - k(F_s/F_{st}). \qquad (4)$$

In our case, by assuming $k = 1$, measurements should be affected by a maximum error of ~11%. The absorption coefficient can then be evaluated by dividing A_s by the optical path length.

D.   Scattering Angular Distribution Measurement

The experimental arrangement for measuring the angular dependence $P(\cos\theta)$ of light scattered by tissue sample is shown in Fig. 3. The laser beam was delivered as above. The sample was positioned at the center of a 20-cm diam cylindrical tank filled with distilled water. A photodiode, with 1-cm^2 active area, was mounted on the rotary stage, which was manually rotated around the sample. A 2-mm diam pinhole restrained the measured scattered light within 2×10^{-4} sr. The measurements were performed at angles between 5 and 45° and from 135 to 150° with the sample fixed at 90° with respect to the laser beam. For the intermediate angles, the sample was rotated at 45°. No azimuthal φ angle dependence of scattering was assumed. Refraction effects due to the tissue–glass–water interfaces were not taken into account for we considered the tissue refractive index close to that of

water.[15] To minimize the multiple scattering effect, samples with a thickness of 25 μm were used. Scattering due to the dummy sample was insignificant with respect to that of tissue; thus this background was not considered. To describe conveniently $P(\cos\theta)$ data by an analytical expression and to fill the gap of the data near 0 and 180°, experimental results were fitted with the Henyey-Greenstein $g_{H\text{-}G}$ function. That function has been used to describe light scattering[16] and characterize a phase function

$$p(\cos\theta) = (1 - g^2)/(1 + g^2 - 2g\cos\theta)^{3/2}, \qquad (5)$$

where g is the average cosine of scattering.

III.   Results

Typical on-axis attenuation results for liver, lung, and uterus are reported in Fig. 4. Data refer to samples from four different subjects, and the values are the means of at least three measurements at different sites on each specimen. A least-squares fit to the data from each separate sample showed a nearly perfect linear relationship, thus indicating the validity of Beer's law at least for those thicknesses. Each least-squares fit had a regression coefficient of >0.95. Great variability was found from subject to subject as indicated by the different slopes of the data. The extinction coefficient was evaluated by averaging the individual slopes. Experimental values of attenuation coefficients of the remaining tissues are reported in Table I.

Figure 5 reports experimental measurements of the absorbance of three different tissues. Data are expressed according to Eq. (4) and as a function of sample thickness. The straight lines are the least-squares fits to the data of each different subject. The regression coefficient for each fit was >0.93. The good linear correlation between absorbance and sample thickness allowed us to estimate the absorption coefficient of each sample from the slope of the data fitted lines. It has to be noted that evaluation of the absorption coefficient being performed on the sample thickness rather than on the optical path length gives an overestimate of the actual absorption coefficient value. A Monte Carlo model is being developed to calculate the path length of photons in passing through a thin specimen. Preliminary results show that the path length is ~15–40% longer than sample thickness, being that this correction factor is not linearly dependent on sample thickness.

As in the case of extinction measurements, there was a great variability from subject to subject. The indicated absorption coefficient values in Fig. 5, and in Table I for the other investigated human tissues, were calculated by averaging the slope of all the subjects. As a result of data variability, the standard deviation related to the absorption coefficient evaluation was very high, thus suggesting that any theoretical correction being applied [i.e., Eq. (2) or (3)] should have only minimal relevance. The result obtained for breast samples (<0.2 cm^{-1}) should be considered only as indicative, since in our experimental conditions the minimum detectable relative difference of photodiode

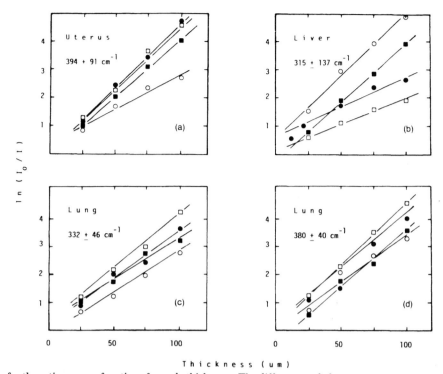

Fig. 4. Attenuation for three tissues as a function of sample thickness. The different symbols represent measurements from specimens of different subjects. Each datum is the mean of at least three measurements at different sites of each sample. The straight lines are the least squares fits for each subject. The extinction coefficient was evaluated by averaging the individual slopes: (a)–(c) attentuation at 635 nm; (d) attenuation at 515 nm.

readings (i.e., $1 - F_s/F_{st}$) was within the noise fluctuation ($\pm 10^{-3}$).

The scattering coefficient was evaluated by simply averaging the differences between extinction and absorption coefficients, which were calculated from the individual subjects. The corresponding values are reported in Table I.

The results of the scattering phase function for liver, lung, and uterus are shown in Fig. 6. Measurements were performed at 635 nm. For each tissue two separate subjects were used. A linear combination of two Henyey-Greenstein functions was used to fit and normalize experimental data. Fitting results (solid lines in Fig. 6) indicated that tissue scattering may be well described by a superimposition of two $g_{\text{H-G}}$ phase functions, one characterized by a forward-directed scattering component and the other by a backward-directed component, with the main contribution due to the former. The resulting average cosine of scattering (Table I) was nearly the same (~0.7) for the three tissues. The scattering diagram for the remaining tissues was not measured.

IV. Discussion

To our knowledge, very few complete-set data on optical characteristics of human tissues have been established. As a consequence, comparison between our results and those previously reported has been

Table I.   Experimental Values of Tissue Optical Parameters

Tissue	Wavelength (nm)	Extinction coeff. (cm^{-1}) ± SD	Absorption coeff. (cm^{-1}) ± SD	Scattering coeff. (cm^{-1}) ± SD	Average cosine $\bar{g}$
Breast	635	395 ± 35	<0.2	395 ± 35	
Dermis	635	246 ± 21	1.8 ± 0.2	244 ± 21	
Liver	635	315 ± 137	2.3 ± 1.0	313 ± 136	0.68
	515	304 ± 21	18.9 ± 1.7	285 ± 20	
Lung	635	332 ± 46	8.1 ± 2.8	324 ± 46	0.75
	515	380 ± 40	25.5 ± 3.0	356 ± 39	
Muscle	515	541 ± 45	11.2 ± 1.8	530 ± 44	
Uterus	635	394 ± 91	0.35 ± 0.1	394 ± 91	0.69

395 ± 137

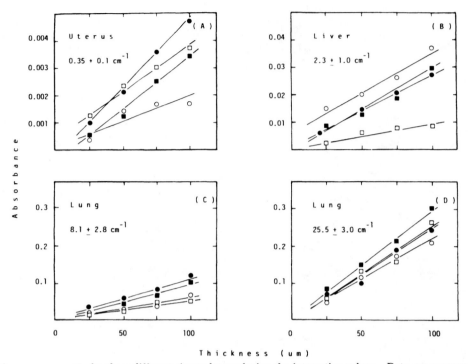

Fig. 5. Absorption measurements for three different tissues by employing the integrating sphere. Data are expressed as the relative difference between the readings when the primary beam is incident on the standard (Fst) or the sample (Fs) for different thicknesses. The different symbols represent measurements from specimens of different subjects. The straight lines are the least-squares fit for each subject. The absorption coefficient was evaluated by averaging the individual slopes. (A)–(C) measurements at 635; (D) measurements at 515 nm.

necessarily limited or extended to similar mammalian tissues or based on extrapolation of other optical properties, like the effective attenuation coefficient Σ_{eff}, which is the most frequently reported. From Ref. 2, Σ_{eff} is defined as

$$\Sigma_{eff} = [3(\Sigma_a)^2 + 3\Sigma_a\Sigma_s(1-g)]^{1/2} \qquad (6)$$

where Σ_a and Σ_s are the absorption and scattering coefficients, respectively, and g is the average cosine of scattering.

Attenuation measurement results obtained in the narrow beam geometry confirm that soft mammalian tissues are characterized by an extinction coefficient at 630 nm in the range of hundreds of cm^{-1}, as recently reported by Jacques et al.[15] for human dermis (190 cm^{-1}) and Flock et al.[11] for chicken (345 cm^{-1}) and bovine muscle (328 cm^{-1}). At 515 nm there is no evidence due to great subject to subject variability of a substantially different extinction value except due to absorption. The good straight-line fit to the data suggests that multiple scattering events have not been detected in our experimental conditions. Actually, the mean free path is in the range of 20–50 μm (which is of the order of magnitude of cell diameter), so that in the 100-μm sample thickness from two to five scattering events do occur.

For breast tissue we found an extinction coefficient of 395 cm^{-1}, which is very close to the 25-μm mean free path (at 700 nm) reported by Crilly.[17] For human dermis, we measured 246 cm^{-1}, while Jacques et al.[15] and Jacques and Prahl[10] reported values of 187 cm^{-1} for human and 280 cm^{-1} for mouse dermis (at 488 nm), respectively. In the optical properties the table reported in the review article by Wilson and Patterson,[2] extinction coefficient values of 65 and 18 cm^{-1} are ascribed to human dermis at 630 nm. Our coefficient for human muscle, i.e., 541 cm^{-1} at 515 nm, is close to that reported by Flock et al.[11] for chicken and bovine muscle, whereas in Table 3 from Ref. 2, 4.1 and 8.3 cm^{-1} were, respectively, reported. For liver and lung only Σ_{eff} values were available from the literature. Values ranging from 8.1 to 13 cm^{-1} for liver and 11 cm^{-1} for human lung were reported.[2] By applying Eq. (6) to our data, Σ_{eff} values of 26.6 and 46.5 cm^{-1} (at 635 nm) were, respectively, evaluated for liver and lung. Comparison with data on the uterus can generally be made from results reported in Ref. 18. Evaluation of light transmission, under the hypothesis that a purely exponential decrease governed by Σ_{eff} (i.e., Beer's law) should exist, shows that 50% is transmitted after a thickness of the uterine wall of 0.6 mm. This value is

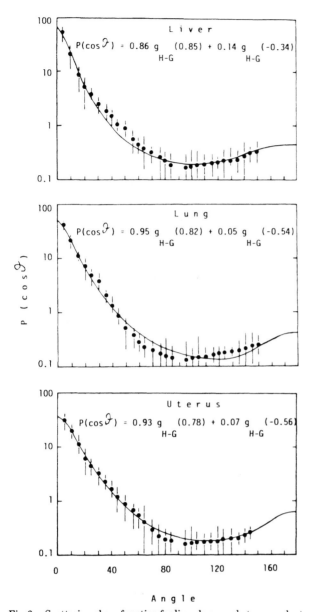

Fig. 6. Scattering phase function for liver, lung, and uterus evaluated at 635 nm. Experimental points have been fitted and normalized by using a linear combination of two Henyey-Greenstein functions. The solid line represents the fitting results.

reasonably comparable with the 28 and 36% transmissions measured in mammalian uterus.

Absorption measurements evidenced a large variation from tissue to tissue of the absorption coefficient values ranging from <0.2 to 25 cm^{-1}. This fact is easily explainable due to the different blood content which still remained in the sliced samples. By using a conventional spectrophotometer, transmittance measurements performed on the most vascularized samples (e.g., liver and lung) indicated the presence of two prominent shoulders at 580 and 420 nm, which are the typical absorbing wavelengths of hemoglobin. In the

case of human dermis, the only available comparable tissue, the evaluated absorption coefficient is between those reported by other authors (from 1 to 5 cm^{-1}).[2,15]

Although the linearity showed by absorbance data vs sample thickness can, in the first approximation, justify evaluation of the absorption coefficient from the straight-line slope, the actual path length of primary photons in passing through sample remains undetermined. From scattering angular dependence measurements, the average cosine of scattering was evaluated in ~0.7. This means that the average path length of photons will be somewhat more than sample thickness, and consequently the absorption coefficient should decrease by the same amount. Thus the overall uncertainties in performing an absorption direct measurement approach and the great variability of samples from subject to subject make it difficult to evaluate the absorption coefficient with great accuracy. However, integrating sphere in-cavity measurements[19] make it possible to estimate reasonably the absorption coefficient of samples with a large scattering coefficient.

Scattering angular distribution measurements have shown that human soft tissue is characterized by a nonisotropic scattering pattern. Nevertheless, our $\bar{g}$ values are somewhat lower than those recently reported for dermis (0.82)[15] and muscle (0.96).[11] Under the hypotheses that cells and their internal structures can be approximated by spherical particles and that the main contribution to scattering is due to the cell envelope, it follows that the diffraction peak due to human tissue cells, which are >7 μm, was not included in the scattering measurement. To consider the diffraction peak as part of scattered light, $\bar{g}$ should be replaced by $g' = \frac{1}{2}(1 + \bar{g})$. In this case, g' increases to 0.85. To evaluate further whether tissue scattering measurements were somehow consistent with other reported data, the scattering phase function of a 1% solution of human blood was determined. Results, not shown, evidenced that scattering was characterized by a $\bar{g}$ value of 0.845 corresponding to a g' of 0.92. This result is in reasonable agreement with that reported by Flock et al.[11] and Steinke and Shepherd,[20] considering that the measurement is strongly dependent by experimental arrangement and physiological conditions.[20]

Our evaluated extinction coefficients are in reasonable agreement with those reported by other authors who employed similar direct methods for attenuation measurement, whereas they are ~1 order of magnitude greater than those evaluated by indirect methods, e.g., derived from transmittance and reflectance measurements, or by using a collimated optical fiber coupled to a photodetector to evaluate the decrease in light flux with depth for in situ measurements.[21] The possible explanations are related to the fact that, in the case of implanted fiber, probe angular response was not perfectly matched to the tissue scattering pattern, e.g., the N.A. of optical fiber was not small enough to reject all the forward scattered light, or that theoretical models used to evaluate optical parameters from reflectance and transmittance measurements were not directly pertinent to the geometry of irradiation or to the scattering pattern, as Welch et al.[4] have pointed out.

V. Conclusions

Although the method we employed is not applicable *in vivo*, the different optical parameters of several human tissues have been evaluated at least as far as the order of magnitude is concerned. The great variability in our experimental data and the investigation performed at only two wavelengths do not allow us to stress either the trend of optical parameters in a function of wavelengths or that human tissues can be characterized by precisely defined constants. Whereas it is reasonable to assume that the scattering coefficient and scattering phase function are only slightly dependent on wavelengths in the visible range, this is not true for the absorption coefficient, since tissue blood content and/or specific absorbing pigments play the main role in determining tissue characteristics. This fact should be kept in consideration while performing the evaluation of light flux distribution in depth. Since space irradiance is greatly dependent on albedo, especially for values close to 1 (as human tissues have), a small variation in the absorption coefficient value could result in a great modification of the light propagation pattern. More effort should, therefore, be made to determine more precisely the absorption coefficient and how it is related to blood flow content.

This work was partially supported by grant 87.01591.44 from the Consiglio Nazionale delle Ricerche, Rome, Italy.

References

1. T. J. Dougherty, "Photodynamic Therapy (PDT) of Malignant Tumors," CRC Crit. Rev. Oncol. Hematol. **2**, 83–115 (1984).
2. B. C. Wilson and M. S. Patterson, "The Physics of Photodynamic Therapy," Phys. Med. Biol. **31**, 327–360 (1986).
3. J. P. A. Marijnissen and W. M. Star, "Quantitative Light Dosimetry In Vitro and In Vivo," Lasers Med. Sci. **2**, 235–242 (1987).
4. A. J. Welch, G. Yoon, and M. J. C. van Gemert, "Practical Models for Light Distribution in Laser-Irradiated Tissue," Lasers Surg. Med. **6**, 488–493 (1987).
5. W. M. Star, J. P. A. Marijnissen, and M. J. C. van Gemert, "Light Dosimetry in Optical Phantoms and in Tissues. 1: Multiple Flux and Transport Theory," Phys. Med. Biol. **33**, 437–454 (1988).
6. A. L. McKenzie, "Can Diffusion be Assumed in Correcting for Oblique Incidence in Laser Photodynamic Therapy?," Phys. Med. Biol. **31**, 285–290 (1986).
7. P. Kubelka, "New Contributions to the Optics of Intensely Light Scattering Material. Part I," J. Opt. Soc. Am. **38**, 448–457 (1948).
8. S. Chandrasekhar, *Radiative Transfer* (Dover, New York, 1960).
9. B. C. Wilson and G. Adam, "A Monte Carlo Model for the Absorption and Flux Distributions of Light in Tissue," Med. Phys. **10**, 824–830 (1983).
10. S. L. Jacques and S. A. Prahl, "Modelling Optical and Thermal Distributions in Tissue During Laser Irradiation," Lasers Surg. Med. **6**, 494–503 (1987).
11. S. T. Flock, B. C. Wilson, and M. S. Patterson, "Total Attenuation Coefficients and Scattering Phase Functions of Tissues and Phantom Materials at 633 nm," Med. Phys. **14**, 835–841 (1987).
12. F. Grum and R. J. Becherer, *Optical Radiation Measurement Vol. 1, Radiometry* (Academic, Orlando, 1979), pp. 292–293.
13. J. A. Jacquez and H. F. Kuppenheim, "Theory of the Integrating Sphere," J. Opt. Soc. Am. **45**, 460–470 (1955).
14. D. G. Goebel, "Generalized Integrating-Sphere Theory," Appl. Opt. **6**, 125–128 (1967).
15. S. L. Jacques, C. A. Alter, and S. A. Prahl, "Angular Dependence of He–Ne Laser Light Scattering by Human Dermis," Lasers Med. Sci. **1**, 309–333 (1987).
16. H. C. van de Hulst, *Multiple Light Scattering: Tables, Formulas, and Applications. Vol. 2* (Academic, New York, 1980), pp. 303–330.
17. R. Crilly, "A Study of the Optical Properties of Soft Tissue in the Near Infra-Red," 1986 AAPM Annual Meeting, Abstract, Med. Phys. **13**, 603 (1986).
18. S. L. Jacques, D. R. Weaver, and S. M. Reppert, "Penetration of Light into the Uterus of Pregnant Mammals," Photochem. Photobiol. **45**, 637–641 (1987).
19. P. Elterman, "Integrating Cavity Spectroscopy," Appl. Opt. **9**, 2140–2142 (1970).
20. J. M. Steinke and A. P. Shepherd, "Comparison of Mie Theory and the Light Scattering of Red Blood Cells," Appl. Opt. **27**, 4027–4033 (1988).
21. J. P. A. Marijnissen and W. M. Star, "Phantom Measurements for Light Dosimetry using Isotropic and Small Aperture Detectors," in *Porphyrin Localization and Treatment of Tumors* D. R. Doiron and C. J. Gomer, Eds. (Alan R. Liss, New York, 1984), pp. 133–148.

Reprinted with permission from *Applied Optics,* Vol. 28(12), pp. 2297-2303
(June 15, 1989). ©1989 Optical Society of America.

Refractive index of some mammalian tissues using a fiber optic cladding method

Frank P. Bolin, Luther E. Preuss, Roy C. Taylor, and Robert J. Ference

The index of refraction n of the many mammalian tissues is an important but somewhat neglected optical constant. Archival and oral papers have quoted the use of values of n for tissue generally ranging from 1.35 to 1.55. However, these values are frequently without experimental basis. They have arbitrarily used values near that of water, which is a major component of mammalian tissue, or have calculated a theoretical n from the weighted elemental composition of tissue. Since these values have not been precise and little information is available on specific indices for each tissue, a study was undertaken to develop a simple, rapid, and reliable method for the experimental determination of n. This was done using the ubiquitous quartz optical fiber. By substituting the usual cladding found on commercial quartz optics by the tissue in question and utilizing the principle of internal reflection, the value of n for the specific tissue can be calculated. This is done by utilizing the known indices for air and quartz and measuring the angle of the emergent cone of light from the output of the optical fiber. A number of indices for mammalian tissue (bovine, porcine, canine, and human) have been determined at 632.8 nm. With few exceptions, for tissues at this wavelength, n was in the 1.38–1.41 range. The species type did not appear to be a factor. Bovine muscle showed normal dispersion characteristics through the visible wavelengths. The denaturation of tissue was shown to alter significantly the refractive index.

I. Introduction

The optical properties of human tissues have assumed increased importance in the past decade due to the growing application of light in medicine and surgery. The laser is a ubiquitous tool for the surgeon, and both coherent and incoherent light is extensively used in treatment and diagnosis.

Optical properties of tissue such as reflection, scattering, and absorption coefficients, scattering phase functions, and irradiance levels (light dosage) at tissue depth are under active investigation. These are important quantities necessary to describe the transport and intensity of light through tissue. Despite the fact that the index of refraction for individual tissues enters into important determinations of reflectivity, angular change in beam direction at tissue interfaces, or into an optical fiber detector's acceptance angle in tissue, little experimental attention has been granted to the measurement of each tissue's index of refraction (n).

A striking paucity of archival reports exists on the measurement methods for n in tissues. For that matter, specific values of n are lacking for most mammalian tissues. A few authors have quoted values of n but frequently without attribution. Values given generally range from the n for water (presumably chosen because it is the major constituent of tissue) to indices slightly higher than 1.500. The lack of measurement reports for tissue n is due to its daunting optical characteristics, which render nonapplicable the use of the traditional physical methods for the experimental determination of the index. Tissue samples are optically turbid, highly scattering, nonhomogeneous, plastic, and changing during extended *in vitro* assay (e.g., desiccating or leaking fluids). The standard physical methods used for transparent, or translucent solids and liquids, which depend on the assay of refraction angles at plane-parallel interfaces, prismatic dispersion, interferometry, and light velocity determinations, among others, are not practical with this difficult material.

The aim of this study was to develop and test a device which would provide the index for various tissue samples. The criteria chosen were that assay would be rapid, use a small sample, be simple mechanically, optically, and electronically, utilize ordinary devices found at the tissue optic's bench, use no complex mathematical analysis, and be simple in calibration.

The authors are with Henry Ford Hospital, Department of Radiation Oncology, Radiation Physics Research Laboratory, 2799 West Grand Boulevard, Detroit, Michigan 48202.

Received 15 December 1988.
0003-6935/89/122297-07$02.00/0.
© 1989 Optical Society of America.

The literature describes methods which may be adapted for the determination of tissue n. Fresnel reflection methods are especially useful.[1] Meyer and Eesley[2] have used the internal Fresnel reflection principle in studies on liquids during their solidification and have successfully followed the change in n during the phase change. Their system determines n below and above the fiber core's index by measuring the backreflected beam in the optical fiber. It requires a high level of sophisticated instrumentation. Thung et al.[3] have determined n of various liquids using the principle of optical frequency reflectometry and light response in a bent optical fiber. Takeo and Hattori[4] have also used a bent fiber system for index measurements in opaque liquids. Kumar et al.[5] developed a multimode tapered optical fiber as a sensing element. This technique measured n at values below that of the core. Leupacker and Penzkofer[6] and Lu and Penzkofer[7] reported the measurement of n in highly absorbing dyes and other opaque liquids, utilizing the Fresnel reflection principle. All involve complex assembly of optical devices using the reflection at the air–surface interface to calculate n. The last two methods do not depend on the use of optical fibers. None meets the criteria which we set up: simplicity of operation and instrumentation as well as low cost.

II. Methods

The method which was developed rests on a simple concept: that the cone of light issuing from an optical fiber is dependent on the indices of the cladding material, quartz, and air into which the cone of light emerges. The commercial cladding on a 1000-μm optical fiber is stripped from the fiber, and the tissue for which the index is to be measured is substituted for the cladding. With the index for air and the quartz fiber known, and the emitted angular light distribution measured at the optical fibers' output, the expression for the fiber's numerical aperture can be used to solve for tissue n utilizing the expression[8]

$$n_s = \mathrm{SQR}\{n_q^2 - [n_0 \sin(\theta)]^2\},\qquad(1)$$

where θ is the half-angle of the emergent cone, n_q is the optical fiber's index, n_s is the index of refraction for the tissue, n_0 is the index of refraction for air. The method requires (for a given instrumental setup) calibration against material of a known index. The calibration is required to establish the fractional peak height position at which the emergent cone angle θ is measured.

The use of Eq. (1) requires the validity of geometrical optics in this system. In addition, for this equation to yield proper results, it is necessary that the mode volume of the fiber be filled. A highly efficient diffuser is used to accomplish this. The use of a large diameter optical fiber ensures that geometrical optics can be applied to this situation. The use of very small fibers (diameter of $\lesssim 5$ μm) would severely limit the modes of light which could propagate through the fiber. In that case, the output intensity would consist of a number of overlapping peaks, and measurement could be severely position dependent. In addition, a significant portion of the power could be propagated through the clad-

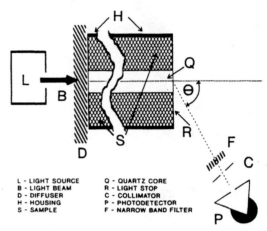

Fig. 1. Schematic of experimental setup for determining index of refraction. A bare quartz fiber is placed in a cladding of substance to be measured. The angular light output distribution is measured, and the index is determined from mathematical laws relating to refractive indices.

ding. The fiber diameter below which electromagnetic waveguide theory must be applied is an order of magnitude below 5 μm.[9]

These problems are avoided by the use of a moderately large diameter fiber. With the larger fiber the number of free-space modes N accepted by the fiber is

$$N \approx 2a^2\pi^2(n1^2 - n2^2)/\lambda^2,\qquad(2)$$

where a is the fiber diameter, λ is the wavelength, and $n1$ and $n2$ are the indices of the core and cladding.[10] With 633-nm light, the number of modes supported by the fiber is ~1.9×10^6 for tissue cladding. The average fractional power propagated through the cladding is

$$P_2/P = 4N^{-1/2}/3,\qquad(3)$$

where P_2 is the power transported in the core, P is the total power, and N is the number of free-space modes.[11] From the above numbers we see that this works out to an approximate fractional value of 0.001. These numbers justify the geometric approach used in the method presented here.

A schematic of the device is given in Fig. 1. The light source L can be a laser or incandescent source. A Jodon 2-mW He–Ne laser, model HN2HF, was used for studies done at 632.8 nm. Narrowband filters F can be used with coherent light sources (Oriel Corp. interference filters with a 10-nm bandwidth at half-height). The optical fiber Q is Quartz Products 1000-μm fused quartz core model PCS1000W $n = 1.457$ at 630 nm. The fiber length was 10 cm. Light diffusion is accomplished at D (Oriel Corp. true Lambertian opal glass diffuser model 48020). There is no optical coupling between the diffuser plate and optical fiber. The end cleaved fibers are polished to a 300-nm finish by standard techniques. Silicon stripper model P/N45-14, General Fiberoptics, was used to remove the cladding. The optic and tissue sample S are housed concentrically, as shown, in a blackened cylindrical tube H with thin lighttight closures R at each end through which the optic protrudes. The polished ends are coincident with the closure surface. This system is aligned on a central axis as shown. We found that good results may be obtained with modest instrumental fabrication and ordinary care in maintaining the optical axis. The dispersion angle of the emitted light is read by a collimated detector P', mounted on a goniometer. The detector collimator aperture was 1 mm. A Hamamatsu model R928 PMT with a response from 185 to 930 nm or an Oriel Corp. model 70 radiometer/photometer is used. The goniometer table allows 1° increments with 6' of accuracy. The detector may be swung through a 90° arc on either side of the system central axis.

The light cone exiting from the optical fiber does not exhibit a sharp cutoff. Thus the measurement is arbitrary and will be dependent on the device geometry. Figure 2 is a plot of the light dispersion from an optical fiber for which the cladding is fresh whole human blood, done in the setup described in Fig. 1 using 632.8-nm laser light. The lack of a sharp cutoff is evident and points out the fact that before measuring tissue or unknowns, it was first necessary to determine the proper method of establishing θ. Similar fiber output curves were found at other wavelengths across the spectrum from 400 to 700 nm. This departure from a sharp cutoff profile was not unexpected. It is known, for example, that diffraction, striae, and surface irregularities can affect the N.A. of the fiber.[12] In practice, the working N.A. is often taken to be defined by the position where the output profile falls to 50% (or other arbitrary criterion figure) of its maximum value.[13] Another consideration is the effect of skew rays. These are rays whose passage through the fiber is not restricted to a single plane. The effect of these rays is to broaden the output profile predicted by Eq. (1). One set of experimental and theoretical data on skew rays reported by Allan shows a broadened profile somewhat similar to those we observed.[14]

Since the output from the optical fiber was Gaussianlike (see Fig. 2), the divergence angle was at first arbitrarily defined as full width at half-maximum (FWHM) of the profile of the light beam. In this case, θ is then established as the angle fixed by one-half of that full width value. However, since this fixing of θ is arbitrary, it might not have given the proper results when used to determine the index. Hence the following calibration procedure was undertaken:

(a) A series of standards of known indices, sucrose solutions, were used as the cladding on a quartz fiber.

(b) The angular output profile of the divergent light was measured.

(c) A quadratic curve of the form $A\theta^2 + B\theta + C = \ln(I_\theta)$ was used to fit the beam profile data, and the curve maximum was determined.

(d) 2θ was calculated from the curve as its profile width on the plot at the following four fractions of peak intensity: $1/2$, $1/e$, $1/e^2$, and $1/e^3$.

(e) The refractive index of each sucrose solution was calculated from Eq. (1) using each of the four values of θ.

(f) The resultant value of the refractive index corresponding to each θ value was compared with the known

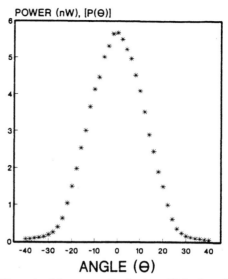

Fig. 2. Example of the output distribution of light through a fiber optic using the setup from Fig. 1. Here human blood is used as the fiber cladding. It is evident that the distribution shows no sharp cutoff but instead assumes an approximately Gaussian form.

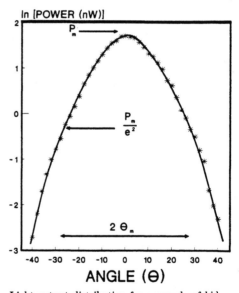

Fig. 3. Light output distribution for a sample of kidney tissue. The value of θ at (peak intensity)/e^2 used in expression (1) obtained for this kidney tissue gives an index value of 1.38 for this sample.

value of index based on the solution concentration level.

For our device design, the optimal measurement position for 2θ was $1/e^2$. Using nine sucrose concentrations, from 0 to 70%, the $1/e^2$ position gave a mean error of 0.2%. This is less than other systematic errors inherent in the calibration. The value $1/e^2$ was used throughout our measurement of n.

Figure 3 is an example of curve fitting done in this study to obtain the value for 2θ. The fraction of the peak height equivalent to $1/e^2$ fit best for our system geometry. However, other fiber lengths and device

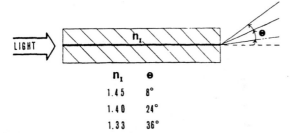

n_1	θ
1.45	8°
1.40	24°
1.33	36°

Fig. 4. Output angle of light from the fiber optic depends on the index of refraction of the cladding as well as the core and surrounding medium. With a quartz core, the output angle in air is shown for several indices associated with biological materials such as water (n_x = 1.330), muscle (n_x = 1.400), and lipid (n_x = 1.45). The range of angle shown provides the measurement system with good sensitivity.

geometries may require a different fraction of peak height to obtain the correct θ value.

The system's sensitivity may be assessed by comparing values of θ in the range of n expected for tissue. If one sets the tissue's lower limit for n at 1.330 (water) and an upper limit of 1.450 (adipose tissue), the corresponding θ values will range from 36 to 8°, a θ range of 28°. This is shown in Fig. 4. With a goniometer positioning accuracy of 6' the sensitivity of the system is thus found to be good.

The use of a short length of fiber (10 cm) provides strength, resistance to bending, and some convenience. However, a question arises as to whether proper mode stripping can be done by this length of fiber. If we assume mode filling by proper use of a diffuser, apply the Fresnel laws of reflection,[15] and use an expression for the number of reflections per unit length of fiber,[16] we can determine whether light which is not totally internally reflected can propagate through the fiber with a resultant broadening of the output pattern. Assuming a core index of 1.457 and a cladding index of 1.41 (tissue), the calculated half-angle θ is ~21.5°. Light entering at greater angles undergoes between twenty-six and thirty reflections with a power reflection coefficient, which is 0.73 at 21.6° but falls rapidly to 0.148 at 24°. The resultant attenuation of these modes is a minimum of −25 dB at 21.6°, falling to −56 dB at 21.7°, and dropping to increasingly low levels as θ increases. This should provide adequate mode stripping for this experimental system.

Although it can be accomplished if great care is taken, it is difficult to place whole tissue in intimate contact about the optical fiber so that it serves as a continuous cladding without damaging the fiber. Tissue homogenization in a moderate speed blender solves this problem. The use of homogenization was resorted to, because on several occasions we noted a change in output pattern when the same tissue sample was more tightly packed. Concern arose, however, as to whether such homogenization alters the index.

Table I summarizes a multisample study in which the twelve samples from a uniform single tissue block were measured individually for n, each in the whole and then in the homogenized state. Average n for the twelve whole tissues was 1.413 and for the same samples, homogenized, was 1.414. The standard deviation was 0.005 for whole tissue and 0.006 for the homogenized sample. Since any difference between the whole and homogenized tissue index was negligible and less than other errors encountered in handling tissue samples, all the index determinations using this method have been carried out with homogenized tissue.

In a test of the method's precision, index determinations were repeated 10 times on a 30% sucrose solution at 590 nm, and ten repeats were also done on a skeletal muscle sample at 630 nm. The average value for n of the sucrose was 1.368 with a standard deviation of 0.0001. The average muscle index was 1.392 with a standard deviation of 0.001.

These repeat experiments required a measurable time period to accomplish. Since the values did not drift during the time of the tissue tests, the precision experiment also shows that the homogenized tissue is not subject to a component segregation around the optic, which would be expected to change the index with time. In any event, there should be little effect from such segregation. Liquid expressed from the homogenate would be a mixture of intracellular and extra cellular fluids, which most probably has an index closely resembling that of the overall tissue.

A further concern is whether homogenization can completely avoid coupling errors. Lack of intimate contact between the tissue cladding and fiber core (as little as a half-wavelength gap) can impair the mode stripping efficiency of the core–cladding system. However, the rapid attenuation of unwanted light (noted above) works in the experimenter's favor. Light rays which encounter an air gap while traveling through the fiber will be totally reflected instead of losing some of their power in transmission. Nevertheless, we estimate that even with as much as 50% of the core contacting air instead of tissue, there should still

Table I. Effects of Homogenization on the Determination of n

Sample	Whole tissue	Homogenized tissue
1	1.416	1.421
2	1.419	1.417
3	1.420	1.410
4	1.409	1.416
5	1.412	1.415
6	1.410	1.414
7	1.416	1.418
8	1.413	1.413
9	1.415	1.403
10	1.416	1.415
11	1.400	1.402
12	1.413	1.415
	n_1 = 1.413	n_2 = 1.414
	s_1 = 0.005	s_2 = 0.006
	N_1 = 12	N_2 = 12

Note: This table shows the results of an experiment designed to determine the effects of tissue homogenization on the index of refraction. Twelve samples from the same block of tissue were measured before and after homogenizing; n_1 and n_2 are the averaged values of the whole and homogenized tissue samples, and s_1 and s_2 are the respective standard deviations. No significant difference was apparent.

be sufficient attenuation of light at unwanted angles. The same consideration holds for light rescattered from the tissue back into the core.

Bending of the fiber can affect the output cone of light. The effect depends on the ratio of the fiber diameter to the radius of curvature.[17] Since the 1000-μm fiber used is rather stiff, we estimate that any bending in our setup would have a minimum radius of ~20 cm. The worst possible effect would be in adipose tissue, where bending of this amount would decrease the θ_{max} by ~0.2°. The homogenized tissue is soft and easily packed. In any case, packing was done carefully to avoid perturbations from such an effect.

III. Results and Discussion

This experimental system was applied to various mammalian tissues from four species: bovine, porcine, canine, and human. It was found that in some cases significant differences occur from the commonly assumed value of ~1.400. The variation in refractive index was considered under four aspects: (a) sample-to-sample variation; (b) differing tissue types; (c) species effect; (d) changes with wavelength. These represent some of the most commonly encountered variants in the tissue optics field. The sample-to-sample variance was estimated for the case of bovine muscle tissue. Seventeen samples were obtained and measured for the index of refraction. Each sample was obtained from a different animal. All were of striated skeletal muscle. Figure 5 presents the results of this experiment in bar graph form. The heavy horizontal line is drawn at the average values, $n = 1.412$. The standard deviation was 0.006. This represents a reasonably small variation for the change between individuals and easily lies within the 1.400–1.410 range, which has been used or assumed by various groups in recent years.

Specimens of various tissue types from several species were obtained and the refractive index measured. Figure 6 summarizes the results. In this figure, note first the relationship between the different tissue types. The one value which stands out is that for adipose tissue, $n = 1.455$. This, although significantly higher than the other values shown here, is reasonable, since its high lipid content brings it into the range of other documented substances of similar composition. For example, the published refractive index of castor oil is 1.477, and that of linseed oil is 1.480.[18] Most of the other tissues measured in the 1.390–1.410 range. Two tissues which tended to have low refractive indices were liver (average 1.380) and lung (1.380 average). Apart from the bovine muscle, only three to seven individual samples (in the case of human, one to two) were measured to obtain the average represented by the bar. Thus there remains some statistical uncertainty as to whether the liver and lung are actually low compared with the other tissue or whether their values can be accounted for by sampling error.

The other aspect to be considered in Fig. 6 is the fact that four different species are represented. In the present state of our experimentation, it appears that no significant species variation can be seen. For example, human kidney has the highest nonadipose val-

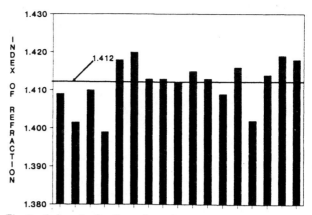

Fig. 5. Index of refraction values of seventeen samples of bovine striated muscle. Samples represent tissue from individual animals. The average, 1.412, is indicated by the horizontal line. The standard deviation was 0.006.

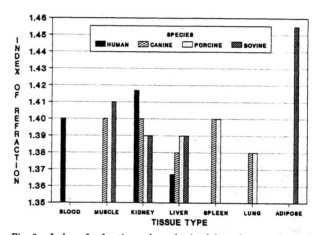

Fig. 6. Index of refraction values obtained from four species and various tissues. The values represent averages of between three and seven trials. The human tissue values represent one to two trials.

ue on the chart ($n = 1.417$); yet human liver yielded the lowest of all values at $n = 1.367$. Examination of the other species values shows no trend. The tentative conclusion at this stage is that no significant species effect is in evidence.

It is important to know what the effects of change of wavelength are on the tissue's index of refraction. Although most treatment and research on PDT and tissue optics are done at 630 nm, other wavelengths are being actively considered. We obtained two samples of bovine from separate animals, and after calibrating with sucrose solutions across the spectrum we used a sequence of narrow bandpass filters to measure the refractive index over the 390–700-nm range. The results are shown in Fig. 7. The index exhibits a definite downward trend in both samples, decreasing from 1.430 to 1.380 in one sample, while falling from 1.420 to 1.395 in the other. Note that both samples give approximately the same value at 630 nm, ~1.400. This decrease in refractive index with increasing wave-

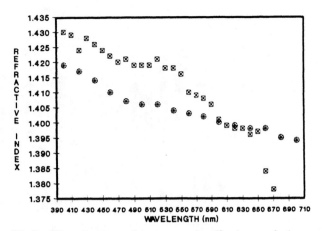

Fig. 7. Dispersion curves from two samples of bovine muscle tissue. The samples are denoted by the two symbol types. The downward trend in index is typical of many substances.

length is typical for more common optical materials,[19] Thus it is not surprising that tissue would also exhibit this behavior. What remains is to quantify accurately dispersion values for other species and tissues.

Another possible parameter that can affect the index of refraction is a denaturation of the tissue. To test this hypothesis, we made measurements on two samples of egg white before and after coagulation. Coagulation was accomplished by heating in a double boiler until thickening was evident. Table II shows that in both cases the index increased substantially. This effect could be an important consideration in estimating light penetration during treatment in which such changes may take place.

IV. Conclusion

This tissue refractive index measurement method has proved its value for determination of the indices for a number of individual mammalian tissue types. It is a relatively simple and fast technique, and it may be applied with both laser light or incoherent broadband sources, such as incandescents. Polychromatic light combined with sequential narrowband filtration can provide tissue dispersion curves of n for the visible band and into the near IR band. If the filtration is sufficiently narrow, that is, with a bandpass profile of ~1 nm at FWHM, the method will delineate chromophore absorption effects in the dispersion plot across the visible and near IR region. The method will allow for determinations of n made out to 2 or 3 μm with currently available cores. The use of optical fibers with higher n allows for determinations on tissues with

indices at 1.500 and above. Our studies to date have been done over the visible band. Determinations at 632.8 nm for several lean well-vascularized tissues with high scattering and absorption properties show most n values to range between 1.390 and 1.410, the exceptions being adipose at 1.455, and liver and lung which had values less than or equal to 1.39. Repeated measurements on specimens from bovine individuals gave an average $n = 1.412$ with a standard deviation of 0.006. No significant difference between species was observed. Dispersion curves of bovine muscle showed a gradual downward trend with increasing wavelength. Coagulation of egg white increased its index substantially.

These values for the tissue's index show some divergence from indices reported by others. For example, Takatani and Graham attempted a theoretical prediction using the weighted n values for the primary compounds which make up tissue. Their results gave a range for tissue n from 1.47 to 1.49.[20] On the other hand, Jacques et al.,[21] again using a predictive method based on the water content of tissue, calculated $n = 1.37$ for tissue. Parrish et al.[22] reported a value of $n = 1.55$ for *stratum corneum*. The variations here strongly point out the need for careful experimental values to be obtained since predictive methods seem to give a range too large for use. The large value quoted for the *stratum corneum* substantiates the fact that a particular tissue type can have an index far outside the 1.4–1.45 range seen for many tissues in our study.

The method reported here has the advantage of ease of setup and operation using ordinary laboratory equipment found at the biophysical research bench where studies involve the tissue's optical characteristics. It suffers from the disadvantage of placing an upper limit on detectable n with quartz cores. However, most tissues fall below this value and are, therefore, measurable by this technique.

This work was supported in part by the NIH under grant 5-RO1-CA33727.

References

1. W. G. Driscoll, Ed., *Handbook of Optics* (McGraw-Hill, New York, 1978), Chap. 10.
2. M. S. Meyer and G. L. Eesley, "Optical Fiber Refractometer," Rev. Sci. Instrum. **58**, 2047–2048 (1987).
3. T. T. Thung, S. K. Teo, F. V. C. Mendis, and B. Van Sel, "Refractometry Through Optical Frequency Domain Reflectometry," Electron. Lett. **21**, 613–614 (1985).
4. T. Takeo and H. Hattori, "Optical Fiber Sensor for Measuring Refractive Index," Jpn. J. Appl. Phys. **21**, 1509–1512 (1982).
5. A. Kumar, T. V. B. Subbrahmanyarm, A. D. Sharma, K. Thyagarajan, G. P. Pal, and I. C. Goyal, "Novel Refractometer Using a Tapered Fiber Optic," Electron. Lett. **20**, 534–535 (1984).
6. W. Leupachur and A. Penzkofer, "Refractive-Index Measurement of Absorbing Condensed Media," Appl. Opt. **23**, 1554–1557 (1984).
7. Y. Lu and A. Penzkofer, "Optical Constants Measurements of Strongly Absorbing Media," Appl. Opt. **25**, 221–225 (1986).
8. W. Allan, *Fibre Optics* (Plenum, London, 1979), p. 8.
9. R. Tiedeken, *Fibre Optics and Its Applications* (Focal Press, London, 1972), p. 21.
10. Ref. 8, p. 196.
11. Ref. 8, p. 197.

Table II.	Effect of Coagulation on Index of Egg White	
Trial	n, Liquid	n, coagulated
1	1.321	1.388
2	1.326	1.374

Note: Resultant effect of denaturation (coagulation) in two samples of egg white. The significant increase in the index carries implications for light transport in high temperature conditions.

12. W. Siegmund, "Fiber Optics," in *Handbook of Optics*, W. Driscoll and W. Vaughan, Eds. (McGraw-Hill, New York, 1978), p. 13–6.

13. W. Siegmund, "Fiber Optics," in *Handbook of Optics*, W. Driscoll and W. Vaughn, Eds. (McGraw-Hill, New York, 1978), pp. 13–21.

14. Ref. 8, p. 28.

15. F. Jenkins and H. White, *Fundamentals of Optics* (McGraw-Hill, New York, 1976), p. 524.

16. Ref. 8, p. 10.

17. Ref. 8, p. 19.

18. N. Lange, *Handbook of Chemistry* (McGraw-Hill, New York, 1967), pp. 780–782.

19. Ref. 15, p. 476.

20. S. Takatani and M. D. Graham, "Theoretical Analysis of Diffuse Reflectance from A Two-Layer Tissue Model," IEEE Trans. Biomed. Eng. **BME-26,** 656–664 (1979).

21. S. Jacques, C. Alter, and S. Prahl, "Angular Dependence of HeNe Laser Light Scattering by Human Dermis," Lasers Life Sci. **1,** 309–333 (1987).

22. J. Parrish, R. Anderson, F. Urbach, and D. Pitts, *UVA* (Plenum, New York, 1978), p. 63.

Reprinted with permission from *Lasers in Surgery and Medicine,* Vol. 9,
pp. 148-154 (1989). ©1989 Wiley-Liss division of John Wiley & Sons, Inc.

Light Distributions in Artery Tissue:
Monte Carlo Simulations for Finite-Diameter Laser Beams

Marleen Keijzer, MSc, Steven L. Jacques, PhD, Scott A. Prahl, PhD, and Ashley J. Welch, PhD

Department of Dermatology, Wellman Laboratory, Harvard Medical School, Massachusetts General Hospital, Boston (M.K., S.L.J.), and Department of Electrical and Computer Engineering, Biomedical Engineering Program, The University of Texas at Austin, Austin (S.A.P., A.J.W.)

Finite-width light distributions in arterial tissue during Argon laser irradiation (476 nm) are simulated using the Monte Carlo method. Edge effects caused by radial diffusion of the light extend ±1.5 mm inward from the perimeter of a uniform incident beam. For beam diameters exceeding 3 mm the light distribution along the central axis can be described by the one-dimensional solution for an infinitely wide beam. The overlapping edge effects for beam diameters smaller than 3 mm reduce the penetration of the irradiance in the tissue. The beam profile influences the light distribution significantly. The fluence rates near the surface for a Gaussian beam are two times higher on the central axis and decrease faster radially than for a flat profile. The diverging light from a fiber penetrates tissue in a manner similar to collimated light.

Key words: absorption, aorta, dosimetry, fiber optics, lasers, photometry, random walk, scattering, radiation

INTRODUCTION

When using laser light in medical treatments, the rates of photochemical and thermal reactions depend on the light dose in the tissue. The distribution of the light within the tissue must be estimated from the irradiance delivered at the surface. To predict the internal light dose in turbid tissue an understanding of radiative transport in scattering media is required.

The most commonly used description of light propagation in highly scattering media is the equation of transfer [1]. This equation has only been solved for a one-dimensional geometry. Two- and three-dimensional solutions require a serious restriction of the angular distribution of the scattered light [2]. Examples of approximations that provide three-dimensional light distributions are the diffusion approximation [3,4] and the seven-flux model [5].

When treating the highly forward-directed light scattering characteristic of tissues [6,7], the validity of the diffusion approximation is suspect [8]. The transition from a collimated laser beam, incident at the surface, to a diffuse flux, deeper in the tissue, occurs in the first several hundred microns of tissue. This is the region that is most important for many laser/tissue interactions yet where the light distributions are the least accurately described by diffusion theory [9].

An alternative to solving the equation of

Accepted for publication December 15, 1988.

Scott A. Prahl is now at the Experimental Laser Unit, Academic Medical Center, 1105 AZ Amsterdam, the Netherlands.

Ashley J. Welch is the Marion E. Forsman Centennial Professor of Electrical and Computer Engineering and Biomedical Engineering.

Steven L. Jacques and Marleen Keijzer are now at the Laser Biology Research Laboratory, Box 17, MD Anderson Cancer Center, 1515 Holcombe Blvd., Houston, TX 77030. Address reprint requests there.

TABLE 1. Optical Parameters, Artery Media, 476 nm

μ_a = 6/cm	Absorption coefficient
μ_s = 414/cm	Scattering coefficient
μ_t = 420/cm	Total attenuation coefficient, $\mu_a + \mu_s$
g = 0.91	Mean cosine of the scattering angle
n = 1.37	Index of refraction

transfer is to simulate light propagation in a scattering medium with the Monte Carlo method [10–12]. Each photon out of a large sample is followed on its random walk until it is absorbed. The total light distribution is estimated from the resulting distribution of absorbed photons. With the Monte Carlo method, light transport can be calculated without approximating the tissue geometry or the angular distribution of light. The exact scattering properties can be simulated as well as the internal reflection at mismatched boundaries.

This paper presents a Monte Carlo simulation for the light distribution in human aorta irradiated with argon laser light (476 nm). The optical properties of normal human aorta at other wavelengths will be published elsewhere [13]. The effect of the beam diameter on the internal light distribution is discussed. The light distributions associated with a uniform beam, a Gaussian beam, and the slightly diverging light from an optical fiber are compared.

MATERIALS AND METHODS
Optical Parameters

The optical parameters used are those of the media of normal human aorta at 476 nm. The absorption coefficient, μ_a, the scattering coefficient, μ_s, and the mean cosine of the scattering angle, g, are listed in Table 1. The total attenuation coefficient, μ_t, is defined as the sum of μ_a and μ_s. The sample is 1.5 mm thick and is surrounded by air. The index of refraction of the sample is assumed to be 1.37 [7].

The optical parameters were obtained experimentally from one sample using the method of Jacques and Prahl [7], modified to include the delta-Eddington approximation of the scattering function [14]. The total attenuation coefficient, μ_t, was obtained by measuring on-axis transmission through thin sections of media (10–50 μm). Integrating sphere measurements of the total transmission and total reflection of the full-thickness sample yielded the remaining optical parameters.

Monte Carlo Method

In the Monte Carlo program, photons are multiply scattered as they propagate through the tissue until they are absorbed. Photons enter the tissue at a single point on the surface. The initial direction of the photons is sampled from the angular distribution of the incident beam. The advantage of having the photons entering through a single point is that the result constitutes a spatial impulse response, which can be convolved over any profile of the incident beam, thus eliminating the need for many lengthy Monte Carlo simulations.

The path of a photon in a scattering medium consists of steps of varying length between interaction sites and angles of deflection for scattering events. Every step length and scattering angle is sampled from its respective distribution (see below). To reduce the number of photons needed to estimate the actual light distribution, weighted photons are used. At each interaction site, μ_a/μ_t of the weight of the photon is deposited as absorbed energy, after which the photon is scattered into a new direction. When the weight of the photon has been reduced to 1/20,000th of its initial weight, the photon is "killed," and a new one is launched. (Instead of one photon losing weight to absorption along its path, the process can be thought of as a bundle of photons leaving a trail of absorbed photons behind.) When the photon hits the tissue/air boundary, part of the photon's weight is transmitted into the air according to Fresnel's laws for unpolarized light. The remaining weight is internally reflected and continues its random walk. The results presented are obtained by launching 20,000 photons.

Below, the random walk of the photons is described in more detail.

Sampling random variables. The principle of the Monte Carlo method is well described by Cashwell and Everett [15]. To determine the random walk of a photon, certain random variables, such as the path length between two scattering events or the scattering angle, must be assigned values at every interaction site. The values of the variable are chosen randomly from the distribution of the variable in the following way.

Define p(x) as the probability density function of a random variable x (a≤x≤b), where

$$\int_a^b p(x)\,dx = 1. \tag{1}$$

Then the sample, x_{rnd}, of the random variable x is

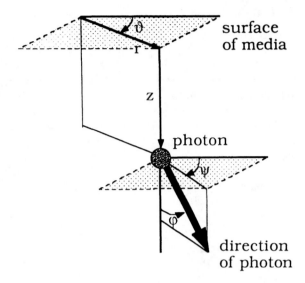

surface
of media

photon

direction
of photon

Fig. 1. Coordinates for random walk. $0 \leq r$, $0 \leq \vartheta \leq 2\pi$, $0 \leq z \leq$ sample thickness, $0 \leq \varphi \leq \pi$, $0 \leq \psi \leq 2\pi$.

simulated by choosing a random number, RND, from a uniform distribution $0 \leq$ RND ≤ 1 and requiring

$$RND = \int_a^{x_{rnd}} p(x)\, dx. \qquad (2)$$

Equation 2 is applied to a particular random variable, x, and rearranged, yielding x_{rnd} as a function of RND.

Coordinates. The coordinate system for the Monte Carlo simulation is shown in Figure 1. The position of the photons, **r**, is described in cylindrical coordinates, (r, ϑ, z) $(0 \leq r,\ 0 \leq \vartheta \leq \pi,$ $0 \leq z \leq$ medium thickness), and the direction of the photons is described in spherical coordinates, (φ, ψ) $(0 \leq \varphi \leq \pi,\ 0 \leq \psi \leq 2\pi)$.

The photons migrate in three dimensions. However, we consider cylindrically symmetric geometries, and therefore the ϑ-dependence of the absorption can be ignored. The tissue is divided into a two-dimensional array in r and z, which specifies element volumes in which the absorbed weights of the propagating photons are recorded. These element volumes are logarithmically scaled: small near the source and large far from the source.

Random walk. Every generated path length between interaction sites, L ($L \geq 0$), is calculated from a random number, RND, as described above. The probability density function, p(L), of the path length is

$$p(L) = \mu_t\, e^{-\mu_t L}, \qquad (3)$$

where p(L) satisfies the normalization of equation 1. Substitution of equation 3 into equation 2 yields an expression for the path length sample, L_{rnd}:

$$L_{rnd} = -\ell n(1 - RND)/\mu_t. \qquad (4)$$

In this way L_{rnd} is selected by RND, which is generated by a random number generator.

The photon is displaced from the old position, (r, ϑ, z), over distance L (which is sampled by L_{rnd}), in direction (φ, ψ). The coordinates of the new position, (r', ϑ', z'), are

$$r' = (r^2 + 2rL\sin\varphi\cos(\psi - \vartheta) + (L\sin\varphi)^2)^{1/2}$$

$$\vartheta' = \begin{cases} \vartheta + a\sin(L\sin\varphi\sin(\psi - \vartheta)/r'), \\ \qquad\qquad \text{for } L\sin\varphi\cos(\pi - \psi + \vartheta) \leq r \\[6pt] \vartheta + \pi + a\sin(L\sin\varphi\sin(\psi - \vartheta)/r'), \\ \qquad\qquad \text{for } L\sin\varphi\cos(\pi - \psi + \vartheta) > r \end{cases}$$

$$z' = z + L\cos\varphi. \qquad (5)$$

At the new position, μ_a/μ_t of the weight of the photon is deposited in an element of the absorption array. The photon is then scattered with μ_s/μ_t of its former weight. We assume that the angle of deflection has a Henyey-Greenstein distribution [16], which, as Jacques et al [17] have demonstrated, well describes the light scattering in tissues:

$$p(\varphi_s) = \tfrac{1}{2}\,(1 - g^2)/(1 + g^2 - 2\,g\cos\varphi_s)^{3/2}$$

$$p(\psi_s) = \tfrac{1}{2\pi}, \qquad (6)$$

where φ_s is the polar scattering angle ($0 \leq \varphi_s \leq \pi$), and ψ_s is the azimuthal scattering angle ($0 \leq \psi_s \leq 2\pi$). Probability density functions $p(\varphi_s)$ and $p(\psi_s)$ satisfy equation 1. Substitution of equations 6 into equation 2 yields relations to obtain the scattering angle samples ($\varphi_{s\,rnd}$, $\psi_{s\,rnd}$):

$$\varphi_{s\,rnd} = a\cos\left(\frac{1}{2g}\Big[1 + g^2 - \Big(\frac{1 - g^2}{1 - g + 2gRND}\Big)^2\Big]\right)$$

$$\psi_{s\,rnd} = 2\pi RND. \qquad (7)$$

The deflection angle, (φ_s, ψ_s), is specified by the samples $\varphi_{s\ rnd}$ and $\psi_{s\ rnd}$. From the old direction, (φ, ψ), the photon is scattered over angle (φ_s, ψ_s) into direction (φ', ψ') according to the following relations [10]:

$$\varphi' = \mathrm{acos}(\cos\varphi_s \cos\varphi - \sin\varphi_s \sin\varphi \cos\psi_s)$$

$$\psi' = \begin{cases} \psi + \mathrm{atan}(\sin\varphi_s \sin\psi_s/\alpha), & \text{for } \alpha > 0 \\[2ex] \psi + \mathrm{atan}(\sin\varphi_s \sin\psi_s/\alpha) \pm \pi, & \text{for } \alpha < 0, \end{cases}$$

where $\alpha = \cos\varphi_s \sin\phi + \sin\phi_s \cos\psi_s \cos\varphi$. (8)

If a photon strikes the surface, part of its weight is transmitted into the air according to Snell's law and Fresnel's equations for unpolarized light. The amount transmitted through the surface is added to the total reflection or total transmission. The remaining fraction of the photon is internally reflected and continues its random walk.

Spatial Impulse Response. The method yields the rate of energy deposition, $Q(\mathbf{r})$, in W/cc per unit of incident power (in W), that enters the sample through a single point on the surface. In other words, $Q(\mathbf{r})$ has unit 1/cc. The corresponding fluence rate distribution, the spatial impulse response, $G(\mathbf{r})$, is coupled to the rate of energy deposition, $Q(\mathbf{r})$, by the absorption coefficient, μ_a:

$$Q(\mathbf{r}) = \mu_a\, G(\mathbf{r}). \quad (9)$$

Therefore, the unit of the spatial impulse response in the tissue, $G(\mathbf{r})$, is $1/cm^2$, which allows the spatial impulse response to be convolved against an incident beam (see equation 10). This convolution yields $\Psi(\mathbf{r})$, the total fluence rate, in W/cm^2.

Two spatial impulse responses are used: one for collimated light incident perpendicularly to

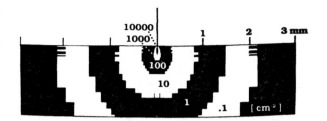

Fig. 2. Spatial impulse response, $G(\mathbf{r})$ in cm^{-2}, light distribution induced by a collimated ray through a point on the surface of tissue with parameters of Table 1. The light penetrates to form a narrow cylinder, then rapidly diffuses into a hemispherical pattern.

the surface and one for divergent light from a fiber with a numerical aperture of 0.26. The spatial impulse response, $G(\mathbf{r})$, for human aorta irradiated by a collimated 476-nm ray is given in Figure 2. The fluence rate directly under the beam is orders of magnitude higher than next to it. However, because of the large differences in volumes, the total amount of light scattered away from the central axis is far greater than the collimated light on axis.

Finite beam convolution. The light distribution in the tissue, $\Psi(\mathbf{r})$, caused by a beam with an arbitrary irradiance profile, $E(r, \vartheta)$ in W/cm^2, is obtained by convolving the spatial impulse response, $G(\mathbf{r})$, with the source:

$$\Psi(r, \vartheta, z) =$$

$$\int_0^{2\pi}\!\!\int_0^\infty E(r', \vartheta')\, G(\sqrt{r^2 + r'^2 - 2rr'\cos(\vartheta - \vartheta')}, z)\, r'dr'd\vartheta'.$$

$$(10)$$

$E(r, \vartheta)$ is constant over the beam area for a flat beam profile. $E(r, \vartheta)$ is proportional to $\exp(-2(r/R_1)^2)$ for a Gaussian beam with a $1/e^2$ radius R_1.

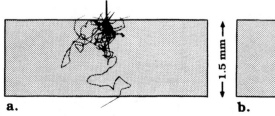 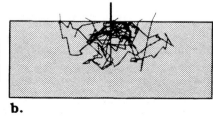

Fig. 3. Monte Carlo simulations of the propagation of photons in human aorta (30 photons shown). The internal light distribution is influenced by the scattering function. **a:** Henyey-Greenstein function, where $g = 0.91$, $\mu_s = 414$/cm. **b:** Isotropic scattering function where the similarity relation is conserved: $g = 0$, $\mu_s = 37.3$/cm.

RESULTS
Influence of the Scattering Function

The paths of 30 photons, generated by the Monte Carlo program, are projected on the $\varphi = 0$ plane in Figure 3. For reasons of clarity, the photons in Figure 3 are multiply scattered without losing weight until a single absorption event terminates propagation.

The consequences of changing the optical scattering parameters can directly be visualized with the Monte Carlo method. In Figure 3a, the photons are scattered according to the Henyey-Greenstein function (equations 6). In Figure 3b, the scattering function in tissue is approximated by an isotropic function (g = 0), according to the similarity relation. The similarity relation asserts that the penetration of light through a scattering media will remain constant, if the "reduced scattering coefficient," $\mu_s(1-g)$, is conserved [18, Chapter 14]. Therefore the scattering coefficient for the isotropic function in Figure 3b is chosen: $\mu_s' = \mu_s(1-g)$. The scattering angles in Figure 3b are much bigger, but more importantly, the whole pattern is wider. For a finite-diameter incident beam this pattern will result in a light distribution that is lower directly under the beam but spread out wider compared to the light distribution calculated with an anisotropic scattering function, as in Figure 3a.

Therefore, the details of the scattering function do influence the light distributions of beams of finite diameter. The Monte Carlo technique enables the Henyey-Greenstein function to be used, rather than an approximation.

Effect of the Beam Diameter

Light distributions in arterial tissue in air for three diameters (200 μm, 1 mm, and 4 mm) of a uniform incident beam are shown in Figure 4. The incident irradiance in each figure is 1 W/cm^2. Back-scattered light augments the incident beam, yielding an internal fluence rate that exceeds the irradiance delivered at the surface. Directly under the incident beam, the light is still rather forward directed, as shown by the large radial gradient in fluence rate at the edge of the beam. Farther away from the source, the light is more diffuse.

Radial diffusion creates edge effects that extend $\pm$1.5 mm from the perimeter of the incident beam inward. The light distribution associated with the 4 mm-wide beam (Fig. 4c) has a central cylinder of 1 mm diameter that is unaffected by

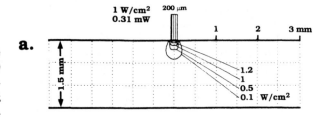

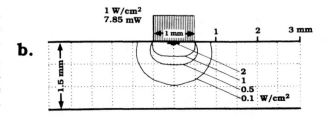

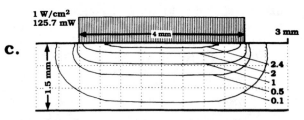

Fig. 4. Distributions of 476 nm light in human aorta for flat, collimated incident beams with different diameters (**a:** 200 μm; **b:** 1 mm; **c:** 4 mm). The power density of the incident beam is 1 W/cm^2. As shown in c, the edge effects extend $\pm$1.5 mm from the perimeter of the beam inward, leaving a central cylinder of 1 mm diameter with a one-dimensional light distribution. The edge effects overlap in the center for beam diameters smaller than 3 mm, which decreases the penetration of light (a,b).

the edge effects. Within this central cylinder, the fluence rates are the same as for an infinitely wide flat beam. When the incident beam is narrower than 3 mm, the edge effects overlap, decreasing the fluence rates in the center (Fig. 4a,b).

The maximum fluence rate is obtained on axis, below the surface. The depth of the maximum depends on the diameter of the incident beam. The maximum fluence rate for beam diameters over 3 mm is obtained at a depth of about 35 μm (Fig. 4c). As the beam diameter is decreased, the maximum moves toward the surface (Fig. 4a,b).

The magnitude of the maximum fluence rate also depends on the beam diameter. The maximum fluence rate for the 4 mm beam is almost 2.5

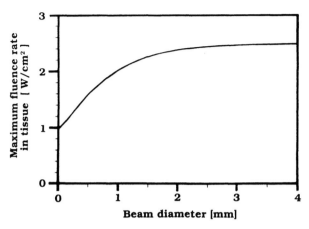

Fig. 5. Maximum fluence rate in the tissue as a function of the beam diameter. As the beam diameter decreases, the edge effects caused by scattering overlap, yielding lower fluence rates within the tissue. The position of the maximum is about 35 μm under the surface for beam diameters over 3 mm and moves toward the surface for decreasing diameters (476 nm, 1 W/cm^2 collimated beam with a flat profile, incident on human aorta).

W/cm^2 (Fig. 4c). The maximum value for the 1 mm beam is 2 W/cm^2 (Fig. 4b) and for the 200 μm beam is 1.2 W/cm^2 (Fig. 4a). The magnitude of the maximum fluence rate depends on the beam diameter, as summarized in Figure 5. The maximum for the limit of a 0-diameter beam has the same magnitude as the incident irradiance, i.e., 1 W/cm^2.

The sample is surrounded by air. Internal reflection, caused by mismatched boundaries, increases the fluence rate near the surface almost to the subsurface maximum. However, for a sample of aorta submerged in water the fluence rate at the surface is about 20% lower than the subsurface maximum for broad beams.

Gaussian Beam

In Figure 4 the beam profile is flat. The light distribution induced by a beam with a Gaussian profile, with a $1/e^2$ diameter of 1 mm, is shown in Figure 6. The total beam power is 7.85 mW, which matches the power of the 1 mm flat beam in Figure 4b. The whole pattern for the Gaussian profile is rounder than the one for the flat profile. The maximum lays nearer to the surface and is less wide. The maximum fluence rate is 4 W/cm^2, twice as high as the one for a flat profile. The profile of the incident beam strongly influences the radial light distribution in the tissue.

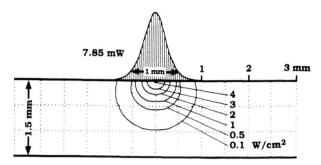

Fig. 6. Distribution of 476 nm light in human aorta for a collimated beam of 7.85 mW with a Gaussian profile ($1/e^2$ diameter of 1 mm). Compare this distribution to the distribution associated with a flat profile as in Figure 4b.

Optical Fiber

Another means of delivery is an optical fiber. Instead of being perfectly collimated, the light coming out of a fiber has an angular distribution. The light distribution in the tissue calculated for a 200 μm diameter fiber with NA = 0.26, positioned just above the surface of the tissue, is shown in Figure 7. The angular distribution of the source is approximately Gaussian, with a standard deviation of 11 degrees [19].

Comparison of Figure 7 to Figure 4b demonstrates that the divergence of the fiber light has little effect on the light distribution in highly scattering tissue. There is additional radial broadening and reduced penetration, but the differences are not significant (the maximum difference is 0.08 W/cm^2). The distributions are even more similar for the case of a fiber in contact with the tissue, as index matching decreases the numerical aperture of the fiber.

DISCUSSION

Since the Monte Carlo program does not approximate the angular distribution of the light or the scattering function, light transport can be calculated with any required accuracy, even near sources and boundaries. (Elsewhere will be published a demonstration of the accuracy of the Monte Carlo method in predicting measured light distributions [13, 20].) Furthermore, no restrictions are placed on the geometry of tissue and incident beam. Inhomogeneities such as blood vessels imbedded in tissue and the layered structure of skin can be included in a straightforward manner. One can simulate any laser beam profile

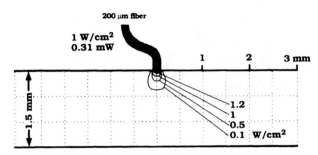

Fig. 7. Distribution of 476 nm light in human aorta for an optical fiber with NA = 0.26 and a diameter of 200 μm. The source is 1 W/cm², 0.31 mW. Compare this distribution for a divergent beam to the distribution induced by a collimated beam as in Figure 4a.

and the dispersion of the light from any fiber tip, either positioned inside the tissue or outside.

Monte Carlo calculations take too long to be used for immediate calculations during an experiment or treatment. However, the results of the calculations for a range of optical parameters can be stored for quick recall during procedures.

By comparing light distributions calculated with approximations to the transport equation (e.g., the diffusion equation) with the results of the Monte Carlo calculations, the former methods can be tested, and their systematic errors can be specified. Thus, light propagation models can be tested for their ability to obtain the tissue optical properties [e.g. 7] and to predict light distributions.

The results presented demonstrate that the internal light dose strongly depends on the diameter and the profile of the incident beam. Broad beams, for example surface irradiation during photodynamic therapy with conventional light sources or expanded laser beams, are well described by the one-dimensional solution (the central cylinder in Fig. 4c). However, narrow laser beam and optical fiber delivery require consideration of the beam diameter dependence of the internal light dose.

ACKNOWLEDGMENTS

This work was funded in part by the National Institutes of Health, grant AM25395-08, the Office of Naval Research under contract #N00014-86-K-00116 and #N00014-86-K-0875 and the Whitaker Health Sciences Fund.

REFERENCES

1. Chandrasekhar S: "Radiative Transfer." London: Oxford Univ. Press, 1950.
2. Case KM, Zweifel PF: "Linear Transport Theory." Reading, MA: Addison-Wesley, 1969.
3. Ishimaru A: "Wave Propagation and Scattering in Random Media," Volume 1. New York: Academic Press, 1978.
4. Keijzer M, Star WM, Storchi PRM: Optical diffusion in layered media. Appl Optics 1988; 27:1820–1824.
5. Yoon G, Welch AJ, Motamedi M, van Gemert MCJ: Development and application of three-dimensional light distribution model for laser irradiated tissue. IEEE J Quantum Electron 1987; QE-23:1721–1733.
6. Flock ST, Wilson BC, Patterson MS: Total attenuation coefficients and scattering phase functions of tissues and phantom materials at 633 nm. Med Phys 1987; 14:835–841.
7. Jacques SL, Prahl SA: Modeling optical and thermal distributions in tissue during laser irradiation. Lasers Surg Med 1987; 6:494–503.
8. Furutsu K: Diffusion equation derived from space time transport equation. J Opt Soc Am [A] 1980; 70:360–366.
9. Ishimaru A, Kuga Y, Cheung R L-T, Shimizu K: Scattering and diffusion of a beam wave in randomly distributed scatterers. J Opt Soc Am [A] 1983; 73:131–136.
10. de Belder M, de Kerf J, Jespers J, Verbrugge R: Light diffusion in photographic layers: Its influence on sensitivity and modulation transfer. J Opt Soc Am [A] 1965; 55:1261–1268.
11. Witt AN: Multiple scattering in reflection nebulae I-IV. Astroph J [Suppl] 1977; 55:1–36.
12. Wilson BC, Adam G: A Monte Carlo model for the absorption and flux distributions of light in tissue. Med Phys 1983; 10:824–830.
13. Keijzer M, Richards-Kortum RR, Jacques SL, Feld M: Fluorescence spectroscopy of turbid media: Autofluorescence of human aorta (in preparation).
14. Joseph JH, Wiscombe WJ: The Delta-Eddington approximation for radiative flux transfer. J Atm Sci 1976; 33:2452–2459.
15. Cashwell ED, Everett CJ: "A Practical Manual on the Monte Carlo Method for Random Walk Problems." New York: Pergamon, 1959.
16. Henyey LG, Greenstein JL: Diffuse radiation in the galaxy. Astroph J 1941; 93:70.
17. Jacques SL, Alter CA, Prahl SA: Angular dependence of HeNe laser light scattering by human dermis. Lasers Life Sci 1987; 1:309–333.
18. van de Hulst HC: "Multiple Light Scattering," Volume II. New York: Academic Press, 1980.
19. Schroeder G: "Technische Optik." Wuerzburg: Vogel, 1984.
20. Jacques SL, Keijzer M, Marijnissen H, Star WM: Light distributions in phantom tissues: Theory meets experiment (in preparation).

Light propagation in multilayer scattering media: modeling by the Monte Carlo method

I. V. Yaroslavskiĭ and V. V. Tuchin

Saratov State University
(Received 9 September 1991)
Opt. Spektrosk. **72**, 934–939 (April 1992)

This paper describes a version of the Monte Carlo method for modeling optical radiation propagation in biological tissues and scattering media, based on the use of Green's functions for the response of the medium to a unit of external action. The algorithm makes it possible to take into account the multilayer nature of the medium, the finite size of the incident beam, and light reflection and refraction at the layer interfaces. The results of a calculation for biological tissues are presented.

INTRODUCTION

The Monte Carlo method (MCM) is widely used to numerically solve problems of optical radiation-transport theory[1,2] in different scientific areas (astrophysics, atmospheric and oceanic optics, and optical technology). Applications of the MCM to the optics of biological tissues have been successfully developed in recent years;[3-6] this development is related to the increasing use in medicine of lasers for diagnostics and therapy[7] (by the need for reliable layer dosimetry of laser radiation and by the prospects for optical tomography).

The place of the MCM among the methods for solving problems in radiation-transport theory is determined by the possibility of using it for media of arbitrary configuration and with any boundary conditions. The penalty for this advantage is that much more computer time is needed. Although the evolution of hardware and software in computer engineering has decreased the role of the time factor,

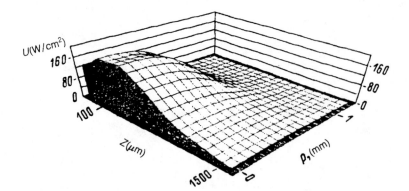

FIG. 1. Total irradiance distribution inside a medium with the optical parameters given in Table I, for an incident beam with a Gaussian profile (initial radius 0.5 mm, power 1 W). z—depth, ρ—distance from beam axis.

development of practical systems that provide, for example, radiation dosimetry for laser therapy requires efficient, comparatively simple, and reliable MCM algorithms.

In this paper, we present a version of the MCM that is a further development of the approach described in Refs. 4 and 5 and can be used to solve a wide range of problems in optical technology and biological optics.

SETTING UP THE PROBLEM

The fundamental equation of radiation transport for monochromatic light in the stationary case has the form[8]

$$\frac{\partial I(\mathbf{r},\mathbf{s})}{\partial s} = -kI(\mathbf{r},\mathbf{s}) + \frac{k_s}{4\pi}\int_{4\pi} I(\mathbf{r},\mathbf{s}')p(\mathbf{s},\mathbf{s}')d\omega', \quad (1)$$

where $I(\mathbf{r},\mathbf{s})$ is the radiant intensity at point $\mathbf{r}$ in direction $\mathbf{s}$, k_s is the scattering coefficient, k_a is the absorption coefficient, $k = k_a + k_s$ is the extinction coefficient, $\Lambda = k_s/k$ is the single-scattering albedo, and $p(\mathbf{s},\mathbf{s}')$ is the scattering phase function. It is assumed that there are no radiation sources inside the medium.

If the radiation-transport process is studied in the region $G \subset R^3$, while ∂G is the boundary of the region, the boundary conditions on ∂G can be written in the general form[9]

$$I(\mathbf{r},\mathbf{s})|_{(\mathbf{sn})<0} = S(\mathbf{r},\mathbf{s}) + \hat{R}I(\mathbf{r},\mathbf{s})|_{(\mathbf{sn})>0}, \quad (2)*$$

where $\mathbf{r} \in G$, $\mathbf{n}$ is the outward normal to G, $S(\mathbf{r},\mathbf{s})$ is the radiant intensity of the incident light, and $\hat{R}$ is the reflection operator. In the presence of light-reflecting and -refracting surfaces in region G, conditions similar to Eq. (2) should be written for each of them.

As a rule, it is not function $I(\mathbf{r},\mathbf{s})$ itself that is of practical interest but integrals of it over certain regions of phase space $(\mathbf{r},\mathbf{s})$. For example, in optical radiation-dosimetry problems in biological tissues, such a quantity is the total irradiance at a point,

$$U(\mathbf{r}) = \int_{4\pi} I(\mathbf{r},\mathbf{s})d\omega. \quad (3)$$

For optical probing of light-scattering objects, the measured quantity is often the distribution function of the radiation leaving the surface of the medium,

$$\Phi(\mathbf{r}) = \int_{(\mathbf{gn})>0} I(\mathbf{r},\mathbf{s})(\mathbf{sn})d\omega, \quad (4)$$

where $\mathbf{r} \in G$.

The algorithm described below is directed toward the calculation of these quantities, but other functionals of $I(\mathbf{r},\mathbf{s})$ can be found similarly.

STATISTICAL MODELING ALGORITHM

The algorithm presented here is designed for calculations of the quantities $U(\mathbf{r})$ and $\Phi(\mathbf{r})$ for a planar, multi-

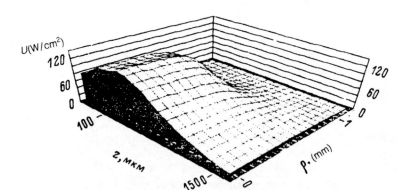

FIG. 2. Same as Fig. 1 for a beam with a rectangular profile.

116

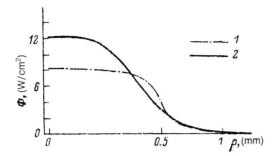

FIG. 3. Radial distribution of diffusely reflected radiation for different profiles of the incident beam (initial radius 0.5 mm, power 1 W). 1—rectangular profile; 2—Gaussian profile.

layered light-scattering and absorbing medium on one of whose surfaces optical radiation is incident. It is assumed here that the solid-angle scattering of the incident radiation can be represented in factorized form,

$$S(\mathbf{r},\mathbf{s}) = A(\mathbf{s})E(\mathbf{r}), \qquad (5)$$

where $A(\mathbf{s})$ describes the angular distribution of a unit power source.

Each ith layer is characterized by the following set of parameters: k_{ai}, k_{si}, $p_i(\theta_s)$ [$\theta_s = \arccos(\mathbf{ss'})$ is the scattering angle], thickness t_i, and the refractive index n_i of the filling medium. Because of the assumed constancy of the optical properties of each layer on a plane parallel to the interfaces between the layers, the problem possesses symmetry with respect to a shift in this plane. This makes it possible in the statistical modeling to ignore the spatial distribution of the incident radiation $E(\mathbf{r})$ and to consider a point source located at the origin of coordinates, with an angular radiation distribution $A(\mathbf{s})$. It is possible in this way to obtain the Green's functions for the response of the medium to an external point action, $G(\mathbf{r})$, $G_T(\mathbf{r})$, and $G_R(\mathbf{r})$, which describe the total illuminance distribution in the medium and the surface distributions of the transmitted and reflected radiation, respectively. The functions $U(\mathbf{r})$, $\Phi_T(\mathbf{r})$, and $\Phi_R(\mathbf{r})$ (where subscript T refers to transmitted and R to reflected light) can be calculated from the integrals

$$U(x,y,z) = \iint G(x',y',z)E(x-x',y-y')dx'dy', \quad (6)$$

$$\Phi_i(x,y) = \iint G_j(x',y')E(x-x',y-y')dx'dy', \quad (7)$$

where $i = R, T$; and x, y, z are the Cartesian coordinates of point $\mathbf{r}$ (the z axis is perpendicular to the boundary and is oriented away from the illuminated surface, into the medium).

It is assumed in what follows that the incident beam has radial symmetry, i.e., $E(x,y) = E(\rho)$ ($\rho = \sqrt{x^2+y^2}$). Then it is convenient to use cylindrical coordinates (ρ,z,θ), where θ is the azimuthal angle in the xy plane. In these coordinates, Eq. (6) becomes

$$U(\rho,z) = \int_0^\infty G(\rho',z)$$
$$\times \left[\int_0^{2\pi} E\big((\rho'^2 + \rho^2 - 2\rho\rho' \cos\theta)^{1/2}\big)d\theta \right]\rho'd\rho'. \qquad (8)$$

Equation (7) is written similarly.

The statistical modeling of the photon motion can be immediately carried out as follows: The (ρ,z) region of interest to us [$0 \leqslant z \leqslant t$, $t = \Sigma_{i=1}^N t_i$ is the total thickness, N is the number of layers, $0 \leqslant \rho \leqslant \rho_{max}$, and ρ_{max} is chosen so that the part of the radiation incident beyond a cylinder of radius ρ_{max} is negligible] is broken up into the cells (i,j). Each photon is characterized by three coordinates and two angles φ and ψ, which determine the direction of its motion (φ is measured from the positive z direction and ψ from the positive x direction in the xy plane). Initially the photon is placed at the origin of coordinates, an initial weight equal to W_0 is attributed to it, and its random direction is determined in accordance with $A(s)$ from

$$\alpha = \int_{x_{min}}^{x_{rnd}} p(x)dx, \qquad (9)$$

where α is a random number uniformly distributed in the interval $(0,1)$; $p(x)$ is the probability density function of the random quantity x, x_{min} is the minimum value of x, and x_{rnd} is the value of x to be chosen. Methods for solving Eq. (9) are quite well developed.[1,2] The values of all the other random quantities needed for modeling the photon motion are also generated by Eq. (9).

When the photon's direction of motion has been determined, the path length of the photon is calculated at the given step of the modeling. If the point on which the photon should be incident is in the same layer as the initial point, the photon is displaced to that point. Otherwise the reflection probability of the photon from the interface of the layers is determined from the Fresnel formulas, and an event consisting of the reflection of the photon is worked out. If the photon crosses an interface, its new direction (the refraction) is calculated, and the part of the path length remaining after crossing the interface is changed to

$$L' = Lk_l/k_m \qquad (10)$$

where L and L' are the old and new remaining parts of the path length, respectively. The photon passes from layer l to layer m.

Furthermore, a part of the photon's weight proportional to $(1-\Lambda)$ is assigned to cell Q_{ij} of an array that characterizes the absorbed energy distribution in the medium. The subscripts i and j are calculated from the current coordinates of the photon. The value of the photon scattering angle is then generated and the procedure is repeated.

When the weight of the photon has decreased to a given small value, the roulette procedure of Ref. 4 is carried out. If, at a subsequent step of the modeling, the photon goes beyond the boundary of the medium, part of its weight proportional to the transmission coefficient of the corresponding boundary is assigned to cell Q_{Ti} (transmis-

117

TABLE I. Optical parameters of biological tissue at 633-nm wave-length.

Layer	k_a (cm^{-1})	k_s (cm^{-1})	g*	n	t(cm)
Epidermis	35.0	480.0	0.79	1.55	0.0065
Dermis	2.7	187.0	0.82	1.55	0.125
Subcutaneous fatty tissue	0.2	20.0	0.80	1.45	0.032
Vessel wall	6.0	414.0	0.91	1.37	0.061
Blood	25.0	400.0	0.98	1.33	0.64

*g is the mean cosine of the scattering angle.

sion) or cell Q_{Ri} (reflection) of the array. Subscript i is determined by the current coordinate ρ.

When this procedure has been carried out for a large enough number of photons N_p, the Green's functions for the response of the medium are calculated from

$$G_{ij} = \frac{Q_{ij}}{N_p V_{ij} k_{aij} W_0},\qquad(11)$$

$$C_{li} = \frac{Q_{li}}{N_p S_i W_0}, \quad l = R, T,\qquad(12)$$

where V_{ij} is the volume of cell (i,j), k_{aij} is the absorption coefficient of the layer that cell (i,j) belongs to, and S_i is the area of the ring corresponding to distance ρ.

Then, using Eqs. (6) and (7), the irradiance distribution inside the medium and the transmitted and reflected radiation distribution are calculated from a given profile of the incident beam.

EXAMPLE: A CALCULATION FOR BIOLOGICAL TISSUES

As an example of the use of the algorithm, the results of modeling the propagation of beams with Gaussian and rectangular profiles in a medium consisting of five layers (of biological tissues) are shown in Figs. 1–3. This problem was solved in terms of the development of a method of transcutaneous laser irradiation of blood (radiation wavelength 633 nm).[10,11] The optical parameters of the biological tissues were taken from the literature[12] and are given in Table I.

The Henyey–Greenstein function

$$p(\theta_s) = \frac{(1-g^2)}{2(1+g^2-2g\cos\theta_s)^{3/2}}.\qquad(13)$$

was used as the scattering phase function for all the layers. It was assumed that the original beams were collimated and were perpendicular to the surface of the medium,

$$A(s) = \delta(s - s_z),\qquad(14)$$

where s_z corresponds to the positive z direction. In this case, for a beam with a Gaussian profile,

$$E_g(\rho) = E_{g0} \exp(-2(\rho/R_0)^2),\qquad(15)$$

where $E_{g0} = 2P/(\pi R_0^2)$, P is the power, and R_0 is the original beam radius. For a beam with rectangular profile,

$$E_f(\rho) = \begin{cases} 0, & \rho > R_0, \\ E_{f0}, & \rho \leqslant R_0, \end{cases}\qquad(16)$$

where $E_{f0} = P/(\pi R_0^2)$.

Figure 3 shows the effect of the incident beam shape on the radial distribution of the reflected light. Transmitted radiation is virtually absent in this case.

The algorithm presented here was successfully used to model light propagation in biological tissues[10,11,13] when solving a number of optical radiation-dosimetry problems for laser therapy. The results were in satisfactory agreement with experiment.[10,11] Using this algorithm made it possible to analyze the dependence of the illuminance distribution inside the tissue from the width, shape, and angular distribution of the incident beam, and the radiation dose into the tissue was optimized on the basis of these calculations. The dependence of the output signal (of the transmitted or reflected radiation) on the geometrical parameters of the initial beam and on the structure of the object can likewise be studied for the laser diagnostics of biological tissues or scattering media. Nephelometry (including polarization nephelometry),[7] Doppler anemometry,[7,14] and determination of the optical parameters of a medium from the radial distribution function of reflected light[3] can serve as examples of such diagnostics.

The authors thank S. R. Utz for fruitful discussions and M. Keiser for collaboration.

---

*The Russian notation for scalar product is retained here: the scalar product of vectors **a** and **b** is (**ab**).

[1]S. M. Ermakov and G. A. Mikhailov, *A Course in Statistical Modeling* (Moscow, 1982).

[2]I. M. Sobol, *Numerical Monte Carlo Methods* (Moscow, 1973).

[3]R. A. J. Groenhuis, H. A. Ferwerda, and J. J. Ten Bosch, Appl. Opt. **22**, 2456 (1983).

[4]S. A. Prahl, M. Keijzer, S. L. Jacques, and A. J. Welch, SPIE Ins. Ser. **IS5**, 102 (1989).

[5]M. Keijzer, S. L. Jacques, S. A. Prahl, and A. J. Welch, Las. Surg. Med. **9**, 148 (1989).

[6]B. C. Wilson and G. Adam, Med. Phys. **10**, 824 (1983).

[7]A. V. Priezzhev, V. V. Tuchin, and L. P. Shubochkin, *Laser Diagnostics in Biology and Medicine* (Moscow, 1989).

[8]S. Chandrasekhar, *Radiative Transfer* (Oxford U. P., 1950; Moscow, 1953).

[9]T. A. Germogenova, *Local Properties of the Solutions of Transport Equations* (Moscow, 1986).

[10]I. V. Yaroslavskiĭ, V. V. Tuchin, S. R. Utz, D. A. Kedrov, and E. Yu. Osintsev, in *Abstracts of Reports of the All-Union Conference on New Methods of Monitoring the Laser Irradiation of Blood and of Estimating the Efficiency of Laser Therapy* (Novosibirsk, 1990), pp. 35 and 69.

[11]S. R. Utz, V. V. Tuchin, I. V. Yaroslavsky *et al.*, in *Abstracts of the Fifth International Congress of the ELA* (Graz, 1990), p. 24.

[12]M. J. C. Van Gemert, S. L. Jacques, H. J. C. M. Sterenborg, and W. M. Star, IEEE Trans. Biomed. Eng. **BM-36**, 1146 (1989).

[13]V. A. Medvedev, V. V. Tuchin, and I. V. Yaroslavsky, Paper 1422-10 at the International Conference on Biomedical Optics 91 (Los Angeles, 1991).

[14]H. W. Jentink, F. F. M. de Mul, R. G. A. M. Hermsen, R. Graf, J. Greve, Appl. Opt. **29**, 2371 (1990).

Reprinted with permission from *Applied Optics*, Vol. 32(4), pp. 426–434
(February 1, 1993). ©1993 Optical Society of America.

Condensed Monte Carlo simulations for the description of light transport

R. Graaff, M. H. Koelink, F. F. M. de Mul, W. G. Zijlstra, A. C. M. Dassel,
and J. G. Aarnoudse

A novel method, condensed Monte Carlo simulation, is presented that applies the results of a single Monte Carlo simulation for a given albedo $\mu_s/(\mu_a + \mu_s)$ to obtaining results for other albedos; μ_s and μ_a are the scattering and absorption coefficients, respectively. The method requires only the storage of the number of interactions of each photon with the medium. The reflectance and transmittance of turbid slabs can thus be found from a limited number of condensed Monte Carlo simulations. We can use an inversion procedure to obtain the absorption and scattering coefficients from the total reflectance and total transmittance of slabs. Remitted photon densities from a semi-infinite medium as a function of the distance between the light source and the detector for all albedos can be found even from the results of a single condensed Monte Carlo simulation. The application of similarity rules may reduce further the number of Monte Carlo simulations that are needed to describe the influence of the distribution of scattering angles on the results.

Key words: Multiple scattering, biological tissue, Monte Carlo simulations, similarity rules, transmittance, reflectance.

1. Introduction

A large number of studies have been published in the past decade in which light propagation within turbid biological media, e.g., blood and human skin, plays an important role.[1–6] Light propagation in turbid media can be characterized by an absorption coefficient μ_a, a scattering coefficient μ_s, and a phase function, which is the distribution of scattering angles per scattering event.[7–9] The symbols Σ_a and Σ_s are also in use for these properties. The phase function is often characterized by the asymmetry factor g, which is defined as the average cosine of the scattering angles. All properties mentioned are wavelength dependent.

Many *in vitro* measurements were performed in order to obtain values of μ_a, μ_s, and g. A recent review is given by Cheong *et al.*[10] These properties often were obtained simultaneously from measurements of T_{tot}, R_{tot}, and T_{coll}, the total transmission, total reflection, and collimated transmission, respectively. Subsequently theoretical models for light propagation in turbid media had to be applied in order to relate the measured light intensities to the fundamental properties of the sample. In some studies distributions of scattering angles from optically thin samples were determined with a goniometer.

Such methods as two- and four-flux Kubelka–Munk models and the diffusion approximation of the transport theory have been applied often to this aim since the numerical solutions can be obtained fast.[7,8,11–13] However, the accuracy is restricted to cases where photon path lengths are not too small and where the reduced scattering coefficient μ_s' $[\equiv \mu_s(1 - g)]$ is much larger than the absorption coefficient μ_a.

Numerical solutions of transmission and reflection, found by application of the transport equation without the restrictions of the diffusion approximation, are more accurate than the solutions of diffusion-approximation two- and four-flux models but can be applied in only relatively simple configurations.[9,14–17] For slabs accurate models such as the adding–doubling method can be applied, which takes a large number of fluxes into account.[18–20] Subsequently one can use tabulated results of total transmission

R. Graaff is with the Center for Biomedical Technology, A. C. M. Dassel and J. G. Aarnoudse are with the Department of Obstetrics and Gynecology, and W. G. Zijlstra is with the Department of Pediatrics, the University of Groningen, Oostersingel 59, 9713 EZ Groningen, The Netherlands. M. H. Koelink and F. F. M. de Mul are with the Department of Applied Physics, University of Twente, 7500 AE Enschede, The Netherlands.

Received 15 November 1991.
0003-6935/93/040426-09$05.00/0.

and total reflection for inversion techniques to obtain the scattering and absorption coefficient for the given distribution of scattering angles for which the simulation has been applied.

It should be noted that the results of *in vitro* measurements on tissue slabs may not provide accurate predictions of the absorption and scattering coefficients and of the phase function *in vivo*, since, e.g., the variation may occur between subjects and tissues as well as with the location within the tissue. This is discussed in more detail elsewhere.[21] The venous and arterial blood volumes *in vivo* are also subject to change.

In several biomedical applications changes in the absorption coefficients μ_a are determined *in vivo* at several wavelengths. Our interest is in the description of laser Doppler flowmetry[22,23] and reflection pulse oximetry.[17,24,25] Other applications are near-IR spectroscopy,[26,27] dental research,[28] and photodynamic therapy.[29,30] In many of the applications described above, the sample is illuminated by a point source or pencil beam at the origin. The optical properties of the tissue must be obtained from the intensity remitted by the tissue as a function of the distance from the origin.

Transport theory in the diffusion approximation has been applied widely to the configuration with pencil-beam illumination so that the density of remitted photons, which depends on the distance along the surface, can be described. The results are applied so that the absorption and scattering properties from the reflection from turbid media can be predicted, if we assume a homogeneous finite, semi-infinite medium,[30–35] of layered structures.[36,37] However, the assumptions of the diffusion approximation have been recognized as one of the main drawbacks of this calculation method.[37]

Monte Carlo simulations have often been avoided in searches for solutions for the transmission and reflection from slabs of turbid materials, probably because of the large amount of simulation time that is needed. Simulation results for each combination of the albedo, $c \equiv \mu_s/(\mu_a + \mu_s)$, and the slab thickness are needed for inversion calculations with a given phase function. The Monte Carlo technique combined with an inversion technique has been applied by several authors.[20,38,39]

The Monte Carlo simulation technique has also been applied to the configuration with illumination at the origin by a point source or pencil beam.[22,23,28,40,41] Monte Carlo simulations can be performed for any configuration,[40,42] but again they consume a great amount of calculation time, especially if the influence from the variation of optical and geometrical properties has to be investigated.

A new method for the determination of the optical properties of tissue slabs is described in Section 3. We show that the results of a single Monte Carlo simulation, performed for a given phase function, can be used for various values of the albedo. With the present approach we introduce the condensed Monte

Carlo simulation. An inversion technique is given in Section 4.

We show that condensed Monte Carlo simulations can also be applied to the interpretation of *in vivo* measurements at the tissue surface as a function of the distance from the origin. As in the case of the determination of diffuse reflection and diffuse transmission from slabs, a method is described in Section 3 for condensing the results of a Monte Carlo simulation on a semi-infinite medium so that the results can also be applied to replacing simulations for other values of the albedo.

The validity of similarity rules for slabs and the semi-infinite medium is investigated in Section 5. One can apply similarity relations to combine variables with a negligible loss of accuracy. When applicable they can reduce further the number of variables needed for the description of light propagation as well as the number of condensed Monte Carlo simulations.

2. Theory for Monte Carlo Simulations

The intensity decay of a collimated beam of photons in a turbid medium equals the probability $p_t(z)$ that a photon has a free path with a length z:

$$p_t(z) = \frac{I(z)}{I(0)} = \exp(-\mu_a z)\exp(-\mu_s z)$$

$$= \exp[-(\mu_a + \mu_s)z] = \exp(-\mu_t z). \qquad (1)$$

$I(z)$ is the intensity at a distance z from the location where the beam enters the medium (Fig. 1); μ_a and μ_s are the absorption and scattering coefficient of the medium, whereas μ_t $(\equiv \mu_a + \mu_s)$ is the transport coefficient.

The chance that a photon travels within the collimated beam to a distance between z and $z + dz$ can be found by the differentiation of Eq. (1):

$$p_t(z) - p_t(z + dz) = \mu_t \exp(-\mu_t z)dz. \qquad (2)$$

These photons can be absorbed or scattered. The

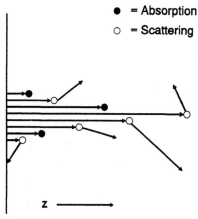

Fig. 1. Intensity decay of a collimated beam caused by absorption and scattering.

scattered fraction equals

$$p_s(z) - p_s(z + \mathrm{d}z) = \mu_s \exp(-\mu_t z)\mathrm{d}z, \qquad (3)$$

which is a fraction c $(= \mu_s/\mu_t)$, the albedo, of the photons that leave the collimated beam.

It might appear as if the decision for absorption is made at the scattering centers. However, this is not true, since it should be noticed that the mean free path between scattering interactions in a Monte Carlo simulation is given by

$$\langle l_s \rangle = \frac{\int_0^1 l\,\mathrm{d}p_s(l)}{\int_0^1 \mathrm{d}p_s(l)} = \frac{\int_0^\infty l\mu_s \exp(-\mu_t l)\mathrm{d}l}{\int_0^\infty \mu_s \exp(-\mu_t l)\mathrm{d}l}, \qquad (4)$$

where l is the path length between two interactions. Substitution of the analytical expressions for both integrals yields

$$\langle l_s \rangle = \frac{\mu_s/\mu_t{}^2}{\mu_s/\mu_t} = \frac{1}{\mu_t} = \langle l_t \rangle. \qquad (5)$$

For an absorption-free medium the average distance between scattering interactions equals $1/\mu_s$. However, if absorption occurs, this mean free path decreases and the chance for interaction increases according to Eq. (5). This occurs because the probability of scattering at longer distances is more decreased by the absorption term $\exp(-\mu_a z)$ in Eq. (1) than at shorter distances.

The intensity decay of a collimated beam in a turbid medium has much in common with the free path length between interactions in Monte Carlo simulations. Therefore in Monte Carlo simulations we simulate the distribution of photon path lengths following from Eq. (2) by choosing random values for each free path length l_t between interactions of the photon during its course through the medium:

$$l_t = \frac{1}{\mu_t} \ln(\epsilon). \qquad (6)$$

The random number ϵ is chosen to be between 0 and 1.[32] The chance that the photon is not absorbed during interaction is c. Therefore we choose a new random number to determine whether the photon has been absorbed or scattered. In the latter case a scattering angle is chosen from the phase function,[22] and a new free path length is determined. All processes are repeated until the photon either is absorbed or leaves the medium. However, if the number of interactions is too high, the photons are terminated in our algorithms, e.g., in the present study when 20,000 interactions are exceeded.

We used Fresnel's law to calculate the possibility of reflection and refraction for each collision of a photon path with an interface. For each of these collisions we used a random number to decide between reflection and refraction. The surface-roughness influ-ence is neglected in that case. Therefore for tissue–air or tissue–water interfaces these rules are only approximate. However, other algorithms can be implemented in the future, e.g., by introducing uncertainty in the angle between the photon path and interface.

3. Condensed Monte Carlo Simulations

A. Theoretical Considerations

Since Monte Carlo simulations may be time-consuming, investigating whether Monte Carlo simulations can be obviated by using the results of other Monte Carlo simulations is interesting. In this section we investigate whether the results of Monte Carlo simulations can be stored so that the results can be used again if the results are needed for the same phase function but for different values of μ_t and c. Two cases are studied: Monte Carlo simulations for the photon density remitted by a semi-infinite medium as a function of the distance between the source and the detector and Monte Carlo simulations for the calculation of optical properties from the reflection and transmission of slabs.

It is obvious that Monte Carlo results can be used again in situations with the same phase function and albedo but where μ_t is different from the simulated value $(\mu_{t,\mathrm{sim}})$ if geometric dimensions can be scaled. For the case of a semi-infinite medium illuminated at the origin, as shown in Fig. 2(a), scaling applies to the distance $r(i)$ where the simulated photon leaves the medium, if it is not absorbed. For each photon this implies that

$$r(i)\mu_t = r_{\mathrm{sim}}(i)\mu_{t,\mathrm{sim}}, \qquad (7)$$

where $r(i)$ is the distance from the origin where photon (i) leaves the medium and $r(i)\mu_t$ represents the same distance in units of the mean free path. Therefore, the relative reflectance $R(r)$, defined as the fraction of all photons remitted by the medium per unit of area at a distance r, is not only introduced here, but also a dimensionless relative reflectance $R_{dl}(\mu_t r)$ is. The latter is defined as the fraction of all injected photons remitted per unit of mean free path squared at a dimensionless distance $\mu_t r$ from the origin. The relationship between both relative reflectances is given by

$$R_{dl}(\mu_t r) = R(r)/\mu_t{}^2. \qquad (8)$$

The values for the dimensionless relative reflectance can be obtained from Monte Carlo simulations by the calculation of

$$R_{dl}[\mu_t r(j)] \equiv R_{dl}(j) = \frac{N(j)}{N_{\mathrm{tot}} A_{dl}(j)}, \qquad (9)$$

where $N(j)$ is the number of photons that escape at a distance $\mu_t r(j)$ and N_{tot} is the total number of photons launched. $A_{dl}(j)$ is the dimensionless area of escape:

$$A_{dl}(j) = \pi[r_{\mathrm{outer}}{}^2(j) - r_{\mathrm{inner}}{}^2(j)]\mu_t{}^2, \qquad (10)$$

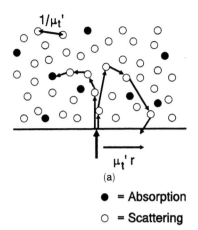

● = Absorption

○ = Scattering

(a)

● = Absorption

○ = Scattering

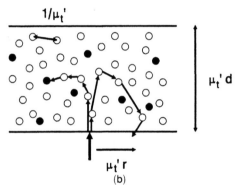

(b)

Fig. 2. Monte Carlo simulations used to predict the relative reflectance expressed per unit of mean free path squared at the surface of a semi-infinite medium with known absorption and scattering coefficients as a function of $\mu_t r$ (a). For finite slabs the results are also a function of $\mu_t d$ (b).

which is the jth annulus with inner and outer radii that are close to $r(j)$. Thus the dimensionless relative reflectance as a function of $\mu_t r$ given per unit of mean free path squared does not depend on μ_t.

For the case where transmission and diffuse reflectance of a slab are studied, the slab thickness d should be scaled too:

$$\mu_t d = \mu_{t,\text{sim}} d_{\text{sim}}, \qquad (11)$$

as shown in Fig. 2(b). In principle a different Monte Carlo simulation is needed for each value of $\mu_t d$. In this respect Monte Carlo simulations on slabs differ from Monte Carlo simulations on semi-infinite media.

As for the question of whether Monte Carlo results, which are performed with an albedo c_{sim}, can also be used again for a lower albedo, it should be noted that the chance that a photon found in the original Monte Carlo simulation, performed with c_{sim}, is not absorbed for a lower albedo c depends on the number of

interactions $N(i)$ within the turbid medium:

$$p(i) = (c/c_{\text{sim}})^{N(i)}. \qquad (12)$$

It should be noted further that the mean free path between scattering interactions is given by $1/\mu_t$ and not by $1/\mu_s$, as shown in Eq. (5). The distribution of free path lengths between interactions therefore does not depend on changes in the albedo as long as μ_t is kept constant. Therefore results for the same value of μ_t but for other values of the albedo can be obtained quickly if the number of interactions within the simulated turbid medium $N(i)$ has been stored for each photon path for which the photon has not been absorbed. For the remitted photon in Fig. 2(a) $N(i) = 4$.

In the case of reflection from a semi-infinite medium a value for $r(i)$ must be available for each photon path too. For slabs it must be known for each photon path if it contributes to reflection or to transmission.

B. Verification of the Theory

To support our theoretical considerations two different Monte Carlo simulations with 30,000 photons have been performed with different absorption chances. In one simulation this chance was set at 0.00001, and thus $c_{\text{sim},1} = 0.99999$; in the other simulation the absorption chance per interaction was 0.005, and thus $c_{\text{sim},2} = 0.995$. Isotropic scattering was simulated, and the number of interactions as well as the position where the photon leaves the medium have been stored for each photon path.

The results of both simulations were used for predictions at lower values of the albedo. Figure 3 shows the results. Each symbol in Fig. 3 represents 600 photon paths selected in order of increasing distance of remission. All data points with the same symbols were based on the same set of photon paths. No differences but statistical noise in the calculated relative reflectance have been observed. The smaller number of symbols at greater distances from the origin for the results based on the simulation with

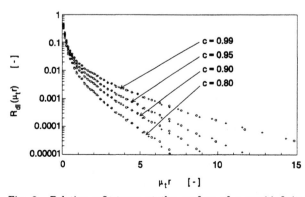

Fig. 3. Relative reflectance at the surface of a semi-infinite medium as a function of $r\mu_t$ for different values of the albedo c. The relative reflectances were derived from two different condensed Monte Carlo simulations: ○, $c_{\text{sim}} = 0.995$, +, $c_{\text{sim}} = 0.99999$. Isotropic scattering, $n_{\text{refr}} = 1.4$.

$c_{\mathrm{sim}} = 0.995$ shows that the number of photon paths that leave the medium at greater distances is smaller in that simulation; this is caused by the higher probability of absorption during simulation. The average number of interactions per photon path is much smaller for the second simulation as well. The computing time needed for the second simulation was therefore much smaller: 3 h instead of half a week.

The values for total transmission and total reflection, which are determined with the condensed results of Monte Carlo simulation, have also been compared with the data given by Prahl.[20] An example of Henyey–Greenstein scattering with $g = 0.875$ is given in Table 1.

We conclude that the results of Monte Carlo simulations can be used again in situations with different values of μ_t and c if the distances can be scaled, if $c \leq c_{\mathrm{sim}}$, and if the positions and the number of interactions are stored for all the photons of interest. For $c > c_{\mathrm{sim}}$ the formula has to be used with care, since the contribution of many photons may be calculated from a single photon path.

4. Inversion of Results from Monte Carlo Simulations

The absorption and scattering coefficients of turbid media are often determined from slabs of the medium. In many cases the sample is kept in place between glass slides. The values of diffuse reflectance, total transmission, and collimated transmission are determined experimentally. Tissue properties are calculated from these measurements.

Prahl has used an inversion method to obtain the absorption and scattering coefficients by interpolation from the tabulated values of total transmission and diffuse reflection with given values of g, $\mu_t d = 2^n$, and the albedo, which is based on adding–doubling results.[20] Van der Zee et al.[39] have applied a similar method, that is based on tabulated results from Monte Carlo simulations.

However, since total reflection and total transmission can be calculated quickly from condensed Monte Carlo simulations for given values of c_{sim} and $\mu_t d$, we decided to develop an inverse procedure based on Monte Carlo simulations. Further simplification appeared to be possible since transmission and reflec-

tion data are calculated from only the number of interactions that are the same for many photons. Therefore the condensed Monte Carlo results for slabs have been tabulated as a function of the number of interactions, as shown in Table 2. Transmission without interactions corresponds to collimated transmission, whereas reflection without interaction corresponds to specular reflection.

Total transmission and reflection for other values of the albedo can be found with

$$T_{\mathrm{tot}} = \sum_{j=0}^{N_{\mathrm{table}}} N_{\mathrm{trans}}(j)\left(\frac{c}{c_{\mathrm{sim}}}\right)^j, \qquad (13)$$

$$R_{\mathrm{tot}} = \sum_{j=0}^{N_{\mathrm{table}}} N_{\mathrm{refl}}(j)\left(\frac{c}{c_{\mathrm{sim}}}\right)^j, \qquad (14)$$

where N_{table} is the maximum number of interactions within the table.

Monte Carlo simulations were performed for Henyey–Greenstein scattering with $g = 0.875$ and optical thicknesses $\mu_t d = 1, 2, 4, 8,$ and 16. It is possible to create a table for different values of the albedo, between which interpolation is performed. However, our calculations are performed for each new estimate of the albedo. Figures 4 and 5 show some results from these tables. The albedo in these figures is given as a reduced albedo, $c' \equiv \mu_s'/\mu_t'$, with $\mu_t' = \mu_a + \mu_s'$, for the purposes described in Section 5.

Figure 4 shows that it is possible to base an interpolation method on the assumption that the values of the logarithm of T_{tot} between two values of $\mu_t d$ are located at straight lines when they are plotted as a function of $\mu_t d$. The dotted curves in Fig. 4 are spline functions that indicate where the deviations caused by linear interpolation occur. For greater values of $\mu_t d$ the T_{tot} slope becomes constant and the deviations disappear.

From Fig. 5 we can see that a similar method also can be used for the logarithm of $R_{\mathrm{tot}} + T_{\mathrm{tot}}$ for slab

Table 1. Total Reflection and Total Transmission for Slabs with Henyey–Greenstein Scatterers between Glass Slides, $g_{HG} = 0.875$, $c = 0.99$[a]

	R_{tot}		T_{tot}	
$\mu_t d$	This Work	Prahl[20]	This Work	Prahl[20]
1.00	0.123	0.127	0.855	0.849
2.00	0.169	0.170	0.779	0.777
4.00	0.231	0.234	0.654	0.649
8.00	0.290	0.287	0.475	0.473
16.00	0.311	0.307	0.282	0.280

[a]Refractive indices are 1.4 for the slab, 1.5 for the glass slides, and 1.0 outside the slab. Results are from condensed Monte Carlo simulations ($N_{\mathrm{tot}} = 30{,}000$ photons, $c_{\mathrm{sim}} = 0.99999$) and from adding–doubling calculations by Prahl.[20]

Table 2. Number of Photons Transmitted and Reflected After j Interactions with the Medium[a]

j	N_{trans}	N_{refl}
0	10,199	1311
1	1452	1739
2	1145	1292
3	1043	1088
4	859	848
5	741	777
6	606	596
7	513	529
8	431	426
9	370	362
10	302	269
—	—	—
—	—	—
53	0	1

[a]Refractive index (air/glass/sample/glass/air): 1.0/1.5/1.4/1.5/1.0. Isotropic scattering. Sample: $\mu_t d = 1$; $c_{\mathrm{sim}} = 0.99999$; $N_{\mathrm{tot}} = 30{,}000$.

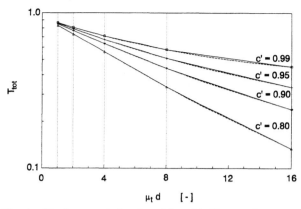

Fig. 4. Total transmission for slabs with Henyey–Greenstein scatterers ($g = 0.875$) between glass slides as a function of slab thickness. Calculations for reduced albedo $c' = 0.99$, 0.95, 0.90, and 0.80. Refractive index (air/glass/sample/glass/air): $1.0/1.5/1.4/1.5/1.0$.

thicknesses for which Monte Carlo results have been derived. The range in Fig. 4 and 5 is used most often for analyzing the scattering and absorption properties of tissue slabs. In Fig. 5 deviations caused by linear interpolation occur for relatively low albedos. For thicker slabs some deviation will also occur for the higher albedos, since for large slabs $R_{tot} + T_{tot}$ becomes almost independent of the slab thickness. Therefore it is possible that the resolution between tables with subsequent values of $\Sigma_t'd$ must be chosen smaller in that range so that the desired accuracy with the present interpolation method is obtained.

An iterative procedure was introduced for solving c and $\mu_t d$. A value for $\mu_t d$ is calculated for the given value of T_{tot} and an estimate of c. We applied a similar procedure to obtain a value for $\mu_t d$ based on the given value of $R_{tot} + T_{tot}$ and the same estimate of c. Both values for $\mu_t d$ are different when the estimate for c differs from the correct value. Therefore calculations are repeated for other values of the

albedo until both calculated values of $\mu_t d$ are the same.

5. Similarity Relations

The application of Monte Carlo simulations with a phase function that differs from the actual phase function is possible if a similarity is assumed:

$$\mu_a = \mu_{a,\text{sim}}, \tag{15}$$

$$\mu_s' = \mu_s(1 - g) = \mu_{s,\text{sim}}(1 - g_{\text{sim}}), \tag{16}$$

where the sim subscript is used for the values of the asymmetry factor and the absorption and scattering coefficients in the Monte Carlo simulation.[9] Equations (15) and (16) are often explained by the addition of purely forward scattering to isotropic scattering. However, the addition of the possibility of exact forward scattering does not change the photon paths. Therefore Eqs. (15) and (16) cannot provide information about the influence on light propagation of different phase functions with the same anisotropy factor.

When the similarity is applied, a reduced dimensionless relative reflectance $R_{dl}'(\mu_t'r)$ can be defined as the photon fraction escaping per reduced mean free path squared with

$$R_{dl}'(\mu_t'r) \equiv R(r)/(\mu_t')^2. \tag{17}$$

The relative reflectances remitted at the surface of the semi-infinite medium with matched boundary conditions can also be predicted by diffusion theory. At greater distances from the origin,

$$R(r) = \text{const} \exp(-\alpha r)/r^2, \tag{18}$$

as given by Schmitt et al.[37] and Patterson et al.[44] The attenuation coefficient for the diffusion approximation α_{diff} is given by

$$\alpha_{\text{diff}} = (3\mu_a\mu_t')^{1/2}. \tag{19}$$

When we plot $(\mu_t'r)^2 R_{dl}'(\mu_t'r)$ logarithmically as a function of $\mu_t'r$, a linear relationship at greater distances is expected from diffusion theory from Eq. (18), which should not depend on g. Therefore we have decided to present the results of Monte Carlo simulations in this section in such a way.

Figure 6 shows the dimensionless relative reflectances for semi-infinite media illuminated by a pencil beam at the origin for $c' = 0.99$ and $c' = 0.80$. The results are shown for Henyey–Greenstein scattering with four different values of the anisotropy factor g. These results show clearly that the similarity between results with high values of g is stronger than when they are compared with isotropic scattering.

For $\mu_t'r < 1.0$ the similarity is weaker, even for $c' \approx 1.0$. Within that range Bolt and Ten Bosch[45] were able to discriminate between latex solutions with different values of g by presenting measured results as in Fig. 6.

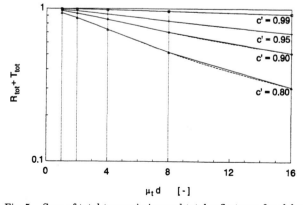

Fig. 5. Sum of total transmission and total reflectance for slabs with Henyey–Greenstein scatterers ($g = 0.875$) between glass slides as a function of slab thickness. Calculations for reduced albedo $c' = 0.99$, 0.95, 0.90, and 0.80. Refractive index (air/glass/sample/glass/air): $1.0/1.5/1.4/1.5/1.0$.

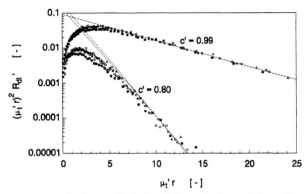

Fig. 6. Similarity test for reduced dimensionless relative reflectances at the surface of a semi-infinite medium as a function of $r\mu_t'$ for different values of the reduced albedo c'. The dimensionless relative reflectances were multiplied by $(r\mu_t')^2$ and were derived from condensed Monte Carlo simulations with different phase functions: Henyey–Greenstein scattering with ■, $g_{HG} = 0$, △, $g_{HG} = 0.75$, ○, $g_{HG} = 0.875$, ◇, $g_{HG} = 0.95$, $n_{refr} = 1.4$. The dotted lines indicate the slope predicted by Eq. (18).

The slope predicted by diffusion theory for $c' = 0.99$ and according to Eqs. (17)–(19) has been added also in Fig. 6. In this case the slope seems to be predicted accurately. However, for $c' = 0.80$ the slope predicted from the diffusion theory, $\alpha_{diff}/\mu_t' = 0.7746$, deviates from the Monte Carlo data. One explanation for this is that α_{diff} is not predicted accurately enough for this value of c'. Therefore more accurate values of α for calculating the slopes have been obtained; they are based on the rigorous method described earlier[43] when it is applied to Henyey–Greenstein scattering. For the $c' = 0.80$ case the slopes for isotropic scattering and highly forward scattering are $\alpha/\mu_t' = 0.7104$ and $0.737 < \alpha/\mu_t' < 0.741$ for $g_{HG} = 0$ and $0.75 < g_{HG} < 0.95$, respectively. A difference remains between the predicted slope and the Monte Carlo results.

For $c' > 0.99$ we also found increasing deviations between the predicted slope and Monte Carlo results: for $c' = 0.999$ the slope is ∼0.025 steeper than the α/μ_t' slope for $g = 0$ as well as for $g_{HG} = 0.875$. Because these deviations occur for both values of g, we conclude that the similarity between the Monte Carlo solutions holds also for $c' \approx 1.0$. Any influence on the slope from photon termination for these large values of c' can be excluded, since the chance that photons will have more than 20,000 interactions is only $c^{20,000} = 2 \times 10^{-9}$. Nor can the deviations be caused by differences between the rigorous values for α and α_{diff}, since these values can be neglected for $c' \approx 1.0$. Therefore we suspect that there is an effect on the slope from internal reflections that has not been taken into account in Eq. (18).

The validity of the similarity rules as shown in Eqs. (15) and (16) has also been investigated for optically thin slabs, as shown in Tables 3 and 4. These tables have been obtained by interpolation between Monte Carlo results for different slab thicknesses, as shown

Table 3. Total Transmission T_{tot} for Optically Thin Slabs between Glass Slides Investigated for Henyey–Greenstein Scattering with $g = 0.875$, $g = 0.75$, and $g = 0^a$

$\Sigma_t'd$	c'	T_{tot} ($g = 0.875$)	T_{tot} ($g = 0.75$)	T_{tot} ($g = 0$)	Error (%)
1.0	0.99	0.583	0.583	0.623	+7
	0.95	0.524	0.523	0.566	+8
	0.90	0.470	0.469	0.517	+10
	0.80	0.402	0.401	0.457	+14
2.0	0.99	0.453	0.452	0.472	+4
	0.95	0.346	0.347	0.371	+7
	0.90	0.267	0.269	0.298	+12
	0.80	0.184	0.188	0.224	+22

^{a}Refractive index (air/glass/sample/glass/air): 1.0/1.5/1.4/1.5/1.0. The indicated error is introduced when results for high values of g are compared with results for isotropic scattering, $g = 0$.

for $g = 0.875$ in Figs. 4 and 5. In the latter case

$$\mu_t d = (\mu_a/\mu_t' + \mu_s'/[(1 - g)\mu_t'])\mu_t'd = (1 + 7c')\mu_t'd.$$

(20)

The validity of the similarity between highly forward scattering and isotropic scattering appears to be restricted in that case, even if the amount of absorption can be neglected. However, the results in Tables 3 and 4 for $g_{HG} = 0.875$ and $g_{HG} = 0.75$ differ by only a few pecentage points. The error increases for increasing absorption.

It has already been shown by van de Hulst that turbid slabs with Henyey–Greenstein scatterers and large values of g are not described effectively by isotropic scattering with the same value of μ_s', especially in the range where the diffusion approximation is not valid.[9] However, the similarity between Henyey–Greenstein scattering results remarkably improves when we compare the results for values of g_{HG} above 0.75. Our previous studies on the attenuation coefficient α in infinite media have confirmed this finding for Rayleigh–Gans scattering.[17,43]

From Fig. 6 and Tables 3 and 4 we conclude that

Table 4. Total Reflection R_{tot} for Optically Thin Slabs between Glass Slides Investigated for Henyey–Greenstein Scattering with $g = 0.875$, $g = 0.75$, and $g = 0^a$

$\Sigma_t'd$	c'	R_{tot} ($g = 0.875$)	R_{tot} ($g = 0.75$)	R_{tot} ($g = 0$)	Error (%)
1.0	0.99	0.379	0.380	0.342	−10
	0.95	0.315	0.318	0.285	−10
	0.90	0.257	0.260	0.235	−10
	0.80	0.183	0.179	0.172	−6
2.0	0.99	0.470	0.471	0.454	−4
	0.95	0.358	0.359	0.349	−3
	0.90	0.274	0.275	0.271	−2
	0.80	0.185	0.187	0.187	+1

^{a}Refractive index (air/glass/sample/glass/air): 1.0/1.5/1.4/1.5/1.0. The indicated error is introduced when results for high values of g are compared with values for isotropic scattering, $g = 0$.

the similarity between results of two phase functions is much better if the values of g are not too different and if the absorption coefficient is much smaller than the reduced scattering coefficient.

6. Conclusions

It has been shown that we can apply the results of a single Monte Carlo simulation to generate results quickly for a large range of values of the albedo. This enables calculations of absorption and scattering properties from given reflectance and transmission data by inversion techniques applied to condensed Monte Carlo results.

Accurate values of the phase function are often not available in biomedical applications because of the variation between subjects. However, in the case of similarity the μ_s' and μ_a values can be predicted from *in vitro* measurements of the total transmission and total reflection of slabs. It is recommended that phase functions be applied that are similar to that in the sample, since predictions with Monte Carlo simulations have been shown to be most accurate if the phase function resembles the phase function of the scatterers within the sample.

To estimate the error if μ_a and μ_s' are derived from thin slabs, we suggest that these properties be predicted with two phase functions, e.g., the expected distribution of scattering angles and isotropic scattering.

The concept of condensed Monte Carlo simulations that is presented here can probably be applied also to analysis of time-resolved spectroscopy, since the number of interactions can be used to estimate the lengths of photon paths within the medium.

The condensed Monte Carlo technique has been shown to be consistent with other results. We have applied it to obtain the optical properties of the skin *in vivo*,[21] and it is used by us to analyze reflection pulse oximetry.[24]

References

1. J. D. Hardy, H. T. Hammel, and D. Murgatroyd, "Spectral transmission and reflectance of excised human skin," J. Appl. Physiol. **9**, 257–264 (1956).
2. W. G. Zijlstra and G. A. Mook, *Medical Reflection Oximetry* (Van Gorcum, Assen, The Netherlands, 1962).
3. R. R. Anderson and J. A. Parrish, "Optical properties of human skin," in *The Science of Photomedicine*, J. D. Regan and J. A. Parrish, eds. (Plenum, New York, 1982), pp. 147–194.
4. R. F. Bonner and R. Nossal, "Principles of laser Doppler flowmetry," in *Laser Doppler Blood Flowmetry*, A. P. Shepherd and P. A. Öberg, eds. (Kluwer, Boston, Mass., 1990), pp. 17–45.
5. B. C. Chance, "Optical method," Ann. Rev. Biophys. Biochem. **20**, 1–28 (1991).
6. L. E. Preuss and A. E. Profio, "Optical properties of mammalian tissue: introduction by the feature editors," Appl. Opt. **28**, 2207–2209 (1989).
7. K. M. Case and P. F. Zweifel, *Linear Transport Theory* (Addison-Wesley, Reading, Mass., 1967).
8. A. Ishimaru, *Wave Propagation and Scattering in Random Media* (Academic, New York, 1978).
9. H. C. van de Hulst, *Multiple Light Scattering* (Academic, New York, 1980).
10. W. F. Cheong, S. A. Prahl, and A. J. Welch, "A review of the optical properties of biological tissues," IEEE J. Quantum Electron. **26**, 2166–2185 (1990).
11. P. Kubelka and F. Munk, "Ein Beitrag zur Optik der Farbanstriche," Z. Tech. Phys. **12**, 593–601 (1931).
12. R. P. Hemenger, "Optical properties of turbid media with specularly reflecting boundaries: applications to biological problems," Appl. Opt. **16**, 2007–2012 (1977).
13. W. M. Star, J. P. A. Marijnissen, and M. J. C. Van Gemert, "New trends in photobiology," J. Photochem. Photobiol. B **1**, 149–167 (1987).
14. R. G. Giovanelli, "Reflection by semi-infinite diffusers," Opt. Acta **2**, 153–162 (1955).
15. J. R. Mika, "Neutron transport with anisotropic scattering," Nucl. Sci. Eng. **11**, 415–427 (1961).
16. K. Klier, "Absorption and scattering in plane parallel turbid media," J. Opt. Soc. Am. **62**, 882–885 (1972).
17. R. Graaff, J. G. Aarnoudse, F. F. M. de Mul, and H. W. Jentink, "Light propagation parameters for anisotropically scattering media, based on a rigorous solution of the transport equation," Appl. Opt. **28**, 2273–2279 (1989).
18. H. C. van de Hulst, "Asymptotic fitting, a method for solving anisotropic transfer problems in thick layers," J. Comput. Phys. **3**, 291–306 (1968).
19. P. S. Mudgett and L. W. Richards, "Multiple scattering calculations for technology," Appl. Opt. **10**, 1485–1502 (1971).
20. S. A. Prahl, "Calculation of light distributions and optical properties of tissue," Ph.D. dissertation (University of Texas at Austin, Austin, Tex., 1988).
21. R. Graaff, A. C. M. Dassel, M. H. Koelink, F. F. M. de Mul, J. G. Aarnoudse, and W. G. Zijlstra, "Optical properties of human dermis *in vitro* and *in vivo*," Appl. Opt. **32**, 435–447 (1993).
22. H. W. Jentink, F. F. M. de Mul, R. G. A. M. Hermsen, R. Graaff, and J. Greve, "Monte Carlo simulations of laser Doppler blood flow measurements in tissue," Appl. Opt. **29**, 2371–2381 (1990).
23. M. H. Koelink, F. F. M. de Mul, J. Greve, R. Graaff, A. C. M. Dassel, and J. G. Aarnoudse, "Monte Carlo simulations and measurements of signals in laser Doppler flowmetry on human skin," in *Time-Resolved Spectroscopy and Imaging of Tissues*, B. Chance, ed., Proc. Soc. Photo-Opt. Instrum. Eng. 63–72 (1991).
24. R. Graaff, A. C. M. Dassel, J. G. Aarnoudse, W. G. Zijlstra, P. Heida, F. F. M. de Mul, M. H. Koelink, and J. Greve, "Biophysical aspects of reflection pulse oximetry," in *Proceedings of the Fourth International Conference on Fetal and Neonatal Physiological Measurements*, H. N. Lafeber, J. G. Aarnoudse, and H. W. Jongsma, eds. (Elsevier, Amsterdam, 1991).
25. R. Graaff, J. G. Aarnoudse, J. R. Zijp, P. M. A. Sloot, F. F. M. de Mul, J. Greve, and M. H. Koelink, "Reduced light scattering properties for mixtures of spherical particles: a simple approximation derived from Mie calculations," Appl. Opt. **31**, 1370–1376 (1992).
26. B. Chance, S. Nioka, J. Kent, K. McCully, M. Fountain, R. Greenfeld, and G. Holtom, "Time-resolved spectroscopy of hemoglobin and myoglobin in resting and ischemic muscle," Anal. Biochem. **174**, 698–707 (1988).
27. D. T. Delpy, M. Cope, P. van der Zee, S. Arridge, S. Wray, and J. Wyatt, "Estimation of optical path length," Phys. Med. Biol. **33**, 1433–1442 (1988).
28. R. A. J. Groenhuis, J. J. Ten Bosch, and H. A. Ferwerda, "Scattering and absorption of turbid materials determined from reflection measurements. II: Measuring method and calibration," Appl. Opt. **22**, 2463–2467 (1983).
29. W. M. Star and J. P. A. Marijnissen, "Calculating the response of isotropic light dosimetry probes as a function of the tissue refractive index," Appl. Opt. **28**, 2288–2291 (1989).

30. R. Bays, L. Winterhalter, H. Funakubo, Ph. Monnier, M. Savary, G. Wagnières, D. Braichotte, A. Châtelain, H. van den Bergh, L. Svaasand, and C. W. Burckhardt, "Clinical optical dose measurement for PDT: invasive and noninvasive techniques," in *Future Trends in Biomedical Applications of Lasers,* L. O. Svaasand, ed., Proc. Soc. Photo-Opt. Instrum. Eng. **1525,** 397–408 (1991).

31. L. Reynolds, C. Johnson, and A. Ishimaru, "Diffuse reflectance from a finite blood medium: applications to the modeling of fiber optic catheters," Appl. Opt. **15,** 2059–2067 (1976).

32. R. A. J. Groenhuis, H. A. Ferwerda, and J. J. Ten Bosch, "Scattering and absorption of turbid materials determined from reflection measurements. I: theory," Appl. Opt. **22,** 2456–2462 (1983).

33. J. M. Schmitt, J. D. Meindl, and F. G. Mihm, "An integrated circuit-based optical sensor for *in-vivo* measurement of blood oxygenation," IEEE Trans., Biomed. Eng. **BME-33,** 98–107 (1986).

34. S. Takatani, H. Noda, H. Takano, and T. Akutsu, "A miniature hybrid reflection type optical sensor for measurement of hemoglobin content and oxygen saturation of whole blood," IEEE Trans., Biomed. Eng. **BME-35,** 187–198 (1988).

35. J. M. Steinke and A. P. Shepherd, "Diffusion model of the optical absorbance of whole blood," J. Opt. Soc. Am. A **5,** 813–822 (1988).

36. S. Takatani and M. D. Graham, "Analysis of diffuse reflectance from a two layer tissue model," IEEE Trans. Biomed. Eng. **BME-26,** 656–664 (1979).

37. J. M. Schmitt, G. X. Zhou, E. C. Walker, and R. T. Wall, "Multilayer model for photon diffusion in skin," J. Opt. Soc. Am. A **7,** 2141–2153 (1990).

38. V. G. Peters, D. R. Wyman, M. S. Patterson, and G. L. Frank, "Optical properties of normal and diseased human breast tissues in the visible and near infrared," Phys. Med. Biol. **35,** 1317–1334 (1990).

39. P. van der Zee, M. Essenpreis, D. T. Delpy, and M. Cope, "Accurate determination of optical properties of biological tissues using a Monte Carlo inversion technique," in *Proceedings of the Topical Meeting on Atmospheric, Volume, and Surface Scattering and Propagation* A. Consortini, ed. (ICO Secretariat, Florence, Italy, 1991), pp. 125–128.

40. J. M. Maarek, G. Jarry, B. de Losnac, A. Lansiart, and B. M. Hung, "A simulation method for the study of laser transillumination of biological tissues," Ann. Biomed. Eng. **12,** 281–284 (1984).

41. R. F. Bonner, R. Nossal, S. Havlin, and G. H. Weiss, "Model of photon migration in turbid biological media," J. Opt. Soc. Am. A **4,** 423–432 (1987).

42. S. L. Jacques and M. Keijzer, "Dosimetry for lasers and light in dermatology: Monte Carlo simulations of 577-nm pulsed laser penetration into cutaneous vessels," in *Lasers in Dermatology and Tissue Welding,* O. T. Tan, R. A. White, and J. V. White, eds., Proc. Soc. Photo-Opt. Instrum. Eng. **1422,** 2–13 (1991).

43. R. Graaff, J. G. Aarnoudse, F. F. M. de Mul, and H. W. Jentink, "Improved expression for anisotropic scattering in absorbing media," in *Scattering and Diffraction,* H. A. Ferwerda, ed., Proc. Soc. Photo-Opt. Instrum. Eng. **1029,** 103–110 (1989).

44. M. S. Patterson, E. Schwartz, and B. C. Wilson, "Quantitative reflection spectrophotometry for the noninvasive measurement of photosensitizer concentration in tissue during photodynamic therapy," in *Photodynamic Therapy: Mechanisms,* P. Dougherty, ed., Proc. Soc. Photo-Opt. Instrum. Eng. **1065,** 115–122 (1989).

45. R. A. Bolt and J. J. Ten Bosch, "A method for measuring position-dependent volume reflection," Appl. Opt. (to be published).

Reprinted with permission from *IEEE Journal of Quantum Electronics*, Vol. 26(12),
pp. 2166-2185 (December 1990). ©1990 IEEE.

A Review of the Optical Properties of Biological Tissues

WAI-FUNG CHEONG, SCOTT A. PRAHL, AND ASHLEY J. WELCH, SENIOR MEMBER, IEEE

Abstract—A comprehensive compilation of published optical properties (absorption, scattering, total attenuation, effective attenuation, and/or anisotropy coefficients) of various biological tissues at a variety of wavelengths is presented. The theoretical foundations for most experimental approaches are outlined. Relations between Kubelka–Munk parameters and transport coefficients are listed. The optical properties of aorta, liver, and muscle at 633 nm are discussed in detail.

I. INTRODUCTION

THE propagation of laser light in tissue is a question of growing concern in many medical applications. Numerous models that predict fluence rates in tissue, or reflection and transmission of light by tissue have been developed. The accuracy of these models ultimately depends upon how well the optical properties of the tissue are known. Optical parameters are obtained by converting measurements of observable quantities (e.g., reflection) into parameters which characterize light propagation in tissue. The conversion process is based on a particular theory of light transport in tissue.

In past years, a host of investigators have reported values for the total attenuation coefficient, the effective attenuation coefficient, the effective penetration depth, the absorption and scattering coefficients, and the scattering anisotropy factor for a variety of tissues at a variety of light wavelengths. The majority of these results are based upon approximations to the radiative transport theory (e.g., diffusion theory). Yet sufficient variations in 1) model assumptions (e.g., isotropic–anisotropic scattering or matched–mismatched boundaries), 2) measurement techniques, 3) experimental apparatus, 4) calibration schemes, and 5) biological heterogeneities exist that efforts to extract average values for different tissue types is complicated. Regardless of these problems, there is a need to consolidate what has already been measured, and the main thrust of this paper is to present a summary of reported optical measurements. All published (within the authors' awareness) optical properties of tissue are gathered into this single compilation.

Manuscript received February 2, 1990; April 20, 1990. This work was supported in part by the Office of Naval Research under Contract N000014-86-K-0875 and by the Albert and Clemmie Caster Foundation, and was done at the University of Texas at Austin.

W.-F. Cheong was with the Biomedical Engineering Program, University of Texas at Austin, Austin, TX 78712. She is now with the Department of Dermatology, Boston University School of Medicine, Boston, MA 02118.

S. A. Prahl is with the Wellman Laboratories of Photomedicine, Harvard Medical School, Massachusetts General Hospital, Boston, MA 02114.

A. J. Welch is with the Department of Electrical and Computer Engineering, University of Texas at Austin, Austin, TX 78712.

IEEE Log Number 9040290.

A brief description of the radiative transport equation which is basic to all the light propagation models, and its associated parameters appears in Section II. Various solutions are presented to show how optical properties can be determined from using different measurements. Section III compares the Kubelka–Munk coefficients and the transport coefficients. Section IV provides specific descriptions of several methods used to determine optical properties. Section V discusses the measured optical properties for three selected tissue groups at 633 nm.

II. LIGHT PROPAGATION MODELS

Most of the recent advances in describing the transfer of laser energy in tissue are based upon transport theory. This theory is preferred in tissue optics instead of analytic approaches using Maxwell equations because of inhomogeneity of biological tissue. According to transport theory, the radiance $L(r, s)$ ($W \cdot m^{-2} \cdot sr^{-1}$) of light at position r traveling in a direction of the unit vector s is decreased by absorption and scattering but it is increased by light that is scattered from s' directions into the direction s. The radiative transport equation which describes this light interaction is [1]

$$s \cdot \nabla L(r, s) = -(\mu_a + \mu_s)L(r, s)$$
$$+ \mu_s \int_{4\pi} p(s, s')L(r, s') \, d\omega' \quad (1)$$

where $\mu_a(m^{-1})$ is the absorption coefficient, $\mu_s(m^{-1})$ is the scattering coefficient, $\mu_t(m^{-1})$ is the attenuation coefficient, $d\omega'$ is the differential solid angle in the direction s', and $p(s, s')$ is the phase function. The total attenuation coefficient is

$$\mu_t = \mu_a + \mu_s. \quad (2)$$

The phase function describes the angular distribution for a single scattering event. For tractability, the phase function is usually assumed to be a function only of the angle between s and s'. If the integral of the phase function is normalized to equal one, then $p(s, s')$ is the probability density function for scattering from direction s' to direction s,

$$\int_{4\pi} p(s, s') \, d\omega' = 1 \quad (3)$$

Usually the form of the phase function is not known. In these cases the phase function is usually characterized by a single parameter g called the average cosine of the phase function g,

$$g = \int_{4\pi} p(s, s')(s \cdot s') \, d\omega'. \qquad (4)$$

This parameter is sometimes called the anisotropy coefficient. It is a measure of the asymmetry of the single scattering pattern; g approaching 1, 0, and -1 describes extremely forward, isotropic, and highly backward scattering, respectively.

Formulation of the transport equation assumes that each scattering particle is sufficiently distant from its neighbors to prevent interactions between successive scattering effects. In theory, these scatterers and absorbers must be uniformly distributed throughout the medium. Fluorescence and polarization events are neglected. Until recently, most tissue optics studies considered only steady-state (time-independent) transport of light.

Calculations of light distribution based on the radiative transport equation require knowledge of the absorption and scattering coefficients, and the phase function. Yet to arrive at these parameters, one must first have a solution of the radiative transport equation. Because of the difficulty of solving the transport equation exactly, several approximations have been made regarding the representation of the radiance and/or of the phase function. Forms of these approximate solutions for calculating light distribution within tissues are dependent upon the type of irradiance (diffuse or collimated) and the optical boundary conditions (matched or unmatched indexes of refraction). Fortunately, two simple solutions of the transport equation exist that provide expressions for the unscattered transmission and for the asymptotic fluence rate deep in a bulk tissue (far from light sources and boundaries).

A. Unscattered Transmission

Unscattered light is attenuated exponentially following Beer's law. For light passing through a slab of tissue with thickness t and having no reflections at the surface, the transmission is given by

$$T_c = e^{-\mu_t t} \qquad (5)$$

where T_c is the unscattered transmission (sometimes also referred to as the collimated or the primary transmission). Thus the total attenuation coefficient can be obtained from a tissue sample using

$$\mu_t = -\frac{1}{t} \ln T_c. \qquad (6)$$

If measurements of T_c are made when surface reflections are present, e.g., in air, corrections are required for the reflections at all mismatched surfaces. For a tissue sample placed between glass or quartz slides, the collimated beam is reflected at the air–slide, slide–tissue, tissue–slide, and slide–air interfaces. If the sample is only a few optical depths thick, multiple internal reflections must be considered. A net reflection coefficient for an air–glass–tissue layer is given by [2]

$$r = \frac{r_g + r_t - 2r_g r_t}{1 - r_g r_t} \qquad (7)$$

where the Fresnel reflections at the air–glass and glass–tissue interfaces are r_g and r_t, respectively. The measured transmission T is

$$T = \frac{(1 - r)^2}{1 - r^2 T_c^2} \, T_c. \qquad (8)$$

Equation (8) is first solved for T_c, before using (6) to calculate μ_t.

B. Asymptotic Fluence Rate

In tissue regions far from light sources and boundaries, the fluence rate ($W \cdot m^{-2}$) decays exponentially. This is the dominant mode of propagation in an unbounded medium [3] and is often called the diffusion mode. The rate of decay is called the effective attenuation coefficient (μ_{eff}) or the diffusion exponent. An expression for this asymptotic fluence rate is

$$\Phi(z) \sim (\text{constant}) e^{-\mu_{eff} z} \qquad (9)$$

In this paper, μ_{eff} will always refer to the *measured* rate of decay of the fluence in this diffusion region. An approximate relation for the effective attenuation coefficient in terms of the absorption, scattering, and anisotropy scattering coefficients is given below.

C. Diffusion Theory

The radiance in (1) can be separated into unscattered and scattered components

$$L(r, s) = L_c(r, s) + L_d(r, s). \qquad (10)$$

The unscattered portion (L_c) contains all light that has not interacted with the tissue. It satisfies Beer's law and the transmission equation (5). The scattered portion contains all light that has been scattered at least once and can be expressed exactly with an infinite sum of Legendre polynomials. However, the diffusion approximation truncates this sum to the first two terms (an isotropic and a slightly-forward directed term). This approximation simplifies the transport equation to the more tractable diffusion equation [4]

$$(\nabla^2 - \kappa^2)\Phi(r) = -Q_0(r) \qquad (11)$$

where $\Phi(r)$ is the total scattered (diffuse) fluence rate given by

$$\Phi(r) = \int_{4\pi} L_d(r, s) \, d\omega. \qquad (12)$$

The source term $Q_o(r)$ is generated by scattering of collimated normal irradiation

$$Q_o(r) = -3\mu_s[\mu_a + \mu_s(1 - g) + \mu_t g]$$
$$\cdot (1 - r_s)F_o(r) \exp(-\mu_t z). \qquad (13)$$

Here F_0 is the irradiance ($W \cdot m^{-2}$). The constant κ in (11) is an approximation of the actual measured effective attenuation coefficient μ_{eff} when absorption is dominated by scattering.

$$\kappa^2 = 3\mu[\mu_a + (1 - g)\mu_s]. \qquad (14)$$

130

For diffuse irradiances, Q_o is typically set to zero because the diffuse incidence is introduced in the boundary conditions. The accuracy of the diffusion equation is affected by the ratio of scattering to absorption, the scattering anisotropy, and the distance from light sources and boundaries [5].

Several phase functions are compatible with the diffusion approximation: the isotropic [6], the delta–isotropic, the Eddington [7], and the delta–Eddington [8]. These functions are approximations of the actual phase function for tissue, e.g., the Henyey–Greenstein function for dermal and aortic tissues [2], [9]. In the diffusion approximation, the delta–Eddington phase function is the best function for simulating light transport in tissues characterized by Henyey–Greenstein scattering [10]. If g_{HG} is the average cosine of the Henyey–Greenstein phase function [3], then the diffusion equation for a delta–Eddington phase function is found by making the following substitutions in (11).

$$\frac{g_{HG}}{(1 + g_{HG})} \rightarrow g \qquad (15a)$$

$$\mu_s(1 - g_{HG}^2) \rightarrow \mu_s. \qquad (15b)$$

The solution of the diffusion equation (1) for the total fluence rate in a finite parallel slab is [4]

$$\Phi_{total}(z) = a_1 \exp(\kappa z) + a_2 \exp(-\kappa z) + a_3 \exp(-\mu_t z). \qquad (16)$$

For a finite slab under plane collimated irradiation, Ishimaru provides values for a_1, a_2, and a_3 [4] for matched boundaries. In the case of a semi-infinite slab a_1 must equal zero; values for a_2 and a_3 have been evaluated by Phahl, based on the delta–Eddington approximation, for a uniform collimated irradiance F_0 for matched and mismatched boundary conditions [2].

The dominant term in (16) for large z in a semi-infinite slab yields the following approximate relation for the measured effective attenuation coefficient

$$\mu_{eff} \approx \kappa \qquad \text{if } \mu_a \ll \mu_s. \qquad (17)$$

The accuracy of this relation decreases with decreasing ratios of scattering to absorption and increasing anisotropy (see Table 23 in van de Hulst [4]) and fails completely when absorption dominates scattering (since both the limiting form of (16) changes and the diffusion approximation itself is inaccurate).

Expressions for light flux solutions of the diffusion equation (11) are

$$F_+(z) = \frac{a_1}{4}[1 - h\kappa]e^{\kappa z} + \frac{a_2}{4}[1 + h\kappa]e^{-\kappa z}$$

$$+ \left\{ \frac{a_3}{4}[1 + h\mu_t] \right.$$

$$\left. + \frac{\mu_s g(1 - r_s)F_0}{2[\mu_a + (1 - g)\mu_s]} \right\} e^{-\mu_t z} \qquad (18a)$$

$$F_-(z) = \frac{a_1}{4}[1 + h\kappa]e^{\kappa z} + \frac{a_2}{4}[1 - h\kappa]e^{-\kappa z}$$

$$+ \left\{ \frac{a_3}{4}[1 - h\mu_t] \right.$$

$$\left. - \frac{\mu_s g(1 - r_s)F_0}{2[\mu_a + (1 - g)\mu_s]} \right\} e^{-\mu_t z} \qquad (18b)$$

$$F_d(z) = F_+(z) - F_-(z). \qquad (18c)$$

$F_+(z)$ and $F_-(z)$ are the forward and backward diffuse fluxes, respectively, and $F_d(z)$ is the net scattered flux along the direction of irradiation. The coefficient h is

$$h = 2/3[\mu_a + \mu_s(1 - g)]. \qquad (19)$$

For a semi-infinite slab, both the fluence rate and the fluxes have the same exponential behavior for large z:

$$F_\pm(z) \sim \frac{a_2}{4}[1 \pm h\kappa]e^{-\kappa z} \qquad \text{if } \mu_a \ll \mu_s. \qquad (20)$$

Consequently, for highly scattering biological tissues, interstitial measurements of either fluence rate by isotropic detectors or flux by flat cut fibers placed deep inside the tissue permits evaluation of κ as suggested by (16) and (20) [11]–[14].

The reflection and transmission of a slab of thickness t with index matched boundaries in the diffusion approximation are given by [2], [4], [15], [16]

$$R = -\frac{\mu_s g}{[\mu_a + (1 - g)\mu_s]} + \frac{h}{2}\{a_1\kappa - a_2\kappa - a_3\kappa\} \qquad (21a)$$

$$T = \frac{\mu_s g}{[\mu_a + (1 - g)\mu_s]} e^{-\mu_t t}$$

$$- \{a_1\kappa e^{\kappa t} - a_2\kappa e^{-\kappa t} - a_3\mu_t e^{-\mu_t t}\}. \qquad (21b)$$

The total transmission is $T_t = T + T_c$, where T_c is given by (5).

Measurements of diffuse reflection (R), total transmission (T_t), and unscattered transmission (T_c) provide sufficient information for uniquely determining three optical parameters (μ_a, μ_s, g). However, if only diffuse reflection and total transmission measurements are available, only absorption (μ_a) and reduced scattering [$\mu_s' = \mu_s(1 - g)$] coefficients can be calculated. The anisotropy (g) has been incorporated into μ_s' by the similarity relations $\mu_a' = \mu_a$ and $\mu_s'(1 - g') = \mu_s(1 - g)$. Anisotropic scattering is reduced to isotropic scattering by setting $g' = 0$ and so $\mu_s' = (1 - g)\mu_s$ [3], [17].

Some diffusion models incorporate index mismatched boundaries, scattering anisotropy, and tissue layers with varying optical properties. However, these models lead to complicated relations for reflection and transmission, and the optical properties cannot be directly expressed in terms of the reflection and transmission. Iterative methods (discussed in the next section) are used to determine optical properties using such models.

Several models proposed for modeling the propagation of laser light in tissue are listed in Table I along with the optical parameters required by each model. In particular, when a one-dimensional geometry is a reasonable representation, then the adding–doubling method [18]–[19] provides an accurate solution of transport equation for any phase function. This method permits modeling of anisotropically scattering, internally reflecting, and arbitrarily thick, layered media with relatively fast computations [3].

D. Kubelka–Munk Theory

The Kubelka–Munk theory describes the propagation of a uniform, diffuse irradiance through a one-dimensional isotropic slab with no reflection at the boundaries [20], [21]. This model is equivalent to a diffusion model having a forward and backward peaked phase function [3]. The Kubelka–Munk expressions for reflection and transmission of *diffuse* irradiance on a slab of thickness t are

$$R = \frac{\sinh(S_{KM}yt)}{x\cosh(S_{KM}yt) + y\sinh(S_{KM}yt)} \quad (22a)$$

$$T = \frac{y}{x\cosh(S_{KM}yt) + y\sinh(S_{KM}yt)} \quad (22b)$$

where A_{KM} and S_{KM} are the Kubelka–Munk absorption and scattering coefficients and have units of inverse length (m^{-1}). The parameters x and y are found using (23c). The advantage of the Kubelka–Munk model is that the scattering and absorption coefficients may be directly expressed in terms of the measured reflection and transmission

$$S_{KM} = \frac{1}{yt}\ln\left[\frac{1 - R(x - y)}{T}\right] \quad (23a)$$

$$A_{KM} = (x - 1)S_{KM} \quad (23b)$$

$$x = \frac{1 + R^2 - T^2}{2R}; \quad y = +\sqrt{x^2 - 1}. \quad (23c)$$

The simplicity of the Kubelka–Munk model has made it a popular method for measuring the optical properties of tissue. Unfortunately, the assumptions of isotropic scattering, matched boundaries, and diffuse irradiance are atypical of the interaction of laser light with tissue. Despite attempts to extend the Kubelka–Munk model to collimated irradiance [16], [22], [23] and anisotropic scattering [15], [22], [25], this method remains a poor approximation for laser light propagation in tissue [24].

III. Transport and Kubleka–Munk Coefficients

Nearly all optical properties can be separated into either transport (μ_a, μ_s, g) or Kubelka–Munk (A_{KM}, S_{KM}) coefficients, based on the theory used to obtain them. Not surprisingly, transport properties correspond to theories based on the transport equation (e.g., the diffusion equation). Kubelka–Munk properties are obtained using (23) above.

TABLE I
CONVERSION FORMULAS RELATING KUBELKA–MUNK TO TRANSPORT COEFFICIENTS

Author	η	χ or χ' [1]	Restrictions [2]
Klier[3] [26]	$\dfrac{(1-\varphi)(1-a)}{(1+\varphi)\xi}$	$-\dfrac{a}{2\xi}\left(1-\dfrac{1}{\varphi}\right)$	*Isotropic scattering,*
van Gemert & Star[4] [27]	$\dfrac{(1-\varphi)(1-a')}{(1+\varphi)\xi}$	$-\dfrac{a'}{2\xi}\left(1-\dfrac{1}{\varphi}\right)$	*Anisotropic scattering; delta-isotropic phase function*
van Gemert & Star [27]	$\dfrac{1}{2}+\dfrac{1}{4}(1-a')$	$\dfrac{4}{3}+\dfrac{38}{45}(1-a')$	*Anisotropic scattering, assumes $\mu_s \gg \mu_a$*
Meador & Weaver [25]	$\dfrac{1}{2}+\dfrac{1}{4}(1-a)$	$\dfrac{4}{3}+\dfrac{38}{45}(1-a)$	*Isotropic scattering; Delta-Eddington phase function (four moments)*
Meador & Weaver [25]	$\dfrac{1}{2}$	$\dfrac{4}{3}+\dfrac{20}{45}(1-a)$	*Isotropic scattering, Delta-Eddington phase function (two moments)*
Brinkworth [28,29]	$\dfrac{1}{2}$	$\dfrac{4}{3}+\dfrac{80}{45}(1-a)$	*Isotropic scattering, Eddington phase function*

1   χ for isotropic and χ' for anisotropic scattering; $a = \mu_s/(\mu_s + \mu_a)$ and $a' = \mu_s(1-g)/[\mu_s(1-g) + \mu_a]$
2   All formulas assume index matched boundaries
3    $(\varphi^2 - 1)/2\varphi = (1 + R^2 - T^2)/2R$, and $\varphi = [\xi + \ln(1-\xi)]/[\xi - \ln(1-\xi)]$
4    $(\varphi^2 - 1)/2\varphi = (1 + R^2 - T^2)/2R$, and $\mu_s(1-g)/[\mu_s(1-g) + \mu_a] = [\xi + \ln(1-\xi)]/[\xi - \ln(1-\xi)]$

Transport coefficients can be derived from the collision of a plane wave with a particle [4]. Some of the wave is scattered, some is absorbed, and some is undisturbed. The absorption (σ_a) and scattering (σ_s) cross sections (m^2) for tissue are ill-defined, because the particles are not separated from one another. Consequently, with the notable exception of blood [4], these cross sections are not well defined and measured. However, the *volumetric* absorption and scattering coefficients (m^{-1}) can be defined by using (ρ) the average density of particles per unit volume of tissue (m^{-3}). The scattering coefficient is $\mu_s = \rho\sigma_s$ and the absorption coefficient is $\mu_a = \rho\sigma_a$. Note that the phase function is not involved in the description of the absorption and scattering coefficients.

The Kubelka–Munk parameters are defined by (22) and (23) above. In the given formulation, the fraction of light scattered forward is equal to the fraction scattered backward. Since the Kubelka–Munk formulas are based on a forward- and backward-peaked phase function, the equal scattering assumption is equivalent to assuming equal magnitudes for the phase function peaks. If these peaks had different magnitudes (as they should for anisotropic scattering), then two unequal scattering coefficients would result. The Kubelka–Munk scattering coefficients are thus dependent on the scattering anisotropy (or phase function) of the tissue.

A large number of investigators have used Kubelka–Munk theory to obtain optical properties. In response to this, several authors have attempted to relate the Kubelka–Munk coefficients to transport coefficients using the following relations [4], [25]–[29]:

$$\mu_a = \eta A_{\mathrm{KM}} \tag{24a}$$

$$\mu_s = \chi S_{\mathrm{KM}} \tag{24b}$$

$$\mu_s(1 - g) = \chi' S_{\mathrm{KM}} \tag{24c}$$

Table I provides expressions for η and χ (or χ'). Only the relations of Klier [26] or van Gemert and Star [27] generate transport coefficients which lead to light distributions that agree with distributions based on exact solutions to the transport equation. Van Gemert and Star extend the isotropic relations of Klier to include anisotropic scattering. Both papers provide graphs of η and χ (or χ') as functions of $\mu_a/(\mu_s + \mu_a)$ and $A_{\mathrm{KM}}/S_{\mathrm{KM}}$. The usefulness of these relations is compromised because internal reflection in the slab is neglected. Such internal reflection effects can dramatically change the measured reflection and transmission [2]. A final set of transformations by Star is $A_{\mathrm{KM}} = 2\mu_a$ and $S_{\mathrm{KM}} = \{3\mu_s(1 - g) - \mu_a\}/4$ [30].

IV. Measurement of Optical Properties

A number of methods have been proposed for measuring the optical properties of tissues. These can be separated into two classes: *direct* and *indirect*. In *direct* techniques, optical properties are found using nothing more complicated than Beer's law. Unscattered transmission measurements [31], effective attenuation measurements [11]–[14], and goniophotometric measurements of the single scattering phase function [2], [9], [58] are direct techniques. In *indirect* techniques, a theoretical model of light scattering is used. Indirect techniques can be subdivided into iterative and noniterative methods. A *noniterative* method uses equations in which the optical properties are explicitly given in terms of the measured quantities. The Kubelka–Munk and three-flux models are noniterative, indirect methods. In indirect *iterative methods*, the optical properties are implicitly related to measured quantities. The values for the optical properties are iterated until the calculated reflection and transmission match the measured values. These methods are the most cumbersome to use, but the optical model employed can be much more sophisticated than in the noniterative methods.

A. Direct Methods

Direct techniques do not depend on any specific model to obtain the optical parameter from measurements. Two optical parameters that are not dependent upon any specific model are the total attenuation coefficient μ_2 and the effective attenuation coefficient μ_{eff}. These parameters are determined using the following methods.

1) The total attenuation coefficient μ_t is obtained from measurements of unscattered transmission using (6), as

depicted in Fig. 1(a). Thin slabs are employed [31]. Experimental data are most affected by beam geometry, sample characteristics, detection schemes, and multiple reflections at boundaries. This measurement is conceptually simple, but difficult to implement because of problems in separating on-axis scattered light from unscattered light.

2) The effective scattering coefficient (μ_{eff}) or effective penetration depth ($\partial_{\mathrm{eff}} = 1/\mu_{\mathrm{eff}}$), is estimated from fluence rate measured by interstitial detectors and using (16) and (19), as depicted in Fig. 1(b) [11]–[14], [32]–[36]. This is the simplest and most commonly determined parameter (see Tables III and IV). Fiberoptic detectors must be located inside the diffusion region of irradiated bulk samples, far from sources and boundaries. It is crucial that the measurement field be in the diffusion region. Otherwise the orientation of the fiber with respect to incoming beam [9], [34], and its numerical aperture (flat cut versus isotropic fibertips [37]–[39]) will introduce measurement errors.

B. Noniterative Indirect Methods

Such approaches require simple expressions relating the optical properties to measured transmission and reflection (e.g., Kubelka–Munk equations). It is not surprising that the two methods presented involve using (23).

1) The first method employs calculations of Kubelka–Munk absorption and scattering coefficients (A_{KM}, S_{KM}) from measurements of diffuse reflection and transmission for diffuse irradiance, and use of (23), as depicted in Fig. 1(c). This method is strongly limited because a perfectly diffuse irradiating source is not readily available.

2) The second method utilizes determination of absorption, scattering, and anisotropy coefficients from diffuse transmission and reflection measurements using relations derived by van Gemert et al. [16]. Kubelka–Munk coefficients are first computed, then transformed into transport coefficients, and finally combined with a measurement of unscattered transmission to yield the three optical coefficients. The same limitations of method 1) apply here. Relations which correct for mismatched boundaries are also available [40].

Other noniterative methods have also been used. An example is the combination of the absorbance of a sample placed in an integrating sphere and angular phase function measurements [41]–[43]. Marijnissen et al. [37] combined measurements of angular radiance patterns with measurements of μ_{eff} to deduce μ_a, μ_s, and g. Yoon [9] used asymptotic measurements of total diffuse transmission for different sample thicknesses with collimated transmission and goniophotometric studies to obtain optical properties.

More recent methods include pulsed photothermal radiometry (PPTR) [44], photoacoustic effects [45], and time-of-flight (TOF) studies [46]. However, PPTR and photoacoustic methods have been demonstrated only for measuring absorption coefficient. These three newer techniques are noninvasive and therefore show promise for *in vivo* determination of optical properties.

133

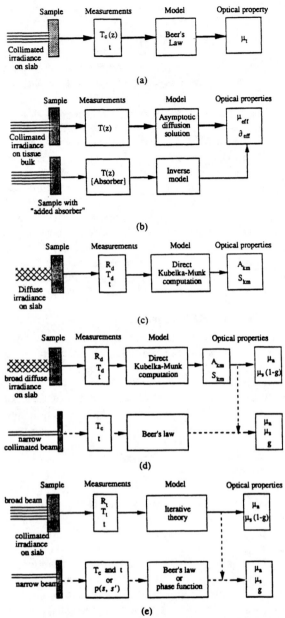

Fig. 1. Measured values from the unscattered transmission T_c, through a sample of thickness t are analyzed using Beer's law to provide estimates of the total attenuation coefficient (μ_t). (b) Interstitial measurements of fluence rate (or flux) inside a sample with or without an added absorber yield an estimate of the effective attenuation coefficient (μ_{eff}) or the effective penetration depth ($\partial_{eff} = 1/\mu_{eff}$). (c) Measurements of diffuse reflection R_d, and diffuse transmission T_d, and sample thickness t, for diffuse irradiance are used in (22) to compute Kubelka-Munk absorption A_{KM} and scattering S_{KM} coefficients. (d) Measurements of diffuse reflection and transmission for diffuse irradiance lead to Kubelka-Munk coefficients; these are then converted to transport parameters. When collimated transmission is available, μ_a, μ_s, and g can be calculated. (e) If only total reflection and transmission are available, the absorption coefficient μ_a and reduced scattering coefficient $\mu_s (1 - g)$ can be determined with an iterative light transport model. An additional measurement (collimated transmission or the phase function) permits separate estimation of μ_a, μ_s, and g.

C. Iterative Indirect Methods

Unlike noniterative techniques, iterative procedures can use complicated solutions to the transport equations. Examples are diffusion theory, adding-doubling models [2],

and Monte Carlo [47]. Typically, μ_a and $\mu_s (1 - g)$ can be obtained if only total reflection and transmission are measured as shown in Fig. 1(e). If a third measurement of either the unscattered transmission or the phase function is available, then values for μ_a, μ_s, and g [or $p(s, s')$] can be determined. Iterative solutions usually include corrections for mismatched boundary conditions and/or for multiple layers. These methods often require two or more of the following measurements on a sample of known uniform thickness:

1) total (or diffuse) transmission for collimated or diffuse irradiance;
2) total (or diffuse) reflection for collimated or diffuse irradiance;
3) absorbance of the sample, placed inside an integrating sphere;
4) unscattered (collimated) transmission for collimated irradiation; and
5) angular distribution of emitted light from an irradiated sample.

Any three measurements from 1) to 5) would be sufficient to determine the three optical properties.

D. Sources of Errors

Computed values for the optical coefficients are inevitably prone to errors in all (or any) of the following:

1) physiological condition of the biological sample-hydration level, homogeneity, species variability, frozen-unfrozen state, *in vivo-in vitro*, fixed-unfixed, surface smoothness of the sample slabs;
2) irradiation geometry;
3) boundary index matching-mismatching;
4) orientation of detecting interstitial fibers with respect to source fiber;
5) numerical apertures of the sensing fibers;
6) angular resolution of the photodetectors;
7) separation of forward scattered light from unscattered light; and
8) theory used for the inverse problem.

These are important factors to consider when comparing optical properties obtained by different investigators.

V. DISCUSSION

In recent years, many measurements of optical properties have been made. These optical properties can be used in the models listed in Table II. Tables III and IV are extensive lists of scattering, absorption, and anisotropy coefficients based on the transport theory. Table III lists the *in vitro* results, and Table IV tabulates optical properties measured *in vivo*. Each entry is accompanied by a brief description of the tissue preparation, sample geometry, experimental measurements and underlying theory. Kubelka-Munk coefficients are collected in Table V. Not all measurements listed in Tables III-V are discussed because of the wide variety of techniques and methods used. Instead, we concentrate on measurements of aorta, liver, and muscle at 633 nm and of liver tissue at 1060 nm.

A. Aorta

Aorta is a turbid tissue composed of interwoven elastin and collagen fibers, arranged in a trilayer structure of intima, media, and adventitia. Its appearance ranges from opaque white (porcine) to a pinkish-white in cadaveric samples.

Cadaveric aorta samples used by Yoon [9] were stripped to different thicknesses leaving mostly the intimal and media layers. Maintaining these samples in saline altered their hydration states. Keijzer et al. [48] froze samples to make microtome cuts. Despite these differences in sample preparation, Keijzer measured a scattering coefficient of 315 cm^{-1} and an anisotropy factor of 0.87 for normal media at 633 nm. These values agree closely with Yoon's values of $\mu_s = 310$ cm^{-1} and $g = 0.90$. In contrast, Keijzer's absorption coefficient of 2.3 cm^{-1} is higher than the $\mu_a = 0.52$ cm^{-1} value obtained by Yoon. If $\mu_a = A_{KM}/2$, then the A_{KM} values by van Gemert et al. [49] and Oraevsky et al. [50] for normal aorta are in closer agreement with the result by Yoon. Differences in treatment of internal reflections at the sample boundaries undoubtedly affected the computed absorption coefficients. Yoon fitted the asymptotic portion of a plot of diffuse transmission versus sample thickness to an equation that was independent of the tissue index of refraction, thus eliminating any need for boundary corrections. Keijzer, however, assumed a value for the refractive index to enable the inverse delta–Eddington program to correct for internal reflections. Another likely source for the descrepancy, was that by soaking the samples in saline, Yoon removed any remaining blood in the aorta sample, thereby reducing the measured absorption coefficient.

B. Liver

Unlike the aorta, liver tissues contain a dense population of erythrocytes within a vacuolar mesh of connective tissue and capillary beds. Absorption coefficients for liver range from 2.3–3.2 cm^{-1} at 633 nm. These are higher than those of other soft tissues. The reported absorption coefficients for liver agree within the errors introduced by interspecies variations. They also match the 1.3–2.7 cm^{-1} obtained for oxygenated whole blood by Pedersen et al. [51] and Reynolds et al. [52]. By comparison, the 6.5 cm^{-1} value for murine livers by Parsa using the delta-Eddington method is very high [53]. Here, index mismatching has been iteratively corrected in the inverse programs using assumed values for refractive indexes; Karagiannes et al. [54] adopted a similar approach. Marchesini et al. [43] and Andreola et al. [42] have not offered any clear details regarding their management of this problem. However, they did correct their absorbance measurements for multiple reflections associated with the integrating sphere, a correction ignored by other investigators. Without correction, the measured absorbance (or reflectance and transmission) exceeds the true absorbance.

TABLE II
FLUENCE MODELS WITH ASSOCIATED OPTICAL PARAMETERS

OPTICAL MODEL	OPTICAL COEFFICIENTS
I FLUX MODELS	
1. 2-Flux Kubelka-Munk (Kubelka [20-21])	A_{KM} and S_{KM}
2. 3-Flux (Atkins [22], van Gemert [16])	μ_a, μ_s, and g
3. 7-Flux (Yoon [9])	μ_a, μ_s, and g
II DIFFUSION MODELS	
1. Asymptotic (Svaasand [11], Profio [67]) Slab Symmetric sphere: Circular solid cylinder	μ_{eff} or $\partial_{eff} (= 0/\mu_{eff})$
2. Eddington (Ishimaru [4])	μ_a, μ_s, and g
3. Delta-Eddington (Joseph [8], Prahl [21])	μ_a, μ_s, g' and f
III. P_n APPROXIMATION (Bell & Glasstone [68])	μ_a, μ_s, and $p(s,s')$
IV DISCRETE ORDINATE (Houf [69])	μ_a, μ_s, and $p(s,s')$
V. ADDING–DOUBLING (van de Hulst [18], Plass [19], Prahl [21])	μ_a, μ_s and $p(s,s')$
VI. MONTE CARLO (Wilson [70], Keijzer [71])	μ_a, μ_s, and $p(s,s')$

Scattering coefficients of 313 and 414 cm^{-1} were obtained, respectively, by Marchesini et al. [43] and Andreola et al. [42] for human liver at 633 nm. The scattering coefficient of 313 cm^{-1} is characteristic of values for soft tissues. However, Marchesini obtained a reduced scattering coefficient $\mu_s(1 - g)$ of 100.6 cm^{-1} that is significantly above the 5.23 cm^{-1} value reported by Kariagannes et al. [54] for bovine tissues and the 7.2 cm^{-1} value for murine samples measured by Parsa et al. [53]. This difference can be attributed to the measured anisotropy factor of 0.65 by Marchesini; it is substantially lower than reported values of 0.95 for rat liver by Parsa et al. [53] or values ranging 0.97 to 0.99 for blood by several authors [31], [55]-[57]. The coefficients determined by Marchesini also resulted in an approximate penetration depth of 33 μm. This suggests that two or more scattering events occurred within the 20–100 μm thick samples used in his goniometric studies to find the anisotropy factor. Jacques et al. [58] have demonstrated that the apparent anisotropy factor decreases as skin samples become thicker.

Measurements of effective attenuation coefficients (and effective penetration depths ∂_{eff}) are done in tissues far from sources and boundaries using isotropic detectors and/or flat cut fibers. These results should be functionally independent of detector geometry. Yet, measurements using the three orthogonal detectors described by Svaasand et al. [11] produced different attenuation coefficients for each detector. This suggests the measurements were made in regions with nonisotropic radiance distributions. The use of isotropic detectors [37]-[39], [59] may minimize these errors by recording an average and direction-independent signal. Also, measured μ_{eff} and calculated κ would not agree if (15a) is used outside its range of validity. Higher

TABLE III
Optical Properties of Tissues *In Vitro*

Tissue	λ (nm)	μt (cm⁻¹)	μa (cm⁻¹)	μs (cm⁻¹)	μs(1-g) (cm⁻¹)	g	μeff (cm⁻¹)	Tissue Preparation	Sample Geometry	Experimental Method	Theory	Reference
Adipose												
Bovine	632.8	—	—	—	—	—	3.4	———	thick slab	total T using interstitial fiber detectors	diffusion theory	Preuss 1982 [13]
Porcine	630	376 (69)a	—	—	—	0.77	—	ground, frozen & sliced	very thin slab	direct T measurement, μt; goniophotometry	Beer's Law, Mie theory	Flock 1987 [31]
Aorta												
Human	632.8	316	0.52	316	41.0	0.87	—	freshly excised, kept in saline.	thin slab	diffuse T measurement, phase function with goniophotometry	asymptotic diffusion, Henyey-Greenstein (H-G) phase function	Yoon 1987 [9]
Human: Intima	476	252	14.8	237	45.0	0.81	—	excised, frozen & sliced	very thin slab	total T and R, unscattered T measurements	diffusion theory (Delta-Eddington)	Keijzer 1989 [48]
	580	191	8.9	183	34.8	0.81	—					
	600	182	4.0	178	33.8	0.81	—					
	633	175	3.6	171	25.7	0.85	—					
Human: Media	476	252	7.3	410	45.1	0.89	—	excised, frozen & sliced	very thin slab	total T and R, unscattered T measurements	diffusion theory (Delta-Eddington)	Keijzer 1989 [48]
	580	191	4.8	331	33.1	0.90	—					
	582	182	2.5	323	35.5	0.89	—					
	633	312	2.3	310	31.0	0.90	—					
Human: Adventitia	476	252	18.1	267	69.4	0.74	—	excised, frozen & sliced	very thin slab	total T and R, unscattered T measurements	diffusion theory (Delta-Eddington)	Keijzer 1989 [48]
	580	191	11.3	217	49.9	0.77	—					
	600	182	6.1	211	46.4	0.78	—					
	633	201	5.8	195	37.1	0.81	—					
Human	1060	—	2.0	—	—	—	—		thick slab	magnitude of acoustic signal	photoacoustic	MacLeod 1988 [45]
Biliary Caculi (Gallstones)												
Pigment Stones	351	—	102 (16)	—	—	—	—	dehydrated, embedded in plastic, and sliced	~1 mm slab	thermal time response	pulsed photothermal radiometry	Long 1987 [44]
	488	—	179 (28)	—	—	—	—					
	580	—	125 (29)	—	—	—	—					
	630	—	85 (11)	—	—	—	—					
	1060	—	121 (12)	—	—	—	—					
Cholesterol Stones	351	—	88 (7)	—	—	—	—	dehydrated, embedded in plastic, and sliced	~1 mm slab	thermal time response	pulsed photothermal radiometry	Long 1987 [44]
	488	—	62 (15)	—	—	—	—					
	580	—	36 (7)	—	—	—	—					
	630	—	44 (10)	—	—	—	—					
	1060	—	60 (9)	—	—	—	—					

† R = Reflectance, T = Transmission
a (± SD) standard deviation

TABLE III
Optical Properties of Tissues *In Vitro* (*Continued*)

Tissue	λ (nm)	μt (cm⁻¹)	μa (cm⁻¹)	μs (cm⁻¹)	μs(1-g) (cm⁻¹)	g	μeff (cm⁻¹)	Tissue Preparation	Sample Geometry	Experimental Method	Theory	Reference
Bladder												
Canine	630	59.6	0.6	59.0	8.85	0.85	—	——	spherical	μa & radiance pattern with flat cut fibers; μeff with isotropic detectors	numerical transport solution by van de Hulst	Star 1987 [72]
Canine	633	52.0	1.25	50.8	2.54	0.95	—	excised and kept in saline	slab	diffuse R and T; axial transmission to get μt	3-flux model, transform KM to transport coeff.	Splinter 1989 [73]
Canine	632.8	45.1	1.10	44.0	3.52	0.92	—	~1 day post-resection, saline	slab	diffuse R and T; axial transmission to get μt	3-flux model, transform KM to transport coeff.	Cheong 1987 [74]
Human	632.8	89.4	1.40	88.0	3.52	0.96	—	~1 day post-resection, saline	slab	diffuse R and T; axial transmission to get μt	3-flux model, transform KM to transport coeff.	Cheong 1987 [74]
Human	633	30.7	1.40	29.3	2.64	0.91	—	excised and kept in saline	slab	diffuse R and T; axial transmission to get μt	3-flux model, transform KM to transport coeff.	Splinter 1989 [73]
Whole Blood												
Human HbO₂, Hct=0.41	685	1416	2.65	1413	—	0.99	—	diluted	——	radial distribution of reflection	transport theory	Pedersen 1976 [51]
Human HbO₂, Hct=0.41	665 / 960	1247 / 508	1.30 / 2.84	1246 / 505	6.11 / 3.84	0.995 / 0.992	— / —	non-hemolyzed, heparinized	cuvette	absorbance as function of sample thickness, angular light distribution	Mie theory	Reynolds 1976 [52]
Human Hb, Hct=0.41	665 / 960	514 / 670	4.87 / 1.68	509 / 668	2.49 / 5.08	0.995 / 0.992	— / —					
Human	633	29.0	—	—	—	0.974	—	diluted, non-hemolyzed	cuvette	unscattered T goniophotometry	Beer's Law Mie theory	Flock 1987 [31]
Canine	632.8 / 660 / 800	— / — / —	— / — / —	— / — / —	— / — / —	0.9845 / 0.9840 / 0.980	— / — / —	heparinized	cuvette	goniophotometry	2-parameter phase function by Reynolds & McCormick [57]	Steinke [56]

137

TABLE III
OPTICAL PROPERTIES OF TISSUES *IN VITRO* (*CONTINUED*)

Tissue	λ (nm)	μt (cm⁻¹)	μa (cm⁻¹)	μs (cm⁻¹)	μs(1-g) (cm⁻¹)	g	μeff (cm⁻¹)	Tissue Preparation	Sample Geometry	Experimental Method	Theory	Reference
Brain Calf	633 1064 1320	— — —	0.19 0.36 0.84	— — —	6.6 6.7 5.4	— — —	3.4[b] 2.5[b] 4.0	frozen sections, post mortem	thin slab on glass slides	total T and diffuse R	numerical iteration of 2-parameter phase fn. similarity transform	Karagiannes 1989 [54]
Brain Bovine	630	—	—	—	—	—	2.5	*post mortem*	*in situ*	direct T with interstitial fiberoptic detectors	diffusion theory	Doiron 1983 [12]
Feline	488 514.5 630	— —	— —	— —	— —	— — —	10.9 13.3 5.3-8.9	*post mortem*	*in situ*	direct T with interstitial fiberoptic detectors	diffusion theory	Doiron 1983 [12]
Porcine	633	1037[c]	0.26	1037[c]	57.0	0.945[d]	6.7	—	thick slab *in situ*	direct T	diffusion theory "added absorber"	Wilson 1986 [14]
	633	—	—	—	—	—	4.3-14.2	*post mortem*	*in situ* thick slab (~40-50 mm)	direct T using two interstitial fiberoptic detectors	diffusion theory	Wilson 1985 [35]
	630	—	0.64	—	52.0	—	—	—	thick slab	direct T using interstitial fiber detectors	diffusion theory	Preuss 1982 [13]
	630	687	—	—	—	0.945	—	frozen & then thawed	thin slab	unscattered T; phase function with goniophotometry	Beer's Law for μt; Mie theory	Flock 1987 [31]
Human: adult	488 514 660 1060	— — — —	— — — —	— — — —	— — — —	— — — —	14.0-25.0 14.0-16.7 7.0-12.5 2.3-3.4	*1-2 days post mortem*, no fix, no irrigation of blood vessel	bulk tissue (250 cm³), *in situ*	total attenuation using interstitial source and fiberoptic detectors	spherical diffusion theory	Svaasand & Ellingsen 1983 [75]
	630	—	0.3-1.0	—	30.0-40.0	—	8.3	*post mortem*	slab	diffuse R and T; unscattered T	Kubelka-Munk to transport	Sterenborg 1988 [66]
Human: neonate	488 514 660 1060	— — — —	— — — —	— — — —	— — — —	— — — —	5.9-7.9 5.8-9.0 2.5-3.3 1.1-1.4	1-2 days post-mortem, no fix, no irrigation of blood vessel	bulk tissue, (250 cm³), *in situ*	total attenuation using interstitial source and fiberoptic detectors.	spherical diffusion theory	Svaasand 1983 [75]
Human: White matter Grey matter	633 633	52.6 62.8	1.58 2.63	51.0 60.2	2.04 7.22	0.96 0.88	— —	excised and kept in saline	thin slab	diffuse R and T; unscattered T	3-flux model KM to transport	Splinter 1989 [73]

b Experimental measurement using interstitial fiberoptic detectors
c Calculated from g (ref. 31, Flock) and μt(1-g)
d From reference [31], Flock 1987

TABLE III
OPTICAL PROPERTIES OF TISSUES *IN VITRO* (*CONTINUED*)

Tissue	λ (nm)	μ_t (cm⁻¹)	μ_a (cm⁻¹)	μ_s (cm⁻¹)	$\mu_s(1-g)$ (cm⁻¹)	g	μ_{eff} (cm⁻¹)	Tissue Preparation	Sample Geometry	Experimental Method	Theory	Reference
Brain												
Canine												
White matter	633	92.2	2.02	90.2	6.31	0.93	—	excised and kept in saline	thin slab	diffuse R and T; unscattered T	3-flux model, transform KM to transport coeff.	Splinter 1989 [73]
Grey matter	633	58.0	1.65	56.3	1.97	0.97	—					
Brain Tumors												
Tumors	630	—	—	—	—	—	3.8-8.3	30-60 min. post-resection	*in situ*	direct T with interstitial fiberoptic detectors	spherical diffusion theory	Svaasand 1985 [77]
— glioma	630	—	5.0	—	7.0	—	—	*post mortem*	thin slab	diffuse R, diffuse T, unscattered T	transform KM into transport coefficients	Sterenborg 1988 [66]
— melanoma	630	—	—	—	8.0	—	—					
Breast Tissue												
Human: Fibrous	514	202	—	—	—	—	—	freshly resected	thin slab (~20μm) between glass	unscattered plus some (<0.8°) scattered T	Beer's law	Key 1988 [78]
	633	189	—	—	—	—	—					
	1060	165	—	—	—	—	—					
Human: Fatty	514	775	—	—	—	—	—	freshly resected	thin slab (~20μm) between glass	unscattered plus some (<0.8°) scattered T	Beer's law	Key 1988 [78]
	633	676	—	—	—	—	—					
	1060	524	—	—	—	—	—					
Human	635	—	≤ 0.2	395(35)ᵃ	—	—	—	frozen sections	very thin slab between glass	absorbance in integrating sphere, unscattered T from goniophotometry	Beer's law	Marchesini 1989 [43]
Heart												
Endocardium	1060	—	0.07	136	—	0.973	—	excised and kept in saline	thin slab	simultaneous diffuse R and T; unscattered T	3-flux model, transform KM to transport coeff.	Splinter 1989 [80]
Epicardium	1060	—	0.35	167	—	0.983	—	excised and kept in saline	thin slab	simultaneous diffuse R and T; unscattered T	3-flux model, transform KM to transport coeff.	Splinter 1989 [80]
Kidney												
Human	630	—	—	—	—	—	4.0	*post mortem*	thin slab	unscattered T	Beer's law	Eichler 1977 [33]
Bovine	630	—	—	—	—	—	7.9	———	*in situ*, thick slab	direct T using interstitial fiber detectors	diffusion theory	Preuss 1982 [13]
Kidney												
Porcine (cortex)	630	—	—	—	—	—	4.8	*post mortem*	*in situ*	direct T using interstitial fiberoptic detectors	diffusion theory	Doiron 1983 [12]

ᵃ (± SD) standard deviation

139

TABLE III

OPTICAL PROPERTIES OF TISSUES *IN VITRO* (*CONTINUED*)

Tissue	λ (nm)	μ_t (cm⁻¹)	μ_a (cm⁻¹)	μ_s (cm⁻¹)	$\mu_s(1-g)$ (cm⁻¹)	g	μ_{eff} (cm⁻¹)	Tissue Preparation	Sample Geometry	Experimental Method	Theory	Reference
Liver												
Bovine	630	—	—	—	—	—	8.1	———	*in situ*, thick slab	direct T measurement with interstitial fiber detectors	diffusion theory	Preuss 1982 [13]
	633	—	3.21	—	5.23	—	6.8b	frozen sections, *post mortem*	thin slab between glass	total T and diffuse R	diffusion theory 2-parameter phase function	Karagiannes, 1989 [54]
	1064	—	0.53	—	1.76	—	3.2b					
	1320	—	0.70	—	1.2	—	2.0					
Human	630	—	—	—	—	—	11.0	*post mortem*	thin slab	unscattered T	Beer's law	Eichler 1977 [33]
	630	—	3.2	414	—	0.95e	—	*post mortem*	thin slab (0.05-0.2 mm)	absorbance in integrating sphere; goniophotometry	Beer's law	Andreola 1988 [42]
	635	315	2.3	313	—	0.68	26.6	frozen sections	thin slab between glass	absorbance in integrating sphere, unscattered T from goniophotometry	Beer's law	Marchesini, 1989 [43]
	515	304	18.9	285	—	—	—					
Murine (albino)	488	—	12.2	173.5	—	0.93	29.9	fresh and frozen sections	thin slab between glass slides	total T and total R, unscattered T	diffusion theory (Delta-Eddington)	Parsa 1989 [53]
	633	—	6.5	143.7	—	0.95	16.3					
	800	—	5.7	97.0	—	0.94	14.0					
	1064	—	5.9	60.9	—	0.92	13.8					
	1320	—	6.6	44.2	—	0.91	14.5					
	2100	—	27.2	24.5	—	0.80	51.2					
Porcine	630	—	—	—	—	—	13.0	*post mortem*	*in situ*	direct T using interstitial fiberoptic detectors	diffusion theory	Doiron 1983 [12]
	630	—	2.7	—	17.0	—	—	———	*in situ*	direct T	diffusion theory	Wilson 1986 [34]
Rabbit	630	—	—	—	—	—	12.5	*post mortem*, surface moist	*in situ* ~15 mm thick	direct T using interstitial fiberoptic detectors	diffusion theory	Wilson 1985 [35]
	1060	—	10.0	—	—	—	—	———	thick slab	magnitude of acoustic signal	photoacoustic	MacLeod 1988 [45]
Lung												
Human lung substance, deflated	633	—	—	—	—	—	11.0	*post mortem*	*in situ*	direct T using interstitial fiberoptic detectors	diffusion theory	Doinon 1982 [62]
Squamous cell Carcinoma	633	—	—	—	—	—	6.3	*post mortem*	*in situ*	— as above —	— as above —	Doiron 1983 [12]
Bronchial mucosa	633	—	—	—	—	—	9.1	*post mortem*	*in situ*	— as above —	— as above —	Doinon 1982 [62]
Human: normal	630	—	8.4	35.9	—	0.95e	—	frozen, rehydrated	thin slab (0.05-0.2 mm)	absorbance in integrating sphere; goniophotometry	Beer's law	Andreola 1988 [42]

b Experimental measurement using interstitial fiberoptic detectors
e Averaged value

TABLE III
OPTICAL PROPERTIES OF TISSUES *IN VITRO* (*CONTINUED*)

Tissue	λ nm	μ_t cm⁻¹	μ_a cm⁻¹	μ_s cm⁻¹	$\mu_s(1-g)$ cm⁻¹	g	μ_{eff} cm⁻¹	Tissue Preparation	Sample Geometry	Experimental Method	Theory	Reference
Lung												
Human: normal	635 515	332 380	8.1 25.5	324 356	— —	0.75 —	— —	frozen sections	thin slab between glass slides	absorbance in integrating sphere, unscattered T from goniophotometry	Beer's law	Marchesini 1989 [43]
Muscle												
Bovine	633	8.30	0.40	7.9	5.53	0.30	2.7	chopped	thick slab	μ_t & radiance pattern with flat cut fibers; μ_{eff} with isotropic detectors	transport theory	Marijnissen 1987 [38]
	633	121[c]	1.50	119[c]	7.0	0.941[d]	6.2	————	thick slab	direct T	diffusion theory "added absorber"	Wilson 1986 [14]
Bovine	630	—	—	—	—	—	5.6	*post mortem*	*in situ*	direct T using interstitial fiberoptic detectors	diffusion theory	Doiron 1983 [12]
	630	—	—	—	—	—	6.9	*post mortem*	*in situ*	direct T measurement with interstitial fiber detectors	diffusion theory	Preuss 1982 [13]
	630	328 (37)[a]	—	—	—	0.941	—	ground, frozen & thawed	thin slab	direct T measurement; phase function with goniophotometry	Beer's law for μ_t Mie theory	Flock 1987 [31]
Bovine	630	—	3.5	45.0	—	—	5.9	————	bulk	isodoses recorded on photographic film, contours yield μ_{eff}	diffusion theory	McKenzie 1988 [39]
	630	—	—	—	—	—	4.3-5.6	————	————	———	diffusion theory	Bolin 1987 [63]
Bovine	633 1064 1320	— — —	1.7 1.2 2.3	— — —	4.4 2.8 2.4	— — —	3.9[b] 2.3[b] 5.6	frozen sections, *post mortem*	thin slab between glass slides	total T and diffuse R	Numerical iterations, 2-parameter phase func., similarity transform	Karagiannes 1989 [54]
Chicken	633	4.30	0.17	4.1	3.3	0.20	1.34	chopped	*in situ*	μ_t & radiance pattern with flat cut fibers; μ_{eff} with isotropic detectors.	transport theory	Marijnissen & Star 1985 [59]
Chicken	633	230[c]	0.12	229[c]	8.0	0.965[d]	1.7	resected & coarsely ground	thick slab	direct T	diffusion theory "added absorber"	Wilson 1986 [14]

[c] calculated from g [ref.31] and $\mu_s(1-g)$
[d] From reference [31], Flock 1987
[a] (± SD) standard deviation
[b] Experimental measurement using interstitial fiberoptic detectors

141

TABLE III
Optical Properties of Tissues *In Vitro* (*Continued*)

Tissue	λ nm	μt cm⁻¹	μa cm⁻¹	μs cm⁻¹	μs(1-g) cm⁻¹	g	μeff cm⁻¹	Tissue Preparation	Sample Geometry	Experimental Method	Theory	Reference
Muscle												
Chicken	630	345 (42)[a]	—	—	—	0.965	—	ground, frozen & then thawed	thin slab	direct T measurement; phase function with goniophotometry	Beer's law Mie theory	Flock 1987 [31]
Human	515	541	11.2	530	—	—	—	frozen sections	thin slab between glass slides	absorbance with integrating sphere, unscattered T from goniophotometry	total attenuation	Marchesini 1989 [43]
Porcine	633	41.0	1.0	40.0	1.2	0.97	—	fresh & frozen sections	thin slab	total T and diffuse R	Monte Carlo	Wilksch 1984 [47]
	1060	—	2.0	—	—	—	—	—	thick slab	magnitude of acoustic signal	photoacoustic	MacLeod 1988 [45]
Rabbit	630	—	—	—	—	—	1.1-1.5	post mortem	in situ	direct T using interstitial fiberoptic detectors	spherical diffusion theory	Doiron 1983 [12]
	514.5	—	—	—	—	—	2.0-2.5	post mortem	in situ, bulk	— as above —	— as above —	Doiron 1982 [62]
Rabbit	630 514	— —	— —	— —	— —	— —	2.7-12.5 3.7-10.0	moist surface	in situ, thick ~30-40 mm	direct T measured interstitially	diffusion theory	Wilson 1985 [35]
Skin												
Human dermis	630	243	1.8	—	—	—	—	excised flaps	thin slab 0.05-0.2 mm	absorbance in integrating sphere; goniophotometry	Beer's law	Andreola 1988 [42]
Human dermis (Caucasian)	633	190	2.7	187	35.5	0.81	—	bloodless, 85% hydration, fresh & frozen	thin slab between glass	goniophotometry; total R and total T	diffusion theory Henyey-Greenstein phase function	Jacques 1987 [58]
Human dermis	635	—	1.8	244	—	—	—	frozen sections	thin slab between glass slides	absorbance in integrating sphere, unscattered T from goniophotometry	Beer's law	Marchesini 1989 [43]
Murine dermis (albino)	488	242	2.8	239	62	0.74	—	Fresh whole dermis	thin slab between glass slides	total R and total T; unscattered T	diffusion theory	Jacques 1987 [15]
Human stratum corneum	193	—	6000	—	—	—	—	frozen sections	thin slab	unscattered T as function of thickness	Beer's law	Watanabe 1988 [79]

[a] (± SD) standard deviation

142

TABLE III
OPTICAL PROPERTIES OF TISSUES *IN VITRO* (*CONTINUED*)

Tissue	λ (nm)	μt (cm⁻¹)	μa (cm⁻¹)	μs (cm⁻¹)	μt(1-g) (cm⁻¹)	g	μeff (cm⁻¹)	Tissue Preparation	Sample Geometry	Experimental Method	Theory	Reference
Tumors												
Rat prostrate tumor (R3327-AT)												
	633	271	0.49	270.	8.1-5.4	.97-.98	3.6-2.9	excised, frozen & sectioned	thin slab (120 μm)	absorbance in integrating sphere; goniophotometry	diffusion theory	Arnfield 1988 [41]
Rat rhabdomyosarcoma												
	630	—	1.1	—	7.0	—	—	freshly excised	thin slab	diffuse R and T	KM converted to transport coefficients using equations [ref. 16]	van Gemert 1985 [81]
	514	—	2.3	—	11.1	—	—					
	405	—	42.9	—	24.8	—	—					
Human intracranial tumors (meningiomas, astrocytomas, glioblastomas)												
	488	—	—	—	—	—	7.1-20.0	freshly resected	tissue vol. ≈5-10 cm³, *in situ*	*in situ* T with embedded fiberoptic detectors.	diffusion theory	Svaasand 1985 [77]
	514	—	—	—	—	—	7.1-20.0					
	635	—	—	—	—	—	5.9-3.9					
	1060	—	—	—	—	—	3.3-1.9					
Rabbit VX2	630	628(106)ᵃ	—	—	—	0.639	—	ground, frozen & then thawed	thin slab	direct T measurement; phase function with goniophotometry	Beer's Law Mie theory	Flock 1987 [31]
Murine sarcoma	630	—	—	—	—	—	2.3	*post mortem*	*in situ*	direct T using interstitial fiberoptic detectors orientated in 3 directions	diffusion theory	Doiron 1982 [62]
	514.5	—	—	—	—	—	4.8					
Murine fibrosarcoma	630	—	—	—	—	—	4.4-9.8	———	———	direct T with interstitial fiberoptics	Beer's law	Driver 1988 [36]
Uterus												
Human	635	394	0.35	394	—	0.69	—	frozen sections	thin slab between glass slides	absorbance in integrating sphere, unscattered T from goniophotometry	Beer's law	Marchesini 1989 [43]

ᵃ (± SD) standard deviation

Optical Properties of Tissues *In Vivo*

Tissue	λ (nm)	μt (cm⁻¹)	μa (cm⁻¹)	μs (cm⁻¹)	μs(1-g) (cm⁻¹)	g	μeff (cm⁻¹)	Tissue Preparation	Sample Geometry	Experimental Method	Theory	Reference
Brain												
Human	630	—	—	—	—	—	2.2-3.7	*in situ*	intact, spherical field	direct T measured during PDT, interstitially; irradiated with embedded inflated balloon light source	diffusion theory spherical solution	Wilson 1986 [82]
	630	—	—	—	—	—	4.8-10.0	*in situ*	intact	— as above —	— as above —	Muller 1986 [83]
Porcine	630	—	—	—	—	—	3.7-4.5	*in situ*	intact spherical field	direct T with distance from irradiation surface, interstitial fiberoptic detectors	diffusion theory	Wilson 1985 [35]
Brain tumors	630	—	—	—	—	—	2.4	*in situ*	intact	direct T at different distances from interstitial spherical source, post-PDT	diffusion theory spherical solution	Wilson 1986 [82]
	630	—	—	—	—	—	2.2-6.6	*in situ*	intact	— as above —	— as above —	Muller 1986 [83]
Cat	631 577 545 405-410	— — — —	— — — —	— — — —	— — — —	— — — —	5.0-9.8 25.9 34.4 44.1	*in situ*	intact organ	direct T using interstitial fiberoptic detectors	diffusion theory	Doiron 1982
Liver												
Rabbit	630	—	—	—	—	—	9.0-25.0	*in situ*	intact	direct T with distance from irradiation surface, interstitial	diffusion theory	Wilson 1985 [35]
Muscle												
Rabbit	630 514	— —	— —	— —	— —	— —	2.6-4.8 4.5-6.3	*in situ*	intact bulk ~30-40 mm	direct T using interstitial fiberoptic detectors	diffusion theory	Wilson 1985 [35]
	630 514.5	— —	— —	— —	— —	— —	1.6-2.3 4.8-7.7	*in situ*	intact	direct T using interstitial fiberoptic detectors	diffusion theory	Doiron 1983, 1982
Tumors												
Human retinoblastoma in athymic mice	488/514 630 668 1064	— — — —	— — — —	— — — —	— — — —	— — — —	6.25 3.03 2.8 1.3	*in situ*	intact tissue	direct T measured with ball-tipped fiberoptics connected distally to photodiode	diffusion theory	Svaasand 1989 [76]
Mammary carcinoma in C3H/HEJ mice	488/514 630 668 1064	— — — —	— — — —	— — — —	— — — —	— — — —	9.1 5.0 4.3 2.7	*in situ*	intact tissue	direct T measured with ball-tipped fiberoptics connected distally to photodiode	diffusion theory	Svaasand 1989 [76]
B16 melanotic melanoma in C57/B16 mice	630 668 1064	— — —	— — —	— — —	— — —	— — —	20.0 20.0 5.0	*in situ*	intact tissue	direct T measured with ball-tipped fiberoptics connected distally to photodiode	diffusion theory	Svaasand 1989 [76]

TABLE V
KUBELKA–MUNK COEFFICIENTS *IN VITRO*

Tissue	λ	Σ [f]	A_{km}	S_{km}	Tissue Preparation	Sample Geometry	Reference
	nm	cm^{-1}	cm^{-1}	cm^{-1}			
Aorta (human)							
Normal	514.5	22.1	11.1(2.7)[a]	11.0(0.8)	Cadaver specimens;	slabs	van Gemert, 1985 [49]
	633	8.1	1.8(.9)	6.3(1.4)			
	1060	3.7	0.9(.3)	2.8(2.0)			
Normal	633	8.2[h]	2.0	16.0	Cadaver specimens	slabs	Oraevsky, 1988 [50]
	488	20.0[h]	7.8	21.7	2-6 hours *post mortem*		
Blood							
Human	514	140	125	15.0		cuvettes	van Gemert, 1985 [49]
	633	4.0	1.0	3.0		cuvettes	
	1060	7.0	4.0	3.0		cuvettes	
Plaque							
Human	514.5	37.0	18.0	19.0	Cadaver specimens	slabs	van Gemert, 1985 [49]
	633	14.0	2.0	12.0	(heterogenous plaque)		
	1060	3.7	1.4	2.3			
Fibrous	633	10.1[h]	2.5	19.2	Cadaver specimens	slabs	Oraevsky, 1988 [50]
	488	30.1[h]	16.6	19.0	2-6 hours *post mortem*		
Skin (human)							
Dermis	630	65.0	5.0	60.0	Frozen sections	slabs	Anderson, 1981 [84]
Dermis [g]	415	—	20.0	138		slabs	van Gemert, 1986 [85]
	500	—	11.3	90.8			
	540	—	9.0	78.0			
	577	—	7.5	69.0			
	694	—	6.8	55.3			
	1060	—	6.0	35.0			
Dermis (breast & abdominal skin)	630	60.0	20	40	In 60°C water to separate dermis from epidermis	slabs	Wan, 1981 [86]
Epidermis [g]	415	—	51.7	44.0		slabs	van Gemert, 1986 [85]
	500	—	36.7	36.7			
	540	—	33.3	33.3			
	577	—	30.0	30.0			
	694	—	26.7	24.0			
	1060	—	20.0	16.0			

[f] Total attenuation coefficient $\Sigma = A_{km} + S_{km}$

[a] (± SD) standard deviation

[h] Effective attenuation coefficient $= \sqrt{(A_{km}^2 + 2A_{km} S_{km})}$

[g] Absorption and scattering coefficients derived from original spectra produced by Wan et. al [86] and Anderson et. al [84], and compiled in figure 1 of reference [85]; tabulated values are digitized from plots in this figure 1.

μ_{eff} values were obtained directly from interstitial fluence measurements [12], [13], [33]–[35] than those calculated from μ_a and $\mu_s(1 - g)$ parameters for bovine (Karagiannes), human (Marchesini), and murine (Parsa) livers.

At 1060 nm, absorption coefficients of 10 cm^{-1} for rabbit liver by MacLeod *et al.* [45] using photoacoustic spectroscopy and 0.53 cm^{-1} for bovine liver by Karagiannes using diffuse reflection and transmission are reported. The 10 cm^{-1} value seems high, even allowing for biological variations among species, since it is about twice the 5.5 cm^{-1} value obtained for arterial clots by Cheong [60]. A possible cause is the 1 cm spatial resolution in the photoacoustic studies. Another possibility is the inclusion of scattering effects in the absorbance measurements. Scattering redistributes the light over a broader tissue volume, effectively increasing the pathlength for optical absorption, and hence a larger absorption coefficient would be measured. In fact, examination of Table III reveals that absorption parameters measured by photoacoustic means are generally higher than those made with other techniques.

C. Muscle

Bovine muscles absorb more light at 633 nm ($\mu_a = 1.5$–3.5 cm^{-1}) than the whiter chicken muscles (0.17–0.12 cm^{-1}) but less than the better perfused human muscles (11.2 cm^{-1}). Marijnissen et al. [37] report an absorption coefficient of 0.4 cm^{-1} for bulk bovine muscle; this is significantly less than the 1.5 cm^{-1} from Wilson et al. [14] using the "added absorber" technique, or the 3.5 cm^{-1} value from McKenzie [39] based on fitting isodose contours on exposed photographic films to diffusion theory. These variations are typical of optical properties reported by different authors. Both Marijnissen and McKenzie used isotropic sensors in their measurements. Wilson used finite aperture detectors. Nevertheless, a large difference exists between the results by Marijnissen and the values by McKenzie. The absorption coefficients by Wilson and Marijnissen are more consistent and are typical of soft tissues at 633 nm. Marchesini's [43] direct measurement of absorbance of a sample placed inside an integrating sphere yielded a high value of 11.2 cm^{-1} for human tissues. Absorbance determined in this way is generally overestimated because scattering increases the average photon pathlength.

Marchesini et al. reported a scattering coefficient of 530 cm^{-1}, which is higher than other values in Table III. The 4.1 and 7.9 cm^{-1} values reported for bovine and chicken muscle by Marijnissen et al. [59] are extremely low. Star et al. attributes this to large detecting apertures [61]. In early studies it was not realized that tissues were highly forward scattering, as shown later by the 0.97 and 0.94 reported for g by Wilksch et al. [47] and Flock et al. [31], respectively. However, early measurements of the effective attenuation coefficient seem more reliable because they compare well with calculated values based on later measurements of μ_a and $\mu_s(1 - g)$.

Noticeable variations are present among the listed reduced scattering coefficients. The "added-absorber" technique produced $\mu_s(1 - g)$ values of 7.0 and 8.0 cm^{-1} for bovine and chicken muscles, respectively, at 633 nm. These are higher than those obtained using total diffuse and transmission measurements [42], [54] and from fluence measurements with isotropic detectors [58]. Ironically, the low anisotropy factor of 0.3 and scattering coefficient of 7.9 cm^{-1} for bovine muscle by Marijnissen is the reason that his value for $\mu_s(1 - g)$ was comparable with other values listed in Table III.

Diffusion theory [13], [62], [63] and the "added absorber" technique [14] were used to estimate the effective attenuation coefficient from interstitial light measurements in bovine muscles. They yielded values of 4.3–6.9 cm^{-1} which are higher than the 2.7 cm^{-1} obtained by Marijnissen and Star [37] using isotropic detectors. The 3.9 cm^{-1} reported by Kariagannes is within the range of the above two sets of results.

Doiron reports that rabbit muscle in vivo attenuates more 630 nm light than in vitro samples. Doiron measured values of 1.6–2.3 cm^{-1} in vivo but 1.1–1.5 cm^{-1} in vitro for the effective attenuation coefficient [12]. These differences might be due to perfusion of the in vivo samples. However, effective attenuation measurements of 2.6–4.8 cm^{-1} in vivo and 2.7–12.5 cm^{-1} post mortem by Wilson [35] did not exhibit any such difference in attenuation.

D. General Observations

This paper has emphasized the importance of matching experimental conditions with the theoretical model used to determine the optical properties. Reliability of optical properties depends on both theoretical and experimental techniques. For example, Kubelka–Munk measurements are questionable because the theoretical model is flawed and the experimental measurements are difficult to perform properly (infinite irradiation width, small diffuse reflection signal, and difficulty obtaining uniformly diffuse irradiances). Judgements of experimental accuracy are difficult, because many different tissue preparations and measurement parameters are involved. Preuss and Bolin [64] have reported a 39% and a 160% change in transmission from prefreezing at 488 and 515 nm, respectively. Such changes may translate into significant errors in the computed optical properties.

In this compilation, most measurements used a laser source. Little has been presented about optical properties measured as a function of wavelength using a spectrophotometer. There are optical property spectra for murine skin [15], cadaveric aorta [48], [65], murine liver [53], and human brain [66]. In the past, spectrophotometric data suffered from several errors. Typically, Beer's law was used to analyze transmission measurements, which is inapplicable if the samples scatter light or if the sample thickness is greater than the average scattering distance. When both spectrophotometric transmission and reflection data were available, Kubelka–Munk theory was used. Usually the data was not corrected for mismatched boundary conditions or pseudo-collimation of the irradiation source. Prahl [2] has described a procedure for matching spectrophotometer measurements to iterative computations of reflection and transmission to obtain μ_a and $\mu_s(1 - g)$. Undoubtedly careful calibration and use of the spectrophotometer with an integrating sphere can produce absorption and reduced scattering coefficients as a function of wavelength.

VI. Conclusion

Optical properties of biological tissues are vital to dosimetry studies. An up-to-date compilation of existing absorption, scattering, and anisotropy parameters accompanied by their associated theory and macroscopic measurements have been presented. Broad ranges in optical properties for any specific tissue are frequent, indicating the sensitivity and vulnerability of such measurements to variations in samples, detection apparatus, boundary conditions, and the governing light propagation model. The reliability of the reported values can be compromised by any of these factors.

Acknowledgment

The authors acknowledge all investigators whose work contributed to this review, and in particular thank W. Star for his "effective" remarks.

REFERENCES

[1] S. Chandrasekhar, *Radiative Transfer*. New York: Dover, 1960.
[2] S. A. Prahl, "Light transport in tissue," Ph.D. dissertation, Univ. Texas at Austin, 1988.
[3] H. C. van de Hulst, *Multiple Light Scattering, Volume 2*. New York: Academic, 1980.
[4] A. Ishimaru, *Wave Propagation and Scattering in Random Media, Volume 1*. New York: Academic, 1978.
[5] W. M. Star, "Comparing the P3-approximation with diffusion theory and with Monte Carlo calculations of light propagation in a slab geometry," *Proc. SPIE*, vol. IS5, Dosimetry of Laser Radiation in Medicine and Biology, G. J. Müller and D. H. Sliney, Eds., pp. 146–154, 1989.
[6] H. C. van de Hulst, *Multiple Light Scattering, Volume 1*. New York: Academic, 1980.
[7] E. P. Shettle and J. A. Weinman, "The transfer of solar irradiance through inhomogeneous turbid atmospheres evaluated by Eddington's approximation," *J. Atmos. Sci.*, vol. 27, pp. 1048–1055, 1970.
[8] J. H. Joseph, W. J. Wiscombe, and J. A. Weinman, "The delta-Eddington approximation for radiative flux transfer," *J. Atmos. Sci.*, vol. 33, pp. 2452–2459, 1976.
[9] G. Yoon, "Absorption and scattering of laser light in biological media—Mathematical modeling and methods for determining optical properties," Ph.D. dissertation, Univ. Texas at Austin, 1988.
[10] S. A. Prahl, J. W. Valvano, M. J. C. van Gemert, and A. J. Welch, "Boundary conditions and phase functions in the diffusion approximation of the radiative transport equation," *Appl. Opt.*, 1990 (submitted).
[11] L. O. Svaasand, D. R. Doiron, and A. E. Profio, "Light distribution in tissue during photoradiation therapy," USC Instit. Phys. Imaging Sci., USC-IPIS 900-02, 1981.
[12] D. R. Doiron, L. O. Svaasand, and A. E. Profio, "Light dosimetry in tissue applications to photoradiation therapy," in *Porphyrin Photosensitization*, D. Kessel and T. J. Dougherty, Eds. New York: Plenum, 1983, pp. 63–75.
[13] L. E. Preuss, F. P. Bolin, and B. W. Cain, "Tissue as a medium for laser light transport—Implications for photoradiation therapy," *Proc. SPIE*, vol. 357, Lasers in Surgery and Medicine, M. Berns, Ed., pp. 77–84, 1982.
[14] B. C. Wilson, M. S. Patterson, and D. M. Burns, "Effect of photosensitizer concentration in tissue on the penetration depth of photoactivating light," *Lasers Med. Sci.*, vol. 1, pp. 235–244, 1986.
[15] S. L. Jacques and S. A. Prahl, "Modeling optical and thermal distributions in tissue during laser irradiation," *Lasers Surg. Med.*, vol. 6, pp. 494–503, 1987.
[16] M. J. C. van Gemert, A. J. Welch, W. M. Star, M. Motamedi, and W. F. Cheong, "Tissue optics for a slab geometry in the diffusion approximation," *Lasers Med. Sci.*, vol. 2, pp. 295–302, 1987.
[17] G. Yoon, S. A. Prahl, and A. J. Welch, "Accuracies of the diffusion approximation and its similarity relations for laser irradiated biological media," *Appl. Opt.*, vol. 28, pp. 2250–2255, 1989.
[18] H. C. van de Hulst, *A New Look at Multiple Scattering*. New York: NASA Instit. Space Studies, 1962.
[19] G. N. Plass, G. W. Kattawar, and F. E. Catchings, "Matrix operator theory of radiative transfer. 1: Rayleigh scattering," *Appl. Opt.*, vol. 12, pp. 314–329, 1973.
[20] P. Kubelka, "New contributions to the optics of intensely light-scattering materials. Part I," *J. Opt. Soc. Amer.*, vol. 38, pp. 448–457, 1948.
[21] P. Kubelka, "New contributions to the optics of intensely light-scattering materials. Part II: Nonhomogeneous layers," *J. Opt. Soc. Amer.*, vol. 44, pp. 330–335, 1954.
[22] J. T. Atkins, "Optical properties of turbid materials," in *The Biologic Effects of Ultraviolet Radiation (with Emphasis on the Skin)*, F. Urbach, Ed. Oxford: Pergamon, 1969, pp. 141–150.
[23] F. Kottler, "Turbid media with plane-parallel surfaces," *J. Opt. Soc. Amer.*, vol. 50, pp. 483–490, 1960.
[24] P. S. Mudgett and L. W. Richards, "Multiple scattering calculations for technology," *Appl. Opt.*, vol. 10, pp. 1485–1502, 1971.
[25] W. E. Meador and W. R. Weaver, "Diffusion approximation for large absorption in radiative transfer," *Appl. Opt.*, vol. 18, pp. 1204–1208, 1979.
[26] K. Klier, "Absorption and scattering in plane parallel turbid media," *J. Opt. Soc. Amer.*, vol. 62, pp. 882–885, 1972.
[27] M. J. C. van Gemert and W. M. Star, "Relations between the Ku-belka–Munk and the transport equation models for anisotropic scattering," *Lasers Life Sci.*, vol. 1, pp. 287–298, 1987.
[28] B. J. Brinkworth, "On the theory of reflection by scattering and absorbing media," *J. Phys. D: Appl. Phys.*, vol. 4, pp. 1105–1106, 1971.
[29] B. J. Brinkworth, "Interpretation of the Kubelka-Munk coefficients in reflection theory," *Appl. Opt.*, vol. 11, pp. 1434–1435, 1972.
[30] W. M. Star, J. P. A. Marijnissen, and M. J. C. van Gemert, "Light dosimetry in optical phantoms and in tissues: I. Multiple flux and transport theory," *Phys. Med. Biol.*, vol. 33, pp. 437–454, 1988.
[31] S. T. Flock, B. C. Wilson, and M. S. Patterson, "Total attenuation coefficients and scattering phase functions of tissues and phantom materials at 633 nm," *Med. Phys.*, vol. 14, pp. 835–841, 1987.
[32] B. C. Wilson, M. S. Patterson, and S. T. Flock, "Indirect versus direct techniques for the measurement of the optical properties of tissues," *Photochem. Photobiol.*, vol. 46, pp. 601–608, 1987.
[33] J. Eichler, J. Knof, and H. Lenz, "Measurements on the depth of penetration of light $(0.35-1.0 \ \mu m)$ in tissue," *Rad. Environ. Biophys.*, vol. 14, pp. 239–242, 1977.
[34] B. C. Wilson and M. S. Patterson, "The physics of photodynamic therapy," *Phys. Med. Biol.*, vol. 31, pp. 327–360, Apr. 1986.
[35] B. C. Wilson, W. P. Jeeves, and D. M. Lowe, "*In vivo* and *post mortem* measurements of the attenuation spectra of light in mammalian tissues," *Photochem. Photobiol.*, vol. 42, pp. 153–162, 1985.
[36] I. Driver, J. W. Feather, P. R. King, and D. Gibson, "*In vivo* light dosimetry in interstitial photoradiation therapy (PRT)," *Proc. SPIE*, Int. Soc. of Opt. Eng. OE'Lase 88, M. Berns, Ed., pp. 98–102, 1988.
[37] J. P. A. Marijnissen and W. M. Star, "Phantom measurements for light dosimetry using isotropic and small aperture detectors," in *Porphyrin Localization and Treatment of Tumors*, D. R. Doiron and C. J. Gomer, Eds. New York: Alan R. Liss, pp. 133–148, 1984.
[38] J. P. A. Marijnissen and W. M. Star, "Quantitative light dosimetry *in vitro* and *in vivo*," *Lasers Med. Sci.*, vol. 2, pp. 235–242, 1987.
[39] A. L. McKenzie and P. O. Byrne, "Can photography be used to measure isodose distribution of space irradiance for laser photoradiation therapy?" *Phys. Med. Biol.*, vol. 33, pp. 113–131, 1988.
[40] G. H. M. Gjisbers, M.S. thesis, Eindhoven Univ., Eindhoven, The Netherlands, 1985.
[41] M. R. Arnfield, J. Tulip, and M. S. McPhee, "Optical propagation in tissue with anisotropic scattering," *IEEE Trans. Biomed. Eng.*, vol. 35, pp. 372–381, 1988.
[42] S. Andreola, A. Bertoni, R. Marchesini, and E. Melloni, "Evaluation of optical characteristics of different human tissues *in vitro*," *Lasers Surg. Med.*, vol. 8, p. 142 (abstract), 1988.
[43] R. Marchesini, A. Bertoni, S. Andreola, E. Melloni, and A. E. Sichirollo, "Extinction and absorption coefficients and scattering phase functions of human tissues *in vitro*," *Appl. Opt.*, vol. 28, pp. 2318–2324, 1989.
[44] F. H. Long, N. S. Nishioka, and T. F. Deustch, "Measurement of the optical and thermal properties of biliary calculi using pulsed photothermal radiometry," *Lasers Surg. Med.*, vol. 7, pp. 461–466, 1987.
[45] J. S. MacLeod, D. Blanc, and M. J. Colles, "Measurement of the optical absorption coefficients at 1.06 μm of various tissues using the photoacoustic effect," *Lasers Surg. Med.*, vol. 8, p. 143 (abstract), 1988.
[46] M. S. Patterson, B. Chance, and B. C. Wilson, "Time resolved reflectance and transmittance for the non-invasive measurement of tissue optical properties," *Appl. Opt.*, vol. 28, pp. 2331–2336, 1989.
[47] P. A. Wilksch, F. Jacka, and A. J. Blake, "Studies of light propagation in tissue," in *Porphyrin Localization and Treatment of Tumors*, D. R. Doiron and C. J. Gomer, Eds. New York: Alan R. Liss, 1984, pp. 149–161.
[48] M. Keijzer, R. R. Richards-Kortum, S. L. Jacques, and M. S. Feld, "Fluorescence spectroscopy of turbid media: autofluorescence of the human aorta," *Appl. Opt.*, vol. 28, pp. 4286–4292, 1989.
[49] M. J. C. van Gemert, R. Verdaasdonk, E. G. Stassen, G. A. C. M. Schets, G. H. M. Gijsbers, and J. J. Bonnier, "Optical properties of human blood vessel wall and plaque," *Lasers Surg. Med.*, vol. 5, pp. 235–237, 1985.
[50] A. A. Oraevsky, V. S. Letokhov, S. E. Ragimov, V. G. Omel'Yanenko, A. A. Belyaev, B. V. Shekhonin, and R. S. Akchurin, "Spectral properties of human atherosclerotic blood vessel walls," *Lasers Life Sci.*, vol. 2, pp. 275–288, 1988.
[51] G. D. Pedersen, N. J. McCormick, and L. O. Reynolds, "Transport calculations for light scattering in blood," *Biophys. J.*, vol. 16, pp. 199–207, 1976.

[52] L. O. Reynolds, C. C. Johnson, and A. Ishimaru, "Diffuse reflectance from a finite blood medium: Applications to the modeling of fiber optic catheters," *Appl. Opt.*, vol. 15, pp. 2059-2067, 1976.

[53] P. Parsa, S. L. Jacques, and N. S. Nishioka, "Optical properties of rat liver between 350 and 2200 nm," *Appl. Opt.*, vol. 28, pp. 2325-2330, 1989.

[54] J. L. Karagiannes, Z. Zhang, B. Grossweiner, and L. I. Grossweiner, "Applications of the 1-D diffusion approximation to the optics of tissues and tissue phantoms," *Appl. Opt.*, vol. 28, pp. 2311-2317, 1989.

[55] G. Mie, "Pioneering mathematical description of scattering by spheres," *Ann. Phys.*, vol. 25, p. 337, 1908.

[56] J. M. Steinke and A. P. Shepherd, "Diffusion model of the optical absorbance of whole blood," *J. Opt. Soc. Amer.*, vol. 5, pp. 813-822, 1988.

[57] L. O. Reynolds and N. J. McCormick, "Approximate two-parameter phase function for light scattering," *J. Opt. Soc. Amer.*, vol. 70, pp. 1206-1212, 1980.

[58] S. L. Jacques, C. A. Alter, and S. A. Prahl, "Angular dependence of HeNe laser light scattering by human dermis," *Lasers Life Sci.*, vol. 1, pp. 309-333, 1987.

[59] J. P. A. Marijnissen, W. M. Star, J. L. van Delft, and N. A. P. Franken, "Light intensity measurements in optical phantoms and *in vivo* during HpD photoradiation treatment using a miniature light detector with isotropic response," in *Photodynamic Therapy of Tumors and Other Diseases*, G. Jori and C. Perria, Eds. Padova, Italy: Libreria Progetto, 1985, pp. 387-390.

[60] W. F. Cheong, "Photo-thermal processes in tissue irradiated by Nd : YAG laser (1.06 μm, 1.32 μm)," Ph.D. dissertation, Univ. Texas at Austin, Dec. 1990.

[61] W. M. Star, J. P. A. Marijnissen, and M. J. C. van Gemert, "Light dosimetry: Status and prospects," *J. Photochem. Photobiol. B: Biology*, vol. 1, pp. 149-167, 1987.

[62] D. R. Doiron, L. O. Svaasand, and A. E. Profio, "Wavelength and dosimetry considerations in photoradiation therapy (PRT)," *Proc. SPIE*, vol. 357, Lasers in Surgery and Medicine, M. Berns, Ed., 1982.

[63] F. P. Bolin, L. E. Preuss, R. C. Taylor, and T. S. Sandu, "A study of the three-dimensional distribution of light (632.8 nm) in tissue," *IEEE J. Quantum. Electron.*, vol. QE-23, pp. 1734-1738, 1987.

[64] L. E. Preuss and F. P. Bolin, "Letter to the editor," *Lasers Life Sci.*, vol. 1, pp. 335-336, 1987.

[65] S. A. Prahl, A. J. Welch, M. P. Sartori, P. D. Henry, R. Roberts, G. L. Valderrama, K. Y. Jong, and M. J. Berry, "Optical properties of normal human aorta from 200 to 2200 nanometers," *Lasers Surg. Med.*, vol. 8, p. 142 (abstract), 1988.

[66] H. J. C. M. Sterenborg, M. J. C. van Gemert, W. Kamphorst, J. G. Wolbers, and W. Hogervorst, "The spectral dependence of the optical properties of the human brain," *Lasers Med. Sci.*, vol. 4, pp. 221-227, 1989.

[67] A. E. Profio and D. R. Doiron, "Transport of light in tissue in photodynamic therapy," *Photochem. Photobiol.*, vol. 46, pp. 591-599, 1987.

[68] G. I. Bell and S. Glasstone, *Nuclear Reactor Theory*. Malabar, FL: Robert E. Krieger, 1985.

[69] W. G. Houf and F. P. Incorpera, "An assessment of techniques for predicting radiation transfer in aqueous media," *J. Quantum Spec. Rad. Trans.*, vol. 23, pp. 101-115, 1980.

[70] B. C. Wilson and G. Adam, "A Monte Carlo model for the absorption and flux distributions of light in tissue," *Med. Phys.*, vol. 10, pp. 824-830, 1983.

[71] M. Keijzer, S. L. Jacques, S. A. Prahl, and A. J. Welch, "Light distributions in artery tissue: Monte Carlo simulations for finite-diameter laser beams," *Lasers Surg. Med.*, vol. 9, pp. 148-154, 1989.

[72] W. M. Star, J. P. A. Marijnissen, H. Jansen, M. Keijzer, and M. J. C. van Gemert, "Light dosimetry for photodynamic therapy by whole bladder wall irradiation," *Photochem. Photobiol.*, vol. 46, pp. 619-624, 1987.

[73] R. Splinter, W. F. Cheong, M. J. C. van Gemert, and A. J. Welch, "*In vitro* optical properties of human and canine brain and urinary bladder tissues at 633 nm," *Lasers Surg. Med.*, vol. 9, pp. 37-41, 1989.

[74] W. F. Cheong, M. Motamedi, and A. J. Welch, "Optical modeling of laser photocoagulation of bladder tissue," *Lasers Surg. Med.*, vol. 7, pp. 72 (abstract), 1987.

[75] L. O. Svaasand and R. Ellingsen, "Optical properties of human brain," *Photochem. Photobiol.*, vol. 38, pp. 293-299, 1983.

[76] L. O. Svaasand, C. J. Gomer, and A. E. Profio, "Laser-induced hyperthermia of ocular tumors," *Appl. Opt.*, vol. 28, pp. 2280-2287, 1989.

[77] L. O. Svaasand and R. Ellingsen, "Optical penetration in human intracranial tumors," *Photochem. Photobiol.*, vol. 41, pp. 73-76, 1985.

[78] H. Key, P. C. Jackson, and P. N. T. Wells, "Light scattering and propagation in tissue," *Poster Presentation, World Cong. Med. Phys., Bioeng.*, San Antonio, TX, Aug. 1988.

[79] S. Watanabe, T. J. Flotte, D. J. McAuliffe, and S. L. Jacques, "Putative photoacoustic damage in skin induced by pulsed ArF excimer laser," *J. Invest. Derm.*, vol. 90, pp. 761-766, 1988.

[80] R. Splinter, *Poster Presentation, Future Directions Lasers in Surg., Med., Eng. Foundat.* Florida, Feb. 1989.

[81] M. J. C. van Gemert, M. C. Berenbaum, and G. H. M. Gijsbers, "Wavelength and light-dose dependence in tumor phototherapy with hematoporphyrin-derivative," *Brit. J. Cancer*, vol. 52, pp. 43-49, 1985.

[82] B. C. Wilson, P. J. Muller, and J. C. Yanche, "Instrumentation and light dosimetry for intra-operative photodynamic therapy (PDT) of malignant brain tumors," *Phys. Med. Biol.*, vol. 31, pp. 125-133, 1986.

[83] P. J. Muller and B. C. Wilson, "An update on the penetration depth of 630 nm light in normal and malignant human brain tissue *in vivo*," *Phys. Med. Biol.*, vol. 31, pp. 1295-1297, 1986.

[84] R. R. Anderson and J. A. Parrish, "The optics of human skin," *J. Invest. Dermatol.*, vol. 77, pp. 13-19, 1981.

[85] M. J. C. van Gemert, A. J. Welch, and A. P. Amin, "Is there an optimal laser treatment for portwine stains?" *Lasers Surg. Med.*, vol. 6, pp. 76-83, 1986.

[86] S. Wan, R. R. Anderson, and J. A. Parrish, "Analytical modeling for the optical properties of the skin with *in vitro* and *in vivo* applications," *Photochem. Photobiol.*, vol. 34, pp. 493-499, 1981.

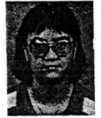

Wai-Fung Cheong was born in Malaysia. She received the B.Sc.(Hons.) degree in physics from the University of Malaya in June 1979 and the Diploma in education in December 1979. She was with Texas Tech University, Lubbock, as a Rotary Foundation Graduate Fellow, where she received the M.E. degree in clinical engineering in 1982.

In 1984 she began her doctoral studies at the University of Texas, Austin. She is currently a Research Assistant with special interests in the theoretical and empirical determination of laser–tissue interactive mechanisms, applied specifically to photocoagulation in urological oncology and laser angioplasty.

Scott A. Prahl, for a biography, see this issue, p. 2304.

Ashley J. Welch (M'66–SM'79), for a biography and photograph, see this issue, p. 2239.

Reprinted with permission from *Applied Optics*, Vol. 32(4), pp. 559-568
(February 1, 1993). ©1993 Optical Society of America.

Determining the optical properties of turbid media by using the adding–doubling method

Scott A. Prahl, Martin J. C. van Gemert, and Ashley J. Welch

A method is described for finding the optical properties (scattering, absorption, and scattering anisotropy) of a slab of turbid material by using total reflection, unscattered transmission, and total transmission measurements. This method is applicable to homogeneous turbid slabs with any optical thickness, albedo, or phase function. The slab may have a different index of refraction from its surroundings and may or may not be bounded by glass. The optical properties are obtained by iterating an adding-doubling solution of the radiative transport equation until the calculated values of the reflection and transmission match the measured ones. Exhaustive numerical tests show that the intrinsic error in the method is < 3% when four quadrature points are used.

1. Introduction

This paper introduces a practical way to determine the optical properties of scattering and absorbing materials. These properties are obtained by repeatedly solving the radiative transport equation until the solution matches the measured reflection and transmission values. The advantages over existing methods are increased accuracy and flexibility in modeling turbid samples with intermediate albedos, mismatched boundary conditions, and anisotropic scattering. The primary disadvantage is that this method is entirely numerical. For brevity this method is called inverse adding–doubling (IAD): inverse implies a reversal of the usual process of calculating reflection and transmission from optical properties, and adding–doubling indicates the method used to solve the radiative transport equation. The IAD algorithm and theory are described in this paper; an experimental implementation is presented in the companion paper.[1]

The optical properties of biological tissue are important for photodynamic therapy and diagnostic techniques.[2] Typically optical properties are obtained by using solutions of the radiative transport equation that express the optical properties in terms of readily measurable quantities.[3] These solutions are either exact or approximate and correspond to the direct or indirect methods described by Wilson *et al.*[4] Direct methods place stringent constraints on the sample to match the assumptions made for the exact solution. For example, the direct method used by Flock *et al.*[5] required thin samples in which multiple scattering could be ignored. Indirect methods relax the sample constraints but require approximations that are often invalid for tissue samples (e.g., nearly isotropic scattering or no internal reflection at the boundaries). The theory used in indirect methods usually falls into one of three categories: Beer's law, Kubelka–Munk, or the diffusion approximation.

Beer's law neglects scattering and is inappropriate for thick scattering materials. The Kubelka–Munk method and variants[6–12] are still used[13,14] but are limited in their accuracy.[11,15] Methods based on the diffusion approximation or a similar approximation (e.g., uniform radiances over the forward and backward hemispheres) tend to be more accurate than the Kubelka–Munk method.[16,17] Techniques using the diffusion approximation include pulsed photothermal radiometry,[18] time-resolved spectroscopy,[19] radial reflectance spectroscopy,[20] weak localization,[21] and an iterative technique that uses reflection and transmission measurements.[22] These methods remain popular because they are easy to use, place relatively minor constraints on the type of sample, and are amenable to analytic manipulation. However, the diffusion approximation assumes that the internal

S. A. Prahl is with the Department of Electrical Engineering and Applied Physics, Oregon Graduate Institute, Beaverton, Oregon 97006. M. J. C. van Gemert is with the Laser Center, Academic Medical Center, Amsterdam, The Netherlands. A. J. Welch is with Biomedical Engineering, University of Texas at Austin, Austin, Texas 78712.

Received 8 January 1992

0003-6935/93/040559-10$05.00/0.

© 1993 Optical Society of America.

radiance is nearly isotropic, and consequently it is inaccurate when scattering is comparable with absorption.[23]

The adding–doubling method is a general, numerical solution of the radiative transport equation.[24] The adding–doubling method[25] was chosen because it is sufficiently fast that iterated solutions are possible on current microcomputers and sufficiently flexible that anisotropic scattering and internal reflection at the boundaries may be included. Other accurate solutions of the radiative transport equation such as Chandrasekhar's X and Y functions,[26] discrete ordinates,[27] Monte Carlo models,[28–30] invariant embedding,[31] or successive orders[24] are too slow or insufficiently flexible to incorporate the necessary boundary conditions needed for turbid materials with mismatched boundaries.

The IAD method consists of the following steps: (1) Guess a set of optical properties. (2) Calculate the reflection and transmission by using the adding–doubling method. (3) Compare the calculated values with the measured reflection and transmissions. (4) Repeat until a match is made. The set of optical properties that generates reflection and transmission values matching the measured values is taken as the optical properties of the sample. The results obtained with the IAD method are accurate for all optical properties and can be made arbitrarily precise at the cost of increased computation time. Furthermore, by avoiding an analytical solution, it is possible to incorporate the necessary corrections for measurements made directly with integrating spheres[32] (see Section 3.F). Such corrections are usually quite awkward to implement because the magnitude of the correction depends on the optical properties of the sample measured.

2. Adding–Doubling Method

A. Definitions

The optical properties of a turbid medium are characterized by the absorption coefficient μ_a, the scattering coefficient μ_s, and the single-scattering phase function $p(\theta)$. The reciprocal of the absorption (scattering) coefficient is the average distance a photon will travel before being absorbed (scattered) by the medium. Two dimensionless quantities that characterize light propagation in a turbid medium are the albedo a and the optical thickness τ. These are defined as

$$a = \frac{\mu_s}{\mu_s + \mu_a}, \qquad \tau = d(\mu_s + \mu_a),$$

where d is the physical thickness of the slab.

The single-scattering phase function $p(\theta)$ describes the amount of light scattered at an angle θ from the incoming direction. The phase function is often expressed in terms of the cosine of this scattering angle $\nu = \cos\theta$. The phase function is normalized so that its integral over all directions is unity:

$$\int_{4\pi} p(\nu)d\omega = 2\pi \int_{-1}^{1} p(\nu)d\nu = 1,$$

where $d\omega$ is a differential solid angle. The functional form of the phase function in tissue is usually not known. However, research by Jacques *et al.*[33] and Yoon *et al.*[34] have shown that a Henyey–Greenstein function approximates single-particle light scattering in human dermis and aorta at 633 nm. Consequently this phase function is used in all calculations in this paper:

$$p(\nu) = \frac{1}{4\pi} \frac{1 - g^2}{(1 + g^2 - 2g\nu)^{3/2}}.$$

The Henyey–Greenstein phase function depends on only the anisotropy coefficient g, defined as

$$g = \int_{4\pi} p(\nu)\nu d\omega = 2\pi \int_{-1}^{1} p(\nu)\nu d\nu.$$

Consequently g is the average cosine of the scattering angle. When $g = 0$, scattering is equally probable in all directions. Typical values for tissues in the red region of the spectrum are $g \approx 0.8$,[2] which is moderately forwardly directed.

Reflection and transmission are relative to the normal irradiance on the sample surface and vary between zero and one. The total reflection R_T is all light specularly reflected and backscattered by the sample. The total transmission T_T is all the light that passes through the sample and includes any light traveling through the sample without being scattered. This unscattered light is denoted T_C, because for collimated irradiance on a sample the light passing directly through the sample is often called the collimated transmission. For a nonabsorbing sample $R_T + T_T = 1$.

B. Theory

The doubling method was introduced by van de Hulst for solving the radiative transport equation in a slab geometry.[35] The advantages of the adding–doubling method are that only integrations over angle are required, physical interpretation of results can be made at each step, the method is equivalent for isotropic and anisotropic scattering, and results are obtained for all angles of incidence used in the integration.[36] The disadvantages are that (a) it is slow and awkward for calculating internal fluences, (b) it is suited to a layered geometry with uniform irradiation, and (c) it is necessary that each layer have homogeneous optical properties. For determining optical properties using only reflection and transmission, internal fluences are not needed, so disadvantage (a) is not a problem. Disadvantages (b) and (c) place restrictions on the sample geometry—the samples must be uniformly illuminated, homogeneous slabs. The adding–doubling method is well suited to iterative problems because it provides accurate total reflection and transmission calculations with relatively few quadrature points. The method is fast for small numbers of quadrature points, and consequently iteration is practical.

In all calculations that follow the following assumptions are made: the distribution of light is independent of time, samples have homogeneous optical properties, the sample geometry is an infinite plane-parallel slab of finite thickness, the tissue has a uniform index of refraction, internal reflection at boundaries is governed by Fresnel's law, and the light is unpolarized. A nonabsorbing layer with a different index of refraction may be present at the boundaries (glass slide).

The doubling method assumes that the reflection $R(\nu, \nu')$ and transmission $T(\nu, \nu')$ for light incident at an angle ν and exiting at an angle ν' is known for one layer. The reflection and transmission of a slab that is twice as thick is found by juxtaposing two identical slabs and adding the reflection and transmission contributions from each slab.[25] The reflection and transmission for an arbitrary slab are calculated first by finding the reflection and transmission for a thin starting slab with the same optical properties (e.g., by using single scattering) and then by doubling until the desired thickness is reached. The adding method extends the doubling method to dissimilar slabs. Thus slabs with different optical properties can be placed adjacent to one another to simulate layered media or internal reflection caused by index-of-refraction differences.

C. Internal Reflection and Boundary Conditions

Internal reflection at the boundaries (caused by mismatched indices of refraction) was included in the calculation by adding an additional layer for each mismatched boundary. The reflection and transmission of this layer equaled the Fresnel reflection and transmission for unpolarized light incident on a plane boundary between two transparent media with the same indices of refraction. If $r(\nu_i)$ is the unpolarized Fresnel reflection for light incident from a medium with the index of refraction n_1 on a medium with an index of refraction n_2 at an angle from the normal with the cosine equal to ν_i, the reflection and transmission operators for the boundary slab are

$$R_{\text{bndry}}(\nu_i, \nu_j) = \frac{r(\nu_i)}{2\nu_i}\delta_{ij}, \quad T_{\text{bndry}}(\nu_i, \nu_j) = \frac{1 - r(\nu_i)}{2\nu_i}\left(\frac{n_1}{n_0}\right)^2\delta_{ij},$$

$$(1)$$

where δ_{ij} is the Kronecker delta function. The square of the ratio of the indices of refraction is due to the n^2 law of radiance,[37] which accounts for the difference in radiances across an index-of-refraction mismatch. The factor of $2\nu_i$ is included for uniformity with van de Hulst's definition of the reflection function.[24] Note finally that the transmission and reflection of the boundary layer were zero and one, respectively, for light that is incident at angles exceeding the

critical angle for total internal reflection. Both operators are diagonal because light is specularly reflected and the angle of incidence equals the angle of reflection.

By sandwiching a tissue sample between glass or quartz plates, we can minimize the usual irregularities in the tissue surface, and the Fresnel reflection is a good approximation. To account for a nonabsorbing boundary with a different index of refraction, we must include all the multiple internal reflections.[2] For example, if ν_i is the cosine of the angle of incidence from the turbid slab (index n_s) onto a glass slide (index n_g), the cosine of the angle inside the glass slide (ν_g) is determined by using Snell's law:

$$n_g(1 - \nu_g{}^2)^{1/2} = n_s(1 - \nu_i{}^2)^{1/2}, \qquad \nu_i < \nu_c,$$

where ν_c is the cosine of the critical angle for total internal reflection. When $r_i = r(\nu_i)$ is defined as the unpolarized Fresnel reflection coefficient for light passing from the slab into glass and $r_g = r(\nu_g)$ is for light passing from glass to air, the net reflection coefficient that should be used in Eqs. (1) is

$$r(\nu) = \begin{cases} \dfrac{r_1(\nu_i) + r_g(\nu_g) - 2r_1(\nu_i)r_g(\nu_g)}{1 - r_1(\nu_i)r_g(\nu_g)} & \text{if } \nu_i < \nu_c \\ 1 & \text{if } \nu_i \geq \nu_c \end{cases}.$$

This value for $r(\nu)$ accounts for the extra reflections within the glass slide. Finally, since light is refracted at the boundary, we must be sure that the incident and reflected fluxes are identified with the proper angles.

The reflection and transmission functions for the thin starting layers were obtained by the diamond initialization method.[38] The optical thickness for the starting layers was based on the smallest quadrature angle as suggested by Wiscombe.[39] The Henyey–Greenstein phase function was used for all calculations. We avoided phase-function renormalization by always using the $\delta - M$ method, which facilitates accurate calculations with highly anisotropic phase functions.[40]

The adding–doubling method is based on the numerical integration of functions with quadrature:

$$\int_0^1 f(\nu, \nu')d\nu' = \sum_{k=1}^{N} H_k f(x_k).$$

The quadrature points x_k and weights H_k are chosen so that the integral is approximated exactly for a polynomial of order $2N - 1$ (or possibly $2N - 2$, depending on the quadrature method). Using N quadrature points (Gaussian quadrature) is equivalent to the spherical harmonic method of order P_{N-1},[41] i.e., four quadrature points correspond to the P_3 method. The choice of quadrature methods is described in Section 3.

The total internal reflection caused problems by changing the effective range of integration. Usually adding–doubling integrals range from 0 to 1, since the angle varies from $\pi/2$ to 0 and therefore the cosine varies from 0 to 1. We used numerical quadrature in calculating the integrations, and the quadrature angles were optimized for this range. If the cosine of the critical angle is denoted by v_c, then for a boundary layer with total internal reflection the effective range of integration is reduced down to v_c to 1 (because the rest of the integration range is now 0). To maintain integration accuracy, we separated the integral into two parts, and each is evaluated by quadrature over the specified subrange:

$$\int_0^1 A(v, v')B(v', v'')\mathrm{d}v'$$

$$= \int_0^{v_c} A(v, v')B(v', v'')\mathrm{d}v' + \int_{v_c}^1 A(v, v')B(v', v'')\mathrm{d}v'.$$

Here $A(v, v')$ and $B(v, v')$ represent reflection or transmission functions, and, if either is identically zero for $v < v_c$, then the integration range is reduced. The calculations in this paper used Gaussian quadrature[42] for the range from 0 to v_c, and thereby calculations at both end points were avoided. (In particular the angle $v = 0$ is avoided, which may cause division by zero.) Radau quadrature was used for the range from v_c to 1, because one quadrature angle may be specified.[43] Normal irradiance corresponds to $v = 1$, and if this angle is specified, interpolation between quadrature points is not needed to obtain reflection and transmission for normal unscattered irradiance. Interpolation can be a significant source of error. The number of quadrature points are divided evenly between 0 to v_c and v_c to 1. Since the quadrature methods work well with even numbers of quadrature points, this dictates that the quadrature points should be chosen in multiples of four. Radau quadrature was used when there was no critical angle.

3. Iteration Process

The iteration process consists of finding optical properties that generate the measured reflection and transmission values. This section begins by showing that a unique solution to the inverse problem exists, and then the simplifications that are necessary when one or more of the experimental measurements is missing are described. Finally three components of the iteration process are given: (1) the function that defines the distance the calculated values are from the measure values, (2) the initial set of optical properties guessed, and (3) the algorithm used to minimize this function.

A. Uniqueness

The iteration method implicitly assumes that a unique combination of the albedo, the optical depth, and the anisotropy is determined by a set of reflection and transmission measurements. Clearly, if a sample is so thick that an accurate unscattered transmission measurement cannot be made, there are more unknowns than observations. Even when all the mea-

surements are available, it is not obvious that a unique set of optical properties (a, τ, g) exists for any set of measurements (R_T, T_T, T_C). For example, increasing the albedo of a sample will increase its total reflection and decrease its total transmission—but so will increasing the optical thickness of the sample. Uniqueness is demonstrated for two cases: fixed unscattered transmission and fixed scattering anisotropy. The former is representative when (R_T, T_T, T_C) are all known; the latter applies when the unscattered transmission measurement is unavailable and a fixed value for the scattering anisotropy must be assumed.

The dependence of the total transmission and total reflection on the anisotropy and albedo is shown in Fig. 1. The bold (a, g) grid was computed with the unscattered transmission fixed at 10% ($T_C = 0.1$), and the boundaries of the sample were matched with its environment. The intersection of the measured total reflection and total transmission grid lines determines a unique albedo and anisotropy.

In Fig. 2 the dependence of the total transmission and the total reflection on the reduced albedo and reduced optical thickness is shown. Scattering in the medium is assumed to be isotropic ($g = 0$), and the index of refraction is 1.4.[44] Again, any nonzero reflection and transmission measurement yields a unique value for the reduced scattering and absorption coefficient. Figure 2 is quite useful for obtaining quick estimates of the optical properties of a sample. For example, if $R_T = 0.4$ and $T_T = 0.2$, then $a \approx 0.96$ and $\tau \approx 7$. If the thickness of the sample is 0.4 mm and the scattering anisotropy is assumed to be ≈ 0.8, using the similarity relations (see below) will fix the optical properties at $(\mu_a, \mu_s, g) \approx (0.7\,\mathrm{mm}^{-1}, 17\,\mathrm{mm}^{-1}, 0.8)$.

C. Simplification

The three measurements usually available are the total reflection, the total transmission, and the unscat-

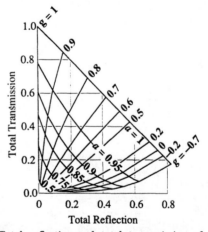

Fig. 1. Total reflection and total transmission of an index-matched slab ($n = 1$) as a function of the albedo a and anisotropy g for a fixed unscattered transmission value of 10%. Each point on the bold (a, g) grid corresponds to a unique (R_T, T_T) pair.

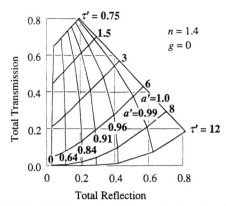

Fig. 2. Total reflection and total transmission of a slab as a function of the reduced albedo a' and reduced optical thickness τ'. Isotropic scattering is assumed as well as an index of refraction mismatch ($n = 1.4$). Each point on the (a', τ') grid corresponds to a unique (R_T, T_T) pair.

tered transmission. It is assumed that the unscattered reflection from each surface is equal to the Fresnel reflection for the unpolarized light that is normally incident on the sample. From the unscattered transmission T_C, we may immediately calculate the optical thickness τ by solving

$$T_C = \frac{(1 - r_{s1})(1 - r_{s2})\exp(-\tau)}{1 - r_{s1}r_{s2}\exp(-2\tau)}, \qquad (2)$$

where r_{s1} and r_{s2} are the primary reflections for light that is normally incident on the front and back surfaces of the slab. If glass slides are present, the specular reflection coefficients r_{s1} and r_{s2} should include multiple internal reflections in the slide (see Subsection 2.C). Once the optical thickness is known, only the albedo and anisotropy remain to be determined. They are varied until the calculated reflection and transmission match the measured values.

When the only measurements available are the total reflection and transmission, as might happen for a thick sample in which an accurate unscattered transmission measurement cannot be made, only two optical parameters can be determined. Typically a value for the scattering anisotropy is assumed, and the albedo and optical thickness are calculated based on this assumed value. The accuracy of say fluence calculations when these values are used (based on similarity) is unknown.

If only one measurement is available, the sample is usually too thick for a transmission measurement to be made. In this case the optical thickness of the sample is assumed to be infinite, and again a fixed value for the scattering anisotropy is chosen. The reduced albedo can now be calculated. This is a simple one-parameter minimization problem, and convergence is robust and rapid.

C. Metric

When the reflection and transmission for a particular set of optical properties are calculated, a definition of how far these values are from those measured is

needed. Several metrics were tried, but one based on a sum of relative errors worked best:

$$M(a, \tau, g) = \frac{|R_{\text{calc}} - R_{\text{meas}}|}{R_{\text{meas}} + 10^{-6}} + \frac{|T_{\text{calc}} - T_{\text{meas}}|}{T_{\text{meas}} + 10^{-6}}.$$

Here R_{meas} and T_{meas} are the measured reflection and transmission for scattered light. The factor of 10^{-6} is included to prevent division by zero when the reflection or transmission is zero. Note that the measurement errors for reflection and transmission are assumed to be equal for this metric. If this is not true, suitable modifications are necessary.

D. Inverse Method

The iteration method uses an N-dimensional minimization algorithm based on the downhill simplex method of Nelder and Mead.[45] One implementation of this method (AMOEBA) varies the parameters from $-\infty$ to ∞.[42] Since the anisotropy, albedo, and optical depth have fixed ranges, they are transformed into a computation space. For example, the transformation function for the albedo is

$$a_{\text{comp}} = \frac{2a - 1}{a(1 - a)}.$$

Thus, as a_{comp} varies from $-\infty$ to ∞, the albedo a varies from 0 to 1. The transformation for the anisotropy g (which varies from -1 to 1) is

$$g_{\text{comp}} = \frac{g}{1 + |g|}.$$

The transformation for the optical thickness τ (which varies from 0 to ∞) is

$$b_{\text{comp}} = \ln(\tau).$$

We can easily invert these relations to obtain relations for the optical properties in terms of the computation values. We made all calculations by using the real values: the transformed values were used only by the simplex method for choosing the next iteration point. Typical convergence was in 20–30 iterations.

E. Initial Values

The starting set of optical properties affects both the rapidity of convergence and the convergence to the correct values. Clearly, with a better first guess, fewer subsequent iterations are needed. Poor guesses have the added disadvantage that the minimization algorithm may converge to a relative rather than the global minimum. Since the global minimum corresponds to the unique solution described above, local minima must be guarded against. Fortunately they are easily detected by examining the magnitude of the minimum. If the magnitude exceeds a small tolerance (typically 10^{-3}), the minimum is a local one and the iteration process must be restarted with a better initial guess. If necessary,

$$\frac{P_r}{P} = \frac{\gamma_1[R_c(1 - \gamma_2 R_d) + \gamma_3 R_{cd}](1 - \gamma_4 R_d) + \gamma_1 \gamma_3 \gamma_4 T_d(T_{cd} + \gamma_5 T_C)}{(1 - \gamma_4 R_d)(1 - \gamma_6 R_d) - \gamma_4 \gamma_6 T_d^{\ 2}},$$

one or two restarts suffice to reach the global minimum.

Generating an initial set of approximately correct optical properties for any reflection and transmission combination is difficult. We can use the similarity relations[46] to facilitate picking starting values by relating (a, τ, g) to the reduced optical properties $(a', \tau', g' = 0)$:

$$a' = \frac{a(1 - g)}{1 - ag}, \qquad \tau' = (1 - ag)\tau. \qquad (3)$$

The inverse relations are

$$a = \frac{a'}{1 - g + a'g}, \qquad \tau = \tau' + \frac{a'\tau'g}{1 - g}. \qquad (4)$$

Now only two parameters need to be found (a', τ') for a combination (R_T, T_T). For example, originally the Kubelka–Munk relations were used to obtain these values for initial guesses.[47] Unfortunately these values were often worse than using just a fixed guess $(a', \tau', g) = (0.5, 1, 0.2)$ to begin all iterations. A good starting set of starting values is based on a crude fit of the reflection and transmission values of Fig. 2. The formula for the reduced albedo is

$$a' = \begin{cases} 1 - \left(\dfrac{1 - 4R_d - T_T}{1 - T_T}\right)^2 & \text{if } \dfrac{R_d}{1 - T_T} < 0.1 \\ 1 - \dfrac{4}{9}\left(\dfrac{1 - R_d - T_T}{1 - T_T}\right)^2 & \text{if } \dfrac{R_d}{1 - T_T} \geq 0.1. \end{cases}$$

The formula for the reduced optical thickness is

$$\tau' = \begin{cases} \dfrac{-\ln T_T \ln(0.05)}{\ln R_T} & \text{if } R_d \leq 0.1 \\ 2^{1 + 5(R_d + T_T)} & \text{if } R_d > 0.1. \end{cases}$$

Once we obtain τ by using Eq. (3), and a' and τ' have been calculated as above, Eqs. (1) and (2) can be used to generate a single set of starting values (a, τ, g). This is the only time the similarity relations are used in the IAD method.

F. Integrating-Sphere Correction

Total transmission and reflection are usually measured with integrating spheres. Interaction between the sample and spheres makes the detected signal no longer proportional to the sample reflection or transmission.[32] For example, when a double-integrating-sphere arrangement is used, the power on the wall of the reflectance sphere P_r, normalized to the incident power P is[32]

where the γ_i values depend on only the geometry and reflectivity of the integrating spheres, and various R and T values correspond to different types of reflection and transmission by the sample. A similar formula holds for the normalized power on the transmission sphere wall. Once the integrating spheres have been characterized (i.e., the γ_i values are known), we can calculate the normalized powers on the walls of the integrating sphere by using reflection and transmission values obtained with the adding–doubling method. The IAD algorithm calculates the normalized powers in the spheres and matches them to the detected powers (rather than matching reflection and transmission directly).

4. Accuracy of the Method

This section addresses the question: If R_T, T_T, and T_C are known exactly, what is the maximum possible error in the derived optical properties caused by the inverse adding–doubling method? The error analysis must be made numerically, because analytical expressions for light propagation in anisotropic media with mismatched boundaries are not available. The numerical tests are designed to find the accuracy of the inverse algorithm as functions of both the optical properties and the reflection and transmission of the sample. Implicit are checks on (a) the convergence of the inverse algorithm to the global minimum, (b) the termination criterion for stopping the iteration procedure, (c) the choice of starting parameters, and (d) the effect of using small numbers of quadrature points. This last test is particularly important, since the method would be useless (too slow) if small errors could be achieved only by using many quadrature points.

Generating a set of accurate testing values presented a problem, since accurate tabulated values for mismatched boundaries with anisotropic scattering could not be found in the literature. Consequently, after demonstrating that our adding–doubling implementation reproduced the published values for matched boundaries[24,46] exactly, we used Monte Carlo to verify a few mismatched cases. This confirmed the boundary condition algorithm. Finally, we compared 36- and 48-quadrature-point adding–doubling calculations. The 36-point calculation was always correct to at least 0.1%. The 48-point calculation was used for the test data and was constrained to include only samples with reduced optical thicknesses of > 0.25 and optical thicknesses of < 32. The rationale was that when $\tau' < 0.25$ either the sample does not multiply scatter and therefore a simpler algorithm should be used, or the sample does multiply scatter, but because of the highly anisotropic nature of each scattering event, the separation of T_C from scattered light would be extremely difficult. The second criterion ($\tau < 32$) ensured that the sufficient collimated transmitted light passed through the sample so that it could be measured [$T_C > \exp(-32) \sim 10^{-14}$]. The IAD method works for any optical thickness, but it becomes progressively less accurate outside this range.

All samples assume slabs with an index of refraction of 1.4 relative to the environment. Results for the index-matched samples indicate that the error in the IAD method is approximately half of those presented here for the mismatched case. This is caused by total internal reflection of light at quadrature angles that are greater than the critical angle (one-half of the total number, see Subsection 2.C). The slabs are not sandwiched by glass: calculations with a sample between glass slides do not alter the mismatched ($n = 1.4$) results significantly and are omitted for brevity.

In all calculations the scattering phase function used was the Henyey–Greenstein phase function. Despite the limited experimental evidence that this phase function is appropriate for tissues, errors arising from an inappropriate phase function should be small, since different phase functions with equivalent g values and different higher-order moments generate nearly equal reflection and transmission values.[46]

The absolute error is defined as the difference between the true or accurate values and those calculated with the inverse adding–doubling method:

$$\Delta a' = |a_{\text{true}}' - a_{\text{calc}}'|. \qquad (5)$$

The relative percentage error is the absolute error divided by the true value and multiplied by 100. The absolute errors in the scattering and absorption coefficients are proportional to the physical thickness of the sample and consequently are not particularly useful. The relative errors for μ_a and μ_s can also be obtained despite the fact that only dimensionless optical parameters are used by noting that the physical thickness cancels:

$$\frac{\Delta\mu_a}{\mu_a^{\text{true}}} = 100\left[1 - \frac{(1 - a_{\text{calc}})\tau_{\text{calc}}}{(1 - a_{\text{true}})\tau_{\text{true}}}\right],$$

$$\frac{\Delta\mu_s}{\mu_s^{\text{true}}} = 100\left(1 - \frac{a_{\text{calc}}\tau_{\text{calc}}}{a_{\text{true}}\tau_{\text{true}}}\right). \qquad (6)$$

B. Variation with Optical Properties

The sensitivity of the inverse adding–doubling method to the optical properties of a sample was evaluated by using a data set consisting of reflection and transmission values for 11 reduced albedos spaced so that $(1 - a_{\text{true}}')^{1/2} = (0, 0.1, \ldots, 1)$, 10 anisotropies spaced similarly (0, 0.19, 0.36, 0.51, 0.64, 0.75, 0.84, 0.91, 0.96, 0.99), and 14 reduced optical depths (listed in Table 1). Thus for each pair (a', τ') there were 10 different values of g that all corresponded to more or less equal values of R_T, T_T. There was a total of 1540

Table 1. Maximum Errors in the Calculated Reduced Optical Thickness τ' for any Albedo or Anisotropy as a Function of the True Reduced Optical Thickness[a]

τ'	Maximum Absolute Errors			Maximum Relative Errors		
	Diffusion	4	8	Diffusion	4	8
1/4	0.04	0.02	0.01	16	9	4
3/8	0.03	0.02	0.01	9	6	3
1/2	0.03	0.02	0.01	5	5	2
3/4	0.03	0.03	0.01	3	3	1
1	0.04	0.03	0.01	4	3	1
3/2	0.07	0.03	0.01	5	2	1
2	0.2	0.04	0.02	11	2	.8
3	0.2	0.04	0.02	7	1	.6
4	0.3	0.05	0.02	8	1	.6
6	0.6	0.1	0.04	10	1	.6
8	0.9	0.2	0.05	11	2	.6
12	1.5	0.3	0.09	12	2	.7
16	2	0.4	0.1	13	2	.7

[a]The calculated values were obtained by using a δ-Eddington approximation (diffusion) or the IAD method with four or eight quadrature points.

different combinations of a_{true}, τ_{true}, g_{true}. For each combination accurate reflection and transmission (R_T, T_T, T_C) values were calculated. The optical properties were found by using the IAD method with four and eight quadrature points. Diffusion equation results were obtained by using the same iteration algorithm but by replacing the adding–doubling calculation with a δ-Eddington diffusion approximation.[22,48]

The spacing in the reduced albedo was based on the observation that reflection and transmission are quite sensitive to changes in the reduced albedo when it is near unity. The anisotropy was chosen to vary in a similar manner for the same reason. Completely forward scattering ($g = 1$) was omitted because it corresponds to the nonscattering case. The nonscattering ($a = 0$) and nonabsorbing ($a = 1$) cases were both included. The range of the reduced optical thickness was chosen because of the natural advantage of making calculations for optical thicknesses that vary by a factor of 2 when the adding–doubling technique is used.

The variation in IAD accuracy with reduced optical thickness is tabulated in Table 1 and displayed in Fig. 3. The maximum relative error for a fixed τ' is the greatest error in a calculated value of τ' for any albedo and scattering anisotropy. The relative error decreases as the number of quadrature points increases. When $1 \leq \tau' \leq 16$ the maximum relative error when four quadrature points are used is $<2\%$. Surprisingly the diffusion approximation works best for $\tau' \approx 1$ but when only the relative error is considered. Table 1 shows that the maximum absolute error $\Delta\tau'$ monotonically increases with τ' for the diffusion approximation as well as the four- and eight-quadrature-point IAD calculations.

The variation in the relative error in the scattering

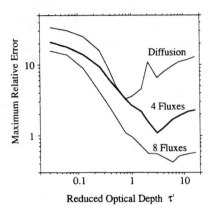

Fig. 3. Maximum error in the calculated reduced optical thickness τ' for any anisotropy and any albedo by using the diffusion approximation and the IAD method with four and eight quadrature points.

coefficient was evaluated for changes in the reduced optical thickness, the reduced albedo, and the scattering anisotropy when only four quadrature points were used. In Fig. 4 the maximum relative error in the calculated scattering coefficient is plotted as a function of the three dimensionless quantities a', τ', and g. As expected the accuracy in determining μ_s increases as the scattering increases (i.e., as $a' \to 1$). The increased scattering implies more uniform internal radiance distributions, which in turn are more accurately approximated than highly anisotropic internal radiance by four-quadrature-point distributions. Errors in the scattering coefficient do not depend strongly on either the reduced optical thickness or the scattering anisotropy. The maximum relative error never exceeds 6% for positive albedos.

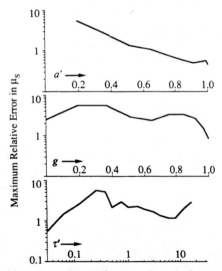

Fig. 4. Maximum relative error in the calculated scattering coefficient as a function of the reduced albedo a', the reduced optical thickness τ', and the scattering anisotropy g by using the IAD method with four quadrature points and mismatched boundaries $n = 1.4$.

B. Variation with Reflection and Transmission

The accuracy of the inverse adding–doubling method varies with the reflection and transmission of the sample. To quantify the maximum error for specific reflection and transmission values another paired set of a_{true}, τ_{true}, g_{true} and R_T, T_T, T_C were generated. In this set the total reflection and total transmission were spaced evenly (in 0.05 increments). By permitting the unscattered transmission to take on different values, 10 different sets of a_{true}, τ_{true}, g_{true} were obtained for each pair (R_T, T_T). The maximum relative error in the absorption coefficient, the scattering coefficient, and the scattering anisotropy was calculated by using the IAD method with four quadrature points.

Figure 5 shows a contour plot of the maximum relative error in the calculated absorption coefficient as a function of total reflection and total transmission. The maximum relative error in the absorption coefficient (assuming $\mu_a > 0$ or $R_T + T_T < 1$) was 10%. The $R_T + T_T = 0$ case is omitted because $\mu_a = 0$ for conservative scattering and the relative error is infinite in this case. For the majority of R_T, T_T combinations the maximum error is 2–3%. The error is greatest when the total transmission is highest, which corresponds to samples that absorb only a small fraction of the light.

Figure 6 shows a contour plot of the maximum relative error in the scattering coefficient as a function of the total reflection and total transmission. In contrast to the error in the absorption coefficient the error for the scattering coefficient is greatest when little light is reflected by the sample. The error drops sharply with increasing reflection values. The maximum error is always <2% for any nonzero value of μ_s. The $\mu_s = 0$ case is omitted for the same reason that conservative scattering is avoided in Fig. 5. The larger relative errors seen in Fig. 4 all correspond to the very small reflection values indicated by the black area in Fig. 6.

Figure 7 shows a contour plot of the maximum

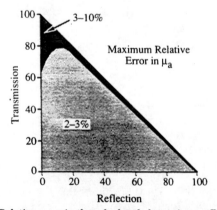

Fig. 5. Relative error in the calculated absorption coefficient as a function of reflection and transmission. The IAD method was used with four quadrature points, and the slab had mismatched boundaries.

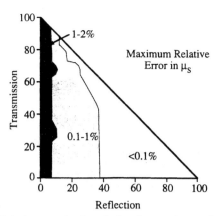

Fig. 6. Relative error in the calculated scattering coefficient as a function of reflection and transmission. The IAD method was used with four quadrature points, and the slab had mismatched boundaries.

absolute error in the scattering anisotropy as a function of total reflection and total transmission. The error is always < 0.03 for all the cases in which the scattering coefficient is nonzero. When the scattering coefficient is zero, no scattering takes place and any measurement will not give information on the shape of the scattering event. These cases correspond to total reflection values that are equal to the unscattered reflected light.

Typically the errors resulting from the IAD method will be much smaller than those resulting from experimental uncertainties. For example, assume that the measurements $R_T = 0.264$, $T_T = 0.261$, and $T_C = 5.91 \times 10^{-5}$ are known with a 1% uncertainty. The relative errors resulting from the IAD method are 0.04% for μ_s, 1% for μ_a, and 0.1% for g. However, perturbing the reflection and transmission values by 1% and re-solving for the optical properties result in errors of 0.4% for μ_s, 17% for μ_a, and 0.4% for g or approximately an order of magnitude larger than the errors inherent in the IAD method itself. Such error estimates are necessary because of the

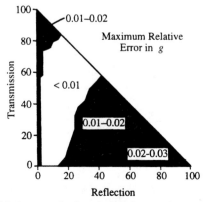

Fig. 7. Relative error in the calculated scattering anisotropy as a function of reflection and transmission. The IAD method was used with four quadrature points, and the slab had mismatched boundaries.

nonlinear relationship between reflection and transmission and the intrinsic optical properties. A primary goal of this study was to develop an accurate method of computing optical properties, so that such estimates can be made without introducing errors caused by the calculation itself.

In practice the two most common sources of experimental errors are (1) loss of light from the edges of the sample (which thereby invalidates the one-dimensional assumptions and underestimating both R_T and T_T) and (2) collecting scattered light in the unscattered transmission measurement (which thereby overestimates T_C). The first problem manifests itself in spuriously high absorption values, and the latter case leads to optical properties that depend on the thickness of the sample. These problems are discussed at length in the experimental implementation of this technique.[1]

5. Conclusions

The inverse adding–doubling method translates total reflection, total transmission, and unscattered transmission measurements into scattering, absorption, and scattering anisotropy values. The method is applicable when the one-dimensional radiative transport equation adequately describes the propagation of light through the sample. Using only four quadrature points, the IAD method generates optical properties (μ_a, μ_s, g) that are accurate to 2–3% for most reflection and transmission values. Higher accuracy is achieved by using more quadrature points, but it requires increased computation time. The validity of the IAD method for samples in which ($\mu_a \approx \mu_s$) is especially important since other methods (e.g., those based on the diffusion approximation) are known to fail in this regime. Furthermore both anisotropic phase functions and Fresnel reflection at boundaries are accurately approximated, and therefore the IAD method is well suited to measurements involving biological tissues sandwiched between glass slides. A computer implementation of the inverse adding–doubling method is available from the authors.

This work was supported by the Office of Naval Research Contract N00014-86-K-0117 and the National Institutes of Health grant 5R01AR25395-11.

References

1. J. W. Pickering, S. A. Prahl, N. van Wieringen, J. B. Beek, H. J. C. M. Sterenborg, and M. J. C. van Gemert, "Double-integrating-sphere system for measuring optical properties of tissue," Appl. Opt. **32**, 399–410 (1993).
2. W. F. Cheong, S. A. Prahl, and A. J. Welch, "A review of the optical properties of biological tissues," IEEE J. Quantum Electron. **26**, 2166–2185 (1990).
3. M. S. Patterson, B. C. Wilson, and D. R. Wyman, "The propagation of optical radiation in tissue II. Optical properties of tissues and resulting fluence distributions," Lasers Med. Sci. **6**, 379–390 (1991).
4. B. C. Wilson, M. S. Patterson, and S. T. Flock, "Indirect versus

direct techniques for the measurement of the optical properties of tissues," Photochem. Photobiol. **46**, 601–608 (1987).

5. S. T. Flock, B. C. Wilson, and M. S. Patterson, "Total attenuation coefficients and scattering phase functions of tissues and phantom materials at 633 nm," Med. Phys. **14**, 835–841 (1987).

6. P. Kubelka, "New contributions to the optics of intensely light-scattering materials. Part I," J. Opt. Am. **38**, 448–457 (1948).

7. P. Kubelka, "Errata: new contributions to the optics of intensely light-scattering materials," J. Opt. Soc. Am. **38**, 1067 (1948).

8. P. Kubelka, "New contributions to the optics of intensely light-scattering materials. Part II: Nonhomogeneous layers," J. Opt. Soc. Am. **44**, 330–335 (1954).

9. J. T. Atkins, "Optical properties of turbid materials," in *The Biologic Effects of Ultraviolet Radiation (With Emphasis on the Skin)*, F. Urbach, ed. (Pergamon, London, 1969), pp. 141–149.

10. S. Q. Duntley, "The optical properties of diffusing materials," J. Opt. Soc. Am. **32**, 61–70 (1942).

11. A. L. Lathrop, "Diffuse scattered radiation theories of Duntley and of Kubelka–Munk," J. Opt. Soc. Am. **55**, 1097–1104 (1965).

12. B. L. Diffey, "A mathematical model for ultraviolet optics in skin," Phys. Med. Biol. **28**, 647–657 (1983).

13. G. M. LaMuraglia, M. R. Prince, N. S. Nishioka, S. Obremski, and R. Birngruber, "Optical properties of human arterial thrombus, vascular grafts, and sutures: implications for selective laser thrombus ablation," IEEE J. Quantum Electron. **26**, 2200–2206 (1990).

14. A. Vogel, C. Dlugos, R. Nuffer, and R. Birngruber, "Optical properties of human sclera, and their consequences for transscleral laser applications," Lasers Surg. Med. **11**, 331–340 (1991).

15. P. S. Mudgett and L. W. Richards, "Multiple scattering calculations for technology," Appl. Opt. **10**, 1485–1502 (1971).

16. J. Reichman, "Determination of absorption and scattering coefficients for nonhomogeneous media. 1: Theory," Appl. Opt. **12**, 1811–1815 (1973).

17. W. G. Egan, T. W. Hilgeman, and J. Reichman, "Determination of absorption and scattering coefficients for nonhomogeneous media. 2: Experiment," Appl. Opt. **12**, 1816–1823 (1973).

18. S. A. Prahl, I. A. Vitkin, B. C. Wilson, and R. R. Anderson, "Determination of optical properties of turbid media using pulsed photothermal radiometry," Phys. Med. Biol. **37**, 1203–1217 (1992).

19. M. S. Patterson, B. Chance, and B. C. Wilson, "Time resolved reflectance and transmittance for the noninvasive measurement of tissue optical properties," Appl. Opt. **28**, 2331–2336 (1989).

20. M. S. Patterson, E. Schwartz, and B. C. Wilson, "Quantitative reflectance spectrophotometry for the noninvasive measurement of photosensitizer concentration in tissue during photodynamic therapy," in *Photodynamic Therapy: Mechanisms*, T. J. Dougherty, ed., Proc. Soc. Photo-Opt. Instrum. Eng. **1065**, 115–122 (1989).

21. K. M. Yoo, F. Liu, and R. R. Alfano, "Angle and time resolved studies of backscattering of light from biological tissues," in *Laser–Tissue Interaction*, S. L. Jacques, ed., Proc. Soc. Photo-Opt. Instrum. Eng. **1202**, 260–271 (1990).

22. S. L. Jacques and S. A. Prahl, "Modeling optical and thermal distributions in tissue during laser irradiation," Lasers Surg. Med. **6**, 494–503 (1987).

23. G. Yoon, S. A. Prahl, and A. J. Welch, "Accuracies of the diffusion approximation and its similarity relations for laser irradiated biological media," Appl. Opt. **28**, 2250–2255 (1989).

24. H. C. van de Hulst, *Multiple Light Scattering* (Academic, New York, 1980), Vol. 1.

25. G. N. Plass, G. W. Kattawar, and F. E. Catchings, "Matrix operator theory of radiative transfer. 1: Rayleigh scattering," Appl. Opt. **12**, 314–329 (1973).

26. S. Chandrasekhar, *Radiative Transfer* (Dover, New York, 1960), Chap. 8.

27. S. E. Orchard, "Reflection and transmission of light by diffusing suspensions," J. Opt. Soc. Am. **59**, 1584–1597 (1969).

28. B. C. Wilson and G. Adam, "A Monte Carlo model for the absorption and flux distributions of light in tissue," Med. Phys. **10**, 824–830 (1983).

29. S. A. Prahl, M. Keijzer, S. L. Jacques, and A. J. Welch, "A Monte Carlo model of light propagation in tissue," in *Dosimetry of Laser Radiation in Medicine and Biology*, G. J. Müller and D. H. Sliney, eds., Proc. Soc. Photo-Opt. Instrum. Eng. **ISO 5**, 102–111 (1989).

30. S. T. Flock, M. S. Patterson, B. C. Wilson, and D. R. Wyman, "Monte Carlo modeling of light propagation in high scattering tissue—I: Model predictions and comparison with diffusion theory," IEEE Trans. Biomed. Eng. **BME-36**, 1162–1168 (1989).

31. R. Bellman and G. M. Wing, *An Introduction to Invariant Imbedding* (Wiley, New York, 1975).

32. J. W. Pickering, C. J. M. Moes, H. J. C. M. Sterenborg, S. A. Prahl, and M. J. C. van Gemert, "Two integrating spheres with an intervening scattering sample," J. Opt. Soc. Am. A **9**, 621–631 (1992).

33. S. L. Jacques, C. A. Alter, and S. A. Prahl, "Angular dependence of HeNe laser light scattering by human dermis," Lasers Life Sci. **1**, 309–333 (1987).

34. G. Yoon, A. J. Welch, M. Motamedi, and M. C. J. V. Gemert, "Development and application of three-dimensional light distribution model for laser irradiated tissue," IEEE J. Quantum Electron. **QE-23**, 1721–1733 (1987).

35. H. C. van de Hulst, *A New Look at Multiple Scattering*, Tech. Rep. (NASA Institute for Space Studies, New York, 1962).

36. W. M. Irvine, "Multiple scattering in planetary atmospheres," Icarus **25**, 175–204 (1975).

37. R. Priesendorfer, *Hydrologic Optics* (U.S. Department of Commerce, Washington, D.C., 1976), Vol. 1.

38. W. J. Wiscombe, "On initialization, error and flux conservation in the doubling method," J. Quant. Spectrosc. Radiative Transfer **16**, 637–658 (1976).

39. W. J. Wiscombe, "Doubling initialization revisited," J. Quant. Spectrosc. Radiat. Transfer **18**, 245–248 (1977).

40. W. J. Wiscombe, "The delta-M method: rapid yet accurate radiative flux calculations for strongly asymmetric phase functions," J. Atmos. Sci. **34**, 1408–1422 (1977).

41. K. M. Case and P. F. Zweifel, *Linear Transport Theory* (Addison-Wesley, Reading, Mass., 1967), Chap. 8, p. 226.

42. W. H. Press, B. P. Flannery, S. A. Teukolsky, and W. T. Vetterling, *Numerical Recipes: The Art of Scientific Computing* (Cambridge U. Press, New York, 1986), Chap. 10, p. 289.

43. F. B. Hildebrand, *Introduction to Numerical Analysis* (Dover, New York, 1974), Chap. 8.

44. F. P. Bolin, L. E. Preuss, R. C. Taylor, and R. J. Ference, "Refractive index of some mammalian tissues using a fiber optic cladding method," Appl. Opt. **28**, 2297–2303 (1989).

45. J. A. Nelder and R. Mead, Comput. J. **7**, 380 (1965).

46. H. C. van de Hulst, *Multiple Light Scattering* (Academic, New York, 1980), Vol. 2. Chap. 14.

47. M. J. C. van Gemert and W. M. Star, "Relations between the Kubelka–Munk and the transport equation models for anisotropic scattering," Lasers Life Sci. **1**, 287–298 (1987).

48. J. H. Joseph, W. J. Wiscombe, and J. A. Weinman, "The delta-Eddington approximation for radiative flux transfer," J. Atmos. Sci. **33**, 2452–2459 (1976).

Reprinted from *Lasers and Medicine,* Proc. SPIE Vol. 1353, pp. 97-102 (1989).
©1989 SPIE.

New optical effects in the human hard tooth tissues

G.B.Altshuler, V.N.Grisimov

Leningrad Institute of Fine Mechanic and Optics,
Department of Quantum Electronics,
I Leningrad Medical Institute, Department of
Therapeutic Stomatology, Leningrad, USSR

ABSTRACT

The results of the investigations of light propagation in the human hard tooth tissues are represented. It is shown that apart from light scattering the novel effect of waveguide light propagation from the enamel surface to the tooth cavity is taken place. The trajectories of light flows are the same that the directions of enamel prisms and dentinal tubules orientations. Anomal optical properties of the tooth are shown to be explained by the waveguide-scattering media model which is developed in this paper.

The development of biophysics, wide application of laser medicine techniques need for more detail investigation of light propagation in human organism tissues. Up to last years such works were made in optical properties of eyes mainly. In this paper the results of first investigations of laser radiation propagation in human tooth tissues are represented. The novel effect of waveguide propagation of light in hard tooth tissues is reported.

It is well known that human tooth consists of three main parts (fig.1): enamel, dentin and pulp. Tooth enamel forms external surface of the dental crown is up to 1.7 mm thick in the direction normal to this surface and consists of various apatites among which the main part (75%) is hydroxiapatite $Ca_{10}(PO_4)_6(OH)_2$. Hydroxiapatite microcrystals form so-called enamel prisms in the form of cut-cylindrical fibers with 4-6 μm transverse dimension oriented normally to the tooth surface. The full length of these prisms exceed the enamel thickness due to prism curvature. Interprism space is filled with the enamel liquor and is up to 0.2% enamel volume. Dentin as the main part of the crown and tooth root is less mineralized than enamel. It consists of 70-72% unorganic substances that in enamel too and 28-30% organic substances and water. The dentin thickness depends on the dental form and human age and is about 1.5-5 mm. The main dentin substance is transpierced dentinal tubules which density varies from $3 \cdot 10^4$ mm^{-2} near the enamelodentine border up to $7.5 \cdot 10^4$ mm^{-2} near the pulpodentine border. The dentinal tubule diameter is about 1-5 μm. Dentinal tubules are filled with processes of odontoblasts - pulp external layer cells. Orientation of enamel

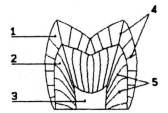

Fig.1.Dental crown.
1 - Enamel
2 - Dentin
3 - Pulp
4 - Enamel prism orientation
5 - Dentin tubule orientation

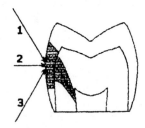

Fig.2a.Light propagation under the incidence of the laser beam on the crown equator.

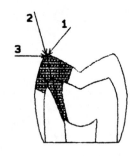

Fig.2b.Light propagation under the incidence of the laser beam on the crown tuber apex.

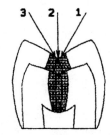

Fig.2c.Light propagation under the incidence of the laser beam on the fissure.

Table

Tooth tissues	Transmission		Anisotropy of transmission
	$T\parallel$	$T\perp$	
Enamel (sample type)	0.05(I)	0.03(II)	1.7
Dentine (sample type)	0.12(III)	0.004(IV)	30.

160

prisms and dentinal tubules is shown at fig.1 . Tooth pulp represents the cribriform tissue with blood vessels and nervules.

Naturally such tooth structure is rather rough. It describes only the elements which make the main contribution to optical properties of tooth.

We studied the propagation of laser radiation (λ=0.628, 0.514, 0.488 nm). In experiments the collimated laser beams with 1mm in diameter were used. The propagation of light in enamel and dentin have been studied throuth the light scattering patterns registered on the frontally and sagitally sawn teeth.

Thus, we discovered that the light flow in tooth can be divided to oriented and diffused components. In enamel the diffused component is well observed, but weak oriented component cannot be neglected. In dentin both components are presented and oriented component of light flow propagates along the dentinal tubules.

Fig.2a,b,c show the traces of oriented light component. The direction of light propagation in the tooth is independent upon the incident angle (1,2,3) of the light on enamel. Every point of the enamel surface as it shown on fig.1 is optically conjugated whith point on the tooth cavity surface. So, tooth is the progective optical system which transports the image from enamel surface to the surface of tooth cavity.

The orientation of light propagation in the hard tooth tissues may be explained by optical waveguide presence. The orientation of these waveguides correlates with tooth hard tissue structures one. These waveguides may be enamel prisms in enamel and dentinal inertubules areas in dentin. Actually, the orientation of these structures correlates with the direction of light wave propagation in the tooth, their density (and refractive index[1]) is higher than in external space and at last their cross-section correlate (for visible light) with the singlemode optical waveguides ones.

To demonstrate the waveguide light propagation effect in the hard tissues of the tooth the following experiment was performed. Plane parallel thin samples from enamel and dentin of four types have been manufactured:
type I   - enamel plates is normal to the enamel prisms
                orientation
type II   - enamel plates is parallel to the enamel prisms
                orientation
type III - dentin plates is normal to the dentinal tubules
                orientation
type IV   - dentin plates is parallel to the dentinal tubules
                orientation

Thickness of plates was 1 mm. The plates of type III being in contact with mira the effect of image transportation from one surface of the plate to another have been observed. Therefore the waveguide character of light propapagation in dentin was demonstrated. In other plates this effect was not observed.

The presence of closely packed collinear waveguides in scattering medium must cause a significant anisotropy of its transparency. The maximum transparency is observed if light propagates along the waveguides.

The anisotropy of transparency of wavaguided-scattering medium may be estimated as follows. Let such medium be consists of closely packed collinear waveguides and scattering particles and has an evenly distributed absorption. Then the transmission of sample for collimated propagating normally to the waveguides laser beam is

$$T\perp = \exp(- k_1 l - k_2 l - \sigma N l) \qquad (1)$$

where: l - thickness of sample
     k_1 - index of sample absorption
     k_2 - index of light scattering on the particles
     σ - effective cross-section of light scattering on the single waveguide oriented normally to the beam
     N - number of waveguides per unit volume

Transmission of sample for laser beam propagating along the waveguide axes approximately is

$$T\| = \exp[- k_1 l - k_2 (1 - \xi) l] \qquad (2)$$

where
$$\xi = \begin{cases} (\vartheta_v / \vartheta_p)^2 & \vartheta_v < \vartheta_p \\ 1 & \vartheta_v > \vartheta_p \end{cases}$$

ϑ_v - aperture angle of the waveguide
ϑ_p - beam angle of forward-scattering on the particle
    In (2) we proposed that scattered on the particles light may be waveguided. The portion of this light is defined by ξ. If $\vartheta_v > \vartheta_p$ the scattered light waveguided totally.

According to (1,2) the anisotropy of transmission is

$$T\|/T\perp = \exp[(k_2 \xi + \sigma N) l] \qquad (3)$$

Values of $T\|$ and $T\perp$ we measured on the four types of samples with 1 mm thickness pointed above. The collimated 1 mm in diameter laser beam propagated normally to the plate surface. The photometer with the same aperture was taken in to contact with the opposite side of the samples. In the table the typical values of $T\|$ and $T\perp$ for $\lambda = 0.63$ μm under the Fresnel losses being taken into account are represented.

162

It is ought to be mentioned that represented values T∥, T⊥ are the average ones for 10 samples. The deviation is less than 30% .

Thus, in the tooth dentin one can observe the great anisotropy of light transmission which may be described by the waveguide-scattering model of the medium. Transmission anisotropy of enamel also may be explained by waveguide effects which are weaker than in dentin.

It should be mentioned too that if incipient caries have taken place the light propagation in tooth changed cardinally. Light is scattered in the porous area of enamel[2] and the pulp surface optically conjugated with the porous area become near totally isolated of light radiation. This 'shadow' effect is of interest to consider with caries pathogenesis.

Human tooth is an unique example of scattering medium. Among the artificially materials as it was shown[3] microporous glass has the same properties. It is a surprise that the light from the enamel surface is concentrated with the waveguides to the tooth cavity. Thus, the hard human tooth tissue is the natural optical phocon transporting the light to the pulp.

So, the main novel properties of the human tooth optics founded out of our investigations are:
- the direction of light propagation in the tooth is independent upon the incident angle of the light on enamel
- in the hard tooth tissues the light propagates along the direction of enamel prisms and dentinal tubules orientation
- every point of enamel surface is optically conjugated with the definite point of the tooth cavity surface
- tooth dentin is able to translate the optical image along the direction of dentinal tubules orientation
- hard tooth tissues have a 'great' anisotropy of light transmission
- the presence of incipient caries on the tooth enamel leads to the darkening of the definite area of the tooth cavity surface and pulp.

We don't know what is the relation between these novel effects and tooth caries resistance, what's the role of high tooth transparency. We know that the greater prevalence of caries on the Earth correlates with the lower insolation level. Our rezults make one think.

REFERENCES

1. B.Houwink, "The Index of Refraction of Dental Enamel Apatite", Brit. dent. J.,vol.135,No.12,pp.472-475,1974.
2. J.Brinkman, J.J.ten Bosch, P.C.F.Borsboom, "Optical Quantitation of Natural Caries in Smooth Surfaces of Extracted Teeth", Caries Res., vol.22,No.5,pp.257-262,1988.
3. G.B.Altshuler et.al., Optika i spektr. (USSR), vol.65,No.5, pp.995-998,1988.

Reprinted from *Applied Optics*, Vol. 31(30), pp. 6535-6546 (October 20, 1992).

Use of polarized light to discriminate short-path photons in a multiply scattering medium

J. M. Schmitt, A. H. Gandjbakhche, and R. F. Bonner

We describe a method for discriminating short- and long-path photons transmitted through a multiply scattering medium that is based on the relationship between the polarization states of the incident and forward-scattered light. Results of Monte Carlo simulations and experiments show that if the scattering anisotropy of the scatterers is sufficiently small, absorbing barriers embedded in optically dense suspensions of polystyrene spheres can be resolved with good contrast by selectively detecting a component of the scattered-light intensity that has preserved its incident circular polarization state.

The principles of operation of a polarization-modulation system capable of measuring small polarization fractions are explained. Using this system we were able to measure polarized light in a depolarized background over 1000 times as large.

Key words: Polarization, imaging, multiple scattering.

1. Introduction

After undergoing a sufficiently large number of collisions, photons propagating in a multiply scattering medium lose all memory of their initial polarization states. The length of the path over which a photon becomes depolarized depends on whether it is initially linearly or circularly polarized, the number of collisions that it experiences, and the scattering anisotropy of the particles with which it interacts. From earlier studies[1,2] it is known that a surprisingly large number of scattering events is required to randomize the polarization of a circularly polarized wave, compared with the number required to randomize its direction of propagation in a medium composed of particles that scatter light anisotropically. In contrast, relatively few scattering events are required to randomize circular polarization in an isotropically scattering medium, or to randomize linear polarization in an anisotropically scattering medium. Proposed applications of polarization effects in multiply scattering media include the size estimation of aerosols by using lidar[3] and the characterization of Mie scatterers in turbid suspensions by using quasielastic light scattering.[1,4]

Results of these earlier studies suggested to us that the dependence of the polarization state of multiply scattered light on the collision histories of individual photons may permit short- and long-path photons emerging from a medium to be discriminated. The discrimination of multiply scattered photons based on total path length has already been demonstrated by using time-of-flight spectrophotometry.[5-7] Recently, crude images of absorbers embedded in multiply scattering media have been made by time-gated imaging systems by employing delayed-coincidence,[8,9] optical heterodyne,[10] and second-harmonic-generation cross-correlation techniques.[11] These imaging systems are expensive, however, and the response time of currently available detectors restricts practical applications to measurements over relatively long optical distances.

In this paper we describe a polarization-encoding method that we have devised for the selective detection of multiply forward-scattered photons transmitted through a medium. Briefly, an optically dense medium is illuminated with a light beam whose polarization alternates rapidly between right and left circular polarization states (or between orthogonal linear polarization states); using a synchronous detection scheme, we measure the difference between the intensities of the oppositely polarized light emerging from the medium. If the single-scattering anisotropy of the scatterers is sufficiently small, this method permits absorbing barriers embedded in the medium

All the authors are with the National Institutes of Health, Bethesda, Maryland 20892. J. M. Schmitt is with the Biomedical Engineering and Instrumentation Program, National Center for Research Resources, Room B2S245, Building 10; A. H. Gandjbakhche is with the Physical Sciences Laboratory, Division of Computer Research and Technology, Room 2007, Building 12A; R. F. Bonner is with the Biomedical Engineering and Instrumentation Program, National Center for Research Resources, Room 3W13, Building 13.

Received 09 July 1991.

that are invisible under transillumination to be resolved with good contrast, because long-path scattered photons are rejected. In Section 2, we first consider some theoretical aspects of the propagation of unpolarized and polarized light beams in a multiply scattering medium. A simple Monte Carlo model is described that permits the propagation of an unpolarized or circularly polarized beam to be evaluated as a function of the volume fraction, total cross sections, and angular scattering functions of spherically symmetric scatterers. We then give results of simulations that compare beam spreading in suspensions of polystyrene spheres of different sizes. In Section 3 the experimental apparatus and the principles on which it is based are explained. A brief description is given of the photoelastic modulation system that we employed to obtain high sensitivity to the polarized component of the predominantly unpolarized scattered light transmitted through a sample. Results of transmission measurements made through suspensions of polystyrene spheres containing embedded absorbers are presented to demonstrate the effects of the single-scattering anisotropy and the concentration of the particles on the rejection of long-path scattered photons. Some implications of this study pertaining to time-of-flight imaging are also discussed.

2. Theory

Most previous analyses of polarized-light propagation in a multiply scattering medium have been made by incorporating the full matrix description of the single-scattering phase function into the transport equation.[12–14] Analytical solutions of the transport equation for polarized light have been obtained for only a few special cases (e.g., a plane wave of infinite extent incident upon a volume of isotropic, scatterers).[15] In this section we introduce a numerical approach based on Monte Carlo simulations for analyzing the diffusion of a circularly polarized light beam in a multiply scattering medium. A simple two-state model is used to describe the polarization transformation that occurs when a photon collides with a scatterer. The simulation method and its underlying principles discussed in this section provide a qualitative basis for understanding the experimental results presented in Section 4. In particular, we use the simulation results to show that the trajectories of the photons that propagate through a dense optical medium and emerge in their original polarization state differ from those that emerge in the opposite polarization state.

A. Effects of Single Scattering on Circular Polarization

Consider a monochromatic plane wave incident upon a spherically symmetric scatterer, as shown in Fig. 1. The polarization state of the incident wave can be

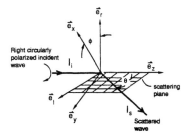

Fig. 1. Geometrical relationship between a circularly polarized plane wave incident on a single scatterer and the scattered wave. The directions of propagation of the incident and scattered waves define the scattering plane, which is aligned parallel to the orientation of one of the orthogonal electric-field vectors that characterize the polarization of the incident wave.

represented by the Stokes vector,[16]

$$\mathbf{I}_i = \begin{bmatrix} I_i \\ Q_i \\ U_i \\ V_i \end{bmatrix}, \qquad (1)$$

where

$$I_i = \langle E_x E_x^* + E_y E_y^* \rangle,$$
$$Q_i = \langle E_x E_x^* - E_y E_y^* \rangle,$$
$$U_i = \langle E_x E_y^* + E_y E_x^* \rangle,$$
$$V_i = \langle E_x E_y^* - E_y E_x^* \rangle.$$

Here E_x and E_y refer to the orthogonal components of the electric field that we take to be directed along the x and y axes, respectively, and $\langle \rangle$ denotes the time average of the bracketed quantity. Upon scattering by a particle, the incident wave generally becomes elliptically polarized. The relationship between the polarization state of the incident and scattered waves at any angle θ in the scattering plane (see Fig. 1) can be described by a 4×4 amplitude-scattering matrix for a spherically symmetric, optically inactive particle,[16]

$$\mathbf{I}_s = \begin{bmatrix} S_{11}(\theta) & S_{12}(\theta) & 0 & 0 \\ S_{12}(\theta) & S_{11}(\theta) & 0 & 0 \\ 0 & 0 & S_{33}(\theta) & S_{44}(\theta) \\ 0 & 0 & -S_{44}(\theta) & S_{33}(\theta) \end{bmatrix} \mathbf{I}_i, \qquad (2)$$

where $\mathbf{I}_s$ is the Stoke's vector representing the polarization state of the scattered wave. The subscript matrix elements are given by

$$S_{11}(\theta) = \tfrac{1}{2}(|S_2|^2 + |S_1|^2),$$

$$S_{12}(\theta) = \tfrac{1}{2}(|S_2|^2 - |S_1|^2),$$

$$S_{33}(\theta) = \tfrac{1}{2}(S_2^* S_1 + S_2 S_1^*),$$

$$S_{34}(\theta) = \tfrac{1}{2}(S_2^* S_1 - S_2 S_1^*),$$

which are functions of the scattering parameters S_1 and S_2 that define the relationship between the transverse components of the scattered and incident electric fields:

$$\begin{bmatrix} E_{xs} \\ E_{ys} \end{bmatrix} = \frac{\exp[ik(r-z)]}{-ikr} \begin{bmatrix} S_2 & 0 \\ 0 & S_1 \end{bmatrix} \begin{bmatrix} E_{xi} \\ E_{yi} \end{bmatrix}.$$

Here r and z are the distances of the observation point from the origin measured along the $\hat{e}_r$ and $\hat{e}_z$ axes (Fig. 1 geometry) and k is the wave number in the medium surrounding the particle. To obtain the scattering matrix elements in Eq. (2), one can expand the matrix parameters S_1 and S_2 as a series and compute them at different scattering angles by upward recursion, according to the Mie theory.[17]

For the special case of a right circularly polarized incident wave, the relationship between the polarization states of the incident and scattered waves is given by

$$\mathbf{I}_s = \begin{bmatrix} S_{11}(\theta) & S_{12}(\theta) & 0 & 0 \\ S_{12}(\theta) & S_{11}(\theta) & 0 & 0 \\ 0 & 0 & S_{33}(\theta) & S_{44}(\theta) \\ 0 & 0 & -S_{44}(\theta) & S_{33}(\theta) \end{bmatrix} \begin{bmatrix} 1 \\ 0 \\ 0 \\ 1 \end{bmatrix} I_0$$

$$= \begin{bmatrix} S_{11}(\theta) \\ S_{12}(\theta) \\ S_{44}(\theta) \\ S_{33}(\theta) \end{bmatrix} I_0. \tag{3}$$

In Eq. (3) I_0 is a scalar value equal to the time-averaged intensity of the incident beam. Note that if none of the amplitude-scattering matrix elements is zero, the scattered wave is elliptically polarized. The circularly polarized component of the scattered intensity can be determined as a function of θ from the light intensities scattered in a particular direction that pass through a pair of circular polarization analyzers,

$$\mathbf{I}_R = \frac{1}{2} \begin{bmatrix} 1 & 0 & 0 & 1 \\ 0 & 0 & 0 & 0 \\ 0 & 0 & 0 & 0 \\ 1 & 0 & 0 & 1 \end{bmatrix} \mathbf{I}_s = \frac{1}{2} \begin{bmatrix} S_{11}(\theta) + S_{33}(\theta) \\ 0 \\ 0 \\ S_{11}(\theta) + S_{33}(\theta) \end{bmatrix} I_0, \tag{4}$$

$$\mathbf{I}_L = \frac{1}{2} \begin{bmatrix} 1 & 0 & 0 & -1 \\ 0 & 0 & 0 & 0 \\ 0 & 0 & 0 & 0 \\ -1 & 0 & 0 & 1 \end{bmatrix} \mathbf{I}_s = \frac{1}{2} \begin{bmatrix} S_{11}(\theta) - S_{33}(\theta) \\ 0 \\ 0 \\ S_{11}(\theta) - S_{33}(\theta) \end{bmatrix} I_0, \tag{5}$$

where $\mathbf{I}_R$ and $\mathbf{I}_L$ are the Stoke's vectors for the light transmitted by the right and left circular polarizers, respectively, which are represented here by their respective 4×4 polarization-transformation matrices.[16] The difference between the first elements of the Stoke's vectors $\mathbf{I}_R$ and $\mathbf{I}_L$, normalized by the total

intensity, gives the fraction of circular polarization of the scattered wave:

$$F_c(\theta) = \frac{1}{2} \frac{S_{11}(\theta) + S_{33}(\theta) - [S_{11}(\theta) - S_{33}(\theta)]}{S_{11}(\theta)}$$

$$= \frac{S_{33}(\theta)}{S_{11}(\theta)}. \tag{6}$$

This quantity varies between $+1$ in the exact forward direction ($\theta = 0°$) and -1 in the exact backward direction ($\theta = 180°$), regardless of particle size; negative values signify a reversal of helicity between the incident and scattered waves.

Figure 2 shows F_c as a function of scattering angle for polystyrene spheres with diameters of 0.22, 0.48, 1.03, and 2.0 μm in water. To generate the curves, we calculated the scattering-matrix elements $S_{11}(\theta)$ and $S_{33}(\theta)$ of the spheres by using Mie theory[16] at a wavelength of 632.8 nm. The spheres were treated as nonabsorbing (relative refractive index = 1.59/1.33 = 1.196). For reference, the value of the average cosine of the scattering angle, g, for each sphere (also calculated by using Mie theory) is shown on each plot. For the spherical scatterers with diameters less than the wavelength of light [see Figs. 2(a) and 2(b)], the dependence of F_c on θ appears to be similar: The helicity of the incident wave tends to be preserved for scattering in the forward hemisphere and reversed for scattering in the backward hemisphere. For the smallest sphere shown (0.22-μm diameter), the Mie-derived curve is approximately the same as that expected for a Rayleigh scatterer [see the dashed curve in Fig. 2(a)], which is described by $F_c = 2 \cos\theta/(1 + \cos^2\theta)$. In the Rayleigh limit $F_c = 0$ at $\theta = 90°$ because the scattered electric-field vector is 100% linearly polarized perpendicular at this angle. As the size of the sphere increases the angle at which the helicity reverses becomes larger, indicating that for scattering at large angles, particles with high g values preserve the polarization of the incident wave better than particles with low g values. Under experimental conditions, the interference structure evident in the curves for the 1.03- and 2.0-μm spheres would normally be smeared by small variations in the diameter of the spheres or by the nonmonochromaticity of the light source.

B. Multiple Scattering—Monte Carlo Simulations

Methods

If the Stokes vector transformations resulting from each scattering event are known, the polarization state of light scattered multiple times by a volume of particles can be determined by using the Monte Carlo method. The simulation technique that we have developed to study the propagation of circularly polarized light in a multiply scattering medium is based on a simple modification to a conventional Monte Carlo method used by others to simulate unpolarized light propagation.[18,19] In our simulations, a photon is considered to be either completely right circularly

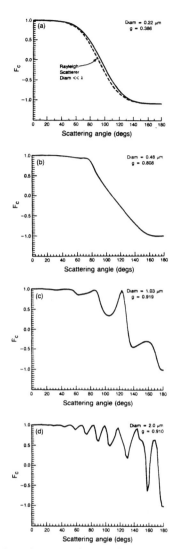

Fig. 2. Circular polarization fraction F_c of light scattered from a polystyrene sphere in water as a function of the polar scattering angle θ: (a) 0.22-μm-diameter sphere (solid curve) and Rayleigh scatterer (dotted curve), (b) 0.48-μm-diameter sphere, (c) 1.03-μm-diameter sphere, and (d) 2.0-μm-diameter sphere. Curves are symmetrical about the direction of propagation of the incident wave (0°); F_c is displayed over only one hemisphere. Curves pertain to right circularly polarized light (633 nm) incident on a nonabsorbing sphere.

polarized (+1 state) or completely left circularly polarized (−1 state). Depending on the angle at which it is scattered, the photon either preserves or reverses its helicity at each collision site. If the polar scattering angle θ exceeds a threshold angle θ_t, then the photon's helicity is flipped; otherwise, its helicity remains the same as before the collision. In our simulations, θ_t was set equal to the angle at which $F_c = 0$, which is determined from the amplitude-scattering matrix of a sphere (see Subsection 2.A). This choice for the threshold angle is somewhat arbitrary; however, the use of more complicated integrated parameters did not seem justified, considering the simplicity of the model and the uncertainty

concerning the shape of the aggregate scattering function of a mixture of polystyrene spheres that had a distribution of sizes. The angle θ was randomly drawn from a cumulative probability-density function, given by

$$\cos(\theta) = \frac{1 + g^2 - (1 - g^2)^2}{2g(1 - g + 2gR)^2}, \quad 0 < \theta < \pi, \quad (7)$$

where g is the average cosine of the scattering angle of the scatterer (also called the asymmetry parameter) and R is a uniformly distributed random variable, $0 \le R \le 1$. This function is based on the Henyey–Greenstein approximation,[20] which has been shown to provide a valid representation of the single-scattering phase functions of anisotropic scatterers in clouds[18] and in biological tissues.[21] The azimuthal angle was selected according to $\phi = 2\pi R'$, where R' is a uniformly distributed random variable between 0 and 1 (distinct from the random variable from which the scattering angle θ was calculated). The length of the path traversed by a photon between collisions, L, was treated as a random variable drawn from an exponential distribution, according to $L = (-1/\Sigma_s)\ln(R'')$; the variable R'' was selected randomly from numbers between 0 and 1, and the macroscopic scattering coefficient (mm^{-1}), Σ_s, was defined as

$$\Sigma_s = \frac{\sigma_s}{v_i} V_f. \quad (8)$$

Here σ_s and v_i are the optical cross section and volume, respectively, of a single particle and V_f is the volume fraction of the particles in the medium. For these simulations the scattering particles were taken to be polystyrene spheres with the same characteristics as those in Subsection 2.A, and the optical cross sections and asymmetry parameters of the spheres were calculated by using Mie theory.

The simulated photons were permitted to migrate within a volume enclosed by completely absorbing walls on all sides. Figure 3 shows the model geometry. Right circularly polarized (state = +1) photons

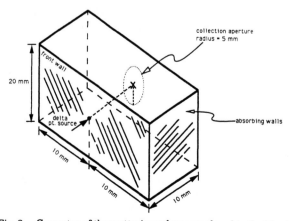

Fig. 3. Geometry of the scattering volume employed in the Monte Carlo simulations.

167

were launched into the medium from the center point of the entrance wall perpendicular to the surface, and the scattered photons that exited the medium through a 5-mm-radius aperture concentric with the beam axis were collected. All emerging photons were recorded, regardless of the angle at which they emerged with respect to the exit wall. The number and the polarization states ($+1$ or -1) of the collected photons were recorded as a function of the radial distance from the center of the aperture at which they exited. The polarized component of the transmitted intensity was determined by subtracting the number of photons that exited in the -1 state from those that exited in the $+1$ state; the total transmitted intensity was taken as the total number of exiting photons, regardless of the polarization state. To obtain enough transmitted photons to generate a single intensity profile having an acceptably low statistical uncertainty, we launched $2 \times 10^5 - 9 \times 10^6$ photons, depending on the optical thickness of the simulated medium.

Results

Results of simulations that were carried out to study the spreading of a collimated (delta) beam of photons in the volume are presented in Figs. 4–7.

Figures 4(a) and 4(b) show normalized intensity profiles in the exit plane for the total and circularly polarized intensities, respectively, as a function of the dimensionless optical thickness τ of a medium composed of 0.22-μm-diameter polystyrene spheres ($g = 0.386$). In this paper we define the optical thickness as $\tau = \Sigma_s d$, where d is the distance between the entrance and exit walls (fixed at 10 mm for these simulations). Comparing the curves in Fig. 4(a) with those in Fig. 4(b), we see that the radial spread of the polarized component is less than or equal to that of the total intensity at all optical thicknesses. As τ increases and consequently the average number of scattering events experienced by a photon increases, the total intensity becomes more diffuse; in contrast, the polarized component remains confined to a narrow zone about the beam-propagation axis, and the width of the radial profile appears to decrease slightly as τ increases. Thus, in a medium in which scattering anisotropy is low, the simulations show that the polarization-maintaining photons tend to migrate along paths closer to the propagation axis than those that undergo a polarization change.

The relationship between the diffusion of the total and helicity-preserving photon flux is markedly different in a medium of large-diameter spheres (diameter of 1.03 μm, $g = 0.919$) that scatter light anisotropically, as shown in Figs. 5(a) and 5(b). In this case, both the total intensity and the polarized component of the total intensity become more diffuse as τ increases; the spreading of the polarized component and total time-averaged intensity is nearly identical at all optical thicknesses. The effect of scattering anisotropy on beam diffusion can be seen more clearly in Fig. 6, which compares the half-width $W_{0.5}$ of the radial intensity distributions in the exit plane (de-

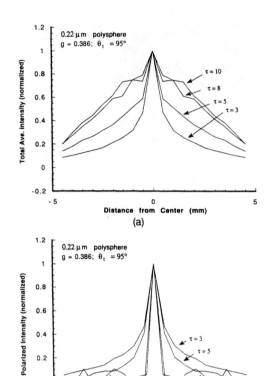

Fig. 4. Radial intensity profiles at the exit aperture of a multiply scattering medium composed of 0.22-μm-diameter polystyrene spheres at different optical thicknesses determined by the Monte Carlo method: (a) total average intensity and (b) circularly polarized component of total intensity. Each curve is shown normalized to the intensity value at the center of the aperture.

fined as the radial distance between the points in the plane of the exit aperture at which the photon flux falls to one half of its maximum value) for the simulated media composed of the small-diameter (0.22-μm) and large-diameter (1.03-μm) spheres. In the medium of 1.03-μm spheres, the spatial spreading of the unpolarized intensity component approaches a limiting value as the optical thickness increases, as seen in earlier simulation studies.[18] Because an impractically long time would have been required to perform the simulations, values of $W_{0.5}$ for the polarized and unpolarized intensities scattered through the medium containing the 0.22-μm spheres are not plotted in Fig. 6 above $\tau = 10$. Presumably, $W_{0.5}$ for the unpolarized intensity also reaches the same limiting value as that for the medium containing the large-diameter spheres.

Figure 7 shows the fraction of circular polarization of the total transmitted intensity calculated over the entire 5-mm aperture as a function of τ. The circular polarization fraction plotted in this figure is defined as the difference between the number of photons that emerged in the $+1$ and -1 states divided by the total number of photons that emerged. From Figs. 6 and 7 we can see that the degree of circular

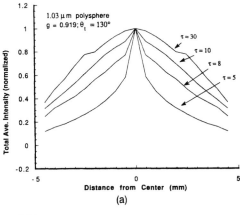

(a)

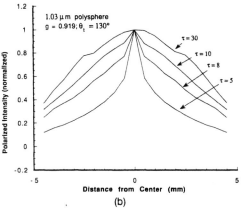

(b)

Fig. 5. Radial intensity profiles at the exit aperture of a multiply scattering medium composed of 1.03-μm-diameter polystyrene spheres at different optical thicknesses determined by the Monte Carlo method: (a) total average intensity and (b) circularly polarized component of total intensity. Each curve is shown normalized to the intensity value at the center of the aperture.

polarization of the total transmitted intensity is much greater for the anisotropically scattering medium than for the nearly isotropically scattering medium at the optical thicknesses that yield equivalent $W_{0.5}$ values.

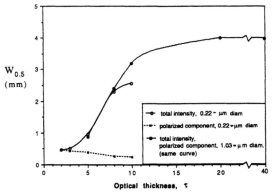

Fig. 6. Beam width at half-maximum determined by the Monte Carlo method at the exit aperture of a multiply scattering medium composed of polystyrene spheres of different sizes. The optical thickness, $\tau = \Sigma_s d$, has not been scaled to reflect the effect of the anisotropy of scattering on the optical density of the simulated medium.

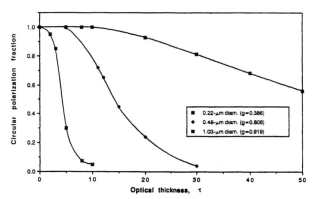

Fig. 7. Fraction of circular polarization of the total flux of photons collected through the aperture of the simulated scattering medium versus optical thickness τ, for three different sizes of scattering particles.

In summary, these simulations show that the trajectories of a subpopulation of photons that maintain their original circular polarization states by means of a sequence of forward-scattered collisions substantially differ from the trajectories of the total population. If the scattering anisotropy of the medium is sufficiently small, the helicity-preserving photons tend to migrate along paths close to the beam-propagation axis. These observations and others based on the simulation results will be discussed in Section 4 in the context of the experimental results.

3. Experimental Methods

In this section we explain the principles of operation of the experimental apparatus that we used to measure polarized light in a background of depolarized light. We then describe a series of experiments in which absorbing barriers embedded in optically dense solutions were imaged by using the apparatus.

A. Apparatus and Polarization Optics

Figure 8 is a schematic of the experimental setup that we used to measure polarized light transmitted through multiply scattering samples. The geometrical arrangement of the polarization optics is shown in detail in Fig. 9. The component designations in the following paragraphs pertain to those in Figs. 8 and 9.

Before impinging upon the photoelastic modulator, PEM (Hinds Model PEM-80 FSA), the laser beam (intensity = I_0) is linearly polarized by polarizer P1. Treating P1 as ideal, we can describe the beam at the output of the polarizer by the Stokes vector[22]

$$\mathbf{S}_1 = I_0 \begin{bmatrix} 1 \\ 1 \\ 0 \\ 0 \end{bmatrix}. \qquad (9)$$

The modulator element introduces a variable retardance δ at its resonant frequency ω, thereby causing the polarization of the beam exiting the modulator to

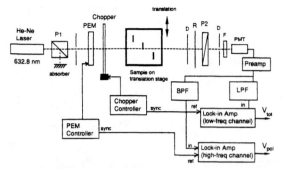

Fig. 8. Schematic of experimental apparatus for measuring unpolarized and polarized light transmitted through multiply scattering samples containing absorbers: P1, polarization-splitting cube; R, $\lambda/4$ retarder (Polaroid); P2, linear polarizer (Polaroid); F, interference filter (633 nm, 10-nm passband); LPF, dc 1-kHz low-pass filter; BPF, 35- to 50-kHz bandpass filter. In some of the experiments (see text in Subsection 3A) R was placed before the PEM in the beam path.

alternate between right and left circular polarization states. At the output of the modulator, the Stokes parameters of the beam are given by:

$$\mathbf{S}_2 = I_0 \begin{bmatrix} 1 & 0 & 0 & 0 \\ 0 & \cos\delta & 0 & -\sin\delta \\ 0 & 0 & 1 & 1 \\ 0 & \sin\delta & 0 & \cos\delta \end{bmatrix} \mathbf{S}_1 = I_0 \begin{bmatrix} 1 \\ \cos\delta \\ 0 \\ \sin\delta \end{bmatrix}. \quad (10)$$

The 4×4 matrix in Eq. (10) describes the transformation produced by a retarder with its fast axis oriented at 45° with respect to that of the linear polarizer P1, as shown in Fig. 9. For the modulator that we employed, the retardation δ varies sinusoidally as a function of time at a frequency $f = \omega/2\pi = 42$ kHz according to

$$\delta = \delta_0 \cos(\omega t), \quad (11)$$

where δ_0 is the peak amplitude of the retardation, which is a variable under the control of the experimenter. By expanding $\cos\delta$ and $\sin\delta$ in terms of Bessel functions,

$$\cos\delta = \cos(\delta_0 \cos\omega t) = J_0(\delta_0) - 2J_2(\delta_0)\cos(2\omega t)$$
$$+ 2J_4(\delta_0)\cos(4\omega t) + \ldots, \quad (12)$$

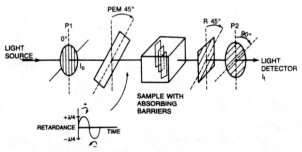

Fig. 9. Drawing showing the orientations of the polarizing elements in the experimental setup of Fig. 8.

$$\sin\delta = \sin(\delta_0 \cos\omega t) = 2J_1(\delta_0)\cos(\omega t)$$
$$- 2J_3(\delta_0)\cos(3\omega t) + \ldots, \quad (13)$$

we can see that the polarization state of the light incident on the sample, represented by $\mathbf{S}_2$, alternates sinusoidally with time between right and left circularly polarized states at the fundamental frequency ω and its odd harmonics [see Eq. (13)].

If no sample is present, the Stokes parameters of the light impinging on the detector can be found simply by forming the product of the matrices that describe the transformations by the quarter-wave retarder R and the linear polarizer P2, which together function as a circular polarization analyzer:

$$\mathbf{S}_3 = \begin{bmatrix} 1 & -1 & 0 & 0 \\ -1 & 1 & 0 & 0 \\ 0 & 0 & 0 & 0 \\ 0 & 0 & 0 & 0 \end{bmatrix} \begin{bmatrix} 1 & 0 & 0 & 0 \\ 0 & 0 & 0 & -1 \\ 0 & 0 & 1 & 0 \\ 0 & 1 & 0 & 0 \end{bmatrix} \mathbf{S}_2$$

$$= \frac{1}{2} \begin{bmatrix} 1 + \sin\delta \\ -(1 + \sin\delta) \\ 0 \\ 0 \end{bmatrix} I_0. \quad (14)$$

The photomultiplier tube (PMT), which we assume to be insensitive to polarization, produces a signal proportional to the intensity I_t, which equals the magnitude of the first element of $\mathbf{S}_3$ from Eq. (14):

$$I_t = \frac{I_0}{2}(1 + \sin\delta)$$

$$= \frac{I_0}{2}(1 + 2J_1(\delta_0)\cos(\omega t) - 2J_3(\delta_0)\cos(3\omega t) + \ldots)$$

$$(15)$$

Here $\sin\delta$ has been replaced with its Bessel function expansion from Eq. (13).

A voltage proportional to the magnitude of the ac component of I_t (labeled V_{pol} in Fig. 8) at the primary frequency was produced by a lock-in amplifier preceded by a filter having a narrow passband centered on 42 kHz. To simplify analysis, we set the magnitude of the peak retardance δ_0 introduced by the PEM equal to 2.404 rad ($\approx 138°$), where $J_0(\delta_0) = 0$; at this retardance value the time average of $\cos\delta$ at the fundamental frequency equals zero [see Eq. (12)]. The amplitude of V_{pol} is proportional to the difference between the right and left circularly polarized components of the scattered intensity detected by the PMT. A voltage proportional to the dc component of I_t (labeled V_{tot} in Fig. 8) was obtained by chopping the beam at 700 Hz and synchronously detecting a signal at the output of the photomultiplier at this frequency. The voltage V_{tot} was used to measure the total (polarized plus unpolarized) time-averaged light intensity detected by the PMT.

In one of our experiments, we used this same

apparatus to irradiate samples with light whose polarization varied sinusoidally between two perpendicular linear polarization states. This irradiation was accomplished by making a simple modification to the setup shown in Fig. 8: The quarter-wave retarder was placed between polarizer P1 and the modulator instead of between the sample and polarizer P2. With this modification, V_{pol} becomes a measure of the difference between the orthogonally oriented linearly polarized components of the scattered intensity detected by the PMT.

With no sample present, the polarization of the received light is nearly 100% modulated, yielding $V_{pol} \approx V_{tot}$. By placing a multiply scattering sample between the modulator and the analyzer, we cause the depolarization of the scattered light, thus reducing V_{pol} relative to V_{tot}. For optically thick samples, $V_{pol} \ll V_{tot}$. In our experiments, the ratio V_{pol}/V_{tot} provided us with a measure of the polarization fraction of the multiply scattered light, referred to as "F" in later paragraphs.

In all experiments, a pair of iris diaphragms (each labeled D in Fig. 8) was employed to permit only forward-scattered light transmitted through the back wall of the sample cuvette within a solid angle of $\sim 5°$ to strike the PMT. We arranged the detection optics in this way to reduce the effect of linearly polarized light on the V_{pol} signal. The probability of converting a circularly polarized wave scattered by a symmetrical particle located near the optical axis to a linearly polarized wave having a given angle of orientation is equal to the probability of converting it to a linearly polarized wave having the orthogonal orientation. The small-aperture azimuthally symmetric detector that we employed in our experiments captures, on average, almost equal numbers of photons in one or the other of the two orthogonal linear polarization states. Consequently, the effects of circular-to-linear scattering transformations on the measurements should be almost canceled, and the ratio V_{pol}/V_{tot} measured by the apparatus should provide a good measure of the fraction of the total intensity of circularly polarized light transmitted through the sample that maintains its original helicity. As the density of scatterers in the samples increases, the incident intensity that maintains its original polarization state becomes an increasingly smaller fraction of the background-depolarized intensity; hence synchronous detection is essential to obtain an adequate signal-to-noise ratio in optically thick samples.

B. Scattering Samples

The multiply scattering samples consisted of suspensions of polystyrene spheres (PolySciences, Inc.) in distilled water, in which three black plastic absorbing barriers were embedded. Figure 10 shows the construction and dimensions of the sample container and absorbing barriers. All surfaces of the glass container, except the entrance and exit surfaces, were coated with black tape to reduce internal reflections. The container was filled with a mixture containing

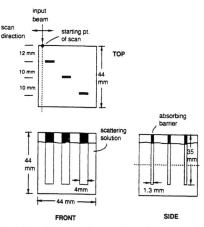

Fig. 10. Drawing of the sample container showing the positions of the embedded absorbing strips. The container walls were made of optical-quality glass and the absorbers were constructed from black plastic.

polystyrene spheres with mean diameters of 0.1, 0.22, or 1.03 μm at a predetermined volume concentration. The macroscopic scattering coefficient of each mixture was calculated according to Eq. (8), using Mie theory to calculate σ_s, as in the Monte Carlo simulations described in Subsection 2.B.

C. Measurement Procedure

The sample container was positioned relative to the modulated beam and detector as shown in Fig. 8. Each series of transmission measurements was made by manually translating the sample containing the fixed absorbing barriers in 1 mm steps, while recording the amplitude of the total intensity (V_{tot}) and polarization (V_{pol}) voltages at each position. The starting point and direction of the scan is marked on the drawing of the sample container in Fig. 10. The voltages were acquired simultaneously and averaged for a period of 20 s by a computer-controlled data-acquisition system. A complete scan consisted of 35 measurements made at points across the width of the container. The first scan in a series was made on a sample at its highest volume concentration, and subsequent scans were made after the sample was diluted with water.

4. Experimental Results

Figures 11(a), 11(b), and 11(c) show the scan profiles that we measured for the mixtures containing polystyrene spheres with diameters of 0.1, 0.22, and 1.03 μm, respectively. Results are shown for three optical thicknesses. For ease of comparison, the total intensity signal (V_{tot}) and circular polarization (V_{pol}) signals are shown superimposed and normalized to their values at a single point in the scan. Also shown on each scan is the fraction of polarization, F, measured over the entire aperture of the detector at the scan position to which all values were normalized.

For the optically dense mixtures containing the 0.1-μm-diameter and 0.22-μm-diameter spheres, it is evident that the resolving power of the circularly

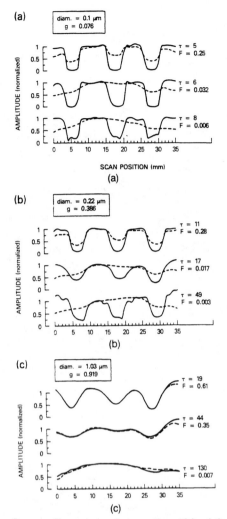

(a)

diam. = 0.1 μm
g = 0.076

τ = 5
F = 0.25

τ = 6
F = 0.032

τ = 8
F = 0.006

SCAN POSITION (mm)

(a)

(b)

diam. = 0.22 μm
g = 0.386

τ = 11
F = 0.28

τ = 17
F = 0.017

τ = 49
F = 0.003

(b)

(c)

diam. = 1.03 μm
g = 0.919

τ = 19
F = 0.61

τ = 44
F = 0.35

τ = 130
F = 0.007

(c)

Fig. 11. Scan profiles measured across the width of the sample container, for a suspension of (a) 0.1-μm-diameter spheres, (b) 0.22-μm-diameter spheres, and (c) 1.03-μm-diameter spheres. To generate the profiles, we recorded the voltages V_{pol} (solid curves) and V_{tot} (dashed curves) each time the sample was translated 1 mm; an interpolating curve was drawn through the measured points. In this series of experiments V_{pol} was a measure of the circularly polarized fraction of the total intensity. Each curve is shown normalized to the voltage measured at the 12-mm scan position (midway between two of the absorbing strips). The fraction of polarization, $F = V_{pol}/V_{tot}$, determined at this point is displayed beside each profile.

polarized intensity component is markedly greater than that of the total intensity [see Figs. 11(a) and 11(b)]. At the highest optical thickness shown for the sample containing the 0.1-μm-diameter spheres ($τ = 8$, $g = 0.076$), none of the absorbing barriers—not even those closest to the front and back walls of the sample container—is discernible from the V_{tot} scan profiles. In contrast, the barriers are seen clearly in the V_{pol} scan profile; at this optical thickness, a reduction of approximately a factor of 5 in the amplitude of V_{pol} was produced by a scan across an absorbing barrier.

Consistent with the simulation results [see Fig.

4(b) and Fig. 6], the radial spread of the polarized intensity component in the samples containing the 0.1-μm-diameter sphere remained small compared with the width of the laser beam (measured Gaussian half-width = 0.4 mm), regardless of the optical thickness. Therefore in this case the beam width limited the resolution of barriers. In contrast, the radial spread of the total intensity was limited by the width of the laser beam only at very low optical thicknesses (below approximately $τ = 4$) and increased rapidly with the volume fraction of the spheres until a limiting value was reached. These observations agree qualitatively with the simulation results for the small-diameter spheres shown in Fig. 4(a). Note also that at the higher optical densities, the amplitude of V_{tot} decreased at the ends of the scan as a result of absorption by the side walls of the sample container, but the amplitude of V_{pol} did not. In other experiments in which measurements were performed in a sample container with partially reflecting sides (results not shown), the baseline of the V_{tot} increased close to the side walls, but again the V_{pol} scans were unaffected.

Similar results were obtained for the suspensions containing the 0.22-μm-diameter spheres, but the contrast and sharpness of the edges of the absorbing barriers were somewhat degraded. As shown by the dotted-curve scans in Fig. 11(b), the resolution of the barriers in the average-intensity scan rapidly deteriorated above $τ = 11$. According to the simulation results for scatterers of this size [Figs. 4(a) and 6], the transition to diffuse scattering is expected to occur within a somewhat lower range of optical thicknesses ($5 < τ < 10$). The half-width of radial spread of the average intensity measured at the exit of the sample was found to reach a limiting value of 4 mm for $τ \geq 17$. As shown by the V_{tot} curves in Fig. 11(b) that were measured on the two most dense samples, this radial spread is sufficient to obscure the barriers almost completely.

In accordance with observations made earlier in the paper that were based on the simulation results (Section 2), the improvement in the resolution of the absorbers in these nearly isotropically scattering media was found to be inversely related to the polarization fraction. Although most of the polarization-maintaining photons captured by the detector travelled along trajectories close to the propagation axis, these photons constituted only a small fraction of the total number emerging from the optically dense samples. For example, at the highest optical thickness at which our measurements were made on the sample containing the 0.22-μm-diameter spheres ($τ = 49$), the polarization fraction was only ~0.3% [see Fig. 11(b)]; therefore, scatter reduction was obtained at the expense of the amplitude of the V_{pol} signal.

The scan profiles obtained from anisotropically scattering samples (1.03-μm-diameter spheres, $g = 0.919$) are shown in Fig. 11(c). In this case, the selection of the circular polarization-maintaining photons did not significantly improve visualization of the absorbers; the measured V_{tot} and V_{pol} scan profiles are nearly the same. The radial spread of the average and polarized intensities measured at the exit of the sample as a function of optical thickness behaved as expected based on the simulated results: At very low optical thicknesses ($\tau < 3$) the point-spread function was determined by the beam diameter, and as τ was increased both the polarized and unpolarized intensity distributions broadened. When τ exceeded ~ 7, the half-width of the distributions increased rapidly, reaching a limiting value of ~ 4 mm. The range of optical thicknesses over which the scattering became diffuse was predicted accurately by the Monte Carlo simulations (see Fig. 6). As we conjectured earlier (Subsection 2.B), the limiting half-width of the radial distributions for the media containing the 0.22-μm and 1.03-μm spheres were found to be the same (4 mm).

These data support our assertion, based on the simulation results in Subsection 2.B, that a large fraction of photons that stray off the beam-propagation axis after many collisions with anisotropically scattering particles retain their original polarization state. Thus short- and long-path forward-scattered photons cannot be effectively differentiated on the basis of their circular polarization states.

A short-path and a long-path photon can be differentiated to some extent, however, on the basis of whether it maintains its original linear polarization state, as shown by the scan profiles in Fig. 12. To perform these scans, we modified the experimental setup to make V_{pol} proportional to the difference between the orthogonally oriented linearly polarized components of the scattered intensity, as we discussed in Subsection 3.A. The resolution of the absorbing barriers was found to be improved at all optical thicknesses measured, but a progressive blurring and contrast degradation is evident at the highest optical thicknesses. Note that the scan profiles in Fig. 12 are asymmetrical because the absorbers closest to the front wall of the sample container caused a greater reduction in V_{tot} than the absorber located at the same distance from the back wall. At the highest optical thickness ($\tau = 103$), the absorbing barrier closest to the exit wall is discernible neither in the V_{pol} profile nor in the V_{tot} profile. The improved scatter rejection evident in the V_{pol} scan profiles in Fig. 12 compared with those in Fig. 11(c) can be explained by the fact that fewer off-axis scattering events are required to randomize linear polarization than are required to randomize circular polarization, because linear polarization is altered by azimuthal rotations resulting from scattering collisions but circular polarization is not.[23] Therefore the effective path length required to randomize the polarization of a linearly polarized photon is shorter than that of a circularly polarized photon.

5. Discussion

In many optical remote-sensing applications, multiple scattering results in a loss of information because of the randomization of the direction and polarization of the incident light wave. We have shown in this study that information regarding the direction of the propagation of a multiply scattered light beam can be recovered by selectively detecting a component of the scattered photon flux that has maintained its initial polarization state. Using the relatively inexpensive apparatus described in this paper, we have been able to measure polarization fractions as small as 1×10^{-3} at equivalent isotropic optical thicknesses as large as 10 in a nonabsorbing medium. (Over this optical distance, an average of ~ 17 collisions per photon in a volume of nearly isotropically scattering particles, $g = 0.4$, or ~ 100 collisions per photon in a volume of highly anisotropically scattering particles, $g = 0.9$, would be expected to occur.) To obtain an acceptable signal-to-noise ratio for measurements at greater optical distances, we would require gated photon counting and integration. In our research, we have been concerned with measurements on biological tissues in which the mean-free path for photons is typically 10–100 μm in the 600- to 1300-nm-wavelength range.[24] Our results indicate that circularly polarized light should be measurable in tissues 1–10 mm thick by using the experimental setup described in this paper. Therefore, as currently implemented, our polarization-detection method is only applicable to thin-tissue sections.

The ability to selectively detect polarized light transmitted through or re-emitted from a multiply scattering medium by using a relatively inexpensive apparatus provides the basis for several potential applications. The measurement of the optical activity of chemical compounds, such as glucose, in skin tissue or whole blood is one possible application. In addition, our polarization-encoding scheme should be useful for reducing the inaccuracy introduced by multiple scattering in the measurement of the single-scattering cross section of thin-tissue slices. Unfortunately, because scattering in most tissues is highly anisotropic (typically, $0.75 \leq g \leq 0.9$),[24] we expect

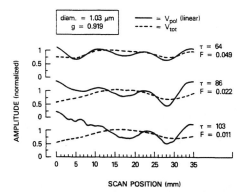

Fig. 12. Scan profiles measured across the width of the sample container containing a suspension of 1.03-μm-diameter spheres. The scan profiles shown here were made in the same way as those in Fig. 11, except in this series of experiments V_{pol} was a measure of the linearly polarized fraction of the total intensity.

that, based on the experimental results presented in Section 4, short-path photon flux cannot be discriminated effectively by using circularly polarized incident light and that discrimination can only be accomplished to a limited extent by using linearly polarized incident light.

The strong dependence of spatial resolution on scattering anisotropy that was found in the imaging experiments reported in this paper suggests that scattering anisotropy may also play an important role in quasiballistic time-resolved imaging. Using time-resolved imaging systems employing collimated sources and detectors arranged in a coaxial configuration, other investigators have demonstrated that spatial resolution can be improved by gating early-arriving photons.[8] The effect of scattering anisotropy on resolution, however, has not been studied. Our results suggest that a substantial fraction of the photons traversing an optically thin medium of anisotropic scatterers can experience a sequence of low-angle (polarization-maintaining) scattering events that cause them to stray off axis during part of their trajectories before being captured by a collimated detector. This experience results in the degradation of the spatial resolution. In contrast, in a medium having the same effective optical thickness but consisting of nearly isotropic scatterers ($0 < g < 0.4$), the loss of spatial resolution caused by off-axis scattering is much reduced. These observations suggest that the spatial resolution of a time-of-flight imaging system designed to discriminate quasiballistic photons may depend on the scattering function of the individual particles comprising the medium. This theory is substantiated by results of an earlier study in which pulse broadening was measured in suspensions of particles of different sizes.[25]

In studies of light transmission through nearly isotropically scattering media, such as noctilucent clouds and some types of smog, the methods demonstrated in this paper may be useful for locating absorbing gases or other substances. Given a sufficiently accurate model, we see that the measurement of the asymmetry parameter of a volume of random scatterers on the basis of the radial spread of a circularly polarized light beam versus that of an unpolarized beam may be feasible, provided that the diameter of the scatterers is smaller than the light wavelength. Although not addressed in this study, the discrimination or short- and long-path photons backscattered from an optically dense media should also be possible by using the experimental setup described in Section 2. With the apparatus set up to measure circular polarization in the backscattering mode, the V_{pol} signal would respond to the flux of photons that have undergone a reversal in helicity, thereby discriminating against long-path forward-scattered photons. This arrangement would be most appropriate for sensing the properties of dense concentrations of anisotropic scatterers.

In future studies, we plan to investigate the propagation of linearly polarized photons in a multiply scattering medium more thoroughly. Of considerable interest is the effect of multiple scattering by a mixture of optically active and optically inactive particles. For these studies a more elaborate simulation method than the approximate method that we employed in this paper—perhaps one incorporating the complete 4×4 Stokes vector transformation matrix of the individual scatterers—will be required.

References

1. F. C. MacKintosh, J. X. Zhu, D. J. Pine, and D. A. Weitz, "Polarization memory of multiply scattered light," Phys. Rev. B **40**, 9342–9345 (1989).
2. K. M. Yoo and R. R. Alfano, "Time-resolved depolarization of multiple backscattered light from random media," Phys. Lett. A **142**, 531–536 (1989).
3. M. J. McCormick, "Particle-size-distribution retrieval from backscattered polarized radiation measurements: a proposed method," J. Opt. Soc. Am. A **7**, 1811–1816 (1990).
4. D. J. Pine, D. A. Weitz, J. X. Zhu, and E. Herbolzheimer, "Diffusing-wave spectroscopy: dynamic light scattering in the multiple scattering limit," J. Phys. (Paris) **51**, 2101–2127 (1990).
5. K. Shimuzu, A. Ishimaru, L. Reynolds, and A. P. Bruckner, "Backscattering of a picosecond pulse from densely distributed scatterers," Appl. Opt. **18**, 3484–3488 (1979).
6. D. T. Delpy, M. Cope, P. Van der Zee, S. Arridge, S. Wray, and J. Wyatt, "Estimation of optical pathlength through tissue from direct time of flight measurement," Phys. Med. Biol. **33**, 1433–1442 (1988).
7. B. Chance, J. Leigh, H. Miyake, D. Smith, S. Nioka, R. Greenfield, M. Finlander, K. Kaufmann, W. Levy, M. Young, P. Cohen, H. Yoshioka, and R. Boretsky, "Comparison of time-resolved and -unresolved measurements of deoxyhemoglobin in brain," Proc. Natl. Acad. Sci. U.S.A. **85**, 4971–4975 (1988).
8. J. C. Hebden, R. A. Kruger, and K. S. Wong, "Time-resolved imaging through a highly scattering medium," Appl. Opt. **30**, 788–794 (1991).
9. S. Andersson-Engels, R. Berg, and S. Svanberg, "Time-resolved transillumination for medical diagnostics," Opt. Lett. **15**, 1179–1181 (1990).
10. M. Toida, M. Kondo, T. Ichimura, and H. Inaba, "Two-dimensional coherent detection imaging in multiple scattering media based on the directional resolution capability of the optical heterodyne method," Appl. Phys. B **52**, 391–394 (1991).
11. K. M. Yoo, Q. R. Xing, and R. R. Alfano, "Imaging objects hidden in highly scattering media using femtosecond second-harmonic-generation cross-correlation time gating," Opt. Lett. **16**, 1019–1021 (1991).
12. C. E. Siewert, "On the equation of transfer relevant to the scattering of polarized light," Astrophys. J. **245**, 1080–1086 (1981).
13. I. Kuscer and M. Ribaric, "Matrix formalism in the theory of diffusion of light," Opt. Acta **6**, 42–51 (1959).
14. R. L. T. Cheung and A. Ishimaru, "Transmission, backscattering, and depolarization of waves in randomly distributed spherical particles," Appl. Opt. **21**, 3792–3798 (1982).
15. S. Chandresekhar, *Radiative Transfer* (Oxford U. Press, New York, 1950).
16. C. F. Bohren and D. R. Huffman, *Absorption and Scattering of Light by Small Particles* (Wiley, New York, 1983), pp. 46–53.
17. C. F. Bohren and D. R. Huffman, *Absorption and Scattering of Light by Small Particles* (Wiley, New York, 1983), pp. 82–129.
18. E. A. Bucher, "Computer simulation of light pulse propagation for communicating through thick clouds," Appl. Opt. **12**, 2391–2400 (1973).

19. S. T. Flock, M. S. Patterson, B. C. Wilson, and D. R. Wyman, "Monte Carlo modeling of light propagation in highly scattering tissues—I: model predictions and comparison with diffusion theory," IEEE Trans. Biomed. Eng. **36,** 1162–1167 (1989).

20. L. Henyey and J. Greenstein, "Diffuse radiation in the galaxy," Astrophys. J. **93,** 70–83 (1941).

21. S. T. Flock, B. C. Wilson, and M. S. Patterson, "Total attenuation coefficients and scattering phase functions of tissues and phantom materials at 633 nm," Med. Phys. **14,** 835–841 (1987).

22. W. A. Shurcliff, *Polarized Light* (Harvard U. Press, Cambridge, Mass., 1962).

23. F. C. MacKintosh and S. John, "Diffusing-wave spectroscopy and multiple scattering of light in correlated random media," Phys. Rev. B **40,** 2383–2406 (1989).

24. W. F. Cheong, S. A. Prahl, and A. J. Welsh, "A review of the optical properties of biological tissues," IEEE J. Quantum Electron. **26,** 2166–2185 (1990).

25. Y. Kuga, A. Ishimaru, and A. Bruckner, "Experiments on picosecond pulse propagation in a diffuse medium," J. Opt. Soc. Am. **73,** 1812–1815 (1983).

Reprinted with permission from *Physics in Medicine and Biology,* Vol. 33(12), pp. 1433-1442 (1988). ©1988 IOP Publishing Ltd.

Estimation of optical pathlength through tissue from direct time of flight measurement

D T Delpy, M Cope, P van der Zee, S Arridge, Susan Wray† and J Wyatt‡

Departments of Medical Physics, †Physiology and ‡Paediatrics, University College London, 1st Floor, Shropshire House, 11-20 Capper Street, London WC1E 6JA, UK

Received 20 May 1988, in final form 22 July 1988

Abstract. Quantitation of near infrared spectroscopic data in a scattering medium such as tissue requires knowledge of the optical pathlength in the medium. This can now be estimated directly from the time of flight of picosecond length light pulses. Monte Carlo modelling of light pulses in tissue has shown that the mean value of the time dispersed light pulse correlates with the pathlength used in quantitative spectroscopic calculations. This result has been verified in a phantom material. Time of flight measurements of pathlength across the rat head give a pathlength of 5.3 ± 0.3 times the head diameter.

1. Introduction

Changes in cerebral oxygenation and metabolism have for a long time been monitored by optical techniques. Such measurements rely upon oxygen dependent absorption changes that occur in tissue caused by natural chromophores, e.g. haemoglobin in the red blood cell and cytochromes a, b, and c in the cell mitochondrial membrane. Because of the intense absorption of visible light by these chromophores, optical monitoring has only been possible using reflected light from the exposed cerebral cortex. However, in 1977 Jöbsis showed that by using near infrared light (NIR), tissue absorption fell sufficiently for transillumination of the intact head of the cat to be possible. In this spectral region (700-1300 nm), the oxygen dependent absorption of haemoglobin is still observable, together with an oxygenation dependent absorption arising from cytochrome aa_3. By measuring absorption changes at several wavelengths it has been possible to monitor continuously the cerebral oxygenation state in many animals (Piantadosi *et al* 1986, Hazeki *et al* 1987) and by operating in reflection mode, on the human adult (Fox *et al* 1985, Ferrari *et al* 1986a) and newborn infant (Brazy *et al* 1985, Ferrari *et al* 1986b). Technical developments of the instrumentation have now made it possible to measure absorption changes across a total of 10 optical densities (OD) equivalent to 8-9 cm of brain tissue (Cope and Delpy 1988). With such instruments it is possible to transilluminate the head of most preterm infants (Wyatt *et al* 1986).

It has previously been demonstrated (Cope *et al* 1988) that when transilluminating a thick section of a highly scattering medium, it is still possible to apply a simple Beer–Lambert calculation to convert the measured variations in attenuation to changes in the absolute concentration of chromophore. However, the optical pathlength used in the calculation must be increased to take into account the effects of multiple scattering. Tissue is an effective multiple scatterer of light, and the pathlength of the light in the tissue is normally unknown. For this reason, most published observations have been of a qualitative nature. When measuring in transillumination mode, it is, however, possible to know the minimum optical pathlength (i.e. the inter-optode spacing), and hence place an upper limit on the calculated chromophore concentrations. In studies in human neonates, it has been shown that several NIR monitored indices of cerebral oxygen can be quantitated by using additional independently monitored physiological data (Wyatt *et al* 1986, Delpy *et al* 1987, Cope *et al* 1988). Further, in recent studies in rats, the optical pathlength has been estimated by monitoring the height of the water absorption peak at 975 nm and assuming a value for the average water content of brain tissue (Wray *et al* 1988). Calculations based upon this method indicate an average optical pathlength across the rat head that is approximately 4.3 times the inter-optode spacing.

The developments of the synchronously pumped dye laser and the synchroscan streak camera now make possible the generation of intense picosecond duration pulses of light and their detection at very low intensity with approximately 10 picosecond resolution. Using this equipment the time of flight and temporal dispersion of light pulses through a multiple scattering medium can be studied. The transit times (t) of the photons can be converted into distance travelled through the medium (d) using the formula

$$d = \frac{ct}{n} \tag{1}$$

where n is the refractive index of the medium and c the velocity of light in a vacuum. For water ($n = 1.33$) the conversion factor is $0.225\ \text{mm ps}^{-1}$ and for tissue ($n = 1.40$, see discussion) the conversion factor is $0.214\ \text{mm ps}^{-1}$. Multiple scattering effects are studied by observing the extra distance travelled by the photons compared with the physical distance across the medium. The 10 ps time resolution corresponds to a spatial resolution of 2.14 mm in the tissue.

2. Modelling light transport in tissue

The measured attenuation of light across the head is a complex function of detector and transmitter geometry, head shape and the scattering and absorption properties of the tissues. Let us assume that the attenuation, in optical density, can be expressed as a modified Beer–Lambert equation

$$\text{Attenuation(OD)} = -\log(I/I_0) = B\mu_a d_p + G \tag{2}$$

where I is the transmitted intensity, I_0 the input light intensity, B is a pathlength factor dependent upon the absorption and scattering coefficients μ_a and μ_s and the scattering phase function; G is an unknown geometry dependent factor, and d_p is the inter-optode distance between source and detector, i.e. the smallest value possible in equation (1).

The validity of equation (2) will depend on how much B varies with the attenuation and scattering coefficients and phase function. It is this question that is addressed in this paper.

To investigate the relationship between attenuation and the transit time of light pulses through tissue, a Monte Carlo model of light transport in tissue has been used (van der Zee and Delpy 1987). This model incorporates an experimentally measured scattering phase function for *in vitro* rat brain measured at 783 nm (van der Zee and

Delpy 1988). The broadening of a spatial delta function input beam of light as it passes through a scattering medium is normally described by the point spread function (PSF). In a similar manner the temporal distribution of light intensity resulting from a spatial and temporal delta function input as it passes through a scattering medium may be described by the temporal point spread function (TPSF). This TPSF will vary with exit position. The TPSF referred to in this paper is integrated over the exit surface area and all exit angles. We implicitly assume in the following that this function is radially symmetric. It should be noted that the origin of the time axis occurs as the light pulse first enters the scattering medium. In this study, the integrated TPSF was modelled for a tissue slab of 1 cm thickness. In the literature, absorption coefficients are usually quoted to base 10 because of the relation to optical density, whilst scattering coefficients are usually to base e, because of their probabilistic definition. Although potentially confusing this is the convention adopted here. Absorption coefficients (base 10) of 0.456, 0.334, 0.263, 0.217, 0.0867 and 0.0434 cm^{-1} and scattering coefficients (base e) of 100, 80, 60, 40 and 20 cm^{-1} were simulated, encompassing the values quoted in the literature for brain tissue (Svaasand and Ellinsen 1983).

Figure 1 shows the calculated attenuation in OD as a function of absorption coefficient for several different scattering coefficients. The simulation is for a delta function input beam at normal incidence. Transmitted light is integrated over the exit surface. The attenuation can be seen to be a non-linear function of absorption, the greatest deviation from linearity occurring at low absorption and high scattering values. This and the normally unknown geometry factor preclude the use of a simple pathlength factor B for a given scattering coefficient. However, in most *in vivo* spectroscopy measurements, one is interested in relating a *change* in a measured attenuation to a *change* in absorption. For this purpose the slope, δOD$/\delta\mu_a$ over the chosen range of scattering and absorption coefficients is required. This parameter we will call the differential pathlength factor, or DPF.

Figure 2 illustrates the modelled integrated TPSFs for a scattering coefficient of 60 cm^{-1} and absorption coefficients of 0.0434, 0.217 and 0.456 cm^{-1}, respectively. It

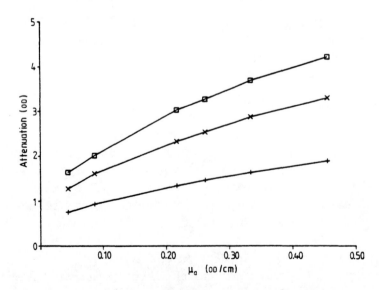

Figure 1. Monte Carlo simulation of attenuation against absorption for light transmitted through a 1 cm slab of brain tissue. Scattering coefficients: +, 20 cm^{-1}; ×, 60 cm^{-1}; □, 100 cm^{-1}.

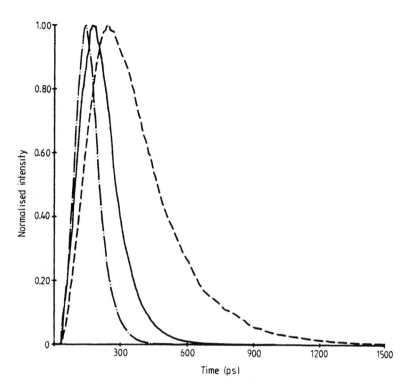

Figure 2. Monte Carlo simulation of the integrated time point spread functions (TPSF) resulting from a normally incident delta function input pulse transmitted through a 1 cm slab of brain tissue. The simulation is for a scattering coefficient of 60 cm^{-1} and absorption coefficients of: - - -, 0.0434 cm^{-1}; ——, 0.217 cm^{-1}; — · —, 0.456 cm^{-1}.

can be seen that there is considerable time dispersion of the pulse and hence a variation in the pathlength of the detected light. The question therefore arises as to whether some parameter, derived from the integrated TPSF, can be found to correlate with the DPF. Using the Monte Carlo data, the change in transmitted intensity (in optical densities) corresponding to known changes in absorption coefficient has been calculated, and its correlation with the integrated TPSF examined. The integrated TPSF for each data point was analysed and the pathlengths equivalent to the mean of the profile and the 5%, 25%, 50%, 75% and 95% of cumulative intensity calculated. Both the mean and the 50th percentile were found to correlate well with the DPF. The mean was chosen to make it easier in the future to include higher moments in a more sophisticated analysis of the TPSF. The result for the mean is illustrated in figure 3(a).

3. Model verification

The model predictions were verified on a tissue phantom composed of polystyrene-latex particles in water and an infrared absorbing dye using the experimental system shown in figure 4. A mode locked krypton ion laser (Coherent K3000) produces ~100 ps pulses at a repetition rate of 76 MHz. These were used both to trigger the synchroscan streak camera (Hamamatsu C1587, M1955), and to pump the ultrafast dye laser (Coherent CR701-3 with Oxazine 750 dye). The output pulses from the dye laser had an autocorrelation width of 6 ps. A beam splitter and monomode optical fibre took a time reference to the edge of the streak camera entry slit, with a variable time delay. The main beam was adjusted to enter the centre of the streak camera entry

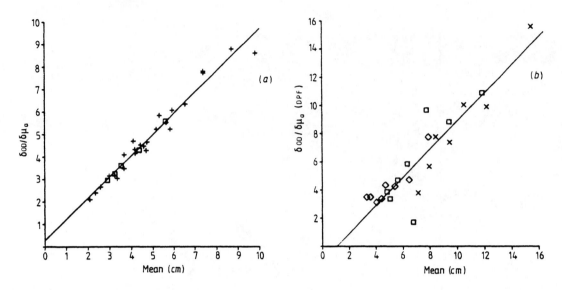

Figure 3. A comparison of modelled and measured phantom results. (*a*) The mean of the integrated TPSFs is expressed as an equivalent distance in centimetres using equation (1) and a refractive index of 1.4. +, data generated with the brain scattering phase function for $\mu_s = 20, 40, 60, 80, 100$ cm^{-1} and $\mu_a = 0.0434$, 0.0867, 0.217, 0.263, 0.334, 0.456 cm^{-1}. The full curve is the regression line, with a slope of 0.94 ± 0.04 and an intercept of 0.28 ± 0.20. □, data generated with the scattering phase function of the phantom material for a scattering coefficient of 60 cm^{-1} and absorption coefficients of 0.043, 0.0867, 0.217, 0.263, 0.334, 0.456 cm^{-1}. (*b*) The DPF plotted against the mean of the integrated TPSF for the phantom. The original mixture ($\times$) contained 2.5% by volume of 1.0 μm diameter polystyrene latex spheres, and 6.7% by volume of 0.05 μm diameter particles, suspended in water. The other concentrations were obtained by 50% (□) and 25% (◇) dilution of this mixture. The full curve is the regression line with a slope of 1.00 (± 0.10) and an intercept of -1.08 (± 0.77). The DPF was calculated by dividing attenuation change by absorption coefficient step. The mean value plotted is the average value of the two integrated TPSFs on either side of the step.

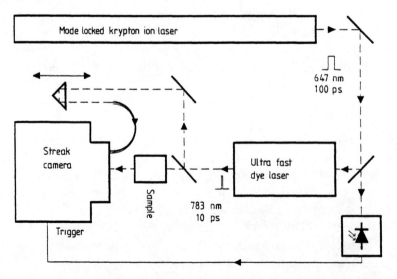

Figure 4. Experimental apparatus for the measurement of integrated TPSFS.

slit. Samples were placed in the main beam and the TPSFs recorded by averaging 128 TV frames. Integrated TPSFs were calculated by summing over the area of the streak camera slit, excluding the time reference. The spatial variation of the TPSF had a full width half maximum less than the 12 mm entry slit size for the sample with maximum scattering and minimum absorption. The input power of the beam was monitored continuously (Coherent 212). Sample attenuation by the phantom was measured using a 1 cm^2 area silicon photodiode (RS Components) placed against the exit side. To correspond with the Monte Carlo model, a cell of 1 cm thickness and a wavelength of 783 nm were employed.

Two sizes of particles were used in the phantom in an attempt to reproduce the scattering phase function of brain tissue. The diameters of the particles were 1.00 μm ($\pm$0.03 μm) and 0.05 μm ($\pm$0.002 μm). The absolute concentrations used gave integrated TPSFs in the range of the Monte Carlo model and the *in vivo* experiments (see later). Variation in scattering coefficient was performed by volumetric dilution of the mixture. The original mixture contained 6.7% by volume of the smaller particles and 2.5% by volume of the larger particles. The total volume of phantom material was 40 ml. Absorption changes were obtained by adding 0.3 ml aliquots of concentrated infrared dye solution (ICI S109564), producing steps in absorption coefficient of 0.053 cm^{-1} up to 0.424 cm^{-1}, i.e. about three times the expected *in vivo* value (Cope *et al* 1988). Experimental results are shown in figure 3(b), and can be seen to be in reasonable agreement with the model predictions. Several explanations are possible for the minor differences between the experimental and modelled results. In particular, the cell size employed is finite (6 cm $\times$ 6 cm), and the acceptance angle and slit width of the streak camera system is limited. Therefore the TPSF cannot be integrated over all space. It is intended to extend the Monte Carlo model to simulate these finite limits. In addition the scattering phase function of the phantom is not identical to that used in the model. The effect of this small difference in phase function was checked by repeating the Monte Carlo calculations for a scattering coefficient of 60 cm^{-1} using the scattering phase function of the phantom material calculated from Mie theory (Bohren and Huffman 1983). These data are also shown in figure 3(a). The effect of the slight difference in phase function on the relationship is negligible.

4. Optical pathlength in the brain

The implications of the model predictions have been studied in a series of experiments to measure the integrated TPSF for the transilluminated rat brain. Nine adult Wistar rats (mean weight 288 g) were studied. Following anaesthesia (Urethane 36% w/v intraperitoneal, 5 m kg^{-1}) the temporoparietal muscles were reflected, the skull exposed and cleared of residual surface tissue. A tracheostomy allowed easy manipulation of inspired gas concentrations and a femoral artery was cannulated for blood sampling. The animal was placed in front of the streak camera in the sample position shown in figure 4, the head being immobilised in a stereotactic frame. Pulses of light from the dye laser were incident on the skull diametrically opposite the streak camera entry slit. Sample attenuation caused by the rat's head was monitored using a 1 mm diameter optical fibre and photomultiplier tube (Hamamatsu R928) in place of the silicon photodiode used experimentally on the model verification. Measurements were made and arterial blood samples taken with the animal breathing 100%, 21% and 12% oxygen (balance N$_2$) and 90% oxygen with 10% carbon dioxide. Further measurements were taken immediately upon death by N$_2$ inspiration, 15 min post mortem and finally approximately 22 h post mortem. The rat head diameter was measured at the end of each experiment.

Figure 5 shows the integrated TPSFs for one rat (head diameter 15 mm) together with the input pulse at time zero. It can be seen that as predicted by the Monte Carlo model, considerable temporal dispersion occurred due to multiple scattering of the light in the brain tissue. The overall pulse shape and position showed small changes over a wide range of optical absorption caused by variation in average oxygen saturation (i.e. inspired oxygen concentration (FiO_2) = 100% and FiO_2 = 12%) or cerebral blood volume (i.e. when inspired CO_2 concentration ($FiCO_2$) = 10%). The data for all animals averaged over equivalent states are shown in table 1. The overall mean of the integrated TPSFs is equivalent to a distance travelled of 5.3($\pm$0.3) times the head diameter. The means of the integrated TPSFs for post mortem tissue (measured at 20 °C following 22.4$\pm$3.7 h storage at 4 °C) were similar to those obtained at an FiO_2 of 100%.

In a final series of studies the effect of the skull on light scattering and on the average pathlength was investigated since it had been conjectured that some transmitted light may be 'guided' through the skull or between dura and skull and hence not traverse the brain tissues. To examine the effect of light scattering by the skull, in one animal small holes (3 mm diameter) were drilled on either side of the skull following the post mortem integrated TPSF measurement. A further time resolved intensity profile was then obtained with the input laser beam incident directly on the brain tissue and the streak camera focused onto the exposed brain at the far side. No significant difference in the time profiles was observable. In another post mortem animal a small section of bone was carefully removed from the top of the skull, and the brain was

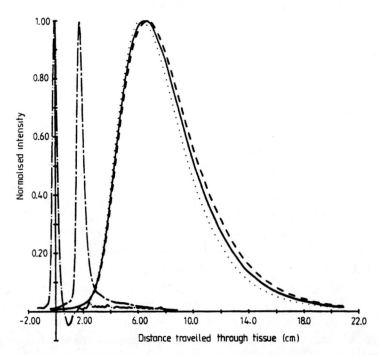

Figure 5. Integrated TPSFs in equivalent distance ($n = 1.4$) measured *in vivo* across a rat head. The input pulse (from the time reference) (— · —) is at the origin and coincides with light first entering the head. Three similar integrated TPSFs show the effect of changes in brain oxygenation. The profiles become narrower as the inspired gas mixture is varied from 100% O_2 (- - -), through 21% O_2 (——) to 12% O_2 (. . . . .), balance N_2. This decrease in cerebral oxygenation produced an increase in absorption in brain tissue (deoxygenated haemoglobin absorbs more than oxygenated haemoglobin at 783 nm). The remaining profile (— – —) shows the result with the brain removed and the skull filled with silicone oil ($n = 1.4$).

Table 1. A table of parameters derived from the integrated TPSFs measured experimentally on nine rat heads. The tabulated values are dimensionless. Parameters displayed correspond to the distance ($n = 1.4$) where 5%, 50% and 95% of the total intensity has been received together with the mean, normalised for the distance across the head. The mean distance across the rat heads (including skull) was 1.46 cm (±0.05). The table shows the values and standard deviations taken over all animals for equivalent states, i.e. the four different inspired gas mixtures and three post mortem states. The final column is an average over all the seven states.

Average (all animals)	100% O_2	10% CO_2 90% O_2	21% O_2 79% N_2	12% O_2 88% N_2	0 min post mortem	15 min post mortem	22 h	Average over all data
5th percentile	2.61	2.57	2.55	2.50	2.43	2.60	2.87	2.59
50th percentile	5.07	4.98	4.95	4.78	4.60	4.83	5.18	4.91
95th percentile	9.62	9.47	9.40	9.04	8.68	8.96	9.41	9.23
Mean	5.43	5.35	5.31	5.12	4.93	5.16	5.52	5.26
Standard deviation								
5th percentile	0.27	0.25	0.28	0.26	0.24	0.22	0.30	0.28
50th percentile	0.24	0.24	0.25	0.25	0.24	0.26	0.41	0.31
95th percentile	0.23	0.31	0.28	0.27	0.26	0.34	0.52	0.44
Mean	0.23	0.24	0.24	0.24	0.24	0.26	0.41	0.31

extracted. The empty skull was then filled with a viscous silicone oil ($n = 1.402$), the bone replaced and the integrated TPSF measured (figure 5). The pulse broadening was <10% of that observed with the brain present. The possibility of light 'channelling' through the bone of the skull was then checked by replacing the silicone oil with water containing a strong absorber (India ink). Under these circumstances very strong attenuation was observed across the head, greater than 6 optical densities compared with the presence of brain in the skull. It thus appears that the skull and dura make negligible contribution to the integrated TPSF observed across the head.

5. Discussion

The integrated TPSF for the rat head shows the considerable degree of multiple scattering that occurs in brain tissue. The first detected photons to emerge from the head (represented by the point when 5% of the cumulative intensity has been reached) appear on average to have travelled 2.6 (±0.3) times the head diameter. The final photons to emerge (the point when 95% of the cumulative intensity has been reached) appear to have travelled 9.2(±0.4) times the head diameter.

The differential pathlength factor derived from the integrated TPSF is 5.3 ± 0.3 times the head diameter. This value is slightly larger than that obtained using the previously described technique of water absorption measurements which was 4.34 ± 0.44 (Wray et al 1988). There may be a number of reasons for this discrepancy. First, the time of flight technique relies on a value for the refractive index of brain tissue. The refractive index will lie between the value of 1.33 for water and 1.55 for fat or concentrated protein solutions (Bennett et al 1951). The value of 1.4 used in this paper is an estimate based on values reported for rat gut (Gahn and Witte 1986). An accurate value for brain tissue refractive index is being sought. Second, the pathlength factor was measured at 783 nm using time of flight techniques, and between 940 to 1050 nm using the water absorption technique. The results in this paper show that there is a variation in differential pathlength factor with absorption and scattering. The DPE increases with increasing scattering and decreases with increasing absorption. Therefore we would predict the DPF at 975 nm to be lower than that at 783 nm since tissue

183

absorption is higher at 975 nm and in general scattering decreases with increasing wavelength.

In previous animal studies we have occasionally noted a considerable transient increase in transmitted light intensity upon death. This effect could not be correlated with absorption changes due to blood deoxygenation and blood volume decrease as it has also been observed in fluorocarbon exchange-transfused rats (unpublished observations). In these studies, the observed increase in transmitted light intensity at death was not accompanied by the increase in mean time expected with a simple decrease in absorption. We believe this can only be explained by a decrease in tissue scattering, the cause of which is unknown. The transient increase in transmitted intensity (and associated shortening of the integrated TPSF) persisted only for 1.0–1.5 min after death. The integrated TPSF for the brain tissue 22 h post mortem gave a slightly increased average DPF of 5.5 ± 0.4, although this value still lay within the range obtained in the living animal.

6. Conclusions

We have introduced the idea of the temporal point spread function (TPSF) of light propagating through tissue together with the differential pathlength factor (DPF) relating changes in measured attenuation to variations in absolute absorption. A Monte Carlo simulation has shown that the mean of the integrated TPSF is in excellent agreement with the DPF. This simulation has been verified experimentally on a phantom with known optical properties. Integrated TPSFs measured across the rat head show a mean value for the DPF of 5.3 ± 0.3 times the head diameter. The maximum variation in the DPF was 0.5 (or 9%) for a wide range of cerebral oxygenation states. The effect of the skull on the DPF is small.

Knowledge of the optical pathlength will permit quantitation of cerebral oxygenation data derived from NIR spectroscopy. Future studies of the way in which the DPF varies with changes in tissue attenuation will further improve quantitation. Additional analysis of the TPSF may also permit direct *in vivo* measurement of tissue absorption and scattering coefficients (Shimizu *et al* 1979) and eventually lead to NIR imaging through tissues (Arridge *et al* 1986, Takiguchi *et al* 1986).

Acknowledgments

This work was carried out with funding provided by The Wellcome Trust, MRC, SERC and Hamamatsu Photonics KK. The authors also wish to thank Dr B Vincent and Dr K Ryan, Department of Physical Chemistry, University of Bristol for the generous supply of polystyrene-latex particles.

Résumé

Estimation du parcours optique dans les tissus par la mesure directe du temps de vol.

La quantification des données spectroscopiques du proche infrarouge dans un milieu diffusant tel que les tissus, nécessite la connaissance du parcours optique dans le milieu. Ce parcours peut maintenant être estimé directement à partir du temps de vol d'impulsions lumineuses de quelques picosecondes. La modélisation par Monte Carlo des impulsions lumineuses dans les tissus a montré que la valeur moyenne du temps des impulsions lumineuses disposées est corrélée avec le parcours utilisé dans les calculs de spectroscopie quantitative. Ce résultat a été vérifié sur fantôme. Les mesures par temps de vol du parcours au travers de la tête de rat donnent un parcours de $5,3 + 0,3$ fois le diamètre de la tête.

Zusammenfassung

Bestimmung der optischen Weglänge in Gewebe durch direkte Flugzeitmessungen.

Die Quantifizierung spektroskopischer Daten im nahen Infrarot in einem Streumedium wie z.B. Gewebe erfordert die Kenntnis der optischen Weglänge des betreffenden Mediums. Diese kann jetzt direkt bestimmt werden aus der Flugzeit von pikosekundenlangen Lichtpulsen. Die Monte Carlo-Simulation von Lichtpulsen in Gewebe hat gezeigt, daß der Mittelwert der Lichtpulse mit der Weglänge korreliert ist, die in quantitativen spektroskopischen Berechnungen verwendet wird. Dieses Ergebnis wurde in einem Phantommaterial verifiziert. Flugzeitmessungen der Weglänge entlang eines Rattenkopfes ergeben eine Weglänge von 5.3 ± 0.3 mal dem Kopfdurchmesser.

References

Arridge S R, Cope M, van der Zee P, Hillson P J and Delpy D T 1986 Visualisation of the oxygenation state of brain and muscle in newborn infants by near infra-red transillumination *Information Processing in Medical Imaging*, ed. S L Bacharach (New York: Martinus Nijhoff) pp 155-76

Bennett A H, Osterburg H, Jupnitz H and Richards O W 1951 *Phase Microscopy* (New York: Wiley)

Bohren C F and Huffman D R 1983 *Absorption and Scattering of Light by Small Particles* (New York: Wiley Interscience)

Brazy J E, Lewis D V, Mitnick M H and Jöbsis F F 1985 Noninvasive monitoring of cerebral oxygenation in preterm infants: Preliminary observations *Paediatrics* **75**(2) 217-25

Cope M and Delpy D T 1988 System for long term measurement of cerebral blood and tissue oxygenation on newborn infants by near infrared transillumination *Med. Biol. Eng. Comput.* **26**(3) 289-94

Cope M, Delpy D T, Reynolds E O R, Wray S, Wyatt J S and van der Zee P 1988 Methods of quantitating cerebral near infrared spectroscopy data *Adv. Exp. Med. Biol.* **222** 183-90

Delpy D T, Cope M C, Cady E B, Wyatt J S, Hamilton P A, Hope P L, Wray S and Reynolds E O R 1987 Cerebral monitoring in newborn infants by magnetic resonance and near infrared spectroscopy *Scand. J. Clin. Lab. Invest.* **47 Suppl.** 188 9-17

Ferrari M, Zanette E, Giannini I, Sideri G, Fieschi C and Carpi A 1986a Effects of carotid artery compression test on regional cerebral blood volume, haemoglobin oxygen saturation and cytochrome -c- oxidase redox level in cerebrovascular patients *Adv. Exp. Med. Biol.* **200** 213-22

Ferrari M, De Marchis C, Giannini I, Nicola A, Agostino R, Nodari S and Bucci G 1986b Cerebral blood volume and haemoglobin oxygen saturation monitoring in neonatal brain by near infrared spectroscopy *Adv. Exp. Med. Biol.* **200** 203-12

Fox E, Jöbsis F F and Mitnick M H 1985 Monitoring cerebral oxygen sufficiency in anaesthesia and surgery *Adv. Exp. Med. Biol.* **191** 849-54

Gahn T and Witte S 1986 Measurement of the optical thickness of transparent tissue layers *J. Microsc.* **141** 101-10

Hazeki O, Seyama A and Tamura M 1987 Near infrared spectrophotometric monitoring of haemoglobin and cytochrome aa_3 *in vivo*, *Adv. Exp. Med. Biol.* **215** 283-9

Jöbsis F F 1977 Non invasive, infrared monitoring of cerebral and myocardial oxygen sufficiency and circulatory parameters *Science* **198** 1264-7

Piantadosi C C, Hemstreet T M and Jöbsis F F 1986 Near infrared spectrophotometric monitoring of oxygen distribution to intact brain and skeletal muscle tissue *Critical Care Med.* **14** (8) 698-706

Shimizu K, Ishimaru A, Reynolds L and Bruckner A P 1979 Backscattering of a picosecond pulse from densely distributed scatterers *Appl. Opt.* **18** 3484-8

Svaasand L O and Ellinsen R 1983 Optical properties of human brain *Photochem. Photobiol.* **38** 293-9

Takiguchi Y, Aoshima S, Tsuchiya Y and Hiruma T 1986 Laser pulse tomography using a streak camera *Proc. Int. meeting on Image Detection and Quality, Paris, July 16-18*

van der Zee P and Delpy T 1987 Simulation of the point spread function for light in tissue by a Monte Carlo model *Adv. Exp. Med. Biol.* **215** 179-92

van der Zee P and Delpy D T 1988 Computed point spread functions for light in tissue using a measured volume scattering function *Adv. Exp. Med. Biol.* **222** 191-8

Wray S, Cope M, Delpy D T, Wyatt J S and Reynolds E O R 1988 Characterisation of the near infrared absorption spectra of cytochrome aa_3 and haemoglobin for the non-invasive monitoring of cerebral oxygenation *Biochim. Biophys. Acta* **933** 184-92

Wyatt J S, Cope M, Delpy D T, Wray S and Reynolds E O R 1986 Quantitation of cerebral oxygenation and haemodynamics in sick newborn infants by near infrared spectroscopy *Lancet* **8515** 1063-1066

Reprinted with permission from *Applied Optics,* Vol. 28(12), pp. 2331-2336
(June 15, 1989). ©1989 Optical Society of America.

Time resolved reflectance and transmittance for the non-invasive measurement of tissue optical properties

Michael S. Patterson, B. Chance, and B. C. Wilson

When a picosecond light pulse is incident on biological tissue, the temporal characteristics of the light backscattered from, or transmitted through, the sample carry information about the optical absorption and scattering coefficients of the tissue. We develop a simple model, based on the diffusion approximation to radiative transfer theory, which yields analytic expressions for the pulse shape in terms of the interaction coefficients of a homogeneous slab. The model predictions are in good agreement with the results of preliminary *in vivo* experiments and Monte Carlo simulations.

I. Introduction

The rapidly increasing use of light in diagnostic and therapeutic medicine has created the need to determine noninvasively the optical properties of living tissue. These properties may be of intrinsic interest; for example, changes in the optical absorption coefficient can be related to blood oxygenation and tissue metabolism.[1,2] Alternatively, the optical properties may be required to calculate the distribution of light in the tissue during, for example, photodynamic therapy[3] or laser surgery.[4] Many papers have been devoted to the measurement of the optical properties of excised tissue specimens, and the detection of diffusely reflected or transmitted light has been studied as a means of monitoring blood oxygenation *in vivo*.[5] More recently, Groenhuis *et al.*,[6] Bonner *et al.*,[7] and Steinke and Shepherd[8] have studied the relationship between the absorption and scattering coefficients of tissue and the spatial dependence of diffuse reflectance near a finite light source. Such measurements may be useful for noninvasive optical characterization, but absolute measurements of reflectance must be made at several locations.

The temporal spreading of a short light pulse as it propagates through a scattering medium also contains information about the optical interaction coefficients. Such measurements have long been of interest in atmospheric research; for example, Weinman and Shipley[9] used the time dependence of a transmitted pulse to deduce the optical thickness of clouds. Theoretical studies of light pulse propagation in multiple scattering media based on the diffusion approximation have been published by Ishimaru[10] and Furutsu.[11] Shimizu *et al.*[12] measured the time resolved reflectance of a plane wave from suspensions of microspheres and suggested that this technique might be used to determine the optical properties of random media such as tissue.

We propose a practical *in vivo* technique in which a short light pulse is produced on the tissue surface by a small source, such as a laser beam or optical fiber, and a small detector some distance away is used to measure the time resolved pulse. Two geometries are considered: a semi-infinite medium which represents measurements made on the surface of a large volume and a finite slab representing reflectance or transmittance measurements on smaller organs. A simple model based on the time dependent diffusion equation is introduced which allows calculation of the pulse shape at any point on either face of the slab. The predictions of the model are shown to be in good agreement with Monte Carlo simulations performed by us and other investigators. We show that in certain conditions the absorption and scattering coefficients can be expressed as functions of simple descriptors of the pulse shape: the time of maximum signal and the decay constant at long times. The pulse shape recorded from the calf muscle of a human volunteer is accurately

B. Chance is with University of Pennsylvania, Department of Biochemistry/Biophysics, Philadelphia, Pennsylvania 19104; the other authors are with Hamilton Regional Cancer Centre, 711 Concession Street, Hamilton, Ontario L8V 1C3, Canada.

Received 15 November 1988.

0003-6935/89/122331-06$02.00/0.

© 1989 Optical Society of America.

predicted by the model, and the derived absorption and scattering coefficients are similar to published values for excised muscle tissue. If economical pulsed light sources can be used, this method offers the potential for fast simple noninvasive determination of tissue optical properties.

II. Theory

The geometry of the problem is illustrated in Figs. 1(a) and 1(b). A narrow collimated pulsed light beam is normally incident on the surface of a semi-infinite [Fig. 1(a)] or finite [Fig. 1(b)] homogeneous tissue slab. We will assume that the diffuse photon fluence rate $\phi(\mathbf{r},t)$ satisfies the diffusion equation

$$\frac{1}{c}\frac{\partial}{\partial t}\phi(\mathbf{r},t) - D\nabla^2\phi(\mathbf{r},t) + \mu_a\phi(\mathbf{r},t) = S(\mathbf{r},t), \qquad (1)$$

where c is the speed of light in the tissue, D is the diffusion coefficient,

$$D = \{3[\mu_a + (1 - g)\mu_s]\}^{-1}, \qquad (2)$$

μ_a is the linear absorption coefficient, μ_s is the linear scattering coefficient, g is the mean cosine of the scattering angle, and $S(\mathbf{r},t)$ is the photon source. This equation can be derived from the radiative transfer equation, and its application to light propagation in turbid media has been discussed by many investigators including Ishimaru.[13] The fluence rate can be accurately calculated using Eq. (1) if $\mu_a \ll (1 - g)\mu_s$ and if the point of interest is far from sources or boundaries. The first condition is generally true for soft tissues in the 650–1300 nm range. Strictly speaking, the second condition is violated in calculating the reflectance and transmittance, but even here we will show that accurate estimates of the relative (rather than absolute) quantities can be obtained.

For a short pulse from an isotropic point source, $S(\mathbf{r},t) = \delta(0,0)$, it may be shown[14] that in an infinite medium the solution of Eq. (1) is

$$\phi(\mathbf{r},t) = c(4\pi Dct)^{-3/2}\exp\left(-\frac{r^2}{4Dct} - \mu_act\right). \qquad (3)$$

We can use this Green's function to solve the problem posed in Fig. 1(a) by making two further assumptions. First, we assume that all the incident photons are initially scattered at a depth

$$z_0 = [(1 - g)\mu_s]^{-1} \qquad (4)$$

so that the actual source term becomes the simple delta function described above. This localization of the first interactions will not produce inaccuracies if we are interested in the fluence rate far from the source or at times long after pulse incidence. We must also specify a boundary condition at the tissue surface. Duderstadt and Hamilton[15] have shown that a useful approach is to set the diffuse fluence rate to zero at an extrapolated boundary some distance beyond the actual surface. For example, if the interface is between tissue and a nonscattering medium with the same index of refraction, this extrapolated boundary is located at $z = -(0.7104) 3 \cdot D$.[13] Hemenger[16] has shown that a mismatch in the index of refraction at the surface, for

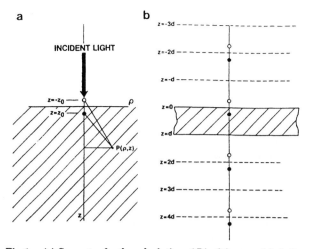

Fig. 1. (a) Geometry for the calculation of $R(\rho,t)$ for a semi-infinite homogeneous medium. The incident pencil beam is assumed to create an isotropic photon source at depth z_0, indicated by the filled circle. The boundary condition $\phi(\rho,0,t) = 0$ can be met by adding a negative source indicated by the open circle. (b) Geometry for the calculation of the time resolved reflectance and transmittance from a homogeneous slab. The boundary conditions $\phi(\rho,0,t) = 0$ and $\phi(\rho,d,t) = 0$ can be met by adding an infinite series of dipole photon sources. The first four are shown in this illustration.

example, an air–tissue interface, can be accounted for by changing this extrapolation length. For our application, where observations are made at a large distance compared with the extrapolation length, we have found that the pulse shape is insensitive to the exact location of the extrapolated boundary. Hence, for simplicity, our second assumption is that $\phi(\mathbf{r},t) = 0$ on the physical boundary $z = 0$. As discussed by Eason et al.,[17] this boundary condition can be met by adding a negative or image source of photons to the infinite medium problem as shown in Fig. 1(a). The fluence rate per incident photon can then be written in cylindrical coordinates as the sum of contributions from the two sources:

$$\phi(\rho,z,t) = c(4\pi Dct)^{-3/2}\exp(-\mu_act)\left\{\exp\left[-\frac{(z - z_0)^2 + \rho^2}{4Dct}\right]\right.$$
$$\left. - \exp\left[-\frac{(z + z_0)^2 + \rho^2}{4Dct}\right]\right\}. \qquad (5)$$

We wish to know the number of photons reaching the surface per unit area per unit time $|\mathbf{J}(\rho,0,t)|$, which can be calculated from Fick's law[15]:

$$\mathbf{J}(\rho,0,t) = -D\nabla\phi(\rho,z,t)|_{z=0}, \qquad (6)$$

which leads to the final expression for the reflectance $R(\rho,t)$:

$$R(\rho,t) = |\mathbf{J}(\rho,0,t)|$$
$$= (4\pi Dc)^{-3/2}z_0 t^{-5/2}\exp(-\mu_act)\exp\left(-\frac{\rho^2 + z_0^2}{4Dct}\right). \qquad (7)$$

For the case where $\rho^2 \gg z_0^2$ we also note that

$$\frac{d}{dt}\log_e R(\rho,t) = -\frac{5}{2t} - \mu_a c + \frac{\rho^2}{4Dct^2} \cdot \qquad (8)$$

The observation that

$$\lim_{t\to\infty}\frac{d}{dt}\log_e R(\rho,t) = -\mu_a c \qquad (9)$$

leads to the suggestion recently made by Chance *et al.*[18] that the absorption coefficient of the tissue can be determined from the asymptotic slope of the $\log_e R(\rho,t)$ vs t curve. (The speed of light depends on the index of refraction n of the tissue which is known to a few percent. We assume that $n = 1.4$,[19] so that $c = 0.214$ mm ps^{-1}.)

The transport scattering coefficient $(1 - g)\mu_s$ can also be determined from the $\log_e R(\rho,t)$ vs t curve by noting that at t_{max}, the time of maximum detected signal, the slope is zero. Solving Eq. (8) yields the expression

$$(1-g)\mu_s = \frac{1}{3\rho^2}(4\mu_a c^2 t_{max}^2 + 10ct_{max}) - \mu_a. \qquad (10)$$

Thus we see from Eqs. (9) and (10) that the optical properties of a semi-infinite slab of tissue could in principle be obtained by measuring the diffusely reflected light some distance from the source as a function of time. A superior signal-to-noise would be obtained by integrating the reflected light over some larger area. As an illustration of the potential of this method, we can integrate $R(\rho,t)$ over the entire surface to obtain $R(t)$:

$$R(t) = \int_0^\infty R(\rho,t)2\pi\rho d\rho$$

$$= (4\pi Dc)^{-1/2}z_0 t^{-3/2}\exp(-\mu_a ct)\exp\left(-\frac{z_0^2}{4Dct}\right). \qquad (11)$$

This expression agrees with the prediction of Ito and Furutsu[20] that for a nonabsorbing medium the total diffuse reflectance should depend on $t^{-3/2}$.

An important question is how measurements of the diffusely reflected light are affected by a finite tissue volume. A related question is whether a simple model can yield results for the time resolved transmittance through a tissue volume. Such measurements have been made for rat brains by Delpy *et al.*[19] and have been shown to carry information about the tissue optical properties. We will consider the simplest case: a finite tissue slab of thickness d illustrated in Fig. 1(b). Here we have an additional boundary where the condition $\phi(\rho,d,t) = 0$ must apply. This condition can be met by adding two sources near $z = 2d$ as shown, but then the boundary condition at $z = 0$ is violated for $t > 2d/c$. Both boundary conditions can be met at all times only by adding an infinite number of dipole sources as shown in Fig. 1(b). In practice, the number of sources required depends on the optical properties of the slab and the maximum time at which the reflectance or transmittance must be calculated.

Following the same development as above, it can be shown that, where three dipoles are retained, the reflectance $R(\rho,d,t)$ is given by

$$R(\rho,d,t) = (4\pi Dc)^{-3/2}t^{-5/2}\exp(-\mu_a ct)\exp\left(-\frac{\rho^2}{4Dct}\right)$$

$$\times\left\{z_0\exp\left(-\frac{z_0^2}{4Dct}\right) - (2d - z_0)\exp\left[-\frac{(2d - z_0)^2}{4Dct}\right]\right.$$

$$\left. + (2d + z_0)\exp\left[-\frac{(2d + z_0)^2}{4Dct}\right]\right\}. \qquad (12)$$

The spatial integral analogous to Eq. (11) can also be computed, and we have

$$R(d,t) = (4\pi Dc)^{-1/2}t^{-3/2}\exp(-\mu_a ct)$$

$$\times\left\{z_0\exp\left(-\frac{z_0^2}{4Dct}\right) - (2d - z_0)\exp\left[-\frac{(2d - z_0)^2}{4Dct}\right]\right.$$

$$\left. + (2d + z_0)\exp\left[-\frac{(2d + z_0)^2}{4Dct}\right]\right\}. \qquad (13)$$

The transmittance $T(\rho,d,t)$ calculated by retaining four dipoles is

$$T(\rho,d,t) = (4\pi Dc)^{-3/2}t^{-5/2}\exp(-\mu_a ct)\exp\left(-\frac{\rho^2}{4Dct}\right)$$

$$\times\left\{(d - z_0)\exp\left[-\frac{(d - z_0)^2}{4Dct}\right]\right.$$

$$- (d + z_0)\exp\left[-\frac{(d + z_0)^2}{4Dct}\right]$$

$$+ (3d - z_0)\exp\left[-\frac{(3d - z_0)^2}{4Dct}\right]$$

$$\left. - (3d + z_0)\exp\left[-\frac{(3d + z_0)^2}{4Dct}\right]\right\}, \qquad (14)$$

and the spatially integrated transmittance is just

$$T(d,t) = (4\pi Dc)^{-1/2}t^{-3/2}\exp(-\mu_a ct)$$

$$\times\left\{(d - z_0)\exp\left[-\frac{(d - z_0)^2}{4Dct}\right]\right.$$

$$- (d + z_0)\exp\left[-\frac{(d + z_0)^2}{4Dct}\right]$$

$$+ (3d - z_0)\exp\left[-\frac{(3d - z_0)^2}{4Dct}\right]$$

$$\left. - (3d + z_0)\exp\left[-\frac{(3d + z_0)^2}{4Dct}\right]\right\}. \qquad (15)$$

A quantity of interest in *in vivo* transmission spectroscopy is the mean distance traversed by photons before exit.[19] An analytical expression for this quantity can be derived from Eq. (15) for the slab geometry. The mean path length $\langle ct \rangle$ is given by

$$\langle ct \rangle = (4\mu_a D)^{-1/2}\frac{(d - z_0)\exp(2z_0\sqrt{\mu_a/D}) - (d + z_0)}{\exp(2z_0\sqrt{\mu_a/D}) - 1}, \qquad (16)$$

where the integrals have been evaluated using the solutions of Gradsteyn and Ryzhik.[21]

III. Materials and Methods

The predictions of the diffusion model were compared with data from three sources: experimental results reported by Chance et al.,[18] Monte Carlo simulation performed by the authors using a code developed by Flock et al.,[22] and Monte Carlo results published by Delpy et al.[19]

The experimental arrangement has been described in detail elsewhere.[18] Briefly, a pulsed dye laser generated 6-ps pulses at 760 nm, which were incident on the calf of a human volunteer. Scattered light was collected at a distance of 40 mm from the source using a 3-mm diam fiber optic bundle in contact with the skin. The detector was a two-stage microchannel plate tube, and the pulse shape was recorded using standard time resolved photon counting methods. The time resolution of the system, as determined by the full width at half-maximum of the directly detected pulse, was 150 ps.

Results for spatially integrated time resolved reflectance were obtained using a Monte Carlo code described by Flock et al.[22] This program allows anisotropic light scattering where the angular dependence of the scattering is described by the analytical Henyey-Greenstein phase function.[23] The cumulative path length traveled by each photon before escape is scored so that the time resolved reflectance can be examined.

For time resolved transmittance we used the results of Delpy et al.[19] Their Monte Carlo code computes the spatially integrated transmittance through a slab. The program incorporates an experimentally determined phase function measured for rat brain tissue at 783 nm.

IV. Results and Discussion

Figure 2 shows the logarithm of the signal detected *in vivo* vs time. The optical properties of the muscle could be obtained by fitting the data to Eq. (7), but Eqs. (9) and (10) allow a simple determination of the absorption and transport scattering coefficients. From the asymptotic slope we calculated that $\mu_a = 0.0176$ mm^{-1}, and, using this value and the time of maximum signal, Eq. (10) gave the value $(1-g)\mu_s = 0.85$ mm^{-1}. These results are in good agreement with the values of $\mu_a = 0.023 \pm 0.004$ and $(1-g)\mu_s = 0.85 \pm 0.08$ published by Wilson et al.[24] for excised bovine muscle. Given that our experiment was performed *in vivo* and that two different species were involved, this agreement may be fortuitous and further studies are clearly required. Nonetheless, this preliminary result shows that the derived coefficients for muscle tissue are reasonable. Using the calculated values, Eq. (7) was used to generate the complete pulse shape, and, as shown in Fig. 2, the agreement with experiment is quite good.

A comparison of Monte Carlo simulations of spatially integrated time resolved reflectance with Eq. (11) is presented in Fig. 3. The tissue was a semi-infinite slab with the same properties as those deduced for the calf muscle discussed above. In the simulation we used a value of $g = 0.95$ as reported for bovine muscle at 630

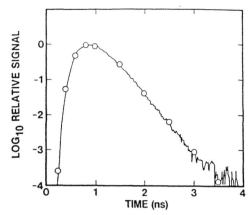

Fig. 2. Experimentally recorded reflectance signal from the calf muscle of a human volunteer at 760 nm is indicated by the solid line. The detector fiber bundle was positioned 40 mm from the pulsed laser source. The open circles show the pulse shape predicted by the diffusion model expression of Eq. (7) normalized to the peak value.

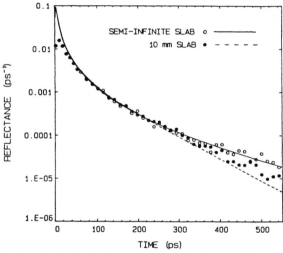

Fig. 3. Monte Carlo (symbols) and diffusion model (smooth curves) calculation of $R(t)$, the spatially integrated time resolved reflectance, from a semi-infinite tissue slab and a slab 10 mm thick. The optical properties of the slab are typical of human skeletal muscle at 760 nm. The diffusion model results have been matched to the Monte Carlo data at 50 ps. Note that the units of $R(t)$ are ps^{-1} as $R(t)$ is the number of photons reaching the surface per unit time per incident photon.

nm by Flock et al.[25] The diffusion model predictions have been normalized to the Monte Carlo data at 50 ps, and the agreement between the two is excellent out to 550 ps where the statistical uncertainties in the Monte Carlo data become large. At times shorter than 25 ps there is considerable discrepancy between the two. This is not surprising as photons exiting at these early times have not undergone multiple large angle scattering and their behavior is inadequately described by diffusion theory. Because of the uncertainty due to the finite number of photon histories the data are only shown out to 550 ps. At this time the asymptotic slope $-\mu_a c$ has not been attained. Substitution in Eq. (11)

shows that at 4 ns the slope would be within 10% of its terminal value for this particular sample. While μ_a can thus be readily determined from spatially integrated measurements, a close inspection of Eq. (11) shows that the shape of such curves is relatively insensitive to the scattering properties of the medium. Spatially resolved measurements, such as that presented in Fig. 2, are superior if information about $(1-g)\mu_s$ is desired. Of course, if μ_a is determined from a time resolved measurement, $(1-g)\mu_s$ could be calculated from some other noninvasive probe, such as the total (spatially integrated, temporally integrated) reflectance which in the diffusion limit depends only on $\mu_a/(1-g)\mu_s$ and the index of refraction.[26]

Also shown in Fig. 3 is the reflectance predicted from Eq. (12) for a slab of identical tissue 10 mm thick along with the results of the Monte Carlo simulation for this geometry. As expected, the loss of photons from the back surface causes the reflectance observed at the front surface to decrease more rapidly with time, although the diffusion model predicts a larger effect than observed in the Monte Carlo simulation. This simple illustration shows that finite tissue geometries can have a significant effect on the observed signal if the observation time is long enough. Caution must, therefore, be exercised in applying simple relations like Eq. (9) to observations made on smaller tissue volumes such as the organs of small animals.

Finally, in Fig. 4 we show that the simple diffusion model is also quite successful in predicting the total time resolved transmittance through a tissue slab as calculated by a Monte Carlo simulation of photon transport. The Monte Carlo results were taken from Delpy et al.[19] and apply to a 10-mm slab of tissue for which $\mu_a = 0.00434$ mm^{-1} and $\mu_s = 6$ mm^{-1}. An experimental phase function[27] which has an anisotropy parameter, $g = 0.72$ was used in their simulation. A parameter of considerable interest is the mean path length traveled by photons before leaving the rear surface. From the results of Delpy et al.[19] shown in Fig. 4, we calculated this to be 80.6 mm. The analytic expression of Eq. (16) gives a result of 77.6 mm, an error of only 3.7%. The shape of the transmitted pulse is strongly influenced not only by μ_a but also by $(1-g)\mu_s$. Such integrated measurements thus have the potential for deducing both optical coefficients.

V. Conclusions

The purpose of this paper has not been to test exhaustively the capability of time resolved reflectance and transmittance measurements for the deduction of tissue optical properties. Rather, the potential of this novel technique has been illustrated by Monte Carlo simulations and preliminary *in vivo* measurements. A simple model based on the diffusion approximation to the radiative transfer equation has been used to derive analytic expressions for the temporal and spatial dependence of diffusely transmitted and reflected light. These expressions have been shown to predict the detected pulse shape quite accurately for optical properties typical of tissue in the so-called therapeutic window of 650–1300 nm. A limitation of the model is

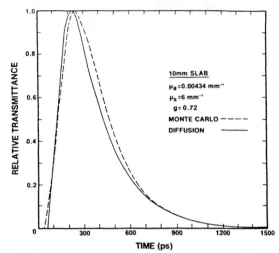

Fig. 4. Comparison of the predictions of the diffusion model (solid line) and Monte Carlo (dashed line) results of Delpy et al.[19] for the spatially integrated time-resolved transmittance through a 10-mm tissue slab. Each curve has been normalized at its peak value.

the remaining ambiguity between g and μ_s, as only the product $(1-g)\mu_s$ can be obtained. Some of this ambiguity might be resolved by examining the behavior of the reflectance at very early times where we have shown diffusion theory to be inadequate. The technical demands of such measurements are higher, but time resolution of the order of a picosecond is within current capabilities. The sort of measurements described in this paper require resolution of the order of 100 ps where off-the-shelf hardware is quite adequate. At some wavelengths, practical systems could incorporate pulsed laser diodes which would greatly reduce the cost and complexity of the light source. Further modeling and experimentation are also required to study the influence of more realistic geometries on the observed signals.

The full potential of time resolved measurements has not been completely explored. Besides the possibility of picosecond work, the interesting problem of spatial location of an optical inhomogeneity in, say, the brain or breast may be aided by studying the time behavior of scattered light. Here numerical solutions of the diffusion equation may provide an alternative to time-consuming Monte Carlo simulations. Much more work needs to be done to explore fully the dimension added by time resolution, but we have shown that such measurements are already capable of noninvasively probing the optical properties of living tissue.

The authors are grateful to Stephen Flock for providing the Monte Carlo results. This work was financially supported by the National Cancer Institute of Canada.

Michael Patterson and B. C. Wilson also work in the Departments of Radiology and Physics of McMaster University.

References

1. M. Tamura, O. Hazeki, S. Nioka, B. Chance, and D. Smith, "Simultaneous Measurements of Tissue Oxygen Concentration and Energy State by Near-Infrared and Nuclear Magnetic Resonance Spectroscopy," in *Chemoreceptors and Reflexes in Breathing*, S. Lahiri, Ed. (Oxford U.P., New York, in press 1989).

2. M. Cope and D. T. Delpy, "System for Long-Term Measurement of Cerebral Blood and Tissue Oxygenation on Newborn Infants by Near Infrared Transillumination," Med. Biol. Eng. Comput. **26**, 289–294 (1988).

3. B. C. Wilson and M. S. Patterson, "The Physics of Photodynamic Therapy," Phys. Med. Biol. **31**, 327–360 (1986).

4. S. L. Jacques and S. A. Prahl, "Modeling Optical and Thermal Distributions in Tissue During Laser Irradiation," Lasers Surg. Med. **6**, 494–503 (1987).

5. F. F. Jobsis, "Noninvasive, Infrared Monitoring of Cerebral and Myocardial Oxygen Sufficiency and Circulatory Parameters," Science **198**, 1264–1267 (1977).

6. R. A. J. Groenhuis, J. J. Ten Bosch, and H. A. Ferwerda, "Scattering and Absorption of Turbid Materials Determined from Reflection Measurements. 2: Measuring Method and Calibration," Appl. Opt. **22**, 2463–2467 (1983).

7. R. F. Bonner, R. Nossal, S. Havlin, and G. H. Weiss, "Model for Photon Migration in Turbid Biological Media," J. Opt. Soc. Am. A **4**, 423–432 (1987).

8. J. M. Steinke and A. P. Shepherd, "Diffuse Reflectance of Whole Blood: Model for a Diverging Light Beam," IEEE Trans. Biomed. Eng. **BME-34**, 826–834 (1987).

9. J. A. Weinman and S. T. Shipley, "Effects of Multiple Scattering on Laser Pulses Transmitted Through Clouds," J. Geophys. Res. **77**, 7123–7128 (1972).

10. A. Ishimaru, "Diffusion of a Pulse in Densely Distributed Scatterers," J. Opt. Soc. Am. **68**, 1045–1050 (1978).

11. K. Furutsu, "On the Diffusion Equation Derived from the Space–Time Transport Equation," J. Opt. Soc. Am. **70**, 360–366 (1980).

12. K. Shimizu, A. Ishimaru, L. Reynolds, and A. P. Bruchner, "Backscattering of a Picosecond Pulse from Densely Distributed Scatterers," Appl. Opt. **18**, 3484–3488 (1979).

13. A. Ishimaru, *Wave Propagation and Scattering in Random Media* (Academic, New York, 1978), pp. 175–190.

14. S. Chandrasekhar, "Stochastic Problems in Physics and Astronomy," Rev. Mod. Phys. **15**, 1–88 (1943).

15. J. J. Duderstadt and L. J. Hamilton, *Nuclear Reactor Analysis* (Wiley, New York, 1976), pp. 140–144.

16. R. P. Hemenger, "Optical Properties of Turbid Media with Specularly Reflecting Boundaries: Applications to Biological Problems," Appl. Opt. **16**, 2007–2012 (1977).

17. G. Eason, A. Veitch, R. Nisbet, and F. Turnbull, "The Theory of the Backscattering of Light by Blood," J. Phys. D **11**, 1463–1479 (1978).

18. B. Chance, S. Nioka, J. Kent, K. McCully, M. Fountain, R. Greenfeld, and G. Holtom, "Time Resolved Spectroscopy of Hemoglobin and Myoglobin in Resting and Ischemic Muscle," Anal. Biochem. **174**, 698–707 (1988).

19. D. T. Delpy, M. Cope, P. van der Zee, S. Arridge, S. Wray, and J. Wyatt, "Estimation of Optical Pathlength Through Tissue from Direct Time-of-Flight Measurements," Phys. Med. Biol. **33**, 1433–1442 (1988).

20. S. Ito and K. Furutsu, "Theory of Light Pulse Propagation Through Thick Clouds," J. Opt. Soc. Am. **70**, 366–374 (1980).

21. I. S. Gradsteyn and I. M. Ryzhik, *Table of Integrals, Series and Products* (Academic, New York, 1980), p. 340.

22. S. T. Flock, M. S. Patterson, and B. C. Wilson, "Monte Carlo Modelling of Light Propagation in Highly Scattering Tissues. I. Model Predictions and Comparison with Diffusion Theory," IEEE Trans. Biomed. Eng. 1989, in press.

23. L. G. Henyey and J. L. Greenstein, "Diffuse Radiation in the Galaxy," Astrophys. J. **93**, 70–83 (1941).

24. B. C. Wilson, M. S. Patterson, S. T. Flock, and J. D. Moulton, "The Optical Absorption and Scattering Properties of Tissues in the Visible and Near-Infrared Wavelength Range," in *Light in Biology and Medicine, Vol. 1* R. H. Douglas, J. Moan, and F. Doll'Acqua eds. (Plenum, New York, 1988) pp. 45–52.

25. S. T. Flock, B. C. Wilson, and M. S. Patterson, "Total Attenuation Coefficients and Scattering Phase Functions of Tissues and Phantom Materials at 633 nm," Med. Phys. **14**, 835–841 (1987).

26. B. C. Wilson and M. S. Patterson, "The Determination of Light Fluence Distributions in Photodynamic Therapy," in *Photodynamic Therapy of Neoplastic Disease*, D. Kessel, Ed. (CRC Press, Cleveland, 1989), in press.

27. P. van der Zee and D. T. Delpy, "Computed Point Spread Functions for Light in Tissue Using a Measured Volume Scattering Function," Adv. Exp. Med. Biol. **222**, 191–197 (1988).

Reprinted with permission from *IEEE Transactions on Biomedical Engineering*,
Vol. 36(12), pp. 1155-1161 (December 1989). ©1989 IEEE.

Time-Resolved Reflectance Spectroscopy in Turbid Tissues

STEVEN L. JACQUES

Abstract—Monte Carlo simulations illustrate how various absorption μ_a and scattering μ_s coefficients influence time-dependent reflectance $R(t)$ from a semi-infinite homogeneous turbid tissue following an impulse of narrow-beam irradiation. The tissue absorption coefficient μ_a in cm^{-1} can be obtained from measurements of $R(t)$ after the first 20–200 ps (depends on μ_s) following an impulse by the expression: $\mu_a = -(n/c) d \ln [R(t)]/dt - 3n/2ct$ where n is the tissue-refractive index and c is the *in vacuo* speed of light. Early data in the first 20–200 ps do not conform to this expression or to diffusion theory. Monte Carlo simulations allow study of the early $R(t)$ behavior. The volume of tissue involved in a measurement is specified by a volume radius r that approximately equals $(6Dtc/n)^{1/2}$ where t is the time of measurement and D is the optical diffusion constant $D = (3\mu_s(1 - g))^{-1}$. At 50 ps and typical values of $\mu_s = 100$ cm^{-1} and anisotropy equal to 0.9, r equals 5 mm. The upper limit for measurable μ_a values is limited by how quickly the reflectance signal is attenuated, and is estimated for current streak camera technology to be $\mu_a \leq 21$ cm^{-1}, assuming several measurements are taken over a dynamic range of two orders of magnitude within a 10 ps period.

INTRODUCTION

THE development of femtosecond (fs) and picosecond (ps) laser systems is opening a broad range of potential applications of ultrashort laser pulses and ultrafast phenomena in medicine. Diagnostic applications of such laser sources include time-resolved fluorescence [1] and reflectance spectroscopy [2], [3]. This paper discusses the advantages and limits of time-resolved reflectance measurements for spectroscopy, particularly when made at the tip of a catheter. Time-resolved Monte Carlo simulations are presented to illustrate the measurement principles and to characterize the deviation of early measurements from the predictions of diffusion theory. A simple expression is presented for calculation of the absorption coefficient from time-resolved reflectance measurements.

BACKGROUND

Before the methods of simulation are presented, some background information is useful. This includes, first, the optical properties of tissue; second, the basics of conventional steady-state reflectance spectroscopy; third, the basics of time-resolved reflectance spectroscopy; and finally, a review of recent contributions to the theory.

Manuscript received February 24, 1989; revised April 21, 1989.
The author is with the Laser Biology Research Laboratory, University of Texas/M.D. Anderson Cancer Center, Houston, TX 77030.
IEEE Log Number 8931099.

Tissue Optical Properties

The absorption coefficient μ_a in cm^{-1} indicates the frequency of absorption events and the mean-free path (mfp) that a photon travels before absorption occurs is equal to $1/\mu_a$. Values of μ_a for tissue range from 0.1 to 10 000 cm^{-1} (mfp of 10 mm–1 μm) over the ultraviolet (UV), visible, and near-infrared (IR) wavelength ranges. The scattering coefficient μ_s in cm^{-1} indicates the frequency of scattering events, and the mean-free path between scattering events is equal to $1/\mu_s$. Values of μ_s in tissue range from 10 to 1000 cm^{-1} (mfp of 1 mm–10 μm).

When a scattering event occurs, the trajectory of the photon is deflected by an angle θ. This random deflection is not isotropic, but rather is forward directed. Such forward-directed anisotropic scattering is less effective in altering the photon's trajectory. The scattering function $p(\theta)$ for tissues has been experimentally shown [4]–[6] to be well described by the Henyey–Greenstein function [7], which approximates Mie scattering. Light transport theory has been developed for astrophysical, atmospheric, and marine optics and describes an anisotropy parameter g for scattering which equals the average cosine of the deflection angle: $\langle \cos \theta \rangle$. Typical tissues have g values in the range of 0.7–0.95 (note: $\cos 45° = 0.71$, $\cos 18° = 0.95$).

For wavelengths in the "therapeutic window" between 600 and 1300 nm [8], hemoglobin and melanin pigments do not absorb strongly, and the deepest light penetration into tissue is possible. A typical turbid tissue in the "therapeutic window" might have optical properties of μ_a equal to 1 cm^{-1}, μ_s equal to 100 cm^{-1}, and g equal to 0.9. To facilitate the following discussion, these parameters will be assumed as representative values and are summarized in Table I.

Conventional Reflectance Spectroscopy

Transmission spectroscopy allows specification of the concentration of a chromophore in a medium by measurement of the attenuation of transmitted light T due to absorption over a known path length L. For a nonscattering solution in a cuvette, the path length is the cuvette thickness. The absorption coefficient μ_a in cm^{-1} is simply calculated:

$$\mu_s = \rho_a \sigma_a = \frac{-\ln (T)}{L}. \tag{1}$$

TABLE I
NOMENCLATURE AND TYPICAL TISSUE OPTICAL PARAMETERS AT WAVELENGTHS IN THE
"THERAPEUTIC WINDOW"

Term	Symbol	Typical Value for Tissue and Units
Absorption Coefficient	μ_a	1 cm^{-1}
Scattering Coefficient	μ_s	100 cm^{-1}
Anisotropy, $\langle \cos \theta \rangle$	g	0.9 (note: cos (26°) = 0.9)
Scattering Deflection Angle	θ	
Tissue Index of Refraction	n	1.37 ($\approx$ 80 percent water content)
Speed of Light in Vacuum	c	2.98 × 10^{10} cm/s
Speed of Light in Tissue	c/n	2.18 × 10^{10} cm/s

The absorption coefficient is related to the number density of the chromophore ρ_a in cm^{-3} and the optical cross-sectional area of the chromophore σ_a in cm^2 (notation of Ishimaru [9]).

Reflectance spectroscopy relies on multiple scattering in the turbid tissue to deflect each photon's trajectory and allow the light to return to the surface for escape and detection. The path length of each photon that successfully escapes the tissue as observable reflectance is not the same. Some photons enter the tissue and are immediately scattered and escape. Other photons wander through the tissue for some time before they migrate to the surface and escape. Therefore, the L is not a single value, but a distribution of path lengths [3], [10], [11], and μ_a cannot be calculated by simply substituting R for T in (1).

Monte Carlo simulations have shown that there is a unique relationship between the total reflectance R_t and the dimensionless ratio of effective scattering to absorption $\mu_s(1 - g)/\mu_a$ in a semi-infinite homogeneous tissue (author, unpublished study). Patterson *et al.* [12] have recently used diffusion theory to derive this relation in an analytic form that is accurate at high albedos when reflectance exceeds ≈ 0.60 and is approximate at lower albedos. This relationship allows one-to-one mapping between observed R_t and the ratio $\mu_s(1 - g)/\mu_a$ for a particular matched or mismatched surface-boundary condition. Therefore, steady-state reflectance measurements can specify the dimensionless ratio $\mu_s(1 - g)/\mu_a$, but not the absolute values of μ_a and $\mu_s(1 - g)$ in specific units.

A second independent measurement is required to specify separately the two unknowns μ_a and $\mu_s(1 - g)$. Radiative transport theory [9], [13] is used for the analysis. Using *in vitro* tissue samples, measurements of both total reflectance R_t and total transmission T_t can be made with integrating spheres to yield the tissue optical properties using diffusion theory [14]. Such measurements would not be possible *in vivo* at the tip of a catheter. The optical properties of a homogeneous tissue can be specified by measurements of the radial dependence of reflectance $R(r)$ where r is radial position ($R_t = \int R(r)2\pi r\,dr$) [15]. This latter technique is applicable *in vivo* when there is sufficient lateral room for measuring $R(r)$, for example, on the surface of an exposed tissue or organ.

Interpretation of $R(r)$ measurements at the tip of a catheter can be problematic. The deduction of μ_a depends on the spacing of the fibers at the catheter tip and the orientation of the fibers with respect to the tissue. These geometric factors determine the form of the radiative transport equations that should be used in the data analysis. Therefore, uncertainty in fiber separation or catheter placement yields uncertainty in the analysis. Time-resolved measurements of reflected light offer an alternative that may avoid these difficulties during catheter-based reflectance spectroscopy.

Time-Resolved Reflectance Spectroscopy

Time-resolved reflectance spectroscopy measures the escape of light as observable reflectance $R(t)$ versus time. Consider $R(t)$ to be the probability density function for escape at a given time t for a single photon. The behavior of an ensemble of photons will also conform to $R(t)$. The probability $R(t)$ can be separated into two independent probabilities: $S(t)$ and $e^{-\mu_a ct/n}$. The term $S(t)$ represents the probability that scattered light will reach the tissue surface and escape in the absence of tissue absorption. The details of scattering mean-free path, anisotropy, and orientation of the incident beam are contained in this term. The term $e^{-\mu_a ct/n}$ represents the probability of transmission without absorption over a path length L equals ct/n where c is the *in vacuo* speed of light and n is the tissue refractive index. The path length is proportional to the time of observed escape regardless of the particular path in the tissue. This latter fact is the major feature of time-resolved measurements. The $R(t)$ is written

$$R(t) = S(t)e^{-\mu_a ct/n} \qquad (2)$$

where

$$R_t = \int_0^\infty R(t)\,dt.$$

The absorption coefficient μ_a can be directly deduced from (2):

$$\mu_a = -\frac{n}{c}\left[\frac{d\ln[R(t)]}{dt} - \frac{d\ln[S(t)]}{dt}\right]. \qquad (3)$$

The $S(t)$ term eventually stabilizes as the rate of change of the light distribution in the tissue slows, and its time derivative becomes negligible (analogous to how thermal diffusion from a point-source impulse of heat is initially rapid, but slows as a Gaussian heat distribution broadens).

193

Then, the rate of decrease in $\ln[R(t)]$ can directly specify μ_a:

$$\mu_a \rightarrow -\frac{n}{c} \frac{d \ln[R(t)]}{dt} \quad \text{as } t \rightarrow \infty. \quad (4)$$

This report considers the time delay required for $S(t)$ to stabilize, so that (4) will reliably yield the absorption coefficient. Because the details of $S(t)$ become neglible after a sufficient time delay, time-resolved reflectance may avoid the problems of geometry and orientation encountered during steady-state measurements of $R(r)$.

Recently, Chance and co-workers at the University of Pennsylvania [2] have applied (4) to time-resolved measurements of light escaping from the cranium after each pulse of radiation from a free-running mode-locked/dye laser system. The absorption coefficients were deduced at 760 and 790 nm in order to specify the level of hemoglobin oxygenation in the brain despite considerable light scattering by the brain and skull. Similar measurements have been developed by Delpy *et al.* at the University College of London [3], with the goal of monitoring neonatal brain oxygenation.

Theory

Two approaches toward the problem have been pursued: 1) approximate analytical descriptions based on diffusion theory, and 2) exact solutions based on Monte Carlo simulations.

Diffusion Theory: Experiments on propagation of short laser pulses through atmospheric clouds illustrated the problem of temporal dispersion in turbid media [16], [17]. Ishimaru developed a time-dependent diffusion equation that describes the transmission of short laser pulses through such media [18]. Time-resolved measurements of the reflectance and transmission of ps pulses through well-defined turbid media (microsphere suspensions) documented how optical properties affect the temporal dispersion of ultrashort pulses [19], [20].

Recently, Patterson *et al.* [21], [22] have used diffusion theory to describe the escape of light as a function of time t and radial position r after an impulse of narrow-beam irradiance is delivered to a semi-infinite tissue:

$$R(r, t) = (4\pi Dc/n)^{-3/2} z_0 t^{-5/2}$$
$$\cdot \exp\left[-\left(\frac{r^2 + z_0^2}{4Dct/n}\right)\right] e^{-\mu_a ct/n} \quad (5)$$

where $D = [3(\mu_a + \mu_s(1 - g))]^{-1}$ is the optical diffusion length and $z_0 = [\mu_s(1 - g)]^{-1}$ is the *effective* mean-free path between scattering sites. The derivation invokes a simplifying approximation at the surface boundary (assumes that the fluence rate at the surface $\phi(0, t)$ is zero, which is imposed by including a negative source of photons outside the tissue at a height of z_0). Patterson *et al.* [21] have shown that (5) can be scaled to match the shape of experimental *in vivo* measurements of $R(r, t)$ on the human cranium.

The time derivative of the natural logarithm of $R(r, t)$ can be expressed

$$\frac{d}{dt} \ln[R(r, t)] = -\mu_a \frac{c}{n} - \frac{5}{2t} + \frac{r^2 + z_0^2}{4Dct^2/n}$$
$$\rightarrow -\mu_a \frac{c}{n} \quad \text{as } t \rightarrow \infty. \quad (6)$$

Therefore, the absorption coefficient can be determined from the asymptotic slope of $\ln[R(r, t)]$ versus time, as before in (4).

Patterson *et al.* [21] also point out that the reduced scattering coefficient $\mu_s(1 - g)$ is related to the time t_{max} at which a maximum in $R(r, t)$ occurs at radial position r:

$$\mu_s(1 - g) = \frac{1}{3r^2}\left[\frac{4\mu_a c^2 t_{max}^2}{n^2} + \frac{10ct_{max}}{n}\right] \quad (7)$$

where $r \gg z_0$. Therefore, time-resolved measurements can also yield the scattering properties of a tissue. Wilson *et al.* [22] have experimentally explored the behavior of such $R(r, t)$ measurements in phantom model tissues using photon-counting techniques. They have explored how anisotropy and albedo influence $R(r, t)$.

Bonner *et al.* and Nossal *et al.* have treated the migration of photons through tissues in an approximate form using lattice models to yield the time-resolved $R(r, t)$ [23], [24]. The lattice spacing is set equal to z_0 [see (5)]. The method, like diffusion theory, assumes that sufficient time has elapsed to randomize the propagation of photons before significant absorption has occurred. The solutions are essentially equivalent to those of diffusion theory.

Patterson *et al.* [21] integrated $R(r, t)$ over r to yield $R(t)$:

$$R(t) = \int_0^\infty R(r, t) 2\pi r \, dr = (4\pi Dc/n)^{-1/2} z_0 t^{-3/2}$$
$$\cdot \exp\left(-\frac{z_0^2}{4Dct/n}\right) e^{-\mu_a ct/n}. \quad (8)$$

The collected terms in (8) which multiply $e^{-\mu_a ct/n}$ correspond to the term $S(t)$ in (2):

$$S(t) = (4\pi Dc/n)^{-1/2} z_0 t^{-3/2} \exp\left(-\frac{z_0^2}{4Dct/n}\right). \quad (9)$$

In the above expression, $S(t)$ depends on D, which includes μ_a. Diffusion theory becomes reliable if $\mu_s(1 - g) \gg \mu_a$, in which case the value of D approaches $(3\mu_s(1 - g))^{-1}$ and $S(t)$ becomes independent of μ_a, consistent with the separation of variables of scattering and absorption in (2). Ito and Furutsu, in their study of pulse propagation through clouds, predicted that $R(t)$ in lossless media, i.e., $S(t)$, would behave as $t^{-3/2}$ [25].

The error in calculated μ_a that occurs with the use of (4) is identical to the second term on the right-hand side of (3), and is derived from (9):

$$\text{error} = \frac{n}{c} \frac{d \ln[S(t)]}{dt} = \frac{3n}{2ct} - \frac{z_0^2}{4D(ct/n)^2}. \quad (10)$$

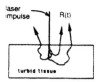

Fig. 1. Model simulation by the Monte Carlo method. An impulse of laser irradiation is delivered as an arbitrarily narrow beam perpendicular to a semi-infinite homogeneous tissue. Photons migrate through the tissue according to the rules of radiative transport. Photons escape at the surface as $R(t)$ in units of s^{-1}, and have traveled a total path length $L = ct/n$.

Monte Carlo Simulations: Monte Carlo simulations offer exact time-resolved solutions to the radiative transport equation by simulating the exact photon movement in terms of μ_a, μ_s, and $p(\theta)$. Simulations can treat the early reflectance events that occur before photon migration has become random. Delpy *et al.* [3] have used time-resolved Monte Carlo methods to explore absorption spectroscopy where delivery and collection fibers are widely spaced. Jacques [26] has used Monte Carlo methods to simulate time-resolved light distributions within turbid tissues as fs and ps laser pulses propagate in order to understand how scattering affects the light dosimetry for single-photon and two-photon photochemical reactions. Flock provided a time-resolved Monte Carlo simulation of $R(t)$ for comparison to diffusion theory [21].

In this paper, time-resolved Monte Carlo simulations yield the total $R(t)$ from a semi-infinite medium of homogeneous tissue after an impulse of perpendicular narrow-beam irradiance (Fig. 1). The results specify how the dynamics of $S(t)$ in (2) will affect the calculation of μ_a using (4).

METHODS

The time-resolved Monte Carlo simulation of photon movement has been described elsewhere [26]. Each photon is launched into the tissue with an initial weight of unity. As it propagates through the tissue in variable steps of free path between scattering sites, the weight of the photon is decreased by 1) tissue absorption, and 2) surface losses due to escape, which accumulate as total reflectance R_t. The photon weight at any given time t is given by $(1 - R_t)e^{-\mu_a ct/n}$. At each scattering site, the photon's trajectory is deflected according to a scattering function $p(\theta)$ that is defined by the Henyey-Greenstein function and characterized by its g value. Whenever the photon strikes the air/tissue surface, a fraction f of the photon weight escapes according to Fresnel's law for randomly polarized light to contribute to the observable reflectance at t, and the remaining fraction $1 - f$ is internally reflected back into the tissue and continues to propagate. The computer simulation program accumulates such contributions to escape in an array $R[i]$ with the programming statement

$$R[i] \leftarrow R[i] + \frac{f(1 - R_t)e^{-\mu_a ct/n}}{N} \qquad \text{where } i = \frac{t}{\Delta t} \tag{11}$$

where N is the total number of photons in the simulation (n equaled 10^4–10^5) and Δt is the time resolution of the numerical method ($\Delta t = 5$ ps). The accumulated total reflectance for each photon R_t, which can vary between 0 and 1, is set equal to zero before the launch of each photon (specular reflectance contributes to R_t at launch), and is updated after each escape event at the surface by the programming statement

$$R_t \leftarrow R + f(1 - R)e^{-\mu_a ct/n}. \tag{12}$$

After all N photons have been launched, the values of $R(t)$ are calculated from the array values of $R[i]$:

$$R(t) = \frac{R[i]}{\Delta t} \qquad \text{where } i = \frac{t}{\Delta t} \tag{13}$$

where is expressed in units of s^{-1}.

RESULTS

In Fig. 2 (upper) is shown the escape of light from tissues with various scattering coefficients: μ_s equals 1, 10, 100, and 1000 cm^{-1} ($\mu_a = 1$ cm^{-1}, $g = 0.9$, air/tissue interface, $n = 1.37$). Increasing μ_s greatly increases the initially observed reflectance in the first 20–200 ps (lines are hand drawn). However, at later times after 20–200 ps, the escape of light is less affected by μ_s, and the slope approaches the curve (lines are calculated) $kt^{-3/2}e^{-\mu_a ct/n}$ where k is a scaling factor that varies with μ_s ($k = 10^{-6.12}$, $10^{-5.43}$, $10^{-5.60}$, $10^{-5.99}$ for $\mu_s = 1, 10, 100, 1000$ cm^{-1}, respectively). Indeed, the highest value of escape at later times occurs for $\mu_s = 10$ cm^{-1}, i.e., a $\mu_s(1 - g)/\mu_a$ ratio of unity. Higher μ_s causes too much initial scattering, and lower μ_s yields too weak scattering.

In Fig. 2 (lower) is shown the influence of absorption. Increasing the absorption coefficient μ_a increases the magnitude of the slope of $\ln[R(t)]$ versus time. After the early reflectance (lines are hand drawn), $R(t)$ behaves as the curve (lines are calculated) $kt^{-3/2}e^{-\mu_a ct/n}$ where $k = 10^{-5.60}$ for all μ_a values. Measurement of the slow attenuation of escaping light after the initial rapid expansion of the light distribution in the tissue offers a sensitive indicator of μ_a. The higher the μ_a value to be measured, however, the shorter is the time available for reliable measurement before attenuation extinguishes the signal.

In Fig. 3, μ_a values are deduced by (4) (the derivative was specified by linear regression of $\ln[R(t)]$ versus t over five data near each time point, $t \pm 10$ ps) and plotted time for μ_a values equal to 1, 2, and 3 cm^{-1}. During the first ≈ 30 ps, the calculated μ_a rises quickly from a negative value. Thereafter, the calculated μ_a is artifactually high due to the influence of $S(t)$ [see (2) and (3)], but the error decreases with time in a predictable manner. A single empirical curve fits all the Monte Carlo data regardless of the absorption coefficient: calculated $\mu_a = 3n/2ct - C_1 \exp(-t/\tau_1) - C_2 \exp(-t/\tau_2)$ where C_1, τ_1, C_2, τ_2 are 120, 5.44 ps, 0.835, and 55.4 ps, respectively. The upper solid line indicates the behavior predicted by diffusion theory using (8) and (9). After ≈ 50

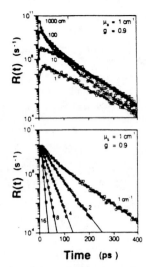

Fig. 2. Influence of scattering and absorption on the escape of light from a typical tissue following an impulse of light. Upper figure: The scattering coefficient is varied (μ_s = 1, 10, 100, 1000 cm^{-1}), while the absorption coefficient (μ_a = 1 cm^{-1}) and anisotropy ($\langle\cos(\theta)\rangle$ or g = 0.9) are held constant. Note the strong influence of μ_s on $R(t)$ during the first 50 ps (lines are hand drawn). Later, the slopes become similar and $R(t)$ behaves (lines are calculated) as $kt^{-3/2}e^{-\mu_a ct/n}$ where k is a scaling constant that varies with μ_s (k = 10$^{-6.12}$, 10$^{-5.43}$, 10$^{-5.60}$, 10$^{-5.99}$ for μ_s = 1, 10, 100, 1000, respectively). Lower figure: The absorption coefficient is varied (μ_a = 1, 2, 4, 8, 16 cm^{-1}), while the scattering (μ_s = 100 cm^{-1}) and anisotropy (g = 0.9) are held constant. After the early reflectance (lines are hand drawn), the behavior of $R(t)$ approaches (lines are calculated) the curve $kt^{-3/2}e^{-\mu_a ct/n}$ where k = 10$^{-5.60}$. (Monte Carlo simulations for semi-infinite slab of tissue.)

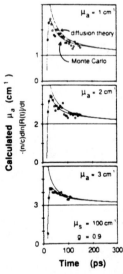

Fig. 3. Calculated absorption coefficient based on the slope of $\ln[R(t)]$ versus time. During the initial phase of rapid redistribution of light within a turbid tissue following an impulse, the calculated μ_a values obtained from the expression $-(n/c)\,d\ln[R(t)]/dt$ are artifactually too high. Monte Carlo simulations indicate the calculated μ_a values versus time for (a) μ_a = 1 cm^{-1}, (b) μ_a = 2 cm^{-1}, and (c) μ_a = 3 cm^{-1}. A single empirical curve fits all Monte Carlo results for the particular scattering properties (μ_s = 100 cm^{-1}, g = 0.9) regardless of the true μ_a: calculated $\mu_a = 3n/2ct - C_1 \exp(-t/\tau_1) - C_2 \exp(-t/\tau_2)$ where C_1, τ_1, C_2, τ_2 are 120, 5.44 ps, 0.835, 55.4 ps, respectively. For comparison, the calculated μ_a values based on diffusion theory predictions of $R(t)$ are also shown.

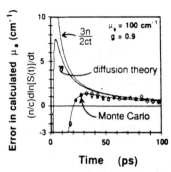

Fig. 4. The error in calculated absorption coefficient. The error in calculated μ_a values based on $-(n/c)\,d\ln[R(t)]/dt$ is equal to the term $(n/c)\,d\ln[S(t)]/dt$ where $S(t)$ is the probability that scattered light will reach the tissue surface and escape at time t in the absence of tissue absorption. This error approaches zero at later times. The error based on Monte Carlo simulations is shown as symbols (μ_a = 1, 2, 3 cm^{-1} depicted as boxes, triangles, and crosses, respectively). The error predicted by diffusion theory is also shown. For the particular scattering properties in this example (μ_s = 100 cm^{-1}, g = 0.9), after $\approx$ 50 ps, the error is well described by the $3n/2ct$ curve which is independent of tissue optical properties. As μ_s increases, the error more quickly approaches the $3n/2ct$ curve, and as μ_s decreases, there is a longer delay before convergence (not shown).

ps, there is only a slight difference between calculated μ_a values derived from Monte Carlo simulation and diffusion theory. At 200 ps, both methods are in close agreement and overestimate the true μ_a by 0.34 cm^{-1}. These results only hold for the particular scattering properties of this example (μ_s = 100 cm^{-1}, g = 0.9).

In Fig. 4, the error in the μ_a value calculated by (4) is plotted versus time. This error is equal to $(n/c)\,d\ln[S(t)]/dt$, as discussed in (3). The Monte Carlo data (μ_a = 1, 2, 3 cm^{-1} depicted as boxes, triangles, and crosses, respectively) are plotted as $-(n/c)\,d\ln[R(t)]/dt - \mu_a$ to yield the error. For comparison, the error based on the diffusion theory prediction of $R(t)$ is also shown (10). After $\approx$ 50 ps, both Monte Carlo and diffusion theory results closely approach the $3n/2ct$ curve, which is independent of tissue optical properties. Monte Carlo simulations (not shown) indicate that higher scattering coefficients cause the error to approach the $3n/2ct$ curve more quickly, and lower scattering coefficients delay the convergence. For example, for μ_s equal to 1000 and 1 cm^{-1}, the delay is approximately 20 and 200 ps, respectively.

DISCUSSION

As the narrow impulse of collimated light enters the tissue, it expands into a distribution of diffuse light, a "glowball." The dynamics of the light distribution can be considered in terms of two phases.

Phase I—The Initial Rapid Expansion into a Glowball: This phase occurs in the first few hundred ps for our typical turbid tissue, and the dynamics of collected light are dominated by the term $S(t)$ in (2).

Phase II—The Subsequent Extinction of the Glowball: This phase occurs after the expansion of the glowball has slowed and $S(t)$ has stabilized. The dynamics of collected light become dominated by the steady rate of light absorption, the term $e^{-\mu_a ct/n}$ in (2). To the observer, the glowball stops expanding and simply extinguishes, as if someone turned off a dimmer switch. It is possible to deduce the absorption coefficient directly from the slope $d \ln[R(t)]/dt$, regardless of the amount of light scattering. Time-resolved reflectance offers an opportunity to simplify absorption spectroscopy in turbid tissues.

According to diffusion theory, the error in calculated μ_a using (4) decreases with time proportional to $1/t$. The term $z_0^2/(4D(ct/n)^2)$ in (10) influences the early error behavior, but becomes small after the first 20–200 ps for typical tissue optical properties (this time delay depends on scattering properties). Thereafter, the error is adequately described by the $3n/2ct$ term which is independent of tissue optical properties. Therefore, correction of the error becomes simple after 20–200 ps, and the combination of (3) and (10) can reliably yield μ_a:

$$\mu_a = -\frac{n}{c}\frac{d\ln[R(t)]}{dt} - \frac{3n}{2ct}. \qquad (14)$$

The details of the early error behavior depends on the tissue optical properties and on the details of the mismatched boundary condition, i.e., the refractive indexes of the external media and tissue and the roughness of the tissue surface. Monte Carlo simulations are in progress to fully characterize the parameters that specify $R(t)$ during the first 20–200 ps when diffusion theory is inadequate.

The volume of tissue involved in the measurement increases with time as the light diffuses through the tissue. The use of (14) assumes that this volume is composed of tissue with homogeneous, isotropic optical properties. The volume of tissue that must meet this criteria is specified by a volume radius r that approximately equals $(6Dtc/n)^{1/2}$ where t is the time of measurement (based on three-dimensional random walk theory). For $t = 50$ ps and typical values of $\mu_s = 100$ cm^{-1} and $g = 0.9$, r equals ≈ 5 mm. Measurements at later times will involve increasingly larger tissue volumes.

Catheter-based reflectance spectroscopy will measure the optical absorption coefficient of a tissue volume at the catheter tip. Reliable measurements of larger tissue volumes are possible in organs (e.g., brain, liver, kidney) and tumors. To deduce the μ_a in smaller tissue volumes ($r < 5$ mm) requires the use of the early reflectance data prior to 50 ps. Such measurements would be useful in measuring blood and clots within vessels, the superficial walls of the gastrointestinal and esophageoal tracts, or the first mm of tissue at a catheter tip which receives strong therapeutic laser irradiation. A more sophisticated analysis and better understanding of the effects of boundary conditions, fiber geometry, and tissue heterogeneities on such measurements must be developed before catheter-based time-resolved reflectance spectroscopy can be applied to small tissue volumes. Monte Carlo simulations are well suited for this purpose.

Another limit occurs at high values of μ_a. The extinction of the light may become so rapid that insufficient time is available for reliable measurements. For example, consider measurements of $R(t)$ using a streak camera, with a 1 ps time resolution that allows ten measurements within a 10 ps period. The data that can be acquired within a sampling time of a few seconds may extend over a dynamic range of two orders of magnitude. Suppose that $R(t)$ can be measured over two orders of magnitude within a time period t_m to allow reliable calculation of the slope $d \ln[R(t)]/dt$. The required t_m depends on the absorption coefficient: $t_m = \ln[10^2]n/c\mu_a$. For $t_m = 10$ ps, the upper limit to μ_a is 21 cm^{-1}. Therefore, measurements of μ_a in the "therapeutic window" of 600–1300 nm are possible, but measurements may become difficult in the shorter visible and UV wavelengths where hemoglobin, melanin, and protein are strongly absorbing or in the longer near-IR wavelengths where tissue water is strongly absorbing.

ACKNOWLEDGMENT

Thanks to M. Keijzer and S. Flock, University of Texas M. D. Anderson Cancer Center, for critical review of the manuscript; to S. Prahl and A. J. Welch, University of Texas at Austin, for continued collaboration on Monte Carlo simulations; to B. Wilson, S. Madsen, and M. Patterson of Hamilton Regional Cancer Centre, Ontario, P. Young, Massachusetts Institute of Technology, and Y. Hefetz, Massachusetts General Hospital, for discussions and ongoing collaborative experiments on time-resolved reflectance measurements; to B. Chance, University of Pennsylvania, and D. Delpy, University College of London, and their colleagues whose experimental work first motivated us all.

REFERENCES

[1] R. Alfano, Ed., *Biological Events Probed by Ultra-Fast Laser Spectroscopy*. New York: Academic, 1982.
[2] B. Chance, J. S. Leigh, J. Miyake, D. S. Smith, S. Nioka, R. Greenfeld, M. Finander, K. Kaufmann, W. E. Levy, M. Young, P. Cohen, H. Yoshioka, and R. Boretsky, "Comparison of time-resolved and -unresolved measurements of deoxyhemoglobin in brain," *PNAS*, vol. 85, pp. 4971–4975, 1988.
[3] D. M. Delpy, M. Cope, P. van der See, S. Arridge, S. Wray, and J. Wyatt, "Estimation of optical pathlength through tissue from direct time-of-flight measurements," *Phys. Med. Biol.*, vol. 33, pp. 1433–1442, 1988.
[4] S. L. Jacques, C. A. Alter, and S. A. Prahl, "Angular dependence of HeNe laser light scattering by human dermis," *Lasers Life Sci.*, vol. 1, pp. 309–333, 1987.
[5] S. T. Flock, B. C. Wilson, and M. S. Patterson, "Total attenuation coefficients and scattering phase functions of tissues and phantom materials at 633 nm," *Med. Phys.*, vol. 14, pp. 835–841, 1987.
[6] G. Yoon, A. J. Welch, M. Motamedi, and M. C. J. van Gemert, "Development and application of three-dimensional light distribution model for laser irradiated tissue," *IEEE J. Quantum Electron.*, vol. QE-23, pp. 1721–1733, 1987.
[7] L. G. Henyey and J. L. Greenstein, "Diffuse radiation in the galaxy," *Astrophys. J.*, vol. 93, pp. 70–83, 1941.
[8] J. A. Parrish, "New concepts in therapeutic photomedicine: Photochemistry, optical targeting and the therapeutic window," *J. Invest. Dermatol.*, vol. 77, pp. 45–50, 1981.
[9] A. Ishimaru, *Wave Propagation and Scattering in Random Media, Vol. I*. New York: Academic, 1978.
[10] R. F. Bonner, R. Nossal, S. Havlin, G. H. Weiss, "Model for photon migration in turbid biological media," *J. Opt. Soc. Amer. A*, vol. 4, pp. 423–432, 1987.

[11] R. Nossal, J. Kiefer, G. H. Weiss, R. Bonner, H. Taitelbaum, and S. Havlin, "Photon migration in layered media," *Appl. Opt.*, vol. 27, pp. 3382-3391, 1988.

[12] M. S. Patterson, E. Schwartz, and B. C. Wilson, "Quantitative reflectance spectrophotometry for the noninvasive measurement of photosensitizer concentration in tissue during photodynamic therapy," in *Proc. SPIE*, Los Angeles, CA, 1989.

[13] H. C. van de Hulst, *Multiple Light Scattering, Vol. II*. New York: Academic, 1980.

[14] S. L. Jacques and S. A. Prahl, "Modeling optical and thermal distributions in tissue during laser irradiation," *Lasers Surg. Med.*, vol. 6, pp. 494-503, 1987.

[15] R. A. J. Groenhuis, J. J. Ten Bosch, and H. A. Ferwerda, "Scattering and absorption of turbid materials determined from reflection measurements. 2. Measuring method and calibration," *Appl. Opt.*, vol. 22, pp. 2463-2467, 1983.

[16] J. A. Weinmann and S. T. Shipley, "Effects of multiple scattering on laser pulses transmitted through clould," *J. Geophys. Res.*, vol. 77, pp. 7123-7128, 1972.

[17] E. A. Bucher and R. M. Lerner, "Experiments on light pulse communication and propagation through atmospheric clouds," *Appl. Opt.*, vol. 12, pp. 2401-2414, 1973.

[18] A. Ishimaru, "Diffusion of a pulse in densely distributed scatterers," *J. Opt. Soc. Amer.*, vol. 68, pp. 1045-1050, 1978.

[19] K. Shimizu, A. Ishimaru, L. Reynolds, and A. P. Breuckner, "Backscattering of a picosecond pulse from densely distributed scatterers," *Appl. Oct.*, vol. 18, pp. 3484-3488, 1979.

[20] Y. Kuga, A. Ishimaru, and A. P. Bruckner, "Experiments on picosecond pulse propagation in a diffuse medium," *J. Opt. Soc. Amer.*, vol. 73, pp. 1812-1815, 1983.

[21] M. S. Patterson, B. Chance, and B. C. Wilson, "Time resolved reflectance and transmittance for the noninvasive measurement of tissue optical properties," *App. Opt.*, vol. 28, 1989.

[22] B. Wilson, T. Park, Y. Hefetz, M. Patterson, S. Madsen, and S. Jacques, "The potential of time-resolved reflectance measurements for the noninvasive determination of tissue optical properties," in *Proc. SPIE*, Los Angeles, CA, 1989.

[23] R. F. Bonner, R. Nossal, and G. H. Weiss, "A random walk theory of time-resolved optical absorption spectyroscopy in tissue," in *Proc. Workshop Photon Migration in Tissue*, B. Chance, Ed. New York: Plenum, 1989.

[24] R. Nossal, R. F. Bonner, and G. H. Weiss, "The influence of path length on remote optical sensing of properties of biological tissue," *Appl. Opt.*, 1989.

[25] S. Ito and K. Furutsu, "Theory of light pulse propagation through thick clouds," *J. Opt. Soc. Amer.*, vol. 70, pp. 366-374, 1980.

[26] S. L. Jacques, "Time-resolved propagation of ultra-short laser pulses within turbid tissues," *Appl. Opt.*, vol. 28, 1989.

Steven L. Jacques, for a photograph and biography, see this issue, p. 1154.

Reprinted with permission from *Journal of the Optical Society of America B,* Vol. 7(8), pp. 1685-1693 (August 1990). ©1990 Optical Society of America.

Biological materials probed by the temporal and angular profiles of the backscattered ultrafast laser pulses

K. M. Yoo, Feng Liu, and R. R. Alfano

Institute for Ultrafast Spectroscopy and Lasers, Department of Physics, The City College of New York, New York, New York 10031

Temporal and angular profiles of backscattered pulses are introduced as a practical, novel, and noninvasive technique to probe biological materials. The optical properties of these materials are quantitatively measured in terms of two scattering-length scales: the transport mean free path and the absorption length of the light. We show that these two scattering lengths can be directly determined from an analysis of the temporal or the angular profile of the backscattered pulse intensity. Experimental results for transient light backscattering from eye, heart, lung, and breast tissues, and from a tooth and a leaf, are presented.

Ultrafast laser pulses in the femtosecond (10^{-15} sec) and picosecond (10^{-12} sec) time domains can be routinely generated with the current state of ultrafast laser technology.[1] Ultrafast streak-detection technology has made possible time-resolved detection on the picosecond and femtosecond time scales.[2,3] The combination of these two state-of-the-art technologies will most likely find a wide range of novel applications in medical diagnosis and material analysis in the near future. The gross optical properties of biological materials can be quantitatively measured in terms of two scattering parameters: the transport mean free path and the absorption lengths of the light traveling in the medium. These parameters can be in turn used to determine the state of the biological material. The absorption length l_a is the distance over which the light propagates in the medium before it is absorbed. This length depends on the chemical composition of the medium i.e., the absorption cross section and the concentration of the absorbing molecules present in the medium. Thus a change in absorption length may indicate a change in chemical composition of the biological material. The transport mean free path l_t is the mean distance over which the light travels between scattering. In a random medium, l_t is simply related to $1/n\sigma_m$, where n is the number density and σ_m is the momentum-exchange scattering cross section of the particle or cell. The σ_m depends on the size of the particle relative to the wavelength of light and the refractive index of the particle. If the arrangement of the particles in the medium is correlated, the light may not be scattered so much as it would be in a completely random medium. This reduction in scattering is due to the correlation of the phase of the scattered light, which reduces the amount of scattering. The light will have a longer transport mean free path in a medium in which the particles are correlated. A change in the state of the material, such as dehydration, would result a change in number density, particle size, particle–particle correlation, and aggregation of particles into a larger particle. These changes would result in different l_t.

The parameters l_t and l_a can be obtained from the transmission technique by either a continuous wave[4-6] or an ultrafast laser pulse.[7,8] The main disadvantages of the transmission technique are the following: (1) it requires a measurement of the thickness of the sample, (2) it may not be feasible for bulk samples because the transmitted energy can become too weak to be detected, and (3) it measures the average properties of the slab through which the light propagates rather than the optical properties over a thin penetration depth. These disadvantages do not exist when the backscattering technique is used. The backscattering geometry has the potential to be a noninvasive technique. Diffuse reflectance spectroscopy[9] has been widely used in the past to determine the absorption spectra of absorbing random media. However, it is extremely difficult to obtain quantitatively the scattering and absorption lengths simultaneously by using the diffuse reflectance technique. The temporal profile of the backscattered pulse[10-16] can be used to determine the scattering parameters of random media. In this paper we show the capability of the present state-of-the-art ultrafast laser technologies to probe biological media in which the photon transport mean free path and the absorption length are obtained from the temporal or the angular profile of a backscattered ultrafast pulse.

In a highly scattering medium, light propagation may be described as diffusive. The intensity of the backscattered light may be obtained by using the diffusion approximation. The temporal profile of a backscattered pulse is determined by the diffusion coefficient $D_0 = vl_t/3$ and the absorption coefficient $\gamma_a = v/l_a$, where v is the effective speed of the wave in the medium. The expression for the intensity of the scattered pulse in the multiple-scattering regime is[10]

$$I(\hat{s}, t) = \int_0^\infty \mathrm{d}t' R(\hat{s}, t')[1 + \exp(-D_0 q^2 t')]$$

$$\times \exp(-\gamma_a t')I_0(t - t'), \qquad (1)$$

where $I_0(t - t')$ is the incident pulse and $R(\hat{s}, t')$ is the response function of the random medium. In the diffusion approximation, one can write

$$R(\hat{s}, t') = \alpha \frac{1}{\sqrt{2\pi}} \exp(D_0 t'/2l_t{}^2) D_{-3}[2D_0 t'/l_t{}^2]^{1/2}, \quad (2)$$

where α is a proportional constant, l_t is the transport mean free path, and $D_{-3}(x) = u(5/2, x)$ is the parabolic cylinder (Weber) function. The coherent interference arising from time-reversal symmetry is taken into account by the factor $\exp(-D_0 q^2 t')$ in Eq. (1), where $q = 2\pi \sin \theta/\lambda$ and θ is the angle between the direction of the scattered light $\hat{s}$ and the incident light. For a finite detecting time resolution, the measured intensity of the backscattered pulse is a convolution of Eq. (1) with the response function $r(t - t')$ of the detecting instrument and is given by

$$I_m(\hat{s}, t) = \int_{-\infty}^{\infty} dt' r(t - t') I(\hat{s}, t'). \quad (3)$$

In this paper the backscattered pulses are computed for comparison with experimental data. The profiles have been convoluted with the temporal response of the streak camera, which is 8 psec full width at half-maximum (FWHM) with a Gaussian profile.

The backscattered light from discrete random media has been found to exhibit the phenomenon of weak localization,[17-27] which arises from the coherent interference between the scattered light and its time-reversed counterpart in the random medium. This interference enhances the intensity of the light scattered in the backward direction within a small angular spread. In the exact backward direction the intensity of the scattered light is nearly twice the diffuse intensity. The intensity decreases to a constant value (equal to diffuse intensity) as the angle of the scattered light increases.

The profile of the angular distribution of scattered light intensity about the backward direction, known as the coherent peak, depends on the transport mean free path l_t and the absorption length l_a of the light in the medium. The angular width of the coherent peak can be directly related to l_t by $\lambda/2\pi l_t$, where λ is the wavelength. The line shape of the coherent peak can be quantitatively described by[20-22]

$$\alpha(\theta) = \frac{3}{16\pi} \left\{ 1 + 2\frac{z_0}{l_t} + \frac{1}{(1 + ql_t)^2} \left[1 + \frac{1 - \exp(-2qz_0)}{ql_t} \right] \right\}, \quad (4)$$

where θ is the angle of the scattered light measured from the exact backward direction, $q = 2\pi\theta/\lambda$, and z_0 is determined by the boundary condition (in a plane interface, $z_0 \approx 0.7l$).

In the case of an absorbing medium, the light that undergoes a long scattering path in the medium will be attenuated. The light scattered through longer path lengths contributes to a narrow portion of the coherent peak near $\theta = 0$.[22,23,27] Cutting off the portion of scattered light that has followed a long scattering path, as would occur in an absorbing medium, reduces the height of the coherent peak. In an absorbing medium q is given by

$$q = (q^2 + q_a{}^2)^{1/2}, \quad (5)$$

where

$$q_a{}^2 = 3/(l_a l). \quad (6)$$

The above description of coherent backscattering has been successfully applied to discrete random media. Biological tissues, by contrast, are a mixture of continuous and discrete components, which may differ somewhat from discrete random media. However, the average scattering characteristics of either kind of medium can be described by the transport mean free path and the absorption length. Thus one would expect Eqs. (4)–(6) to hold for the backscattering of light from biological tissues.

The measured angular profile of the backscattered light is a convolution of Eq. (4) with the angular response of the detection system and is given by

$$\alpha_m(\theta) = \int_{\infty}^{-\infty} d\theta' \alpha(\theta') r(\theta - \theta'), \quad (7)$$

where $r(\theta - \theta')$ is the angular response function of the measuring system.

Equation (1) implies that the temporal profile of the backscattered pulse is determined by both the transport mean free path l_t and the absorption length l_a. For large l_t, the time interval between scattering events is large. Thus the temporal profile of the backscattered pulse from a long l_t medium will be broader than from a short l_t medium. As an illustration, the temporal profiles of the backscattered pulses are computed from Eq. (1) and plotted in Fig. 1(a) for $l_t = 50$, 500, 5000, and 50 000 μm and $l_a = \infty$, which is the case for a nonabsorbing medium. The pulse broadens as l_t increases. Figure 1(b) shows the corresponding cases of Fig. 1(a) when the temporal profile is convoluted with the impulse response of the detecting system. For a short transport mean free path, for example, $l_t = 300$ μm, the full width at $1/e$ of the maximum scattered pulse intensity is approximately a picosecond. The scattered pulse profile at early times is similar to the impulse-response function. Comparing the pulse profiles of Figs. 1(a) and 1(b), one finds that the observed profiles at early times are greatly affected by the instrumental response for a short l_t medium. The full width at $1/e$ maxima computed for l_t range from 10 to 10,000 μm and are plotted in Fig. 1(c). The full width at $1/e$ maximum of the temporal profile for $l_t = 50$ μm is 0.2 psec.

Although the temporal profiles at early times are significantly affected by the instrumental response, the presence of a long tail at later times in the temporal profile helps us to determine the value of l_t for values as short as 50 μm. The weight of the high-intensity scattering at early times, which is governed mainly by the time resolution of the streak camera, can be significantly deemphasized by taking the logarithm of the intensity $I(t)$ in the curve-fitting process. That is, fitting the curve of $\log I(t)$ versus time t could significantly improve our estimation of l_t compared with fitting $I(t)$ versus t directly, especially for short l_t. A faster time-resolution detecting system is necessary for probing media with shorter l_t values. A time response in the subpicosecond regime is now available from a single-shot streak camera. Improved time resolution but with lower sensitivity can also be achieved by using a cross correlation or a Kerr gate technique. Nevertheless, the

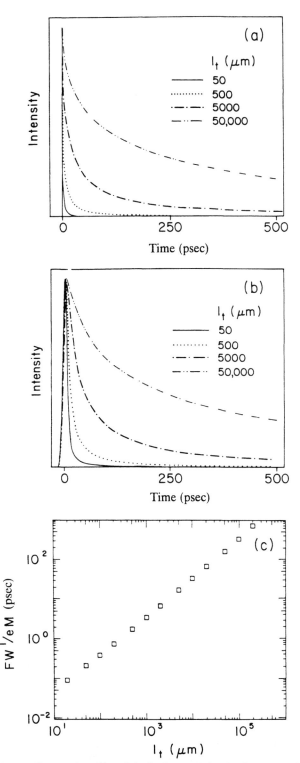

Fig. 1 Temporal profiles of the backscattered pulse for values of l_t = 50, 500, 5000, and 50 000 μm computed (a) from Eq. (1); (b) from Eq. (3), i.e., convolution of Eq. (1) with 8 psec FWHM. There is no absorption. (c) Log–log plot of full width at $1/e$ maxima of the backscattered pulse computed from Eq. (1) for various values of l_t.

present synchroscan streak camera with an 8-psec response is capable of studying biological materials. As we shall show below, the l_t for most biological materials is longer than 100 μm.

In an absorbing medium, light that undergoes a long scattering path length or that emerges from the medium at later times has a higher probability of being attenuated. The reduction in intensity at later times depends on the absorption length. Figure 2(a) illustrates the temporal profile predicted with different absorption lengths l_a of 500, 2000, 5000, and 50 000 μm, given that l_t = 200 μm. A semilog plot of the scattered intensity from Fig. 2(a) is plotted in Fig. 2(b) and shows that the temporal profiles at later times are linear. The gradient of the linear slope at later times indicates the absorption length.

As we mentioned above, the intensity of the backscattered light around the backward direction is enhanced because of coherent interference between the scattered light and its time-reversed counterpart. Figure 3 illustrates the salient features of the angular profiles of the coherent peak for various values of l_t. The angular width of the coherent peak becomes narrower as l_t increases, as illustrated in Fig. 3(a) for l_t = 50, 500, and 5000 μm. The possibility of measuring larger l_t from the coherent peak may be restricted by the angular divergence of the laser and the nonideal nature of the detecting system. For the

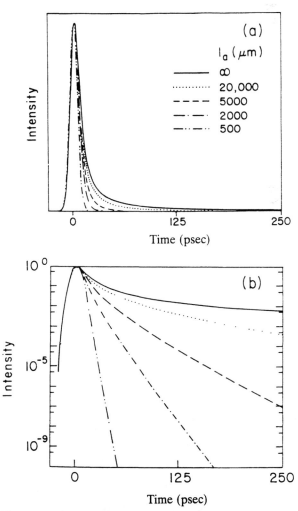

Fig. 2. (a) Temporal profiles of the backscattered pulse computed from Eq. (1) for values of l_a = $-\infty$, 20 000, 5000, 2000, and 500 μm. l_t = 200 μm. The impulse response of the detection is 8 psec FWHM. (b) Semilog plot of (a).

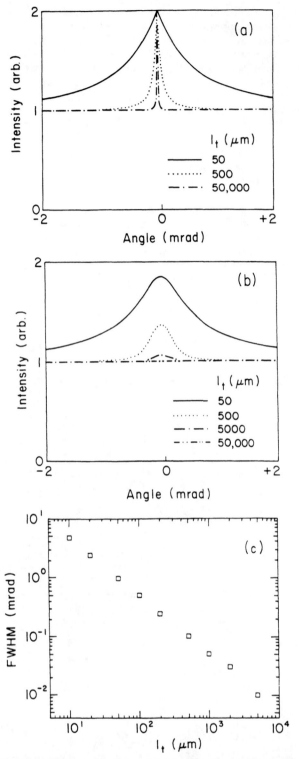

combination of the divergence of the laser and the instrument response of the lens collecting system and the streak camera. Figure 3(b) shows the convoluted angular profiles for the corresponding cases in Fig. 3(a). The angular profile with angle less than 0.3 mrad is significantly modified by the instrumental response. When $l_t = 5000$ μm, the FWHM of the coherent peak is 0.01 mrad. The intensity of the scattered light within this narrow coherent peak is smeared over an angle of 0.3 mrad. The height of the measured coherent peak is significantly reduced, and one could hardly see it. To illustrate the experimental limitation, the FWHM of the coherent peak for l_t ranging from 10 to 10 000 μm is plotted in Fig. 3(c). As discussed above, for a 4-mm-diameter beam at $\lambda = 620$ nm the diffraction is 0.2 mrad, which limits our ability to measure a medium with l_t larger than 500 μm or an angular width of less than 0.1 mrad FWHM.

Figure 4(a) illustrates the salient features of the angular profiles of the coherent peak for various values of $l_a = 20\,000$, 5000, 2000, and 500 μm. The height of the coherent peak is reduced as the absorption length of the medium decreases. This reduction can be understood

Fig. 3. Angular profile of the coherent peak of the backscattered light from nonabsorbing media with values of $l_t = 50$, 500, and 5000 μm, computed from (a) Eq. (4); (b) Eq. (7), which convolutes Eq. (4) with 0.3 mrad FWHM. (c) Log–log plot of the FWHM of the coherent peak for various l_t.

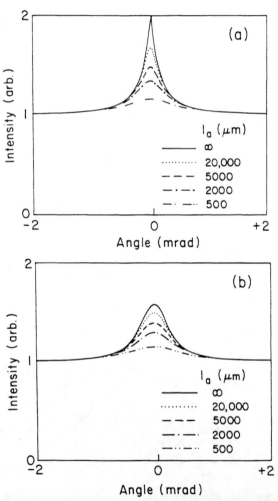

Fig. 4. (a) Angular profile of the coherent peak of the backscattered light from absorbing media with various l_a and with $l_t = 200$ μm. (b) Convolution of (a) with 0.3 mrad FWHM angle response obtained by using Eq. (7).

laser used here the beam diameter is $d = 4$ mm, the wavelength is $\lambda = 620$ nm, and the angular diffraction $1.2\lambda/d$ is 0.2 mrad FWHM. In our experimental setup, we measure the angle response to be 0.3 mrad FWHM, which is a

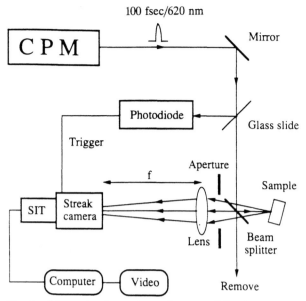

100 fsec/620 nm

Fig. 5. Schematic of experimental setup. SIT, silicon intensified target.

from the fact that the light that undergoes a long scattering path and contributes to the central portion of the coherent peak is being removed by absorption. The modification of the coherent peaks due to an instrumental response of 0.3 mrad FWHM is shown in Fig. 4(b) for the corresponding cases in Fig. 4(a).

The limitations in measuring l_t that are due to finite time response and angle response of the instrument are complementary. The 8-psec time response limits our capability to determine l_t for values smaller than 50 μm from fitting the temporal profile. With an angle response of 0.3 mrad one can easily determine l_t equal to or smaller than 50 μm from fitting the angular profile of the backscattered light. However, with this angle response one cannot determine l_t values greater than 500 μm. But this large l_t can be determined from the temporal profile of the scattered pulse.

A schematic diagram of the experimental setup is shown in Fig. 5. Ultrafast laser pulses of 100 fsec (repetition rate 82 MHz, $\lambda = 620$ nm, spectral bandwidth 15 nm, beam diameter 3 mm, beam power 10 mW) were generated from a colliding-pulse mode-locked dye laser (CPM).[1] The laser beam was collimated and incident upon the biological tissues after reflection from a beam splitter. The light scattered from the sample around the backward direction was angularly resolved by a 500-mm focal-length lens. The detector (Hamamatsu streak camera) was placed at the focal plane of the lens. Each position on the face of the detector corresponds to a given scattering angle. The temporal and angular information for the scattered pulse from the tisue was acquired simultaneously. Each datum was acquired over a time duration of 15 sec. In the angular profile measurement, the polarization of the scattered light parallel to the incident light is measured.

We illustrate several examples of temporal and angular profiles of ultrafast laser pulses backscattered from different biological media, showing the versatility of the method.

Figure 6 illustrates the backscattered pulse at an angle of 3° from two different tissues in the heart: the fat tissue deposited upon the heart and the heart tissue itself. Their temporal profiles are different, and one can easily distinguish between them. The temporal profile of the fat is shorter but with a longer tail, indicating shorter l_t and longer l_a. These are reasonable because the fatty portions are white and absorb light less strongly than heart tissue, which contains strongly absorbing hemoglobin.

Figure 7 plots a series of backscattered pulses at an angle of 3° from different portions of a human canine tooth. The scattered pulse from the top portion of the

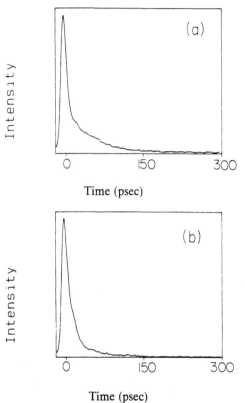

Fig. 6. Temporal profiles and backscattered pulses at an angle of 3° from (a) fatty and (b) muscle tissue of a heart.

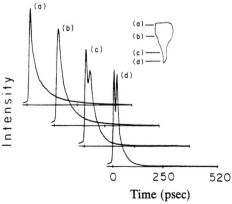

Fig. 7. Temporal profiles of backscattered pulses at an angle of 3° from different portions of a tooth.

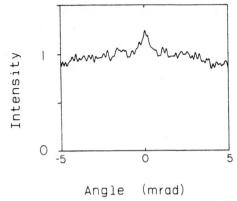

Fig. 8. Angular profiles of total time-integrated backscattered pulses from a tooth.

tooth is plotted in curve (a). From fitting of the temporal profile to the theory, we obtain $l_t = 3.2 \pm 2$ mm and $l_a = 85 \pm 5$ mm. The uncertainty provided is uncertainty in fitting the experimental curve. The temporal profiles from the root of the tooth show a double peak and a much shorter tail. The short tail indicates that the scattered light is being cut off at some later time because of the finite thickness of the tooth; the light scattered out from the other side will be lost. Because of refractive-index mismatch at the second tooth–air interface, light is reflected, and part of it is scattered and is detected by the streak camera as a second peak. The temporal distance between the two peaks can be used to estimate the optical thickness or the refractive index of the medium. The presence of second peak shows that ultrafast laser pulses can penetrate deep into the tooth or bone, indicating the possibility of using ultrafast technologies to probe a cavity in a tooth. The angular profile of the total time-integrated backscattered light from the tooth is presented in Fig. 8.

The backscattered intensity at an angle of 3° of a laser pulse as a function of time, for a clear, a partially cataracted, and a severely cataracted eye lens are shown in Figs. 9(a), 9(b), and 9(c), respectively. The cataracts are artificially induced in the bovine eye lens by submerging the eye in a saline solution containing hydrogen peroxide. The two peaks displayed in Figs. 9(a) and 9(b) arise from scattering off the front and the back interfaces between the eye lens and the saline solution. The temporal separation δt between these two peaks is approximately 40 psec. The thickness of the lens d can be computed from this time separation as $d = c\,\delta t/2n_g$, where c is the speed of light and n_g is the refractive index of the lens. The thickness of the lens is computed to be approximately 4 mm, which is in fair agreement with the actual lens thickness.

In a clear eye, there is little scattering in the lens. Only scattering at the interfaces is observed, as shown by the two clear peaks in Fig. 9(a). As the eye develops a cataract, some of the light is scattered inside the eye lens. This scattering reduces the ratio of the intensity of the back to the front peak, as illustrated in Fig. 9(b). This decrease in ratio is a measure of the extent of scattering in the lens and hence increasing opacity owing to formation of cataracts. For a severely cataracted eye, the light undergoes multiple scattering, and the diffusion approximation

for light scattering holds. The experimental data in Fig. 9(c) can be fitted to the theory. The best fit between eperiment and theory is plotted in Fig. 10. The transport mean free path and the absorption length are found to be 200 ± 50 μm and 30 ± 5 mm, respectively. The absorption length is 150 times longer than the transport mean free path. This measurement shows that the attenuation due to absorption is significantly smaller than that due to scattering at $\lambda = 620$ nm.

Figure 11 shows the angular distribution of the total time-integrated scattered laser intensity from human breast tissue. The coherent peak is clearly seen. A similar effect but with a wider coherent peak was observed in human benign lung tissue, which is shown in Fig. 12. The transport mean free path l_t, and the absorption length l_a can be obtained by fitting the experimental data with Eqs. (4)–(7) convoluted with the angular resolution of detection. For the breast tissue, the best fit to the experimental data of the coherent peak occurs when $l_t = 250 \pm 30$ μm and $l_a = 4000 \pm 1000$ μm. In the case of lung tissue, $l_t = 80 \pm 20$ μm and $l_a = 3000 \pm 1000$ μm for the best fit. The theoretical fits are traced by smooth

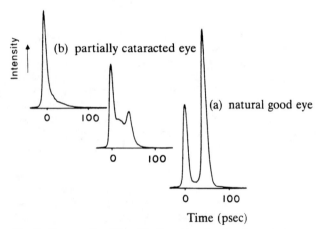

Fig. 9. Temporal profiles of backscattered pulses from eye lenses with different characteristics.

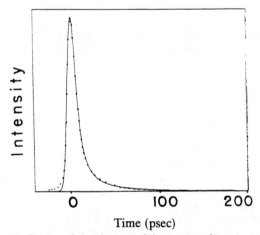

Fig. 10 Fitting of the theory (solid curve) to the experimental data (dotted curve) for a severely cataracted eye.

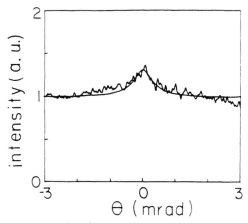

Fig. 11. Angular distribution of total time-integrated intensity of light backscattered from human breast tissue. The solid curve is the theoretical fit from Eq. (1).

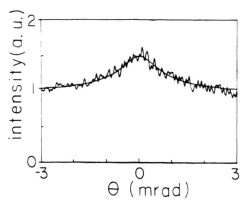

Fig. 12. Angular distribution of total time-integrated backscattered pulse intensity from human lung tissue. The solid curve is the theoretical fit from Eq. (1).

solid curves in the figures. The coherent peak for lung tissue is broader than that of breast tissue, which shows that lung tissue is a stronger light-scattering medium than breast tissue. Quantitatively, the light has a shorter l_t in lung tissue ($l_t = 80$ μm) than in breast tissue ($l_t = 250$ μm).

It has been shown that the coherent peak becomes narrower as the light scatters through a longer distance in a random medium.[20,23,27] This is also observed in biological tissue, which is shown by an example for light scattering in cancerous lung tissue. The intensity and the line shape of the coherent peak of the scattered light at various times after the incident pulse are plotted in Fig. 13. The intensity of the peak compared with the constant background is less than a factor of 2. One of the primary reasons is the finite angular resolution of the detecting system. Note that in Fig. 13 the coherent peak disappears at times greater than 22 psec. At times greater than 22 psec the angular width of the coherent peak is estimated to be less than 0.4 mrad. This angular width is comparable with the angular resolution of our detecting system, and thus the coherent peak is not observed.

The temporal profiles of the backscattered pulse at two angular regions, coherent (at 0 mrad) and diffuse (at 3 mrad) regions, for normal lung and breast tissues are

displayed in Figs. 14 and 15, respectively. The intensity of the scattered light in the coherent region is greater than that in the diffuse region in the early times. The profiles merge at later times. The scattered pulse from the breast

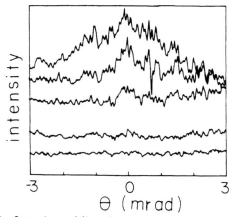

Fig. 13. Intensity and line shape of the coherent peak of the scattered light at various times after the 100-fsec pulse incident upon lung tissue. The selected plots, from top to bottom, are at times 4, 8, 13, 22, and 35 psec.

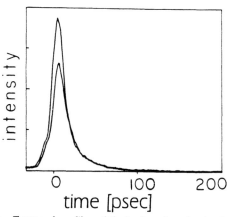

Fig. 14. Temporal profiles of the backscattered pulse from lung cancer tissue. The higher curve is for light scattered at 0 mrad, and the lower one is for 3 mrad.

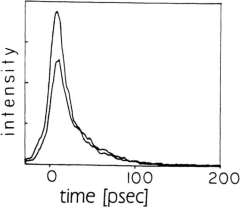

Fig. 15. Temporal profiles of the scattered pulse from breast cancer tissue. The higher curve is for light scattered at 0 mrad, and the lower one is for 3 mrad.

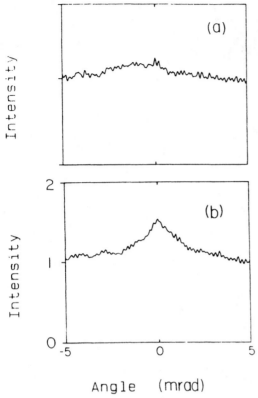

Fig. 16. Angular profiles of the total time-integrated intensity backscattered pulses from a leaf: (a) top portion of a green leaf, (b) leaf with chlorophyll extracted.

free path and the absorption length of the light in tissues have been measured and can be determined from either the line shape of the coherent peak $I(\theta)$ or the temporal profile $I(t)$ of the backscattered pulse. The absorption length can be obtained from the slope of log $I(t)$ versus t at later times. The transport mean free path can be obtained by fitting the log $I(t)$-versus-t curve from which l_t longer than 20 μm can be determined by using an 8-psec impulse-response synchroscan streak camera. The time-resolved backscattering technique using a streak camera and an ultrafast laser will be a versatile probe of biological materials since most materials have l_t longer than 100 μm. The coherent peak can be used to determine l_t when it is shorter than 20 μm. The temporal profile of the back-scattered pulse has the potential to monitor the extent of cataract development in the eye and to differentiate different components and states of biological tissues. Thus the temporal and angular profiles of backscattered light can be used in the medical diagnosis and investigation of biological systems.

ACKNOWLEDGMENTS

Parts of this study were performed in collaboration with R. A. Ahmed, Y. Takiguchi, G. C. Tang, K. Arya, R. M. Klapper, S. Wahl, and J. B. Birman. Their contributions are gratefully acknowledged. This research is supported in part by Hamamatsu Photonics, Mediscience Technology, the Strategic Defense Initative/Office of Naval Research, and the City University Faculty Award Program.

cancer tissue (Fig. 15) is broader than that from the lung cancer tissue (Fig. 14). This indicates the transport mean free path of the light is longer in the breast tissue, which is in qualitative agreement with the results obtained from the line shape of the coherent peak.

The best fit to the experimental data for breast tissue, shown in Fig. 15, occurs when $l_t = 1.6 \pm 0.3$ mm and $l_a = 20 \pm 4$ mm. The best fit for lung tissue is shown in Fig. 14: $l_t = 350 \pm 50$ μm and $l_a = 16 \pm 4$ mm. These lengths are similar to the values obtained in the transmission geometry by Navarro and Profio[4]. However, these lengths are significantly longer than those obtained from the angular line shape, which needs to be addressed and studied further.

Finally, we illustrate an example of using the angular profile of the coherent peak to probe the absorption property of a leaf at 620 nm (see Fig. 16). There is no coherent peak for light backscattered from the green leaf. The chlorophyll of the leaf is then extracted by submerging the leaf in methanol for a day. A coherent peak is then observed. These results are presented in Fig. 16. By fitting this coherent peak, l_t and l_a are found to be equal to 70 ± 15 μm and 1800 ± 400 μm, respectively. The absence of coherent light in the top part of the leaf shows that green leaves absorbs light efficiently at 620 nm. The l_a is approximately 150 ± 50 μm. This approach can be used to measure the absorption spectrum at low levels in highly scattering media.

In conclusion, weak localization of light scattered from biological tissues has been observed. The transport mean

REFERENCES

1. R. L. Fork, B. I. Greene, and C. V. Shank, Appl. Phys. Lett. **38**, 671 (1981).
2. H. R. Dorsinville, R. R. Alfano, and N. H. Schiller, *The Photonics Design and Applications Handbook* (Laurin, Pittsfield, Mass., 1987), p. H-28.
3. K. A. Nelson, D. R. Lutz, M. D. Fayer, and L. Madison, Phys. Rev. B **24**, 3261 (1981).
4. G. A. Navarro and A. E. Profio, Med. Phys. **15**, 181 (1988).
5. A. J. Welch, G. Yoon, and M. J. C. van Gemert, Lasers Surg. Med. **6**, 488 (1987).
6. A. E. Profio, Appl. Opt. **28**, 2216 (1989).
7. J. M. Drake and A. Z. Genack, Phys. Rev. Lett. **63**, 259 (1989).
8. G. H. Watson, P. A. Fleury, and S. L. McCall, Phys. Rev. Lett. **58**, 945 (1987). .
9. W. W. Wendlandt and H. G. Hecht, *Reflectance Spectroscopy* (Interscience, New York, 1966).
10. K. M. Yoo, K. Arya, G. C. Tang, J. L. Birman, and R. R. Alfano, Phys. Rev. A **39**, 3728 (1989).
11. R. Vreeker, M. P. van Albada, R. Sprik, and A. Lagendijk, Phys. Lett. **132**, 516 (1988).
12. K. Shimizu, A. Ishimaru, L. Reynolds, and A. P. Bruckner, Appl. Opt. **18**, 3484 (1979).
13. S. L. Jacques, Appl. Opt. **28**, 2223 (1989).
14. M. S. Patterson, B. Chance, and B. C. Wilson, Appl. Opt. **28**, 2331 (1989).
15. B. Chance, J. S. Leigh, H. Miyake, D. S. Smith, S. Nioka, R. Greenfeld, M. Finander, K. Kaufman, W. Levy, M. Young, P. Cohen, H. Yoshioka, and R. Boretsky, Proc. Natl. Acad. Sci. USA **85**, 4971 (1988).
16. R. A. Elliot, Appl. Opt. **22**, 2670 (1983).
17. Y. Kuga and A. Ishimaru, J. Opt. Soc. Am. A **8**, 831 (1984).
18. M. P. van Albada and A. Lagendijk, Phys. Rev. Lett. **55**, 2692 (1985).

19. P. E. Wolf and G. Maret, Phys. Rev. Lett. **55,** 2696 (1985).
20. E. Akkermans, P. E. Wolf, and R. Maynard, Phys. Rev. Lett. **56,** 1471 (1986).
21. M. J. Stephen and G. Cwilich, Phys. Rev. B **34,** 7564 (1986).
22. P. E. Wolf, G. Maret, E. Akkermans, and R. Maynard, J. Phys. (Paris) **49,** 63 (1988).
23. S. Etemad, R. Thompson, M. J. Andrejco, S. John, and F. C. Mackintosh, Phys. Rev. Lett. **59,** 1420 (1987).
24. S. Etemad, R. Thompson, and M. J. Andrejco, Phys. Rev. Lett. **57,** 1420 (1986).
25. M. Rosenbluh, I. Edrei, M. Kaveh, and I. Freud, Phys. Rev. A **37,** 4458 (1987).
26. M. P. van Albada, M. B. van der Mark, and A. Lagendijk, Phys. Rev. Lett. **58,** 361 (1987).
27. K. M. Yoo, Y. Takiguchi, and R. R. Alfano, IEEE Photon. Tech. Lett. **1,** 94 (1989).

Reprinted with permission from *Optics Letters,* Vol. 16(21), pp. 1632-1634
(November 1, 1991). ©1991 Optical Society of America.

Study of photon migration depths with time-resolved spectroscopy

Weijia Cui, Naiguang Wang, and Britton Chance

Department of Biochemistry and Biophysics, School of Medicine, University of Pennsylvania, Philadelphia, Pennsylvania 19104-6089

Received June 17, 1991

In this study a light-shielding plate with a hole was placed in an intralipid emulsion. The probability distribution for photons emitted from a surface light source, passing through the hole at different depths, and reaching a surface detector at the other side of the plate was experimentally assessed. We provide qualitative verification for a model derived by Weiss *et al.* [J. Mod. Opt. **36,** 349 (1989)] that the migration depths for the measured photons follow a distribution in depth and that this distribution has a maximum probability at a describable depth beneath the surface. This agreement, corroborated by a parallel study, suggests that we may have assessed the maximum migration depth distribution of photons that reached the detector and that the random walk model may describe the maximum migration depth distribution. The experimental results indicate that photons with the same path lengths within the medium reach a wide range of depths and suggest difficulties in resolving optical structure with time-resolved measurement. The results also provide experimental evidence that, for a given source–detector separation, the photons that migrate deeper have longer mean path lengths with larger variation in their path lengths.

Biological tissue presents a layered structure, like the brain covered with skin and skull or muscle covered with skin and fat. Assessing deep-tissue blood perfusion conditions with surface optical measurements is of clinical significance for monitoring and diagnosing purposes. The migration depths of incident photons before they reach the detector determine the possible probing depths within biological tissue.

The migration depths for photons measured at the surface of a semi-infinite turbid medium have been studied with the random walk theory[1] and photon diffusion theory.[2] The study with the random walk theory suggests that the migration depths of photons measured at a given source–detector separation follow a distribution with a maximum probability at a describable depth beneath the medium surface. However, experimental evidence supporting this proposition has not been found in the literature.

Incident photons in a turbid medium undergo multiple scatterings before they reach a detector. The traveling direction of a photon changes randomly with each scattering occurrence. This propagation process makes it difficult to study the propagation paths for individual photons. A question also arises whether photons that migrate deeper should have longer path lengths for a given source–detector separation. This question is related to the possibility of separating the layered biological information from path-length measurements on the surface. (The path length is defined as the length of the travel trace of a photon that reaches the detector.)

In our experiment, photons passing a hole on a light-shielding plate submerged in an intralipid emulsion were measured. The plate prevented any incident photons, except those passing through the hole, from reaching the detector. The measurements taken when the hole was at different depths were related to the random walk model.[1] Moreover, the path lengths of the measured photons were examined at different hole depths. Time-resolved spectroscopy[3] was used in this experiment to measure the path lengths of individual photons within the medium by measuring the traveling time of the photons.

Figure 1 shows the experimental setup. A light-shielding plate was placed between the optical fibers (sending fiber diameter 2.5 mm and detecting fiber diameter 3 mm) with equal distance to the fibers and was perpendicular to the medium surface. The plate prevented incident light from reaching the detecting fiber. A hole (1.5 mm × 5 mm) on the plate selectively admitted photons that had paths intersecting with the hole. The plate was painted black to absorb photons that struck it. The assumptions for this experiment were that the plate would block all the photons except those passing through the hole and that the interactions among the photons were negligible. Thus, by immersing the plate in the intralipid emulsion at different depths (Fig. 1), the photons that passed the hole at different depths were selectively measured.

A Hamamatsu picosecond light pulser (PLP-01) was used to provide the light pulse, with a pulse width of 50 to 60 ps at a wavelength of 670 nm and a peak power of 40 mW. One channel of a Hamamatsu Multianode (MCP-PMTs R1224-03) was used to detect the emergent photons. Time delay of the emerged photons was measured by a Tennelec TAC system and a Nucleus DMR-II digital multiplexer router system (Model 116C).

Figure 2 shows the time-resolved response from 0.5% intralipid emulsion and for 2-cm separation be-

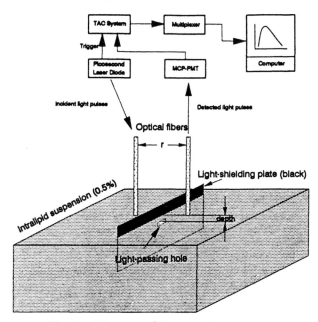

Fig. 1. Diagram of the experiment setup.

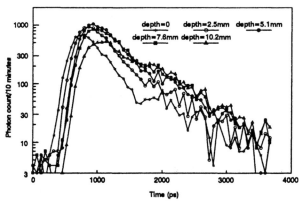

Fig. 2. Time-resolved responses when the hole is at different depths.

the depth of the hole. The integration increased when the hole moved farther from the surface, reaching maximum when the depth was 5.1 mm. It started to decrease when the hole was deeper than 5.1 mm. Figure 3 also shows a simulated photon probability distribution in depth (see below) with the model given by Weiss et al.[1]

The experimental data agree with the simulation data except at shallower depths. The model derived from random walk theory described the possibility of photons at different depths, while the experiment assessed the distribution of the possibility for photons to pass the hole at different depths. The agreement between the experiment and simulation suggests that they are closely related. A parallel study[4] with a different method demonstrated that the possible paths for the measured photons are distributed in a region shaped as a banana, with its two ends connecting the source and detector and its middle portion reaching the deepest. Thus, by moving the hole in depth along the middle line between the fibers, we may assess the maximum migration depth distributions, except that the existence of the plate may change the photon distribution. The light-shielding plate absorbs the photons that strike the plate. Some of the absorbed photons would be scattered to the hole location if the plate was not present. Thus the photons measured at the existence of the plate could be only a part of the photons that might intersect the hole location and end at the detector in the absence of the plate. The maximum probability depth in this experiment (5.1 mm) is comparable with that of a similar measurement (5.4 mm) in a parallel study,[4] suggesting that the distortion of the distribution due to the plate may be insignificant.

The model by Weiss et al.[1] assumes that the migration of the photons is axisymmetric about the incident point. The model developed has two coordinates, the distance from the incident point and the

tween the fibers. The curves in Fig. 2 were obtained when the hole was 0, 2.5, 5.1, 7.6, and 10.2 mm deep, respectively. The FWHM of these curves are shown in Table 1. The depth of the hole was measured from the top of the hole to the surface of the emulsion. The FWHM of the system response to the incident light pulses was 120 ps. Since this study concentrated on the relative intensities and the relative time delays of the photons when the hole was at different depths, only the time-resolved curves from the sample are shown.

Figure 2 shows that the relative peaks of the time-resolved curves vary as the depth of the hole changes. The total photons that passed the hole and reached the detector are proportional to the time integration of the time-resolved curve. As all these measurements were obtained over the same time interval (10 min), with the same incident pulse intensity and the same repetition rate, the integrations for the different curves should represent the possibility of the photons passing the hole at the corresponding depth. Figure 3 shows the integrated values of the time-resolved measurements versus

Table 1. FWHM of Each Curve in Fig. 2

	Depth (mm)				
	0	2.5	5.1	7.6	10.2
FWHM (ps)	499.5	532.8	599.4	632.7	699.3

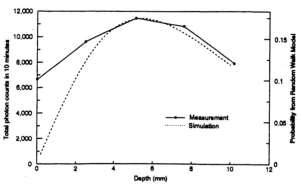

Fig. 3. Integration of the time-resolved responses when the hole is at different depths.

Table 2. MTT of the Photons for Each Curve in Fig. 2

	Depth (mm)				
	0	2.5	5.1	7.6	10.2
MTT (ps)	1047	1143	1247	1331	1492

depth. It describes the migration depth's distribution of the measured photons at all angular directions with the same source–detector separations. For the experimental setup in Fig. 1, we expected that the probability profile measured along the middle line between the light source and detector would approximate the situation described by the model. To assess the distribution in depth, a smaller hole size would be desirable, but that would reduce the measurable light intensity. The choice of the 1.5 mm × 5 mm hole is a compromise between the measurable light intensity and approximation to the two-dimensional situation, which may also introduce deviations between the simulation and experimental data.

The optical parameters used in the simulation may not describe the intralipid emulsion in this experiment, which should further contribute to the deviation between the experimental data and simulation data. Moreover the assumptions for random walk modeling (like the cubic lattice model), isotropic scattering, zero specular reflections on the inner side of the surface, and the absorbing boundary for the medium may also contribute to this deviation. In addition, the depth of the hole in the experiment was measured from the top of the hole, which shifted the experimental curve in Fig. 2 left by 0.5 mm.

Figure 2 also shows that the time-resolved curves delayed more when the hole was deeper. We define the mean travel time (MTT) for each curve as follows:

$$\text{MTT} = \frac{\sum n_i t_i}{\sum n_i}, \qquad (1)$$

where n_i is the number of photons that arrived at the detector at time t_i and t_i is the time relative to the origin on the abscissa of Fig. 2. The MTT's for the different depths are shown in Table 2. The larger MTT for a deeper hole location demonstrated the longer mean path length for the photons that reached deeper.

The large overlap in time for the time-resolved curves demonstrates that individual photons passing the hole do not necessarily have a shorter path length for a lesser depth. The large overlap also indicates that photons with the same path lengths cover a wide depth range, which in turn indicates the difficulties of resolving spatial optical structures using time-resolved measurement. The time-resolved curves with a larger FWHM for deeper hole positions demonstrate more variations in their path lengths.

The random walk model[1] of photon migration depth assumes a lattice model for the medium. The lattice spacing L is defined as the rms distance traveled between successive scattering events.[5] For the assumption that the scattering path lengths are exponentially distributed,

$$L = \sqrt{2}/[(1 - g)\mu_s], \qquad (2)$$

where $(1 - g)\mu_s$ is the backscattering coefficient. μ_a (the absorption coefficient) and $(1 - g)\mu_s$ were suggested to be 0.0026/mm and 0.72/mm,[6] respectively, for a 0.5% intralipid emulsion. From Eq. (2), L is approximately 2 mm.

The parameters used in the model include ρ, the separation between fibers; z, the depth parameter; and u, the absorption parameter. ρ and z were measured in multiples of L and are equal to half the separation and depth measured in millimeters for the 0.5% intralipid emulsion. The absorption probability per L is e^{-u}, where u equals twice the absorption coefficient for this intralipid emulsion. The parameters for the simulation in Fig. 3 were $u = 0.0053$ and $\rho = 10$.

In summary, this study measured the photons passing a hole on a light-shielding plate when the hole was at different depths. This measurement, although not a direct assessment of the maximum migration depth distribution, agrees with the model by Weiss et al., provides qualitative verification to the model's expectation, and suggests that the model may describe the maximum migration depth of the measured photons. The theoretical study suggests that the maximum probability depth is a function of the source–detector separation and the optical properties of the medium.[1] This study also provides evidence that measured photons have longer mean path lengths with larger variations, if they reach greater depths, and suggests that resolution of spatial optical structure may be difficult with time-resolved measurements.

Weijia Cui is now with the BOC Group, Technical Center, 100 Mountain Avenue, Murray Hill, New Jersey 07974.

References

1. G. H. Weiss, R. Nossal, and R. F. Bonner, J. Mod. Opt. **36**, 349 (1989).
2. W. Cui, Ph.D. dissertation (Biomedical Engineering Department, Rensselaer Polytechnic Institute, Troy, N.Y., 1990).
3. M. S. Patterson, B. Chance, and B. C. Wilson, Appl. Opt. **28**, 2331 (1989).
4. W. Cui, C. Kumar, and B. Chance, Proc. Soc. Photo-Opt. Instrum. Eng. **1431**, 180 (1991).
5. R. F. Bonner, R. Nossal, S. Havlin, and G. H. Weiss, J. Opt. Soc. Am. A **4**, 423 (1987).
6. M. S. Patterson, J. D. Moulton, B. C. Wilson, and B. C. Chance, Proc. Soc. Photo-Opt. Instrum. Eng. **1203**, 62 (1990).

Reprinted with permission from *Journal of Photochemistry and Photobiology B: Biology,* Vol. 16, pp. 141-153 (1992). ©1992 Elsevier Sequoia S.A.

Time-resolved spectroscopy of the human forearm

Marco Ferrari[a,†], Qingnong Wei[b], Luca Carraresi[b], Roberto A. De Blasi[c] and Giovanni Zaccanti[b]

[a]*Dipartimento di Scienze e Tecnologie Biomediche, Università dell'Aquila, 67100 L'Aquila (Italy) and Laboratorio di Biologia Cellulare, Istituto Superiore di Sanità, 00161 Roma (Italy)*
[b]*Dipartimento di Fisica, Via Santa Marta 3, Università di Firenze, 50139 Firenze (Italy)*
[c]*Istituto di Anestesiologia e Rianimazione, 1 Università di Roma, 00161 Roma (Italy)*

Abstract

For spectroscopic purposes, the forearm is a conveniently large object to be investigated because consistent oxygenation and blood volume changes can be obtained. Human forearm spectral properties were investigated using picosecond near-IR laser spectroscopy. The behaviour of the temporal point spread function in resting conditions and during ischaemia, venous occlusion and exercise is reported. The effect of path length inaccuracy on muscle oxygen consumption, obtained by combining spectral data with the path length, is discussed.

1. Introduction

Near-IR spectroscopy (NIRS), introduced by Jobsis [1], has been successfully employed to monitor changes in the relative amounts of oxyhaemoglobin and deoxyhaemoglobin and near-IR optical imaging using time-resolved methods is currently being investigated by different groups (for a review, see ref. 2). Early cerebral and muscle NIRS measurements, using multi-wavelength photometers, are only qualitative because the mean path length travelled by the photons is unknown. Since the transport of photons through tissue occurs primarily by scattering, the path length is significantly longer than the inter-optode distance. Recently, it has been shown that the tissue path length can be evaluated by measuring the amplitude and phase shift of an amplitude-modulated light source or the time taken for a picosecond light pulse to cross tissue [2]. Data can be obtained by the analysis of the temporal point spread function (TPSF), *i.e.* the temporal response of the tissue illuminated by a picosecond light pulse [3]. The mean path length is calculated from the mean transit time of the pulse. Delpy *et al.* [3] have defined the differential path length factor (DPF), which is calculated by dividing the mean path length by the inter-fibre distance. The DPF was measured on adult forearm, calf and head and was found to be constant when the inter-fibre distance was greater than 25–30 mm [4]. These DPF data are currently used to quantify oxyhaemoglobin/deoxyhaemoglobin measurements and to calculate cerebral blood flow and volume in newborns and adults using commercially available instruments (NIRO 1000/NIRO 500, Hamamatsu Photonics KK, Japan) [5–7]. However, to date, data on the regional path length are scarce and path length variations during various pathophysiological events are not available.

We have previously studied human forearm oxygenation during ischaemia using fast scanning spectroscopy and picosecond near-IR laser spectroscopy [8, 9]. Muscle oxygen consumption was measured by inducing an abrupt flow limitation and evaluating the haemoglobin (Hb) to myoglobin (Mb) desaturation rate [8]. For spectroscopic purposes, the human forearm is a conveniently large object to be investigated because consistent oxygenation and blood volume changes can be easily obtained by graded cuff compression and/or exercise.

The aim of this study was to investigate the behaviour of the forearm TPSF in resting conditions with different geometries of the optode, and dynamically during ischaemia, venous occlusion and voluntary isometric exercise. Variations in the optical density, DPF and slope of the pulse, which is related to the absorption coefficient, were investigated. The effect of DPF inaccuracy on muscle oxygen consumption is discussed.

---

†Author to whom correspondence should be addressed.

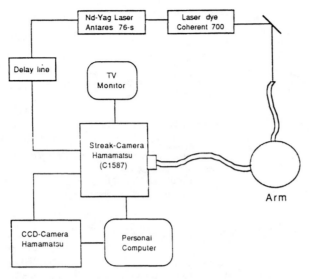

Fig. 1. Experimental set-up for the measurement of the TPSF in human muscle.

2. Materials and methods

Fifteen healthy adult volunteers (male and female) were recruited from the laboratory. The subjects were aged between 21 and 44 years (median, 34 years). Informed consent was obtained from each subject. All measurements were performed on the forearm. A pneumatic cuff was loosely wrapped around the arm. The muscle was illuminated using an optic fibre (length, 70 cm; active diameter, 0.3 cm) with ultrashort light pulses (duration, 4 ps; repetition rate, 76 MHz; wavelengths, 760 and 800 nm) from a Coherent 700 dye laser pumped by a mode-locked Nd–Yag laser (Fig. 1). Wavelengths were selected according to the spectral properties of Hb [8]. The average laser light power was 50–100 mW at the end of the optic fibre which illuminated the forearm. The light emerging from the tissue was collected with an optic fibre (length, 70 cm; active diameter, 0.5 cm) positioned at various distances by a metal holder which maintained a constant geometry throughout all experimental procedures. Light was measured over a 5 s period by a synchroscan streak camera (Hamamatsu Photonics, C1587). The full width at half-maximum of the pulse, measured with this equipment, was about 70 ps when the pulse was transmitted through the fibres. This broadening was due to the dispersion of the fibres. The temporal window of the streak camera was 1500 ps. In the occlusion and exercise protocols, measurements were collected consecutively every 30 s. The same experimental apparatus was been used by several investigators [3, 4].

Typical forearm responses to the light pulse are shown in Figs. 2 and 3. Optical density changes were calculated from the integral of the received pulses. The transit times (t) of the IR photons can be converted into distance travelled through the medium (d) using the formula $d = ct/n$ (c is the speed of light in a vacuum and $n = 1.4$ is the tissue refractive index [10]). The mean path length was calculated from the mean transit time of the photons through the tissue. The DPF was calculated by dividing the mean path length by the inter-fibre distance measured with a caliper. As shown in Figs. 2 and 3 the TPSF intensity is approximately linear with time in a semi-logarithmic plot. We verified that the semi-logarithmic slope was approximately linear by measuring the TPSF with two or three different delays of the streak camera. Combining the two or three TPSFs into a single pulse, the temporal window was 2500–3000 ps and the terminal slope was approximately linear and could be accurately measured. This procedure was performed when the DPF was calculated from the TPSFs as shown in curves c–e of Fig. 3.

The quantity μ_a' was obtained from the pulse $I(t)$ (plotted on a semi-logarithmic scale) as

$$\mu_a' = -\frac{n}{c}\frac{\mathrm{d}}{\mathrm{d}t}\ln I(t) \tag{1}$$

The logarithmic derivative (natural logarithm) was evaluated from the slope of the straight line which best fitted the pulse over a time interval of about 300 ps starting from the time of the half-peak amplitude. As suggested by Chance et al. [11] the

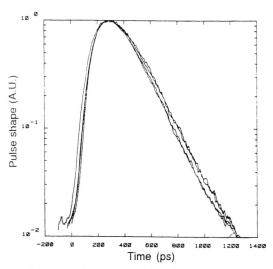

Fig. 2. Temporal point spread functions measured on the proximal forearm brachioradialis muscle at different angles with respect to the arm axis. Curves correspond to the following angles: 45°, 90°, 135° and 310°. Inter-optode distance, 3 cm; wavelength, 800 nm.

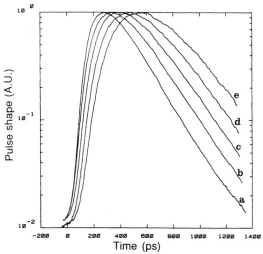

Fig. 3. TPSFs measured with the optic fibres at different distances (d) on the proximal forearm. Curves a–e correspond to d values of 2.0, 2.6, 3.0, 3.5 and 4.2 cm respectively. Wavelength, 800 nm.

slope of the pulse is related to the absorption coefficient μ_a of the medium. Patterson *et al.* [12] showed that

$$\mu_a = \lim_{t \to \infty} - \frac{n}{c} \frac{d}{dt} \ln I(t) \tag{2}$$

From a practical point of view, when typical values for the optical properties of biological tissues in the near-IR are assumed, eqn. (2) is valid only after several nanoseconds from the time of the pulse peak. With our experimental apparatus, it was impossible to measure the pulse during this time interval due to both the available temporal window (approximately 1.5 ns) and the sensitivity of the detector.

Monte Carlo simulations were performed as previously described [9] to explore the discrepancies between μ_a' and μ_a. The forearm was roughly modelled as a cylinder with optical parameters typical for human muscle (absorption coefficient, $\mu_a = 0.15$ cm^{-1}; reduced scattering coefficient $\mu_d = 10$ cm^{-1}). Figure 4(a) shows the TPSF pertaining to different source–receiver distances. Figure 4(b) gives the percentage error (ϵ) in the value μ_a when μ_a' is obtained from these curves

$$\epsilon \, (\%) = \frac{\mu_a - \mu_a'}{\mu_a} \times 100 \tag{3}$$

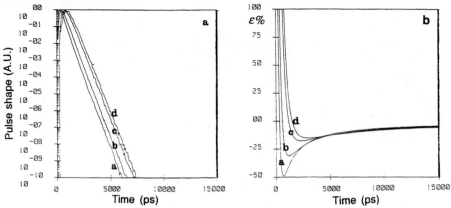

Fig. 4. (a) Monte Carlo simulations of the forearm TPSF for different distances (d) between source and receiver. The forearm was modelled as a cylinder (radius, 4 cm) containing homogeneous diffusers with $\mu_a = 0.15$ cm^{-1} and $\mu_d = 10$ cm^{-1}. Pulse shapes were normalized to the maximum. Curves a, b, c and d correspond to d values of 2, 3, 4 and 5 cm respectively. (b) Percentage error ϵ (eqn. (3)) resulting when the value μ_a', measured from the pulse slope, is considered as the tissue absorption coefficient (μ_a).

The percentage error is more relevant when the distance between source and detector is small (curve a). In particular, for the typical forearm geometry of a source–receiver distance of 3 cm (curve b), the value of μ_a', measured by fitting the signal over a time interval of about 300 ps starting from the time of the half-peak amplitude, overestimated the value of μ_a by less than 30%. The error was around 10% even when the temporal window was 5 ns.

Spectral measurements were made using a fast scanning spectrophotometer (model 6500, NIRSystems, Silver Spring, MD). The spectral analysis procedure has been described elsewhere [8, 13]. Briefly, two optic fibres (length, 200 cm; active diameter, 0.5 cm) were applied 3 cm apart. NIRSystems software was utilized to automatically collect a scan every 5 s. Spectra were analysed according to a modified Lambert–Beer law in order to obtain quantification of Hb changes during the experimental procedures. Difference spectra (ΔA) of the muscle tissue were calculated relative to the pre-ischaemic or pre-exercise period. These were converted into values of muscle absorption coefficient ($\Delta\mu_a$) using $\Delta\mu_a = \Delta A/(Bd)$ where d is the physical separation of the fibres on the skin surface and B is the DPF calculated from the TPSF. Changes in muscle absorption coefficient were assumed to result only from changes in the concentration of oxy-Hb/Mb and deoxy-Hb/Mb. The results were expressed as micromole per litre of tissue (μM l^{-1}). No difference in the absorption spectra of Hb and Mb in the near-IR region have been reported in $vitro$ [14]. In this paper [Hb] and [HbO$_2$] represent the combined concentrations of deoxy-Hb and Mb and oxy-Hb and Mb respectively. The tissue absorption coefficient spectra ($\Delta\mu_a$) were split into Δ[Hb] and Δ[HbO$_2$] using multilinear regression analysis [15] of the Hb and HbO$_2$ spectra [16]. The regression analysis was performed over the wavelength region 750–900 nm with data points at 2 nm intervals. Oxygen consumption (V_{O_2}) was measured by calculating the rate of change of the conversion of oxy-Hb to deoxy-Hb ($i.e.$ 0.5 d(Δ[HbO$_2$] $-$ Δ[Hb])/dt) and taking into account the molecular ratio between Hb and oxygen [17]. V_{O_2} was calculated during voluntary contraction and for the first 60 s of ischaemia when the desaturation process was linear. It was assumed that in this period changes in saturation were mainly due to Hb.

Venous occlusion was performed on seven subjects. After a stabilization period of 5 min, an abrupt flow interruption was achieved using a pneumatic cuff loosely wrapped around the arm. Venous occlusion was obtained by inflating the cuff to a pressure of 40–60 mmHg. The cuff was released 10 min after the occlusion started. Two subjects were initially submitted to 10 min arterial occlusion (cuff pressure, 240–260 mmHg), and later executed an isometric voluntary contraction.

3. Results

Figure 2 shows a typical TPSF measured on the proximal forearm brachioradialis muscle using a laser wavelength of 800 nm. No change in the TPSF was found for

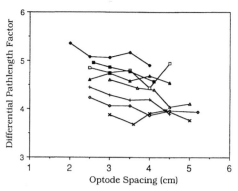

Fig. 5. Values of the DPF *vs.* distance between optic fibres measured on the proximal forearm of eight adult volunteers (three females represented with the filled symbols). Wavelength, 800 nm.

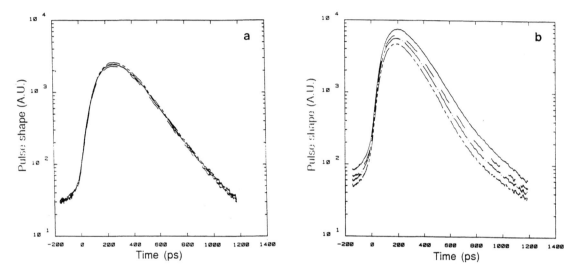

Fig. 6. Typical TPSF values, measured at 800 nm, before and during 10 min forearm arterial (a) and venous (b) occlusion induced by application of a tourniquet: —— before occlusion; – – –, 0.5 min occlusion; – · – 1 min occlusion; – - - –, 2 min occlusion.

a fixed distance between the fibres when the angle with respect to the axis of the arm was changed. The TPSF was modified when the distance between the fibres was changed (Fig. 3). In Figs. 2 and 3 $t = 0$ corresponds to the time of arrival of the pulse peak calculated for the unscattered photons. A reference pulse, measured with the fibres aligned in air, was used to obtain $t = 0$. The inter-subject variations in the DPF are shown in Fig. 5. Each volunteer presented DPF values almost constant beyond an inter-optode spacing of 2.5 cm (Fig. 5). At an inter-optode spacing of 3 cm the DPF measured at 800 nm was 4.3 ± 0.2 (mean $\pm$ standard deviation (SD); $n = 14$), which is very similar to previously reported data [4, 11, 18].

We have previously found consistent changes in the TPSF during 10 min of forearm arterial occlusion using 760 nm laser light, which corresponds to the deoxy-Hb/Mb absorption peak [9]. Conversely, no changes in amplitude and shape were observed using an 800 nm pulse, a wavelength close to the 'in vitro' Hb/Mb isosbestic point (Fig. 6(a)). This indicates that, at least in these experimental conditions, 800 nm is also an isosbestic wavelength 'in vivo' because no significant scattering variations occurred during the 10 min occlusion. However, during venous outflow restriction, an increase in blood volume suddenly occurred, because of the persisting arterial blood inflow, until a steady state was reached. Consistent changes in pulse amplitude and slope were observed during these blood volume changes using 800 nm laser light (Fig. 6(b)).

The time course of the venous occlusion is better represented in Fig. 7 which shows changes in optical density (ΔOD), μ_a' and DPF during venous occlusion and subsequent recovery. A close correlation between all these parameters is evident. In particular, they reach a maximum after only 3 min of occlusion and are unchanged until the cuff is released. After the release, control conditions are quickly reached in

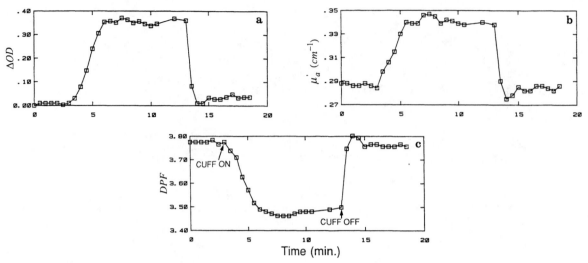

Fig. 7. Time course of ΔOD, μ_a' and DPF measured from the TPSF at 800 nm during 10 min venous occlusion and recovery.

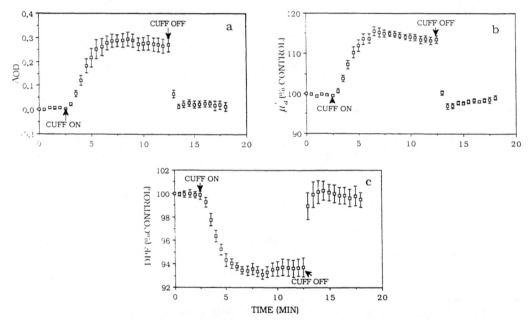

Fig. 8. Time course of ΔOD, μ_a' (% control) and DPF (% control) measured from the TPSF at 800 nm during 10 min venous occlusion and recovery. After 3 min of occlusion a plateau was reached until cuff release. Cuff release was accompanied by a rapid recovery. Means ± standard error; $n = 7$.

a few minutes. The results of the time course of 10 min venous occlusion performed on seven subjects are shown in Fig. 8. After 3 min of occlusion a plateau is reached until cuff release. Cuff release is accompanied by a rapid recovery. The DPF consistently changes during venous occlusion and isometric exercise, which strongly affects muscle oxygenation and haemodynamics. The time course of the DPF changes during isometric voluntary contraction of two volunteers is reported in Fig. 9. A similar time course of ΔOD has recently been reported [19]. The DPF decreases during the contraction time. The DPF recovery phase at the end of exercise is slower than the DPF recovery after venous occlusion (Fig. 8).

Many groups have used DPF values to quantify oxy-Hb/deoxy-Hb measurements as well as to calculate cerebral blood flow and volume [5–7]. We have recently combined spectral information, using fast scanning spectroscopy, with path length data in order to quantify oxy-Hb/Mb and deoxy-Hb/Mb during ischaemia and exercise [8]. Figure 10 reports a typical desaturation pattern during ischaemia (left panel) and two isometric maximal voluntary contractions (right panel) using the DPF value (3.98) measured by

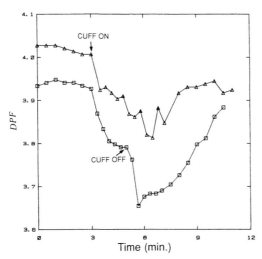

Fig. 9. Time course of DPF changes during isometric voluntary contraction. The strength was 60% of maximum. Inter-optode spacing of 3 cm. Wavelength, 800 nm.

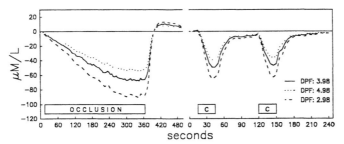

Fig. 10. Typical Hb/Mb deoxygenation slopes during ischaemia (left panel) and two isometric maximal voluntary contractions (right panel) calculated from near-IR spectra and measured DPF (3.98, continuous tracing). The exercise provoked a faster desaturation rate than that occurring in the occlusion without contraction. The use of underestimated (2.98) and overestimated (4.98) DPF values strongly affects the quantitation. The inter-optode spacing was 3 cm (wavelength, 800 nm).

picosecond near-IR laser spectroscopy on the same subject. V_{O_2} was 2.38 μM min^{-1} (100 g)$^{-1}$ during constant tourniquet pressure in resting muscle and was raised to 23.50 μM min^{-1} (100 g)$^{-1}$ during maximal voluntary contraction. Similar V_{O_2} values were obtained using an invasive method [20]. The accurate evaluation of V_{O_2} depends on the precision of the DPF. Figure 5 shows the range of DPF values that can be measured on the forearm. The presently available clinical instruments [5–7] do not measure DPF. As shown in Fig. 10, V_{O_2} values are incorrectly evaluated when underestimated or overestimated DPF data are used for Hb/Mb quantitation.

A further problem that can affect these quantitation procedures is shown in Fig. 11. When the TPSF is measured along the forearm, the TPSF is significantly expanded and the DPF is increased when the bone to muscle ratio is increased in the optical field.

4. Discussion

Skeletal muscle is particularly suited for the investigation of metabolic regulation and oxygen consumption as it shows the highest variability in energy turnover from the resting state to maximal activity among tissues. NIRS has been developed experimentally and clinically to monitor brain and muscle oxygenation non-invasively. Recently NIRS has been employed to measure the rate of muscular oxygen utilization in patients with mitochondrial myopathy [21] and heart failure [22]. These studies only provide a qualitative analysis of Hb/Mb oxygen saturation. The evaluation of saturation changes has been conventionally made considering full saturation during 100% oxygen breathing and complete desaturation after 5–10 min of ischaemia [19]. The new techniques of time- and frequency-resolved spectroscopy allow the measurement of the distribution of optical path lengths in order to quantify the absorption changes of NIRS in tissues [5–8].

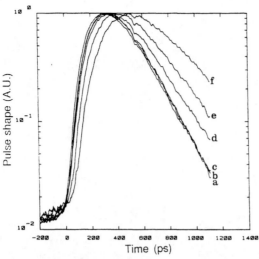

Fig. 11. Temporal point spread functions measured along the forearm with the fibre holder positioned on the proximal brachioradialis muscle and moved distally. Curves a–f correspond to distances d from the elbow of 3, 5, 7, 9, 13 and 14.5 cm respectively. Corresponding DPF values were 4.0, 4.0, 3.9, 4.3, 4.5 and 5.3. The inter-optode spacing was 3 cm (wavelength, 800 nm).

As shown in Fig. 2, using the Hb/Mb isosbestic wavelength, the pulse shape is relatively constant when the position of the fibre holder is changed. The pulse shape changes and the DPF is constant when the distance between the fibres is increased (Fig. 3). The same value of the DPF was obtained for the same subject after several months. However, although the DPF values are very reproducible, Fig. 5 indicates that the range of DPF values found in healthy subjects in resting conditions is broad. These variations may be explained by different tissue blood contents and different tissue scattering properties. Figure 11 clearly indicates the effect of the high scattering properties of bone on the TPSF because the DPF is increased when the muscle layer is very thin.

We have previously reported, using the deoxy-Hb peak wavelength, variations in the TPSF during the consistent changes in forearm oxygenation due to arterial occlusion [9]. In this study, we investigated the TPSF changes of the forearm provoked by venous outflow restriction, a procedure which causes an increase in arm blood volume [19]. Using the isosbestic wavelength of 800 nm [9, 16], a decrease in the DPF and an increase in μ'_a were found. The increase in Hb volume was thought to be responsible for these variations. During venous occlusion the DPF decreased by about 7% (Fig. 8). Isometric exercise was also capable of provoking a similar transient decrease in the DPF (Fig. 9).

No clinical instrument presently available can measure the DPF and quantitation is obtained using literature data [4]. The reported DPF variations and the spectral dependence of the TPSF investigated at University College, London indicate that the accuracy of the clinical measurements is questionable as demonstrated by the results shown in Fig. 10.

We found by Monte Carlo simulations that, for a 3 cm inter-optode distance, the slope overestimated the correct value of μ_a by less than 30% (Fig. 4). This result indicates that the pulse shape information may also be used for IR imaging purposes. Optical imaging in the near-IR is currently being pursued by different groups [2]. However, there are significant technical problems related to the imaging technique which have yet to be solved before it can become a routine clinical tool. Nevertheless, the images of rat brain oxygenation during middle cerebral artery ischaemia, obtained using the dual-wavelength picosecond near-IR laser technique combined with conventional back-projection image reconstruction, are very promising [23].

Acknowledgments

We wish to thank Professor S. Califano, Director of the European Laboratory for Non-Linear Spectroscopy, University of Florence. This research was supported in part by CNR contributions 91.00253.04, 91.02086.11 and 92.01027.04.

References

1 F. F. Jobsis, Non invasive infrared monitoring of cerebral and myocardial oxygen sufficiency and circulatory parameters, *Science, 198* (1977) 1264–1267.

2 B. Chance, in Time resolved spectroscopy and imaging of tissues, *Proc. Soc. Photo-Opt. Instrum. Eng., 1431* (1991).

3 D. T. Delpy, M. Cope, P. van der Zee, S. R. Arridge, S. Wray and J. S. Wyatt, Estimation of optical pathlength through tissue from direct time of flight measurement, *Phys. Med. Biol., 33* (1988) 1433–1442.

4 P. van der Zee, M. Cope, S. R. Arridge, M. Essenspreis, L. A. Potter, A. D. Edwards, J. S. Wyatt, D. C. McCormick, S. C. Roth, E. O. R. Reynolds and D. T. Delpy, Experimentally measured optical pathlengths for the adult head, calf and forearm and the head of the newborn infant as a function of inter optode spacing, *Adv. Exp. Med. Biol.,* in the press.

5 A. D. Edwards, C. Richardson, M. Cope, J. S. Wyatt, D. T. Delpy and E. O. R. Reynolds, Cotside measurement of cerebral blood flow in ill newborn infants by near infrared spectroscopy, *Lancet, 2* (1988) 770–771.

6 J. S. Wyatt, M. Cope, D. T. Delpy, S. Wray and E. O. R. Reynolds, Quantification of cerebral oxygenation and hemodynamics in sick newborn infants by near infrared spectrophotometry, *Lancet, 2* (1986) 1063–1066.

7 J. S. Wyatt, A. D. Edwards, M. Cope, D. T. Delpy, D. C. McCormick, A. Potter and E. O. R. Reynolds, Response of cerebral blood volume to changes in arterial carbon dioxide tension in preterm and term infants, *Pediatr. Res., 29* (1991) 553–557.

8 R. A. De Blasi, E. Quaglia and M. Ferrari, Skeletal muscle oxygenation monitoring by near infrared spectroscopy, *Biochem. Int., 25* (1991) 241–248.

9 M. Ferrari, R. De Blasi, P. Bruscaglioni, M. Barilli, L. Carraresi, M. Gurioli, E. Quaglia and G. Zaccanti, Near infrared time-resolved spectroscopy and fast scanning spectrophotometry in ischemic human forearm, *Proc. Soc. Photo-Opt. Instrum. Eng., 1431* (1991) 276–283.

10 F. Bolin, L. E. Preuss, R. C. Taylor and R. J. Ference, Refractive index of some mammalian tissues using a fiber optic cladding method, *Appl. Opt., 28* (1989) 2297–2302.

11 B. Chance, S. Nioka, J. Kent, K. McCully, M. Fountain, R. Greenfeld and G. Holtom, Time resolved spectroscopy of hemoglobin and myoglobin in resting and ischemic muscle, *Anal. Biochem., 174* (1988) 698–707.

12 M. S. Patterson, B. Chance and B. C. Wilson, Time resolved reflectance and transmittance for the non-invasive measurement of tissue optical properties, *Appl. Opt., 28* (1989) 2331–2336.

13 M. Ferrari, D. A. Wilson, D. F. Hanley, J. F. Hartman, R. J. Traystman and M. C. Rogers, Non invasive determination of venous hemoglobin saturation in the dog by derivative near infrared spectroscopy, *Am. J. Physiol., 256* (1989) H1493–H1499.

14 M. Sassaroli and D. Rousseau, Time dependence of near-infrared spectra of photodissociated hemoglobin and myoglobin, *Biochemistry, 26* (1987) 3092–3098.

15 M. Cope, D. T. Delpy, E. O. R. Reynolds, S. Wray, J. Wyatt and P. van der Zee, Methods of quantitating cerebral near infrared spectroscopy data, *Adv. Exp. Med. Biol., 222* (1988) 183–189.

16 S. Wray, M. Cope, D. T. Delpy, J. S. Wyatt and E. O. R. Reynolds, Characterization of the near infrared absorption spectra of cytochrome a, a_3 and haemoglobin for the non invasive monitoring of cerebral oxygenation, *Biochim. Biophys. Acta, 33* (1988) 184–192.

17 T. R. Cheatle, L. A. Porter, M. Cope, D. T. Delpy, P. D. Coleridge Smith and J. H. Scurr, Near-infrared spectroscopy in peripheral vascular disease, *Br. J. Surg., 78* (1991) 405–408.

18 B. Chance, M. T. Dait, C. Zhang, T. Hamaoka and K. Hagerman, Recovery from exercise-induced desaturation in the quadriceps muscle of elite competitive rowers, *Am. J. Physiol., 262* (1992) C766–C775.

19 N. B. Hampson and C. A. Piantadosi, Near infrared monitoring of human skeletal muscle oxygenation during forearm ischemia, *J. Appl. Physiol., 64* (1988) 2449–2457.

20 O. J. Hartling, H. Kelbaek, T. Gjorup, B. Schibye, K. Klausen and T. Jensen, Forearm oxygen uptake during maximal forearm dynamic exercise, *Eur. J. Appl. Physiol., 58* (1989) 466–470.

21 E. Sobolewski, A. Guyot, M. Fisher, B. Chance and P. L. Peterson, Near infrared reflectance spectroscopy (NIRS) of mitochondrial myopathy, *Neurology, 40* S(1) (1990) 645.

22 J. R. Wilson, D. M. Mancini, K. McCully, N. Ferraro, V. Lanoce and B. Chance, Non invasive detection of skeletal muscle underperfusion with near-infrared spectroscopy in patients with heart failure, *Circulation, 80* (1989) 1668–1674.

23 Y. Shinohara, M. Haida, F. Kawaguchi, Y. Ito and H. Takeuchi, Hemoglobin oxygen-saturation image of rat brain using near infrared light, *J. Cerebral Blood Flow Metab., 11* (1991) S459.

Reprinted with permission from *Optics Letters,* Vol. 18(13), pp. 1092-1094
(July 1, 1993). ©1993 Optical Society of America.

Ultrafast time-gated imaging in thick tissues: a step toward optical mammography

B. B. Das, K. M. Yoo, and R. R. Alfano

*Institute for Ultrafast Spectroscopy and Lasers, Mediphotonic Laboratory, Departments of Physics and Electrical Engineering,
The City College and The Graduate School of The City University of New York, New York, New York 10031*

With an ultrafast time-gated optical detection method, a thin translucent strip of fat (2.5 mm thick) hidden inside a 4-cm-thick tissue is located with millimeter spatial resolution.

Imaging of a translucent (scattering) object hidden in a highly scattering random medium with light is a challenging problem. Conventional transillumination techniques with cw light have been used for many years in an attempt to image growths in a breast.[1-4] However, strong random multiple scattering of light in tissues washes out the shadow and renders these techniques ineffective for imaging breast tumors. The advent of ultrashort pulse lasers and novel time-resolved detection technologies has made it possible to eliminate selectively the multiple scattered light that limits the steady-state transillumination for imaging. Recently, time-resolved transillumination techniques have been used to image opaque[5-10] and partially absorbing[11] objects hidden in various random media.

When ultrashort laser pulses are incident upon a slab of scattering medium the transmitted pulses consist of a ballistic (coherent) component,[12,13] a diffuse component, and a snake component.[5] The intensity of the ballistic component (consisting of photons traveling along the straight-line path) is attenuated exponentially with the thickness of the sample, and this attenuation puts a severe limitation on its practical application, especially for medical imaging. The diffuse component is temporally broadened, as it consists of photons that have been scattered randomly in all directions and have traversed different path lengths. The temporal profile of a diffuse pulse can be approximated by the diffusion theory when the thickness of the sample is many times larger than the transport mean free path (l_t) of the sample. For a narrow beam of ultrashort laser pulses incident at a point on a slab, the temporal profile of a transmitted pulse at a point on the other side of the slab is given by

$$I_d(t) = \frac{1}{4td^2}\exp(-vt/l_a)\sum_1^\infty m\sin\frac{m\pi L}{d}$$
$$\times \exp[-(m\pi)^2 Dt/d^2], \qquad (1)$$

where $d = L + 1.42l_t$, v is the speed of light in the medium, D is the diffusion coefficient, and l_a is the absorption length. The snake component, consisting of the early-arriving photons that have undergone only a few scatterings along quasi-

straight-line paths (zigzag paths slightly off the straight-line path) through the turbid medium, forms the early portion of the diffuse pulse. The snake photons travel slightly off the straight path and, hence, carry information on the optical properties of the medium and any foreign object lying along this path line. Using time-resolved detection techniques, we can separate these snake photons from the diffuse component and use them to construct the image of the foreign object with different optical properties. These methods have potential use in imaging bones, tumors, and other types of diseased tissue that differ from their surrounding medium in optical properties (scattering and absorption coefficients).

In this Letter we demonstrate for what is to our knowledge the first time that a 2.5-mm-thick fat tissue embedded in a 40-mm-thick chicken breast tissue can be located by using state-of-the-art ultrafast time-resolved transillumination techniques. This work shows the potential of current ultrafast optical technologies for imaging breast tumors without x-ray radiation.

The experimental setup has been described in greater detail in our previous Letter.[14] A colliding-pulse mode-locked dye laser was used to produce ultrashort laser pulses of ~100 fs at 620 nm (with an 82-MHz repetition rate and 5-mW power). A part of the incident beam was used to trigger the streak camera with the use of a photodiode. The beam was focused by a long-focal-length lens ($f = 50$ mm) into a small 1-mm-diameter spot on the

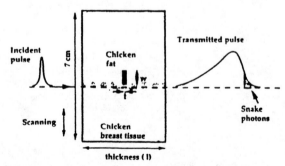

Fig. 1. Cross section of the chicken breast tissue sample in the plane of the scanning with a thin fat strip embedded in it.

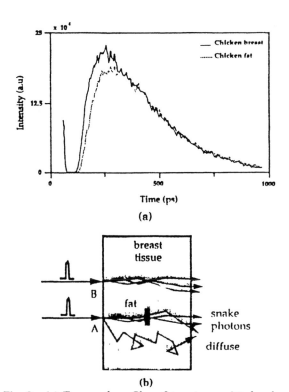

(a)

(b)

Fig. 2. (a) Temporal profiles of two transmitted pulses through the 2.6-cm-thick sample: the dotted curve is for incidence through the center of the fat strip, and the solid curve is at a 5-mm distance from the center. A part of the reference pulse is shown at ~75 ps. (b) Snake photon diagram: the snake photons carry information about the scattering and the absorption properties of the fat tissue when the laser beam is incident at point A, whereas the snake photons at point B do not carry this information.

sample. We prepared two samples of different dimensions by embedding a thin strip of chicken fat in the middle of a thick, smooth chicken breast tissue. We prepared the samples by sandwiching the thin strip of fat between the two soft pieces of chicken breast tissues. We pressed these samples between two parallel glass plates to keep them uniformly thick. The first sample had a 2-mm-thick, 5-mm-wide, and 40-mm-high fat strip embedded in the middle of a 26-mm-thick, 70-mm-wide, and 40-mm-high chicken breast tissue. The error in each dimension is ±0.5 mm. We mounted the sample holder on a translation stage to let the laser beam scan across the fat strip, as is displayed in Fig. 1. The sample was measured at the room temperature, and the transmitted signal was detected by a synchroscan streak camera. Small apertures were used to collect the transmitted photons scattered in the forward direction. These measurements were repeated for the second sample with a 2.5-mm-thick, 7-mm-wide, and 40-mm-high strip of fat inside a 40-mm-thick, 70-mm-wide, and 40-mm-high chicken breast tissue.

The l_t and l_a for the fat and the chicken breast tissues were measured with the pulse transmission technique described in our previous study.[15] The

values for fat and chicken breast tissues are $l_t = 0.58$ mm, $l_a = 139.3$ mm and $l_t = 2.5$ mm, $l_a = 51.7$ mm, respectively.

In order to locate the thin fat tissue inside the breast tissue, we laterally scanned the sample across the laser beam in 1-mm steps from one side of the fat tissue to the other (in 2-mm steps when scanning farther away from the fat). Figure 2(a) displays two temporal profiles of the transmitted pulses propagating through the 26-mm-thick tissue: the dotted curve is for the case when the line of beam incidence passes through the center of the fat strip, and the solid curve is for the case when the line passes ~5 mm away from the center of the strip. Note a significant difference in the intensities of the early parts of the two transmitted signals, whereas the later portions merge with each other. This difference at the early part is due to much stronger scattering in the fat tissue compared with that in the chicken breast tissue. In both tissues, the loss of light that is due to absorption is negligible compared with the loss that is due to scattering. This pronounced intensity difference in the early portion of the profile suggests the suitability of snake photons in obtaining the maximum contrast for imaging.

The schematic diagram in Fig. 2(b) shows the advantage of using snake photons for imaging when the laser beam is incident in the line of the fat tissue (point A) and away from it (point B). The snake photons at point A carry information about the scattering and absorption properties of the fat tissue, whereas the snake photons at point B do not. Most of the late-arriving photons from both points A and B, on the other hand, do not carry information about the fat tissue. The shorter transport mean free path for fat means light is scattered more in fat than in breast tissue. When the laser beam is incident near the fat tissue, a large number of the snake photons are lost owing to this higher scattering in fat, which gives

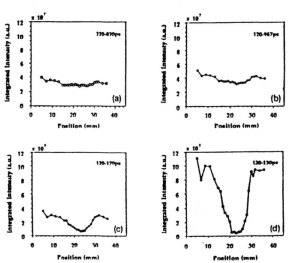

Fig. 3. Time-integrated intensity from the transmitted signal through the 2.6-cm-thick sample at different time gates versus different beam-incidence positions: (a) 220–820 ps, (b) 120–967 ps, (c) 120–170 ps, and (d) 120–130 ps.

221

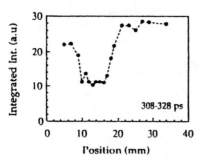

Fig. 4. Time-integrated intensity from the transmitted signal through the 4-cm-thick sample with a 2.5-mm-thick fat strip within a 20-ps window (308–328 ps) versus different beam-incidence positions.

rise to the pronounced difference in the early part, as shown in Fig. 2(a). On the other hand, most of the diffuse photons, traveling around the small fat tissue, are not significantly affected by its presence. So it is the snake photon that is selected to detect the location of the fat inside the breast tissue with maximum contrast

The straight-line propagation time through a 26-mm-thick tissue is ~116 ps. The time-integrated intensities for four different time windows, 220–820, 120–967, 120–170, and 120–130 ps, were calculated from the transmitted signal for various positions of incidence on the sample. The last window captures 10 ps of snake light. We calculated the integrated intensity by summing the transmitted pulse intensity over each time window. The results are plotted in Fig. 3. The integrated intensity with the 220–820-ps time gate [Fig. 3(a)], which collects most of the transmitted pulse except the snake photons, shows almost a straight line without revealing the position of the fat tissue. Figure 3(b) displays the integrated intensity for the whole signal, and this case is equivalent to cw transillumination. The 120–170-ps time gate, which eliminates a significant portion of the diffuse component, displays a dip in the curve at the fat region [Fig. 3(c)]. The resolution is significantly improved, with the 120–130 ps time gate [Fig. 3(d)], by eliminating the late-arriving photons further. By choosing mostly the snake photons (for 10 ps), not only do we correctly predict the location of the fat tissue but the edges of the strip are also resolved. The relatively flat bottom of the curve matches well with the width of the fat strip inside the breast tissue with millimeter resolution.

These measurements were repeated on the 4-cm-thick sample. The diffuse photons start to arrive at ~300 ps. A 20-ps time window (308–328 ps) was used at the early part of the diffuse pulse to collect the snake photons. The time-integrated intensity of light within this window versus the different beam incidence positions is displayed in Fig. 4. As in the

2.6-cm-thick sample, the integrated intensity curve shows a nearly flat line at the region of the fat strip, and it rises almost as a step function once we scan past the edges of the fat strip.

The spatial resolution of this optical approach can be significantly improved by (1) using an infrared laser operated in the 900–1350-nm spectral region, where light scattering is reduced in breast tissues and where the use of chromophores may help improve the image quality, (2) using a more stable laser such as a solid-state laser instead of a dye laser, (3) increasing the sensitivity of detection by using a cooled CCD camera, (4) using a streak camera of 1-ps response instead of the standard 8 ps that we have used, (5) using 5-μm-diameter fibers for light delivery and signal collection, and (6) using the absorption by Hb, HbO$_2$, and H$_2$O in tissues to help reduce the late-arriving photons.

This research may be extended by using a two-dimensional array of fibers to obtain a two-dimensional image of a tumor in a breast. With suitable improvements in optical devices this novel method may lead in the near future to a noninvasive and nonionizing technique for detecting malignant tumors in breast with high spatial resolution.

This research is supported by the Mediscience Technology Corporation and organized research at the City College of the City University of New York.

References

1. D. J. Watmough, Radiology **147**, 89 (1983).
2. G. A. Navarro and A. E. Profio, Med. Phys. **15**, 181 (1988).
3. R. Lafrenuere, F. S. Ashkar, and A. S. Ketcham, Am. Surg. **52**, 123 (1986).
4. E. A. Sickles, Recent Results Cancer Res. **105**, 31 (1987).
5. L. Wang, P. P. Ho, C. Liu, G. Zhang, and R. R. Alfano, Science **253**, 769 (1991).
6. H. Chen, Y. Chen, D. Dilworth, E. Leith, J. Lopez, and J. Valdmanis, Opt. Lett. **16**, 487 (1991).
7. E. N. Leith, C. Chen, H. Chen, Y. Chen, J. Lopez, and P. C. Sun, Opt. Lett. **16**, 1820 (1991).
8. M. D. Duncan, R. Mahon, L. L. Tankersley, and J. Reintjes, Opt. Lett. **16**, 1868 (1991).
9. K. M. Yoo, Q. Xing, and R. R. Alfano, Opt. Lett. **16**, 1019 (1991).
10. S. Anderson-Engels, R. Berg, S. Svanberg, and O. Jarlman, Opt. Lett. **15**, 1179 (1990).
11. J. C. Hebden, R. A. Kruger, and K. S. Wong, Appl. Opt. **30**, 788 (1991).
12. K. M. Yoo and R. R. Alfano, Opt. Lett. **15**, 320 (1990).
13. F. Liu, K. M. Yoo, and R. R. Alfano, Opt. Lett. **16**, 351 (1991).
14. K. M. Yoo, B. B. Das, and R. R. Alfano, Opt. Lett. **17**, 958 (1992).
15. K. M. Yoo, F. Liu, and R. R. Alfano, Phys. Rev. Lett. **64**, 2647 (1990).

Reprinted with permission from *Chemical Physics Letters,* Vol. 166(3), pp. 246-252
(February 23, 1990). ©1990 Elsevier Science Publishers B.V.

FREQUENCY-DOMAIN MEASUREMENTS OF PHOTON MIGRATION IN TISSUES

Joseph R. LAKOWICZ and Klaus BERNDT [1]

Department of Biological Chemistry, School of Medicine, University of Maryland,
660 West Redwood Street, Baltimore, MD 21201, USA

Received 4 December 1989

We report the use of frequency-domain (FD) measurements to characterize time-dependent migration of 620–740 nm photons in tissues, in particular arm and finger. The time dependence of the re-emerged light appears to be characterized by a delay time which depends on path length and detector geometry, a transient-time spread which appears to depend on sample homogeneity, and an exponential decay time which depends on sample absorbance and/or path length. The time delay is revealed by a phase angle exceeding 90°, which is not explainable for directly initiated multi- or single-exponential processes. The transit-time spread is revealed by a frequency-dependent decrease in modulation which is more rapid than for an exponential decay. Potential clinical uses of the FD photon migration measurements are discussed.

1. Introduction

Transmission of long wavelength and/or near infrared light through tissues has been used for physiological studies of bioenergetics [1–3], for trend measurements of hemoglobin, myoglobin and/or tissue oxygenation [4,5] and of cytochrome oxidation [6,7]. A major obstacle to the quantitative use of light transmission in tissues is the unknown pathlength for photon migration and the consequential inability to use the signal levels for quantitation of the absorbing species. An imaginative solution to this problem was recently suggested by Chance and co-workers [8]. These workers noted that following insertion of a picosecond light pulse, the re-emerged light at time t has necessarily traveled a distance $L=ct/n$, where c is the speed of light and n is the refractive index. An exponential time decay was found, and the time axis corresponds to the distance traveled by the scattered light. These results, which also demonstrated the possibility of non-invasive measurements of tissue oxygenation, indicate the potential usefulness of time-dependent measure-

ments of photon migration for clinical sensing.

In the present report we extend the studies of Chance and co-workers [8] to further characterize time-dependent photon migration (TDPM) in tissues. In particular, we used frequency-domain (FD) measurements [9–11], which are known to provide good resolution of complex fluorescence decays. Additionally, because the FD instrumentation can be made small and inexpensive, these studies can assist in the development of clinical applications of time-dependent photon migration. We now describe our initial FD studies of photon migration in tissues.

2. Theory

Consider a highly scattering medium into which one injects a δ-function pulse of light. The theory of photon migration in tissues and turbid media has been presented by several groups [12–17]. Of these, the recent theory of Peterson et al. [15] is of greatest interest because it presents the expressions for time-dependent re-emergent light. However, we used alternative expressions which provide an intuitive representation of time-dependent photon migration. Based upon our present level of experience with FD measurements of light migration, we consider three

[1] Permanent address: Central Institute of Optics and Spectroscopy, Academy of Sciences of the GDR, Rudower Chaussee 6, DDR 1199, Berlin, German Democratic Republic.

processes which affect the time-dependent arrival of scattered light at the detector. First, there is a time delay Δt_L due to the photon traveling a distance L. The time delay can be related to the distance traveled by the photon using the speed of light in tissues, which is expected to be about 23 cm/ps [8]. Due to multiple scattering events the apparent distance is expected to be about 1.5- to several-fold larger than the geometric distance between the source and the detector. Second, the pulse appears to be broadened [18], which we believe is due to various possible path lengths. This is analogous to transit time spread in a photomultiplier tube, and hence we use the term Δt_{ts}. And finally, the emergent light decays exponentially [8,18] due to the Beer–Lambert law, with a decay time τ_D.

We observe the emergent light using the frequency-domain (FD) method. In this case the phase shift of the emergent light is given by

$$\phi_\omega = \arctan(\omega \tau_D) + \omega \Delta t_L . \tag{1}$$

where ω is the circular modulation frequency in rad/ s. The relationship of the phase shift due to τ_D is that known for an exponential process [19]. The phase angle due to the time delay (ϕ_D) is given by $\phi_D = \omega \Delta t_L$ [20], and should not be confused with the approximate expression used elsewhere [21]. Eq. (1) is based on the known dependence of ϕ_ω in the presence of consecutive processes [22]. The modulation is given by

$$m_\omega = m_{ts} m_D . \tag{2}$$

where

$$m_{ts} = (1 + \omega^2 \Delta t_{ts}^2)^{-1/2} . \tag{3}$$

$$m_D = (1 + \omega^2 \tau_D^2)^{-1/2} . \tag{4}$$

Eq. (4) describes the usual relationship between a decay time and demodulation. Eq. (3) is an analogous expression for time dispersion of the incident light [23]. The product is used (eq. (2)) to account for the experimental results, and it is also known that the product is needed to account for consecutive time-dependent events [22]. This suggests that the time dispersion of the incident light should be regarded as occurring prior to arrival of the pulse at the detector. We note that the modulation values are not sensitive to the phase of the scattered light, and

hence not sensitive to Δt_L, so that Δt_L does not appear in eqs. (2)–(4). Since this model appears to account for the data, the parameters τ_D, Δt_L and Δt_{ts} are adequate to describe the re-emerged light. If desired, it should be possible to relate these parameters to those given in ref. [15].

In our initial studies the path lengths are typically in the range of 10–20 mm. Hence, the Δt_L values are expected to be near 88 to 176 ps, assuming a speed of 23 cm/ns [8] and an effective path length of twice the geometric distance between source and collector. It seems probable that Δt_{ts} would be a fraction of Δt_L, and probably near 25% of Δt_L or 20 to 40 ps.

3. Materials and methods

Frequency-domain measurements were performed using the 2 GHz instrument described previously [11], with the following modifications. The externally cross-correlated microchannel plate (MCP) PMT was replaced with a grid-gatable MCP PMT from Hamamatsu, model R2024U. Cross-correlation [24] was accomplished by modulation of the grid, which is behind the photocathode, at frequencies 25 Hz offset from the integer harmonics of the laser pulse repetition frequency. We found it possible to obtain useful modulation to 4.5 GHz [25] and, with appropriate correction procedures, to perform fluorescence measurements over the same range of frequencies [26]. While this grid-modulated PMT does show a wavelength-dependent time response [25], this is not important for scattered light, which is at the same wavelength as the incident light. The light source was a 3.76 MHz train of 5 ps pulses, obtained from the cavity-dumped output of a R6G (560–620 nm) or pyridin 2 (695–770 nm) dye laser, each pumped by a mode-locked argon ion laser. Measurements are possible at all integer multiples of the cavity-dumped frequency, using the harmonic content of the pulse train.

The incident light was directed onto the tissue and collected to the detector using 3 mm diameter fiber optic bundles. The sample consisted of either a finger or forearm. The control measurement was the phase and modulation observed when the two bundles were placed in line without tissue, but separated by a thin diffuser. The distance between the bundle ends ranged from 6 to 18 mm, on the same side of the finger or forearm.

Data were analyzed by a non-linear least-squares algorithm, provided by Dr. Michael L. Johnson of the University of Virginia, Department of Pharmacology. The measured phase (φ_ω) and/or modulation (m_ω) values were compared with the calculated (c) value. The parameter values (t_D, Δt_L and/or Δt_{ts}) were varied to yield the minimum value of χ_R^2,

$$\chi_R^2 = \frac{1}{2} \sum_\omega \left(\frac{\varphi_\omega - \varphi_\omega^c}{\delta\varphi} \right)^2 + \frac{1}{2} \sum_\omega \left(\frac{m_\omega - m_\omega^c}{\delta m} \right), \qquad (5)$$

where ω is the number of degrees of freedom and $\delta\varphi = 0.2°$ and $\delta m = 0.005$ are the uncertainties in the measured quantities.

4. Results

Frequency-dependent phase angles were first measured for 620 nm light migration through a finger, with the fiber bundle ends spaced 18 mm apart (fig. 1). The most striking feature of the data are the phase angles in excess of 90°, in this case extending to about 270°. Phase angles in excess of 90° are not possible for a directly excited exponential process, and can only be explained by consecutive processes [22] or due to time delays such as those due to color effects in photomultiplier tubes [20,21,27]. The need for a delay time Δt_L is illustrated by the inability to fit the data using a single decay time τ_D (dashed line). However, the data are easily fit if the algorithm allows for a time delay (full line). The delay time was found to be about 200 ps. A delay of 78 ps is expected due to the 18 mm path length. The fact that the observed delay time is longer than that due to the spacing between the fibers suggests a complex path for light migration in fingers.

Modulation data for the same finger are shown in fig. 2. The modulation data are not sensitive to the time-delay (phase) of the detected light. Nonetheless, it was not possible to account for the data using a single decay time (dashed line). Remarkably, the frequency-dependent modulation appears to decrease faster than is possible for a single-exponential process. This effect is not possible for a simultaneous multi-exponential process [22]. We reasoned that an effect which decreases the apparent modulation

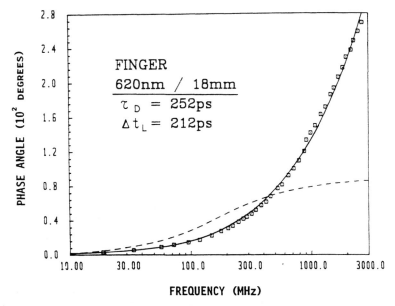

Fig. 1. Representative frequency-dependent phase angles for 620 nm photon migration in a finger. The distance between the fiber ends was 18 mm. – – –, best fit with a single decay time; ———, best fit with the decay time and delay time as variable parameters.

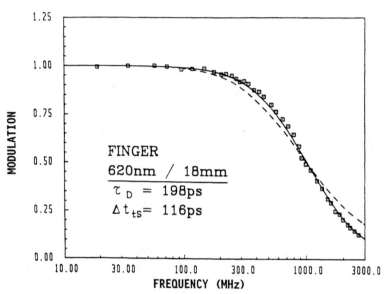

Fig. 2. Representative frequency-dependent modulation data for 620 nm light in a finger, 18 mm between the fiber ends. ---, best fit for a single decay time: ——, best fit with the decay time and transit time spread as variable parameters.

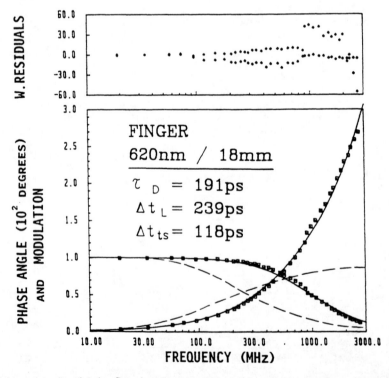

Fig. 3. Combined phase angle and modulation fit to time-dependent 620 nm light migration in a finger. The dashed lines show the best fit with a single decay time, and the solid lines the best fit with τ_D, Δt_L and Δt_{ts} as variable parameters. The upper panel shows the deviations between the data and the best fit parameters, $\tau_D = 191$, $\Delta t_L = 239$, $\Delta t_{ts} = 118$ ps. The residuals are in units of the standard deviation of the phase ($\delta\varphi = 0.2°$) and modulation ($\delta m = 0.005$).

226

of the incident light, independent of the decay time τ_D, could result in such data. In fact, inclusion of a term to account for a transit time spread (eqs. (3) and (4)) allowed us to fit the modulation data (full line). The apparent value of Δt_{ts} is near 100 ps, which corresponds to about 23 mm. Once again, this suggests a complex light migration path in a finger.

We also attempted to simultaneously fit the phase and modulation data (fig. 3). It was impossible to even approximate the data using a single decay time τ_D (dashed line). In contrast, both the phase and the modulation data are reasonably well fit using the three parameter model, τ_D, Δt_L and Δt_{ts}. The deviations (upper panel) are somewhat larger than we are willing to accept in analysis of our fluorescence data, but this simple model provides an intuitive representation of the experimental results.

We performed similar measurements of photon migration in a forearm (fig. 4), in this case using 740 nm. Once again, it was not possible to account for

the data using a single delay time (dashed line), but a reasonable fit was found for the model which also contained a delay time. In this case the apparent value of Δt_{ts} was smaller, and the data could be fit with any value of Δt_{ts} ranging from 0 to 50 ps. This indicates that the value of Δt_{ts} is too small to be detectable with our current instrumentation. In contrast, the data for the finger could not be fit using these values (0–50 ps) for Δt_{ts}. Additionally, the delay time at 740 nm per mm is smaller for the forearm. These combined results suggest a more direct and/or homogeneous light migration path in the forearm, which is reasonable given the absence of nearby bone, tendon and other potentially transparent and/or reflective media.

5. Discussion

Additional experimental results are summarized in table 1. It appears that the delay time Δt_L in-

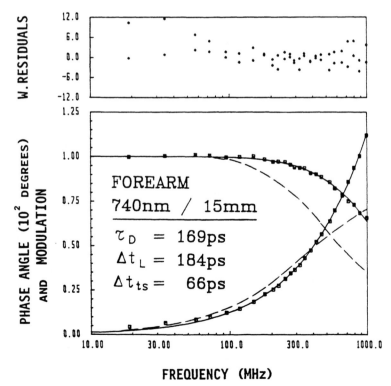

Fig. 4. Combined phase angle and modulation fit to 740 nm photon migration in a forearm. 15 mm between fiber ends. The dashed lines show the best fit with a single decay time, and the solid lines the best fit with τ_D, Δt_L and Δt_{ts} as variable parameters.

Table 1
Parameters describing photon migration in the forearm and finger

	Wavelength (nm)	Distance (mm)	τ_D (ps)	Δt_L (ps)	Δt_{ts} (ps)
forearm	620	6	93	28	0
	620	9	102	58	0
	620	12	111	122	45
	700	9	118	62	0–15
	740	9	123	60	0
	740	12	136	108	42
	740	15	169	184	66
finger	620	6	106	24	0
	620	12	109	151	104
	620	18	191	239	118

creases with distance between the fibers, as is expected for a longer path length. The values of Δt_{ts} appear to be larger in the finger than in the forearm, which is consistent with a more heterogeneous light path in the fingers. The decay times appear to be larger for the longer wavelengths, which is expected if the medium is less absorbing at the longer wavelengths [8,18]. Surprisingly, the decay times appear to increase as the distance between the fibers is increased. This is surprising because we expected the values of τ_D to be determined by the tissue and its absorbance, and not by the detector geometry. However, these effects are understandable if one remembers that there exists in the tissue an ensemble of migrating photons. At any instant the observed intensity is a measure of the surviving photons in the sample, in particular those incident on the detecting fiber. It seems possible that at longer distances one selectively observes photons which have migrated over longer distances. Since the survival of a photon depends upon its time-of-flight, these longer-lived signals may be selectively enriched with photons which have traveled through less optically dense regions of the tissue. Additional experimentation and analysis is required to confirm or refute this speculation.

The present studies must be regarded as preliminary, but this nonetheless suggest the usefulness of frequency-domain methods for studies of time-dependent photon migration in tissues. For clinical sensing of tissue oxygenation it will be necessary to select appropriate wavelengths and/or differential wavelength methods [1–3] to match absorption bands and isosbestic points of hemoglobin and/or cytochromes. Furthermore, the sensitivity of the decay times, delay times and transit time spread to the optical properties of the tissue supports the suggestion by Chance [8] that photon migration might be used for non-invasive imaging of tissues. And finally, the growing availability of laser diodes and the simplicity of the frequency-domain instrumentation should make such applications feasible.

Acknowledgements

The authors thank Dr. Michael L. Johnson, University of Virginia, for providing the computer programs for data analysis, and the support of the Medical Biotechnology Center at the University of Maryland School of Medicine. The authors also express their appreciation to Hamamatsu, Inc. and Mr. David Fatlowitz for the opportunity to perform test measurements using the R2024U photomultiplier tube. Supported by grants DMB-8502835 and DIR-8710401 from the National Science Foundation.

References

[1] B. Chance, Science 120 (1954) 767.

[2] B. Chance, V. Legallair and B. Schoener, Nature 195 (1962) 1073.

[3] B. Chance, J. Biol. Chem. 234 (1959) 3036.

[4] F.F. Jobsis, Science 198 (1977) 1264.

[5] J.W. Seds, R.C. Cefalo, H.J. Proctor and F.F. Jobsis-van der Vliet, Am. J. Obstet. Gynecol. 149 (1984) 679.

[6] F.F. Jobsis-van der Vliet, Advan. Exp. Med. Biol. 191 (1985) 833.

[7] F.F. Jobsis, J.H. Keizer, J.C. Lamanna and M. Rosenthal, J. Appl. Physiol. 113 (1977) 858.

[8] B. Chance, J.S. Leigh, H. Miyake, D.S. Smith, S. Nioka, R. Greenfeld, M. Finander, K. Kaufmann, W. Levy, M. Young, P. Cohen, H. Yoshioka and R. Boretsky, Proc. Natl. Acad. Sci. US 85 (1988) 4971.

[9] E. Gratton and M. Limkeman, Biophys. J 44 (1983) 315.

[10] J.R. Lakowicz and B.P. Maliwal, Biophys. Chem. 21 (1985) 61.

[11] J.R. Lakowicz, G. Laczko and I. Gryczynski, Rev. Sci. Instr. 57 (1986) 2499.

[12] A.J. Welsh, G. Yom and M.J.C. von Gemert, Lasers Surg. Med. 6 (1987) 488.

[13] M. Keijzer, S.L. Jacques, S.A. Prahl and A.J. Welsh, Lasers Surg. Med. 9 (1989) 148.

[14] S.L. Jacques and S.A. Prahl, Lasers Surg. Med. 6 (1987) 494.

[15] M.S. Patterson, B. Chance and B.C. Wilson, Appl. Opt. 28 (1989) 2331.

[16] G.H. Weiss, R. Nossal and R.F. Bonner, J. Mod. Opt. 36 (1989) 349.

[17] R.F. Bonner, R. Nossal, S. Havlin and G.H. Weiss, J. Opt. Soc. Am. 4 (1987) 423.

[18] B. Chance, S. Nioka, J. Kent, K. McCully, M. Fountain, R. Greenfeld and G. Holton, Anal. Biochem. 174 (1988) 698.

[19] J.R. Lakowiz, Principles of fluorescence spectroscopy (Plenum Press, New York, 1983).

[20] K.W. Berndt, H. Durr and D. Palme, Opt. Commun. 47 (1983) 321.

[21] D.M. Jameson and G. Weber, J. Phys. Chem. 85 (1981) 953.

[22] J.R. Lakowicz and A. Balter, Biophys. Chem. 16 (1982) 99.

[23] J. Wilson and J.F.B. Hawkes, Optoelectronics: an introduction (1983) p. 431.

[24] R.D. Spencer and G. Weber, Ann. NY Acad. Sci. 158 (1969) 361.

[25] K.W. Berndt and J.R. Lakowicz, Rev. Sci. Instr., in preparation.

[26] J.R. Lakowicz, K.W. Berndt and I. Gryczynski, Biophys. Chem., in preparation.

[27] D. Phillips, R.C. Drake, D.V. O'Connor and R.L. Christensen, Anal. Instr. 14 (1985) 267.

Reprinted with permission from *Applied Optics,* Vol. 30(31), pp. 4474-4476
(November 1, 1991). ©1991 Optical Society of America.

Frequency-domain reflectance for the determination of the scattering and absorption properties of tissue

Michael S. Patterson, J. David Moulton, Brian C. Wilson,
Klaus W. Berndt, and Joseph R. Lakowicz

M. S. Patterson, J. David Moulton, and B. C. Wilson are with the Hamilton Regional Cancer Centre and McMaster University, 711 Concession Street, Hamilton L8V 1C3, Canada. K. W. Berndt and J. R. Lakowicz are with the Department of Biological Chemistry, School of Medicine, University of Maryland, 660 West Redwood Street, Baltimore, Maryland 21201.

Received 18 December 1990.
0003-6935/92/314474-22$05.00/0.
© 1991 Optical Society of America.

Measurements of the phase and modulation of amplitude-modulated light diffusely reflected by turbid media can be used to deduce absorption and scattering coefficients.

Many diagnostic and therapeutic applications of light in medicine require information about the scattering and absorption properties of tissues. Ideally these data should be acquired noninvasively from measurements of diffusely reflected light. A technique based on the characterization of the temporal spreading of a picosecond pulse caused by propagation along different multiple-scattering paths between source and detector has recently been proposed.[1] It was shown that, if the tissue is homogeneous and semi-infinite in extent, the source and detector are small compared with their separation ρ on the surface, and the pulse can be considered a unit impulse in time, then $R(\rho,t)$, the number of photons backscattered to the surface per unit time and area, is

$$R(\rho, t) = \frac{z_o}{(4\pi Dc)^{3/2}} \, t^{-5/2} \exp\left(-\frac{\rho^2 + z_o^2}{4Dct}\right) \exp(-\mu_a ct), \qquad (1)$$

where

$$z_o = [(1 - g)\mu_s]^{-1}, \qquad (2)$$

$$D \cong [3(1 - g)\mu_s]^{-1} \qquad (3)$$

and μ_a is the tissue absorption coefficient, μ_s is the scattering coefficient, g is the mean cosine of the scattering angle, and c is the speed of light in the tissue. The derivation of Eq. (1) was based on a diffusion model of light propagation, and its validity is limited to wavelengths where $\mu_a \ll (1 - g)\mu_s$. In practice μ_a and the transport-scattering coefficient $\mu_s' = (1 - g)\mu_s$ are estimated by fitting the pulse shape as measured by time-correlated single-photon counting to the expression in Eq. (1). We describe advantages to making such measurements in the frequency domain, present equations relating the amplitude modulation and phase to μ_a and μ_s', show some preliminary data, and suggest a potentially useful combination of frequency-domain and steady-state techniques.

Frequency-domain measurements of modulation M and phase ϕ are well established in fluorescence spectroscopy[2] and should provide information equivalent to that obtained in the time domain. Specific advantages offered by frequency-domain measurements are as follows:

(1) Instrumentation can be considerably cheaper and simpler, particularly if frequencies below 200 MHz are adequate.

(2) The terms μ_a and μ_s' can in principle be calculated from measurements of M and ϕ at a single frequency.

(3) The terms M and ϕ can be measured in a time that is short enough to permit the monitoring of dynamic phenomena such as changes in hemoglobin oxygenation.

(4) The correction for instrument response requires relatively simple arithmetic operations rather than deconvolution.

Analytic expressions for the modulation and phase, derived by the Fourier transformation[3] of Eq. (1) for modulation frequency f, are

$$M(\rho, f) = \frac{(1 + \psi_i^2 + 2\psi_i)^{(1/2)}}{(1 + \psi_\infty)} \exp(\psi_\infty - \psi_i), \qquad (4)$$

$$\phi(\rho, f) = \psi_r - \tan^{-1}\left(\frac{\psi_r}{1 + \psi_i}\right), \qquad (5)$$

where

$$\psi_o = \left\{3[\mu_a + (1 - g)\mu_s](\rho^2 + z_o^2)([\mu_a c]^2 + [2\pi f]^2)^{1/2} c^{-1}\right\}^{1/2}, \qquad (6)$$

$$\psi_r = -\psi_o \sin\left(\frac{\theta}{2}\right), \qquad (7)$$

$$\psi_i = \psi_o \cos\left(\frac{\theta}{2}\right), \qquad (8)$$

$$\theta = \tan^{-1}\left(\frac{2\pi f}{\mu_a c}\right), \qquad (9)$$

$$\psi_\infty = \psi_o(f = 0) = \psi_i(f = 0) = \{3\mu_a[\mu_a + (1 - g)\mu_s](\rho^2 + z_o^2)\}^{1/2}. \qquad (10)$$

For fixed values of ρ and f, the absorption and scattering coefficients can be obtained graphically from plots such as Fig. 1 or more precisely by a multidimensional Newton–Raphson algorithm[4] designed to solve Eqs. (4) and (5). The optimum frequency for measurement of M and ϕ depends somewhat on the optical properties of the tissue as discussed here.

As a preliminary test of the model we acquired phase and modulation data for a tissue-simulating material consisting of a light-scattering lipid emulsion to which increasing

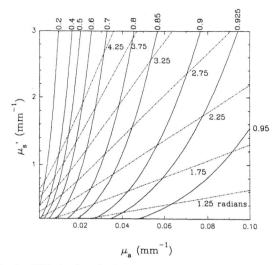

Fig. 1. Diffusion-based calculations of lines of constant modulation (solid) and phase (dashed) for optical properties typical of soft tissues in the red and near infrared. The modulation frequency has been fixed at 400 MHz and the source–detector separation at 50 mm.

amounts of India ink were added. By a narrow beam transmission measurement we determined that $\mu_s = 0.86$ mm^{-1} for the emulsion. Pulsed light (755 nm) was delivered through an optical fiber bundle to the surface of a cylindrical tank (130 mm in diameter) containing the emulsion. Light was collected by another bundle separated by 80 mm on the surface, and the phase and modulation of this light were measured by a cross-correlation technique previously described elsewhere.[2]

For each concentration of added ink, Eqs. (4) and (5) were used to calculate μ_a and μ_s' for frequencies where $0.2 < M < 0.8$. The mean value of the derived parameters was then used to generate the smooth curves shown in Fig. 2. Excellent fits to the experimental data were obtained over the full frequency range. The best estimates of the scattering and absorption coefficients are plotted versus the relative amount of added ink in Fig. 3. The scattering coefficient is seen to be independent of the added absorber, and the derived value $\mu_s' = 0.19$ mm^{-1} is consistent with the measured value $\mu_s = 0.86$ mm^{-1} if $g = 0.78$. While g was not independently measured in this preliminary experiment, values of 0.7–0.8 are typical for such emulsions.[5] The estimated absorption coefficient increases linearly with the amount of added ink as expected. Future experiments will test the ability of the model to provide quantitative estimates of μ_a and μ_s'.

The curves in Figs. 1 and 2 suggest that measurements are best performed at a frequency where the modulation is changing rapidly. For smaller values of ρ and of μ_a and μ_s' that are typical of soft tissues, this frequency may be so high that the use of inexpensive photomultiplier tubes and externally modulated light sources is precluded. A possible solution is to use a gain-modulated avalanche photodiode[6] as a detector and the high-frequency harmonic content of a picosecond pulsed laser diode as a source.

A second solution is to combine a measurement of the phase (which can be readily and accurately determined even at low frequencies[7]) with a steady-state measurement of μ_{eff}, the effective attenuation coefficient. It has been shown that μ_{eff}, which is equal to $[3\mu_a(\mu_a + \mu_s')]^{1/2}$ under the assumptions of diffusion theory, can be determined from

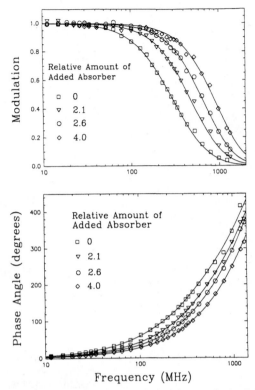

Fig. 2. Plots of phase angle and modulation obtained for a scattering emulsion to which increasing amounts of India ink were added. The smooth curves were generated from solutions to Eqs. (4) and (5) and represent best estimates of the absorption and transport-scattering coefficients.

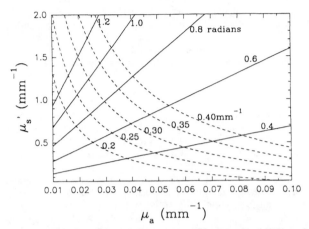

Fig. 4. Calculated lines of constant phase angle (solid) and effective steady-state attenuation coefficient (dashed) in the space defined by the tissue absorption and transport-scattering coefficients. The modulation frequency was fixed at 200 MHz and the source–detector separation (for the frequency domain) at 30 mm.

surements of the phase and the effective attenuation coefficient. This technique would not be limited to wavelengths where diffusion theory is accurate as both ϕ and μ_{eff} can be calculated by more exact radiation transport models or Monte Carlo simulation

The support of the Ontario Laser & Lightwave Research Centre is acknowledged.

noninvasive measurements of the spatial dependence of the diffuse reflectance on the tissue surface.[8] Figure 4 is a graph showing diffusion theory calculations of lines of equal phase angle and μ_{eff} in the optical properties space defined by μ_a and μ_s'. Such plots or iterative numerical techniques could be used to estimate the interaction coefficients from mea-

References

1. M. S. Patterson, B. Chance, and B. C. Wilson, "Time resolved reflectance and transmittance for the non-invasive measurement of tissue optical properties," Appl. Opt. **28**, 2331–2336 (1989).
2. J. R. Lakowicz, G. Laczko, I. Gryczynski, H. Szmacinki, and W. Wiczk, "Gigahertz frequency-domain fluorometry: resolution of complex decays, picosecond processes and future developments," J. Photochem. Photobiol. B: Biol. **2**, 295–311 (1988).
3. I. S. Gradshteyn and I. M. Ryzhik, *Table of Integrals, Series and Products* (Academic, San Diego, Calif., 1980), p. 340.
4. J. D. Moulton, "Diffusion modelling of picosecond laser pulse propagation in turbid media," M. Eng. thesis (McMaster University, Hamilton, Canada, 1990).
5. C. J. M. Moes, M. J. C. van Gemert, W. M. Star, J. P. A. Marijnissen, and S. A. Prahl, "Measurements and calculations of the energy fluence rate in a scattering and absorbing phantom at 633 nm," Appl. Opt. **28,** 2292–2296 (1989).
6. K. W. Brendt, H. Duerr, and D. Palme, "Picosecond laser spectroscopy with avalanche photodiodes," in *Time Resolved Laser Spectroscopy in Biochemistry*, J. R. Lakowicz, ed., Proc. Soc. Photo-Opt. Instrum. Eng. **909**, 209–215 (1988).
7. B. Chance, M. Maris, J. Sorge, and M. Z. Zhang, "A phase modulation system for dual wavelength difference spectroscopy of hemoglobin deoxygenation in tissues," in *Time Resolved Laser Spectroscopy in Biochemistry II*, J. R. Lakowicz, ed., Proc. Soc. Photo-Opt. Instrum. Eng. **1204,** 481–491 (1990).
8. B. C. Wilson, T. J. Farrell, and M. S. Patterson, "An optical fiber-based diffuse reflectance spectrometer for non-invasive investigation of photodynamic sensitizers in vivo," in *Future Directions and Applications in Photodynamic Therapy*, C. J. Gomer, ed. (SPIE Institutes, Bellingham, Wash., 1990), Vol. IS6, pp. 219–232.

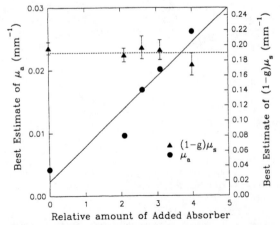

Fig. 3. Plot of the best estimates of absorption and transport-scattering coefficients versus the relative amount of added ink. As expected the estimated values of μ_s' are independent of the amount of added ink while the estimate of μ_a increases linearly.

Reprinted from *Time-Resolved Spectroscopy and Imaging of Tissues*, Proc. SPIE
Vol. 1431, pp. 122-135 (1991). ©1991 SPIE.

DIFFUSION OF INTENSITY MODULATED
NEAR-INFRARED LIGHT IN TURBID MEDIA

Joshua Fishkin, Enrico Gratton, Martin J. vandeVen, William W. Mantulin
Laboratory for Fluorescence Dynamics, Department of Physics,
University of Illinois at Urbana-Champaign, 1110 W. Green, Urbana IL 61801

1.   ABSTRACT

Light propagation in turbid media can be described by photon diffusion. In the
frequency domain, sinusoidally intensity-modulated light gives rise to diffusive
waves which have a coherent front. In a homogeneous medium, the wave front
propagates with a constant phase velocity and the amplitude   attenuates
exponentially as the diffusional wave advances. We have studied the diffusion
approximation to the one-speed linear transport equation with a sinusoidally
intensity modulated point source of particles and performed experiments using
frequency domain detection methods on homogeneous scattering and absorbing
media to test the applicability of the above mentioned transport equation to
photon migration in turbid media. We have used the analytical solutions of the
linear transport equation in homogeneous, infinite media to determine via a
simple analysis of our frequency domain data the linear scattering and
absorption coefficients.

2.   INTRODUCTION

Light propagation in highly scattering, low absorbing media has been described
by the diffusion approximation to the one-speed linear transport equation [1].
This approximation treats the light propagation as a process in which photons
are particles undergoing a large number collisions. It is known that the
accuracy of the predictions of the diffusion-approximation deteriorate as the
absorbing strength of the transporting medium increases. Higher order
approximations to the linear transport equation have been used to obtain a more
accurate description of the particle transport process [1, 2]. Patterson et al. [3]
have developed a model for the propagation of a light pulse through a
homogeneous semi-infinite medium and through a homogeneous slab based on
the diffusion approximation to linear transport theory. Their model yields
expressions for the pulse shape as a function of space and time in terms of the
scattering and absorption coefficients of the medium. These expressions have
been shown to accurately predict the temporal and spatial properties of a light
pulse as it propagates through biological tissue. Lakowicz et al. [4] have
measured the phase shift and demodulation of intensity modulated light as it
passed through biological tissue, however the empirical formulas presented by
Lakowicz do not appear to have been derived from linear transport theory. We
have used linear transport theory to derive the equations describing the
diffusion of light through a homogeneous scattering and absorbing medium
when the light originates from a sinusoidally intensity modulated point source.

We have performed experiments using a highly scattering medium and a fiber
optic illumination system in which the light source is an intensity modulated
laser. We have fit our data to expressions derived from the diffusion
approximation to the one-speed linear transport equation with a sinusoidally
intensity modulated point source of particles. Using frequency domain
detection methods, we have measured the attenuation and phase delay of the
wave front of intensity-modulated light as it propagates in the highly scattering
medium. We have detected the front of the intensity-modulated wave, not the
front of the electromagnetic wave, which is incoherent in our experiments. We
examine intensity-modulation frequencies in the megahertz range rather than
in the 10^{14} Hz range corresponding to visible light. The quantities measured

in our experiments were the DC intensity, AC amplitude, and the phase shift of the detected signal relative to the source. The variable parameters in our experiments were the distance between the source and the detector, the modulation frequency of the source intensity, and the amount of absorber in the scattering medium.

3. THE ONE-SPEED LINEAR TRANSPORT EQUATION

The linear transport equation describes the balance of particles which flow in a certain element of volume, taking into account their velocity and position and their changes due to collisions. The one-speed linear transport equation is given by [2]

$$\frac{\partial \Psi(\mathbf{r},\Omega,t)}{\partial t} + v\Omega \bullet \nabla \Psi + v\sigma(\mathbf{r},v)\Psi = \tag{1}$$

$$q(\mathbf{r},\Omega,t) + \sigma(\mathbf{r},v)c(\mathbf{r},v)\int \Psi(\mathbf{r},\Omega',t)f(\Omega'\bullet\Omega,\mathbf{r},v)d\Omega'$$

It is called the one-speed transport equation because it describes the scattering of particles whose speed v is constant. The terms in the above equation are defined in the following manner:

Ω is a unit vector in the direction of the velocity of a particle.

$\Psi(\mathbf{r},\Omega,t)d^3rd\Omega$ is the expected number of particles in the volume element d^3r about the point $\mathbf{r}$, whose velocity directions lie in the element of velocity direction space $d\Omega$ about Ω, at time t.

$\sigma(\mathbf{r},v)$ is the inverse mean free path or macroscopic cross-section of a particle at $\mathbf{r}$ of speed v.

$c(\mathbf{r},v)$ is the average number of secondary particles per collision produced at $\mathbf{r}$ by a particle of speed v. c=1 for an elastic scattering collision and c=0 for an absorption collision.

$$f(\Omega'\bullet\Omega,\mathbf{r},v) = \frac{\sigma(\Omega'\bullet\Omega,\mathbf{r},v)}{c(\mathbf{r},v)\sigma(\mathbf{r},v)} \tag{2}$$

where $\sigma(\Omega'\bullet\Omega,\mathbf{r},v)v'\Psi(\mathbf{r},\Omega',t)d^3rd\Omega'd\Omega dt$ is the probable number of particles in d^3r at $\mathbf{r}$ emitted into $d\Omega$ at Ω in time dt about t due to collisions taking place at time t induced by particles within $d\Omega'$ at Ω'.

$q(\mathbf{r},\Omega,t)d^3rd\Omega dt$ = the number of particles inserted into d^3r at $\mathbf{r}$ and $d\Omega$ at Ω between t and t + dt.

Note that the density of particles $\rho(\mathbf{r},t)$ is given by the integral of Ψ over all possible directions.

$$\rho(\mathbf{r},t) \equiv \int \Psi(\mathbf{r},\Omega,t)d\Omega \tag{3}$$

The particle current density $\mathbf{J}(\mathbf{r},t)$ is given by the integral of $v\Omega\Psi$ over all possible directions

$$\mathbf{J}(\mathbf{r},t) \equiv v\int \Omega\Psi(\mathbf{r},\Omega,t)d\Omega \tag{4}$$

4. THE DIFFUSION APPROXIMATION

Equation 1 may be solved by the spherical harmonics method [2], which introduces into the transport equation the spherical harmonics expansion of $\Psi(\mathbf{r},\Omega,t)$ and $q(\mathbf{r},\Omega,t)$. The diffusion approximation is simply the first order spherical-harmonics approximation, that is, the expansions of $\Psi(\mathbf{r},\Omega,t)$ and

$q(\mathbf{r},\Omega,t)$ include only those terms with the spherical harmonics $Y_{00}(\Omega)$, $Y_{1-1}(\Omega)$ and $Y_{11}(\Omega)$. In this approximation $\Psi(\mathbf{r},\Omega,t)$ and $q(\mathbf{r},\Omega,t)$ can be written as [2]

$$\Psi(\mathbf{r},\Omega,t) \cong \frac{1}{4\pi}[\rho(\mathbf{r},t) + \frac{3}{v}\mathbf{J}(\mathbf{r},t)\bullet\Omega] \tag{5}$$

$$q(\mathbf{r},\Omega,t) \cong \frac{1}{4\pi}[q_0(\mathbf{r},t) + 3\mathbf{q}_1(\mathbf{r},t)\bullet\Omega] \tag{6}$$

By inserting equations 5 and 6 into equation 1 and integrating over Ω the basic equations of diffusion theory are obtained:

$$\frac{\partial\rho(\mathbf{r},t)}{\partial t} + v\sigma(\mathbf{r},v)[1-c(\mathbf{r})]\rho(\mathbf{r},t) + \nabla\bullet\mathbf{J}(\mathbf{r},t) = q_0(\mathbf{r},t) \tag{7a}$$

$$\frac{1}{3}\nabla\rho(\mathbf{r},t) + \frac{1}{v^2}\frac{\partial\mathbf{J}(\mathbf{r},t)}{\partial t} + \frac{\mathbf{J}(\mathbf{r},t)}{(3vD(\mathbf{r}))} = \mathbf{q}_1(\mathbf{r},t) \tag{7b}$$

where the diffusion coefficient D is given as [2]

$$D(\mathbf{r}) \equiv \frac{1}{(3\sigma(\mathbf{r})[1-c(\mathbf{r})\mu])} \tag{8}$$

Here μ is the average of the cosine of the scattering angle. For isotropic scattering, $\mu = 0$.

5. ISOTROPIC SINUSOIDALLY MODULATED POINT SOURCE IN THE DIFFUSION APPROXIMATION

An isotropic point source of light that is sinusoidally intensity-modulated is given by

$$q_0(\mathbf{r},t) = \delta(\mathbf{r})S(1 + A\exp[-i(\omega t + \varepsilon)]) \tag{9a}$$

$$q_1(\mathbf{r},t) = 0 \tag{9b}$$

where $\delta(\mathbf{r})$ is a Dirac-delta function located at the origin, S (in units of photons/second) is the source strength, A is the modulation of the source, $i = \sqrt{-1}$, ω is the angular modulation frequency, and ε is an arbitrary phase.

We assume the following properties for the systems we examine:

$$\begin{array}{llll} \sigma(\mathbf{r}) & = \text{constant} & || & \text{uniform scattering} \\ c(\mathbf{r}) & = \text{constant} & || & \text{uniform absorption} \\ \mu & = 0 & || & \text{isotropic scattering} \end{array}$$

Under this set of assumptions, the diffusion coefficient is given by

$$D(\mathbf{r}) = \frac{1}{3\sigma} = \text{constant} \tag{10}$$

Substituting equations 9 and 10 into equation 7 and assuming that the solutions of the resulting equation have the form

$$\rho(\mathbf{r},t) = \rho_1(\mathbf{r}) + \rho_2(\mathbf{r})\exp[-i(\omega t + \varepsilon)]) \tag{11a}$$

$$\mathbf{J}(\mathbf{r},t) = \mathbf{J}_1(\mathbf{r}) + \mathbf{J}_2(\mathbf{r})\exp[-i(\omega t + \varepsilon)]) \tag{11b}$$

we obtain the steady-state equations

$$v\sigma(1 - c)\rho_1(\mathbf{r}) + \nabla\bullet\mathbf{J}_1(\mathbf{r}) = S\delta(\mathbf{r}) \tag{12a}$$

$$\mathbf{J}_1(\mathbf{r}) = - \frac{v}{3\sigma}\nabla\rho_1(\mathbf{r}) \tag{12b}$$

and the frequency dependent equations

$$-i\omega\rho_2(\mathbf{r}) + v\sigma(1 - c)\rho_2(\mathbf{r}) + \nabla\bullet\mathbf{J}_2(\mathbf{r}) = SA\delta(\mathbf{r}) \tag{13a}$$

$$\mathbf{J}_2(\mathbf{r}) = - \frac{v}{3\sigma}\left(\frac{1+i\omega/v\sigma}{1+(\omega/v\sigma)^2}\right)\nabla\rho_2(\mathbf{r}) \tag{13b}$$

Since photons photons have a speed $v \approx 10^{11}$ mm/s and for our experiments $\omega \approx 10^9$ rad/s and $\sigma \approx 1$ mm^{-1}, we have $\omega/v\sigma = (10^9$ rad/s$)/[(10^{11}$ mm/s$)(1$ mm$^{-1})] = 0.01 << 1$.

In this case, $\mathbf{J}_2(\mathbf{r})$ may be expressed as

$$\mathbf{J}_2(\mathbf{r}) \cong - \frac{v}{3\sigma}\nabla\rho_2(\mathbf{r}) \tag{14}$$

For an infinite medium, equations 11, 12, 13a, and 14 yield

$$\rho(\mathbf{r},t) = \frac{3\sigma S}{4\pi vr}\exp\left(-r\sigma(3(1-c))^{1/2}\right) +$$

$$\frac{3\sigma SA}{4\pi vr}\exp\left(-r\left(\frac{v^2\sigma^2(1-c)^2+\omega^2}{(v/3\sigma)^2}\right)^{1/4}\cos\left(\frac{1}{2}\tan^{-1}\left(\frac{\omega}{v\sigma(1-c)}\right)\right)\right)$$

$$\exp\left(ir\left(\frac{v^2\sigma^2(1-c)^2+\omega^2}{(v/3\sigma)^2}\right)^{1/4}\sin\left(\frac{1}{2}\tan^{-1}\left(\frac{\omega}{v\sigma(1-c)}\right)\right)-i(\omega t + \epsilon)\right) \tag{15}$$

For a non-absorbing medium, $c = 1$ and equation 15 reduces to

$$\rho(\mathbf{r},t) = \frac{3\sigma S}{4\pi vr} + \frac{3\sigma SA}{4\pi vr}\exp\left(-r\left(\frac{3\omega\sigma}{2v}\right)^{1/2}\right)\exp\left(ir\left(\frac{3\omega\sigma}{2v}\right)^{1/2}-i(\omega t + \epsilon)\right) \tag{16}$$

Examination of equations 15 and 16 reveals some important aspects of the propagation of intensity-modulated light by diffusion: 1) The intensity modulated light maintains coherence i.e. the photon-density wave travels with a constant phase velocity and 2) low frequency waves attenuate less than high frequency waves. For non-absorbing media the photon-density wave for a sinusoidally modulated source at frequency ω has a wavelength (from equation 16) of

$$\lambda = 2\pi\sqrt{\frac{2v}{3\sigma\omega}} \tag{17}$$

and its wave-front advances at constant speed

$$V = \sqrt{\frac{2v\omega}{3\sigma}} \tag{18}$$

Equation 17 describes the wavelength of the intensity-modulated photon density, not the color of the light. For $v \cong 10^{11}$ mm/s, $\omega \cong 10^9$ rad/s, and $\sigma \cong 1$ mm^{-1}, the wavelength λ of the photon-density wave given by equation 17 is on the order of 50 mm and the speed of the wave-front V given by equation 18 is on the order of 10^{10} mm/s. Note that for larger σ, i.e. for a smaller mean free path, λ in equation 17 becomes smaller. This paradoxically means that increased scattering improves the spatial resolving power of the photon-density waves. We also see from equation 17 that the spatial resolving power of the waves is also improved by increasing the modulation frequency of the photon source. The presence of uniform absorption (i.e. c < 1) decreases the spatial resolution by increasing the wavelength of the photon-density wave. The approach of regarding photon transport in highly scattering media as a diffusional process shows that intensity-modulated light waves in very turbid media can be treated in the framework of wave phenomena (equations 15 thru 18). As a consequence, the photon density constitutes a scalar field that is propagating at constant speed in a spherical wave. The intensity of the wave at any given point from a number of point sources or localized absorbers can be calculated by superposition. The exponential decrease of the photon-density wave results in a reduction of interference effects from waves that travel a longer distance. A major difference between normal light optics and diffusional wave optics is the exponential attenuation of a photon-density wave's amplitude as it propagates in a scattering and absorbing medium. There is a practical difference in describing the diffusion of photons in the frequency-domain with respect to its Fourier transform equivalent in the time domain: intensity modulated waves at any frequency propagate coherently, while pulses do not.

Figure 1(a) gives a schematic representation of light intensity measured in response to a very narrow pulse traversing a scattering medium, and figure 1(b) shows the time evolution of the intensity measured when light from a sinusoidally intensity-modulated source traverses the same medium. The quantities that are measured with a frequency domain instrument are shown in Figure 1b, namely the phase lag Φ of the intensity modulated wave relative to the source intensity, the average intensity of the detected signal, i.e. the DC intensity, and the amplitude of the frequency dependent part of the detected signal, i.e. the AC amplitude. The diffusion approximation to the linear

Figure 1 (a) Schematic representation of the time evolution of the light intensity measured in response to a very narrow pulse traversing an arbitrary distance in a scattering and absorbing medium. If the medium is strongly scattering, there are no coherent components in the transmitted pulse. (b) The time evolution of the intensity measured when a wave coming from a sinusoidally intensity modulated source traverses the same medium. The transmitted wave, which retains the same frequency as the incoming wave, is delayed due to the phase velocity in the medium. The reduced amplitude of the transmitted wave arises from attenuation related to scattering and absorption processes. The demodulation is the ratio AC/DC normalized to the modulation of the source.

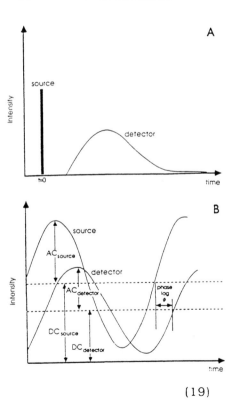

transport equation with a sinusoidally intensity-modulated point source yields expressions containing these experimentally determined quantities which are derived from equation 15. Actually, one measures photon intensity I(r,t) rather than photon density $\rho(\mathbf{r},t)$, where the photon intensity is given by

$$I(\mathbf{r},t) = v\rho(\mathbf{r},t) \tag{19}$$

So, from equations 15 and 19 we have for the phase Φ, DC intensity, and AC part the following relationships:

$$\Phi = r\left(\frac{v^2\sigma^2(1-c)^2+\omega^2}{(v/3\sigma)^2}\right)^{1/4} \sin\left(\frac{1}{2}\tan^{-1}\left(\frac{\omega}{v\sigma(1-c)}\right)\right) - \varepsilon \tag{20}$$

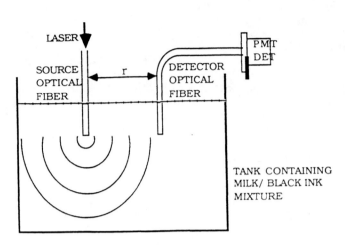

Figure 2. The source and the detector optical fibers point in the same direction. Phase shift, DC intensity, and AC amplitude measurements are made as a function of r and modulation frequency with the optical fibers in this configuration to insure that only scattered photons are detected. The light source was a Spectra Diode Laboratories SDL-2431-H2 diode laser with a 1 m fiber optic pigtail of diameter 100 μm. The average diode current was set at 200mA and sinusoidally modulated with a Marconi Instruments Model 2022A signal generator with its output amplified by a Wideband RF Amplifier Model M502C from RF Power Labs, Inc. The detector fiber has an aperture of 1 mm diameter.

$$\ln[r\ DC] = -r\sigma(3(1-c))^{1/2} + \ln\left(\frac{3\sigma S}{4\pi}\right) \tag{21}$$

$$\ln[r\ AC] = -r\left(\frac{v^2\sigma^2(1-c)^2+\omega^2}{(v/3\sigma)^2}\right)^{1/4} \cos\left(\frac{1}{2}\tan^{-1}\left(\frac{\omega}{v\sigma(1-c)}\right)\right) + \ln\left(\frac{3\sigma SA}{4\pi}\right) \tag{22}$$

The three expressions above are linear functions of the source/detector distance r, but have a more complicated dependence on the modulation frequency ω, the inverse mean free path σ, and the fraction of collisions that do not result in an absorption c. From equations 20, 21, and 22 we see that the linear dependence of Φ, ln[r DC], and ln[r AC] on r of is a necessary (but not sufficient) condition for the validity of the diffusion approximation to the linear transport equation with a sinusoidally intensity modulated point source for the case of photon transport through very turbid media. To test for this condition we have performed measurements of the phase shift Φ, DC intensity, and AC amplitude of light emitted from a sinusoidally intensity modulated source as a function of the distance r between the source and the detector. The measurements were performed on systems in which the light from the sinusoidally intensity modulated source propagated at fixed modulation frequencies in homogeneous scattering solutions containing fixed concentrations of absorber.

6.   MATERIALS AND METHODS

We have studied the photon transport properties of media consisting of 3.78 liters of skim milk containing quantities of black India ink that vary from no ink to 10 microliters of ink. Our light source was a Spectra Diode Laboratories SDL-2431-H2 diode laser with a 1 m fiber optic pigtail of diameter 100 μm. The average diode current was set at 200 mA and sinusoidally modulated with a Marconi Instruments Model 2022A signal generator with its output amplified by a Wideband RF Amplifier Model M502C from RF Power Labs, Inc. In a given experiment, light was transferred from the diode-laser into the skim milk/black ink medium via the optical fiber pigtail of the diode-laser whose end was immersed in the milk solution. The wavelength of the diode-laser light was 810 nm. The light detector was 1mm diameter optical fiber attached to a photomultiplier (Hamamatsu R928). The PMT signals were processed by a cross-correlation electronics system using a digital aquisition system [5]. The end of the detecting fiber was immersed in the milk solution at a distance r from the end of the source fiber as is shown in figure 2. The reason for the relative orientation of the source and the detector optical fibers that are shown in figure 2 is to assure that only the scattered photons are detected. r was varied from 2.5 cm to 9.6 cm in steps of 0.115 cm during the course of an experiment, and the quantities measured as a function of r were phase lag Φ, DC intensity, and AC amplitude (Figure 1(b)). The modulation frequency was fixed for a given set of source/detector distances. Data were acquired at modulation frequencies of 40 MHz and 120 MHz. The phase data were recorded relative to the phase measurement made at the shortest source/detector separation distance, and the DC and AC data were respectively normalized to to the DC and the AC values made at the shortest source/detector separation distance.

7.   RESULTS AND DISCUSSION

Figure 3 shows the phase shift of the signal detected at a distance r from the end of the light source optical fiber versus the distance r between the ends of the source and the detector optical fibers. The data in figure 3 which are fit by the solid lines with the steeper slopes correspond to the skim milk systems containing lesser amounts of black India ink. The correlation coefficients for the linear fits to the phase shift data in figure 3 are close to 1, which indicates that the phase shift data come from a signal that is propagating with a constant phase velocity through the mixtures of skim milk and black ink. Figure 3 also shows that for a given milk/black ink mixture and source/detector separation, the phase shifts measured at a modulation frequency of 120 MHz are greater than the phase shifts measured at a modulation frequency of 40 MHz. The above results are consistent with equation 20. The wavelength and phase velocity of a signal detected in a given milk/black ink mixture at a given modulation frequency can be calculated from the slopes of the solid lines in figure 3. From the linear fits to the phase data acquired at a modulation frequencies of 40 MHz and 120 MHz we have calculated values for the wavelength λ and phase velocity V of a signal propagating through 3.78 L of skim milk containing no ink to 10 μL of black India ink (see Table 1A for the 40 MHz values of λ and V and Table 1B for the 120 MHz values of λ and V).

Figure 4 shows the natural logarithm of the source/detector distance r multiplied by the DC value of the signal detected at distance r from the source versus the source/detector distance r. The data in figure 4 that were fit by the solid lines with the shallower slopes correspond to the skim milk systems containing lesser amounts of black India ink. The correlation coefficients for the linear fits to the data in figure 4 are close to 1, which is consistent with equation 21. Figure 5 shows the natural logarithm of the source/detector distance r multiplied by the AC value of the signal detected at distance r from the source versus the source/detector distance r. The data in figure 5 that were fit by the solid lines with the shallower slopes correspond to the skim milk systems containing lesser amounts of black India ink. The correlation coefficients for the linear fits to the phase data are close to 1, which is consistent with equation 22. The optical properties of the skim milk/black ink medium could be obtained by fitting the data to equation 15, but equations 20, 21, and 22 allow for a simple determination of the scattering and absorption coefficients, which are related to σ and c in the following manner:

$$\sigma = \mu_a + \mu_s \tag{23}$$

$$c = \frac{\mu_s}{\mu_a + \mu_s} \tag{24}$$

where μ_s is the linear scattering coefficient and μ_a is the linear absorption coefficient of the medium. From the ratio of the natural logarithm of the normalized demodulation of the signal

demodulation=[AC$_{detector}$/DC$_{detector}$]/[AC$_{source}$/DC$_{source}$])

to the relative phase shift Φ, we have calculated values for μ_s and μ_a for media consisting of 3.78 L of skim milk containing no ink to 10 μL of black India ink.

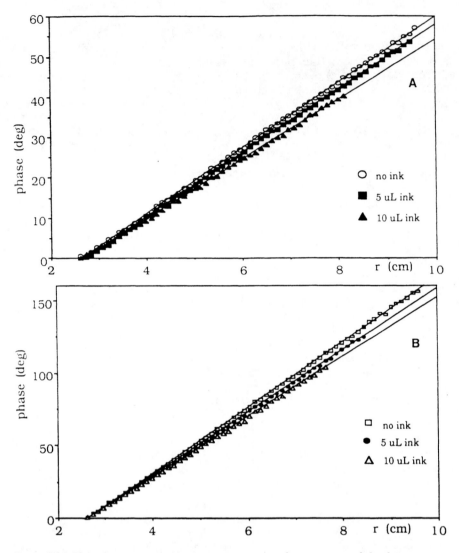

Figure 3 (a) Phase lag vs. source/detector separation r, where source and the detector are immersed in 3.78 L skim milk. The steepest line fits the phase data for 3.78L skim milk containing no ink, the middle line fits the phase data for 3.78 L skim milk containing 5 μL black ink, and the shallowest line fits the phase data for 3.78L skim milk containing 10 μL black ink. The data were collected with the experimental arrangement shown in figure 2. The modulation frequency at which these data were collected was 40 MHz. The correlation coefficients for each of the data fits at this modulation frequency is close to 1. (b) Same as part (a) except that the modulation frequency is 120 MHz. The correlation coefficients for each of the data fits at this modulation frequency is close to 1.

Table 1A ($\omega/2\pi$ = 40 MHz)

	λ (mm)	V (mm/s)
no ink	442	1.77×10^{10}
5 μL black ink	456	1.82×10^{10}
10 μL black ink	489	1.96×10^{10}

Table 1B ($\omega/2\pi$ = 120 MHz)

	λ (mm)	V (mm/s)
no ink	160	1.92×10^{10}
5 μL black ink	168	2.02×10^{10}
10 μL black ink	176	2.11×10^{10}

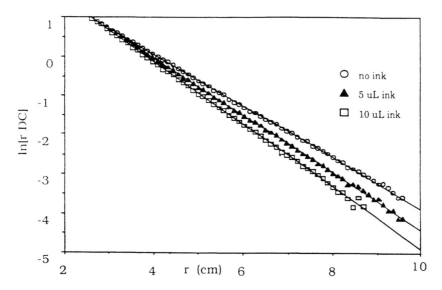

Figure 4. Natural logarithm of r multiplying the normalized DC of the signal detected at distance r from the source versus the source/detector separation r, where r is the distance between a source and a detector that are immersed in the 3.78 L skim milk. The shallowest line fits the intensity data for 3.78 L skim milk containing no black ink, the middle line fits the intensity data for 3.78 L skim milk containing 5 μL of black ink, and the steepest line fits the intensity data for 3.78 L skim milk containing 10 μL black ink. The data were collected with the experimental arrangement shown in figure 2. The correlation coefficients for each of the data fits is close to 1.

The values we calculated for μ_s and μ_a at different concentrations of black India ink are listed in Table 2.

Table 2

	μ_s (mm^{-1})	μ_a (mm^{-1})
no ink	0.50 ~~0.82~~	0.0017
5 μL black ink	0.52 ~~0.84~~	0.0022
10 μL black ink	0.47 ~~0.80~~	0.0024

We believe that if μ_s is a constant as a function of absorber (i.e. black ink concentration) then the absorbing material of the medium is separate from the scattering centers of the medium, whereas if the absorbing medium tends to coat the scatterers, both μ_s and μ_a will be a function of the amount of absorber in the medium. Our values for μ_s and μ_a are not independent of the concentration of black ink, which indicates that some of the ink in the skim milk may be "painting" the milk particles rather being suspended in the solution separately from the milk particles.

8. CONCLUSION

The linear dependence of our measurements of Φ, ln[r DC], and ln[r AC] on r confirm a necessary (but not sufficient) condition for the validity of the diffusion approximation to the one-speed linear transport equation with a sinusoidally intensity modulated point source. While the data we present here does not provide an exhaustive test of the above mentioned diffusion approximation, the linearity of the phase in r demonstrates that the wave front of a sinusoidally intensity modulated wave that is emitted into a highly scattering medium maintains its coherence as it propagates through the scattering medium. The wavelength of the diffusional waves is of the order of 100 mm and their phase velocity is on the order of 10^{10} mm/s in our experiments at 120 MHz. The coherence of the diffusional waves has implications for the imaging of of objects that are immersed in a highly scattering medium -- one may detect the diffraction pattern that a diffusional wave makes after it scatters around a object whose size is of the order of the diffusional wavelength and thereby reconstruct

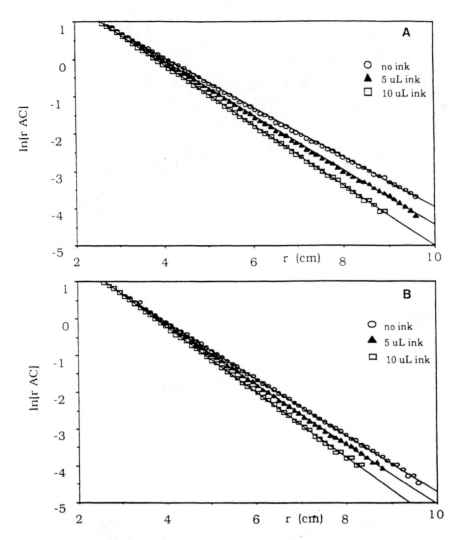

Figure 5 (a) Natural logarithm of r multiplying the normalized AC of the signal detected at distance r from the source versus the source/detector separation r, where r is the distance between a source and a detector that are immersed in the 3.78 L skim milk. The shallowest line fits the intensity data for 3.78 L skim milk containing no black ink, the middle line fits the intensity data for 3.78 L skim milk containing 5 μL of black ink, and the steepest line fits the intensity data for 3.78 L skim milk containing 10 μL black ink. The data were collected with the experimental arrangement shown in figure 2. The modulation frequency at which these data were collected was 40 MHz. The correlation coefficients for each of the data fits at this modulation freque ncy is close to 1. (b) Same as part (a) except that the modulation frequency is 120 MHz. The correlation coefficients for each of the data fits at this modulation frequency is close to 1.

the object from the diffraction pattern. The diffusion approximation appears to have described all the details of our experiments.

9.   ACKNOWLEDGEMENTS

This research was performed in the Laboratory for Fluorescence Dynamics (LFD) in the Department of Physics at the University of Illinois at Urbana-Champaign (UIUC). The LFD is funded by the National Institutes of Health (RR03155 to EG) and UIUC. The authors thank Brett Feddersen and Julie Butzow for help in preparing this paper.

10.   REFERENCES

[1]   Ishimaru, A. *Wave Propagation in Random Scattering Media.* Academic Press, 1978, New York.

[2]   Case, K. M. And P. F. Zweifel. *Linear Transport Theory.* Addison-Wesley Publishing Co., Inc., Reading, MA, Palo Alto, London, Don Mills, Ontario,

1967.

[3] Patterson, M. S., B. Chance and B. C. Wilson. Time resolved reflectance and transmittance for the non-invasive measurement of tissue optical properties. *Appl. Optics 28*, 2223-2229, 1989.

[4] Lakowicz, J. R., K. W. Berndt, M. L. Johnson. Photon Migration In Scattering Media and Tissue. *Proc. SPIE, Time-Resolved Laser Spectroscopy*, J. R. Lakowicz, Ed., *1204*, 468-480, 1990.

[5] Feddersen, B. A., D. W. Piston, E. Gratton. Digital Parallel Aquisition in Frequency Domain Fluorometry. *Rev. Sci. Instrum. 60*, 2929-2936, 1989.

Reprinted from *Annual Conference on Engineering in Medicine and Biology*, pp. 332-333 (1992).

Random Walk Theory Applied to Noninvasive in vivo Optical Measurements of Human Tissue

A. H. Gandjbakhche, J. M. Schmitt, R. Bonner, and R. Nossal

National Institutes of Health, Bethesda, MD 20892

Abstract—Expressions for the photon intensity profile and mean transit time are derived from random walk theory. These differ from previously derived quantities, in that scattering angle anisotropy now is explicitly taken into account. Results are used to determine the scattering and absorption cross-sections of tissues.

I. INTRODUCTION

Noninvasive optical spectroscopy on skin and other external surfaces of tissues offers great potential for clinical screening and continuous monitoring of physiological parameters. Newly developed transit-time techniques enable one to directly measure optical pathlengths, thus facilitating quantitative determination of chromophore concentrations in tissues in which a high degree of multiple scattering occurs. In order to interpret such optical data, and to form the basis for simple quantitative measurements, one needs to develop appropriate models to analyze the migration of photons.

Previously, two theoretical models have been used to describe photon migration: the diffusion approximation of radiative transport theory [1,2] and a random walk model [3,4]. The latter has been used to derive expressions such as the intensity profile and the mean transit time, which can be used to compute optical properties of tissue from appropriate data. By including corrections which take into account the scattering-angle anisotropy of the medium [5,6], the effective scattering coefficient, $\Sigma'_s = (1-g)\Sigma_s$, and the absorption coefficient, Σ_a, of tissue can be inferred. [Here, g represents the coefficient of anisotropy, defined as the mean cosine of the scattering angle.]

II. THEORY

One model that describes photon migration in a turbid medium is based on representing photon movement by a random walk in discrete time on a lattice [3]. We consider the case in which photons impinge upon a homogenous, spatially isotropic, scattering medium at a point on its surface and the sample is considered to be of semi-infinite extent. The expression of interest is the joint probability, $\Gamma(n, \rho)$, that a walker (i.e., photon) emerges at a distance ρ on the surface after n steps. $\Gamma(n, \rho)$, which is derived elsewhere, is given as [3]

$$\Gamma(\rho, n) = \frac{\sqrt{3}}{2}(2\pi n)^{-3/2}(1 - e^{-6/n})e^{-3\rho^2/2n}e^{-\mu n}, \quad (1)$$

where $\rho = (x^2 + y^2)^{1/2}$ is the radial distance from the point of insertion to the point of reemission, expressed in terms of the lattice spacing, which is set equal to the rms distance traveled between successive scattering events. The quantity μ is the absorption per unit scattering length.

The intensity profile, $I(\rho)$, calculated from (1) by integrating over n, is, for large ρ,

$$I(\rho) \sim \frac{\sqrt{6\mu}}{4\pi\rho^2}e^{-2\mu}\exp(-\rho\sqrt{6\mu}) \quad \rho >> 2. \quad (2)$$

Another quantity of interest is the expected number of steps taken by a photon before it is reemitted at the surface, given as

$$\langle n|\rho \rangle \sim 2 + 3\rho/\sqrt{6\mu} \quad \rho >> 2. \quad (3)$$

The variables ρ, n, and μ are expressed in terms of Σ_s, Σ_a, and real distance r and time t, as [3,5,6]

$$\rho = \frac{r\Sigma_s}{\sqrt{2}}, \qquad n = c_T\Sigma_s t, \qquad \mu = \frac{\Sigma_a}{\Sigma_s}, \quad (4)$$

where c_T is the speed of light in the tissue.

Scattering-angle anisotropy can be accounted for by appropriate similarity relationships [5,6]. When the scatterers within the medium are randomly distributed, the scattering lengths can be assumed to be exponentially distributed, which leads [6] to the following scaled variables (*c.f.* (4))

$$\rho^* = \frac{r\Sigma_s(1-g)}{\sqrt{2}(1+g)^{1/2}}, \qquad n^* = \frac{c_T\Sigma_s t(1-g)}{(1+g)},$$
$$\text{and} \qquad \mu^* = \frac{\Sigma_a(1+g)}{\Sigma_s(1-g)}. \quad (5)$$

Hence, (2) and (3) can be written in terms of these scaled variables as

$$\ln[r^2 I(r)] \sim -[3\Sigma_a\Sigma_s(1-g)]^{1/2}r, \quad (6)$$

and

$$\langle \ell | r \rangle \sim [\frac{3\Sigma_s(1-g)}{4\Sigma_a}]^{1/2} r, \qquad (7)$$

where $\ell = c_T t$ is the pathlength. Results of Monte-Carlo simulations have been shown to be in excellent agreement with these expressions [5, 6].

III. MEASUREMENT AND DATA ANALYSIS

The quantities given in (6) and (7) can be determined with a specially configured frequency domain spectrometer [7]. A mode-locked dye laser ($\lambda = 609$ nm) generated narrow light pulses, which were used to illuminate the tissue. The phase and magnitude of the resultant diffusive wave produced in the tissue at 246 MHz were recorded at the surface, using a phase sensitive CCD camera.

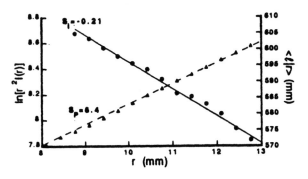

Fig. 1. Intensity profile and pathlength measurements of photons diffusing within a human thumb, as a function of distance between the incident source and the detector. Lines are least-square fits to the data ($R^2 > 0.99$) [solid line corresponds to intensities, dotted line to pathlengths].

For illustration, we examined the optical properties of a human thumb. The intensity profile and the phase shift were obtained as a function of r. Results are presented in

Fig. 1, where the phase shift has been related to the mean transit time and photon pathlength as

$$\Delta\phi \sim [2\pi f]\langle t \rangle = [2\pi f]\langle \ell \rangle / c_T \qquad (8)$$

where f is the modulation frequency. According to (6) and (7), the effective scattering coefficient, $\Sigma_s(1-g)$, and the absorption coefficient, Σ_a, are obtained from these data as

$$\Sigma_s(1-g) = \frac{2}{3}(S_I S_p); \qquad \Sigma_a = S_I/(2S_p), \qquad (9)$$

where S_I and S_p are the absolute values of the slopes obtained from intensity profile and phase shift measurements. We found the values of the cross-sections of the tissue to be $\Sigma_a = 0.016$ mm^{-1} and $\Sigma'_s = (1-g)\Sigma_s = 0.89$ mm^{-1}. Expressions similar to those given in (6) and (7) have been derived for the transmission through a slab of finite thickness. These methods enable us to determine the optical parameters of different types of tissue, both *in vivo* and *in vitro*.

REFERENCES

[1] M. Patterson, B. Chance, and B.C. Wilson, "Time resolved reflectance and transmittance for the noninvasive measurement of tissue optical properties," *Appl. Opt.*, vol. 28, pp. 2331–2336, 1989.

[2] J. M. Schmitt, G. H. Zhou, E. C. Walker, and R. T. Wall, "A multilayer model of photon diffusion in skin," *J. Opt. Soc. Am.*, vol. A 14, pp. 2141–2153, 1990.

[3] R. Bonner, R. Nossal, S. Havlin, and G. H. Weiss, "Model of photon migration in turbid biological tissue," *J. Opt. Soc. Am. A*, vol. 4, pp. 423–432, 1987.

[4] R. Nossal, R. F. Bonner, and G. H. Weiss, "The influence of pathlength on remote sensing of properties of biological tissue," *Appl. Opt.*, vol. 28, pp. 2238–2244, 1989.

[5] A. H. Gandjbakhche, R. Bonner, and R. Nossal, "Scaling relationships of anisotropic random walks," *J. Stat. Phys.*, in press.

[6] A. H. Gandjbakhche, R. Nossal, and R. Bonner, "Scaling relationships for tissue optics," *Appl. Opt.*, in press.

[7] A. Knüttel, J. M. Schmitt, and J. R. Knutson, "Spatial localization of absorbing bodies by interfering diffusive photon-density waves," *Appl. Opt.*, submitted.

Reprinted with permission from *Physics in Medicine and Biology,* Vol. 37(7), pp. 1531-1560 (1992). ©1992 IOP Publishing Ltd.

The theoretical basis for the determination of optical pathlengths in tissue: temporal and frequency analysis

S R Arridge†, M Cope‡ and D T Delpy‡

† Department of Computer Science, University College London, Gower Street, London WC1E 6BT, UK
‡ Department of Medical Physics and Bioengineering, University College London, First Floor Shropshire House, 11–20 Capper Street, London WC1E 6JA, UK

Received 23 December 1991, in final form 5 March 1992

Abstract. A concise theoretical treatment is developed for the calculation of mean time, differential pathlength, phase shift, modulation depth and integrated intensity of measurements of light intensity as a function of time on the surface of tissue, resulting from either the input of picosecond light pulses, or radio frequency-modulated light. The treatment uses the Green's function of the diffusion approximation to the radiative transfer equation, and develops this and its Fourier transform in a variety of geometries. Detailed comparisons are made of several of these parameters in several geometries, and their relation to experimentally measured clinical data. The limitations of the use of phase measurements is discussed.

1. Introduction

Near-infrared (NIR) light in the wavelength range 650 to 1200 nm can penetrate tissues to considerable depths, making it possible to measure the optical absorption properties of intact organs, often in a totally non-invasive manner (Cope and Delpy 1988, Cope 1991). In the NIR region of the spectrum, two important tissue chromophores, haemoglobin and cytochrome aa₃ display oxygenation-dependent spectral changes, and by monitoring these it is possible to calculate the degree of both blood and intracellular oxygenation in intact organs (Wray *et al* 1988). This monitoring method was first employed to observe the oxygenation of the brain of the cat (Jöbsis 1977), but has subsequently been successfully applied to monitoring brain oxygenation in newborn infants (Brazy *et al* 1985, Wyatt *et al* 1986, Edwards *et al* 1988) and adults (Ferrari *et al* 1986), and muscle oxygenation in normal subjects (Hampson and Piantadosi 1988) and those with peripheral vascular disease (Cheatle *et al* 1991).

Tissue is a highly light scattering medium, and the light that is detected in such studies has travelled considerably further through the tissues than the direct distance between the input and output optodes. In order to quantitate spectral information, it is necessary to know this 'optical pathlength', and the way in which it changes with tissue type, wavelength, attenuation and measuring geometry. The question of the optical pathlength is also important in the work that is currently under way into imaging with the transmitted NIR light. Many approaches to the problem of imaging are being pursued. The simplest has been to measure the spatial distribution of light intensity at the object surface, and attempt to use a conventional back-projection reconstruction (Jarry *et al* 1984, Jackson *et al* 1987, Tamura *et al* 1987, Oda *et al* 1991). Alternatively, the concept of using ultra-short light pulses and time gating the detector has been explored, either to detect the few unscattered or 'ballistic' photons (Wang *et al* 1991), or to limit the range of scatter of the detected light (Hebden and Kruger 1990). Unfortunately, when measuring across more than one or two centimetres of tissue, the degree of scattering is so high that the ballistic photons are too few to be usable, and time gating within a narrow window severely reduces the signal-to-noise ratio. Finally, it is possible to incorporate both the spatial and the temporal distribution of the detected light in an imaging scheme (Arridge *et al* 1985, 1991, 1992). Results from both modelled and experimentally measured data indicate that the presence of absorbing centres in a scattering object are more noticeable through their effects upon the light pathlength than on the light intensity distribution at the object surface (Arridge *et al* 1990, 1991, Fishkin *et al* 1991, Berndt and Lakowicz 1991).

It is therefore important both in tissue spectroscopy as well as in imaging to measure not only the transmitted light intensity, but also the mean pathlength. One way of doing this is the 'time-of-flight' method, using ultra-short light pulses and a fast optical detector (Delpy *et al* 1988). Unfortunately the equipment for doing this is at present both bulky and expensive. An alternative methodology has, however, been developed which employs a radiofrequency (RF) modulated light source and phase-sensitive detection of the transmitted light (Chance *et al* 1990, Lakowicz and Berndt 1990). The phase shift of the detected light has been equated to the mean optical pathlength as measured by the 'time-of-flight' method (Patterson *et al* 1990).

In this paper we give a brief explanation of the time and phase measurement techniques, and then develop a theoretical basis for the relation of the mean optical pathlength, as measured by a time-of-flight method, to the phase delay of an intensity-modulated optical carrier. This analysis is carried out using the diffusion approximation to describe light transport in tissue, and relationships are derived for the major tissue geometries of clinical interest.

2. Time and frequency domain measurements

In time domain measurements, a laser-generated light pulse a few picoseconds long is input to the tissues and, as a result of multiple scattering, the light pulse exiting the tissues has a broad distribution of pathlengths, this distribution being termed the temporal point spread function (TPSF). The differential pathlength (DP), defined below in (15), when used in a Beer–Lambert calculation, permits the measured attenuation changes to be converted into the corresponding variations in chromophore concentration. In a previous study we have shown that it is possible to derive this DP value from a measurement of the mean of the TPSF (Delpy *et al* 1988). It has also been shown that the dimensionless differential pathlength factor (DPF) obtained by dividing the DP by the inter optode spacing is almost constant for a given tissue once the inter optode spacing exceeds 2.5 cm. Values for the DPF have been measured for various tissues (Wyatt *et al* 1990, van der Zee *et al* 1992).

In the frequency domain measurement technique, RF intensity-modulated light is input to the tissues, and the phase shift of the emerging light is measured (Chance *et al* 1990). This phase shift is given by the Fourier transform (FT) of the TPSF, which is itself the response function (Green's function) to a delta function input.

It can easily be shown that the information from the picosecond laser and the RF-modulated light source systems are Fourier transforms of each other. A picosecond laser pulse travelling through a multiple-scattering medium undergoes dispersion analogous to that seen in multimode optical fibres where there are multiple paths possible for the light travelling through the fibre. A picosecond laser system with a temporal resolution of 10 ps effectively measures the impulse response of the scattering medium with a limited frequency spectrum from 0 up to 100 GHz at 76 MHz intervals (the laser repetition rate).

In the following we introduce some notation that is more precisely defined in section 3. Since the impulse response of the scattering medium is a Green's function, it will be referred to in this section as a real function $g(t)$. In reality it depends not just on time, but also on space r, and on the position and time of arrival of the input pulse $\delta(r', t')$. Similarly we will define light intensity as a *flux*, $\Gamma(t)$, defined in (12). Consider the effect of passing a sine-wave-modulated light beam through the scattering medium. The intensity of the input beam is given by

$$\Gamma^{(i)}(t) = \Gamma_0(1 + M\,\mathrm{e}^{\mathrm{i}\omega_\mathrm{m}t})\,\mathrm{e}^{\mathrm{i}\omega_\mathrm{c}t} \tag{1}$$

where ω_c, ω_m are the angular frequencies of the carrier light beam and RF modulation respectively. Γ_0 is the average flux and M the depth of modulation.

The optical detector rectifies and low-pass filters the carrier frequency; hence it is only necessary to consider the modulated wave

$$\Gamma^{(i)}(t) = \Gamma_0(1 + M\,\mathrm{e}^{\mathrm{i}\omega_\mathrm{m}t}). \tag{2}$$

The effect of passing $\Gamma^{(i)}(t)$ through the scattering medium is simply given by the convolution of $g(t)$ and $\Gamma^{(i)}(t)$; hence the output beam is given by

$$\Gamma^{(o)}(t) = \frac{1}{\sqrt{2\pi}} \int_{-\infty}^{\infty} \Gamma^{(i)}(t - t') g(t')\,\mathrm{d}t' \tag{3}$$

i.e.

$$\Gamma^{(o)}(t) = \Gamma_0 \frac{1}{\sqrt{2\pi}} \int_{-\infty}^{\infty} g(t')\,\mathrm{d}t' + \Gamma_0 M\,\mathrm{e}^{\mathrm{i}\omega_\mathrm{m}t} \frac{1}{\sqrt{2\pi}} \int_{-\infty}^{\infty} g(t')\,\mathrm{e}^{-\mathrm{i}\omega_\mathrm{m}t'}\,\mathrm{d}t'. \tag{4}$$

Here the first term represents the attenuation of the zero-frequency component and the second term shows that the sine wave modulation will be transmitted through the scattering medium, emerging with a reduced modulation (modulus $\hat{G}(\omega_\mathrm{m})$) and a retarded phase ($\psi = \mathrm{Arg}\,\hat{G}(\omega_\mathrm{m})$) where $\hat{G}(\omega_\mathrm{m})$ is the Fourier transform of $g(t)$ (defined in appendix A, equation (A1)). From the point of view of tissue optical spectroscopy, the most important characteristic of $g(t)$ has been shown to be the mean time delay

$$\langle t \rangle = \int_{-\infty}^{\infty} g(t) t\,\mathrm{d}t \bigg/ \int_{-\infty}^{\infty} g(t)\,\mathrm{d}t \tag{5}$$

and we need to know whether there is a simple relationship between the mean time delay $\langle t \rangle$ and the phase shift of the modulated carrier ψ.

If $g(t)$ represented an attenuating non-dispersive system with a time delay $\bar{t}$ and transmittance T, i.e. $g(t) = T\delta(t - \bar{t})$ then $\langle t \rangle = \bar{t}$ and $\psi = -\omega_\mathrm{m}\bar{t}$, and the time and phase are simply related by the modulation frequency ω_m. Note, however, that ψ must be less than 2π because a real detector cannot differentiate between phase shifts of 0, $2\pi, 4\pi$ etc. Sevick and Chance (1991) have commented that the same simple relationship between $\langle t \rangle$ and ψ can be used for highly dispersive systems such as are found in tissue when the approximation $\mathrm{e}^{\mathrm{i}\omega t} \simeq \mathrm{i}\omega t$ holds. However, most practical measurements report phase shifts in the range of 20° to 60° where this approximation is not valid. There are, however, situations when this relationship can be used at large phase shifts, namely when $g(t)$ is nearly symmetrical.

Consider a highly dispersive system in which $g(t)$ is symmetrical about a mean time $\bar{t}$, i.e. $g(\bar{t}+t) = g(\bar{t}-t)$. When $g(t)$ has this property, $\hat{G}(\omega)$ can be simplified by using two properties of Fourier transforms—firstly by a shift of the time origin from $t = 0$ to $t = \bar{t}$

$$\hat{G}(\omega) = e^{-i\omega\bar{t}} \int_{-\infty}^{\infty} g(t'+\bar{t}) \, e^{-i\omega t'} \, dt' \qquad (6)$$

and secondly by splitting the integral into its real and imaginary parts:

$$\hat{G}(\omega) = \frac{e^{-i\omega\bar{t}}}{\sqrt{2\pi}} \left(\int_{-\infty}^{\infty} g(t'+\bar{t}) \cos(\omega t') \, dt' - i \int_{-\infty}^{\infty} g(t'+\bar{t}) \sin(\omega t') \, dt' \right)$$

$$= \frac{e^{-i\omega\bar{t}}}{\sqrt{2\pi}} \int_{-\infty}^{\infty} g(t'+\bar{t}) \cos(\omega t') \, dt'. \qquad (7)$$

Note that as $g(t)$ is real the result of the integral will also be real, and thus $\psi = \text{Arg}[\hat{G}(\omega)] = -\omega\bar{t}$. However, also note any dispersion will lead to a loss of modulation depth. Hence for all symmetrical $g(t)$, the mean time $\langle t \rangle = \bar{t}$ and ψ are linearly related via the angular frequency ω.

In reality, $g(t)$ is not truly symmetrical. It always appears to exhibit positive skewness and in this case $|\psi| < \omega\bar{t}$ and hence $|\psi|$ under reads the mean time delay of $g(t)$. If $g(t)$ is expressed in terms of its various moments (mean, standard deviation, skew, kurtosis etc) then the difference between $\langle t \rangle$ and ψ can be found in its odd moments. Hence to a first approximation the difference is dependent upon the skewness of $g(t)$.

Figure 1(a) shows an impulse response measured *in vivo* across 4 cm of the adult head using a picosecond laser system (Tsunami, Spectra Physics, USA) and synchroscan streak camera (C1587, Hamamatsu Photonics KK, Japan) with a 10 ps resolution. It illustrates the typical skewness of impulse functions of human tissue. A fast Fourier transform was performed on these data (510 data points at 4.95 ps intervals) after post-padding with zeros up to a total of 4096 data points. This enabled the data in the frequency domain to be interpolated to 50 MHz intervals, as plotted in figure 1(b).

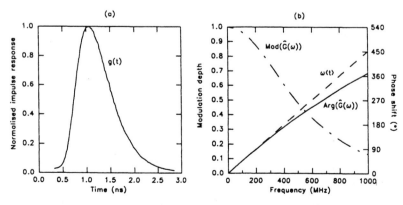

Figure 1. (a) Impulse response measured across 4 cm of adult head at 800 nm with a picosecond laser system and streak camera; (b) Fourier transform of (a) with the phase shift compared to the linear approximation based on the mean time delay of (a).

3. Diffusion model for light transport

The most general model for light transport that may be given is the theory of radiative transfer, or photon transport theory, which has been extensively studied in atmospheric physics (Chandrasekhar 1950, Ishimaru 1978a, van der Hulst 1980), and in neutron transport (Case and Zweifel 1967). It is an integro-differential equation that is complex to model and is very often simplified by an expansion in spherical harmonics (Lewis 1950, Bremmer 1964, Case and Zweifel 1967). The result is a set of $(N+1)^2$ coupled partial differential equations known as the P_N approximation. For odd N, such equations may be reduced to a single $(N+1)$th-order differential equation. For example when $N = 1$, four coupled partial differential equations are required, which reduce to a single diffusion-type expression:

$$(\boldsymbol{\nabla} \cdot \gamma^2 \boldsymbol{\nabla} - \mu_a c)\Phi(\boldsymbol{r}, t) = -q(\boldsymbol{r}, t). \tag{8}$$

Here q is the isotropic source term from the input distribution, μ_a the absorption coefficient, c the velocity of light, Φ the photon density, and $\gamma(\boldsymbol{r})$ is given by

$$\gamma^2 = c/\{3[\mu_a + (1 - \bar{p})\mu_s]\} \tag{9}$$

i.e. γ depends on μ_a, the scattering coefficient μ_s and $\bar{p}$, the average cosine of the phase function. In all the following we implicitly assume that Φ is scaled by $h\nu$, where ν is the frequency of the light and h is Planck's constant, so that the gradient of Φ represents an intensity in the normal way.

For the time-dependent case equation (8) becomes

$$(\boldsymbol{\nabla} \cdot \gamma^2 \boldsymbol{\nabla} - \mu_a c - \partial/\partial t)\Phi(\boldsymbol{r}, t) = -q(\boldsymbol{r}, t). \tag{10}$$

Other suggestions have been made, involving first- and second-order derivatives in space and time (Ishimaru 1978b, Patterson *et al* 1989). P_N approximations for $N > 1$ have also been suggested (Star 1989).

We will consider our basic equation of light transport to be (10) in an isotropic medium:

$$(\gamma^2 \boldsymbol{\nabla}^2 - \mu_a c - \partial/\partial t)\Phi(\boldsymbol{r}, t) = -q(\boldsymbol{r}, t) \tag{11}$$

We will refer to this as the *lossy diffusion equation* and distinguish it from the case where $\mu_a = 0$, the *lossless diffusion equation*, equivalent to the heat conduction equation. We wish to derive the solutions Φ in a volume Ω bounded by a surface $\partial\Omega$, and in particular to look for the *output flux* on the boundary given by

$$\Gamma(\boldsymbol{\xi}, t) = -\gamma^2(\partial/\partial n)\Phi(\boldsymbol{r}, t)|_{\partial\Omega} = -\gamma^2 \hat{\boldsymbol{n}} \cdot \boldsymbol{\nabla}\Phi(\boldsymbol{r}, t)|_{\partial\Omega} \tag{12}$$

where $\boldsymbol{\xi}$ is a point on $\partial\Omega$, and $\hat{\boldsymbol{n}}(\boldsymbol{\xi})$ is the outward surface normal. These time-dependent flux expressions correspond to the measurements of intensity as a function of time that can be made using short-pulsed lasers and streak camera technology.

The source term $q(\boldsymbol{r}, t)$ in (11) represents the form of the input pulse as a function of space and time. In general, the solution for any input pulse can be derived by convolution of $q(\boldsymbol{r}, t)$ with the Green's function for (11) in the appropriate geometry, as used in (3). Then this solution can be substituted into (12) to obtain the flux intensity. We may also be interested in some functional of Γ, such as its temporal integral (for integrated intensity measurements), initial integral up to a time T (representing early light), the log of the slope in the limit (Chance *et al* 1988), or the spatial integral over some measuring window.

We will be concerned with the following quantities:

(i) $\Gamma(\boldsymbol{\xi}, t)$ itself, which is the TPSF, and the integrated intensity (which has units of energy per unit area):

$$E(\boldsymbol{\xi}) = \int_{-\infty}^{\infty} \Gamma(\boldsymbol{\xi}, t) \, dt \tag{13}$$

(ii) the mean time-of-flight:

$$\langle t \rangle(\boldsymbol{\xi}) = \int_{-\infty}^{\infty} t \Gamma(\boldsymbol{\xi}, t) \, dt \Big/ \int_{-\infty}^{\infty} \Gamma(\boldsymbol{\xi}, t) \, dt \tag{14}$$

(iii) the DP:

$$DP(\boldsymbol{\xi}) = -d \ln E(\boldsymbol{\xi})/d\mu_a \tag{15}$$

(iv) the phase as a function of frequency ω:

$$\psi(\boldsymbol{\xi}, \omega) = \mathrm{Arg}\left(\int_{-\infty}^{\infty} \Gamma(\boldsymbol{\xi}, t) \, e^{-i\omega t} \, dt \right). \tag{16}$$

We will develop expressions for these in various geometries, and compare the correlation of (ii), (iii) and (iv).

4. Fourier transform approach

We have already introduced the Fourier transform approach in section 2 as the means of deriving the phase from a given TPSF. As will become apparent in the following, the forms (i)-(iv) above can also be derived concisely by applying Fourier transform techniques to (11). The explicit means of deriving these results from the Fourier transform are given in appendices A and B. However there is a considerable literature on Green's functions in the theory of conduction of heat and we first develop some results that relate this field to our case.

4.1. Relationship to conduction of heat

Carslaw and Jaeger (1986) derive Green's functions and their Laplace transforms for the heat equation, which is (11) with $\mu_a = 0$ i.e. the lossless diffusion equation. We can relate these to the lossy diffusion equation, equation (11), via the following theorem.

Theorem 1. If $g(\boldsymbol{r}, t)$ is a Green's functions of the lossless diffusion equation, then $e^{-\mu_a c t} g(\boldsymbol{r}, t)$ is a Green's function of (11).

Proof. We have:

$$(\gamma^2 \nabla^2 - \partial/\partial t) g(\boldsymbol{r}, t) = \delta(\boldsymbol{r}, t) \tag{17}$$

for any given boundary conditions. Let $T(t)$ be a function of time only. Then

$$(\gamma^2 \nabla^2 - \mu_a c - \partial/\partial t) T(t) g(\boldsymbol{r}, t) = T(t)(\gamma^2 \nabla^2 - \partial/\partial t) g(\boldsymbol{r}, t) - g(\boldsymbol{r}, t)(\partial/\partial t + \mu_a c) T(t). \tag{18}$$

If $T(t) = e^{-\mu_a c t}$ then the second term on the right is always zero. The first term is $T(t)\delta(\boldsymbol{r}, t)$ which is zero, except for when $t = 0$, where $T = 1$. Thus

$$(\gamma^2 \nabla^2 - \mu_a c - \partial/\partial t) \, e^{-\mu_a c t} g(\boldsymbol{r}, t) = \delta(\boldsymbol{r}, t) \tag{19}$$

as required. $\qquad\square$

251

Theorem 2. If $g(t)$ is a Green's function of the lossless diffusion equation, then $\hat{G}(\omega) = (2\pi)^{-1/2}\bar{g}(i\omega)$ where $\hat{G}(\omega)$ is the Fourier transform of $g(t)$ and $\bar{g}(s)$ is the Laplace transform, provided that all poles of $\bar{g}(s)$ lie to the right of $\mathrm{Re}(s) > 0$.

Proof. Since $g(t)$ is a Green's function, we have from physical considerations that $g(t) = 0$ for $t < 0$. Thus

$$\hat{G}(\omega) = \mathscr{F}_{t\to\omega}[g(t)] = \frac{1}{\sqrt{2\pi}} \int_0^\infty g(t)\, \mathrm{e}^{-\mathrm{i}\omega t}\, \mathrm{d}t. \tag{20}$$

But

$$\bar{g}(s) = \mathscr{L}_{t\to s}[g(t)] = \int_0^\infty g(t)\, \mathrm{e}^{-(b+\mathrm{i}\omega)t}\, \mathrm{d}t \tag{21}$$

where b is taken large enough that the integral on the right converges and $s = b + \mathrm{i}\omega$. This defines the Laplace transform whose inverse is

$$g(t) = \mathscr{L}_{s\to t}^{-1}[\bar{g}(s)] = \frac{1}{2\pi\mathrm{i}} \int_{b-\mathrm{i}\infty}^{b+\mathrm{i}\infty} \bar{g}(s)\, \mathrm{e}^{st}\, \mathrm{d}s. \tag{22}$$

We thus have the relation in the theorem provided that $b = 0$ i.e. provided that $g(t)\, \mathrm{e}^{-\mathrm{i}\omega t}$ is integrable in the positive-t domain, or conversely that in the inverse Laplace transform all poles of $\bar{g}(s)$ lie to the right of $\mathrm{Re}(s) > 0$. This will be true for all the Green's functions that we will consider, as can be seen by inspection, and it is a necessary consequence of the physical interpretation of the diffusion equation. $\square$

Corollary. The Fourier transform of the corresponding Green's function for the lossy diffusion equation is $(2\pi)^{-1/2}\bar{g}(\mu_a c + \mathrm{i}\omega)$.

This derives simply from using $b = \mu_a c$ in (21) and the result from theorem 1.

In the following, we will represent the Green's function for (11) as $g_k^{(\Phi)}(\boldsymbol{r}, \boldsymbol{r}', t, t')$, where the subscript k will refer to different geometries, and the result of substituting this into (12) as $g_k^{(\Gamma)}(\boldsymbol{\xi}, \boldsymbol{r}', t, t')$.

4.2. Infinite-medium case

We commence with the Green's function for the photon density in an infinite medium (Carslaw and Jaeger (1986), section 14.1; Patterson *et al* (1989), equation (3)):

$$g_{\mathrm{inf}}^{(\Phi)}(\boldsymbol{r}, \boldsymbol{r}', t, t') = 1/[4\pi\gamma^2(t-t')]^{3/2} \exp\{-[\mu_a c(t-t') + |\boldsymbol{r}-\boldsymbol{r}'|^2/4\gamma^2(t-t')]\} \tag{23}$$

whose Fourier transform is given by applying theorems 1 and 2 to equation (6) of Carslaw and Jaeger (1986), appendix V:

$$\hat{G}_{\mathrm{inf}}^{(\Phi)}(\boldsymbol{r}, \boldsymbol{r}', \omega, t') = \mathrm{e}^{-\mathrm{i}\omega t'}\, \mathrm{e}^{-\alpha|\boldsymbol{r}-\boldsymbol{r}'|}/[2(2\pi)^{3/2}|\boldsymbol{r}-\boldsymbol{r}'|\gamma^2] \tag{24}$$

where $\alpha = (\mu_a c + \mathrm{i}\omega)^{1/2}/\gamma$. This result is derived from first principles in appendix A, and demonstrates the correctness of the use of theorems 1 and 2. The *phase* of this function is just the imaginary part of the exponent:

$$\mathrm{Im}[-(\mu_a c + \mathrm{i}\omega)^{1/2}|\boldsymbol{r}-\boldsymbol{r}'|/\gamma] = -[(\mu_a c)^2 + \omega^2]^{1/4}(|\boldsymbol{r}-\boldsymbol{r}'|/\gamma)\sin[\tfrac{1}{2}(\mathrm{Tan}^{-1}\omega/\mu_a c)] \tag{25}$$

(see equation (A.15)). We may find the corresponding terms for the flux at some radius d from the pulse by substituting (23) into (12). The formulae for $g_{\mathrm{inf}}^{(\Gamma)}(d, t, t')$ and its corresponding Fourier transform are given in table 1, equation (1.1)† and table 2,

---

† See also table 5, for the notation.

Table 1.

Case	Green's function (time domain)	
Infinite medium	$g_{\mathrm{inf}}^{(\Gamma)}(d,t,t') = \{d/[2(4\pi\gamma^2)^{3/2}(t-t')^{5/2}]\}\exp\{-[\mu_a c(t-t') + d^2/4\gamma^2(t-t')]\}$	(1.1)
Semi-infinite half-space	$g_{\mathrm{half}}^{(\Gamma)}(\xi,z_0,t,t') = \{z_0/[(4\pi\gamma^2)^{3/2}(t-t')^{5/2}]\}\exp\{-[\mu_a c(t-t') + \rho^2/4\gamma^2(t-t')]\}$	(1.2)
Infinite slab $0 < z < d$ (evaluated at $z = d$)	$g_{\mathrm{slab}}^{(\Gamma)}(\xi,z_0,t,t') = \dfrac{-\exp\{-[\mu_a c(t-t') + \xi^2/4\gamma^2(t-t')]}{(4\pi\gamma^2)^{3/2}(t-t')^{5/2}} \sum_{n=0}^{\infty}\left[z_{+n}\exp\left(\dfrac{-(z_{+n})^2}{4\gamma^2(t-t')}\right) - z_{-n}\exp\left(\dfrac{-(z_{-n})^2}{4\gamma^2(t-t')}\right)\right]$	(1.3a)
Infinite slab (evaluated at $z = 0$)	$g_{\mathrm{slab}}^{(\Gamma)}(\xi,z_0,t,t') = \dfrac{\exp\{-[\mu_a c(t-t') + \xi^2/4\gamma^2(t-t')]\}}{(4\pi\gamma^2)^{3/2}(t-t')^{5/2}}\left\{z_0\exp\left(\dfrac{-z_0^2}{4\gamma^2(t-t')}\right)\right.$ $\left. + \sum_{n=1}^{\infty}\left[z_{+n'}\exp\left(\dfrac{-z_{+n'}^2}{4\gamma^2(t-t')}\right) - z_{-n'}\exp\left(\dfrac{-z_{-n'}^2}{4\gamma^2(t-t')}\right)\right]\right\}$	(1.3b)
2D circle radius a	$g_{\mathrm{circ}}^{(\Gamma)}(a,r',t,t') = \dfrac{\gamma^2\,\mathrm{e}^{-\mu_a c(t-t')}}{\pi a^2}\sum_{n=-\infty}^{\infty}\cos(n\theta)\sum_{\beta_n}\mathrm{e}^{-\gamma^2\beta_n^2(t-t')}\dfrac{\beta_n J_n(\beta_n r')}{J_{n+1}(\beta_n a)}$	(1.4)
Finite cylinder, radius a, length l	$g_{\mathrm{fcyl}}^{(\Gamma)}(a,r',t,t') = \dfrac{2\gamma^2\,\mathrm{e}^{-\mu_a c(t-t')}}{\pi a^2 l}\sum_{m=1,\mathrm{odd}}^{\infty}\mathrm{e}^{-\gamma^2 m^2\pi^2(t-t')/l^2}\sum_{n=-\infty}^{\infty}\cos(n\theta)\sum_{\beta_n}\mathrm{e}^{-\gamma^2\beta_n^2(t-t')}\dfrac{\beta_n J_n(\beta_n r')}{J_{n+1}(\beta_n a)}$	(1.5)
Infinite cylinder, radius a, $z = z'$	$g_{\mathrm{cyl}}^{(\Gamma)}(a,r',t,t') = \dfrac{\gamma\,\mathrm{e}^{-\mu_a c(t-t')}}{2\pi a^2\sqrt{\pi(t-t')}}\sum_{n=-\infty}^{\infty}\cos(n\theta)\sum_{\beta_n}\mathrm{e}^{-\gamma^2\beta_n^2(t-t')}\dfrac{\beta_n J_n(\beta_n r')}{J_{n+1}(\beta_n a)}$	(1.6)
Sphere, radius a	$g_{\mathrm{sph}}^{(\Gamma)}(a,r',t,t') = \dfrac{\gamma^2\,\mathrm{e}^{-\mu_a c(t-t')}}{2\pi a^2\sqrt{ar'}}\sum_{n=0}^{\infty}\sum_{\beta_{n+1/2}}\mathrm{e}^{-\gamma^2\beta_{n+1/2}^2(t-t')}\dfrac{\beta_{n+1/2}J_{n+1/2}(\beta_{n+1/2}r')}{J_{n+3/2}(\beta_{n+1/2}a)}(2n+1)P_n(\cos\theta)$	(1.7)

Table 2.

Case	Green's function (frequency domain)	
Infinite medium	$\hat{G}_{\mathrm{inf}}^{(\Gamma)}(d,\omega,r') = \mathrm{e}^{-i\omega t'}(1+\alpha d)\,\mathrm{e}^{-\alpha d}/[2(2\pi)^{3/2}d^2]$	(2.1)
Semi-infinite half-space	$\hat{G}_{\mathrm{half}}^{(\Gamma)}(\xi,z_0,\omega,t') = \mathrm{e}^{-i\omega t'}(1+\alpha\rho)z_0\,\mathrm{e}^{-\alpha\rho}/[(2\pi)^{3/2}\rho^2]$	(2.2)
Infinite slab $0 < z < d$ (evaluated at $z = d$)	$\hat{G}_{\mathrm{slab}}^{(\Gamma)}(\xi,z_0,\omega,t') = \dfrac{-\mathrm{e}^{-i\omega t'}}{(2\pi)^{3/2}}\sum_{n=0}^{\infty}\left(\dfrac{z_{+n}}{\rho_{+n}^3}(1+\alpha\rho_{+n})\,\mathrm{e}^{-\alpha\rho_{+n}} - \dfrac{z_{-n}}{\rho_{-n}^3}(1+\alpha\rho_{-n})\,\mathrm{e}^{-\alpha\rho_{-n}}\right)$	(2.3a)
Infinite slab (evaluated at $z = 0$)	$\hat{G}_{\mathrm{slab}}^{(\Gamma)}(\xi,z_0,\omega,t') = \dfrac{\mathrm{e}^{-i\omega t'}}{(2\pi)^{3/2}}\left[\dfrac{z_0}{\rho^3}(1+\alpha\rho)\,\mathrm{e}^{-\alpha\rho} + \sum_{n=1}^{\infty}\left(\dfrac{z_{+n'}}{\rho_{+n'}^3}(1+\alpha\rho_{+n'})\,\mathrm{e}^{-\alpha\rho_{+n'}} - \dfrac{z_{-n'}}{\rho_{-n'}^3}(1+\alpha\rho_{-n'})\,\mathrm{e}^{-\alpha\rho_{-n'}}\right)\right]$	(2.3b)
2D circle radius a	$\hat{G}_{\mathrm{circ}}^{(\Gamma)}(a,r',\omega,t') = \dfrac{\mathrm{e}^{-i\omega t'}}{(2\pi)^{3/2}a}\sum_{n=-\infty}^{\infty}\cos(n\theta)\dfrac{I_n(\alpha r')}{I_n(\alpha a)}$	(2.4)
Finite cylinder, radius a, length l	$\hat{G}_{\mathrm{fcyl}}^{(\Gamma)}(a,r',\omega,t') = \dfrac{\mathrm{e}^{-i\omega t'}}{\pi(2\pi)^{1/2}al}\sum_{m=1,\mathrm{odd}}^{\infty}\sum_{n=-\infty}^{\infty}\cos(n\theta)\dfrac{I_n(\alpha_m r')}{I_n(\alpha_m a)}$	(2.5)
Infinite cylinder, radius a, $z = z'$	$\hat{G}_{\mathrm{cyl}}^{(\Gamma)}(a,r',\omega,t') = \dfrac{\mathrm{e}^{-i\omega t'}}{(2\pi)^{3/2}a^2}\sum_{n=-\infty}^{\infty}\cos(n\theta)\sum_{\beta_n}\dfrac{1}{(\alpha^2+\beta_n^2)^{1/2}}\dfrac{\beta_n I_n(\beta_n r')}{J_{n+1}(\beta_n a)}$	(2.6)
Sphere, radius a	$\hat{G}_{\mathrm{sph}}^{(\Gamma)}(a,r',\omega,t') = \dfrac{\mathrm{e}^{-i\omega t'}}{2(2\pi)^{3/2}\sqrt{a^3 r'}}\sum_{n=0}^{\infty}\dfrac{I_{n+1/2}(\alpha r')}{I_{n+1/2}(\alpha a)}(2n+1)P_n(\cos\theta)$	(2.7)

Table 3.

Case	Phase	
Infinite medium	$\psi_{\text{inf}}^{(\Gamma)}(d) = \tan^{-1}\{Ad\sin(\tfrac{1}{2}\tau)/[1+Ad\cos(\tfrac{1}{2}\tau)]\} - Ad\sin(\tfrac{1}{2}\tau)$	(3.1)
Semi-infinite half-space	$\psi_{\text{half}}^{(\Gamma)}(\rho) = \tan^{-1}\{A\rho\sin(\tfrac{1}{2}\tau)/[1+A\rho\cos(\tfrac{1}{2}\tau)]\} - A\rho\sin(\tfrac{1}{2}\tau)$	(3.2)
Infinite slab	No analytic expression	(3.3)
2D circle, radius a	No analytic expression	(3.4)
Finite cylinder	No analytic expression	(3.5)
Infinite cylinder, radius a, $z=z'$	$\langle\psi\rangle_{\text{cyl}}^{(\Gamma)}(\boldsymbol{a},\boldsymbol{r}') = \tan^{-1}\left[-\sum_{n=-\infty}^{\infty}\cos(n\theta)\sum_{\beta_n}\left(\dfrac{\sin(\tfrac{1}{2}\tau_{\beta_n})}{A_{\beta_n}}\dfrac{\beta_n J_n(\beta_n r')}{J_{n+1}(\beta_n a)}\right)\right] \Big/ \left[\sum_{n=-\infty}^{\infty}\cos(n\theta)\sum_{\beta_n}\left(\dfrac{\cos(\tfrac{1}{2}\tau_{\beta_n})}{A_{\beta_n}}\dfrac{\beta_n J_n(\beta_n r_0)}{J_{n+1}(\beta_n a)}\right)\right]$	(3.6)
Sphere, radius a	No analytic expression	(3.7)

Table 4.

Case	Mean time	
Infinite medium	$\langle t\rangle_{\text{inf}}^{(\Gamma)}(d) = \tfrac{1}{2}d^2[\gamma^2+d(\mu_a c)^{1/2}\gamma]$	(4.1)
Semi-infinite half-space	$\langle t\rangle_{\text{half}}^{(\Gamma)}(\rho) = \tfrac{1}{2}\rho^2[\gamma^2+\rho(\mu_a c)^{1/2}\gamma]$	(4.2)
Infinite slab $0<z<d$ (evaluated at $z=d$)	$\langle t\rangle_{\text{slab}}^{(\Gamma)}(\xi,z_0) = \dfrac{1}{2\gamma^2}\sum_{n=0}^{\infty}\left(\dfrac{z_{+n}}{\rho_{+n}^3}e^{-\sigma\rho_{+n}} - \dfrac{z_{-n}}{\rho_{-n}}e^{-\sigma\rho_{-n}}\right) \Big/ \left[\sum_{n=0}^{\infty}\left(\dfrac{z_{+n}}{\rho_{+n}^3}(1+\sigma\rho_{+n})e^{-\sigma\rho_{+n}} - \dfrac{z_{-n}}{\rho_{-n}^3}(1+\sigma\rho_{-n})e^{-\sigma\rho_{-n}}\right)\right]$	(4.3a)
Infinite slab (evaluated at $z=0$)	$\langle t\rangle_{\text{slab}}^{(\Gamma)}(\xi,z_0) = \dfrac{1}{2\gamma^2}\left[\dfrac{z_0}{\rho}e^{-\sigma\rho} + \sum_{n=1}^{\infty}\left(\dfrac{z_{+n'}}{\rho_{+n'}}e^{-\sigma\rho_{+n'}} - \dfrac{z_{-n'}}{\rho_{-n'}}e^{-\sigma\rho_{-n'}}\right)\right] \Big/ \left[\dfrac{z_0}{\rho^3}(1+\sigma\rho)e^{-\sigma\rho} + \sum_{n=1}^{\infty}\left(\dfrac{z_{+n'}}{\rho_{+n'}^3}(1+\sigma\rho_{+n'})e^{-\sigma\rho_{+n'}} - \dfrac{z_{-n'}}{\rho_{-n'}^3}(1+\sigma\rho_{-n'})e^{-\sigma\rho_{-n'}}\right)\right]$	(4.3b)
2D circle, radius a	$\langle t\rangle_{\text{circ}}^{(\Gamma)}(\boldsymbol{a},\boldsymbol{r}') = \dfrac{1}{2\sigma\gamma^2}\left(\sum_{n=-\infty}^{\infty}\dfrac{r'I_n'(\sigma r')I_n(\sigma a) - aI_n(\sigma r')I_n'(\sigma a)}{I_n^2(\sigma a)}\cos(n\theta)\right) \Big/ \left(\sum_{n=-\infty}^{\infty}\dfrac{I_n(\sigma r')}{I_n(\sigma a)}\cos(n\theta)\right)$	(4.4)
Finite cylinder, radius a, length l	$\langle t\rangle_{\text{fcyl}}^{(\Gamma)}(\boldsymbol{a},\boldsymbol{r}') = \dfrac{1}{2\gamma^2}\left(\sum_{m=1,\text{odd}}^{\infty}\sum_{n=-\infty}^{\infty}\dfrac{r'I_n'(\sigma_m r')I_n(\sigma_m a) - aI_n(\sigma_m r')I_n'(\sigma_m a)}{\sigma_m I_n^2(\sigma_m a)}\cos(n\theta)\right) \Big/ \left(\sum_{m=1,\text{odd}}^{\infty}\sum_{n=-\infty}^{\infty}\dfrac{I_n(\sigma_m r')}{I_n(\sigma_m a)}\cos(n\theta)\right)$	(4.5)
Infinite cylinder, radius a, $z=z'$	$\langle t\rangle_{\text{cyl}}^{(\Gamma)}(\boldsymbol{a},\boldsymbol{r}') = \dfrac{1}{2\gamma^2}\left(\sum_{n=-\infty}^{\infty}\cos(n\theta)\sum_{\beta_n}\dfrac{1}{(\sigma^2+\beta_n^2)^{3/2}}\dfrac{\beta_n J_n(\beta_n r')}{J_{n+1}(\beta_n a)}\right) \Big/ \left[\sum_{n=-\infty}^{\infty}\cos(n\theta)\sum_{\beta_n}\dfrac{1}{(\sigma^2+\beta_n^2)^{1/2}}\dfrac{\beta_n J_n(\beta_n r')}{J_{n+1}(\beta_n a)}\right]$	(4.6)
Sphere, radius a	$\langle t\rangle_{\text{sph}}^{(\Gamma)}(\boldsymbol{a},\boldsymbol{r}') = \dfrac{1}{2\sigma\gamma^2}\left(\sum_{n=0}^{\infty}\dfrac{r'I_{n+1/2}'(\sigma r')I_{n+1/2}(\sigma a) - aI_{n+1/2}(\sigma r')I_{n+1/2}'(\sigma a)}{I_{n+1/2}^2(\sigma a)}(2n+1)P_n(\cos\theta)\right) \Big/ \left(\sum_{n=0}^{\infty}\dfrac{I_{n+1/2}(\sigma r')}{I_{n+1/2}(\sigma a)}(2n+1)P_n(\cos\theta)\right)$	(4.7)

equation (2.1) respectively. Note that $g_{\text{inf}}^{(\Gamma)}$ has the correct dimensions of inverse time and inverse area, as required by our use of Φ as a photon density. We put

$$A = [(\mu_a c)^2 + \omega^2]^{1/4}/\gamma \qquad \tau = \text{Tan}^{-1}(\omega/\mu_a c). \qquad (26)$$

Then (2.1) has phase given by table 3, equation (3.1)†, and using (B3) for $g_{\text{inf}}^{(\Gamma)}$ we obtain the expression for the mean time of flight in table 4, equation (4.1), with the differential pathlength $\text{DP}_{\text{inf}}^{(\Gamma)}$ following from theorem B1 applied to (4.1):

$$\text{DP}_{\text{inf}}^{(\Gamma)} = \tfrac{1}{2}\{cd^2/[\gamma^2 + (\mu_a c)^{1/2}\, d\gamma]\}[1 + (3/c)\mu_a \gamma^2]. \qquad (27)$$

Note that in the results in tables 3 and 4, t' is implicitly assumed to be zero. It is easily verified that the correct result for $t' \neq 0$ is obtained by adding t' to $\langle t \rangle$ and $-\omega t'$ to ψ.

4.3. Other geometries

Solutions for a number of other geometries can be derived in a similar way, starting from the Green's function for the lossless diffusion equation given by Carslaw and Jaeger, using the theorems from section 4.1, and substituting into (12). Results for some geometries are given in tables 1–4, and may be derived for others in a similar way. In this section, we comment briefly on any specific points relevant to particular geometries. In some cases it is of interest to inspect the spatial integral of the results over a plane, representing, for example, the surface of a detecting instrument, which is often considered infinite. The expressions derived are often simpler, but are not necessarily applicable.

Since the detailed derivations may be found in Carslaw and Jaeger (1986) for the heat equation, and related to our cases by the theorems of section 4.1, we will not give them here. However, a few comments on methodology are useful. The solutions are obtained by starting with the solution for the infinite medium and proceeding in one of two ways. The method of images adds a number of auxiliary source terms, outside the domain of the solution Ω, which are the reflections of the source in the boundary $\partial\Omega$, and which ensure that $\Phi = 0$ on $\partial\Omega$. The uniqueness theorem ensures that if this combination of sources produces a valid solution in Ω, then it is the only possible solution. The other solution technique is to seek solutions of the auxiliary equation:

$$(\gamma^2\nabla^2 - \mu_a c - \partial/\partial t)\Psi(\mathbf{r}, t) = 0. \qquad (28)$$

There will be a set of eigenfunctions that satisfy equation (28), and a linear combination of these are chosen in such a way that the composite function $\Phi + \Psi$ satisfies the boundary conditions.

Table 5. Glossary of notation for table 1–4.

$\xi = (x^2 + y^2)^{1/2}$	$\sigma = (\mu_a c)^{1/2}/\gamma$
$\rho = (\xi^2 + z_0^2)^{1/2}$	$\alpha_m = (\alpha^2 + m^2\pi^2/l^2)$
$z_{+n} = (2n+1)d + z_0$	$\sigma_m = (\mu_a c/\gamma^2 + m^2\pi^2/l^2)^{1/2}$
$z_{-n} = (2n+1)d - z_0$	r' is the radial position of the source
$z_{+n'} = 2nd + z_0$	β_n is a positive root of $J_n(\beta_n a) = 0$
$z_{-n'} = 2nd - z_0$	$\beta_{n+1/2}$ is a positive root of
$\rho_{+n'} = (\xi^2 + z_{+n'}^2)^{1/2}$	$J_{n+1/2}(\beta_{n+1/2}a) = 0$
$\rho_{-n'} = (\xi^2 + z_{-n'}^2)^{1/2}$	$A_\beta = [(\mu_a c + \gamma^2\beta_n^2)^2 + \omega^2]^{1/4}/\gamma$
$\alpha = (\mu_a c + i\omega)^{1/2}/\gamma$	$\tau_\beta = \tan^{-1}[\omega/(\mu_a c + \gamma^2\beta_n^2)]$

† See also table 5, for the notation.

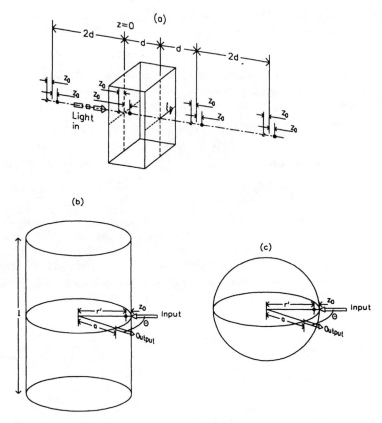

Figure 2. Geometries used for the calculations of integrated intensity, mean time, and phase of a δ-function source in a homogeneous diffusing medium: (a) infinite slab, width d—solution obtained with method of multiple images; (b) finite cylinder length l, radius a; (c) sphere radius a.

4.4. Semi-infinite half-space

The discussion of Patterson *et al* (1989) applies to a semi-infinite space and uses the method of images. This is a common approximation when we are concerned with the measurement of a reflected signal. Photons are assumed to come from an instantaneous point source at a depth $z' = z_0$ below the surface, given by $z_0 = [(1 - \bar{p})\mu_s]^{-1}$. We note that, strictly, the time of this scattering is delayed to $t' = t_0 = z_0/c$ from the time of input of the pulse. In the following $t = t_0$ is taken as zero.

The method of images then puts a negative source of the same strength at a position outside the slab that is the mirror image of the positive source (figure 2(a)). If we put $\xi^2 = (x - x')^2 + (y - y')^2$ we get:

$$g_{\text{half}}^{(\Phi)}(\mathbf{r}, \mathbf{r}', t, t') = \frac{1}{[4\pi\gamma^2(t - t')]^{3/2}} \exp - \left(\mu_a c(t - t') + \frac{\xi^2}{4\gamma^2(t - t')} \right)$$
$$\times [\exp(-(z - z_0)^2/4\gamma^2(t - t')) - \exp(-(z + z_0)^2/4\gamma^2(t - t'))] \tag{29}$$

which is zero on $z = 0$ as required. The Fourier transform of this is then just

$$\hat{G}_{\text{half}}^{(\Phi)}(\mathbf{r}, \mathbf{r}', \omega, t') = [e^{-i\omega t'}/2(2\pi)^{3/2}\gamma^2]\{e^{-\alpha[\xi^2 + (z - z_0)^2]^{1/2}}/[\xi^2 + (z - z_0)^2]^{1/2}$$
$$- e^{-\alpha[\xi^2 + (z + z_0)^2]^{1/2}}/[\xi^2 + (z + z_0)^2]^{1/2}\} \tag{30}$$

which is also zero on $z = 0$ as required. From these the forms for the flux density at $z = 0$ are easily obtained by applying (12) with $\hat{n} = -\hat{z}$ (equations (1.2) and (2.2)). These may be integrated over x and y to give

$$g_{1\text{half}}^{(\Gamma)}(z_0, t, t') = [z_0/\sqrt{4\pi\gamma^2(t-t')^3}] \exp\{-[\mu_a c(t-t') + z_0^2/4\gamma^2(t-t')]\} \tag{31}$$

and

$$\hat{G}_{1\text{half}}^{(\Gamma)}(z_0, \omega, t') = [e^{-i\omega t'}/(2\pi)^{1/2}] e^{-\alpha z_0}. \tag{32}$$

From comparing the form of (2.2) and (2.1) we find

$$\langle t \rangle_{\text{half}}^{(\Gamma)} = \langle t \rangle_{\text{inf}}^{(\Gamma)} \qquad DP_{\text{half}}^{(\Gamma)} = DP_{\text{inf}}^{(\Gamma)} \qquad \psi_{\text{half}}^{(\Gamma)} = \psi_{\text{inf}}^{(\Gamma)}. \tag{33}$$

From (32) we obtain even simpler results:

$$\langle t \rangle_{1\text{half}}^{(\Gamma)} = z_0/[2\gamma(\mu_a c)^{1/2}]$$
$$DP_{1\text{half}}^{(\Gamma)} = \{cz_0/[2\gamma(\mu_a c)^{1/2}]\}[1 + (3/c)\mu_a\gamma^2] \tag{34}$$
$$\psi_{1\text{half}}^{(\Gamma)} = -Az_0 \sin(\tfrac{1}{2}\tau).$$

4.5. Infinite slab $0 < z < d$

The method of multiple images gives an infinite sequence of dipoles:

$$g_{\text{slab}}^{(\Phi)}(\boldsymbol{r}, \boldsymbol{r}', t, t') = \frac{\exp\{-[\mu_a c(t-t') + \xi^2/4\gamma^2(t-t')]\}}{[4\pi\gamma^2(t-t')]^{3/2}} \tag{35}$$

$$\times \sum_{n=-\infty}^{\infty} [\exp(-(z - 2nd - z_0)^2/4\gamma^2(t-t'))$$
$$- \exp(-(z - 2nd + z_0)^2/4\gamma^2(t-t'))]$$

which is zero on $z = 0$ with an odd number of terms, and zero on $z = d$ with an even number of terms. If we take the gradient in the z direction ($-\hat{z}$ for the surface $z = 0$, $+\hat{z}$ for the surface $z = d$) then we obtain (1.3) for both $z = 0$ and $z = d$, and the Fourier transform and mean time are given by (2.3) and (4.3). We may integrate these through x and y to give on $z = d$

$$g_{1\text{slab}}^{(\Gamma)}(d, z_0, t, t') = \frac{-e^{-\mu_a c(t-t')}}{(\gamma^2 4\pi(t-t')^3)^{1/2}} \sum_{n=0}^{n=\infty} [z_{+n} \exp(-z_{+n}^2/4\gamma^2(t-t'))$$
$$- z_{-n} \exp(-z_{-n}^2/4\gamma^2(t-t'))] \tag{36}$$

where $z_{+n} = (2n+1)d + z_0$ and $z_{-n} = (2n+1)d - z_0$. The Fourier transform of this expression is

$$\hat{G}_{1\text{slab}}^{(\Gamma)}(d, z_0, \omega, t') = \frac{-e^{-i\omega t'}}{(2\pi)^{1/2}} \sum_{n=0}^{n=\infty} (e^{-\alpha[(2n+1)d+z_0]} - e^{-\alpha[(2n+1)d-z_0]})$$
$$= \frac{e^{-i\omega t'}}{(2\pi)^{1/2}} \frac{\sinh(\alpha z_0)}{\sinh(\alpha d)} \tag{37}$$

and on $z = 0$

$$g_{1\text{slab}}^{(\Gamma)}(0, z_0, t, t') = \frac{e^{-\mu_a c(t-t')}}{(\gamma^2 4\pi(t-t')^3)^{1/2}} \left\{ z_0 \exp\left(\frac{-z_0^2}{4\gamma^2(t-t')}\right) \right.$$
$$\left. + \sum_{n=1}^{n=\infty} \left[z_{+n'} \exp\left(\frac{-z_{+n'}^2}{4\gamma^2(t-t')}\right) - z_{-n'} \exp\left(\frac{-z_{-n'}^2}{4\gamma^2(t-t')}\right) \right] \right\} \tag{38}$$

where $z_{+n'} = 2nd + z_0$ and $z_{-n'} = 2nd - z_0$. The Fourier transform of this expression is

$$\hat{G}^{(\Gamma)}_{\text{1slab}}(0, z_0, \omega, t') = \frac{e^{-i\omega t'}}{(2\pi)^{1/2}}\left(e^{-\alpha z_0} + \sum_{n=1}^{n=\infty}\left(e^{-\alpha(2nd+z_0)} - e^{-\alpha(2nd-z_0)}\right)\right)$$

$$= \frac{e^{-i\omega t'}}{(2\pi)^{1/2}}\left(e^{-\alpha z_0} - e^{-\alpha d}\frac{\sinh(\alpha z_0)}{\sinh(\alpha d)}\right). \qquad (39)$$

The mean time is obtained, using (B3), on $z = d$:

$$\langle t \rangle^{(\Gamma)}_{\text{1slab}}(d, z_0) = \{1/[2(\mu_a c)^{1/2}\gamma]\}[z_0 \coth(\sigma z_0) - d \coth(\sigma d)] \qquad (40)$$

where $\sigma = \alpha(\omega = 0) = (\mu_a c)^{1/2}/\gamma$. On $z = 0$ the expression is more complex:

$$\langle t \rangle^{(\Gamma)}_{\text{1slab}}(d, z_0) = \{1/[2(\mu_a c)^{1/2}\gamma]\}\{-z_0 e^{-\sigma z_0}\sinh(\sigma d) - z_0 e^{-\sigma d}\cosh(\sigma z_0)$$

$$+ d\, e^{-\sigma d}[\sinh(\sigma z_0) + \coth(\sigma d)\sinh(\sigma z_0)]\}/$$

$$[e^{-\sigma z_0}\sinh(\sigma d) - e^{-\sigma d}\sinh(\sigma z_0)]. \qquad (41)$$

In both cases, we know that, as always, $\text{DP} = [1 + \mu_a/(\mu_a + \mu_s(1-\bar{p}))]c\langle t \rangle$. The phase for this geometry does not have an analytic form, but may be found numerically.

4.6. Two-dimensional circular region (infinite line source in infinite cylinder)

This case is not given explicitly by Carslaw and Jaeger, so we derive it here, and this will serve as an illustration of the general form of the auxiliary equation method. We commence with the two-dimensional form of the infinite-medium Green's function:

$$g^{(\Phi)}_{\text{2D}}(r, r', t, t') = \{1/[4\pi\gamma^2(t-t')]\}\exp\{-[\mu_a c(t-t') + |r-r'|^2/4\gamma^2(t-t')]\} \qquad (42)$$

which has the Fourier transform

$$\hat{G}^{(\Phi)}_{\text{2D}}(r, r', \omega, t') = [e^{-i\omega t'}/(2\pi)^{3/2}\gamma^2]K_0(\alpha|r-r'|) \qquad (43)$$

where K_0 is the modified Bessel function of the second kind of order zero (theorems 1 and 2 applied to Carslaw and Jaeger (1986), Appendix V, equation (23)). The auxiliary equation in the Fourier domain is

$$\left(\frac{\partial^2}{\partial r^2} + \frac{1}{r}\frac{\partial}{\partial r} + \frac{1}{r^2}\frac{\partial^2}{\partial \theta^2} - \alpha^2\right)\hat{H}^{(\Phi)}(r, \omega) = 0 \qquad (44)$$

which has the solutions

$$\hat{H}^{(\Phi)}(r, \omega) = \sum_n^\infty [a_n I_n(r\alpha) + b_n K_n(r\alpha)]\cos(n\theta) \qquad (45)$$

where I_n and K_n are the modified Bessel functions of the first and second kind. The solution is then found by using an addition theorem for Bessel functions (Watson 1944):

$$K_0(\alpha|r-r'|) = \begin{cases} \displaystyle\sum_{n=-\infty}^\infty \cos(n\theta)I_n(\alpha r')K_n(\alpha r) & (r > r') \\[2ex] \displaystyle\sum_{n=-\infty}^\infty \cos(n\theta)I_n(\alpha r)K_n(\alpha r') & (r < r') \end{cases} \qquad (46)$$

and finding the coefficients a_n, b_n so that $\hat{G}_{2D}^{(\Phi)} + \hat{H}^{(\Phi)} = 0$ on the boundary. The only possibility is

$$b_n = 0 \qquad a_n = -I_n(\alpha r') K_n(\alpha a) / I_n(\alpha a) \tag{47}$$

and so:

$$\hat{G}_{circ}^{(\Phi)}(r, r', \omega, t')$$
$$= \frac{e^{-i\omega t'}}{(2\pi)^{3/2}\gamma^2} \sum_{n=-\infty}^{\infty} \cos(n\theta) \frac{I_n(\alpha r')}{I_n(\alpha a)} [K_n(\alpha r) I_n(\alpha a) - I_n(\alpha r) K_n(\alpha a)] \tag{48}$$

for $r > r'$, and the case $r < r'$ is found by interchanging r and r'. Taking the gradient in the radial direction and using (12) we obtain (2.4), where we have used a property of Bessel functions: $[I_\nu(z) K_\nu'(z) - K_\nu(z) I_\nu'(z)] = -1/z$. To obtain the Green's function in the spatial domain we take the inverse Fourier transform of (2.4). The contour is completed in the upper half-plane for $t > t'$ and the only poles are on the imaginary axis at the zeros of $J_n(\alpha a) = 0$. The summation over all these poles, for all Bessel functions, gives (1.4). This will be seen to be just the integral over the z dimension of (1.6). The mean time is then given by (4.4) and the phase must be evaluated numerically.

4.7. Finite cylinder $-l/2 < z < l/2$

In this case (figure 2(b)) we use the auxiliary equation, in the Fourier domain:

$$\left(\frac{1}{r^2} \frac{\partial^2}{\partial\theta^2} + \frac{\partial^2}{\partial r^2} + \frac{1}{r} \frac{\partial}{\partial r} + \frac{\partial^2}{\partial z^2} - \alpha^2 \right) \hat{H}^{(\Phi)}(r, \omega) = 0 \tag{49}$$

which has solutions

$$\hat{H}^{(\Phi)}(r, \omega) = \sum_{m,n}^{\infty} \left[\left[a_{m,n} I_n \left\{ \left[\alpha^2 + \left(\frac{m\pi}{l}\right)^2 \right]^{1/2} r \right\} \right.\right.$$
$$\left.\left. + b_{m,n} K_n \left\{ \left[\alpha^2 + \left(\frac{m\pi}{l}\right)^2 \right]^{1/2} r \right\} \right] \cos(n\theta) \sin\left(\frac{m\pi z}{l}\right). \tag{50}$$

The solution is then found by using an addition theorem for Bessel functions (Watson 1944) and finding the coefficients $a_{m,n}$ $b_{m,n}$ such that $\hat{G}_{inf}^{(\Phi)} + \hat{H}^{(\Phi)} = 0$ on the boundary. Differentiating this gives equation (2.5) and its inverse Fourier transform gives equation (1.5). In these expressions we have assumed that $z = z' = l/2$.

4.8. Infinite cylinder

The expressions for this case may be obtained as the limit $l \to \infty$ of the finite case. We get an integral expression for the result:

$$\hat{G}_{cyl}^{(\Gamma)}(a, r', \omega, t') = \frac{e^{-i\omega t'}}{(2\pi)^{3/2}a^2} \sum_{n=-\infty}^{\infty} \cos(n\theta) \int_0^{\infty} \frac{I_n[(\alpha^2 + y^2)^{1/2} r']}{I_n[(\alpha^2 + y^2)^{1/2} a]} \, dy. \tag{51}$$

Completing the integral in the upper half-plane picks up all the poles of I_n on the imaginary axis, which are just the zeros of $J_n(\alpha a)$, and thus yields (2.6). The same expression is obtained by writing down the Green's function for photon density for a homogeneous cylinder of radius a (Carslaw and Jaeger (1986), section 14.13):

$$g_{cyl}^{(\Phi)}(r, r', t, t') = \frac{-\exp\{-[\mu_a c(t - t') + |z - z'|^2/4\gamma^2(t - t')]\}}{2\pi a^2 \gamma \sqrt{\pi(t - t')}} \sum_{n=-\infty}^{\infty} \cos(n\theta)$$
$$\times \sum_{\beta_n} e^{-\gamma^2 \beta_n^2 (t - t')} \frac{J_n(\beta_n r) J_n(\beta_n r')}{J_{n+1}(\beta_n a)^2} \tag{52}$$

where β_n is a positive root of $J_n(\beta_n a) = 0$, θ is the angular separation of r' and r, and the summations are over all roots of all Bessel functions of the first kind J_n. This is zero on $r = a$, as required. The corresponding Green's function for flux density is given by (1.6) where we have assumed that $z = z'$. The Fourier transform is given by

$$\hat{G}_{\text{cyl}}^{(\Gamma)}(a, r', \omega, t') = \frac{e^{-i\omega t'}}{(2\pi)^{3/2} a^2} \sum_{n=-\infty}^{\infty} \cos(n\theta) \sum_{\beta_n} \frac{e^{-(\alpha^2 + \beta_n^2)^{1/2}|z - z'|}}{(\alpha^2 + \beta_n^2)^{1/2}} \frac{\beta_n J_n(\beta_n r')}{J_{n+1}(\beta_n a)} \tag{53}$$

which simplifies to (2.6) for $z = z'$, and the mean time is given by

$$\langle t \rangle_{\text{cyl}}^{(\Gamma)}(a, r') = \frac{1}{2\gamma^2} \left[\sum_{n=-\infty}^{\infty} \cos(n\theta) \sum_{\beta_n} \left(\frac{1 + (\sigma^2 + \beta_n^2)^{1/2}|z - z'|}{(\sigma^2 + \beta_n^2)^{3/2}} \right) \right.$$

$$\left. \times e^{-(\sigma^2 + \beta_n^2)^{1/2}|z - z'|} \left(\frac{\beta_n J_n(\beta_n r')}{J_{n+1}(\beta_n a)} \right) \right] \Big/$$

$$\left[\sum_{n=-\infty}^{\infty} \cos(n\theta) \sum_{\beta_n} \left(\frac{e^{-(\sigma^2 + \beta_n^2)^{1/2}|z - z'|}}{(\sigma^2 + \beta_n^2)^{1/2}} \right) \frac{\beta_n J_n(\beta_n r')}{J_{n+1}(\beta_n a)} \right] \tag{54}$$

which simplifies to (4.6) for $z = z'$, with the phase given by (3.6).

However, from a computational point of view, the integral expression, equation (51), is possibly easier to compute, since $I_n(x)$ is smooth and $\to (2\pi/x)^{1/2} e^{-x}$ as $x \to \infty$.

4.9. Sphere

In this case (figure 2(c)) we use the auxiliary equation, in the Fourier domain:

$$\left(\frac{\partial^2}{\partial r^2} + \frac{2\partial}{r\partial r} + \frac{1}{r^2 \sin\theta} \frac{\partial}{\partial\theta} \sin\theta \frac{\partial}{\partial\theta} - \alpha^2 \right) \hat{H}^{(\Phi)}(r, \omega) = 0. \tag{55}$$

The solutions of this that are finite at the origin are

$$\hat{H}^{(\Phi)}(r, \omega) = \left(\frac{\pi}{2\alpha r} \right)^{1/2} \sum_{n}^{\infty} a_n I_{n+1/2}(r\alpha) P_n(\cos\theta) \tag{56}$$

where P_n is the Legendre polynomial for order n. From Carslaw and Jaeger (1986), section 14.16,

$$g_{\text{sph}}^{(\Phi)}(r, r', t, t') = \frac{-e^{-\mu_a c(t - t')}}{2\pi a^2 \sqrt{rr'}} \sum_{n=0}^{\infty} \sum_{\beta_{n+1/2}} e^{-\gamma^2 \beta_{n+1/2}^2 (t - t')}$$

$$\times \frac{J_{n+1/2}(\beta_{n+1/2} r) J_{n+1/2}(\beta_{n+1/2} r')}{J_{n+3/2}(\beta_{n+1/2} a)^2} (2n + 1) P_n(\cos\theta) \tag{57}$$

where $\beta_{n+1/2}$ is a positive root of $J_{n+1/2}(\beta_{n+1/2} a) = 0$, θ is the angular separation of r' and r, and the summations are over all roots of all Bessel functions of the first kind of half-integer order $J_{n+1/2}$. This is zero on $r = a$ as required. Taking the gradient of this in the radial direction, and setting $r = a$ leads to (1.7). To obtain the Fourier transform, we write down the result for Φ for $r > r'$, and the case $r < r'$ is found by interchanging r and r':

$$\hat{G}_{\text{sph}}^{(\Phi)}(r, r', \omega, t') = \frac{e^{-i\omega t'}}{2(2\pi)^{3/2} \gamma^2 \sqrt{rr'}} \sum_{n=0}^{\infty} \frac{K_{n+1/2}(\alpha r) I_{n+1/2}(\alpha a) - I_{n+1/2}(\alpha r) K_{n+1/2}(\alpha a)}{I_{n+1/2}(\alpha a)}$$

$$\times (2n + 1) I_{n+1/2}(\alpha r') P_n(\cos\theta). \tag{58}$$

Note that this is zero on $r = a$ as required. For flux density we take $\partial/\partial r$ at $r = a$ to obtain (2.7), where we have used the same property of Bessel functions as in section 4.6. The mean time may then be derived as (4.7). As in the infinite-slab case, the phase may only be derived computationally.

5. Computational considerations

Whereas the expressions in table 1–4 are exact, the evaluation of them presents some computational problems. The infinite-space and infinite-half-space geometries present no difficulties, but all other expressions require summations over infinite series. The number of terms in the series increases with the proximity of r' to the boundary. Since the exact point at which the source is created is to some extent a topic of discussion, we seek only to show the self-consistency of the expressions for $\langle t \rangle$ and ψ. In a subsequent paper we will investigate the variation of the results with this factor, and the dipole limit.

In the case of the infinite slab, the terms in the series decay very rapidly and we found that the series required no more than five terms before becoming smaller than the required precision. For the cylinder and sphere geometries we are summing series of the form

$$\sum_{n=0}^{\infty} F_n(\cos \theta) Q_n$$

where $F_n(\cos \theta) = \cos(n\theta)$ for the cylinder, and the Legendre polynomial $P_n \cos \theta$, for the sphere. For the parameters used here the terms Q_n are very slowly decaying, and the F_n is oscillatory with period of at least N, the number of angular samples. This has the effect that we are subtracting two numbers of nearly equal magnitude with the attendant loss of precision and a number of considerations have to be made:

(i) the terms should be summed from smallest to largest;
(ii) the number of terms must be a multiple of N;
(iii) the working precision must be sufficient to give the requisite final precision.

The last point has meant that we needed a high-precision arithmetic library. The calculations presented in section 6 were carried out at 48 decimal places of precision using the 'Mathematica' package version 2.0 (Wolfram 1991, Wolfram Research Incorporated). This type of precision means that calculations are carried out in an interpretative manner and the computation time is very greatly increased. The results for the sphere and 2D cylinder took about 48 hours each on a Sun Sparc 2 machine. The results for the infinite cylinder involve a double summation that makes the computation almost prohibitively time-consuming. We achieved a slight speed-up by performing a numerical integration of the expression in (51).

It is worth pointing out that the expressions in table 1 for the circle, finite cylinder, and sphere require an extra summation, and also the calculation of multiple roots of Bessel functions. This will increase the computational complexity by an order of magnitude. Furthermore, to compute TPSF curves, these expressions would have to be evaluated at many time points, thus making the overall calculations extremely lengthy. The results presented here thus have a considerable advantage in that they can compute parameters of interest, such as mean time, integrated intensity, phase and modulation depth, by a direct method that is very much faster.

261

6. Results and discussion

Figure 1(b) shows that in frequency domain measurements across several centimetres of tissue, the modulation depth of the light will have fallen to 10% at 1 GHz, which implies that the maximum frequency at which experimental measurements would be possible is approximately 2 GHz (modulation depth $\simeq 1\%$). The linear relationship between phase shift and frequency appears to hold up to 200 MHz, beyond which the measured phase shift noticeably under-reads ωt. Fourier transforms of impulse functions measured across 4 cm of brain tissue and 2 cm of arm tissue showed similar break frequencies for linearity. Hence it is likely that single-frequency phase-shift methods can only be used to measure directly mean time delays of light transmitted through tissue at modulation frequencies up to 200 MHz.

By coincidence 200 MHz is typically the maximum usable frequency of most conventional photomultiplier tubes, and hence modulation frequencies greater than this are rarely employed. Frequencies that have been used for experimental phase shift measurements in tissue have been in the range 50 to 220 MHz (Chance *et al* 1990, Fishkin *et al* 1991).

Using the expressions in tables 1–4, values for various parameters have been calculated for several geometries. Calculations have been performed for the cases of a point source in an infinite slab 50 mm thick (both transmission and reflection), an infinite line source in an infinite cylinder and a point source in a sphere, both 50 mm in diameter. In each case the source was located at a distance 0.5 mm in from the surface, and a refractive index of 1.4 was assumed (Bolin *et al* 1989), so the speed of light was $c = 0.21$ mm ps^{-1}. Values for μ_a of 0.025 mm^{-1} and for μ_s of 2.0 mm^{-1} were used, these being representative of brain tissue (van der Zee *et al* 1991), enabling the results to be compared with the experimentally derived data shown in figure 1. Note that for these values, the correction factor in theorem B1 is 1.012. The results for the infinite slab are shown in figures 3 (transmission) and 4 (reflection), for the cylinder in figure 5 and for the sphere in figure 6.

There are several interesting points to note. Most striking is the remarkable similarity for all geometries of the behaviour of both the phase and modulation depth as a function of frequency for transmission (figures 3, 5 and 6(d)). As frequency rises, the phase angle increases and modulation depth drops. As predicted, at all frequencies, the phase shift underestimates the mean optical pathlength—the difference increasing with frequency—although below 200 MHz the differences are small. This is even true in the circular geometries at an angle of 90° (figures 5 and 6(e)). The data for back-scattered light (figures 4(d), 5(f) and 6(f)) may at first appear unnecessary, since it is well known that the diffusion equation is not valid in this case; however, the results serve to validate the correctness of the derived expressions. The small differences between mean time and phase can be seen more clearly in figures 3, 4, 5 and 6(b) where the ratios of the two at 200 MHz have been calculated as functions of position on the object surface. It can be seen that the magnitude of the difference is $<1\%$ in the worst case. This result validates the application of phase measurement as an indicator of optical pathlength in spectroscopy systems (as long as the measurement frequency is <200 MHz).

A second feature of the results (figures 3, 4, 5 and 6(c)) is the large range in the integrated intensity as a function of position on the exit surface of the object ($>10^{15}$). This result has been predicted previously, as well as observed experimentally (Arridge *et al* 1990). This has implications for attempts to image absorbing centres within tissue,

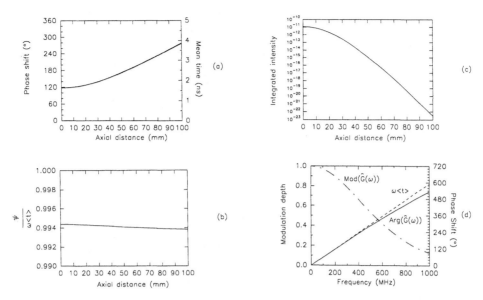

Figure 3. Results for an infinite slab 50 mm thick. (a) Phase shift ψ in degrees and mean time $\langle t \rangle$ in nanoseconds as a function of distance ξ from the input axis, on the transmission side of the slab, at a modulation frequency of 200 MHz; (b) ratio of $\psi/(\omega\langle t \rangle)$ against ξ; (c) integrated intensity E_0 as a function of ξ; (d) ψ (solid), $\omega\langle t \rangle$ (dotted), and modulation depth M (dash-dotted) against frequency in MHz for $\xi = 0$.

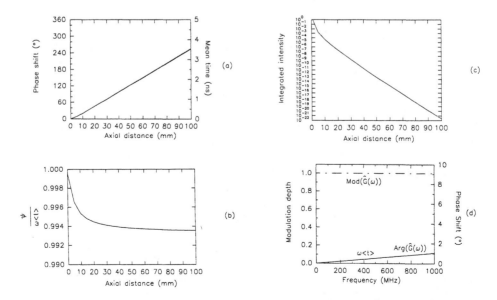

Figure 4. Results as in figure 3, but for an infinite slab 50 mm thick on the reflection side. Note that part (d) corresponds to part (f) in figures 5 and 6.

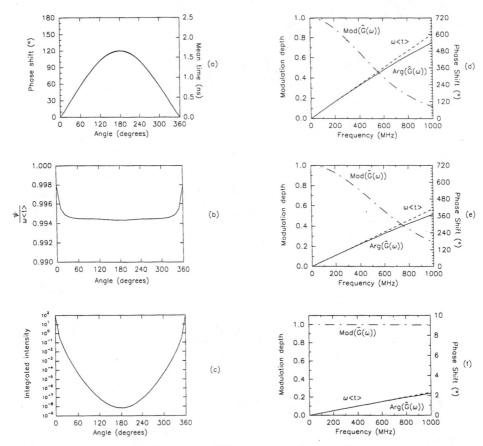

Figure 5. Results for an infinite line source in an infinite cylinder 50 mm in diameter (2D circular case). (a) Phase shift ψ in degrees and mean time $\langle t \rangle$ in nanoseconds as a function of angle θ from the input position, at a modulation frequency of 200 MHz; (b) ratio of $\psi/(\omega\langle t \rangle)$ against θ; (c) integrated intensity E_0 as a function of θ; (d) ψ (solid), $\omega\langle t \rangle$ (dotted), and modulation depth M (dash-dotted) against frequency in MHz for $\theta = 180°$; (e) as (d), but for $\theta = 90°$; (f) as (d), but for $\theta = 0°$.

since any measuring system would have to be designed to work over an enormous dynamic range as well as having a high resolution. Previous results have shown that mean time is a more sensitive indicator of the presence of local variations of absorbance within a scattering media (Arridge *et al* 1991).

In section 2, the relationship between time-resolved and phase-resolved measurements was outlined. Time-resolved measurements can currently be made with a resolution of 8 ps. To obtain similar data, a phase system would have to measure at up to 10 GHz. Such measurements are not yet feasible, and costs would probably limit a bedside measuring system to 200–300 MHz. It would in theory be possible to sample data at several frequencies and then attempt to fit the measurements to a model of the tissue in order to predict the response at all other frequencies. However, this would be difficult to do from the phase data only. It can be seen from the figures that the modulation depth signal shows the greatest change over this frequency range, and it would therefore be essential for phase systems to measure modulation depth also.

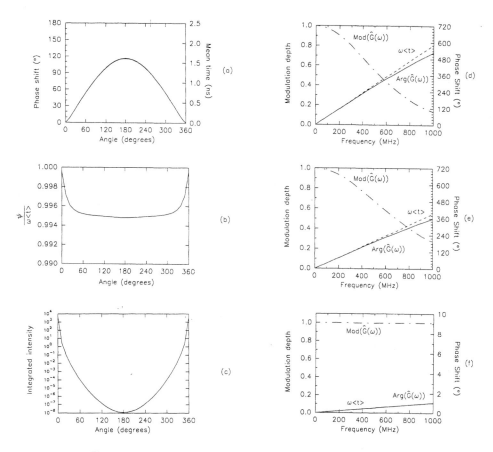

Figure 6. Results for a sphere 50 mm in diameter. (a) Phase shift ψ in degrees and mean time $\langle t \rangle$ in nanoseconds as a function of angle θ from the input position, at a modulation frequency of 200 MHz; (b) ratio of $\psi/(\omega\langle t \rangle)$ to θ; (c) integrated intensity E_0 as a function of θ; (d) ψ (solid), $\omega\langle t \rangle$ (dotted), and modulation depth M (dash-dotted) against frequency in MHz for $\theta = 180°$; (e) as (d), but for $\theta = 90°$; (f) as (d), but for $\theta = 0°$.

In quantitative tissue spectroscopy the geometric distance between the measuring optodes (the chord length in circular geometries) is used together with the DPF to quantitate the optical pathlength. It is therefore useful to examine the relationship between the predicted phase shift, mean time or modulation depth and the chord length for these differing geometries. In figure 7(a), the calculated phase shifts (at 200 MHz) for the sphere, cylinder and slab are plotted as a functions of chord length. As can be seen, there is an almost linear relationship between the two, and the differences between the results for each geometry are small. In figure 7(b) the same cases are plotted for modulation depth against chord length and the same comments apply. In figure 7(c), the DPF for each geometry is plotted as a function of chord length. Note that this DPF is calculated from $\langle t \rangle$ and therefore ignores the correction factor of 1.2% (theorem B1) that would not normally be known in a clinical measurement. This shows more clearly the predicted deviations from linearity of the relationship between mean time and the physical separation of source and detector. Its general form is similar to that predicted by Monte Carlo modelling (van der Zee *et al* 1990), the change in DPF

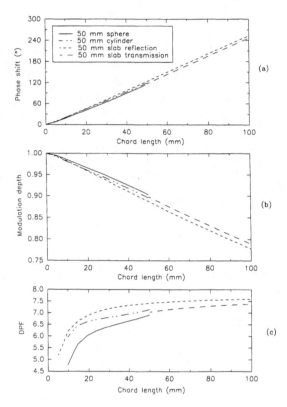

Figure 7. Comparative results for three geometries. (a) Phase shift ψ in degrees as a function of chord distance from source to boundary at 200 MHz. (b) As (a), but for modulation depth. (c) As (a), but for DPF.

being small once the chord length exceeds 25–30 mm. However, both the Monte Carlo and the diffusion equation methods incorrectly model the relationship between the DPF and chord length that has been measured experimentally (van der Zee *et al* 1992). Experimentally, the DPF measured on heads, arms and legs increases with decreasing chord length, although it is approximately constant for chord lengths greater than 3.0 cm. This indicates some inadequacies in these models which may arise from neglecting the effects of collimated sources and detectors, or the multi-layer nature of the tissues.

The experimentally derived data at 4 cm chord length (figure 1(b)) are similar to the theoretical results. The exact magnitude of the phase-shift for the experimental data at 200 MHz (89.2°) and the values from each of the theoretical cases evaluated at 4 cm chord length (slab 97.8°, circle 93.8°, sphere 90.1°) are very similar. The experimental modulation depth is 0.874, and the theoretical predictions are: slab, 0.911; circle, 0.918; and sphere, 0.926. Thus although the phase shift seems to be predicted accurately by the sphere model, the modulation depth is overestimated. To correct this overestimate would entail a broadening of the TPSF without increasing the mean time, by decreasing both scattering and absorption coefficients. Conversely, the infinite slab has predicted the modulation depth quite well but the phase-shift is about 10% too high. In theory we could vary both μ_s and μ_a in order to obtain a best fit for a particular geometry. This provides an advantage over a previously reported method (Madsen *et al* 1991) wherein the correlation of the measured and predicted TPSF was optimized, as our method does not entail either the measurement of TPSFs nor the computationally intensive calculation of the theoretical values.

Possible reasons for any differences are various. Firstly, the geometries of the systems being compared are not the same. The experimental data were obtained at an optical fibre spacing of 4 cm on a head of approximately 16 cm diameter. In addition the head is not homogeneous, with skin, muscle, skull and CSF overlying the brain. Moreover, the values of μ_a and μ_s used in the calculations were from post-mortem measurements on rat brain. In the light of these differences, the correlation between theory and experiment is remarkably good.

7. Conclusions

We have derived a theoretical explanation for the empirical result that was found in our previous study, that the mean time and DP correlate closely. This result is a consequence of the use of the homogeneous diffusion approximation, and is therefore a justification for that approximation. The correlation is independent of any frequency measurements, and it is exact except for the variation of the diffusion coefficient with μ_a. This variation must be small since this is a condition of validity of the diffusion approximation.

We have also shown that in human brain tissue, phase correlates to mean time very closely below 200 MHz. Since phase is much easier to measure at the bedside we envisage that a system measuring phase will be able to generate data that continually monitor optical pathlength, and therefore provide the required information for a modified Beer–Lambert law calculation of relative changes in chromophore concentration. The accuracy with which this method can determine absolute scattering and absorption coefficients of tissue is still uncertain because of the small geometry dependence of the relationships.

This also has an important implication for imaging systems, since we have shown, previously, both that mean-time measurements have a larger signal-to-noise ratio, and that they have better image reconstruction properties. Previous reconstructions of absorbance images have been limited by the difficulty of obtaining these mean-time data, but the analysis presented here shows that these data can be derived from a measurement of the phase shift.

Acknowledgments

This work was supported in part by the SERC, MRC, the Wellcome Trust, the Wolfson Foundation and Hamamatsu Photonics KK. SRA would like to thank R G C Arridge for discussion of the counter integrals in appendix A.

Appendix A. Derivation of the Fourier transform of a Green's function

The Fourier transform (FT) of a function $f(t)$ is defined by

$$\hat{F}(\omega) = \mathscr{F}_{t \to \omega}[f(t)] = \frac{1}{\sqrt{2\pi}} \int_{-\infty}^{\infty} f(t)\, e^{-i\omega t}\, dt \tag{A1}$$

and the inverse transform by

$$f(t) = \mathcal{F}^{-1}_{\omega \to t}[\hat{F}(\omega)] = \frac{1}{\sqrt{2\pi}} \int_{-\infty}^{\infty} \hat{F}(\omega) \, e^{i\omega t} \, dt. \tag{A2}$$

Consider the various functions $g_k^{(\Phi)}$ and $g_k^{(\Gamma)}$ derived from (11). Taking the FT of such functions is rather formidable but it can be done, by considering how they are derived from (11) in the first place, which is by a Fourier transform method. Note that

$$\mathcal{F}_{t \to \omega}[df/dt] = i\omega \hat{F}(\omega). \tag{A3}$$

We put $\Phi = g_{\text{inf}}^{(\Phi)}(r, r', t, t')$, and $q = \delta(r - r', t - t')$ in (11). Then taking the 4D FT $(t \to \omega, r \to k)$ of each side yields

$$-(k^2 \gamma^2 + \mu_a c + i\omega) \hat{G}_{\text{inf}}^{(\Phi)}(k, r', \omega, t') = e^{-i(k \cdot r' + \omega t')} \tag{A4}$$

and applying the inverse FT yields

$$g_{\text{inf}}^{(\Phi)}(r, r', t, t') = \frac{-1}{(2\pi)^4} \int d^3k \int_{-\infty}^{\infty} d\omega \, \frac{e^{i[k \cdot (r-r') + \omega(t-t')]}}{(k^2 \gamma^2 + \mu_a c + i\omega)} \tag{A5}$$

which is the Green's function for infinite space (equation (23)). Thus to obtain the time FT only, i.e.

$$\hat{G}_{\text{inf}}^{(\Phi)}(r, r', \omega, t') = \frac{1}{\sqrt{2\pi}} \int_{-\infty}^{\infty} g_{\text{inf}}^{(\Phi)}(r, r', t, t') \, e^{-i\omega t} \, dt \tag{A6}$$

we need only do the k-integration in (A5), i.e.

$$\hat{G}_{\text{inf}}^{(\Phi)}(r, r', \omega, t') = \frac{-1}{(2\pi)^{7/2}} \int d^3k \, \frac{e^{i[k \cdot (r-r') + \omega(t-t')]}}{(k^2 \gamma^2 + \mu_a c + i\omega)}. \tag{A7}$$

To do this, convert to spherical polars $(d^3k \to k^2 \sin\theta \, dk \, d\theta \, d\phi)$. The ϕ-integral is trivial and so

$$\hat{G}_{\text{inf}}^{(\Phi)}(r, r', \omega, t') = \frac{-e^{-i\omega t'}}{(2\pi)^{5/2}} \int_0^\pi \sin\theta \, d\theta \int_0^\infty k^2 \, dk \, \frac{e^{ik\rho\cos\theta}}{(k^2 \gamma^2 + \mu_a c + i\omega)} \tag{A8}$$

where $\rho = |r - r'|$, and so

$$\hat{G}_{\text{inf}}^{(\Phi)}(r, r', \omega, t') = \frac{e^{-i\omega t'}}{(2\pi)^{5/2} i\rho} \int_0^\infty k \, dk \, \frac{e^{-ik\rho} - e^{ik\rho}}{\gamma^2 (k + i\alpha_+)(k + i\alpha_-)} \tag{A9}$$

where $\alpha^2 = (\mu_a c + i\omega)/\gamma = A^2 e^{i\tau}$, with $A = [(\mu_a c)^2 + \omega^2]^{1/4}/\gamma$ and $\tan(\tau) = \omega/\mu_a c$, and we note that α^2 has two roots: $\alpha_+ = A \, e^{i\tau/2}$ or $\alpha_- = -\alpha_+ = A \, e^{i(\tau/2 + \pi)}$ (see figure A1). In equation (A9) the integrand is even, which allows us to replace the limits of integration by the range $[-\infty, \infty]$ to obtain

$$\hat{G}_{\text{inf}}^{(\Phi)}(r, r', \omega, t') = \frac{e^{-i\omega t'}}{2(2\pi)^{5/2} i\rho} \int_{-\infty}^{\infty} k \, dk \, \frac{e^{-ik\rho} - e^{ik\rho}}{\gamma^2 (k + i\alpha_+)(k + i\alpha_-)}. \tag{A10}$$

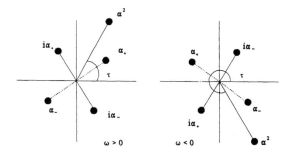

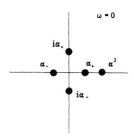

Figure A1. Location of the poles of the integrand of equation (A12) for the cases where $\omega < 0$, $\omega = 0$, and $\omega > 0$.

Furthermore the two exponential terms contribute the same amount to the integral (to see this substitute $k' = -k$); and so

$$\hat{G}_{\text{inf}}^{(\Phi)}(\mathbf{r}, \mathbf{r}', \omega, t') = \frac{e^{-i\omega t'}}{(2\pi)^{5/2} i\rho} \int_{-\infty}^{\infty} k\, dk \frac{e^{ik\rho}}{\gamma^2 (k + i\alpha_+)(k + i\alpha_-)} \tag{A11}$$

leading to

$$\hat{G}_{\text{inf}}^{(\Phi)}(\mathbf{r}, \mathbf{r}', \omega, t') = \frac{e^{-i\omega t'}}{(2\pi)^{5/2} i\rho} \int_{-\infty}^{\infty} dk \frac{e^{ik\rho}}{2\gamma^2} \left(\frac{1}{(k + i\alpha_+)} + \frac{1}{(k + i\alpha_-)} \right). \tag{A12}$$

This has two poles at $k = i\alpha_+$, and $k = i\alpha_-$. The contour is completed in the upper half-plane, so as $k \to i\infty$ the integrand goes to zero. Since the Fourier transform needs to be able to be defined for all ω we consider two cases: for $\omega > 0$ only the pole at $i\alpha_+$ contributes, and for $\omega < 0$ only the pole at $i\alpha_-$ contributes. Thus our required result is

$$\hat{G}_{\text{inf}}^{(\Phi)}(\mathbf{r}, \mathbf{r}', \omega, t') = \begin{cases} e^{-i\omega t'} e^{-\alpha_+ \rho}/[2(2\pi)^{3/2}\rho\gamma^2] & \omega > 0 \\ e^{-i\omega t'} e^{-\alpha_- \rho}/[2(2\pi)^{3/2}\rho\gamma^2] & \omega < 0 \end{cases}. \tag{A13}$$

From figure A1 we have that $\alpha_-(-\omega) = \alpha_+^*(\omega)$, where * indicates complex conjugation. Thus $\hat{G}(\mathbf{r}, \mathbf{r}', -\omega, t') = \hat{G}^*(\mathbf{r}, \mathbf{r}', \omega, t')$ as required by the properties of Fourier transforms. Further, we note that the phase of this function is just the imaginary part 'f the exponent, so

$$\psi_{\text{inf}}^{(\Phi)} = \begin{cases} -A\rho \sin[\tau(\omega)/2] & \omega > 0 \\ A\rho \sin[\tau(-\omega)/2] & \omega < 0 \end{cases} \tag{A14}$$

and therefore the formula

$$\psi_{\text{inf}}^{(\Phi)} = -[(\mu_a c)^2 + \omega^2]^{1/4}(\rho/\gamma)\sin[\tfrac{1}{2}\tan^{-1}(\omega/\mu_a c)] \tag{A15}$$

is correct for all frequencies.

Appendix B. Relationship between $\langle t \rangle$ and DP

We can use some properties of the Fourier transform to obtain some interesting results for the mean time. For any function

$$\int_{-\infty}^{\infty} g(t)\,\mathrm{d}t = \sqrt{2\pi}\,\hat{G}(\omega)\big|_{\omega=0} \tag{B1}$$

$$\frac{\partial}{\partial\omega}\hat{G}(\omega) = \frac{1}{\sqrt{2\pi}}\frac{\partial}{\partial\omega}\int_{-\infty}^{\infty} g(t)\,\mathrm{e}^{-\mathrm{i}\omega t}\,\mathrm{d}t = -\frac{\mathrm{i}}{\sqrt{2\pi}}\int_{-\infty}^{\infty} tg(t)\,\mathrm{e}^{-\mathrm{i}\omega t}\,\mathrm{d}t \tag{B2}$$

and thus

$$\langle t \rangle = \mathrm{i}[(\partial/\partial\omega)\hat{G}(\omega)]_{\omega=0}/[\hat{G}(\omega)]_{\omega=0}. \tag{B3}$$

The denominator in (B3) is just the total intensity integrated through time, E_0. We can also find an expression for the DP. In general,

$$\mathrm{DP} = -(\partial/\partial\mu_a)\ln E_0 = -(\partial/\partial\mu_a)\ln\hat{G}(\omega)\big|_{\omega=0}$$

$$= -(\partial\hat{G}(\omega)/\partial\mu_a)\big|_{\omega=0}/\hat{G}(\omega)\big|_{\omega=0}. \tag{B4}$$

The relationship of DP to mean time can be stated as follows.

Theorem (B1) For any geometry, $\mathrm{DP} = [1 + 2\mu_a\gamma(\partial/\partial\mu_a)(1/\gamma)]c\langle t \rangle$.
Proof. We rewrite the differentials in (B3) and (B4) as functions of α to obtain

$$\frac{\mathrm{DP}}{\langle t \rangle} = -\left(\frac{\partial\hat{G}(\alpha)}{\partial\mu_a}\right)_{\omega=0}\bigg/\mathrm{i}\left(\frac{\partial}{\partial\omega}\hat{G}(\alpha)\right)_{\omega=0} = \left(\frac{-\partial\alpha}{\partial\mu_a}\right)_{\omega=0}\bigg/\mathrm{i}\left(\frac{\partial\alpha}{\partial\omega}\right)_{\omega=0}. \tag{B5}$$

From the definition of α we have:

$$\partial\alpha/\partial\mu_a = c/2\gamma\alpha^2 + \gamma\alpha(\partial/\partial\mu_a)(1/\gamma) \tag{B6}$$

and

$$\partial\alpha/\partial\omega = \mathrm{i}/2\alpha\gamma^2. \tag{B7}$$

At $\omega = 0$ we have $\alpha\gamma = (\mu_a c)^{1/2}$, which gives the result as stated. $\quad\square$

This is not quite the simple result that has previously been stated, i.e. that $\partial(\text{OD})/\partial\mu_a = c\langle t \rangle$, but if plotted for the ranges of μ_a, μ_s that are relevant to tissue, it may approximate it. Notice that γ is likely to be slowly varying in the region where $\mu_s \gg \mu_a$—which is the case in most tissues—and so the second term in (B6) is almost zero. In fact, from (9) and the definition of α the expression simplifies to $[1 + \mu_a/(\mu_a + \mu_s(1 - \bar{p}))]c\langle t \rangle$, which is very close to the desired relation.

Résumé

Bases théoriques de la détermination des trajets optiques dans les tissus: analyse temporelle et fréquentielle.

Les auteurs ont mis au point une méthode théorique concise pour le calcul du temps moyen, du trajet optique différentiel, du décalage de phase, de la amplitude de modulation, et de la valeur intégrée des mesures d'intensité de lumière en fonction du temps à la surface d'un tissu, résultant soit de l'application d'impulsions lumineuses de durées de l'ordre de la picosonde, soit de lumière modulée par radiofréquence. La méthode utilise la fonction de Green établie pour l'Approximation de la diffusion de l'équation de transfert radiatif, et développe cette fonction et sa transformée de Fourier pour des géométries diverses. Des comparaisons détaillées de plusieurs de ces paramètres ont été effectuées dans diverses géométries, tenant compte de leur relation avec les données mesurées en clinique. Let limitations de l'utilisation des mesures de phase sont également discutées.

Zusammenfassung

Theoretische Grundlagen für die Bestimmung optischer Weglängen in Gewebe: Zeit- und Frequenzanalyse.

Eine geeignete Theorie wurde entwickelt für die Berechnung der mittleren Zeit, der differentiellen Weglänge, der Phasenverschiebung, der Modulationstiefe und der integralen Intensität von Messungen der Lichtstärke als Funktion der Zeit auf der Gewebeoberfläche entweder aufgrund der Einwirkung eines Picosekunden-Lichtimpulses oder aufgrund von Hochfrequenz-moduliertem Lich. Bei der theoretischen Behandlung wird die Green's Funktion der Diffusionnäherung an die radiative Transfergleichung sowie ihre Fouriertransformierte in einer Vielzahl von Geometrien verwendet. Für einige dieser Parameter und ihre Beziehung zu experimentell gemessenen klinischen Daten werden für verschiedene Geometrien detailierte Vergleiche angestellt. Die Grenzen der Anwendbarkeit von Phasenmessungen werden diskutiert.

References

Arridge S R, Cope M, van der Zee P, Hillson P J and Delpy D T 1985 Visualisation of the oxygenation state of brain and muscle in newborn infants by near infra-red transillumination *Information Processing in Medical Imaging* ed S L Bacharach (Amsterdam: Martinus Nijhoff) pp 155-176
Arridge S R, van der Zee P, Cope M and Delpy D T 1990 New results for the development of infra-red absorption imaging *Proc. SPIE* **1245** 91-103
—— 1991 Reconstruction methods for infrared absorption imaging *Proc. SPIE* **1431** 204-15
Arridge S R, van der Zee P, Delpy D T and Cope M 1992 Aspects of clinical infrared absorption imaging *The Formation, Handling, and Evaluation of Medical Images* ed A Todd Pokropek and M A Viergever, (Nato ASI Series F) (Heidelburg: Springer) pp 407-18
Berndt K W and Lakowicz J R 1991 Detection and localisation of absorbers in scattering media using frequency domain principles *Proc. SPIE* **1431** 149-58
Bolin F P, Preuss, L E, Taylor R C and Ference R 1989 Refractive index of some mammalian tissues using a fibre optic cladding method *Appl. Opt.* **28** 2297-302
Brazy J E, Lewis D V, Mitnick M H and Jöbsis van der Vliet F F 1985 Noninvasive monitoring of cerebral oxygenation in preterm infants: preliminary observations *Paediatrics* **75** 217-25
Bremmer H 1964 Random volume scattering *Radio Sci. J. Res.* **680** 967-81
Carslaw H S and Jaeger J C 1986 *Conduction of Heat in Solids* 2nd edn (Oxford: Clarendon)
Case M C and Zweifel P F 1967 *Linear Transport Theory* (New York: Addison-Wesley)
Chance B, Nioka S, Kent J, McCully K, Fountain M, Greenfield R and Holtom G 1988 Time resolved spectroscopy of haemoglobin and myoglobin in resting and ischemic muscle *Anal. Biochem.* **174** 698-707
Chance B, Maris M, Sorge J and Zhang M Z 1990 A phase modulation system for dual wavelength difference spectroscopy of haemoglobin deoxygenation in tissue *Proc. SPIE* **1204** 481-91
Chandrasekhar R 1950 *Radiation Transfer* (Oxford: Clarendon)

Cheatle T R, Potter L A, Cope M, Delpy D T, Coleridge-Smith P D and Scurr J H 1991 Near infra-red spectroscopy in peripheral vascular disease *Br. J. Surgery* **78** 405–8

Cope M 1991 The application of near infrared spectroscopy to non-invasive monitoring of cerebral oxygenation in the newborn infant *PhD Thesis* University of London

Cope M and Delpy D T 1988 System for long term measurement of cerebral blood and tissue oxygenation of newborn infants by near infrared transillumination *Med. Biol. Eng. Comput.* **26** 289–94

Delpy D T, Cope M, van der Zee P, Arridge S R, Wray S and Wyatt J 1988 Estimation of optical pathlength through tissue from direct time-of-flight measurement *Phys. Med. Biol.* **33** 1433–42

Edwards A D, Wyatt J S, Richardson C E, Delpy D T, Cope M and Reynolds E O R 1988 Cotside measurement of cerebral blood flow in ill newborn infants by near infrared spectroscopy *Lancet* **ii** 770–1

Ferrari M, Zanette E, Giannini I, Sideri G, Fieschi C and Carpi A 1986 Effects of carotid artery compression test on regional cerebral blood volume, haemoglobin oxygen saturation and cytochrome-c-oxidase redox level in cerebrovascular patients *Oxygen Transport to Tissue VIII* ed I A Longmuir (New York: Plenum) pp 213–22

Fishkin J, Gratton E, van de Ven M J and Mantulin W W 1991 Diffusion of intensity modulated near infrared light in turbid media *Proc. SPIE* **1431** 122–35

Hampson N B and Piantadosi C A 1988 Near-infrared monitoring of human skeletal muscle oxygenation during forearm ischaemia *J. Appl. Physiol.* **64** 2449–57

Hebden J C and Kruger R A 1990 Transillumination imaging performance: a time of flight imaging system *Med. Phys.* **17** 351–6

Ishimaru A 1978a *Wave Propagation and Scattering in Random Media* (New York: Academic)

—— 1978b Diffusion of a pulse in densely distributed scatterers *J. Opt. Soc. Am.* **68** 1045–50

Jackson P C, Stevens P H, Smith J H, Kear D, Key H and Wells P N T 1987 The development of a system for transillumination computed tomography *Br. J. Radiol.* **60** 375–80

Jarry G, Ghesquiere S, Maarek J M, Debray S, Bui-Mong-Hung and Laurent D 1984 Imaging mammalian tissues and organs using laser collimated transillumination *J. Biomed. Eng.* **6** 70–4

Jöbsis F F 1977 Noninvasive, infrared monitoring of cerebral and myocardial oxygen sufficiency and circulatory parameters *Science* **198** 1264–7

Lakowicz J R and Berndt K 1990 Frequency domain measurement of photon migration in tissues *Chem. Phys. Lett.* **166** 246–52

Lewis H W 1950 Multiple scattering in an infinite medium *Phys. Rev.* **78** 526–9

Madsen S J, Patterson M S, Wilson B C, Park Y D, Moulton J D, Jacques S L, and Hefetz Y 1991 Time resolved diffuse reflectance and transmittance studies in tissue simulating phantoms: a comparison between theory and experiment *Proc. SPIE* **1431** 42–51

Oda I, Ito Y, Eda H, Tamura T, Takada M, Abumi R, Nagai K, Nakagawa K, and Tamura M 1991 Non-invasive haemoglobin oxygenation monitor and computed tomography by NIR spectrophotometry *Proc. SPIE* **1431** 284–93

Patterson M S, Chance B and Wilson B C 1989 Time resolved reflectance and transmittance for the non invasive measurement of tissue optical properties *Appl. Opt.* **28** 2331–6

Patterson M S, Moulton J D, Wilson B C and Chance B 1990 Applications of time resolved light scattering measurements to photodynamic therapy dosimetry *Proc. SPIE* **1203** 62–75

Sevick E M and Chance B 1991 Photon migration in a model of the head measured using time and frequency domain techniques: potentials of spectroscopy and imaging *Proc. SPIE* **1431** 84–96

Star W M 1989 Comparing the P3-approximation with the diffusion theory and with Monte Carlo calculations of light propagation in a slab geometry (dosimetry of laser radiation in medicine and biology) *Proc. SPIE* **1035** 146–54

Tamura M, Nomura Y and Hazeki O 1987 Laser tissue spectroscopy—near infrared CT *Rev. Laser Eng.* (*Japan*) **15** 74–82

van der Hulst H C 1980 *Multiple Light Scattering* (New York: Academic)

van der Zee P, Arridge S R, Cope M and Delpy D T 1990 The effect of optode positioning on optical pathlength in near infrared spectsocopy of brain *Adv. Exp. Med. Biol.* **277** 79–84

van der Zee P, Cope M, Arridge S R, Essenpreis M, Potter L A, Edwards A D, Wyatt J S, McCormick D C, Roth S C, Reynolds E O R and Delpy D T 1992 Experimentally measured pathlength for the adult head, calf and forearm and the head of the newborn infants as a function of inter optode spacing *Adv. Exp. Med. Biol.* at press

van der Zee P, Essenpreis M, Delpy D T and Cope M 1991 Accurate determination of the optical properties of biological tissues using a Monte Carlo inversion technique *Proc. ICO Mg on Atmospheric, Volume and Surface Scattering and Propagation* pp 125–8

Wang L, Liu Y, Ho P P and Alfano R R 1991 Ballistic imaging of biomedical samples using picosecond optical Kerr gate *Proc. SPIE* **1431** 97–101

272

Watson G N 1944 *A Treatise on the Theory of Bessel Functions* (Cambridge: Cambridge University Press)

Wolfram S 1991 *Mathematica: a system for Doing Mathematics by Computer* 2nd ed (Redwood, NJ: Addison-Wesley)

Wray S, Cope M, Delpy D T, Wyatt J S and Reynolds E O R 1988 Characterisation of the near infrared absorption spectra of cytochrome aa_3 and haemoglobin for the non-invasive monitoring of cerebral oxygenation *Biochim. Biophys. Acta* **933** 184-92

Wyatt J S, Cope M, Delpy D T, van der Zee P, Arridge S R, Edwards A D and Reynolds E O R 1990 Measurement of optical pathlength for cerebral near infrared spectroscopy in newborn infants *Dev. Neurosc.* **12** 140-4

Wyatt J S, Cope M, Delpy D T, Wray S and Reynolds E O R 1986 Quantitation of cerebral oxygenation and haemodynamics in sick newborn infants by near infrared spectroscopy *Lancet* **ii** 1063-6

Reprinted from *Optical Methods of Biomedical Diagnostics and Therapy,* Proc. SPIE
Vol. 1981, pp. 101-107 (1992). ©1992 SPIE.

Frequency domain measurements of tissue optical parameters:
A theoretical analysis

I. V. Yaroslavsky and V. V. Tuchin

Saratov University, Saratov 410071, Russia

ABSTRACT

A theoretical aspect of frequency domain measurements of tissue optical parameters is considered. In the framework of radiative transfer theory the expressions have been obtained, which describe dependence of modulation M and phase shift $\Delta\Theta$ of scattered radiation on frequency. As an example, the results of processing of experimental data are presented.

1. INTRODUCTION

Determination of tissues optical parameters is an important item both of planning of laser treatment and of diagnostics, based on differences in optical properties of pathological and healthy tissues[1]. Recently, time dependent methods of spectroscopy of turbid media attract attention of many researchers[3-10], particularly as a tool for *in vivo* applications.

Description of the propagation of short laser pulses in tissues with multiple scattering in the framework of rigorous Maxwell's theory meets serious mathematical difficulties[2]. For this reason, the radiative transfer theory (RTT) is widely used. In many cases diffusion approximation of RRT can be applied[2,4-8]. Thus, Patterson et al.[6-8] have obtained the expressions, allowing to calculate the optical parameters of scattering tissues from measurements of time profile of pulses of diffusely scattered light. Good agreement of their theory with experimental data has been reported[6-8]. On the other hand, recently the method of frequency domain measurements has been suggested[9,10] for investigation of photon migration in scattering media. The results of measurements in frequency domain seem to be more convenient for interpretation and can be obtained, using less sophistical apparatus, than ones in time domain[9].

Based on time dependent RTT, we have derived the equations, which describe dependence of modulation coefficient and phase shift of output signal on frequency for the case, when initial radiation is sinusoidally modulated. That allows to calculate the optical parameters of tissues, using frequency domain measurements and least squares method for fitting of experimental data.

2. DEDUCTION OF THE EQUATIONS

Let us separate in time dependent case the radiance $I(\mathbf{r}, \mathbf{s}, t)$ into diffuse component I_d and attenuated incident component I_{ri}:

$$I = I_d + I_{ri}; \quad I_d = I_d(\mathbf{r}, \mathbf{s}, t); \quad I_{ri} = I_{ri}(\mathbf{r}, \mathbf{s}, t),$$

where $\mathbf{r}$ - point vector, $\mathbf{s}$ - unit vector of direction, t - time.

The basis equations of RTT look like[11]:

$$\frac{s\nabla I_d}{k_t} + t_2 \frac{\partial I_d}{\partial t} = -I_d + \frac{\Lambda}{4\pi} \int\limits_{4\pi} \left[\int\limits_{-\infty}^{t} I_d(\mathbf{r}, \mathbf{s}', t') \exp\left(-\frac{t-t'}{t_1}\right) \frac{dt'}{t_1} \right] p(\mathbf{s}, \mathbf{s}') dw' +$$

$$+ \frac{\Lambda}{4\pi} \int\limits_{4\pi} \left[\int\limits_{-\infty}^{t} I_{ri}(\mathbf{r}, \mathbf{s}', t') \exp\left(-\frac{t-t'}{t_1}\right) \frac{dt'}{t_1} \right] p(\mathbf{s}, \mathbf{s}') dw', \qquad (1)$$

$$\frac{s\nabla I_{ri}}{k_t} + t_2 \frac{\partial I_{ri}}{\partial t} = -I_{ri}, \qquad (2)$$

where $k_t = k_a + k_s$ – extinction coefficient, k_a – absorption coefficient, k_s – scattering coefficient, t_1 – lifetime of photon in absorbed state, $t_2 = n/ck_t$ – time of flight of photon between two interaction sites, n – refractive index of tissues, c – light velocity in vacuum, $\Lambda = k_s/k_t$ – albedo of single scattering, $p(\mathbf{s}, \mathbf{s}')$ – scattering phase function.

The boundary conditions can be written as[13]:

$$I_d(\mathbf{r}, \mathbf{s}, t) \Big|_{(\mathbf{sn})<0} = \hat{R} I_d(\mathbf{r}, \mathbf{s}, t) \Big|_{(\mathbf{sn})>0}, \qquad (1')$$

$$I_{ri}(\mathbf{r}, \mathbf{s}, t) \Big|_{(\mathbf{sn})<0} = q(\mathbf{r}, \mathbf{s}, t) + \hat{R} I_{ri}(\mathbf{r}, \mathbf{s}, t) \Big|_{(\mathbf{sn})>0}, \qquad (2')$$

where $\mathbf{n}$ – external normal to medium surface, $q(\mathbf{r}, \mathbf{s}, t)$ – surface distribution of incident radiation, R – operator of reflection on the boundary.

Consider half-infinite medium ($z \geq 0$), illuminated by the source of sinusoidally modulated radiation:

$$q = q_0(1 + \text{Re}(m_0 \exp(i\omega t))), \qquad (3)$$

where $q_0 = q_0(\bar{\rho}, \mathbf{s})$, $\bar{\rho} = ix + jy$, m_0 and $\omega = 2\pi f$ – coefficient and frequency of modulation, respectively. It is naturally to find solution of the problem (1),(1') in the form:

$$I_d = I_{d0}(\mathbf{r}, \mathbf{s}) + \text{Re}(C(\mathbf{r}, \mathbf{s}) \exp(i\omega t)), \qquad (4)$$

where I_{d0} satisfies the time independent transfer equation. Substituting eq. 4 into Eq. 1 and having straightforward solution of the problem (2),(2'), we obtain:

$$\frac{s}{k_t} \nabla C + i t_2 \omega C = -C + \frac{\Lambda}{4\pi} \int\limits_{4\pi} \frac{C(\mathbf{r}, \mathbf{s})}{1 + i\omega t_1} p(\mathbf{s}, \mathbf{s}') dw' +$$

$$+ \frac{\Lambda}{4\pi} \int\limits_{4\pi} m_0 q_0(\bar{\rho}', \mathbf{s}') p(\mathbf{s}, \mathbf{s}') \frac{\exp((k_t z(1 + i t_2 \omega))/\cos\theta)}{1 + i\omega t_1} dw', \qquad (5)$$

where $\bar{\rho}' = ix' + jy'$,

$x = x + z \, tg\theta \cos\psi$, $y' = y + z \, tg\theta \sin\psi$,

θ – polar angle, ψ – azimuthal angle in the plane (x, y).

Thus, the problem of transfer of modulated laser light is reduced to time independent transfer problem in the medium with complex optical parameters:

$$k_s^* = \frac{k_s}{1 + it_1\omega}, \qquad k_a^* = (k_a + k_s)(1 + it_2\omega) - k_s^* \tag{6}$$

Further, we assume that angular distribution of time dependent and time independent parts of diffuse radiation coincide, i.e.:

$$C(\mathbf{r}, \mathbf{s}) = m_d(\mathbf{r}) I_{d0}(\mathbf{r}, \mathbf{s}) \tag{7}$$

This assumption is much more weak, than usually used diffusion approximation.

Consider detector, placed in the area, where attenuated incident radiance I_{ri} is equal to zero. For example, this situation is realized, if detector is placed on the surface of tissue ($z=0$) out of initial beam. Then substituting Eq.7 into Eq.5, we obtain the following equation for m_d:

$$\frac{s}{k_t}(I_{d0}\nabla m_d + m_d \nabla I_{d0}) + (1 + it_2\omega)m_d I_{d0} =$$

$$= \frac{\Lambda m_d}{4\pi(1 + it_1\omega)} \int_{4\pi} I_{d0}(\mathbf{r}, \mathbf{s}') p(\mathbf{s}, \mathbf{s}') dw' \tag{8}$$

Let us define k_m as:

$$k_m = m_d(\mathbf{r})/m_0 \tag{9}$$

Substituting Eq.9 into Eq.8, we derive equation for k_m, which can be solved by the method of characteristics:

$$M = |k_m| = \exp\left(-\frac{H_\tau \omega^2 t_1^2}{1 + t_1^2 \omega^2}\right), \tag{10}$$

$$\Delta\Phi = |\varphi_{k_m}| = \omega\left(\frac{H_\tau t_1}{1 + t_1^2 \omega^2} + t_\tau\right), \tag{11}$$

where $H_\tau = \tau k_s$, $t_\tau = \tau n/c$. Parameter τ can be considered as mean path length of photons in tissue, depending on geometry of experiment.

Eq.10,11 describe dependence of modulation coefficient and of phase shift of scattered laser light on modulation frequency.

3. PROCESSING OF EXPERIMENTAL DATA

We have performed processing of the results of frequency domain measurements, reported in [9,10], using the least squares method.

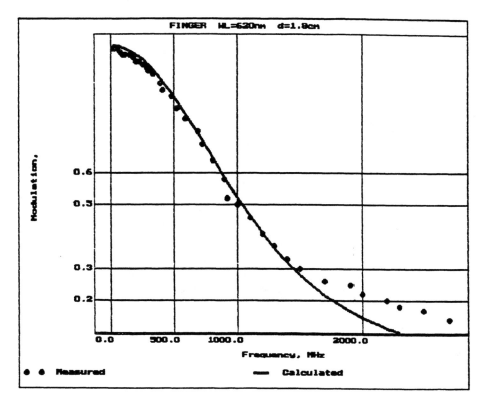

A

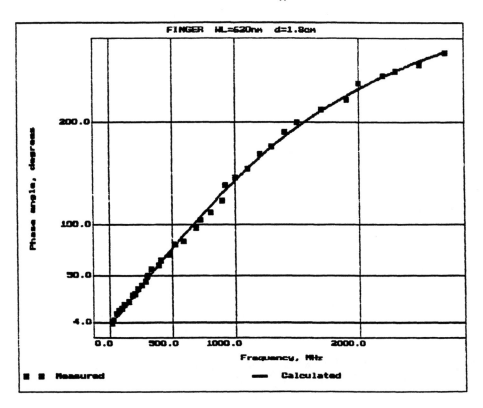

B

Results of experimental data fitting for measurements performed on finger.
Wavelength 620 nm, distance between fiber tips 1.8 cm.

A - modulation coefficient   B - phase shift

The Fig. A and B present the experimental data[9,10] and fitting curves for experiments, which have been done on human finger *in vivo*. We assumed that refractive index of tissue was equal to 1,5. Scattering coefficient k_s, life time t_1 and mean path length τ have been calculated. We have obtained the following meanings: $k_s = 2,49$ cm^{-1}, $t_1 = 5,76 \cdot 10^{-11}$ sec, $\tau = 2,23$ cm. Calculated value of k_s is significantly lower than typical values of k_s for tissues, reported by other investigators[12]. The explanations of this fact can be following: 1) Insufficient accuracy of input data scanning , 2) Influence of attenuated incident radiation reflected from boundaries inside tissue, and 3) Presence of optical unhomogeneties inside tissue. It is clear that more experiments are required for reliable confirmation of Eq. 10,11.

4. CONCLUSION

Presented here method of determination of tissue optical parameters is based directly on time dependent RTT. Assumption on angular structure of scattered light (See Eq. 7) can be still valid even in the cases, when diffusion approximation cannot be used.

Suggested method allows, in principle, to determine life time t_1 that may yield valuable diagnostic information on tissue. On the other hand, mean path length τ is dependent on absorption coefficient k_a, so the meaning of this coefficient can be calculated from frequency domain measurements, using further analysis in the framework of RTT and taking into account the geometry of experiment.

5. REFERENCES:

1. B. C. Wilson, M. S. Patterson, S. T. Flock *Photochem. Photobiol.* vol. 46, N 5. pp. 601-608, 1987.
2. A. Ishimaru *Wave propagation and scattering in random media*, Academic Press, NY, 1978.
3. B. Chance *Optical Method Annu. Rev. Biophys. Biophys. Chem.*, vol. 20, pp. 1-28, 1991.
4. E. M. Sevick, B. Chance, J. Leigh et al., "Quantitation of time-and frequency-resolved optical spectra for determination of tissue oxygenation", *Anal. Biochem*, vol. 195. pp. 330-351, 1991.
5. K. M. Yoo, Feng Liu, and R. R. Alfano, "Photon migration in random media: angle and time resolved studies", *Proc. SPIE*, vol. 1204. pp. 492-497, 1990.
6. S. J. Madsen, M. S. Patterson, B. S. Wilson et al., "Time resolved diffuse reflectance and transmittance studies in tissue simulating phantoms: a comparison between theory and experiment", *Proc. SPIE*, vol. 1431-06, 1991. 7. S. R. Arridge, P. van der Zee, M. Cope, D. T. Delpy, "Reconstruction methods for infra-red absorption unaging", *Proc. SPIE*, vol. 1431-23, 1991.
8. M. S. Patterson, B. Chance, B. C. Wilson, "Time-resolved reflectance and transmittance for the noneinvasive measurement of tissue optical properties", *Appl. Opt.*, vol. 28, pp. 2331-2336, 1989.
9. J. R. Lakowicz, K. W. Berndt, "Frequency-domain measurements of photon migration in tissues", Chem. Phys. Lett., vol. 166, pp. 246-252, 1990.
10. J. R. Lakowicz, K. W. Berndt, M. L. Johnson, "Photon migration in scattering media and tissue", *Proc. SPIE*, vol. 1204, pp. 468-480, 1990.
11. I. N. Minin, *Theory of radiative transfer in planetary atmospheres*, Nauka, Moscow, 1988. (in Russ.)
12. M. J. C. van Gemert, S. L. Jacques, H. J. C. M. Sterenborg, and W. M. Star, "Skin Optics", IEEE Biomedical Engineering, vol. 36, pp. 1146-1154, 1989.
13. T. A. Germogenova, *Local properties of transfer equation solutions*. Nauka, Moscow, 1986 (in Russ.)

Reprinted with permission from *Physical Review Letters,* Vol. 69(18), pp. 2658-2661
(November 2, 1992). ©1992 American Physical Society.

Refraction of Diffuse Photon Density Waves

M. A. O'Leary, [1],[2] D. A. Boas, [1],[2] B. Chance, [2] and A. G. Yodh [1]

[1]*Department of Physics, University of Pennsylvania, Philadelphia, Pennsylvania 19104-6396*

[2]*Department of Biochemistry and Biophysics, University of Pennsylvania, Philadelphia, Pennsylvania 19104-6089*

(Received 10 August 1992)

Experiments are performed which illustrate the properties of damped traveling waves in diffusive media. Our observations demonstrate the manipulation of these waves by adjustment of the photon diffusion coefficients of adjacent turbid media. The waves are imaged, and are shown to obey simple relations such as Snell's law. The extent to which analogies from physical optics may be used to understand these waves is further explored, and the implications for medical imaging are briefly discussed.

The correlation and transport properties of diffuse light have been the subject of intense recent interest [1]. A practical aspect of these problems concerns the potential uses of diffuse light to locate objects embedded within turbid media [2]. By turbid media, we mean any medium in which the transport of light energy density, $U(\mathbf{r},t)$, is governed by the diffusion equation [3], $\partial U/\partial t = D\nabla^2 U$. To this end a variety of probes, including amplitude modulated (AM) continuous-wave laser sources [4], have been employed to study the effects of inhomogeneities on optical path lengths in model biological systems. Interestingly, insertion of the AM light source into any optically dense random medium is accompanied by the generation of a small but measurable traveling wave disturbance of the light energy density which we will hereafter refer to as a *diffuse photon density wave.*

Diffuse photon density waves are scalar, damped, traveling waves. These highly damped traveling waves arise formally in *any* diffusive system that is driven by an oscillating source [5]. Recently the problem has been discussed within the context of diffuse photon transport [6–8]. Fishkin and Gratton, for example [8], have calculated the light energy density, $U(\mathbf{r},t)$, within an optically dense homogeneous media in the presence of a modulated point light source at the origin. They then used the result and the principle of superposition to derive the light energy density in the presence of an absorbing semi-infinite plane. The oscillatory part of the solution for an *infinite,* homogeneous, nonabsorbing dense random media is [6,8]

$$U_{\text{ac}}(\mathbf{r},t) = (A/Dr)\exp\{-k\cos\varphi r\}$$
$$\times \exp\{ik\sin\varphi r - i\omega t\}, \qquad (1)$$

where A is a constant, $D = \frac{1}{3}(c/n)l^*$ is the diffusion coefficient for light in the media, l^* is the photon transport mean free path in the medium, c/n is the speed of light in the medium, ω is the source modulation frequency, and in the absence of absorption [9] $\varphi = \pi/4$ and $k = (\omega/D)^{1/2}$. Although the wave is very rapidly attenuated, it has a well-defined wavelength, amplitude, and phase at all points. Qualitatively, this wavelength corresponds to the root-mean-square displacement experienced by a typical photon during a single modulation period. It can be altered by modifying D or ω.

In this paper we inquire further into the basic properties of these waves. We present experimental observations of circular wave fronts and we examine how these wave fronts propagate from one semi-infinite turbid media to another. Our results *experimentally* demonstrate that a "diffusional index of refraction" is a useful concept for these waves, and that it is possible to manipulate them by controlling the *photon diffusion coefficients* (D) of adjacent turbid media. This may be of considerable importance in biological systems, where the natural curvature of organs such as the brain, heart, or kidney, together with changes of scattering and absorption as in the grey-white matter transition of the brain, can lead to significant modifications of the trajectories of diffuse photons. While the potential for focusing has been noted qualitatively in one early paper [6], to our knowledge the present observations are the first documented experiments of refraction phenomena in a diffusive system. We also discuss briefly the extent to which simple ideas from physical optics, such as Huygen's principle, might be adapted to better understand phase images that can be formed using these waves.

The experimental apparatus is depicted in Fig. 1. The dense random medium we used was a liquid called Intralipid [10]. Intralipid is a polydisperse suspension of particles with an average diameter of ~ 0.4 μm, but a relatively wide range of sizes (i.e., from ~ 0.1 to ~ 1.1 μm). By changing the solution concentration we were able to vary the light diffusion coefficient of the medium. The photon transport mean free path l^* was about 0.2 cm in a 0.5% concentrated solution. Typically we filled a large fish tank (30 cm × 30 cm × 60 cm) with Intralipid. We performed experiments in three geometries. In the first case there was no partition and the sample was homogeneous. In the other two cases, a plane or cylindrical acrylic partition separated two solutions with different concentrations. In our experiments the absorption is very small, the suspensions are dilute, and therefore the diffusion coefficient is inversely proportional to the Intralipid concentration.

Source and detector optical fibers (~ 4 mm in diameter) were immersed in the solution at the same height

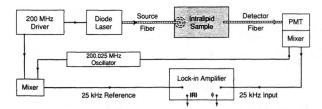

FIG. 1. A known concentration of Intralipid sample fills a glass fish tank. Our source is a diode laser that is amplitude modulated by a 200-MHz driver. Light is delivered into the sample through a source fiber, and picked up by a movable detector fiber. The fibers are pointed in orthogonal directions to minimize gradient systematics. The signal at the photomultiplier tube (PMT) is down-converted to 25 kHz (by modulating a PMT dynode at 200.025 MHz), and then fed into a lock-in amplifier. The 25-kHz lock-in reference signal is derived from the 200-MHz driver by standard mixing techniques. The two-phase lock-in provides amplitude ($|\mathbf{R}|$), and phase (ϕ) output signals.

above the tank floor. The source light was derived from a 3-mW diode laser operating at 816 nm. The diode laser was amplitude modulated at 200 MHz, and the source fiber position was fixed. The detector fiber could be positioned anywhere in the plane, and was connected to a photomultiplier tube on its other end. In order to facilitate the phase and amplitude measurements, both the reference signal from the source and the detected signal were down-converted to 25 kHz by heterodyning with a second oscillator at 200.025 MHz. The low-frequency signals were then measured using a lock-in amplifier. The phase shift (and ac amplitude) of the detected light was measured with respect to the source at each point on a 0.5-cm square planar grid throughout the sample. Constant phase contours were easily determined by linear interpolation of the grid data. The sensitivity of our current apparatus is about 10^5. Since the signal amplitude decays by $> e^{-2\pi}$ in one wavelength, the range of our experiments is limited to slightly more than one wavelength. Nevertheless, it is possible to clearly distinguish the essential physical phenomena in the present experiments.

Our results for the $\sim 0.5\%$ concentrated homogeneous media are exhibited in Fig. 2. Constant phase contours are shown at 20° intervals about the source in Fig. 2. Notice that the contours are circular, and that their radii can be extrapolated back to the source. In the inset of Fig. 2 we plot the phase shift and the quantity $\ln|rU_{ac}(\mathbf{r},t)|$ as a function of radial distance from the source. From these measurements we deduce the wavelength of the diffuse photon density wave (11.2 cm), as well as the photon transport mean free path (~ 0.2 cm), and the photon absorption length (~ 52 cm) [9] in $\sim 0.5\%$ Intralipid at 22 °C. The photon absorption can be attributed almost entirely to water [11].

In Fig. 3 we demonstrate the refraction of these waves

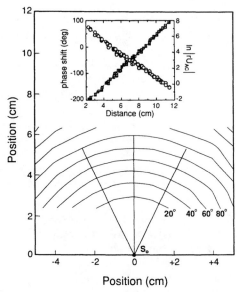

FIG. 2. Constant phase contours shown as a function of position for homogeneous, 0.5% Intralipid solution. The contours are shown in 20° intervals. Inset: The measured phase shift (circles) and $\ln|rU_{ac}(\mathbf{r},t)|$ (squares) are plotted as a function of radial distance from the source S_o.

in three ways. Figure 3 shows constant phase contours (every 20°). This time, however, a plane boundary is introduced separating the lower medium with concentration $c_l \approx 1.0\%$ and light diffusion coefficient D_l from the upper medium with concentration $c_u \approx 0.25\%$ and light diffusion coefficient D_u. The contours below the boundary are just the homogeneous media contours (without

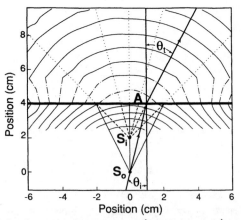

FIG. 3. Constant phase contours (in 20° intervals) as a function of position showing the propagation of a diffuse photon density wave across a planar boundary that separates 1% concentrated Intralipid from 0.25% Intralipid. See text for detailed discussion. S_o, source position; S_i, apparent source position; A, point on boundary; θ_i, angle of incident ray; θ_t, angle of refracted ray. The solid lines are obtained directly from data. The dot-dashed lines are obtained by interpolation over large distances, and are drawn to show the irregularities at large angles.

reflection); they are obtained *before* the partition is introduced into the sample. The contours above the boundary are derived from the diffuse photon density waves transmitted into the less concentrated medium. As a result of our detector geometry, our closest approach to the partition was about 1 cm. We expect a number of general results. First, the wavelength in the less dense medium ($\lambda_u = 14.8$ cm) should be greater than the wavelength of the diffuse photon density wave in the incident medium ($\lambda_l = 8.17$ cm). This was observed. The ratio of the two wavelengths should equal the ratio of the diffusional indices of refraction of the two media. Specifically we found, as expected, that $\lambda_u = \lambda_l (D_l/D_u)^{-1/2} \sim \lambda_l (c_l/c_u)^{1/2}$. Furthermore, we would expect that the apparent source position (S_i), *as viewed from within the upper medium*, should be shifted from the real source position ($S_o = 4.0 \pm 0.2$ cm) by a factor $\lambda_l/\lambda_u = 0.55$. Within the accuracy of this measurement this is what we find. Using the radii from the full contour plots we see that the apparent source position is shifted from 4.0 ± 0.2 to 2.0 ± 0.25 cm.

Finally in Fig. 3 we explicitly demonstrate Snell's law for diffuse photon density waves. This can be seen by following the ray from S_o to the point A at the boundary, and then into the upper medium. The ray in the lower medium makes an angle $\theta_i = 14°$ with respect to the surface normal. The upper ray is constructed in the standard way between the apparent source position S_i, through the point A on the boundary, and into the medium above the boundary [12]. It is perpendicular to the circular wave fronts in the less dense medium, and makes an angle $\theta_t = 26.6°$ with respect to the boundary normal. Within the accuracy of the experiment we see that $\sin\theta_i/\sin\theta_t = 0.54 \approx \lambda_l/\lambda_u$, so that Snell's law accurately describes the propagation of diffuse photon density waves across the boundary. It is interesting to note that the wave fronts become quite distorted when the source ray angle exceeds $\sim 30°$. These irregularities are a consequence of total internal reflection, diffraction, and some spurious boundary effects. We will discuss the phenomena in greater detail in a future paper.

A third important observation we make in this work is presented in Fig. 4. Here we use a circular boundary separating two turbid media to demonstrate that we can alter the curvature of the diffuse photon density wave fronts in analogy with a simple lens in optics. Again two semi-infinite media are separated by a boundary. This time the medium on the right is more concentrated. The constant phase contours of the transmitted wave exhibit a shorter wavelength, and are clearly converging toward some image point to the right of the boundary. The medium on the left (λ_l) has an Intralipid concentration of $\sim 0.1\%$, and the medium on the right (λ_r) has a concentration of $\sim 1.6\%$, and the wavelength ratio was measured to be $\lambda_r/\lambda_l = 3.8 \pm 0.3$. The curved surface has a radius $R = 9.0 \pm 0.4$ cm. The object position (the source) is $S_o = 9.4 \pm 0.3$ cm. The image position was determined

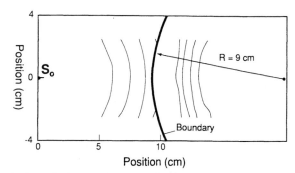

FIG. 4. Refraction by a spherical surface. A curved boundary separates two media of different concentration, and modifies the curvature of an incident diffuse photon density wave. The constant phase contours on the left occur in 20° intervals, and the constant phase contours on the right occur in 40° intervals. The reversal of wave-front curvature is evident.

to be $S_i = 12 \pm 2$ cm. This result deviates somewhat from the well-known paraxial result from geometrical optics for imaging by a spherical refracting surface [12]. The deviation is primarily a result of spherical aberration [12]. The central point remains, however; that is, the curvature of the wave fronts is reversed after traversing the circular boundary.

The experiments depicted in Figs. 2, 3, and 4 indicate that it is possible to exert substantial control over the transport of diffuse light in dense random media. We have clearly demonstrated that the index of refraction of these waves depends on the photon diffusion coefficient or random walk step in these media. Further work remains, not only with regard to analogous optical effects and quantitation, but towards utilizing these waves to image inhomogeneities within turbid media. Work along these lines is under way in our laboratories. Presently, however, we comment on some important ideas from optics that may be of use in considering the scattering and propagation of these waves. In the following discussion we will *ignore the effects of absorption*, and we will assume that the time it takes for light to travel a single random walk step is much shorter than the modulation period as in these studies.

In deriving Eq. (1) from the differential form of Fick's law and photon flux conservation, one finds that the oscillatory part of the light energy density $U_\omega(\mathbf{r})$ obeys the Helmholtz equation, i.e., $(\nabla^2 + k^2)U_\omega(\mathbf{r}) = 0$. The only significant difference in comparison to conventional wave phenomena is that $k^2 = i(\omega/D)$, and therefore k is complex. The spatial part of $U_{ac}(\mathbf{r}, t)$ in Eq. (1) is simply the Green's function solution of the Helmholtz equation with the appropriate k. These similarities suggest that some basic theorems that apply to solutions of the Helmholtz equation will apply to these diffuse photon density waves. For example, one can construct a Kirchhoff integral for these waves [13], using the Green's-function solution. This provides a formal apparatus by which to calculate the wave amplitude and phase at various distances from a "diffracting" aperture. To the extent that the Kirchhoff integral embodies the basic Huygens-Fresnel principle we may envision the contributions of different elements of a scattering surface as arising from *damped*, spherical point sources. This also implies that the focusing of diffuse photon density waves will have the same limitations due to diffraction as in the case of light.

With further improvements in the signal-to-noise ratio we should be able to increase the range of our measurements to several wavelengths. Unfortunately, we still will not be able to take advantage of many of the far-field results often used in optics. Nevertheless, the near-field form of the solution provides a framework by which we can understand the phase and amplitude images formed by scatterers in dense random media. In practical biomedical scenarios we will be looking for distortions of these wave fronts as a result of absorptive and dispersive inhomogeneities within objects such as the human breast. Since the radius of the human breast is reachable within a range of one wavelength, imaging of small breast tumors appears to be feasible. In the present paper we have taken a first step towards this goal by discerning structure within a two-component sample.

We are happy to acknowledge useful conversations with Peter Kaplan, Charles Kane, Tom Lubensky, Michael Cohen, and Dinos Gonatas, as well as the technical assistance of Jian Weng. A.G.Y. gratefully acknowledges partial support from the National Science Foundation through the Presidential Young Investigator program and Grant No. DMR-9003687, and from the Alfred P. Sloan Foundation. B.C. gratefully acknowledges support from HL-44125, ACSBE-B, NS-27346, and Hamamatsu Photonics.

---

[1] See, for example, S. John, Phys. Today **44**, No. 5, 32 (1991); S. Feng and P. A. Lee, Science **251**, 633 (1991); D. J. Durian, D. A. Weitz, and D. J. Pine, Science **252**, 686 (1991), and references therein.

[2] See, for example, imaging overviews in *Future Trends in Biomedical Applications of Lasers*, SPIE Proceedings Vol. 1525 (SPIE–International Society for Optical Engineering, Bellingham, WA, 1991).

[3] A. Ishimaru, *Wave Propagation and Scattering in Random Media* (Academic, New York, 1978), Vol. 1.

[4] See, for example, B. J. Tromberg, L. O. Svaasand, T. Tsay, R. C. Haskell, and M. W. Berns, in *Future Trends in Biomedical Applications of Lasers* (Ref. [2]), p. 52, and references therein.

[5] For an interesting example of a diffusion wave in the context of heat conduction, see A. Sommerfeld, *Partial Differential Equations in Physics* (Academic, New York, 1949), p. 68.

[6] E. Gratton, W. Mantulin, M. J. van de Ven, J. Fishkin, M. Maris, and B. Chance, in *Proceedings of the Third International Conference: Peace through Mind/Brain Science, 1990* (Hamamatsu Photonics KK, Hamamatsu, 1990), p. 183.

[7] A. Knuttel, J. M. Schmidt, and J. R. Knudsen, Appl. Opt. (to be published).

[8] J. Fishkin and E. Gratton, J. Opt. Soc. Am. A (to be published).

[9] For a medium characterized by absorption length l_a, $\tan 2\varphi = (\omega l_a)n/c$. Absorptive corrections to k and D are small for the samples we consider, and can be found in [6,8].

[10] The Intralipid used here can be obtained from Kabi Pharmacia in Clayton, North Carolina.

[11] C. M. Hale and M. R. Querry, Appl. Opt. **12**, 555 (1973).

[12] E. Hecht, *Optics* (Addison-Wesley, Reading, MA, 1987), Chaps. 4–6.

[13] M. Born and E. Wolf, *Principles of Optics* (Pergamon, New York, 1980), Chap. 8.

Reprinted from *Journal of the Optical Society of America A*, Vol. 9(10), pp. 1832-1843
(October 1992).

Interference of diffusive light waves

J. M. Schmitt

*Biomedical Engineering and Instrumentation Program, National Center for Research Resources,
National Institutes of Health, Bethesda, Maryland 20892*

A. Knüttel

*Laboratory of Cardiac Energetics, National Heart, Lung, and Blood Institute, National Institutes of Health,
Bethesda, Maryland 20892*

J. R. Knutson

*Laboratory of Cellular Biology, National Heart, Lung, and Blood Institute, National Institutes of Health,
Bethesda, Maryland 20892*

Received December 6, 1991; revised manuscript received April 21, 1992; accepted May 6, 1992

We examine interference effects resulting from the superposition of photon-density waves produced by coherently modulated light incident upon a turbid medium. Photon-diffusion theory is used to derive expressions for the ac magnitude and phase of the aggregate diffusive wave produced in full- and half-space volumes by two sources. Using a frequency-domain spectrometer operating at 410 MHz, we verify interference patterns predicted by the model in scattering samples having optical properties similar to those of skin tissue. Potential imaging applications of interfering diffusive waves are discussed in the context of the theoretical and experimental results.

1. INTRODUCTION

Since the early 1960's the photon-diffusion model has been used widely to describe light propagation in biological tissues[1,2] and other turbid media.[3] New frequency- and time-domain methods[4–7] for probing the optical properties of turbid materials have stimulated renewed interest in photon diffusion. Recently several investigators demonstrated that a high-frequency, sinusoidally modulated light wave travels in a homogeneous turbid medium at a reduced speed while maintaining a spatially coherent wave front.[8] Coherent propagation of the wave front does not require coherence at optical frequencies. Depending on the absorption and scattering properties of the medium, the wavelength of a diffusely propagating wave can be many times smaller than its free-space wavelength. The wave's amplitude, however, diminishes rapidly with distance away from the source, especially in a medium in which both absorption and scattering are high.

In an earlier experimental study[9] we demonstrated that diffusive photon-density waves can interfere and that, if the sources and detectors are properly configured, this interference permits localization of an absorbing object in a turbid medium. Various ways of exploiting interfering diffusive waves for imaging embedded objects have been proposed.[10] Other investigators have also considered the possibility of diffusive optical imaging based on frequency-domain methods.[11]

In this paper we consider some theoretical aspects of diffusive-light-wave interference. Using a simple photon-diffusion model to determine the complex amplitude of the photon density at points in the illuminated volume, we examine the conditions required for two or more diffusive

waves propagating in a homogeneous random medium to interfere constructively or destructively. Wave interference in regions predicted by the model was verified experimentally by using a phantom with optical properties similar to those of skin tissue.

2. THEORY

A. Single-Point Source in a Full-Space (Unbounded) Region

Consider a single-point source of light in a volume of random scatterers containing no boundaries, as illustrated in Fig. 1(a). The source produces a narrow (delta) pulse of photons that diffuse away in all directions. We assume that the time-dependent photon density $\psi(r, z, t)$ generated in the volume can be described by the diffusion equation[12]

$$\frac{1}{c_n}\frac{\partial}{\partial t}\psi(r, z, t) - D\nabla^2\psi(r, z, t) + \mu_a\psi(r, z, t) = S(r, z, t), \quad (1)$$

where c_n is the velocity of light in the medium, $S(r, z, t)$ is the source function, D is the optical diffusion coefficient, and μ_a is the optical absorption coefficient. Here we employ the similarity relationship $\mu_s' = \mu_s(1 - g)$,[13] where μ_s' is the equivalent-isotropic (transport-corrected) scattering coefficient, and define the diffusion coefficient accordingly as

$$D = [3(\mu_a + \mu_s')]^{-1}. \quad (2)$$

Defined in this manner, D incorporates the effects of the scattering anisotropy of the particles constituting the medium. The mean photon-diffusion length increases with

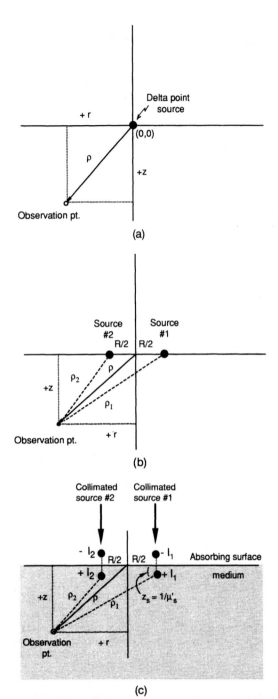

(a)

(b)

(c)

Fig. 1. Coordinate systems and source arrangements for calculating the photon-density wave produced by one or more point sources in a volume of random scatterers. (a) A single source in a medium of infinite extent. (b) Two sources separated by a distance R in a medium of infinite extent. One plane of the cylindrically symmetrical volume is shown. (c) Two collimated beams separated by a distance R incident upon a semi-infinite medium. One plane of the cylindrically symmetrical volume is shown.

g, the average cosine of the angular scattering function of the particles. To obtain valid results using Eq. (1), we will restrict our attention to points several diffusion lengths away from the sources in low-absorption media in which the condition $\mu_a \ll \mu_s'$ is satisfied. The contribution to the total photon flux by short-path (i.e., nondif-

fusive) photons can then be neglected. For an isotropic point source at the origin emitting a delta pulse of intensity I_0 (photons/s) at time $t = 0$, the source function can be written as $S(r, z, t) = I_0 \delta(t = 0)\delta(0, 0)$, and Eq. (1) becomes

$$\frac{1}{c_n}\frac{\partial}{\partial t}\psi(r, z, t) - D\nabla^2\psi(r, z, t) + \mu_a\psi(r, z, t)$$
$$= I_0\delta(t = 0)\delta(0, 0). \quad (3)$$

The Fourier transform of this equation with respect to time,

$$-D\nabla^2\psi(r, z, \omega) + [\mu_a + (i\omega/c_n)]\psi(r, z, \omega) = I_0\delta(0, 0), \quad (4)$$

has the same form as the steady-state (i.e., $\partial/\partial t = 0$) diffusion equation with μ_a replaced by $\mu_a + i\omega/c_n$. The solution of Eq. (4) can then be written as

$$\psi(r, z, \omega) = \frac{I_0}{4\pi D\rho}\exp\left[-\rho\left(\frac{\mu_a}{D} + \frac{i\omega}{Dc_n}\right)^{1/2}\right], \quad (5)$$

where ρ is the radial distance away from the source, given by $\rho = (r^2 + z^2)^{1/2}$, in accordance with the Fig. 1(a) coordinate system. If we apply De Moivre's theorem, we can convert this equation to another form from which the phase and the magnitude of the diffusing wave at a single frequency ω can easily be obtained:

$$\psi(\rho, \omega) = \frac{I_0}{4\pi D\rho}\exp\left\{-a\rho\left[\cos\left(\frac{\theta}{2}\right) + i\sin\left(\frac{\theta}{2}\right)\right]\right\}, \quad (6)$$

where

$$a = \left[\left(\frac{\mu_a}{D}\right)^2 + \left(\frac{\omega}{Dc_n}\right)^2\right]^{1/4},$$

$$\theta = \tan^{-1}[\omega/(\mu_a c_n)].$$

At a single frequency ω, the photon-density wave described by Eq. (6) is composed of a sinusoidally varying (ac) component superimposed upon a nonzero average (dc) component. The magnitude $m_{ac}(\rho)$ and the phase $\phi(\rho)$ of the ac component and the magnitude $m_{dc}(\rho)$ of the dc component are, from the preceding equation,

$$m_{ac}(\rho) = \frac{1}{4\pi D\rho}\exp\left\{-\rho\left[\left(\frac{\mu_a}{D}\right)^2 + \left(\frac{\omega}{Dc_n}\right)^2\right]^{1/4}\right.$$
$$\left.\times\cos\left[\frac{1}{2}\tan^{-1}\left(\frac{\omega}{\mu_a c_n}\right)\right]\right\}, \quad (7)$$

$$\phi(\rho) = \rho\left[\left(\frac{\mu_a}{D}\right)^2 + \left(\frac{\omega}{Dc_n}\right)^2\right]^{1/4}\sin\left[\frac{1}{2}\tan^{-1}\left(\frac{\omega}{\mu_a c_n}\right)\right], \quad (8)$$

$$m_{dc}(\rho) = \frac{1}{4\pi D\rho}\exp\left\{-\rho\left[\left(\frac{\mu_a}{D}\right)^{1/2}\right]\right\}. \quad (9)$$

These equations have been derived previously by Fishkin et al.[8] in terms of a different set of optical constants. For use in later expressions, the magnitudes above have been normalized by setting I_0 equal to 1. Although we express the ac and dc components as separate quantities, they also can be expressed as a ratio (m_{ac}/m_{dc}) analogous to the modulation factor measured by phase fluorometers. In a nonabsorbing medium $(\mu_a = 0)$ a diffusive wave behaves as a spherical wave with a wave front that advances at a constant velocity $v = (2c_n D\omega)^{1/2}$. Therefore at a given frequency its phase increases linearly with the radial distance away from the light source. The wavelength depends on both the frequency and the optical properties of the medium; either an increase in scattering or a decrease in absorption reduces the wavelength. Note that the magnitudes of the ac and dc components of the wave both decrease with the radial distance from the point source in proportion to $\rho^{-1}\exp(-\rho k)$, where k is a constant that is equal to the far-field attenuation coefficient $\alpha = (\mu_a/D)^{1/2}$ at dc and increases with frequency.

B. Interference of Waves in a Full-Space (Unbounded) Region

Building on the results derived for a single source, we now consider the interference of waves generated by two delta point sources separated by a distance R in an unbounded medium. The coordinates of the sources are defined in Fig. 1(b). The intensities of the light pulses and the times at which they are applied are assumed to be different. Therefore, in general, components of the diffusing waves of the same frequency generated by the sources arrive at an arbitrary point $\rho = (r, z)$ in the medium with unequal phases and magnitudes. At frequency ω, the magnitude and the phase of the resultant wave at ρ can be found by adding the complex scalar amplitudes of the individual waves. From Eq. (6) we have

$$\psi_{fs}(\rho, \omega) = \frac{1}{4\pi D}\left(\frac{I_1}{\rho_1}\exp\left\{-a\rho_1\left[\cos\left(\frac{\theta}{2}\right) + i\,\sin\left(\frac{\theta}{2}\right)\right]\right\}\right.$$
$$\left. + \frac{I_2}{\rho_2}\exp\left\{-a\rho_2\left[\cos\left(\frac{\theta}{2}\right) + i\,\sin\left(\frac{\theta}{2}\right) + i\Delta\phi_0\right]\right\}\right),$$
$$(10)$$

where $\psi_{fs}(\rho, \omega)$ represents the photon-density wave at frequency ω (the subscript fs signifies full space, to distinguish this quantity from a similar quantity derived in Section 3 for a half-space volume). I_1 and I_2 are the intensities of the sources, and $\Delta\phi_0$ is the phase delay of source 2 relative to source 1 ($\Delta\phi_0 = 2\pi\omega\Delta t$ rad, where Δt is the difference between the times at which the source light pulses are activated). The distances between ρ and the sources are $\rho_1 = [(r + R/2)^2 + z^2]^{1/2}$ and $\rho_2 = [(r - R/2)^2 + z^2]^{1/2}$. The quantities a and θ are defined as before [see the definitions following Eq. (6)]. The ac magnitude and phase of $\psi_{fs}(\rho, \omega)$ are

$$M_{fs}(\rho, \omega) = \{I_1^2 m_{ac}^2(\rho_1) + I_2^2 m_{ac}^2(\rho_2)$$
$$+ 2I_1 I_2 m_{ac}(\rho_1)m_{ac}(\rho_2)$$
$$\times \cos[\phi(\rho_2) - \phi(\rho_1) + \Delta\phi_0]\}^{1/2},\quad (11)$$

$$\Phi_{fs}(\rho, \omega) = \tan^{-1}[(\{I_1 m_{ac}(\rho_1)\sin[\phi(\rho_1)]$$
$$+ I_2 m_{ac}(\rho_2)\sin[\phi(\rho_2) + \Delta\phi_0]\})/(\{I_1 m_{ac}(\rho_1)$$
$$\times \cos[\phi(\rho_1)] + I_2 m_{ac}(\rho_2)\cos[\phi(\rho_2) + \Delta\phi_0]\})],$$
$$(12)$$

where $m_{ac}(\rho)$ is the single-source full-space magnitude given by Eq. (7). It follows from Eq. (11) that total destructive interference of the two waves at a particular frequency occurs when two conditions are met: $\phi(\rho_2) - \phi(\rho_1) + \Delta\phi_0 = \pm(2n + 1)\pi$ and $m_{ac}(\rho_1) = m_{ac}(\rho_2)$, where

n is an integer greater than or equal to 1. That is, the magnitudes of the waves must be the same, and their phases must differ by an odd multiple of π. To simplify the analysis, $n = 1$ is assumed throughout the rest of this paper, because the wave intensity becomes small at distances greater than a wavelength for the frequencies and the medium properties with which we are concerned. These conditions can be satisfied at any point in the volume by appropriate choices of the magnitude and the delay time of one of the light pulses relative to the other. The ratio of the initial intensities of and the phase difference between the sources required for complete destructive interference at point ρ are

$$(I_2/I_1)^{des} = \frac{\rho_2}{\rho_1}\exp\left(-(\rho_1 - \rho_2)\left[\left(\frac{\mu_a}{D}\right)^2 + \left(\frac{\omega}{Dc_n}\right)^2\right]^{1/4}\right.$$
$$\left.\times\left\{\cos\left[\frac{1}{2}\tan^{-1}\left(\frac{\omega}{\mu_a c_n}\right)\right]\right\}\right),\quad (13)$$

$$\Delta\phi_0^{des} = \pi - (\rho_1 - \rho_2)\left[\left(\frac{\mu_a}{D}\right)^2 + \left(\frac{\omega}{Dc_n}\right)^2\right]^{1/4}$$
$$\times\sin\left[\frac{1}{2}\tan^{-1}\left(\frac{\omega}{\mu_a c_n}\right)\right].\quad (14)$$

For maximum constructive interference to occur, the same conditions must be satisfied, except that the phase of one of the incident light pulses must be shifted such that the waves arrive at ρ in phase, thus requiring that $\Delta\phi_0^{con} = \Delta\phi_0^{des} \pm \pi$.

For a fixed value of $\Delta\phi_0$, Eq. (13) describes a locus of points traced out in the plane of the two sources as I_2/I_1 ranges from 1 to ∞; similarly, for I_2/I_1 fixed, Eq. (14) describes a locus of points in the plane of the two sources at which the ac magnitude of the combined diffusing wave is zero for $-\pi < \Delta\phi_0 < \pi$.

C. Interference of Waves in a Semi-Infinite Region

In most practical situations the incident light emanates from a point on the surface of a scattering material rather than from a point embedded deeply within it; the full-space solutions obtained in Subsection 2.B are applicable only to the latter source configuration. Fortunately, using the method of images,[14,15] we can make minor modifications of the preceding analysis to obtain solutions applicable to photon diffusion in a semi-infinite, cylindrically symmetric region.[16]

Figure 1(c) shows the geometry of the half-space problem. Light from each of the two collimated sources is assumed to become diffused within one transport-corrected scattering length such that the incident photons can be treated as having originated from a depth $z_s = [(1 - g)\mu_s]^{-1}$ below the surface.[12] Assuming that the boundary is totally absorbing, an imaginary equal-intensity, negative photon source (i.e., sink) of photons originating from a point $z = -z_s$ can be added to each of the sources to satisfy the boundary condition at the surface. By superimposing the contributions from the two actual (positive) and the two image (negative) sources, we can obtain the phase and the magnitude at any point in the half-space region. Using the general form of the complex amplitude of a diffusing wave from Subsection 2.A [Eq. (6)], we can derive an expression for the amplitude of the diffusing wave at point

$\rho = (r, z)$ that is valid for $z > 0$. The result is

$$\psi_{hs}(\rho, \omega) = \frac{1}{4\pi D} \left(\frac{I_1}{\rho_1} \exp\left\{ -a\rho_1 \left[\cos\left(\frac{\theta}{2}\right) + i \sin\left(\frac{\theta}{2}\right) \right] \right\} \right.$$
$$- \frac{I_1}{\rho_1{}'} \exp\left\{ -a\rho_1{}' \left[\cos\left(\frac{\theta}{2}\right) + i \sin\left(\frac{\theta}{2}\right) \right] \right\}$$
$$+ \frac{I_2}{\rho_2} \exp\left\{ -a\rho_2 \left[\cos\left(\frac{\theta}{2}\right) + i \sin\left(\frac{\theta}{2}\right) + i\Delta\phi_0 \right] \right\}$$
$$\left. - \frac{I_2}{\rho_2{}'} \exp\left\{ -a\rho_2{}' \left[\cos\left(\frac{\theta}{2}\right) + i \sin\left(\frac{\theta}{2}\right) + i\Delta\phi_0 \right] \right\} \right),$$

$$(15)$$

where $\psi_{hs}(\rho, \omega)$ is the photon-density wave at frequency ω (the subscript hs signifies half-space) and the distances between ρ and the sources are given by

$$\rho_1 = [(r + R/2)^2 + (z - z_s)^2]^{1/2} \qquad (16a)$$

$$\rho_1{}' = [(r + R/2)^2 + (z + z_s)^2]^{1/2} \qquad (16b)$$

$$\rho_2 = [(r - R/2)^2 + (z - z_s)^2]^{1/2} \qquad (16c)$$

$$\rho_2{}' = [(r - R/2)^2 + (z + z_s)^2]^{1/2}. \qquad (16d)$$

The primed terms are associated with the image sources. As in Subsection 2.B, the two sources are assumed to have, in general, different initial intensities ($I_1 \neq I_2$) and an initial phase difference of $\Delta\phi_0$. At frequency ω the photon density varies sinusoidally and has a magnitude given by the real part of the sum of the complex amplitudes of the waves generated by the two sources and their images,

$$M_{hs}(\rho, \omega) = (\{I_1 m_{ac}(\rho_1)\cos[\phi(\rho_1)] - I_1 m_{ac}(\rho_1{}')\cos[\phi(\rho_1{}')]$$
$$+ I_2 m_{ac}(\rho_2)\cos[\phi(\rho_2) + \Delta\phi_0]$$
$$- I_2 m_{ac}(\rho_2{}')\cos[\phi(\rho_2{}') + \Delta\phi_0]\}^2$$
$$+ \{I_1 m_{ac}(\rho_1)\sin[\phi(\rho_1)] - I_1 m_{ac}(\rho_1{}')\sin[\phi(\rho_1{}')]$$
$$+ I_2 m_{ac}(\rho_2)\sin[\phi(\rho_2) + \Delta\phi_0]$$
$$- I_2 m_{ac}(\rho_2{}')\sin[\phi(\rho_2{}') + \Delta\phi_0]\}^2)^{1/2}, \qquad (17)$$

and the phase of the wave relative to source 1 is given by

$$\Phi_{hs}(\rho, \omega) = \tan^{-1}(\{I_1 m_{ac}(\rho_1)\sin[\phi(\rho_1)]$$
$$- I_1 m_{ac}(\rho_1{}')\sin[\phi(\rho_1{}')] + I_2 m_{ac}(\rho_2)\sin[\phi(\rho_2) + \Delta\phi_0]$$
$$- I_2 m_{ac}(\rho_2{}')\sin[\phi(\rho_2{}') + \Delta\phi_0]\}/\{I_1 m_{ac}(\rho_1)\cos[\phi(\rho_1)]$$
$$- I_1 m_{ac}(\rho_1{}')\cos[\phi(\rho_1{}')] + I_2 m_{ac}(\rho_2)\cos[\phi(\rho_2) + \Delta\phi_0]$$
$$- I_2 m_{ac}(\rho_2{}')\cos[\phi(\rho_2{}') + \Delta\phi_0]\}). \qquad (18)$$

These equations are written in terms of the single-source full-space magnitude at the observation point given by Eq. (7), with the distances from the sources defined by Eqs. (16).

As in the full-space case, the diffusive waves generated by sources 1 and 2 undergo complete destructive interference when they arrive at some point in the semi-infinite medium with equal magnitudes and a phase difference of 180°. The ratio of intensities and the phase differences

between the sources required in order to satisfy these conditions at ρ are

$$(I_2/I_1)^{des} = (\{m_{ac}{}^2(\rho_1) + m_{ac}{}^2(\rho_1{}')$$
$$- m_{ac}(\rho_1)m_{ac}(\rho_1{}')\cos[\phi(\rho_1) - \phi(\rho_1{}')]\}/\{m_{ac}{}^2(\rho_2)$$
$$+ m_{ac}{}^2(\rho_2{}') - m_{ac}(\rho_2)m_{ac}(\rho_2{}')$$
$$\times \cos[\phi(\rho_2) - \phi(\rho_2{}')]\})^{1/2}, \qquad (19)$$
$$\Delta\phi_0{}^{des} = \pi - \tan^{-1}(\{m_{ac}(\rho_1)\sin[\phi(\rho_1)]$$
$$- m_{ac}(\rho_1{}')\sin[\rho(\rho_1)]\}/\{m_{ac}(\rho')\cos[\phi(\rho_1)$$
$$- m_{ac}(\rho_1{}')\cos[\phi(\rho_1{}')]\}) - \tan^{-1}(\{m_{ac}(\rho_2)$$
$$\times \sin[\phi(\rho_2)] - m_{ac}(\rho_2{}')\sin[\phi(\rho_2{}')]\}/\{m_{ac}(\rho_2)$$
$$\times \cos[\phi(\rho_2)] - m_{ac}(\rho_2{}')\cos[\phi(\rho_2{}')]\}). \qquad (20)$$

With the intensity ratio set to the value required for complete destructive interference at a given point, maximum constructive interference can be achieved by shifting the phase of source 2 by an additional 180°.

For the more general case of N sources located on the surface of a semi-infinite medium, equations for the magnitude and the phase of the photon-density wave can be obtained by summing the contributions of the individual sources, in a manner analogous to that used to obtain Eqs. (17) and (18).

3. EXPERIMENTAL METHODS

Using a specially designed frequency-domain spectrometer, we measured the magnitude and the phase of the photon-density wave at various points in a scattering medium illuminated by two pulsed laser beams. The experiments were designed to demonstrate the interference of diffusing waves by direct measurement of the two-dimensional distributions of ac magnitudes generated at a particular frequency.

Figure 2 is a simplified block diagram of the spectrometer. A Spectra-Physics mode-locked Nd:YAG laser (Model 3400) synchronously pumped a dye laser that was cavity dumped to produce pulses of ~10-ps duration at a repetition rate of 4.1 MHz. The average power was ~100 mW at 605 nm. A photodiode sampling of the laser's output provided the reference signal, and a beam splitter divided the main intensity-modulated beam into two beams. Both beams were attenuated with a neutral-density filter to ensure operation within the dynamic range of the detection system. The ratio of their intensities was controlled by attenuating one of the beams with a variable neutral-density filter. To set the phase difference between the two beams, we adjusted the path length of one beam by a retroreflecting prism mounted on a rail.

A portion of the scattered photon flux at different points inside the sample was captured by a 625-μm-diameter step-index fiber attached to a multiaxis translation stage. The proximal end of the fiber was aligned perpendicular to the plane of the two input beams. In the regions in which the measurements were made, the gradient of the photon density was assumed to be nearly isotropic and undisturbed by the fiber such that the measured signal could be regarded as proportional to the photon density at the fiber tip. The intensity-modulated light from the

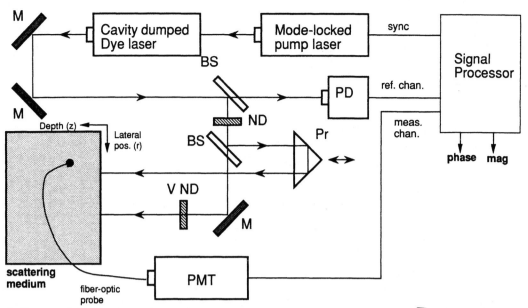

Fig. 2. Block diagram of the experimental setup for measuring interference patterns of diffusive photon-density waves. Component names are abbreviated as follows: M's, mirrors; BS's, beam splitters; PD, photodiode; ND, neutral-density filter; Pr, retroreflecting prism; V ND, variable neutral-density filter; PMT, photomultiplier tube.

distal end of the fiber was detected by the Hamamatsu Model H2431 photomultiplier tube. The photomultiplier tube signal and the reference signal were mixed externally (Minicircuits mixer Model Z) with a high-frequency signal from a synthesizer (Marconi Model 2022 C) down to an intermediate frequency of 200 kHz. After amplification and filtering, both signals were again downconverted to an audio frequency of 40 Hz with the aid of another synthesizer (same model) and again were sharply filtered. This superheterodyne method provides better signal-to-noise-ratio performance than conventional heterodyne methods. The audio-frequency signal was digitized and processed to display magnitude and phase, both normalized to the reference signal. A third synthesizer (PTS Model 250) provided the signal for the mode-locked laser, and its external standard synchronized the other synthesizers.

A liquid scattering phantom consisting of a mixture of whole milk (4% fat content) in water (25%:75%) was used to simulate the optical properties of bloodless skin tissue. The main scattering particles in milk are small casein micelles (0.05–0.3-μm diameter) and large fat globules ($\approx$3-μm diameter). On the basis of results of a separate experiment in which backscattered (dc) intensities were measured for various source–detector distances and background absorbances, the transport-corrected scattering coefficient and the intrinsic absorption coefficient of this mixture were estimated to be 0.75 and 0.004 mm^{-1}, respectively, at 632 nm.[17] By adding food-coloring dye (a mixture of Red Dye No. 3 and Green Dye No. 6), we adjusted the optical absorption in the medium to obtain an estimated total absorption coefficient of 0.01 mm^{-1} at 605 nm, assuming that the intrinsic absorption of the milk solution was the same at this wavelength.

The scattering liquid was contained in an 80 mm (width) $\times$ 60 mm (depth) $\times$ 70 mm (height) black Lucite box. The size of the box was large enough that the effect of its outer walls on the measured intensities could be

neglected. The distance between the tip of the detection fiber and the back (and the side walls) of the chamber always exceeded 20 isotropic mean free paths. To fix the separation of the sources precisely, we made 2-mm-diameter transparent windows in the side of the box through which the beams impinged upon the scattering medium. Each beam was weakly focused to a diameter of approximately 1 mm at the surface of the medium. Except within the small areas occupied by the source windows, the entire inner surface of the box was coated with flat black paint, which reduced specular reflection from the inner surfaces of the box.

At the beginning of each experiment, we nulled the ac signal by adjusting the relative phases and intensities of the beams with the tip of the detector fiber positioned at a predetermined point in the source plane. This point served as the coordinate origin to which all subsequent locations of the fiber were referenced.

4. THEORETICAL AND EXPERIMENTAL RESULTS

Figures 3(a) and 3(b) show the magnitude and the phase of the photon density measured at 410 MHz by the fiber-optic probe at different positions in the experimental scattering medium illuminated by a single beam. The data, acquired from points throughout the sample chamber, are plotted as a function of radial distance from the beam entrance window. At depths greater than approximately 10 mm, the decrease in magnitude was found to be proportional to $\rho^{-1} \exp(-\rho k_1)$, with $k_1 \approx 0.20$ [see Fig. 3(a)]. The phase increased linearly as ρk_2, with $k_2 \approx 5.8°$/mm; thus the wavelength in the medium was approximately $360°/k_2 = 6.2$ cm. In free space, light modulated at 410 MHz has a wavelength approximately 12 times longer (73 cm). As expected, the decrease in magnitude with radial distance near the surface was greater because of light absorption by the black wall of the chamber.

These observations agree with the theoretical results developed in Section 2. By fitting the theoretical magnitude decrease and the phase change given by Eqs. (17) and (18) for the half-space model to the $\rho^{-1} \exp(-\rho k)$ and ρk_2 functional forms, we obtained the following estimates of the absorption coefficients and the scattering coefficients, respectively, of the medium: $\mu_s = 1.1$ mm^{-1} and $\mu_a = 0.008$ mm^{-1}. (The speed of light in the scattering sample was assumed to be $c_n = 0.222$ mm/ps.) These values differ somewhat from those obtained from measurements of re-emitted light (continuous-wave) in a separate experiment ($\mu_s = 0.75$ mm^{-1}; $\mu_a = 0.01$ mm^{-1}; see Section 3). The value of the scattering coefficient derived from the continuous-wave data may be lower because these measurements were carried out at a longer wavelength (632 versus 605 nm in the frequency-domain experiments). Intrinsic absorption at the two wavelengths may have been different as well.

Figure 4 shows the predicted magnitude and phase of a 410-MHz photon-density wave at various points in the experimental medium illuminated by a single beam, assuming the best-fit scattering and absorption coefficients. For comparison, the magnitude and the phase contours predicted by the full-space model [Eqs. (11) and (12)] in

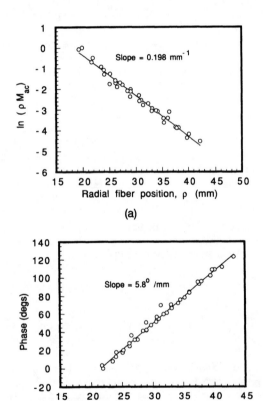

Fig. 3. Magnitude and phase of the photon-density wave produced by a 410-MHz modulated beam incident upon the experimental scattering medium. The data points shown are measurements made throughout the medium at a radial distance greater than 20 mm from the detector at depths greater than 10 mm. (a) Log$_e$ of the product of the ac magnitude and the radial distance between the source and the detector. (b) Measured phase in degrees. All measurements are shown normalized to the value measured at the shortest source–detector separation distance.

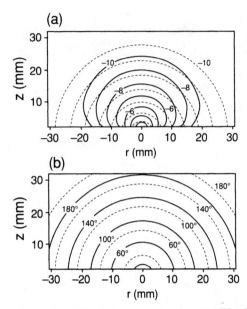

Fig. 4. Calculated phase and magnitude of a 410-MHz photon-diffusion wave generated by a point source in a half-space medium (solid curves) and in the forward hemisphere of a full-space medium (dashed curves). Note the distortion of the spherical wave front caused by the absorbing boundary: (a) isomagnitude contours [$\log_e(m_{ac})$], (b) isophase contours. The model parameters, which were chosen to represent experimental conditions, were as follows: $I_0 = 1$, $C_n = 0.222$ mm/ps, $\omega = 2.58 \times 10^9$ rad, $\mu_s' = 1.1$ mm^{-1}, $\mu_a = 0.008$ mm^{-1}.

the forward hemisphere are shown as dotted curves. Note that the boundary alters the shape of the isomagnitude contours but has little effect on the shape of the isophase contours. At points close to the surface the decrease in the ac magnitude of the photon density with radial distance from the source is steeper than the decrease at points deeper in the medium, as a result of loss of photons at the surface. The phase changes more rapidly close to the boundary in the radial direction as well, because short-path photons are absorbed, thereby increasing the mean path length of the photons that propagate to a given point adjacent to the boundary [(compare the dotted and solid curves in Fig. 4(b)]. As we discuss later in this section, the ratio of the intensities of two sources required for destructive interference to be obtained in superficial regions can be quite large because of this effect.

The set of equations given in Section 2 specifies the regions in a scattering volume within which destructive or constructive interference occurs for two sources having different initial intensities and phases. The contour plots in Fig. 5 show the source-intensity ratios [$(I_2/I_1)^{des}$, solid curves] and the phase differences ($\Delta\phi_0^{des}$, dotted curves) required for destructive interference to be produced at various points in the source plane for the conditions under which one of our experiments was performed. Results are shown for a source separation of 12 mm at a frequency of 410 MHz. The values plotted in Fig. 5(a) were calculated by using Eqs. (19) and (20) (half-space case), and those in Fig. 5(b) were calculated by using Eqs. (13) and (14) (full-space case); in both cases the optical parameters obtained by fitting the single-source experimental data (see above) were used in the calculations. In Fig. 5(b) only the for-

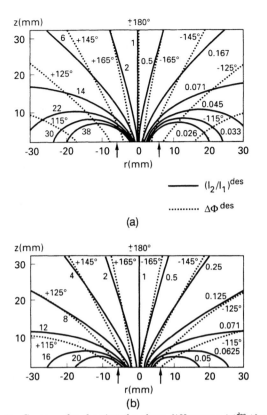

(a)

(b)

Fig. 5. Contour plot showing the phase differences $\Delta\phi^{\text{des}}$ (dotted curves) and source-intensity ratios $(I_2/I_1)^{\text{des}}$ (solid curves) required simultaneously for complete destructive interference at points in the plane of the sources. I_1 is the intensity of source 1, located at $r = -6$ mm; I_2 is the intensity of source 2, located at $r = +6$ mm. The arrows indicate the locations of the sources. The model parameters used were the same as those used to generate Fig. 4 (see the caption to Fig. 4). (a) The semi-infinite medium [from Eq. (13)]. (b) The infinite medium [from Eqs. (19) and (20)]. Only the forward hemisphere is shown.

ward hemisphere is shown. Results for the semi-infinite [Fig. 5(a)] and infinite [Fig. 5(b)] media are presented to illustrate the effect of the absorbing boundary. For a given magnitude ratio and phase difference, the point at which destructive interference occurs is determined by the intersection of the equal-phase-difference (dotted) curves and the equal-intensity-ratio (solid) curves. The points of maximum constructive interference can be found by simply adding 180° to the phase-difference values marked on the plot. When we compare the dotted and the solid contours in the figures, it is apparent that the absorbing boundary affects both the phase difference and the source-intensity ratio required for destructive interference at a given point. The intensity of the source located at the farthest radial distance required for a null to be produced at a point close to the $z = 0$ plane can be substantially greater in the half-space case than in the full-space case. From Fig. 5(b) one can see that, for $r > 2R$ and $r < -2R$, the position of the null point is most sensitive to a change in the intensity of either source and least sensitive to a change in phase. Conversely, close to the midline between the sources ($r = 0$), a change in the phase of either source affects the position of the null point more than does a change in its intensity.

It can also be seen from Fig. 5 that, for a given source-intensity ratio and phase difference, total destructive interference either does not occur at all or occurs at only one point in the plane defined by the sources, except when $I_2 = I_1$ and $\Delta\phi_0 \pm \pi$. In this particular case, complete destructive interference occurs along the entire line $r = 0$, which passes through the origin halfway between the two sources.

Figure 6 is a surface plot of the ac magnitude (410-MHz modulation frequency) measured at various locations in the tissue phantom illuminated by two equal-intensity sources. The data plotted in Fig. 6(a) and 6(b) were obtained with the sources 180° out of phase (destructive-interference condition) and in phase (constructive-interference condition), respectively. Figures 7(a) and 7(b) show the corresponding measured phases. These data provide clear evidence of diffusive-wave interference. In Fig. 8 the magnitude and phase values measured as the detector fiber was moved laterally at a fixed depth are compared with those predicted by diffusion theory [Eqs. (17) and (18)]. The experiments confirmed the

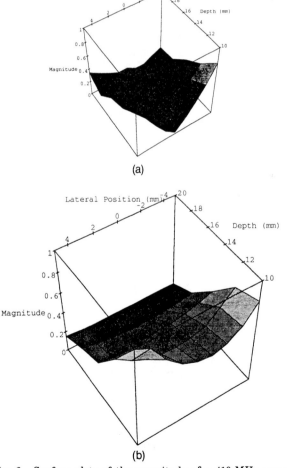

(a)

(b)

Fig. 6. Surface plots of the magnitude of a 410-MHz wave formed by two interfering diffusive waves. Measurements were made with the tip of the detector fiber placed at different positions in the source plane. The interfering waves were produced by equal-intensity beams incident upon the medium at lateral positions $r = -12$ mm and $r = +12$ mm: (a) destructively interfering, (b) constructively interfering.

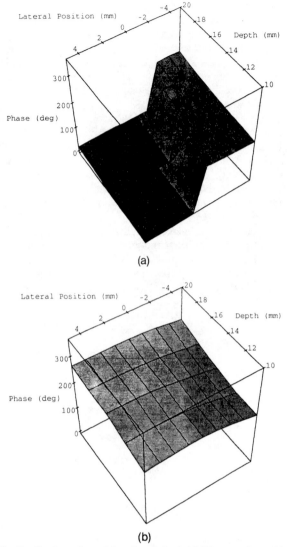

(a)

(b)

Fig. 7. Surface plots of the phase of a 410-MHz wave formed by two constructively interfering diffusive waves. Measurements were made with the tip of the detector fiber placed at different positions in the source plane. The interfering waves were produced by equal-intensity beams incident upon the medium at lateral positions $r = -12$ mm and $r = +12$ mm: (a) destructively interfering, (b) constructively interfering.

large changes, predicted by the theory, in the phase and the magnitude of the photon density along the midline. The asymmetry that is evident in the experimental phase and magnitude curves resulted from a slight lateral misalignment of the fiber tip with respect to the wall of the sample chamber.

Close to a null point located off the midline, partial destructive interference occurs over a broad region extending over approximately one half of the diffusive wavelength. This region becomes more confined as the modulation frequency increases. At a particular frequency its location can be varied by adjusting the ratio of the intensities of the sources. The phase difference between the sources affects mainly the depth of the null within the region. Figure 9 illustrates the shapes of the null regions produced in a simulated medium for a variety of source-intensity ratios and phase differences. The

contour plots in the figure were obtained by plotting M_{hs} from Eq. (17) as a function of r and z, again assuming tissuelike absorption and scattering parameters. In Figs. 9(a), 9(c), and 9(e) the magnitude patterns produced under constructive and destructive conditions are shown superimposed. Note that the regions of partial destructive interference roughly follow the solid-curve contours of Fig. 5(a) and that the constructive and destructive interference patterns differ significantly only in the vicinity of the null point. In Figs. 9(b), 9(d), and 9(f) the ratios of the constructive and destructive magnitudes are plotted to show the differences in the interference patterns more clearly. Combining the ratios of the constructive and destructive magnitudes produced by two pairs of sources, as illustrated in Fig. 9(g), establishes a well-defined region of illumination (ac). These simulations indicate the potential advantages of using multiple sources for imaging ap-

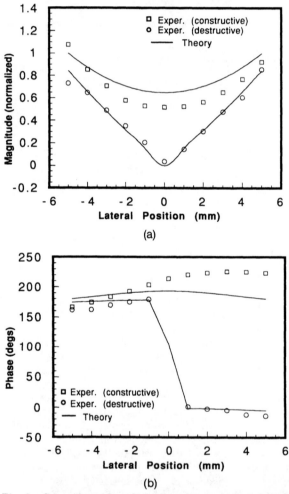

(a)

(b)

Fig. 8. Comparison of predicted magnitudes and phases with those measured at a fixed depth ($z = 12.5$ mm) under constructive- and destructive-interference conditions. The plotted values have been normalized to the average of the values measured at $r = -5$ mm and $r = 5$ mm under constructive-interference conditions. Model parameters for constructive interference: $I_1 = I_2 = 1$, $\Delta\phi = 1$; for destructive interference: $I_1 = I_2 = 1$, $\Delta\phi = 180°$. The remaining parameters were the same as those listed in the caption to Fig. 4. (a) Ac magnitude for the constructive-interference (upper curve) and destructive-interference cases (lower curve). (b) Phases for the constructive-interference (upper curve) and destructive-interference cases (lower curve).

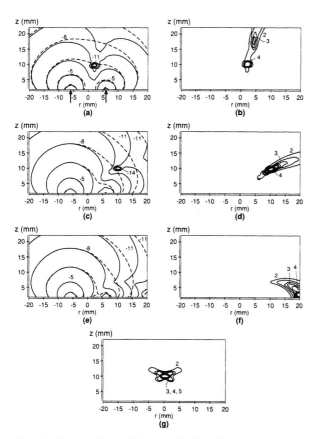

Fig. 9. Constructive- and destructive-interference patterns produced by two 410-MHz sources having different magnitudes and phases, derived by using the half-space model [Eq. (17)]. The contour lines, which connect the points having equal $\log_e$ ac magnitudes, are spaced to show an incremental decrease in photon density equal to $e^{1.5}$. Sources 1 and 2 are located at $r = -6$ mm and $r = +6$ mm, respectively (the arrows indicate the points of entry of the photons), and the model parameters are the same as those listed in the caption to Fig. 4. (a) Destructive conditions (solid curves): $I_2/I_1 = 0.453$, $\Delta\phi = -169.1°$; constructive conditions (dashed curves): $I_2/I_1 = 0.453$, $\Delta\phi = +10.9°$. (b) $\log_e$ ratio of the constructive and destructive magnitudes shown in Fig. 10(a). (c) Destructive conditions (solid curves): $I_2/I_1 = 0.0598$, $\Delta\phi = -135.8°$; constructive conditions (dashed curves): $I_2/I_1 = 0.0598$, $\Delta\phi = +44.2°$. (d) $\log_e$ ratio of the constructive and destructive magnitudes shown in Fig. 10(c). (e) Destructive conditions (solid curves): $I_2/I_1 = 0.0278$, $\Delta\phi = -114.3°$; constructive conditions (dashed curves): $I_2/I_1 = 0.0278$, $\Delta\phi = +65.7°$. (f) $\log_e$ ratio of the constructive and destructive magnitudes shown in Fig. 10(e). (g) Sum of $\log_e$ constructive/destructive ratios produced by two source pairs located symmetrically about the origin (one source pair is centered around $r = +10$ mm and the other around $r = -10$ mm, both with a source separation of 12 mm). Initial intensities and phases for the source pair centered around $r = -10$ mm are the same as those used to generate the plot in Fig. 10(c); the phase and the magnitude of the sources constituting the other pair are interchanged.

plications. The ability to detect, with the use of selective illumination, an isolated fluorescent object (idealized as a point source) embedded in a homogeneous medium depends on the degree to which the combined constructive/destructive magnitude ratios can be confined (assuming that light re-emitted by the object is captured by a large-area detector). However, the computed curves in Fig. 9(g) should not be construed as evidence for the ability to *resolve* two objects finely or to image an extended object with two-source interference methods. The resolution of

multiple embedded objects with the use of frequency-domain techniques depends on crucial factors—in particular, detector geometry and diffraction effects—that this paper does not address.

We experimentally studied the characteristics of the broad null region that the model predicts will be produced if the intensities and phases of the beams are adjusted to produce total destructive interference at a point located a large radial distance away from the beams, close to an absorbing boundary. In this experiment the two beams were separated by 12 mm, and their phases and magnitudes were adjusted to produce a null at a point 2 mm deep inside the experimental medium at a radial position 30 mm from the midline between the points at which the beams impinged upon the medium. The photon density was sampled in the plane of the beams. As a result of partial destructive interference, the magnitude was found to be reduced throughout a broad region close to the surface (near wall) of the medium between the null point and the point at which the nearest beam impinged upon the medium. In Fig. 10 the experimentally measured ac magnitude-versus-depth and phase-versus depth profiles at two lateral positions are compared with those predicted by the photon-diffusion theory. The theoretical predictions agree well with the experimental data, including the odd shape of the region of partial wave destruction. According to the model, the source-intensity ratio and the phase difference required for total destructive interference at the desired point were 23:1 and 112°, respectively. For this set of source parameters, partial destructive interference occurs over a broad region, because the photon-density waves produced by the sources are out of phase at all points along the near wall. At points deeper in the medium (i.e., at increasing values of z), the relative contribution of the source farthest away from the null point becomes greater, and the waves no longer cancel. The large change in phase with depth predicted by the theory and seen in the experiments under destructive-interference conditions manifests the increasing domination of the photon-density wave produced by the source farthest from the null point.

5. DISCUSSION AND CONCLUSIONS

The interference of intensity-modulated light waves in transparent media such as air and glass is a familiar concept on which holography and numerous other optical heterodyning techniques are based. A fact not widely appreciated is that intensity-modulated light waves traveling in a dense medium of random scatters can also interfere, but the nature of the interference is different. This type of interference can be readily understood by treating the propagation of the waves as a diffusive process similar to heat conduction. If this diffusion model is adopted, it follows that diffusive-light-wave interference results from the scalar addition of *photon-density* waves produced by coherently modulated sources. The optical-frequency waves do not add coherently but merely act as carriers of the photon-density fluctuations.

Our theoretical results show that the interference patterns produced by interfering diffusive waves can be complicated. The locations of the regions of partial constructive and destructive interference depend on several variables, including the optical properties of the medium,

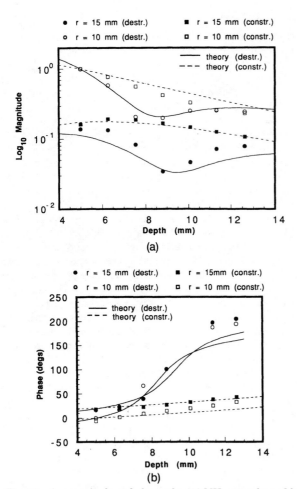

• r = 15 mm (destr.)   ■ r = 15 mm (constr.)
○ r = 10 mm (destr.)   □ r = 10 mm (constr.)
—— theory (destr.)
- - - theory (constr.)

(a)

• r = 15 mm (destr.)   ■ r = 15mm (constr.)
○ r = 10 mm (destr.)   □ r = 10 mm (constr.)
—— theory (destr.)
- - - theory (constr.)

(b)

Fig. 10. Ac magnitude and phase of a 410-MHz wave formed by two interfering diffusive waves plotted as a function of depth into the medium. The two beams, which were incident upon the medium at lateral positions $r = 0$ mm and $r = +12$ mm, were adjusted to produce a null at r (lateral position), z (depth) coordinates $(-30$ mm, 2 mm). The data measured at two lateral positions, $r = 10$ mm and $r = 15$ mm, are compared with theory. The plotted values are shown normalized to the phase and magnitude measured at the depth $z = 5$ mm. Model parameters for constructive interference: $I_2/I_1 = 0.0428$, $\Delta\phi = +67.8°$; for destructive interference: $I_2/I_1 = 0.0428$, $\Delta\phi = -112.2°$; the remaining parameters were the same as those listed in the caption to Fig. 4. (a) Ac magnitude for the constructive-interference and destructive-interference cases. (b) Phases for the constructive-interference and destructive-interference cases. The filled and open squares are experimental values recorded under constructive-interference conditions, and the filled and open circles are experimental values recorded under destructive-interference conditions.

the phases and intensities of the sources, the modulation frequency, and the source-separation distance. With the modulation frequency and source separation fixed, the directionality and ac-magnitude profile of the aggregate diffusive wave can be coarsely adjusted by varying the phases or intensities of the sources. This situation differs in several important respects from the focusing of radiated radio-frequency energy, which can be accomplished by using conventional microwave antenna arrays. Unlike the polarity of radio-frequency waves, the polarity of a diffusive wave can never be negative; the average dc component of a diffusive wave always equals or exceeds one half of its ac component. Therefore the average amount of energy deposited in a given region in a turbid medium cannot be altered by phasing alone. Also, attenuation of diffusive waves is in general much greater than that of microwaves. As a result, interference effects associated with diffusive waves become less pronounced as the distance from the points sources increases. The dependence of the positions of the destructive-interference nulls on the relative intensities of the sources that we demonstrated in our experiments is partly a consequence of the damping of the diffusive waves in the experimental medium. In spite of these differences, however, the concepts underlying the design of microwave arrays may still prove useful in the design of diffusive-wave imaging systems.

For the phase front of a diffusive wave to propagate coherently without distortion, the medium must be homogeneous on a spatial scale of the order of the wavelength of the diffusive wave. Any local variation in the absorption or scattering coefficient will cause refraction or diffraction of the wave. We show that a totally absorbing boundary distorts the shape of the wave front produced by a point source on the boundary. As a result, at points close to the boundary the wavelength is a function of position and direction. We expect that partially reflecting boundaries, which are not considered in this paper, will produce a similar effect. It may be possible to incorporate reflecting boundaries into our model by changing the positions of the image sources to make the photon fluence equal zero on an extrapolated boundary rather than on the physical boundary.[18]

Our simple diffusion model clearly embodies several assumptions. One assumption is that the medium is composed of particles that can be treated as isotropic scatterers. The dominant scatterers at visible and near-infrared wavelengths in many substances, including tissue, are equal to or larger than the wavelength of light and therefore scatter light anisotropically. With appropriate scaling of the scattering coefficient, however, the diffusion approximation still holds, provided that a sufficiently large number of scattering events occur to randomize the direction of propagation of the photons emitted by the sources.[19] This provision imposes a restriction on the minimum distance from the sources at which the expressions derived in this paper are valid. Time-resolved transmission studies[20] have shown that measured values of the mean photon-propagation time deviate from those predicted by the transport-corrected diffusion theory at distances less than 10 equivalent-isotropic scattering lengths away from a collimated source. Therefore the reliability of the model is questionable in this region.

A closely related assumption concerns the polarization state of the source flux, which we neglect in our analysis. On the basis of the results of previous experimental studies,[21] we assume that both the polarization and the wave direction of a collimated source become randomized over comparable optical distances in a dense random medium.

One limitation of the diffusion model that we consider here concerns the modulation frequency. Because the diffusion equation [Eq. (1)] contains no propagation term (it is first order in time), it necessarily fails at short times.[20,22] Therefore when ballistic photons and quasi-ballistic photons, which arrive earlier than predicted by the diffusion equation, constitute a substantial fraction of the photon flux measured at a certain point, then the predicted and the measured values of the phase and the magnitude of a diffusive wave will not agree. Viewed in another way, an increase in modulation frequency and an increase in optical absorption can have analogous effects: both reduce the contribution of long-path, multiply scattered photons to the total photon flux. The diffusion approximation is most accurate when both the absorption coefficient and the modulation frequency are low, namely, $\mu_a \ll \mu_s'$ and $\omega \ll c_n \mu_s'$. For a medium with $\mu_s' = 1$ mm^{-1} and $\mu_a = 0.01 - 0.05$ mm^{-1}, typical values for skin tissue,[17] the diffusion approximation should give good results at modulation frequencies below 20–50 GHz.

In the experiments described in this paper, only two beams were used to generate the interfering diffusive waves. Multiple sources could be used to create better-defined regions of constructive and destructive interference. For example, one can imagine illuminating the surface of a medium with an array of phased sources designed to steer the aggregate wave, in an approach similar to that on which sector-scanning ultrasonic imaging systems are based. The simple diffusion analysis developed in this paper can be used to predict the interference pattern produced by an arbitrary number of point sources. Furthermore, if pulsatile sources are used, information can be obtained from interference patterns produced at multiple frequencies. The problem of arranging sources to produce an optimum illumination pattern at different frequencies for a particular application is more challenging and will be addressed in future publications.

The potential applications of diffusive-wave interference that have been proposed to date pertain to the imaging of fluorescent or absorptive objects embedded in a scattering medium.[9,10] Perhaps the most straightforward application is the localization of a fluorescent marker in a scattering background (e.g., a biological tissue containing a fluorescent contrast agent). This problem was addressed before by the use of a phase-sensitive imaging approach without interference.[23] We are now studying the benefits of using interfering diffusive waves for illumination to permit imaging of a deeply embedded fluorescent object. Any theoretical analysis of this problem must address the effect of the position of a detector on its sensitivity to the fluorescent light re-emitted by the object. If the fluorescent object is small and weakly absorbing, the theoretical results in Section 2 can be extended by using the source–detector reciprocity theorem to estimate the fraction of the total fluorescent light flux that is captured by a detector located on the surface of a half-space medium. One possible approach is the following: Let the complex amplitude of the aggregate light wave generated by N sources illuminating an object located at point ρ_0 in a semi-infinite medium be $\psi_{hs}(\rho_0, \omega)$, which, for the two-source case, is given by Eq. (15). The object re-emits fluorescent light with an ac magnitude proportional to the product of the real part of $\psi_{hs}(\rho_0, \omega)$ and the fluorescence quantum yield η. (For simplicity, we neglect here the phase delay and demodulation resulting from the finite lifetime of the fluorescent emission.) In accordance with the reciprocity theorem, a point detector located at point ρ_d on the surface of the medium can be treated as a dipole source; this detector-turned-source produces a wave with a complex amplitude $\psi_{hs}(\rho_d - \rho_0, \omega)$ at the point ρ_0. The intensity

of the modulated fluorescent light received by the detector is then proportional to $\eta \psi_{hs}(\rho_0, \omega) \psi_{hs}^*(\rho_d - \rho_0, \omega)$. Unfortunately, simple analytical techniques based on the reciprocity theorem cannot be used to solve problems involving highly absorptive or large, irregularly shaped fluorescent objects. To solve such problems, finite-difference, Monte Carlo, or other numerical simulation methods are needed.

REFERENCES

1. R. L. Longini and R. Zdrojkowski, "A note on the theory of backscattering of light by living tissue," IEEE Trans. Biomed. Eng. **BME-15**, 4–10 (1968).
2. A. Ishimaru, "Diffusion of light in turbid material," Appl. Opt. **28**, 2210–2222 (1989).
3. L. F. Gate, "The determination of light absorption in diffusing materials by a photon diffusion model," J. Phys. D **4**, 1049–1056 (1971).
4. B. Chance, S. Nioka, J. Kent, K. McCully, M. Fountain, R. Greenfeld, and G. Holtom, "Time-resolved spectroscopy of hemoglobin and myoglobin in resting and ischemic muscles," Anal. Biochem. **174**, 698–707 (1988).
5. D. T. Delpy, M. Cope, P. Van der Zee, S. Arridge, S. Wray, and J. Wyatt, "Estimation of optical pathlength through tissue from direct time of flight measurement," Phys. Med. Biol. **33**, 1433–1442 (1988).
6. J. R. Lakowicz and K. W. Berndt, "Frequency-domain measurements of photon migration in tissues," Chem. Phys. Lett. **166**, 246–252 (1990).
7. B. Chance, ed., *Photon Migration in Tissues* (Plenum, New York, 1989).
8. J. Fishkin, E. Gratton, M. J. vandeVen, and W. W. Mantulin, "Diffusion of intensity-modulated near-infrared light in turbid media," in *Time-Resolved Spectroscopy and Imaging of Tissues*, B. Chance, ed., Proc. Soc. Photo-Opt. Instrum. Eng. **1431**, 122–135 (1991).
9. A. Knüttel, J. M. Schmitt, and J. R. Knutson, "Spatial localization of absorbing bodies by interfering diffusive photon-density waves," Appl. Opt. (to be published).
10. A. Knüttel and J. R. Knutson, "Methods and apparatus for imaging a physical parameter in turbid media using diffusive waves," U.S. patent application 07/722,823 (May 7, 1991).
11. E. Gratton, W. W. Mantulin, M. J. vandeVen, J. B. Fishkin, M. B. Maris, and B. Chance, "The possibility of a near-infrared optical imaging system using frequency domain methods," in *Proceedings of the Third International Conference on Peace through Mind/Brain Science* (Hamamatsu Corp., Hamamatsu, Japan, 1990), pp. 183–188.
12. M. S. Patterson, B. Chance, and B. C. Wilson, "Time resolved reflectance and transmittance for the noninvasive measurement of tissue optical properties," Appl. Opt. **28**, 2331–2336 (1989).
13. H. C. van de Hulst, *Multiple Light Scattering: Tables, Formulas, and Applications* (Academic, New York, 1980), Vol. 1, Chap. 14, pp. 477–492.
14. R. J. Hirko, R. J. Fretterd, and R. L. Longini, "Diffusion dipole source," J. Opt. Soc. Am. **63**, 336–337 (1973).
15. J. Mathews and R. L. Walker, *Mathematical Methods of Physics* (Benjamin, New York, 1970), p. 245.
16. M. S. Patterson, J. D. Moulton, B. C. Wilson, and B. Chance, "Applications of time-resolved light scattering methods to photodynamic dosimetry," in *Photodynamic Therapy: Mechanisms II*, T. J. Dougherty, ed., Proc. Soc. Photo-Opt. Instrum. Eng. **1203**, 62–75 (1990).
17. J. M. Schmitt, G. X. Zhou, E. C. Walker, and R. T. Wall, "Multilayer model of photon diffusion in skin," J. Opt. Soc. Am. A **7**, 2141–2153 (1990).
18. D. J. Pine, D. A. Weitz, G. Maret, P. E. Wolf, E. Herbolzheimer, and P. M. Chaikin, in *Scattering and Localization of Classical Waves in Random Media*, P. Sheng, ed. (World Scientific, Singapore, 1989).
19. G. Yoon, S. A. Prahl, and A. J. Welch, "Accuracies of the diffu-

sion approximation and its similarity relations for laser irradiated biological media," Appl. Opt. **28**, 2250–2255 (1989).

20. K. M. Yoo, L. Feng, and R. R. Alfano, "When does the diffusion approximation fail to describe photon transport in random media?" Phys. Rev. Lett. **64**, 2647–2650 (1990).

21. J. M. Schmitt, A. H. Gandjbakhche, and R. F. Bonner, "Use of polarized light to discriminate short-path photons in a multiply scattering medium," Appl. Opt. (to be published).

22. K. Furutsu, "Diffusion equation derived from space-time transport equation," J. Opt. Soc. Am. **70**, 360–366 (1980).

23. J. R. Lakowicz and K. W. Berndt, "Lifetime-selective fluorescence imaging using an rf phase-sensitive camera," Rev. Sci. Instrum. **62**, 1727–1734 (1991).

Reprinted with permission from *Physical Review E,* Vol. 47(5), pp. R2999-R3002
(May 1993). ©1993 American Physical Society.

Scattering and wavelength transduction of diffuse photon density waves

D. A. Boas and M. A. O'Leary

Department of Physics and Department of Biochemistry and Biophysics, University of Pennsylvania,
Philadelphia, Pennsylvania 19104-6396

B. Chance

Department of Biochemistry and Biophysics, University of Pennsylvania, Philadelphia, Pennsylvania 19104-6396

A. G. Yodh

Department of Physics, University of Pennsylvania, Philadelphia, Pennsylvania 19104-6396
(Received 22 December 1992)

Experiments are performed that illustrate the scattering and reradiation of damped traveling waves of light energy density from objects within otherwise homogeneous turbid media. We demonstrate that simple diffractive and refractive models can be used to understand the scattering of these waves by absorptive and dispersive spheres. Furthermore, using a fluorescent dye we can reestablish the origin of the diffuse photon density waves, by converting from one optical and diffusive wavelength to another while maintaining phase coherence. The possibilities for precise medical imaging are presented.

Diffuse photon density waves are just beginning to receive attention as a result of intrinsic interest in their phenomenology and because of their propensity to provide information about the dense random media through which they move. Briefly, diffuse photon density waves are scalar, overdamped, traveling waves of light energy density. They will propagate through any medium in which the transport of light energy density, $U(\mathbf{r},t)$, is governed by the diffusion equation [1], $\partial U/\partial t = D\nabla^2 U$, where D is the light diffusion constant in the medium. Examples of such media for visible light include dense colloidal suspensions of micrometer-size spheres, human tissue, paints, foams, and Intralipid. The traveling waves are produced by introducing amplitude modulated light, with source modulation frequency ω, into the optically turbid medium [2-6].

In essence, the introduction of amplitude-modulated light into the turbid medium produces a *macroscopic ripple of brightness* that is *microscopically* composed of individual photons undergoing random walks. The macroscopic disturbance obeys a Helmholtz equation, and therefore has many properties that we normally associate with conventional electromagnetic radiation. In a recent paper, for example, we have demonstrated the refraction of these waves [5]. Other experiments that have been accomplished recently exhibit aspects of simple diffraction [4] and interference [3,7] using these waves.

In this paper we investigate the scattering and reradiation of diffuse photon density waves by obstacles located within otherwise turbid homogeneous media. The reradiation experiments introduce a new and potentially useful physical phenomenon that is brought about through the interaction of these waves with fluorescent scattering inhomogeneities, and the scattering experiments demonstrate the utility of two conceptually simple diffractive and refractive models for wave-front distortion. The measurements span two approaches to the detection of

localized inhomogeneities within optically dense media. At the conclusion of this paper we will comment briefly on the biomedical potential of the two approaches.

In the first set of experiments we have observed the conversion or transduction of a diffuse photon density wave from one *optical and diffusive* wavelength to another. This was accomplished by illuminating an obstacle filled with absorbing dye by a diffuse photon density wave. The dye was chosen to absorb radiation at the source wavelength, and very soon thereafter to *reradiate* photons at a red-shifted energy. Because the dye had a lifetime of less than 1 nsec compared to the 5-nsec period of the source, the reradiated energy was also in the form of a diffuse photon density wave that was readily detected at the red-shifted energy. This phenomenon might be described as a type of "fluorescence" of a diffuse photon density wave. In the process, the inhomogeneity is converted into a *source* of diffuse photon density waves. Localization of the obstacle can be accomplished by determination of the source center from the reradiated wave fronts.

In the second set of experiments we have measured the wave-front distortions that arise when these waves are scattered by purely absorptive or dispersive homogeneous spheres. In general, one would expect both refractive and diffractive processes to affect the scattered wave fronts. Unfortunately, our intuition from conventional optics is of limited applicability, since we must work in the near field. We have found that measurements of wave-front distortions from purely absorbing spheres are well described by a simple diffraction model whereby the diffuse photon density wave is scattered by an absorbing disk of the same diameter. The pure dispersive case is more complex. A ray optic model works well for scatterers characterized by a larger light diffusion constant relative to that of the surrounding turbid medium, but a diffractive model is required in the other limit.

Our scheme for the generation, propagation, and detection of diffuse photon density waves has been described [5]. The diffuse medium is Intralipid solution [8], in which an amplitude-modulated (200-MHz 1-mW diode laser operating at either 780 nm or 816 nm is inserted. In a homogeneous medium, the oscillating part of the light energy density radiated by the source has the form $U(\mathbf{r},t) = (A/Dr)\exp[-k(\cos\phi)r]\exp\{i[k(\sin\phi)r-\omega t]\}$ where A is a constant and $k = (\omega/D)^{1/2}$, and for a medium characterized by absorption length l_a and optical index of refraction n, $\tan 2\phi = (\omega l_a)(n/c)$. Absorptive corrections to k and D are relatively small for the samples we consider.

Light is delivered into the sample through a source fiber and is collected by a movable detector fiber. The oscillating part of the diffuse light energy density is measured by standard phase-sensitive methods. Typically we determine the amplitude and phase of the diffuse photon density wave at the movable detector as a function of its position in the medium. In the present experiments we also introduce spherical obstacles into the medium.

The primary results of our reradiation experiments are shown in Fig. 1. Here the source laser is located at the origin, and a 1.8-cm-diam transparent spherical shell filled with a 0.1% solution of Intralipid is located a distance of 4.5 cm from the source. The surrounding Intralipid has the same concentration, giving a photon diffusion constant $D = 6.0 \times 10^9$ cm²/sec. A biologically useful dye, indocyanine green [9] was dissolved in the spherical shell at a concentration of 0.41 μg/cm³. The indocyanine green absorbed light from the incident diffuse photon density wave at 780 nm, and then emitted photons at 830 nm. The absorption and emission characteristics of the indocyanine green are shown in Fig. 1(a). Since the lifetime of the dye is relatively short (< 1 nsec), the reradiated radiation was also in the form of a diffuse photon density wave. Using spectral filters we separately measured the incident wave at 780 nm in the presence of the obstacle, and the reradiated wave at 830 nm. The latter measurement can in principle have zero background.

In Fig. 1(b) the constant amplitude contours of the diffuse photon density wave at 780 nm are presented at intervals that decrease by a factor of 0.3 with increasing distance from the source. We see that these contours are reasonably circular and can be extrapolated back to the laser source. The small deviations observed are primarily a result of absorption by the obstacle. A similar contour plot of the phase was also measured, and could also be extrapolated back to the laser source. The measured wavelength of the diffuse photon density wave in the homogeneous Intralipid was ~18 cm.

In Fig. 1(c) we exhibit the constant amplitude contours of the wave at 830 nm, and thus demonstrate the diffuse photon density wave character of the reradiated waves. We see clearly that *the reradiated wave originates from within the absorbing obstacle*. From the contours we deduce a source origin of ~4.6 cm. The overall quantum efficiency of the dye from 780 to 830 nm was ~10^{-5}. Similar conclusions could be drawn from the phase contours although the phase data were more sensitive to the small light leakages at 780 nm and were therefore considerably noisier. The diffuse photon density wavelength at 830 nm was measured to be ~27 cm, somewhat larger than the wave at 780 nm reflecting the larger light diffusion constant for 830 nm light in Intralipid. We have also compared reradiated waves from spherical and cylindrical objects. The measurements clearly show that the contours in the case of the cylinder are more elliptical than those of the sphere, thereby demonstrating that the reradiation technique can be sensitive to the shape of the obstacle.

Our scattering experiments fall into two categories. We consider the pure absorptive spheres first (see Fig. 2). We have measured constant phase and amplitude contours for diffuse density waves traveling in different concentrations of Intralipid and then scattering from a 4.0-cm-diam absorptive sphere. The sphere was saturated with ink so that the fraction of incident light at 816 nm transmitted through the sphere was below our detection limit of ~10^{-6}. Nevertheless, we detect robust wave fronts on the other side of the sphere. These wave fronts are formed by the diffraction of the wave around the sphere.

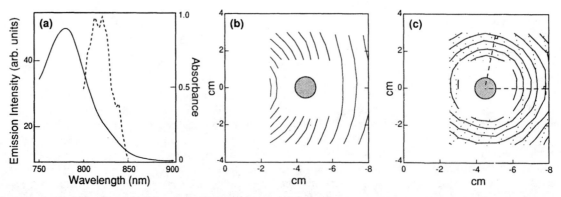

FIG. 1. (a) Indocyanine green absorption (solid line) and emission (dashed line) spectra. The laser radiates at 780 nm. (b) Constant amplitude contours of the incident diffuse photon density wave at 780 nm. (c) Constant amplitude contours at 830 nm (solid lines) clearly exhibiting the reradiated nature of the wave. The dashed lines are the amplitude contours at 780 nm, and the center of the radiator is located by finding the intersection of the lines normal to these contours. The amplitude of the adjacent contours decreases by a factor of 0.3.

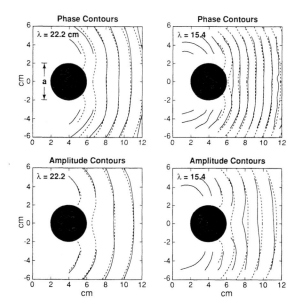

FIG. 2. These plots show the diffraction of a diffuse photon density wave by a spherical absorber ($a = 4.0$ cm). The light source is at the origin and generates a wave with a wavelength of 22.2 cm in the plots on the left, and a wavelength of 15.4 cm in the plots on the right. Our experimental (theoretical) results are the solid (dashed) curves. The phase contours are plotted every 20° and the amplitude contours are plotted in decreasing intervals of e^{-1}.

We have modeled this effect in a simple way. We replaced the sphere by a totally absorbing disk of the same diameter. The disk was chosen to lie in a plane containing the center of the sphere, with surface normal pointing in the z direction. Then we calculated the diffraction from this disk using the standard Kirchoff construction [10] that, as we have discussed previously [5], should apply to these waves, i.e.,

$$U(x_p, y_p = 0, z_p) = \frac{kz_p}{2\pi i} \int_s U(\mathbf{R}_1) \frac{e^{ikR_2}}{R_2^2} \left[\frac{i}{kR_2} + 1 \right] dx \, dy .$$

(1)

The construction is depicted in Fig. 3(a). Here $U(\mathbf{R}_1)$ is the complex amplitude of the light energy density in the plane of the disk, R_1 is the length of the vector from the source at position $\mathbf{R}_s = (x_s = 0, y_s = 0, z_s)$ to a point $\mathbf{A} = (x, y, z = 0)$ on the diffraction plane, and R_2 is the length of the vector going from $\mathbf{A}$ to the detection point $\mathbf{R}_p = (x_p, y_p = 0, z_p)$. The Green's function is derived from the point source solution for diffuse photon density waves in an infinite homogeneous medium [11] so that k is complex.

Our experimental (theoretical) results are the solid (dotted) curves in Fig. 2. We see that our simple model approximates the measured wave-front distortion reasonably well. We note that there are no free parameters in our fit, and that it was important to incorporate the effects of absorptive loss in the Intralipid in order to obtain the best agreement. The model appears to fit the experimental results better for bigger ratios of diffuse photon density wavelength to object diameter. Of course,

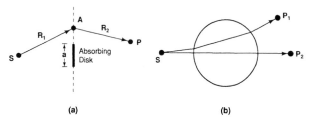

FIG. 3. (a) In our diffraction model the sphere is replaced by an absorbing disk of the same diameter ($a = 4.0$ cm), which lies in a plane through the center of the sphere. R_1 is the distance from the source S to a point $\mathbf{A}$ in the diffraction plane (dashed line) and R_2 is the distance from $\mathbf{A}$ to the image point P. Here we take the z axis to be normal to the diffraction plane, and we let the diffraction plane coincide with the xy plane (i.e., $z = 0$). The wave front at P is calculated by integrating the standard Kirchoff equation over the diffraction plane [11]. (b) In the ray model the wave front is calculated by determining the phase and amplitude of rays, which are refracted through a spherical lens.

our function $U(\mathbf{R}_1)$ in the plane of the disk is only approximately correct as a result of shadowing and diffraction by the front portion of the sphere. A similar effect will modify the scattered wave. Nevertheless, the model captures the qualitative physics of the scattering.

In Fig. 4 we show the constant phase contours (solid line) arising from the scattering of a *nonabsorptive* sphere. The Intralipid surrounding the sphere had the same concentration in both experiments, but the concentration of Intralipid inside the sphere was either smaller [Fig. 4(a)] or larger [Fig. 4(b)] than the surrounding medium. We observe that the patterns are different. Results of our simple modeling of these effects are described below.

One model is derived from ray optics where we simply treated the scatterer like a spherical lens with a different diffusional index of refraction than the surrounding medium. The basic idea of the model is depicted in Fig. 3(b).

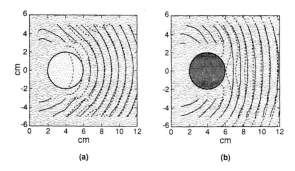

FIG. 4. The scattering of a diffuse photon density waves by purely dispersive spheres. (a) The Intralipid concentration within the spherical shell is 0.125%, less than the surrounding medium. (b) The Intralipid concentration is 2.8%, greater than the surrounding medium. For both, the surrounding Intralipid is the same, the source is located at the origin, and the sphere has a diameter of 4.0 cm and is centered at $x = 4.0$ cm, $y = 0.0$ cm. The phase contours are drawn every 20° for our experimental (solid lines) and theoretical (dashed lines) results. The theoretical results were calculated in (a) by the ray model and in (b) by the diffraction model.

To get the complex wave amplitude we simply kept track of the amplitude and phase for points along the rays emerging from the source. Some of the rays were refracted through the sphere, others were not. This model ignores multiple scattering in the sphere, since the waves are heavily damped.

Again, we do not expect the model to give perfect quantitative agreement with the measurements since diffraction effects are omitted. However, because the rays transmitted through the sphere will have a larger amplitude than pathways around the sphere, we might expect that the ray picture would work well when the diffusional index of refraction of the sphere is less than that of the surrounding Intralipid. This behavior was observed [see Fig. 4(a)]. For near axis rays the model also predicts an apparent source position at $z_s = 3.5$ cm. This is easily verified by standard ray construction techniques.

The ray method did not work well for dense spheres. The dense sphere acts more like an absorber, since the diffuse photon density wave will be significantly attenuated upon traveling through the sphere. For this reason one might expect the purely diffractive model discussed earlier to work better. Indeed, this is what was observed [see Fig. 4(b)].

In the experiments we have described, spatial inhomogeneities of varying nature were detected using diffuse photon density waves. The incident wave fronts were shown to diffract around and refract through objects, and by a clever use of an absorptive dye, new wave fronts were created within the medium by objects that reradiate at different *optical* wavelengths. Practical biomedical imaging systems with diffusing light will take advantage of these types of distortions in order to detect inhomogeneities. The reradiation technique can be applied, since emissive dyes (i.e., contrast agents) are known to be preferentially accumulated at spatial inhomogeneities [12], such as breast tumors and infarcted regions of brain tissue. In this case, the presence of any reradiated wave would signal the existence of the tumor or infarcted region, and the location of its center is reconstructed using the shape of the reradiated wave fronts. We are presently implementing this idea along with delineated antenna arrays of diffuse photon density waves to improve detection capabilities [13]. The diffracted wave fronts can also be used to detect tumors, with or without the use of absorbing dyes. Here the improved sensitivity is achieved through the interference of phased arrays of diffuse light sources [7,13].

We acknowledge useful conversations with Peter Kaplan, Tom Lubensky, K. S. Reddy, and Jack Leigh. A.G.Y. gratefully acknowledges partial support from the National Science Foundation through the Presidential Young Investigator program and Grant No. DMR-9003687, and from the Alfred P. Sloan Foundation. B.C. gratefully acknowledges support from HL-44125, ACSBE-B, NS-27346, NIM Inc., and Hamamatsu Photonics.

[1] A. Ishimaru, *Wave Propagation and Scattering in Random Media* (Academic, New York, 1978), Vol. 1.

[2] E. Gratton, W. Mantulin, M. J. van de Ven, J. Fishkin, M. Maris, and B. Chance, in *Proceedings of the Third International Conference: Peace through Mind/Brain Science,* Hamamatsu, Japan, 1990 (Hamamatsu Photonics, Hamamatsu, 1990), p. 183.

[3] J. M. Schmitt, A. Knuttel, and J. R. Knudsen, J. Opt. Soc. Am. A **9**, 1832 (1992).

[4] J. Fishkin and E. Gratton J. Opt. Soc. Am. A **10**, 127 (1993).

[5] M. A. O'Leary, D. A. Boas, B. Chance, and A. G. Yodh, Phys. Rev. Lett. **69**, 2658 (1992).

[6] See also, for example, B. J. Tromberg, L. O. Svaasand, T. Tsay, R. C. Haskell, and M. W. Berns, in *Proceedings of the SPIE '91 Vol. 1525, Future Trends in Biomedical Applications of Lasers,* Berlin, 1991, edited by S. Jaques (International Society for Optical Engineering, Bellingham, 1991), p. 52, and references therein.

[7] B. Chance, K. Kang, L. He, and J. Weng, in *Proceedings of the International Society on Oxygen Transport to Tissue (ISOTT),* Mainz, Germany, 1992, edited by P. Baupel (Plenum, New York, 1993).

[8] The Intralipid used here can be obtained from Kabi Pharmacia in Clayton, NC.

[9] Indocyanine-green is a water soluable, tricarbocyanine dye. We obtained the dye from Hynson, Wescott & Dunning, Inc., Baltimore, MD 21201.

[10] J. D. Jackson, *Classical Electrodynamics* (Wiley, New York, 1975), Chap. 9.

[11] The Green's function for this problem is derived from a superposition of Green's-function solutions of the Helmholtz equation (i.e., of the form $e^{ikr}/4\pi r$). We chose a superposition to satisfy Dirichlet boundary conditions on our diffraction plane at $z=0$. Therefore, (1) is derived from the integral $\int U(\mathbf{R}_1)(dG_D/dz)dx\,dy$ over the diffraction plane, with $G_D(R,R')=[e^{ikR}/R - e^{ikR'}/R']/4\pi$, where $\mathbf{R}=\mathbf{R}_p - \mathbf{A}$, $\mathbf{R}'=\mathbf{R}_{p'} - \mathbf{A}$, and $\mathbf{R}_{p'}$ is just the image of $\mathbf{R}_p$ reflected about the diffraction plane.

[12] F. W. Flickinger, J. D. Allison, R. Sherry, and J. C. Wright, in *Proceedings of the Society of Magnetic Resonance in Medicine 11th Annual Scientific Meeting,* Berlin, Germany, 1992 (Society of Magnetic Resonance in Medicine, San Francisco, 1992); R. N. Bryan, *ibid.*

[13] M. A. O'Leary, D. A. Boas, B. Chance, and A. G. Yodh, in *SPIE Proceedings of the Biomedical Optics Society,* Los Angeles, 1993, edited by B. Chance and R. Alfano (International Society for Optical Engineering, Bellingham, 1993).

Reprinted with permission from *Journal of the Optical Society of America A*,
Vol. 10(1), pp. 127-140 (January 1993). ©1993 Optical Society of America.

Propagation of photon-density waves in strongly scattering media containing an absorbing semi-infinite plane bounded by a straight edge

Joshua B. Fishkin and Enrico Gratton

*Laboratory for Fluorescence Dynamics, Department of Physics, University of Illinois at Urbana-Champaign,
1110 West Green Street, Urbana, Illinois 61801*

Received March 2, 1992; revised manuscript received May 18, 1992; accepted July 2, 1992

Light propagation in strongly scattering media can be described by the diffusion approximation to the Boltzmann transport equation. We have derived analytical expressions based on the diffusion approximation that describe the photon density in a uniform, infinite, strongly scattering medium that contains a sinusoidally intensity-modulated point source of light. These expressions predict that the photon density will propagate outward from the light source as a spherical wave of constant phase velocity with an amplitude that attenuates with distance r from the source as $\exp(-\alpha r)/r$. The properties of the photon-density wave are given in terms of the spectral properties of the scattering medium. We have used the Green's function obtained from the diffusion approximation to the Boltzmann transport equation with a sinusoidally modulated point source to derive analytic expressions describing the diffraction and the reflection of photon-density waves from an absorbing and/or reflecting semi-infinite plane bounded by a straight edge immersed in a strongly scattering medium. The analytic expressions given are in agreement with the results of frequency-domain experiments performed in skim-milk media and with Monte Carlo simulations. These studies provide a basis for the understanding of photon diffusion in strongly scattering media in the presence of absorbing and reflecting objects and allow for a determination of the conditions for obtaining maximum resolution and penetration for applications to optical tomography.

1. INTRODUCTION

Light diffusion in strongly scattering media is of primary importance in several fields, including spectroscopy of highly turbid media and optical imaging of thick tissues.[1–7] After a few scattering events the light propagation process can be treated as a transport of particles that undergo a large number of collisions, performing a random walk through the scattering medium. This diffusion approximation is valid at distances from the light source much larger than the mean free path for light scattering.[8,9] In a macroscopically uniform medium without boundaries the measurement of the average light intensity at different distances from the source and at different angles cannot separate scattering from absorption properties. For the case of multiple scattering of light, fluctuation correlation spectroscopy has been used largely in the study of optical properties, with an emphasis on the determination of the diffusion coefficient of the scattering particles. A large literature on this subject exists, and for a review we refer to Ref. 1. However, when the problem is the identification of macroscopic regions in the scattering medium with different absorption and transport scattering coefficients, this approach cannot be used. In the present approach we neglect the diffusion of the scattering particles. It has been suggested that the use of short light pulses can provide a better approach to the identification of different macroscopic regions with different optical properties, since the time of photon propagation through a strongly scattering medium is related to the effective optical path, which is dependent on the absorption and transport scattering coefficients of the medium. Time gating makes

possible discrimination between the direct optical path and the longer photon paths, which permits one to isolate regions of the medium with different optical properties. A number of publications have recently appeared on the different aspects of light pulse propagation and reflection, almost exclusively in the time domain.[4,6,10,11]

In this paper we present the complementary frequency-domain approach, and we show that in the frequency domain the problem of light propagation in strongly scattering media can be treated within the familiar framework of wave phenomena. It must be remembered that, in the frequency-domain method, only the front of the photon-density wave is considered, not the optical light front, which is multiply scattered in the diffusion regime. In particular, we derive the Green's function for the diffusion approximation to the Boltzmann transport equation with a sinusoidally modulated point source, and we experimentally verify the basic predictions of the theory. Having in mind the problem of optical imaging of tissues and its application to medicine, we performed a frequency-domain study of the problem of the diffusion of photons in the presence of a semi-infinite absorbing plane bounded by a straight edge. Our aim in studying the effect of the edge on the diffusing photons is to determine systematically the conditions necessary for obtaining the highest spatial resolution by observing how different parameters of the experiment affect the sharpness of the edge. In this paper we present an analytical solution to the edge problem in the frequency domain that is derived from the above-mentioned Green's function, and we verify with experiments the principal features of the solution. Hebden and Kruger have reported preliminary time-domain observations of the effect of an absorbing edge on photon diffusion.[12] We perform frequency-domain Monte Carlo simulations of particles diffusing in a lattice in which we simulate the presence of an absorbing plane bounded by a straight edge to verify the theoretical prediction further and to compare it with experiments.

The detection of unscattered photons in strongly scattering media has also received attention.[13] Of course, if unscattered light can be detected, optical spectroscopy and optical imaging are feasible in the conventional way. However, for most applications to the medical field, the use of unscattered light for optical imaging is restricted to only a few tissues such as the eye or to tissues that are at most a few millimeters thick.[14]

2. ANALYTICAL SOLUTION FOR A UNIFORM INFINITE MEDIUM

An isotropic source of visible or near-infrared light is immersed in a macroscopically homogeneous, strongly scattering medium. It is assumed for this case that the density of photons $U(\mathbf{r}, t)$ and the photon current density $\mathbf{J}(\mathbf{r}, t)$ satisfy the diffusion approximation to the Boltzmann transport equation[1,9,15]:

$$\frac{\partial U(\mathbf{r}, t)}{\partial t} + v\mu_a U(\mathbf{r}, t) + \nabla \cdot \mathbf{J}(\mathbf{r}, t) = q_0(\mathbf{r}, t), \quad (1a)$$

$$\nabla U(\mathbf{r}, t) + \frac{3\partial \mathbf{J}(\mathbf{r}, t)}{v^2 \partial t} + \frac{\mathbf{J}(\mathbf{r}, t)}{vD} = 0, \quad (1b)$$

where v is the speed of a photon in the transporting medium (i.e., water in our experiments), D is the diffusion coefficient, namely,

$$D = \{3[\mu_a + \mu_s(1 - g)]\}^{-1}, \quad (2)$$

μ_a is the linear absorption coefficient (i.e., the inverse of the mean free path for photon absorption, with units of inverse distance), μ_s is the linear scattering coefficient (i.e., the inverse of the mean free path for photon scattering), g is the average of the cosine of the scattering angle, and $q_0(\mathbf{r}, t)$ is the photon source. Equations (1) imply a tremendous simplification. Use of the diffusion approximation to the Boltzmann transport equation means neglect of interference terms arising from the superpositioning of electromagnetic fields. Polarization as a degree of freedom is also neglected. The density of photons and the photon current density can be accurately calculated from the diffusion approximation to the Boltzmann transport equation when the point of interest is far from sources or boundaries and when the ratio $\mu_s/(\mu_a + \mu_s)$ is close to unity, i.e., when the absorption of the medium is low.[15]

In the case of a sinusoidally intensity-modulated point source of light, the photon source is

$$q_0(\mathbf{r}, t) = \delta(\mathbf{r})S\{1 + A \exp[-i(\omega t + \epsilon)]\}, \quad (3)$$

where $\delta(\mathbf{r})$ is a Dirac delta function located at the origin, S is the fluence of the source (in photons per second), A is the modulation of the source, $i = \sqrt{-1}$, ω is the angular modulation frequency of the source, and ϵ is an arbitrary phase. Substituting Eq. (3) into Eq. (1a) and assuming that $U(\mathbf{r}, t)$ and $\mathbf{J}(\mathbf{r}, t)$ have the forms

$$U(\mathbf{r}, t) = [U(\mathbf{r})]_{dc} + [U(\mathbf{r})]_{ac} \exp[-i(\omega t + \epsilon)], \quad (4a)$$

$$\mathbf{J}(\mathbf{r}, t) = [\mathbf{J}(\mathbf{r})]_{dc} + [\mathbf{J}(\mathbf{r})]_{ac} \exp[-i(\omega t + \epsilon)], \quad (4b)$$

we obtain the steady-state equations (i.e., the dc part)

$$v\mu_a[U(\mathbf{r})]_{dc} + \nabla \cdot [\mathbf{J}(\mathbf{r})]_{dc} = S\delta(\mathbf{r}), \quad (5a)$$

$$[\mathbf{J}(\mathbf{r})]_{dc} = -vD\nabla[U(\mathbf{r})]_{dc} \quad (5b)$$

and the frequency-dependent equations (i.e., the ac part)

$$(v\mu_a - i\omega)[U(\mathbf{r})]_{ac} + \nabla \cdot [\mathbf{J}(\mathbf{r})]_{ac} = SA\delta(\mathbf{r}), \quad (6a)$$

$$[\mathbf{J}(\mathbf{r})]_{ac} = -vD\left[\frac{1 + i3\omega D/v}{1 + (3\omega D/v)^2}\right]\nabla[U(\mathbf{r})]_{ac}. \quad (6b)$$

We make the assumption that $\omega D \ll v$, which is equivalent to saying that the wavelength in vacuum of the wave of angular frequency ω is much larger than the distance between the scattering particles in the medium. With this assumption Eq. (6b) reduces to

$$[\mathbf{J}(\mathbf{r})]_{ac} \cong -vD\nabla[U(\mathbf{r})]_{ac}. \quad (7)$$

Eliminating the dependent variable $[\mathbf{J}(\mathbf{r})]_{dc}$ from Eqs. (5), we obtain the steady-state diffusion equation

$$\nabla^2[U(\mathbf{r})]_{dc} - (\mu_a/D)[U(\mathbf{r})]_{dc} = -(S/vD)\delta(\mathbf{r}). \quad (8)$$

Eliminating the dependent variable $[\mathbf{J}(\mathbf{r})]_{ac}$ from Eq. (6a) and expression (7), we obtain the frequency-dependent diffusion equation

$$\nabla^2[U(\mathbf{r})]_{ac} - \left(\frac{v\mu_a - i\omega}{vD}\right)[U(\mathbf{r})]_{ac} = -\frac{SA}{vD}\delta(\mathbf{r}). \quad (9)$$

For an infinite medium, Eqs. (8) and (9) can easily be solved to yield

$$U(\mathbf{r}, t) = \frac{S}{4\pi vDr} \exp\left[-r\left(\frac{\mu_a}{D}\right)^{1/2}\right] + \frac{SA}{4\pi vDr}$$
$$\times \exp\left\{-r\left(\frac{v^2\mu_a{}^2 + \omega^2}{v^2 D^2}\right)^{1/4} \cos\left[\frac{1}{2}\tan^{-1}\left(\frac{\omega}{v\mu_a}\right)\right]\right\}$$
$$\times \exp\left\{ir\left(\frac{v^2\mu_a{}^2 + \omega^2}{v^2 D^2}\right)^{1/4} \sin\left[\frac{1}{2}\tan^{-1}\left(\frac{\omega}{v\mu_a}\right)\right]\right.$$
$$\left. - i(\omega t + \epsilon)\right\}. \quad (10)$$

For a nonabsorbing medium, $\mu_a = 0$, and Eq. (10) reduces to

$$U(\mathbf{r}, t) = \frac{S}{4\pi vDr} + \frac{SA}{4\pi vDr} \exp\left[-r\left(\frac{\omega}{2vD}\right)^{1/2}\right]$$
$$\times \exp\left[ir\left(\frac{\omega}{2vD}\right)^{1/2} - i(\omega t + \epsilon)\right]. \quad (11)$$

Equation (10) is the Fourier transform equivalent of

$$\rho(\mathbf{r}, t) = \frac{1}{(4\pi vDt)^{3/2}} \exp\left(-\frac{r^2}{4vDt} - \mu_a vt\right), \quad (12)$$

which is the time-dependent solution of the diffusion equation as reported by Patterson et al.[6] Here, $\rho(\mathbf{r}, t)$ is the photon density that satisfies the diffusion approximation to the Boltzmann transport equation when the source term is a narrow pulse given by $q_0(\mathbf{r}, t) = \delta(\mathbf{r})\delta(t)$. Examination of Eqs. (10) and (11) shows that the photon density $U(\mathbf{r}, t)$ generated by a sinusoidally intensity-modulated point source immersed in a strongly scattering, infinite medium constitutes a scalar field that is propagating at a constant speed in a spherical wave and attenuates as

$\exp(-\alpha r)/r$ as it propagates. Equations (10) and (12) show the practical difference in describing photon diffusion in the frequency domain with respect to its Fourier transform equivalent in the time domain: the photon density generated by a sinusoidally intensity-modulated source at any given modulation frequency propagates with a single phase velocity, while pulses undergo dispersion owing to the different phase velocity of each frequency component of the pulse.

The approach that regards photon transport in strongly scattering media as a diffusional process shows that light emitted from a sinusoidally intensity-modulated point source in such a medium can be treated within the framework of wave phenomena; we therefore refer to $U(\mathbf{r}, t)$ as a photon-density wave. The study of the propagation, the reflection, and the refraction of these waves becomes a trivial problem. For a nonabsorbing medium the photon-density wave emitted from a source of angular modulation frequency ω has a wavelength, from Eq. (11), of

$$\lambda = 2\pi(2vD/\omega)^{1/2}, \qquad (13)$$

and its wave front advances at constant speed

$$V = (2vD\omega)^{1/2}. \qquad (14)$$

Note that Eqs. (13) and (14), respectively, describe the wavelength and the phase velocity of a photon-density wave, not the wavelength and the phase velocity of the electromagnetic wave, which is multiply scattered for the case of visible and near-infrared light propagating over large distances in strongly scattering media. Sinusoidal modulation of the intensity of a light source in strongly scattering media has the following consequences:

(1) A diffraction pattern caused by an object immersed in a strongly scattering medium should be evident in the presence of a photon-density wave. From the Green's function solution of Eq. (9), we can use the superposition principle to calculate this diffraction pattern caused by the absorbing and/or reflecting object.

(2) An apparent index of refraction of the photon-density wave can be defined as the ratio of the phase velocity of the photon-density wave to the phase velocity of light in vacuum.

(3) The phase velocity is dependent on the modulation frequency of the source but is independent of the distance from the source.

(4) There is an exponential attenuation of the amplitude of a photon-density wave as it propagates in the strongly scattering medium because of the first-order time derivative in Eqs. (1).

Figure 1(a) gives a schematic representation of light intensity measured in response to a narrow pulse emitted into a strongly scattering medium, and Fig. 1(b) shows the time evolution of the intensity measured when light from a sinusoidally intensity-modulated source propagates through the same medium. In Fig. 1(b) the light signal measured by the detector is of the same modulation frequency as that of the light source, but it is shifted in phase and demodulated relative to the light source. The quantities that are measured in a frequency-domain experiment, namely, the phase lag Φ of the signal at the detector relative to the source, the average intensity of the detected signal (i.e., the dc), and the amplitude of the frequency-dependent part of the detected signal (i.e., the ac), are shown in Fig. 1(b). Equation (10) yields expressions for these experimentally determined quantities in a uniform, infinite medium:

$$\Phi = r\left(\frac{v^2\mu_a^2 + \omega^2}{v^2D^2}\right)^{1/4} \sin\left[\frac{1}{2}\tan^{-1}\left(\frac{\omega}{v\mu_a}\right)\right],$$
$$(15)$$

$$\ln[(r)(\mathrm{dc})] = -r\left(\frac{\mu_a}{D}\right)^{1/2} + \ln\left(\frac{S}{4\pi vD}\right), \qquad (16)$$

$$\ln[(r)(\mathrm{ac})] = -r\left(\frac{v^2\mu_a^2 + \omega^2}{v^2D^2}\right)^{1/4}$$
$$\times \cos\left[\frac{1}{2}\tan^{-1}\left(\frac{\omega}{v\mu_a}\right)\right] + \ln\left(\frac{SA}{4\pi vD}\right). \quad (17)$$

The above three expressions are linear functions of the source/detector separation r but have a more complicated

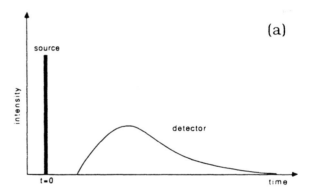

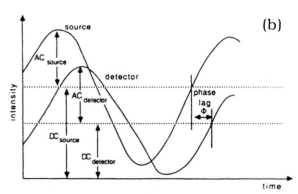

Fig. 1. (a) Schematic representation of the time evolution of the light intensity measured in response to a narrow light pulse traversing an arbitrary distance in a scattering and absorbing medium. If the medium is strongly scattering, there are no unscattered components in the transmitted pulse. (b) Time evolution of the intensity from a sinusoidally intensity-modulated source. The transmitted photon wave retains the same frequency as the incoming wave but is delayed owing to the phase velocity of the wave in the medium. The reduced amplitude of the transmitted wave arises from attenuation related to scattering and absorption processes. The demodulation is the ratio ac/dc normalized to the modulation of the source.

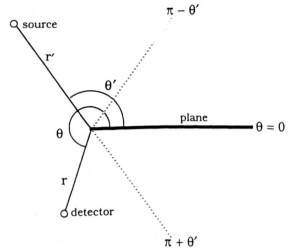

Fig. 2. Cylindrical coordinate system used to describe the configuration of a semi-infinite plane bounded by a straight edge, the point photon source, and the point detector. The edge of the plane lies on the z axis, and the face of the plane is at $\theta = 0$. The coordinates of the point source are (r', θ', z'), and the coordinates of the detector are (r, θ, z).

dependence on ω, v, μ_a, μ_s, and g. Note that the natural logarithm of the demodulation, i.e., $\ln(\mathrm{ac/dc})$, is also linear in r. Thus it is seen that the linear dependence on r of Φ, $\ln[(r)(\mathrm{dc})]$, and $\ln[(r)(\mathrm{ac})]$ is a necessary but not a sufficient condition for the validity of the diffusion approxima-

dinate system with the edge of the semi-infinite plane lying on the z axis and the plane itself at $\theta = 0$. The coordinates of the point source are (r', θ', z'), and the coordinates of the detector are (r, θ, z), as shown in Fig. 2. On inspection of our steady-state and frequency-dependent equations for photon diffusion, i.e., Eqs. (8) and (9), respectively, we see that our physical problem, like the sound-wave problem solved by Carslaw, reduces to the solution of an equation of the form

$$\nabla^2 U + k^2 U = -4\pi\delta(\mathbf{R}) \qquad (18)$$

in the twofold Riemann space described by Carslaw,[16] Sommerfeld,[17] and Jeans,[18] where the source/detector separation R is given by

$$R = [r^2 + r'^2 + (z - z')^2 - 2rr'\cos(\theta - \theta')]^{1/2} \qquad (19)$$

and where U is a function of r, θ, and z and has the following properties:

(1) It is a finite, single-valued, and continuous function of position in the twofold Riemann space.

(2) It has one and only one infinity, this being at the point (r', θ', z') on the first sheet of the Riemann space, with U approximating the function $\exp(-ikR)/R$ as R approaches zero.

(3) It is zero at $r = \infty$.

Carslaw gives two solutions of Eq. (18) in the twofold Riemann space that satisfy the above conditions[16]:

$$U_1(\theta') = \frac{\exp(-ikR)}{R} - \frac{1}{\pi}\cos\left[\frac{1}{2}(\theta - \theta')\right]\int_0^\infty \frac{\exp\{-ik[r^2 + r'^2 + (z - z')^2 + 2rr'\cosh\beta]^{1/2}\}\cosh(\beta/2)\mathrm{d}\beta}{[r^2 + r'^2 + (z - z')^2 + 2rr'\cosh\beta]^{1/2}[\cos(\theta - \theta') + \cosh\beta]}, \qquad (20)$$

$$U_2(\theta') = -\frac{1}{\pi}\cos\left[\frac{1}{2}(\theta - \theta')\right]\int_0^\infty \frac{\exp\{-ik[r^2 + r'^2 + (z - z')^2 + 2rr'\cosh\beta]^{1/2}\}\cosh(\beta/2)\mathrm{d}\beta}{[r^2 + r'^2 + (z - z')^2 + 2rr'\cosh\beta]^{1/2}[\cos(\theta - \theta') + \cosh\beta]}, \qquad (21)$$

tion to the Boltzmann transport equation. We note that we can obtain the optical properties of a macroscopically homogeneous, infinite, strongly scattering medium by fitting the phase, demodulation, and dc intensity data to Eq. (10) to recover μ_a and D.

3. DIFFRACTION BY AN EDGE

We will now use the Green's functions obtained from Eqs. (8) and (9) above to calculate the diffraction and the reflection of photon-density waves from an absorbing and/or reflecting semi-infinite thin plane bounded by a straight edge, the plane being immersed in an infinite, strongly scattering medium. The study of this problem will provide information about how sharply an edge immersed in a highly turbid medium can appear and what parameters affect the sharpness. In performing the calculation to study the effect of an edge on a photon-density wave, we follow the methodology of Carslaw[16] in his study of a point source of sound in the presence of a thin, rigid semi-infinite plane bounded by a straight edge. Carslaw's research on this topic involves an extension of the methodology developed by Sommerfeld[17] in his study of a single point charge in the presence of an uninsulated, semi-infinite conducting plane at zero potential. So, following Sommerfeld and Carslaw, we use a cylindrical coor-

where $U_1(\theta') = U_2(\theta') = (1/2)\exp(-ikR)/R$ when $\theta = \pi + \theta'$ and $U_1(-\theta') = U_2(-\theta') = (1/2)\exp(-ikR)/R$ when $\theta = \pi - \theta'$. Note that U_1 and U_2 are periodic in θ with a period of 4π. With respect to the dc part of the photon density, we compare Eq. (8), the steady-state diffusion equation, with Eq. (18) and write

$$k_{\mathrm{dc}} \equiv -i(\mu_a/D)^{1/2}, \qquad (22)$$

noting that the source strength of Eq. (8) is $-S/vD$ as compared with the source strength of Eq. (18), which is -4π. We then have the two solutions to Eq. (8) in the twofold Riemann space, i.e., $U_{\mathrm{dc1}}(\theta')$ and $U_{\mathrm{dc2}}(\theta')$, these solutions being analogous to $U_1(\theta')$ and $U_2(\theta')$ in Eqs. (20) and (21), respectively, but with the substitution of k_{dc} for k and with an additional pre-exponential factor of $S/4\pi vD$. With respect to the ac part of the photon density, we compare Eq. (9), the frequency-dependent diffusion equation, with Eq. (18) and write

$$k_{\mathrm{ac}} \equiv -i\left(\frac{v\mu_a - i\omega}{vD}\right)^{1/2} \qquad (23)$$

or

$$-ik_{\mathrm{ac}} = -\left(\frac{v^2\mu_a{}^2 + \omega^2}{v^2 D^2}\right)^{1/4}\cos\left[\frac{1}{2}\tan^{-1}\left(\frac{\omega}{v\mu_a}\right)\right] + i\left(\frac{v^2\mu_a{}^2 + \omega^2}{v^2 D^2}\right)^{1/4}\sin\left[\frac{1}{2}\tan^{-1}\left(\frac{\omega}{v\mu_a}\right)\right] \qquad (24)$$

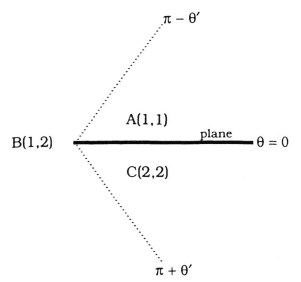

Fig. 3. Division of the physical space into three regions about the semi-infinite plane bounded by a straight edge and the corresponding values of U_1 and U_2 used for $U(\theta')$ and $U(-\theta')$ in each region of the physical space.

and note that the source strength of Eq. (9) is $-SA/vD$. We then have the two solutions to Eq. (9) in the twofold Riemann space, i.e., $U_{ac1}(\theta')$, and $U_{ac2}(\theta')$, which are analogous to $U_1(\theta')$ and $U_2(\theta')$ in Eqs. (20) and (21), respectively, but with the substitution of k_{ac} for k and with an additional pre-exponential factor of $SA/4\pi vD$.

The boundary condition imposed by a semi-infinite absorbing plane is that the photon density U must vanish at $\theta = 0$ and $\theta = 2\pi$. To satisfy this condition, we put poles at (r',θ',z') and $(r',-\theta',z')$ and take the physical space to be the first sheet of the twofold Riemann space, as defined by

$$0 < \theta < 2\pi,$$

and the imaginary space to be the second sheet of the twofold Riemann space, as defined by

$$-2\pi < \theta < 0.$$

Thus

$$\overline{U} = U(\theta') - U(-\theta') \qquad (25)$$

satisfies all the conditions of the physical problem posed by an absorbing plane in a strongly scattering medium, where $U(\theta')$ is the source function and $U(-\theta')$ is the image function.

As shown by Carslaw,[16] care must be taken in the choice of proper values for $U(\theta')$ and $U(-\theta')$ in Eq. (25), the choice of these functions being dependent on the value of θ in the physical space. The physical space is divided into three regions, as shown in Fig. 3. In the region $0 \le \theta < \pi - \theta'$ the values for both $U(\theta')$ and $U(-\theta')$ in Eq. (25) are given by U_1. In the region $\pi - \theta' < \theta < \pi + \theta'$, U_1 is taken for $U(\theta')$ and U_2 is taken for $U(-\theta')$. In the region $\pi + \theta' < \theta \le 2\pi$ the values for both $U(\theta')$ and $U(-\theta')$ are given by U_2. At the coordinate $\theta = \pi - \theta'$, U_1 is taken for $U(\theta')$ and $(1/2)\exp(-ikR)/R$ is taken for $U(-\theta')$, where R is defined in Eq. (19) as the source/detector separation. At the

coordinate $\theta = \pi + \theta'$, $(1/2)\exp(-ikR)/R$ is taken for $U(\theta')$ and U_2 is taken for $U(-\theta')$. Thus the solution to the problem of the absorbing semi-infinite plane takes the following forms (refer to Fig. 3):

Region A:

$$\overline{U}_{dc} = U_{dc1}(\theta') - U_{dc1}(-\theta'), \qquad (26)$$

$$\overline{U}_{ac} = U_{ac1}(\theta') - U_{ac1}(-\theta'); \qquad (27)$$

Region B:

$$\overline{U}_{dc} = U_{dc1}(\theta') - U_{dc2}(-\theta'), \qquad (28)$$

$$\overline{U}_{ac} = U_{ac1}(\theta') - U_{ac2}(-\theta'); \qquad (29)$$

Region C:

$$\overline{U}_{dc} = U_{dc2}(\theta') - U_{dc2}(-\theta'), \qquad (30)$$

$$\overline{U}_{ac} = U_{ac2}(\theta') - U_{ac2}(-\theta'); \qquad (31)$$

At $\pi - \theta'$:

$$\overline{U}_{dc} = U_{dc1}(\theta') - \frac{1}{2}\frac{S}{4\pi vD}\frac{\exp[-R(\mu_a/D)^{1/2}]}{R}, \qquad (32)$$

$$\overline{U}_{ac} = U_{ac1}(\theta') - \frac{1}{2}\frac{SA}{4\pi vD}\frac{\exp(-ik_{ac}R)}{R}; \qquad (33)$$

At $\pi + \theta'$:

$$\overline{U}_{dc} = \frac{1}{2}\frac{S}{4\pi vD}\frac{\exp[-R(\mu_a/D)^{1/2}]}{R} - U_{dc2}(-\theta'), \qquad (34)$$

$$\overline{U}_{ac} = \frac{1}{2}\frac{SA}{4\pi vD}\frac{\exp(-ik_{ac}R))}{R} - U_{ac2}(-\theta'). \qquad (35)$$

We see from Eqs. (26) and (27) that at $\theta = 0$, $\overline{U}_{dc} = 0$ and $\overline{U}_{ac} = 0$ for $0 < r < \infty$, and from Eqs. (30) and (31) we see that at $\theta = 2\pi$, $\overline{U}_{dc} = 0$ and $\overline{U}_{ac} = 0$ for $0 < r < \infty$.

For a reflecting semi-infinite plane the boundary condition is that $(1/r)\partial U/\partial\theta$ must vanish at $\theta = 0$ and $\theta = 2\pi$. This condition is met in a manner that is analogous to the solution for the photon-absorbing plane, the only difference being that for the reflecting plane we add the source function to the image function to satisfy the boundary condition.

Thus

$$\overline{U} = U(\theta') + U(-\theta') \qquad (36)$$

satisfies the boundary condition imposed by a reflecting plane in a strongly scattering medium.

For the case of a semi-infinite plane that has a probability p_{abs} of absorbing a photon that collides with it, the solution of the physical problem is given by

$$\overline{U} = U(\theta') - p_{abs}U(-\theta') + (1 - p_{abs})U(-\theta'). \qquad (37)$$

When $p_{abs} = 1$, Eq. (37) reduces to Eq. (25), the solution for the absorbing plane, and when $p_{abs} = 0$, Eq. (37) reduces to Eq. (36), the solution for the reflecting plane. If some of the light is able to pass through the plane, we add an isotropic source term such as Eq. (10) above at point (r',θ',z') with a coefficient proportional to the transmission probability and we normalize the absorption, reflection, and transmission probabilities.

The phase shift Φ relative to the source, the average (dc) intensity, and the amplitude of the frequency-dependent part of the signal (the ac) are given by

$$\Phi = \tan^{-1}\left[\frac{\text{Im}(\overline{U}_{\text{ac}})}{\text{Re}(\overline{U}_{\text{ac}})}\right], \qquad (38)$$

$$\text{dc} = \overline{U}_{\text{dc}}, \qquad (39)$$

$$\text{ac} = [\text{Re}(\overline{U}_{\text{ac}})^2 + \text{Im}(\overline{U}_{\text{ac}})^2]^{1/2}, \qquad (40)$$

respectively, and

$$\text{demodulation} = \text{ac/dc}, \qquad (41)$$

where $\text{Re}(\overline{U}_{\text{ac}})$ and $\text{Im}(\overline{U}_{\text{ac}})$ are, respectively, the real and the imaginary parts of $\overline{U}_{\text{ac}}$.

4. MONTE CARLO SIMULATION

To confirm further the validity of the analytical solution and to treat problems with more complicated boundary conditions, we implemented a Monte Carlo simulation program to trace individual photon histories. We simulated a point source of photons in a homogeneous cubic lattice in which each cell has a probability for absorption and scattering. We also added a semi-infinite absorbing plane bounded by a straight edge to the homogeneous lattice, where the plane had the thickness of a lattice cell. We performed the simulations by using a random-number generator to sample discrete events from probability distributions derived from the speed of a photon, v, in the scattering medium, the absorption coefficient μ_a, the scattering coefficient μ_s, and the average cosine of scattering angle, g. In a given simulation we built up a time histogram in the three-dimensional lattice by tracing at least 10^6 individual photon histories. We then performed a fast Fourier transform on the time histogram at each point in the lattice to obtain a frequency-domain Monte Carlo simulation, that is, a simulation of an intensity-modulated point source in a strongly scattering medium. The size of the lattice was such that, for the value of μ_a used, no photon escaped the lattice.

5. EXPERIMENTAL APPARATUS AND METHOD

We have studied the photon-transport properties of strongly scattering media through frequency-domain experiments on 3.78 L of skim milk mixed with quantities of black India ink varying from no ink to 2000 μL of ink. We have qualitatively compared the data from the analytical solutions, the Monte Carlo simulations, and the skim-milk experiments.

For the skim-milk experiments our light source was a Spectra Diode Laboratories SDL-2431-H2 diode laser with a 1-m fiber optic pigtail of diameter 100 μm. The average diode current was set at values ranging from 200 to 830 mA and was sinusoidally modulated with a Marconi Instruments Model 2022A signal generator with its output amplified by a Model M502C wideband rf amplifier from RF Power Labs, Inc. In a given experiment, light was transferred from the diode laser into the skim-milk/black-India-ink medium through the optical fiber pigtail of the diode laser, the end of the fiber being immersed in

the milk/black-ink solution. The wavelength of the diode-laser light was 810 nm, and the intensity of the light source was modulated at frequencies ranging from 20 to 120 MHz, the modulation frequency being fixed for a given experiment. The light detector was a 3-mm-diameter optical fiber bundle with one end immersed in the skim-milk solution and the other end attached to a Hamamatsu R928 photomultiplier. The photomultiplier signals were processed by a cross-correlation electronics system using the digital acquisition system described by Feddersen et al.[19] In the course of the skim-milk experiments, care was taken to keep the ends of the source and detector optical fibers as far as possible from the walls of the solution container and from the surface of the solution. The entire setup was completely protected from room light that could influence the dc measurement.

Three types of experiment were performed by the Monte Carlo simulations and the skim-milk/black-India-ink experiments. In one type of experiment we measured the phase shift Φ, the dc intensity, and the ac amplitude of the light intensity [Fig. 1(b) above] at a given modulation frequency as a function of the source/detector separation r to verify the validity of the diffusion approximation result of Eq. (10) above. Here, the phase data were recorded relative to the phase measurement made at the shortest source/detector separation distance, and the dc and ac data were normalized to the respective dc and ac values made at the shortest source/detector separation distance. In the case in which this experiment was performed on skim milk, the end of the detector optical fiber was immersed in the milk at a distance r from the source optical fiber, with the ends of the two fibers pointing in the same direction, as shown in Fig. 4. This orientation of the end of the detector fiber relative to the end of the source optical fiber ensured that only scattered photons were detected. In the skim-milk experiments the source/detector separation was varied from 2.5 to 9.6 cm in increments of 0.115 cm during the course of an experiment. The two other types of experiment were undertaken to verify the validity of Eqs. (26)–(35) above. We measured the effect that an absorbing semi-infinite plane immersed in our scattering media had on the intensity-modulated light. The geometry for these experiments is explained in the caption to Fig. 5. We measured the phase shift Φ, the dc

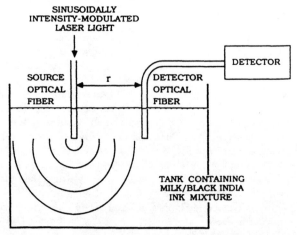

Fig. 4. Schematic of the experimental setup used to test the validity of the diffusion approximation result of Eq. (10) above.

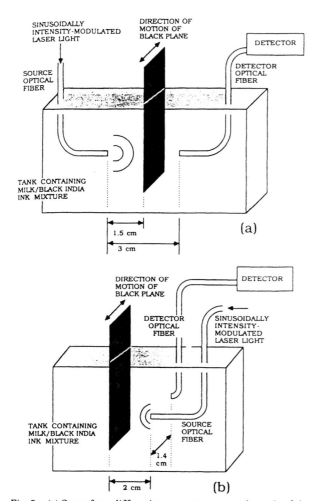

Fig. 5. (a) Setup for a diffraction measurement: the ends of the source and detector optical fibers are set a fixed distance apart (3 cm) on opposite sides of the absorbing plane, the face of the absorbing plane is oriented perpendicularly to the line joining the ends of the source and detector optical fibers, and each point of the face of the plane is equidistant from the end of each optical fiber. Measurements are performed as a function of the position of the edge of the plane relative to the line joining the source and the detector optical fibers. The 0-cm position of the plane edge is defined to be the point where the edge of the plane crosses the line joining the ends of the source and detector optical fibers. (b) Setup for a reflection measurement: same as that in (a), except that now the ends of the source and detector optical fibers are set a fixed distance (1.4 cm) apart on the same side of the absorbing plane, with the ends of the optical fibers pointing in a direction that is perpendicular to the face of the plane. The 0-cm position of the plane edge is defined to be the point where the edge of the plane crosses the line coming from the end of the source optical fiber.

intensity, the ac amplitude, and the demodulation of the signal at a given modulation frequency for each position of the source and detector optical fibers relative to the edge of the plane. The phase data were recorded relative to the phase measurement made when the source and the detector were in their initial positions relative to the edge of the plane, that is, where the plane was far from the source and the detector and the dc intensity, ac amplitude, and demodulation data, respectively, were normalized to the dc intensity, ac amplitude, and demodulation values recorded for the initial position of the source and the detector relative to the edge of the plane.

6. RESULTS OF EXPERIMENTS ON HOMOGENEOUS MEDIA

Figures 6–9 show plots derived from frequency-domain experiments in homogeneous mixtures of skim milk and black India ink and from frequency-domain Monte Carlo simulations. Figure 6 shows the phase shift of the detected sinusoidally intensity-modulated light signal versus the source/detector separation in media of different absorptions μ_a. The linearity of the phase shifts in Fig. 6 with respect to the source/detector separation r is consistent with the predictions of Eq. (15) above, indicating that the photon density generated by a sinusoidally intensity-modulated light source propagates with a single phase velocity through the strongly scattering media. Figure 7 shows phase-shift values at four source/detector separations versus the square root of the modulation frequency of the light intensity. Equation (15) predicts that for $\mu_a = 0$ the phase will increase linearly as the square root of the modulation frequency, which is not the case for the data shown in Fig. 7, owing to μ_a's being equal to 0.000125/mm

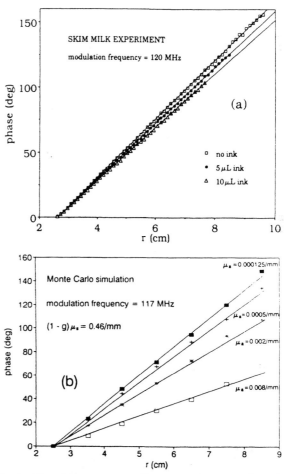

Fig. 6. Phase lag versus source/detector separation r, where the source and the detector are immersed in 3.78 L of skim milk mixed with three amounts of black India ink. The phase data were plotted relative to the phase measured with the shortest source/detector separation. The data were collected at a 120-MHz modulation frequency. The correlation coefficients for the lines fitting data of each milk/ink mixture are equal to 1.000. (b) Frequency-domain Monte Carlo simulation of phase lag versus source/detector separation r for four values of μ_a. The data were plotted relative to the phase at 2.5 cm from the source.

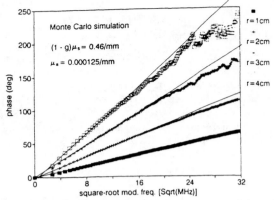

Fig. 7. Frequency-domain Monte Carlo simulation of phase lag versus the square root of modulation frequency. Each set of data was obtained at a fixed source/detector separation.

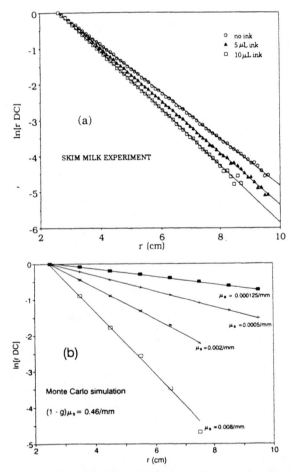

Fig. 8. (a) Natural logarithm of the source/detector separation r multiplying the dc intensity obtained at r, versus r, where the source and the detector are immersed in 3.78 L of skim milk mixed with three amounts of black India ink. The data are normalized to the r dc value at $r = 2.5$ cm. The correlation coefficients for the lines fitting these data are equal to 1.000. (b) Monte Carlo simulation of $\ln(r\ dc)$ versus r for four values of μ_a. The data are normalized to the r dc value at $r = 2.5$ cm.

in this particular frequency-domain Monte Carlo simulation. Figures 8 and 9 report plots of the natural logarithm of the source/detector separation r multiplying the dc intensity and the ac intensity of the detected light signal versus the source/detector separation r in media of

different absorptions μ_a. The linearity of the fits to the data in Figs. 8 and 9 is consistent with the predictions of Eqs. (16) and (17) respectively, as are the decreasing values of the slopes of the linear fits to the data in Figs. 8 and 9 with respect to the increasing media absorption μ_a.

The slopes of the linear fits to the phase-shift data of Fig. 6(a) were used in the calculation (Table 1) of values for the wavelength λ and the phase velocity V of sinusoidally intensity-modulated light at 120-MHz modulation frequency as it propagates in the homogeneous scattering medium (3.78 L of skim milk mixed with no ink to 10 μL of black India ink). Comparing the wavelength and the phase velocity of the 120-MHz light-intensity wave in a vacuum with the wavelength and the phase velocity of the 120-MHz photon-density wave in the skim-milk media,

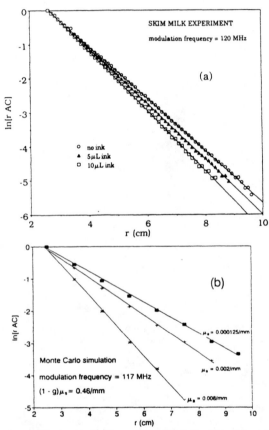

Fig. 9. (a) Natural logarithm of the source/detector separation r multiplying the ac amplitude obtained at r, versus r, where the source and the detector are immersed in 3.78 L of skim milk mixed with three amounts of black India ink. The data are normalized to the r ac value at $r = 2.5$ cm. The correlation coefficients for the lines fitting these data are equal to 1.000. (b) Frequency-domain Monte Carlo simulation of $\ln(r\ ac)$ versus r for three values of μ_a. The data are normalized to the r ac value at $r = 2.5$ cm.

Table 1. Wavelength and Phase Velocity of a Photon Density Wave in 3.78 L of Skim Milk Mixed with Black India Ink[a]

	λ (mm)	V (mm/s)
No ink	160	1.92×10^{10}
5 μL of black ink	168	2.02×10^{10}
10 μL of black ink	176	2.11×10^{10}

[a] $\omega/2\pi = 120$ MHz.

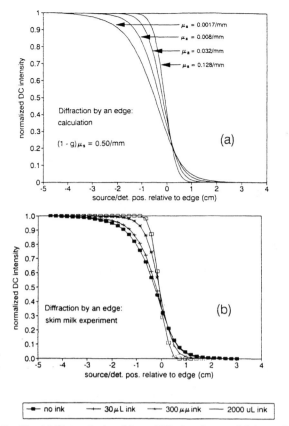

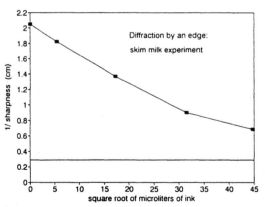

Fig. 10. (a) Plots calculated from diffusion theory of dc intensity at four medium absorptions versus the position of an absorbing edge. (b) Measurement in skim milk mixed with four amounts of black India ink of dc light intensity versus the position of an absorbing edge.

Fig. 11. Inverse sharpness of an edge (the sharpness is the inverse of the distance moved by the edge, relative to the source/detector position, that causes the intensity to decrease from 90% to 10% of the initial value) versus the square root of the volume of black India ink in the skim milk. This figure was derived from the plots in Fig. 10(b).

we see that the wavlength and the phase velocity of the photon-density wave in skim milk are reduced by a factor of the order of 10 relative to the wavelength and the phase velocity, respectively, of the light-intensity wave in a vacuum. The values in Table 1 show that, as the medium absorption increases, the wavelength of the photon-density wave increases, as does the phase velocity. The magnitude of the photon-absorbing properties of a transporting

medium thus has implications for the use of sinusoidally intensity-modulated light in the imaging of objects immersed in strongly scattering media: the effect of increasing the photon-absorbing properties of a scattering medium reduces the resolving power of the frequency-dependent part of the photon density by increasing its wavelength. This result is consistent with Eq. (10) above. Note that Eq. (10) also predicts that increasing the density of scatterers in a transporting medium improves the resolving power of the frequency-dependent part of the photon density by reducing its wavelength. As the results in Section 7 will show, the ability to resolve an object immersed in a highly scattering medium may be improved by

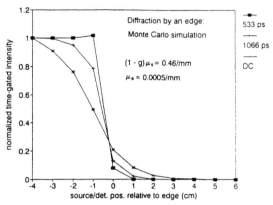

Fig. 12. Monte Carlo simulation of the time-gated intensity versus the position of an absorbing edge.

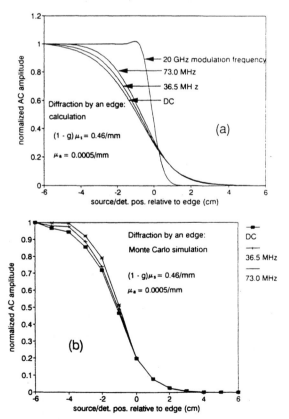

Fig. 13. (a) Plots calculated from diffusion theory of ac amplitude at four modulation frequencies versus the position of an absorbing edge. (b) Frequency-domain Monte Carlo simulation of ac amplitude at three modulation frequencies versus the position of an absorbing edge.

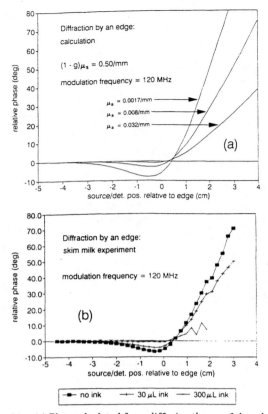

Fig. 14. (a) Plots calculated from diffusion theory of the relative phase at three media absorptions versus the position of an absorbing edge. (b) Measurement in skim milk mixed with three amounts of black India ink of the relative phase versus the position of an absorbing edge.

an increase in the photon-absorption properties of the medium if properties of the dc part (instead of the ac part) of the photon density are used in the imaging process.

7. DIFFRACTION AND REFLECTION BY AN ABSORBING EDGE: SIMULATIONS AND EXPERIMENTS

Figures 10–19 were obtained with the use of the geometry shown in Fig. 5(a) above. Figure 10 shows plots of the normalized dc light intensity of a diffracted signal in scattering media of different absorptions versus the source/detector position relative to an absorbing edge. The plots of Fig. 10(a) are derived from diffusion theory, and the plots of Fig. 10(b) were obtained from the detection of the dc light intensity in skim milk mixed with different amounts of black India ink. The sharpness in the decrease in dc intensity in Fig. 10 increases with increasing photon absorption in the medium, owing to the deletion of photons traveling relatively long path lengths from the source to the detector. We define the sharpness as the inverse of the distance moved by the edge, relative to the source/detector line, that causes a decrease in the intensity from 90% to 10% of its initial value. Increasing absorption leads to a narrowing of the distribution of photon paths from the source to the detector, resulting in a sharpening of the intensity decrease as the edge of the plane cuts into the narrowing bundle of light. Figure 11 shows a plot of inverse sharpness of the decrease in dc in-

tensity versus the square root of the volume of black India ink mixed with skim milk. Note that the inverse sharpness plotted in Fig. 11 appears asymptotically to approach 0.3 cm, which is the diameter of the aperture of the detector optical fiber. Figure 10 shows that when the edge is exactly between the source and the detector, the dc light intensity is less than one half of the maximum. This is a consequence of the diffusion of the photons, which allows for the deletion of photon paths that would have crossed the area occupied by the edge multiple times. Figure 12 shows a Monte Carlo simulation of the normalized time-gated light intensity versus the source/detector position relative to an absorbing edge in a diffraction experiment. The sharpness of the time-gated intensity plot in Fig. 12 increases with the separation of the earlier photons from the rest of the photons, which is a consequence of the earlier photons' traversing a relatively straight path in their movement from the source to the detector (i.e., the earlier photons undergo relatively few collisions). Figure 13 shows plots derived from diffusion theory and from a frequency-domain Monte Carlo simulation of the normalized ac amplitude of the photon density generated by a source that is sinusoidally modulated at different modulation frequencies versus the source/detector position relative to an absorbing edge in a diffraction experiment. The sharpness of the normalized ac amplitude in Fig. 13 increases with increasing modulation frequency. At high modulation frequencies, only those photons traveling a relatively straight path from the source to the detector

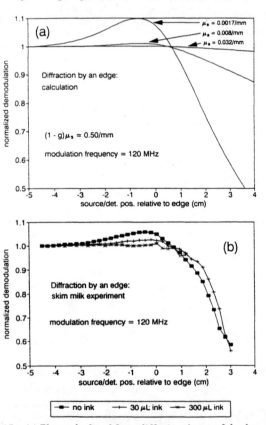

Fig. 15. (a) Plots calculated from diffusion theory of the demodulation at three media absorptions versus the position of an absorbing edge. (b) Measurement in skim milk mixed with three amounts of black India ink of signal demodulation versus the position of an absorbing edge.

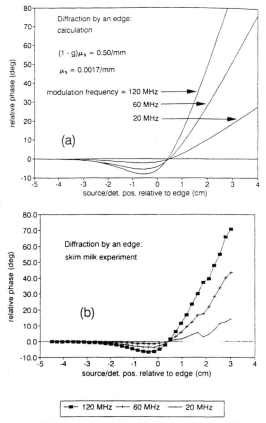

Fig. 16. (a) Plots calculated from diffusion theory of the relative phase at three modulation frequencies versus the position of an absorbing edge. (b) Measurement in skim milk of the relative phase at three modulation frequencies versus the position of an absorbing edge.

survive, owing to the $\exp(-\alpha r)/r$ attenuation of the ac part of the signal. In comparing the plots of Fig. 10 with the plots of Figs. 12 and 13, we can see that the photon-absorption properties of a medium and the time resolution of the scattered photons are analogous insofar as how they affect the resolution of the absorbing edge in the scattering medium. Higher photon absorption in the medium provides sharper resolution of the edge when the dc intensity of the light signal is measured, owing to the deletion from the medium of photons traveling relatively longer path lengths from the source to the detector; faster time gating or higher modulation frequencies provide sharper resolution of the edge in measurements of the time-gated or frequency-dependent part of the signal, owing to the detection of photons undergoing relatively few scattering events. Figures 14 and 15, respectively, show plots of the phase and the demodulation of a diffracted signal at 120-MHz modulation frequency versus the source/detector position relative to an absorbing edge in media of different absorptions. The plots of Figs. 14(a) and 15(a) are derived from diffusion theory, and the plots of Figs. 14(b) and 15(b) were obtained from the detection of a sinusoidally intensity-modulated light signal in skim milk mixed with different amounts of black India ink. Figures 16 and 17, respectively, show plots of the phase and the demodulation of a diffracted signal at different modulation frequencies versus the source/detector position relative to an absorbing edge. The plots of Figs. 16(a) and 17(a) are derived from

diffusion theory, and the plots of Figs. 16(b) and 17(b) were obtained from the detection of a sinusoidally intensity-modulated light signal in skim milk. Figures 18 and 19, respectively, show plots of the phase and the demodulation of a diffracted signal at different modulation frequencies versus the source/detector position relative to an absorbing edge. The plots of Figs. 18(a) and 19(a) are derived from diffusion theory, and the plots of Figs. 18(b) and 19(b) are from a frequency-domain Monte Carlo simulation.

The frequency-resolved plots of Figs. 14–19 show that the phase first decreases as the source and the detector approach the zero position and then sharply increases. The overall magnitude of the effect decreases as the photon absorption within the medium increases. To explain this effect qualitatively, we must consider that at the detector we are measuring the contribution of photons traveling throughout a distribution of paths. As the source and the detector approach the zero position, the field of view becomes occupied by the absorbing edge, and all the longer paths that would have crossed the boundary now occupied by the edge are deleted. This deletion causes an effective advance of the average wave front and an increase in the modulation of the signal. As the source and the detector move closer to the zero position, the phase reaches its minimum value and the modulation reaches its maximum value. When the edge passes the zero position, all the shorter paths are deleted, and the wave front is strongly retarded and demodulated. The addition of ink effectively deletes the longer photon paths, thereby de-

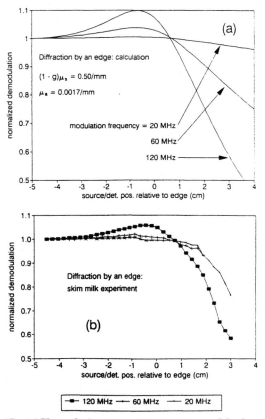

Fig. 17. (a) Plots calculated from diffusion theory of the demodulation at three modulation frequencies versus the position of an absorbing edge. (b) Measurement in skim milk of the signal demodulation at three modulation frequencies versus the position of an absorbing edge.

309

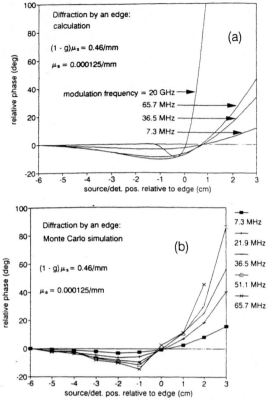

Fig. 18. (a) Plots calculated from diffusion theory of the relative phase at four modulation frequencies versus the position of an absorbing edge. (b) Frequency-domain Monte Carlo simulation of the relative phase at five modulation frequencies versus the position of an absorbing edge.

creasing the overall effect. In the limit of high absorption the phase difference caused by the insertion of the edge becomes small since the effective wave velocity is high.

Figures 20 and 21, respectively, show plots of the phase and the demodulation of a reflected signal at different modulation frequencies versus the source position relative to an absorbing edge. These plots were acquired with the use of the geometry shown in Fig. 5(b) above. The plots of Figs. 20(a) and 21(a) are derived from diffusion theory, and the plots of Figs. 20(b) and 21(b) were obtained from the detection of a sinusoidally intensity-modulated light signal in skim milk. The plots of Figs. 20 and 21 show that the phase decreases as the source approaches the zero position and then reaches a constant value, while the modulation increases and then reaches a constant value. The qualitative explanation of this effect is almost identical to the qualitative explanation of the behavior of the phase and the demodulation in the diffraction experiment, the only difference being that the phase and the modulation reach a constant value in the reflection experiment because the source and the detector are on the same side of the plane; when the edge of the plane passes the source and the detector, the distribution of the photon paths between the source and the detector becomes constant.

8. CONCLUSION

The diffusion approximation to the Boltzmann transport equation fully describes our experiments of propagation of

photons in macroscopically homogeneous infinite media for all the absorptions investigated. The range of absorption and transport scattering coefficients that we have studied is typical of many animal tissues in the near-infrared region.[6] At high absorption or at distances from the light source that are of the order of the mean free path for light scattering, the diffusion approximation should fail.[15] Given the value of $(1 - g)\mu_s$ and the value of μ_a for light of 810-nm wavelength in skim milk, which we determined from our data to be 0.50/mm and 0.0017/mm, respectively, few unscattered photons will survive the transit from the source to the detector when the source/detector separation is of the order of a few centimeters. (Note that for our measurements the minimum source/detector separation was 2.5 cm.) However, at short distances from the source, unscattered photons will contribute to the light intensity. We have performed other experiments, not reported here, in which we have studied the angular dependence of the light intensity in a milk suspension. We have oriented the end of the detector optical fiber either directly toward the source or away from the source, and we have measured the same intensity in the medium within errors. Only when the detector was very close to the source, less than a centimeter for the skim-milk experiment, did we observe a definitive dependence of the light intensity on the orientation of the end of the detector optical fiber relative to the source. The effects on the measured light intensity in the milk suspension that are due to the boundary of the tank containing

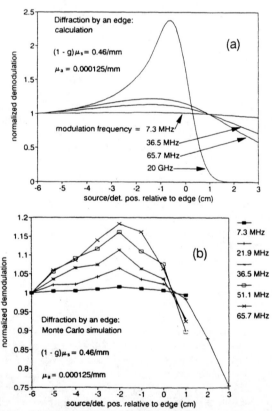

Fig. 19. (a) Plots calculated from diffusion theory of the demodulation at four modulation frequencies versus the position of an absorbing edge. (b) Frequency-domain Monte Carlo simulation of the demodulation at five modulation frequencies versus the position of an absorbing edge.

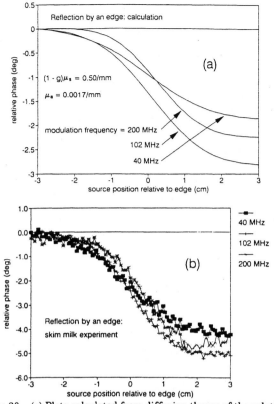

Fig. 20. (a) Plots calculated from diffusion theory of the relative phase at three modulation frequencies versus the position of an absorbing edge. (b) Measurement in skim milk of the relative phase at three modulation frequencies versus the position of an absorbing edge. The light source that was used to generate these data was a synchronously pumped Rhodamine 6G single-jet dye laser that was cavity dumped at 2 MHz. The dye laser was tuned to a wavelength of 690 nm. Apart from the light source, the experimental setup is as described in Section 5.

the milk suspension were also studied; deviations from the expected behavior (based on the diffusion approximation for an infinite medium) were observed, these were due to the light exchange with the room rather than to the presence of the boundaries. The milk suspension acts as a condenser for light, since the photon density is inversely proportional to the photon diffusion coefficient. An optical fiber immersed in the milk suspension measures a higher photon intensity than that measured by the fiber in the room (assuming isotropic illumination).

For the purpose of spectroscopy and the imaging of thick tissues, the scattered light component provides the only contribution of the light transmitted through the sample, since the unscattered component is already strongly attenuated at distances comparable with the mean free path. The amount of the scattered component that is transmitted depends only on the absorption of the sample. To put this scattered component to better use, we superimpose a sinusoidal amplitude modulation upon the intensity of the light source, or we can pulse the light source. The photon-density wave reproduces some of the features of the original electromagnetic wave of wavelength λ and allows for the recovery of the spectroscopic parameters $\mu_a(\lambda)$ and $[1 - g(\lambda)]\mu_s(\lambda)$ from a measurement of the ac phasor. [As was noted by Patterson et al., a limitation of the model based on the diffusion approximation is the ambiguity be-

tween g and μ_s, since only the product $(1 - g)\mu_s$ can be obtained.[6]] However, since the propagation is by diffusion, the amplitude-modulated term attenuates as $\exp(-\alpha r)/r$ as the photon-density wave advances (even with no photon absorption). Consequently the amplitude-modulated term, which carries information on the optical parameters, becomes negligible after propagation through 10–15 cm of scattering medium (with properties similar to those of tissues) at rf modulation. To obtain good spatial resolution, one must increase the amplitude modulation frequency, which also reduces the penetration of the photon-density wave at that modulation frequency. As a consequence of the $\exp(-\alpha r)/r$ attenuation of the ac amplitude, there is a quasi-linear relationship between the wavelength of the photon-density wave and the penetration of the photon-density wave in a strongly scattering medium when $\mu_a = 0$. Given the exponential nature of the attenuation process, there is only a logarithmic advantage in increasing the source intensity.

The edge resolution experiments show that the basic rule that governs the resolution or the sharpness of the edge is the deletion of the longer photon paths. Several processes and measurement protocols can cause the effective deletion of the longer path: photon absorption, high modulation frequency, and faster time gating. The mechanism by which the sharpness of an edge is increased

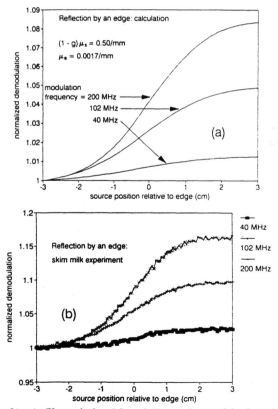

Fig. 21. (a) Plots calculated from diffusion theory of the demodulation at three modulation frequencies versus the position of an absorbing edge. (b) Measurement in skim milk of the signal demodulation at three modulation frequencies versus the position of an absorbing edge. The light source described in the caption to Fig. 20(b) was used in the acquisition of these data, but, apart from the light source, the experimental setup is as described in Section 5.

can easily be explained from the perspective of a bundle of photon paths that join the source to the detector. The thinner the light bundle, the closer the approach to the computer tomography geometry. In practice, the effective light bundle can be made very narrow, of the order of a millimeter for source/detector distances of 3–5 cm and absorption and scattering transport coefficients of the order of those found in animal tissues in the near infrared. The ultimate resolution or sharpness of an edge should not be confused with the detectability of a small object. The detectability is determined by the precision of the phase and demodulation measurement, which can be extremely high.[20] Instead, the sharpness of an edge or the separation of two small objects depends on the optical properties of the medium, modulation frequency, or time gating. Since we have obtained the analytical solution for some typical cases, we understand how the optical properties and modulation frequency or time gating determine the sharpness of an edge.

The measurement of the photon-density wave front provides a simple and powerful method to detect macroscopic inhomogeneities in a scattering medium. An absorbing object causes a wave-front deformation that is easy to measure. We are studying the limit of resolvability of small absorbing objects in highly turbid media.

ACKNOWLEDGMENTS

These experiments and analyses of the data produced were performed at the Laboratory for Fluorescence Dynamics (LFD) in the Department of Physics at the University of Illinois at Urbana-Champaign (UIUC). The LFD and this study are supported jointly by the Division of Research Resources of the National Institutes of Health (RR03155) and UIUC. The authors thank Julie Butzow for help in preparing this paper.

REFERENCES

1. A. Ishimaru, *Wave Propagation and Scattering in Random Media* (Academic, New York, 1978).
2. M. J. Stephen, "Temporal fluctuations in wave propagation in random media," Phys. Rev. B **37**, 1–5 (1988).
3. R. Berkovits and S. Feng, "Theory of speckle-pattern tomography in multiple-scattering media," Phys. Rev. Lett. **65**, 3120–3123 (1990).
4. B. White, P. Sheng, M. Postel, and G. Papanicolaou, "Probing through cloudiness: theory of statistical inversion for multiply scattered data," Phys. Rev. Lett. **63**, 2228–2231 (1989).
5. J. R. Singer, F. A. Grunbaum, P. Kohn, and J. P. Zubelli, "Image reconstruction of the interior of bodies that diffuse radiation," Science **248**, 990–993 (1990).
6. M. S. Patterson, B. Chance, and B. C. Wilson, "Time resolved reflectance and transmittance for the non-invasive measurement of tissue optical properties," Appl. Opt. **28**, 2331–2336 (1989).
7. D. J. Pine, D. A. Weitz, P. M. Chaikin, and E. Herbolzheimer, "Diffusing-wave spectroscopy," Phys. Rev. Lett. **60**, 1134–1137 (1988).
8. P. W. Anderson, "The question of classical localization: a theory of white paint?" Philos. Mag. B **52**, 505–509 (1985).
9. A. Ishimaru, "Diffusion of light in turbid material," Appl. Opt. **28**, 2210–2215 (1989).
10. B. Chance, S. Nioka, J. Kent, K. McCully, M. Fountain, R. Greenfeld, and G. Holtom, "Time-resolved spectroscopy of hemoglobin and myoglobin in resting and ischemic muscle," Anal. Biochem. **174**, 698–707 (1988).
11. B. White, P. Sheng, Z. Q. Zhang, and G. Papanicolaou, "Wave localization characteristics in the time domain," Phys. Rev. Lett. **59**, 1918–1921 (1987).
12. J. C. Hebden and R. A. Kruger, "A time-of-flight breast imaging system: spatial resolution performance," in *Time-Resolved Spectroscopy and Imaging of Tissues*, B. Chance, ed., Proc. Soc. Photo-Opt. Instrum. Eng. **1431**, 225–231 (1991).
13. K. M. Yoo, F. Liu, and R. R. Alfano, "Biological materials probed by the temporal and angular profiles of the backscattered ultrafast laser pulses," J. Opt. Soc. Am. B **7**, 1685–1693 (1990).
14. R. R. Anderson and J. A. Parrish, *The Science of Photomedicine*, J. D. Regan and J. A. Parrish, eds. (Plenum, New York, 1982), Chap. 6, p. 147.
15. K. M. Case and P. F. Zweifel, *Linear Transport Theory* (Addison-Wesley, Reading, Mass., 1967).
16. H. S. Carslaw, "Some multiform solutions of the partial differential equations of physical mathematics and their applications," Proc. London Math. Soc. **30**, 121–161 (1898).
17. A. Sommerfeld, "Über verzweigte Potentiale im Raum," Proc. London Math. Soc. **28**, 395–429 (1897); **30**, 161–163 (1898).
18. J. H. Jeans, *Mathematical Theory of Electricity and Magnetism* (Cambridge U. Press, London, 1933).
19. B. A. Feddersen, D. W. Piston, and E. Gratton, "Digital parallel acquisition in frequency domain fluorometry," Rev. Sci. Instrum. **60**, 2929–2936 (1989).
20. B. Barbieri, F. De Picoli, M. vandeVen, and E. Gratton, "What determines the uncertainty of phase and modulation measurements in frequency domain fluorometry?" in *Time-Resolved Laser Spectroscopy in Biochemistry II*, J. R. Lakowicz, ed., Proc. Soc. Photo-Opt. Instrum. Eng. **1204**, 158–170 (1990).

Reprinted from *Optical Engineering*, Vol. 32(2), pp. 258-266 (February 1993).
©1993 SPIE.

Tissue characterization and imaging using photon density waves

Lars O. Svaasand, MEMBER SPIE
University of Trondheim
Norwegian Institute of Technology
Division of Physical Electronics
Trondheim N-7034, Norway

Bruce J. Tromberg
University of California at Irvine
Beckman Laser Institute and Medical Clinic
1002 Health Sciences Road East
Irvine, California 92715-3054

Richard C. Haskell, MEMBER SPIE
Harvey Mudd College
Physics Department
Claremont, California, 91711

Tsong-Tseh Tsay
Michael W. Berns
University of California at Irvine
Beckman Laser Institute and Medical Clinic
1002 Health Sciences Road East
Irvine, California 92715-3054

Abstract. The optical properties of brain tissues have been evaluated by measuring the phase velocity and attenuation of harmonically modulated light. The phase velocity for photon density waves at 650-nm wavelength has been found to be in the range of 5 to 12% of the corresponding velocity in a nonscattering medium, and the optical penetration depth was in the range 2.9 to 5.2 mm. These results are used to predict the resolution of optical imaging of deep tissue structures by diffusely propagating incoherent photons. The results indicate that structures of a few millimeters in linear dimension can be identified at 10 mm depth provided that proper wavelength and time resolution are selected. This depth can possibly be enlarged to 30 mm in the case of tissues with very low scattering such as in the case of the neonatal human brain.

Subject terms: biomedical optics; tissue optics; optical imaging; time-resolved techniques; frequency-resolved techniques.

Optical Engineering 32(2), 258–266 (February 1993).

1 Introduction

Optical techniques represent a valuable tool for *in vivo* analysis of tissue properties and for imaging of tissue structures.[1,2] Recent developments have emphasized dynamic measurements where either an ultrashort laser pulse or high-frequency amplitude-modulated laser light is launched into the tissue.[3–8] The properties of the transmitted light range from quasi-coherent properties of the almost directly transmitted early part of the light to the almost randomized incoherent extensively scattered late part. This paper considers the advantages as well as the limitations of using diffusely propagating incoherently scattered light for evaluation of tissue properties and for imaging.[6,7,9]

Irridiation with harmonically modulated optical beams will initiate density waves of diffusely propagating photons. The velocity of these waves, which is strongly dependent on the modulation frequency, can typically vary from the velocity of light as an upper limit, down to about 5% of this value in highly scattering tissues. We will also demonstrate that image resolution in the time domain can be significantly improved by receiving only the first part of the diffuse transmitted light and that the resolution can be further improved by using an optical wavelength that is optimally selected with respect to the scattering and absorption coefficient.[3,10–12] This paper, however, will be limited to the diffusion approximation. The propagation of nonscattered or almost nonscattered photons can therefore not be considered within the framework of this theory. Diffusion theory only accounts for heavily scattered photons that propagate with a reduced effective velocity.

2 Optical Properties of Tissues

Biological media have because of their complicated structure very complex irregular optical properties. The optical inhomogeneities are due to differences in the ability for optical polarization as well as in the optical absorption. These differences exist between the cells and their surroundings as well as within each individual cell.

The propagation of light in tissue is strongly influenced by this mechanism; light is very efficiently scattered out of an incident collimated beam. The light will typically be

Paper BM-056 received July 1, 1992; revised manuscript received Nov. 1, 1992; accepted for publication Nov. 1, 1992.

scattered into an almost isotropic distribution within a few millimeters from the source. In some heavy scattering tissues, such as in the case of adult brain tissues, this randomization takes place within a fraction of a millimeter.

The total optical radiation in tissues is therefore composed of waves arriving from different directions with different optical phases. An important question is whether the phase relationships between these various waves are slowly varying or if they vary in a rapid and stochastic manner. The waves subjected to the first condition will add in a partially coherent manner. The total optical power will then be determined by the average value of the square of the total electric field. The power might then be higher or lower than the sum of the optical power in each wave, dependent on whether the waves add constructively or destructively. On the other hand, the waves with rapid and stochastic phase fluctuations will add incoherently. The total optical power will then always be the sum of the power of all participating waves. Light propagating in mammalian tissues will typically loose coherence after a few millimeters from the irradiated surface; the only exception to this rule is ocular media. The incoherent optical power can be characterized by the radiant energy fluence rate defined as the optical energy flux incident on an infinitesimal small sphere divided by the cross-sectional area of that sphere.[13] This case is illustrated by Fig. 1. The photons are scattered in the tissue, and each cell will be irradiated with incoherent light coming from all directions.

3 Propagation of Harmonic Waves

The diffuse scattered optical energy will propagate to distal locations in tissue by a mechanism very much of the same nature as an ordinary diffusion process. The net transport of the diffuse photons will occur only from regions with a high fluence rate to regions with smaller values. The dynamics of this process can conveniently be described by expressing the fluence rate in terms of harmonic waves. These waves, which characterize the temporal and spatial variations in the photon density, can be expressed in the form,[6]

$$\varphi(t,x) \propto \cos(\omega t - k_i x) \exp(-k_r x) , \qquad (1)$$

where $\varphi(t,x)$ is the value of the fluence rate at position x in space at time t.

The waves are characterized by the angular frequency ω, which gives the change in radians per unit time, and by the angular repetency k_i, which gives the change in radians per unit length in space.[13] The relation between the angular frequency and the period in time, T, and the one between the angular repetency and the period in space, i.e., the wavelength λ, are

$$\omega = 2\pi/T , \qquad k_i = 2\pi/\lambda . \qquad (2)$$

The attenuation of the waves is given by the attenuation coefficient k_r. The reciprocal value of this coefficient is equal to the optical penetration depth, δ, corresponding to a decay of the amplitude to $1/e$ or 37% of the initial value.

The propagation of a photon density wave is shown in Fig. 2. The density of the photons is given by the amplitude of the solid curve, and the direction of the individual photons is illustrated by the arrows.

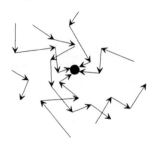

Fig. 1 Propagation of photons in scattering media.

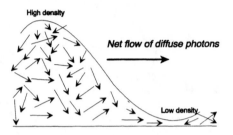

Fig. 2 Representation of photon density wave from high to low fluence rate regions.

4 Propagation of Lossless Waves

Because the photons flow from high- to low-density regions, the net transport of diffuse photons in the positive x-direction will require that the waves are attenuated. The flux of photons in an unattenuated wave during one period in time will result in the same amount in the backward direction as in the forward direction, and the net flux will be zero. The angular repetency k_i and the attenuation coefficient k_r are identically equal in any lossless diffusion process. They can be expressed in the form [see Eq. (13)]

$$k_i = k_r = (\omega/2X)^{1/2} , \qquad (3)$$

where X is the optical diffusivity. Optical diffusivity, in turn, is a function of the familiar optical properties described by the absorption β and effective scattering σ_{eff} coefficients [See Eq. (11)], which are, respectively, the reciprocal average distance between absorption and scattering events.

The diffusive waves are of the evanescent kind, and they are attenuated even in the absence of any loss mechanism. The total attenuation over a distance corresponding to one wavelength λ, since $\lambda = 2\pi/k_i = 2\pi/k_r$, is always equal to $\exp(-2\pi)$. The amplitude of the waves is thus reduced to about 0.2% of the initial value over a distance corresponding to one wavelength. The waves also exhibit frequency dependent phase velocity. This velocity is given by [Eq. (13)]

$$v_{\text{ph}} = \frac{\omega}{k_i} = (2X\omega)^{1/2} . \qquad (4)$$

Under lossless conditions, the phase velocity increase is proportional to the square root of the frequency. The phase velocity is infinitely large for waves of infinite high frequencies. This arises from the fact that the diffusion model is invalid for time scales shorter than the time between several scattering events. The propagation of those photons that only undergo a very limited amount of scattering must be described by the more complete electromagnetic equations.

The propagation of photons from a source can be characterized by a spectrum of harmonic diffusive waves. The high-frequency waves, since they have the highest velocity, will arrive first. But the high-frequency waves are the most heavily attenuated, and a noticeable increase in the photon density will occur only after arrival of waves with more moderate attenuation. This will occur when waves with reciprocal attenuation coefficients comparable to the distance arrive. The frequencies of these waves are given by [Eq. (3)]

$$k_r = \left(\frac{\omega}{2X}\right)^{1/2} \sim \frac{1}{L} , \qquad (5)$$

where L is the distance. The order of magnitude for the time delay of arrival of these waves can therefore be expressed,

$$t_{\text{delay}} = \frac{1}{\omega} \sim \frac{L^2}{X} . \qquad (6)$$

5 Propagation of Waves with Loss

The presence of photon absorption alters the properties of the waves in two significant ways. The absorption will primarily increase the attenuation. But this increased attenuation will, since a steepening of the density profile enhances the diffusion, secondarily result in an increased wave velocity. The absorption mechanism, which is important at all frequencies below the reciprocal optical absorption relaxation time (i.e., $\omega\tau \ll 1$) results in an attenuation and a velocity of the form [Eq. (13)]

$$k_r = \frac{1}{(\tau X)^{1/2}} = \frac{1}{\delta} ,$$

$$v_{\text{ph}} = \frac{\omega}{k_i} = 2\left(\frac{X}{\tau}\right)^{1/2} , \qquad (7)$$

where $\tau = 1/\beta c$ is the absorption relaxation time and $\delta = [3\beta(\beta + \sigma_{\text{eff}})]^{-1/2}$ is the optical penetration depth.

The attenuation and the phase velocity are now frequency independent. This latter property has the important consequence that the velocity of the optical energy is frequency independent and equal to the phase velocity. The time delay for the envelope of an optical pulse to be transported over a distance L is thus [Eq. (7)]

$$t_{\text{delay}} = \frac{L}{2\left(\frac{X}{\tau}\right)^{1/2}} . \qquad (8)$$

The relations between frequency, angular wavenumber (repetency), and attenuation are shown in Fig. 3 [Eq. (13)]. The upper curve in Fig. 3 (series 2) shows the frequency in GHz ($f = \omega/2\pi$) versus the angular wavenumber in inverse meters (i.e., in radians/meter). This curve gives the dispersion relation between frequency and repetency in a region where the presence of loss is important. This curve

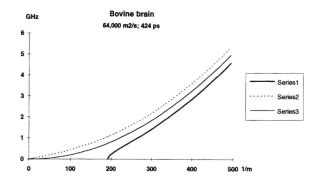

Fig. 3 Relations between frequency, angular wavenumber and attenuation. The optical diffusivity ($X = 64,000$ m^2/s) and the relaxation time ($\tau = 424$ ps) correspond to values for bovine brain measured *ex vivo* at 650-nm wavelength (See Table 1). Series 1, 2, and 3, respectively, correspond to attenuation k_r with loss (lower curve), repetency k_i with loss (upper curve), and the lossless case where $k_r = k_i$ (middle curve).

approaches, as follows from Eq. (13), the lossless case for high frequencies, i.e., for frequencies much higher than the reciprocal relaxation time ($f >> 1/2\pi\tau = 0.38$ GHz). In the low-frequency region, however, the curve approaches zero with a finite angle with the horizontal axis. This finite angle represents the nonzero phase velocity as given by Eq. (7). The lower curve (series 1) gives, correspondingly, the relation between the frequency in GHz and the attenuation coefficient in inverse meters. The attenuation coefficient approaches the finite value of $k_r = 1/\delta$ in the zero frequency limit, whereas in accordance with Eq. (13), k_r approaches the value for the lossless case in the high-frequency limit. The middle curve (series 3) corresponds to the lossless case where the attenuation coefficient k_r and the angular repetency k_i are equal. The phase velocity and the attentuation are in this case, as follows from Eqs. (3) and (4), both approaching zero in the zero frequency limit.

The results from measurements of low-frequency phase velocity and attenuation in various tissues are given in Table 1. These data were acquired using previously described frequency-domain photon migration methods.[14] Briefly, the photon migration instrument is a modified multiharmonic Fourier transform phase and modulation fluorometer (SLM, 48000-medium high frequency, Champaign, Illinois). Light is provided by a water-cooled argon-ion laser (Coherent Innova 90-5) pumping a dye laser. A Pockels cell driven by the amplified output of a harmonic comb generator is used to produce light pulses with high harmonic content. The harmonic comb generator output, in the frequency domain, is a fundamental frequency (typically 5 MHz) and its integer harmonics at 5, 10, and 15 MHz, etc., to 250 MHz. Modulated light is coupled to a 600-μm-diam fused-silica fiber optic probe and directed onto the sample.

A second fused-silica fiber (same dimension) collects the scattered light and transmits it to the measurement photomultiplier tube (Hamamatsu R928). The gain of the photomultiplier tube is modulated by a second harmonic comb generator and driven at the frequency of the Pockels cell plus a small difference frequency (the cross-correlation frequency). The sample's phase and amplitude response at each modulation frequency is contained within the corresponding cross-correlation frequency. Using the multiharmonic tech-

Table 1 Optical properties of tissues.

Tissue	Diffusivity	Relaxation time	Absorption coeff.	Scattering coeff.	Penetration depth	Phase velocity
	X	τ	β	σ_{eff}	δ	v_{ph}
	m^2/s	ps	cm^{-1}	cm^{-1}	mm	$1/c$ *
Bovine brain	64 000	424	0.11	11	5.2	0.12
Ocular sclera, human	26 500	583	0.08	25	3.9	0.06
Corpus callosum, human brain	14 300	583	0.08	50	2.9	0.05

* Relative to velocity of light in a non-scattering medium with the same index of refraction, i.e. $c = 2.14 * 10^8$ m/s, Wavelength 650 nm, Measured ex-vivo

nique, we can acquire phase shifts and demodulations for 50 frequencies (5 to 250 MHz) in a few seconds. Brain data were recorded from fresh refrigerated samples under infinite medium conditions by inserting source and detector fibers into the material. Sclera data were collected under simulated infinite medium conditions by stacking several sections from fresh human globes. The resulting dimensions were approximately 15×15 mm, and boundary effects were minimized by immersing the entire sclera stack in 10% intralipid during measurements. Optical properties were determined from phase and amplitude information fit to a previously described expression [Eq. (13) and Ref. 7] for at least three source/detector separations. The results of Table 1 were found utilizing the technique and equipment as described in an earlier publication.[14]

Table 1 gives six different optical tissue parameters for each tissue. There are, however, only three independent sets of parameters. When the index of refraction is given, the optical properties can be characterized either by the optical diffusivity and relaxation time (X, τ), by the effective scattering and absorption coefficient $(\sigma_{\text{eff}}, \beta)$, or finally by the optical penetration depth and low-frequency phase velocity (δ, v_{ph}). The relations between the optical diffusivity, relaxation time, effective scattering coefficient, and absorption coefficient are given in Eq. (13). The corresponding relations between the optical diffusivity, relation time, penetration depth δ, i.e., the attenuation coefficient in the zero frequency limit, and phase velocity v_{ph}, i.e., the phase velocity in the zero frequency limit, are given in Eq. (7). The data given in Table 1 range from tissues with more moderate scattering, such as in the case of bovine and porcine brain, to intense scattering media, such as the corpus callosum of the human brain.

6 Propagation of Pulsed Optical Power

The propagation of an optical pulse can be represented with a spectrum of harmonic waves, and the high-frequency con-

tent of this spectrum increases with the shortening of the pulse. An infinitesimally short pulse releasing a finite amount of optical energy, i.e., a so-called Dirac or delta pulse, corresponds to an infinitely broad frequency spectrum of harmonic waves. The propagation of such a pulse is illustrated in Fig. 4.

An initial pulse of diffuse photons as shown on the left side in Fig. 4, broadens during propagation as illustrated by the pulse on the right side. The pulse broadening in a diffusion process occurs because the various frequency components of the pulse propagate with different velocities; the high-frequency components generally arrive before those with low-frequency. The time delay for the pulse envelope is also dependent on whether the rather lossless high-frequency waves or the more lossy low-frequency waves are the predominant ones in the broadened pulse. If the high-frequency components are the relevant ones, the delay is approximately given by $t_{\text{delay}} = L^2/X$, where L is the traveled distance [Eq. (6)]. The corresponding time delay for the pulse envelope in the low-frequency case is given by $t_{\text{delay}} = L/v_{\text{ph}}$ [Eq. (8)]. These two mechanisms are of equal importance when

$$\frac{L^2}{X} \sim \frac{L}{2\left(\dfrac{X}{\tau}\right)^{1/2}}$$

or

$$L \sim \frac{1}{2}(X\tau)^{1/2} \sim (X\tau)^{1/2} = \delta \ . \tag{9}$$

The delay time for the arrival of the pulse envelope thus increases quadratically with distance until the pulse has traveled a length approximately equal to the optical penetration

316

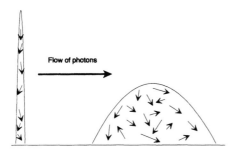

Fig. 4 Representation of pulse broadening during propagation.

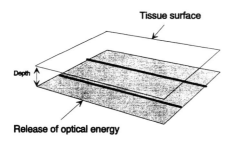

Fig. 5 Initial conditions for Fig. 6 simulations: release of optical energy below tissue surface.

depth. In the case of larger lengths, the delay time increases approximately linearly with traveled distance. The different properties of the various frequency components of an optical pulse have important implications in imaging of tissue structures. This is demonstrated by the series of simulations illustrated in Figs. 5 and 6. Figure 5 describes the model boundary conditions: two parallel absorbing lines, 1 mm in width, 10 mm apart, embedded in tissue at a depth of either 5 or 10 mm below the surface. A Dirac pulse is released below the surface at time $t=0$ in the absorber plane. Infinitely absorbing lines are selected to optimize contrast. Contrast enhancement in real imaging applications would, of course, involve some degree of optical frequency manipulation. In addition, we have necessarily selected relatively simple conditions that do not violate our diffusion theory framework. Thus, the Fig. 6 simulation involves observation of the shadow cast by each line under uniform field illumination. Real systems would employ more complex single- or multiple-point sources at a partially transmitting surface. These source and boundary conditions were intentionally imposed, however, to reveal more clearly the interplay between photon diffusion and spatial contrast.

Figure 6 shows the time development of the fluence rate for various conditions. The fluence rate was calculated from the diffusion equation with boundary solutions for a totally reflecting surface as derived in Sec. 8. The explicit solution for this fluence rate is given by Eq. (23). The vertical axis gives the surface fluence rate in W/m^2. As illustrated in Fig. 5, the optical energy is released in a horizontal layer below the surface. Here, the two black lines intersect at right angles, the marks in the middle of the z axis. The second horizontal axis records time elapsed (picoseconds) after release of a Dirac pulse of 10^4 J/m^2, roughly the maximum energy density that can be released without introducing thermal damage to the tissue.

The case of 5-mm-deep lines is illustrated in Fig. 6(a). The time axis spans from the release of the pulse to the arrival of the pulse envelope [Eq. (8)]. This delay is for bovine brain tissue equal to $t_{delay}=203$ ps for $L=5$ mm. The presence of the two individual lines is now clearly identifiable in the peak of the pulse. The corresponding results for 10-mm-deep lines are shown in Fig. 6(b). Here, the two individual lines are difficult to identify, but the general presence of the absorbing lines is still clearly visible. However, this information is almost completely lost on the tail of the pulse arriving after 814 ps [see Fig. 6(c)]. Clearly, much better resolution is possible if light is collected before the scattering has become too extensive. This can, in principle, be obtained by two different techniques. The first, and rather obvious one, is to receive only the first part of the pulse and reject all light that arrives later. The flank of the pulse arriving after 129 ps contains, as shown in Fig. 6(d), well-defined information on the presence of the two individual black lines. The second method is to shorten the delay of the pulse itself by selecting an optical wavelength with higher loss. As discussed previously, enhancement of the loss will increase the velocity of the pulse envelope. The propagation of a pulse at a wavelength corresponding to $10\times$ higher loss is shown in Fig. 6(e). Under these conditions a pulse delayed only 129 ps contains information regarding individual lines at the peak of the pulse. This technique, of course, has the drawback that the flank of the pulse is somewhat attenuated.

The amount of this loss follows from Figs. 6(d) and 6(e); the maximum value of the fluence rate in Fig. 6(d) is a factor of about 15 larger than the maximum value in Fig. 6(e). The impact of reduced loss is demonstrated by Fig. 6(f). This figure shows the pulse after propagation 10 mm through a medium with the same optical diffusivity as the bovine brain, but with a loss corresponding to the ultimate minimum loss for tissues, i.e., that of sea water. The pulse in the sea waterlike phantom tissue, which has an optical relaxation time of 10 ns and an optical penetration depth of $\delta=25$ mm, will be dominated by the high-frequency waves. The time delay is therefore only dependent on the diffusivity, and the time delay is about $t_{delay}=1563$ ps as given by Eq. (6). The contrast is now very poor, and the presence of the absorbing lines is barely seen in the pulse amplitude.

These results, however, also reveal the limitations of the diffusion approximation. No upper limit exists for the wave velocity within this approximation; waves of infinite high frequencies have infinite high phase velocity. On the other hand, the attenuation of the high-frequency waves are heavily attenuated; waves of infinite high frequencies are infinitely heavily attenuated. This phenomenon is responsible for the nonzero values of the fluence rate at times shorter than the time of flight of nonscattered photons, i.e., $L/c=47$ ps for Figs. 6(b) through 6(f). The diffusion theory based on a multiple scattering process is basically invalid for time scales comparable or shorter than the time of flight of nonscattered photons.

7 Conclusions

The properties of brain tissues reveal that optical imaging of tissue structures is also possible within the framework of diffusely propagating incoherent photons. However, the depth of resolution for time-independent imaging is very limited

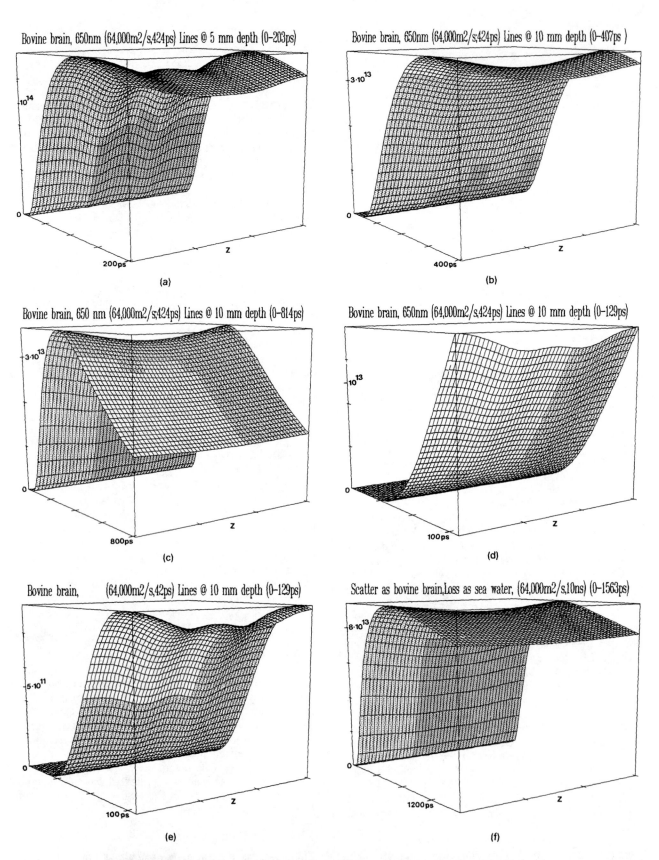

Fig. 6 Optical fluence rate at the tissue surface in W/m² [vertical after release of an optical Dirac pulse of 10,000 J/m² (1 J/cm²)] in the layer embedded into the tissue. Horizontal axes describe time (picoseconds) release of the pulse and the position of two totally absorbing 1-mm lines located in the horizontal plane normal to the z axis.

when optical wavelengths corresponding to maximum penetration are used. This restriction can be improved either by selecting an optical wavelength with higher loss or by using time- or frequency-resolved techniques. The technique of enhancing the optical loss has its limitations because the relevant signal attenuation also is increased, whereas the practical applicability of time-resolved techniques is limited by the availability of inexpensive fast optical equipment. The relevant time and frequency scales are, respectively, 10 to 100 ps and 1 to 10 GHz for imaging of 10- to 30-mm-deep structures. However, the progress of high-speed laser diodes and solid state detectors over the last decade indicates that optical techniques might have significant future applications for *in vivo* spectroscopy and imaging of tissue structures.

8 Appendix

The optical diffusion equation can be expressed[6]

$$X\nabla^2\varphi - \frac{\partial\varphi}{\partial t} - \frac{\varphi}{\tau} = -qc , \qquad (10)$$

where φ is the optical fluence rate, t is time, q is the diffuse photon source density, and c is the velocity of light in the medium. The optical diffusivity X and the absorption relaxation time τ can be expressed[15]

$$X = \frac{c_0}{3[\sigma(1-g)+\beta]n} = \frac{c_0}{3(\sigma_{\text{eff}}+\beta)n} , \qquad (11)$$

$$\tau = \frac{n}{c_0\beta} ,$$

where σ and g are, respectively, the scattering coefficient and the average cosine of the scattering angle. The parameter $\sigma_{\text{eff}} = \sigma(1-g)$ is the effective scattering coefficient, β is the absorption coefficient, and c_0 and n are, respectively, the velocity of light in vacuum and the index of refraction of the medium.

Harmonic solutions of the diffusion equation can be written in the form

$$\varphi \propto \exp[i(\omega t - k_i x)] \exp(-k_r x) , \qquad (12)$$

where k_i and k_r, respectively, are the angular repetency and the attenuation coefficient. The angular frequency is ω, and x is the distance in space. The relation between these quantities follows from substitution of Eq. (12) in Eq. (10)[6]:

$$k_r = \frac{1}{(2X\tau)^{1/2}} \{[1+(\omega\tau)^2]^{1/2}+1\}^{1/2} , \qquad (13)$$

$$k_i = \frac{1}{(2X\tau)^{1/2}} \{[1+(\omega\tau)^2]^{1/2}-1\}^{1/2} ,$$

The 1-D time dependent can be found by expressing the spatial dependence of the solutions in the form

$$\varphi \propto \exp(-kx) . \qquad (14)$$

The Laplace transform of the homogeneous diffusion equation can thus be expressed [Eqs. (10) and (14)]

$$\varphi(x,s)\left(Xk^2 - s - \frac{1}{\tau}\right) = 0 , \qquad (15)$$

where

$$k = \pm \left[\frac{1}{X}\left(s+\frac{1}{\tau}\right)\right]^{1/2} \qquad (16)$$

The boundary condition at a partially transmitting radiative surface can be expressed

$$\frac{X}{c}\frac{\partial\varphi}{\partial x} = A\varphi , \qquad (17)$$

where A is a photon flux transfer coefficient at the surface. This quantity, which is a function of the properties of the tissue and of the surrounding medium, ranges from zero to infinity, respectively, for the totally reflecting and the totally transmitting boundary.

A finite amount of optical energy released in a layer parallel to the surface at a depth of $x = \xi$ gives the following:

$$\frac{X}{c}\frac{\partial\varphi_1}{\partial x} - \frac{X}{c}\frac{\partial\varphi_2}{\partial x} = Q_{\text{pl}} ,$$

$$\varphi_1 = \varphi_2 , \qquad (18)$$

where φ_1 and φ_2, respectively, are the Laplace transforms of the fluence rates at $x = \xi-$ and $x = \xi+$. The quantity Q_{pl} is energy density released per unit area in the layer at time $t = 0$.

The Laplace transform of the solutions can be expressed in the form [Eq. (14)]

$$\varphi(x,s) = C_1 \exp(kx) + C_2 \exp(-kx) \quad \text{for } 0 < x < \xi ,$$

$$\varphi(x,s) = C_3 \exp(-kx) \quad \text{for } x > \xi , \qquad (19)$$

where k is the positive root of Eq. (16). The constants C_1, C_2, and C_3 follow from the boundary conditions given in Eqs. (17) and (18). The solution can then be expressed in the form

$$\varphi(x,s) = \frac{cQ_{\text{pl}}}{2X}\left(\frac{1}{k}\exp(-k|\xi-x|) + \frac{1}{k}\exp[-k(\xi+x)]\right.$$
$$\left. -2\frac{cA}{X}\left\{\frac{1}{k[k+(cA/X)]}\exp[-k(\xi+x)]\right\}\right) . \qquad (20)$$

The time-dependent solution follows from the inverse Laplace transform:

$$\varphi(x,t) = \mathscr{L}^{-1}\varphi(x,s) =$$

$$\left(\frac{1}{2(\pi Xt)^{1/2}}\left\{\exp\left[-\frac{(x-\xi)^2}{4Xt}\right] + \exp\left[-\frac{(x+\xi)^2}{4Xt}\right]\right\}\right.$$

$$-h\exp[h(x+\xi)+h^2Xt]$$

$$\left.\times \text{erfc}\left[\frac{x+\xi}{2(Xt)^{1/2}}+h(Xt)^{1/2}\right]\right)\left[cQ_{\text{pl}}\exp\left(-\frac{t}{\tau}\right)\right] ,$$

$$(21)$$

where $h = Ac/X$ has been substituted.

The term containing the complementary error function can also be written

$$-h \exp[h(x+\xi) + h^2 Xt] \, \mathrm{erfc}\left[\frac{x+\xi}{2(Xt)^{1/2}} + h(Xt)^{1/2}\right] =$$

$$-\frac{h}{(\pi Xt)^{1/2}} \int_0^\infty \exp(-h\alpha) \exp\left[-\frac{(x+\xi+\alpha)^2}{4Xt}\right] d\alpha \quad . \quad (22)$$

The fluence rate due to the release of a uniform energy density Q_{cyl} per unit length of an infinite thin line parallel to the surface at time $t = 0$ can correspondingly be expressed[16]

$$\varphi(x,z,t) = \left\{\exp\left[-\frac{(x-\xi)^2}{4Xt}\right] + \exp\left[-\frac{(x+\xi)^2}{4Xt}\right]\right.$$

$$-\int_0^\infty 2h \exp(-h\alpha) \exp\left[-\frac{(x+\xi+\alpha)^2}{4Xt}\right] d\alpha\bigg\}$$

$$\times \exp\left[-\frac{(z-\zeta)^2}{4Xt}\right]\frac{1}{4\pi Xt}cQ_{cyl}\exp\left(-\frac{t}{\tau}\right) \quad , \quad (23)$$

where the line is oriented parallel to the y-axis and goes through the point given by ($x = \xi$, $z = \zeta$).

Acknowledgments

This work was performed with support from The George Hewitt Foundation for Medical Research, the Office of Naval Research grant #N00014-91-C-0134, and the Department of Energy grant #DE-FG03-91 ER61227. The authors wish to thank Khai Vu, Eric Cho, Matthew McAdams, and Joseph Ahdoot for their contributions.

References

1. S. Ertefai and A. E. Profio, "Spectral transmittance and contrast in breast diaphanography," *Med. Phys.* **12**, 393–400 (1985).
2. G. A. Navarro and A. E. Profio, "Contrast in diaphanography of the breast," *Med. Phys.* **15**, 181–187 (1988).
3. S. Andersson-Engels, R. Berg, S. Svanberg, and O. Jarlman, "Time-resolved transillumination for medical diagnostics," *Opt. Lett.* **15**, 1179–1181 (1990).
4. M. S. Patterson, B. Chance, and B. C. Wilson, "Time-resolved reflectance and transmittance for the non-invasive measurement of tissue optical properties," *Appl. Opt.* **28**, 2331–2336 (1989).
5. K. M. Yoo, Q. Xing, and R. R. Alfano, "Imaging objects hidden in highly scattering media using femtosecond second-harmonic-generation cross-correlation time gating," *Opt. Lett.* **16**, 1019–1021 (1991).
6. L. O. Svaasand and B. J. Tromberg, "On the properties of optical waves in turbid media," in *Future Trends of Biomedical Applications of Lasers, Proc. SPIE* **1525**, 41–50 (1991).
7. B. J. Tromberg, L. O. Svaasand, T. Tsay, R. C. Haskell, and M. W. Berns, "Optical property measurement in turbid media using frequency domain photon migration," in *Future Trends of Biomedical Applications of Lasers, Proc. SPIE* **1525**, 52–58 (1991).
8. E. M. Sevick, B. Chance, J. Leigh, S. Nioka, and M. Maris, "Quantification of time and frequency-resolved optical spectra for the determination of tissue oxygenation," *Anal. Biochem.* **195**, 330–351 (1991).
9. A. E. Profio, "Light transport in tissue," *Appl. Opt.* **28**, 2216–2222 (1989).
10. K. M. Yoo, F. Liu, and R. R. Alfano, "Imaging through a scattering wall using absorption," *Opt. Lett.* **16**, 1068–1070 (1991).
11. J. C. Hebden, R. A. Kruger, and K. S. Wong, "Time resolved imaging through a highly scattering medium," *Appl. Opt.* **30**, 788–794 (1991).
12. J. Fishkin, E. Gratton, M. J. vandeVen, and W. W. Mantulin, "Diffusion of intensity modulated near-infrared light in turbid media," in *Time Resolved Spectroscopy and Imaging of Tissues, Proc. SPIE* **1431**, 122–135 (1991).
13. "Quantities and units of light and related electromagnetic radiations," International Standard ISO 31/6 (1980).
14. B. J. Tromberg, L. O. Svaasand, T. T. Tsay, and C. H. Haskell, "Properties of photon density waves in multiple-scattering media," *Appl. Opt.* (in press).
15. A. Ishimaru, "Diffusion of light in turbid materials," *Appl. Opt.* **28**, 2210–2215 (1989).
16. H. S. Carslaw and J. C. Jaeger, *Conduction of Heat in Solids*, Oxford Science Publication, Oxford, pp. 371 (1959).

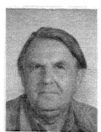

Lars O. Svaasand received the MS degree in electrical engineering and the PhD degree in physical electronics in 1961 and 1974, respectively, from the Norwegian Institute of Technology, University of Trondheim, Norway. He has been a professor of physical electronics at the Division of Physical Electronics, Norwegian Institute of Technology, since 1982, and he served as chairman of the Department of Electrical Engineering and Computer Science at the Institute from 1984 to 1987. He has been a visiting professor at the University of California/Santa Barbara, the University of Southern California School of Medicine, and at the University of California/Irvine. He is a member of the American Physical Society, American Society for Laser Medicine and Surgery, American Society for Photobiology, The New York Academy of Sciences, SPIE, The Norwegian Academy of Technical Sciences, and The Royal Norwegian Society of Sciences. He is also a coeditor of the Journal *Lasers in Medical Science*.

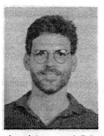

Bruce J. Tromberg is an assistant professor with joint appointments in the departments of Surgery and Physiology-Biophysics at the Beckman Laser Institute and Medical Clinic, University of California/Irvine. He completed his undergraduate studies at Vanderbilt University and was subsequently awarded a Department of Energy Predoctoral Fellowship at Oak Ridge National Laboratory and the University of Tennessee. In 1988 he received a PhD in chemistry, specializing in optical spectroscopy and fiber sensors, and began a Hewitt Foundation Postdoctoral Fellowship at the Beckman Laser Institute. Dr. Tromberg's research interests include the development of noninvasive optical techniques for monitoring physiology in single cells and tissues.

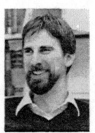

Richard C. Haskell is an associate professor of physics at Harvey Mudd College in California. He received his PhD in nuclear physics from Johns Hopkins University in 1972, after which he devoted six years to laser light scattering studies of skeletal muscle in the Biophysics Department at Johns Hopkins. His current interests in biophysics focus on laser probes of membrane dynamics and laser diagnostics of tissue. Haskell is a member of SPIE, the American Physical Society, and the Biophysical Society.

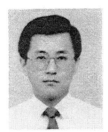 **Tsong-Tseh Tsay** attended the National Cheng Kung University, Taiwan, from 1976 through 1980, receiving a BS degree in physics. He was a graduate student at the University of North Carolina at Chapel Hill, receiving the MS and PhD degrees in biomedical engineering in 1986 and 1990, respectively. Since 1990, he has held a George E. Hewitt Foundation research fellowship position at Beckman Laser Institute and Medical Clinic at the University of California/Irvine. His current research interests include photon migration in tissue, optical spectroscopy, and imaging for biomedical applications.

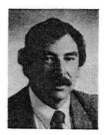 **Michael W. Berns,** the Arnold and Mabel Beckman professor, is president, director, and cofounder of the Beckman Laser Institute and Medical Clinic at the University of California/Irvine. He is also a professor of surgery, cell biology, radiology, and ophthalmology. Dr. Berns earned his bachelor's, master's, and doctorate degrees from Cornell University, Ithaca, New York, where he specialized in genetics, cell biology, and developmental biology. His basic research interests are focused on studies of cell genetics, cellular motility and cell movement, and the development of lasers and computers for biomedical studies. His clinical research involves the use of lasers in cancer, cardiovascular surgery, and vision.

Reprinted with permission from *Lasers in Surgery and Medicine,* Vol. 6, pp. 494-503 (1987). ©1987 Wiley-Liss division of John Wiley & Sons, Inc.

Modeling Optical and Thermal Distributions in Tissue During Laser Irradiation

Steven L. Jacques, PhD, and Scott A. Prahl, BS

Department of Dermatology, Massachusetts General Hospital, Harvard Medical School, Boston (S.L.J.); Biomedical Engineering Program, University of Texas, Austin (S.A.P.)

The propagation of light energy in tissues is an important problem in phototherapy, especially with the increased use of lasers as light sources. Often a slight difference in delivered energy separates a useless, efficacious, or disastrous treatment. Methods are presented for experimental characterization of the optical properties of a tissue and computational prediction of the distribution of light energy within a tissue. A standard integrating sphere spectrophotometer measured the total transmission, T_t, total reflectance, R_t, and the on-axis transmission, T_a, for incident collimated light that propagated through the dermis of albino mouse skin, over the visible spectrum. The diffusion approximation solution to the one-dimensional (1-D) optical transport equation computed the expected T_t and R_t for different combinations of absorbance, k, scattering, s, and anisotropy, g, and by iterative comparison of the measured and computed T_t and R_t values converged to the intrinsic tissue parameters. For example, mouse dermis presented optical parameters of 2.8 cm^{-1}, 239 cm^{-1}, and 0.74 for k, s, and g, respectively, at 488 nm wavelength. These values were used in the model to simulate the optical propagation of the 488-nm line of an argon laser through mouse skin in vivo. A 1-D Green's function thermal diffusion model computed the temperature distribution within the tissue at different times during laser irradiation. In vitro experiments showed that the threshold temperature range for coagulation was 60°-70° C, and the kinetics were first order, with a temperature-dependent rate constant that obeyed an Arrhenius relation (molar entropy 276 cal/mol-°K, molar enthalpy 102 kcal/mol). The model simulation agreed with the corresponding in vivo experiment that a 2-s pulse at 55 W/cm^2 irradiance will achieve coagulation of the skin.

INTRODUCTION

The propagation of light within tissues is an important problem that confronts the dosimetry of therapeutic laser delivery and the development of diagnostic spectroscopy. In the clinical application of photodynamic therapy (PDT) and in other research applications in photobiology, the photon deposition within a tissue determines the spatial distribution of photochemical reactions. When high intensities of light are delivered, eg, during laser irradiation, thermal damage is possible, and the photon deposition becomes the distributed heat source for a thermal diffusion problem. We have developed an animal model (albino BALB/c mouse) for the study of cutaneous tissue responses to thermal damage caused by argon laser irradiation, which yields reproducible, even, full thickness aseptic wounds (R. Granstein, S. Jacques, unpublished study). This paper presents 1) the experimental determination of the threshold temperature range and kinetics for coagulation of mouse skin, and 2) the

experimental specification of the threshold laser irradiance and exposure duration (488 nm) required for photocoagulation of mouse skin in vivo.

Standard spectrophotometric equipment was used for optical measurements on the thin tissue samples. The simple geometry of the in vitro measurement allowed a three-parameter model to uniquely specify the intrinsic optical parameters of the tissue: scattering (s), absorption (k), and anisotropy (g). These intrinsic tissue parameters become available for other more sophisticated models to predict optical distributions in complex geometries. This paper outlines the procedures that computed 1) the optical parameters, s, k, and g, based on experimental measure-

Address reprint requests to Steven L. Jacques, PhD, Wellman Laboratories, Department of Dermatology, Massachusetts General Hospital, Boston, MA 02114.

Accepted for publication September 17, 1986.

ments, 2) the photon deposition within in vivo mouse skin, and 3) the temporal evolution of the temperature distribution within the skin during simulated laser irradiation by the 488-nm argon laser. The procedures presented offer a general approach toward specification of the intrinsic optical properties of thin tissues.

MATERIALS AND METHODS

Tissue

Fourteen 6–8-week-old BALB/c albino mice were sacrificed in pairs, and the fur was plucked from the back. The full thickness skin was excisd from the back in a 2 × 4-cm rectangular sample. The fat layer was removed by scraping with forceps until only the dermis and the thin epidermis remained. Each sample was immediately placed on a glass slide with the dermis against the glass and the epidermis exposed to the air. The loss of moisture across the stratum corneum was minimal. The exposed edges of a sample dried slightly during the experiment, which retarded further water loss. The edges were not involved in the optical measurements. Each sample thickness was determined by micrometer measurements of the tissue between glass slides of known thickness. After optical measurements were made on each sample, the two samples were placed together to provide a thicker tissue specimen for a third optical measurement. Some manipulation was required to remove air bubbles between the samples, which slightly stretched the samples and reduced the net thickness. Micrometer measurements documented the final thickness of the double layer.

Optical Measurements

A standard integrating sphere spectrophotometer (Beckman UV 5270) was used for optical transmission and reflection measurements, as outlined in Figure 1. The integrating sphere was used to measure the total transmission, T_t, and total reflectance, R_t, from the skin sample mounted on the glass slide. The sample was placed at the entry port of the sphere during measurements of T_t. Collimated light directly struck the sample and propagated into the integrating sphere for detection. During measurements of R_t, the sample was removed from the entry port and replaced a removable BaSO$_4$ plate at the back exit port. Collimated light entered the entry port and directly struck the sample positioned at the back exit port, and reflected light was detected within the sphere. As a supplemental measurement to test the predictive ability of the model, the total reflectance with a black backing, R_0, was measured where the tissue sample rested on the blackened surface of a painted glass slide or on an agar gel containing black India ink. These absorbing boundaries eliminated internal reflectance at

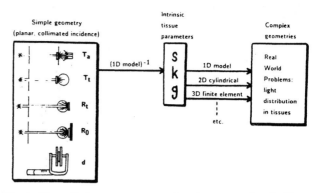

Fig. 1. The optical measurements conducted on mouse dermis. The on-axis transmission, T_a, was made with the standard spectrophotometer configuration. The integrating sphere was used for measurements of total transmission, T_t, total reflection, R_t, and total reflection with a black backing, R_0. The 1-D diffusion approximation solution to the transport equation [Ishimaru, 1978] provided the theoretical model.

the dermis/glass/air interface on the back side of the sample.

Removal of the integrating sphere assembly allowed measurements of the on-axis transmission, T_a, by placement of the sample over the standard exit port. Collimated light struck the sample, but only light that continued to propagate on-axis beyond the sample was detected. To determine the solid angle of collection by the detector, measurements were made on a 2-mm thickness of Teflon, which yielded a perfectly diffuse transmission pattern as verified by angular scattering experiments not presented here. The on-axis transmission, T_a, was 0.08% ± 0.01% (SD for five wavelengths, 486–490 nm). The total transmission, T_t, measured with the integrating sphere was 27.0% ± 0.1%. The ratio T_a/T_t was 0.00296. This ratio is a function of the half-angle, θ, off the central axis for collection of light:

$$T_a/T_t = 1/(2\pi R^2) \int_0^\theta 2\pi R \sin(\theta)\cos(\theta)\,R\,d\theta = \frac{\sin^2(\theta)}{2}$$

or

$$\theta = \arcsin([2T_a/T_t]^{1/2}), \qquad (1)$$

where the $\cos(\theta)$ term is introduced to account for Lambert's law of cosines [see Sliney and Wolbarsht, 1980], which describes the observation of light from a diffuse planar light source. According to equation 1, the ratio T_a/T_t, 0.00296, corresponds to a 4.4° half-angle θ of collection off the central axis, or 0.039 steradians of solid angle. (The concept of solid angle is valid only for a point source of light, so an approximation is made here when we treat the diffuse light transmitted by the Teflon slab as a point source.)

A portion of the measured T_a is due to diffuse light transmission. The ratio, b, equal to T_a/T_t that was observed for the Teflon slab was 0.00296. Therefore, we assumed that 0.296% of the total transmitted light, T_t, would be collected in the T_a measurement but should not be considered as collimated transmission, T_c. The following relation was used to calculate the measured T_c minus the contribution from T_t:

$$\text{measured } T_c = (T_a - bT_t)/(1 - b) \qquad (2)$$

The ratio T_c/T_a was 0.93 ± 0.08 over 21 measurements, which indicated that this was a minor correction.

The value for T_c included the effects of specular reflectance, R_s, at discontinuities in refractive index. The R_s is $(n_2-n_1)^2/(n_2+n_1)^2$ between two media with indices of refraction n_1 and n_2. In general, the refractive index of tissue varies between 1.33 and 1.5 for water contents between 100% and 0% [Bausch and Lomb]. The n for dry stratum corneum at the skin surface is about 1.45 [Solan et al, 1977], appropriate for a 30% water content. Therefore, the R_{s1} at the air/epidermis interface was assumed to be 3.4%. This neglected the effects of surface roughness. At the back of the tissue, collimated light encounters a wet dermis/glass/air interface. The n for wet dermis (about 70% water content), glass, and air are 1.38, 1.55, and 1, respectively. Because multiple reflections occur between the tissue/glass and glass/air interfaces, the net reflectance from this interface is given:

$$R_{s2} = 1 - (1 - R_1)(1 - R_2)[1 + \sum_i R_1^i R_2^i] \qquad (3)$$

where R_1 is the dermis/glass reflectance 0.3%, and R_2 is the glass/air reflectance 4.7%. The net R_{s2} is 5.0%. Therefore, the value for T_c, was corrected for specular reflectances:

$$\text{actual } T_c = (\text{measured } T_c)/(1 - R_{s1})(1 - R_{s2}) \qquad (4)$$

In summary, a measured T_a was corrected by equation 2 to account for the contribution from T_t and yield the measured T_c, then equation 4 accounted for specular reflectances to yield the actual T_c.

The observed values T_t and R_t also included the effects of specular reflectance, and were related to the diffuse transmission and reflectance, T_d and R_d, as discussed in Appendix I.

The internal reflectance r_i of diffuse light at the air/epidermis and the dermis/glass/air interfaces must also be considered. Although the front and surfaces should exhibit different values for r_i, the differences were expected to be small, based on an analysis using the Fresnel equations (calculations not shown). The measurements, T_t, R_t, and R_0 from 91 various experiments with full

thickness skin, isolated dermis, and hydrated dermis were introduced into Kottler's formulae to specify a mean value for r_i [Kottler, 1960]. This value was used in the following propagation model.

Optical Propagation Model

The one-dimensional (1-D) diffusion approximation solution to the transport equation [Ishimaru, 1978] provided a means 1) to compute the expected T_d and R_d, given a choice of s, k, and g, and 2) to compute the distribution of light within the tissue. An initial choice of s, k, and g, was made, and the expected T_d and R_d were calculated. Comparison with the observed T_d and R_d allowed an improved choice of s, k, and g. Iteration of this choice/comparison/improved choice algorithm converged quickly to a unique set of s, k, and g values. The choices of s and k always met the constraint that $s + k$ equaled γ, the attenuation constant for collimated light:

$$T_c = e^{-\gamma d} \quad \text{or} \quad \gamma = -\ln(T_c)/d \qquad (5)$$

where d was the sample thickness in cm. The implementation of the 1-D solution is presented in Appendix I. In the appendix the absorption coefficient k is denoted $\rho\sigma_a$, the scattering coefficient s is denoted $\rho\sigma_s$, and the attenuation constant γ is denoted $\rho\sigma_t$, to be consistent with the notation of Ishimaru [1978].

Thermal Diffusion Model

The optical distribution obtained for the best choice of s, k, and g multiplied by the absorption coefficient, k, yielded the spatial distribution of photon deposition in W/cc, which is the distributed heat source for a thermal diffusion problem. A one-dimensional Green's function for thermal diffusion in a wet tissue was convolved against the spatial distribution of photon deposition within the tissue to yield the temperature distribution within the tissue as a function of time (see Appendix II). The Green's function was based on the following assumed values: 0.80 cal/g-°C for heat capacity, C, 1.09 g/cc for density, ρ, and 1.01×10^{-3} cm²/s for diffusivity, α, which are all based on the expected values for a tissue with 70% water content, W, according to the review of Takata et al [1977; see Welch, 1984], and assuming a density of 1.3 g/cc for dry tissue:

$$C = [0.37 + 0.67W/\rho](\text{cal/g}-{}^0\text{c})$$
$$\alpha = [0.133 + 1.36W/\rho] \times 10^{-3}] \ (\text{cm}^2/\text{s}) \qquad (6)$$
$$\rho = [1.3 - 0.3W] \ (\text{g/cc})$$

Temperature Threshold for Thermal Coagulation

To determine the threshold temperature for tissue coagulation, three full thickness skin samples were each marked with a 3 × 3 grid of black points separated 1 cm apart. The grid was easily documented by making a photocopy of the tissue sample held on the outer surface of a petri dish. The samples were immersed for 10 s in a well-stirred water bath at a known temperature, removed to the petri dish, and again photocopied. This procedure was repeated for increasing water bath temperatures. When the threshold temperature for coagulation was reached, the spacing between the grid points suddenly decreased. To determine the kinetics of coagulation, 18 skin samples from six mice were repeatedly immersed for 10-s periods in the water bath at one of three temperatures, 62°C, 64°C, or 66°C (six samples per temperature tested). The degree of coagulation in the direction of lateral orientation across the back of the mouse as a function of time was recorded.

Argon Laser Experiments

Three anesthetized animals (BALB/c mice, 6–8 weeks old, 0.8% chloral hydrate, 0.1 ml per 10 g body weight) were the subjects of argon laser irradiation at 488 nm wavelength. The ambient skin temperature was 29° ± 1°C, as measured by thermocouple. Laser light was transmitted through 4 feet of 600-μm diameter optical fiber, and focused through a ×10 objective lens to yield a 3-mm diameter image of the fiber tip on the animal's back. This method of optical delivery produced a very flat field. The irradiance of the spot could be adjusted up to 60 W/cm^2 by controlling the electrical discharge current in the laser. The laser light was delivered in either 1/2-s or 1-s pulses by a timed shutter at increasing irradiances until thermal coagulation of the skin was observed.

RESULTS
Optical Measurements

The total transmission, T_t, total reflection, R_t, and total reflection with a black backing, R_0, are shown in Figure 2A for wavelengths from to 350 to 800 nm, and the on-axis transmission, T_a, is shown in Figure 2B. At shorter wavelengths absorption was significant, and all measurements decreased. Some blood remained in this fresh tissue specimen, as indicated by absorption centered at 418 nm and 540–580 nm. At 488 nm there was only a slight contribution to the absorbance by the blood, and dermal absorbance was the dominant site of photon deposition. The following results consider only the data at 488 nm, as listed in Table I.

The calculated values for the intrinsic optical parameters, s, k, and g, based on the γ, T_t, and R_t values, are summarized in Table II. The ability to determine k was sensitive to thin spots in the dermis that occasionally

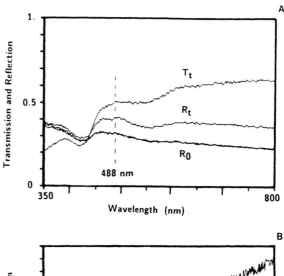

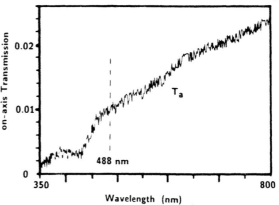

Fig. 2. The spectrophometric data from 350–800 nm for one of the mouse skin samples. **A**: The total transmission, T_t, the total reflection, R_t, and the total reflection with a black backing, R_0. Two R_0 scans are plotted, one for a black painted glass slide backing and the other for an India ink/agar backing, but they are indistinguishable. **B**: The on-axis transmission, T_a.

occurred during preparation. The determination of s and g were less sensitive to such problems in technique.

To illustrate how the s, k and g parameters were calculated, Figure 3 plots as R_t versus T_t both the measured data and the expected values based on the different choices of s, k, and g. The graph is appropriate for a tissue thickness of 116 μm (average single skin thickness) and a wavelength of 488 nm. The grid is based on a γ value of 242 cm^{-1}, and shows constant g lines at various k and constant k lines at various g. The mouse skin values are those expected for a tissue that is 116 μm thick, according to Figure 4 (below). There is a unique choice for s, k, and g, which corresponds to mouse skin. The curve in the grid that corresponds to $g = 0$ indicates the behavior of purely isotropic scattering media. Mouse skin scatters light in a more strongly forward direction, which increases T_t and decreases R_t. (The negative reflec-

TABLE I. Summary of Measurements on Mouse Skin

No.	d	T_a	T_t	R_t	R_0
1	123	.0121	.525	.440	.283
2	161	.0198	.578	.341	.256
1 + 2	199	.0033	.360	.491	.438
3	80	.0546	.629	.241	.123
4	132	.0457	.6782	.229	.137
3 + 4	134	.0168	.567	.321	.170
5	101	.0257	.587	.281	.150
6	80	.0796	.713	.205	.094
5 + 6	164	.0123	.479	.338	.197
7	96	.1689	.689	.252	.125
8	100	.2307	.681	.254	.142
7 + 8	152	.0629	.591	.288	.176
9	118	.0703	.702	.234	.135
10	133	.0823	.687	.275	.150
9 + 10	211	.0189	.588	.347	.225
11	117	.0517	.648	.283	.175
12	119	.1673	.706	.224	.140
11 + 12	185	.0380	.585	.304	.228
13	126	.0311	.632	.274	.184
14	132	.0683	.726	.246	.123
13 + 14	232	.0087	.5038	.363	.253

No., specimen No. (double layers indicated by sum); d, tissue thickness (μm); T_a, on-axis transmission, within 4.4° half angle of acceptance; T_t, total transmission, collected by integrating sphere; R_t, total reflection, collected by integrating sphere; R_0, R_t for tissue with a black backing.

TABLE II. Summary of Calculated Intrinsic Optical Parameters

No.	s	k	g
1	361	1.1	.66
2	241	2.0	.74
1 + 2	298	3.0	.58
3	350	7.0	.78
4	228	2.9	.84
3 + 4	303	3.3	.76
5	354	5.3	.78
6	304	4.2	.84
5 + 6	264	4.7	.71
7	173	2.5	.67
8	135	2.7	.57
7 + 8	175	3.4	.69
9	218	1.4	.80
10	181	1.1	.75
9 + 10	187	1.2	.75
11	246	2.3	.76
12	141	2.4	.72
11 + 12	172	2.5	.72
13	270	3.0	.80
14	199	0.8	.82
13 + 14	206	2.3	.73
Mean	238	2.8	.74
SD	67	1.5	.07

No., specimen No. (double layers indicated by sum); s, scattering coefficient (cm^{-1}); k, absorption coefficient (cm^{-1}); g, anisotropy.

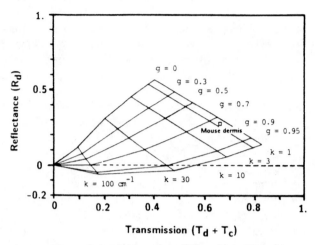

Fig. 3. Diffuse reflectance, R_d, versus diffuse plus collimated transmission ($T_d + T_c$) at 488 nm. The values for mouse skin expected for a 116-μm tissue thickness are mapped as a single point. The grid indicates the theoretical values for R_d and ($T_d + T_c$) for a range of values for absorption, k, scattering, s, and anisotropy, g. This grid meets the constraints: $k + s = 242$ cm^{-1}, and thickness, d, equals 116 μm, which was the average dermal thickness.

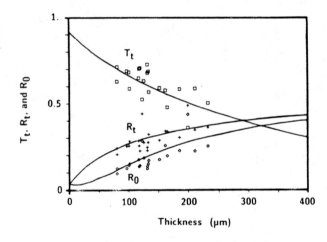

Fig. 4. The measurements on mouse skin at 488 nm, plotted as a function of sample thickness. The total transmission, T_t (□), total reflectance, R_t (+), and total reflectance with a black backing, R_0 (◇), are shown.

tance indicated by the grid for very anisotropic media [g close to 1] are expected. The diffusion approximation assumes that light distribution is nearly uniform. For highly anisotropic media, the boundary conditions cannot satisfy the constraints that light be both nearly uniform and highly anisotropic, and the model breaks down.)

The measured values for T_t, R_t, and R_0 are plotted in Figure 4 as a function of sample thickness, d. The theoretical curves for T_t, R_t, and R_0, as calculated by the 1-D model, using the average values for s, k, and g in

Table II are plotted as solid lines. To compute R_0, the internal reflection, R_i, at the inner boundary was set to equal zero. The black backing during the R_0 measurement absorbed any light that reached the back of the tissue, and decreased the observed R_t since there was no longer internal reflectance at the back interface. There was no difference in R_0 measurements made with a black painted glass slide versus an agar gel containing India ink. Since the R_0 measurements were not used to deduce the s, k, and g values, the agreement of the theoretical curve and the observed R_0 data constitutes a test of the predictive ability of the model.

Predicted Optical and Thermal Distributions In Vivo

The distributions of optical fluxes in vivo as calculated by the 1-D model using the average values of s, k, and g in Table II are plotted in Figure 5. The internal

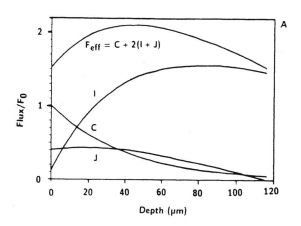

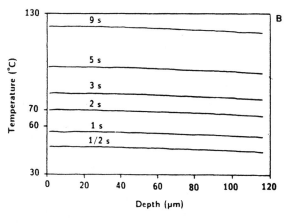

Fig. 5. The calculated distribution of optical fluxes and temperatures within mouse skin during argon laser irradiation. A: The collimated flux, C, the forward diffuse flux, I, the backward diffuse flux, J, and the total effective flux, $F_{eff} = C + 2(I + J)$, which contributes to heating. B: The calculated distribution of temperatures versus tissue depth during argon laser irradiation in vivo at 55 W/cm². The temperature profiles at 0.5, 1, 2, 3, 5, and 9 s are shown. Initial skin temperature was 29°C.

reflectance from the inner skin surface was assumed to be zero, which was an approximation since there was actually some reflectance from the deeper tissues. The incident collimated flux, C, attenuated quickly, and the $1/e$ depth equaled 40 μm. The forward diffuse flux, I, increased to a maximum near an 80-μm depth. The backward diffuse flux, J, increased steadily toward the tissue front surface. The total effective flux, F_{eff} in W/cm², which contributed to heating, equaled $C + 2(I + J)$. (See Appendix I.) F_{eff} achieved a maximum value at a depth of 45 μm that was more than twice the incident collimated flux, F_0. At the surface, F_{eff} exceeded F_0 by 52%. (F_0 equal to 55 W/cm².)

The distribution of temperature in vivo during argon laser irradiation was calculated (see Appendix II) based on the predicted optical flux distribution in Figure 5A. The temperatures at 0.5, 1, 2, 3, 5, and 9 s of laser irradiation are plotted in Figure 5B. Thermal diffusion distributed the absorbed laser energy, and a subsurface maximum in temperature was not obvious. The dermis was relatively evenly heated to 70°C by 2 s of laser irradiation. After 5–9 s of irradiation, temperatures were in the neighborhood of 100–120°C.

Thermal Coagulation

Coagulation of in vitro skin occurred above 60°C, as indicated by the contraction of the tissue and as documented by the decrease in grid spacing. The kinetics of coagulation were first order, as shown in Figure 6 in which the grid spacing, x, in cm is plotted versus time of

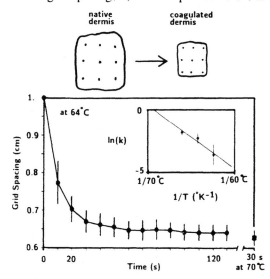

Fig. 6. The thermal coagulation of mouse skin at 64°C. The spacing between grid points drawn on a skin sample decreased with repeated 10-s immersions. The mean grid spacing for six specimens is plotted versus accumulated time of immersion, and standard deviations are shown. **Insert**: the first order rate constants, k (s⁻¹), for coagulation at 62°C, 64°C, and 66°C are plotted versus inverse temperature. The slope yields a molar enthalpy of 102 kcal/mol and the y-intercept at infinite temperature yields a molar entropy of 296 cal/mol-°K.

immersion, t. The grid spacing decreased with time of immersion:

$$x = [1 - (1 - x_{max})(1 - e^{-kt})] \text{ (cm)} \quad (7)$$

where x_{max} is the grid spacing after maximum coagulation, and k is a first-order rate constant, in s^{-1}. The same x_{max} was achieved after several repeated exposures at 62, 64, or 66°C. Subsequent 30-s exposure to a 70°C bath did not cause significant further coagulation. Table III summarizes the data. The rate constant, k (s^{-1}), increased with temperature according to an Arrhenius relationship (see insert, Fig. 6):

$$\ell n(k) = \Delta S/R + \Delta H/RT \quad (8)$$

where molar entropy, ΔS, equaled 297 cal/mol-°K and molar enthalpy, ΔH, equaled 102 kcal/mol.

Experimental Argon Laser Photocoagulation

The threshold for photocoagulation of mouse skin in vivo by CW argon laser irradiation was a 1.5-s pulse at 55 W/cm^2, which produced a whitening of the skin owing to the increased scattering of coagulated dermis. A 2-s pulse at this irradiance reliably achieved coagulation. Obvious contraction of the skin site began at this time. If the laser irradiation was delivered continuously, a sudden explosive vaporization occurred at 5–10 s, which according to Figure 5b was when temperatures exceeded 100°C. Onset of this explosive event was variable.

DISCUSSION

This method for experimental specification of the intrinsic transport parameters for a tissue is appropriate for thin specimens. It is necessary for sufficient light to penetrate the specimen so that a reliable measurement of T_a is made. The acceptance angle for the T_a measurement on this spectrophotometer was ±4.4°. There is a degree of arbitrariness and oversimplification in choosing to call light accepted within this angle "on-axis," and to call all transmitted light not collected "diffuse." A laser beam does not immediately become "diffuse" after a single scattering event, according to goniometric studies of the angular dependence of dermal scattering (S. Jacques. unpublished study). How different would the calculated s, k, and g values be if a spectrophotometer with a larger or smaller acceptance angle was used? The limits of this approach toward specification of tissue optical parameters are currently under study. However, at this time we feel that these concerns will not prove serious, and the method offers a simple approach using equipment widely available.

The optical distribution within the tissue showed a maximum total flux at a depth of 45 μm beneath the skin surface. However, the thermal diffusion throughout the dermal thickness of 116 μm was rapid, and the temperature distribution was quite even. Such uniform heating can achieve a controlled coagulation, which offers a reliable wound model for tissue-response studies.

The kinetics of coagulation are temperature dependent. The rate constant becomes very slow below 60°C and very fast above 70°C. Within this threshold temperature range the coagulation process takes seconds. and there is ample opportunity for changes in optical properties to occur, which would alter the photon deposition. For example, a recent report describes how thermal coagulation affects the optical properties of aorta by doubling reflectance and halving transmission [Gourgouliatos et al, 1986]. Work continues on the optical changes that occur during dermal coagulation and on how to incorporate such changes into the simulation of laser irradiation of tissue.

ACKNOWLEDGMENTS

We thank Martin van Gemert, Willem Star. Wai Fung Cheong, Norm Nishioka, and Rox Anderson for many important discussions; A.J. Welch and John Parrish for their interest and facilitation in the collaboration of our laboratories; Rick Granstein for help with the in vivo argon irradiation experiments; Susan Clegg for help with the optical measurements; and Kosta Zinis for help with the in vitro thermal coagulation experiments. The latter three persons continue in the mouse skin studies. which will be reported in more complete form.

This work was supported by NIH grant AM25395-08. O.N.R. Contract #N001486K0017, and the Arthur O. and Gullan M. Wellman Foundation.

REFERENCES

Abramowitz M. Stegun IA. eds.: "Handbook of Mathematical Functions." eq. 7.4.32, New York: Dover Publications Inc.. 1972. p 303.

TABLE III. Thermal Coagulation of Mouse Skin

T	x_{max}	$x_{70°}$	k
62°C			
Average	.648	.638	.036
SD	.045	.022	.026
64°C			
Average	.645	.628	.109
SD	.025	.026	.037
66°C			
Average	.661	.635	.116
SD	.064	.041	.037

Six samples at each temperature (three samples per mouse). T, water bath temperature (°C): x_{max}. grid spacing after maximum coagulation (cm); $x_{70°}$. grid spacing after 30 s at 70°C (cm); k, first-order rate constant (s^{-1}).

Bausch and Lomb: "Refractive Index and Percent Dissolved Solids Scale." Analytic Systems Division (S-5195 0675).

Birngruber R: Thermal modeling in biological tissues. In Hillenkamp F, Pratesi R, Sacchi CA (eds): "Lasers in Biology and Medicine." New York and London: Plenum Press, 1980.

Carslaw HS, Jaeger JC: "Conduction of Heat in Solids." Oxford: Clarendon Press, 1973.

Gourgouliatos ZF, Welch AJ, van Gemert MCJ: Behavior of optical properties of tissue (transmittance and reflectance) as a function of temperature (abstract). Lasers Surg Med 6:166, 1986.

Groenhuis RAJ, Ferwerda HA, Ten Bosch JJ: Scattering and absorption of turbid materials determined from reflection measurements. Applied Optics 22:2456–2462, 1983.

Ishimaru A: "Wave Propagation and Scattering in Random Media."

New York: Academic Press, 1978.

Kottler F: Turbid media with plane-parallel surfaces. J Optical Soc 50:483–490, 1960.

Sliney D, Wolbarsht M: "Safety with Lasers and Other Optical Sources: A comprehensive handbook." New York: Plenum Press, 1980, p 22.

Solan JL, Laden K: Factors affecting the penetration of light through stratum corneum. J Soc Cosmet Chem 28:125–137, 1977.

Takata AN, Zaneveld L, Richter W: Laser-induced thermal damage in skin. USAF School of Aerospace Med., Brooks AFB, TX. Rep. SAM-TR-77-38, 1977.

Welch AJ: The thermal response of laser irradiated tissue. IEEE J Quantum Electronics QE-20:1471–1481, 1984.

APPENDIX I. One Dimensional Optical Propagation

The transport equation with no internal sources is (the notation and derivation in this appendix closely follow that by Ishimaru [1978]):

$$s \cdot \nabla I(r,s) = -\rho\sigma_t I(r,s) + \frac{\rho\sigma_t}{4\pi} \int_{4\pi} p(s,s')\, I(r,s')\, d\omega'$$

where $I(r,s)$ is the total specific intensity (W/cm^2/sr) at position r in the direction of the unit vector s and $d\omega'$ is the differential solid angle in the direction s'. The total scattering coefficient $\rho\sigma_t$ is the sum of the absorption and scattering coefficients, which are denoted by $\rho\sigma_a$ and $\rho\sigma_s$, respectively. The phase function $p(s,s')$ represents the fraction of light scattered from the direction s into the direction s'.

The total intensity $I(r,s)$ is split into collimated $I_{ri}(r)$ and diffuse $I_d(r,s)$ portions.

$$I(r,s) = I_{ri}(r) + I_d(r,s)$$

Assuming that the collimated beam is uniform and normal to the surface of the slab, then

$$I_{ri}(r) = F_0\, e^{-\rho\sigma_t z}\, \delta(\omega_s \cdot \omega_z)$$

where z is a unit vector in the direction of increasing z (normal and into the slab). F_0 has units of W/cm^2 and $\delta(\omega_s \cdot \omega_z)$ is a solid angle delta function with units of sr^{-1}.

The diffusion approximation expresses the diffuse intensity as the sum of an isotropic part $U_d(r)$ and an anisotropic part $F_d(r) \cdot s$:

$$I_d(r,s) = U_d(r) + \frac{3}{4\pi} F_d(r) \cdot s$$

where

$$U_d(r) = \frac{1}{4\pi} \int_{4\pi} I_d(r,s)\, d\omega, \quad F_d(r) = \int_{4\pi} I_d(r,s)(S \cdot Z)\, d\omega.$$

In a slab of infinite extent in the x and y directions, the specific intensity cannot depend on x or y (for symmetry reasons). By making the above substitutions the transport equation reduces to the photon diffusion equation,

$$\frac{d^2 U_d(z)}{dz^2} - \kappa_d^2 U_d(z) = -Q_0 e^{-\rho\sigma_t z} \qquad \text{(A1)}$$

where $\rho\sigma_{tr} = \rho\sigma_s(1-g) + \rho\sigma_a$ is the transport coefficient. $Q_0 = (3/4\pi)F_0(\rho\sigma_s\rho\sigma_{tr} + \rho\sigma_s\rho\sigma_t g)$, and $\kappa_d^2 = 3\rho\sigma_a\rho\sigma_{tr}$. The anisotropy coefficient g (equivalent to the $\bar{\mu}$ of Ishimaru) is defined as the average cosine of the phase function

$$g = \frac{1}{4\pi\omega_0} \int_{4\pi} p(s',s)\, (s \cdot s')\, d\omega, \quad \text{where } \omega_0 = \frac{\rho\sigma_s}{\rho\sigma_t}$$

The treatment of boundary conditions follows Groenhuis et al [1983] who assumed that the diffuse flux moving in the Z direction downward from the top surface was equal to the reflection of diffuse flux moving upward. Thus, if $\mu = s \cdot z$ and r_i is the internal reflection coefficient, then at the top surface

$$\int_{\substack{2\pi \\ \mu > 0}} I_d(r,s)\, (s \cdot z)\, d\omega = r_i \int_{\substack{2\pi \\ \mu < 0}} I_d(r,s)\, (s \cdot z)\, d\omega,$$

which reduces to the mixed inhomogeneous boundary condition

$$U_d(z) - h'\frac{dU_d(z)}{dz} + \frac{Q_1'(z)}{2\pi} = 0; \text{ @ } z = 0. \quad \text{(A2.1)}$$

A similar boundary condition is found for the bottom surface,

$$U_d(z) + h'\frac{dU_d(z)}{dz} - \frac{Q_1'(z)}{2\pi} = 0; \text{ @ } z = d, \quad \text{(A2.2)}$$

where

$$h' = \frac{1 + r_i}{1 - r_i} \cdot \frac{2}{3\rho\sigma_{tr}} \quad \text{and} \quad Q_1'(z) = \frac{1 + r_i}{1 - r_i} \cdot \frac{g\rho\sigma_s F_0}{\rho\sigma_{tr}} e^{-\rho\sigma_t z}.$$

The r_i used to calculate h' in A2.1 (top surface) may be chosen to be different than the r_i used for h' in A2.2 (bottom surface).

Solutions to (A1) subject to boundary conditions (A2) are given by Ishimaru, except that his $Q_1(z)$ and h are replaced by $Q_1'(z)$ and h'.

$$U_d(z) = Ae^{-\rho\sigma_t z} + C_1 e^{\kappa_d z} + C_2 e^{-\kappa_d z} \quad \text{(A3)}$$

where $A = -Q_0/[(\rho\sigma_t)^2 - \kappa_d^2]$. C_1 and C_2 can be found by substituting (A3) into (A2) and solving the resulting pair of linear simultaneous equations for C_1 and C_2:

$$C_1(1 - h'\kappa_d) + C_2(1 + h'\kappa_d)$$
$$= -A(1 + \rho\sigma_t h') - (1/2\pi)Q_1'(0),$$

$$C_1(1 + h'\kappa_d)e^{\kappa_d d} + C_2(1 - h'\kappa_d)e^{-\kappa_d d}$$
$$= -A(1 - \rho\sigma_t h')e^{-\rho\sigma_t d} + (1/2\pi)Q_1'(d).$$

Once C_1 and C_2 are known, then $U_d(z)$ may be calculated from (A3). The total intensity (W/cm^2) at a depth z is given by

$$I_{total}(z) = 4\pi U_d(z) + F_0 e^{-\rho\sigma_t z}. \quad \text{(A4)}$$

The product of the absorption coefficient $\rho\sigma_a$ and $I_{total}(z)$ yields the photon deposition in W/cc.

The distribution of light may also be discussed in terms of the collimated, forward diffuse, and backward diffuse fluxes, C, I, and J, respectively, which are expressed in W/cm^2 rather than the units W/cm^2-sr that are used for U_d. The definitions of these fluxes are given:

$$C = F_0 e^{-\rho\sigma_t z}$$

$$I = 2\pi(U_d/2 + B)$$

$$J = 2\pi(U_d/2 - B)$$

where

$$B = h(-\rho\sigma_t Ae^{-\rho\sigma_t z} + \kappa_d[C_1 e^{\kappa_d z} - C_2 e^{-\kappa_d z}])/2$$

The total effective flux, F_{eff} in W/cm^2, which contributes to heating, equals $C + 2(I + J)$, and is identical to I_{total} given in (A4). The factor of 2 accounts for the average double pathlength traveled by diffuse light compared to collimated light.

The diffuse transmission and reflection are given:

$$T_d = I(z = d)/F_0 \quad \text{(A5)}$$
$$R_d = J(z = 0)/F_0$$

Finally, the experimentally observed T_t and R_t values are given:

$$T_t = (1 - R_{s1})[T_d + (1 - R_{s2})T_c] \quad \text{(A6)}$$
$$R_t = R_{s1} + (1 - R_{s1})R_d$$

where R_{s1} and R_{s2} are the specular reflectances at the front and back surfaces, respectively, of the tissue sample, and T_c is the collimated transmission equal to $F_0 e^{-\rho\sigma_t d}$.

The implementation of the inverse model (model^{-1}) iteratively compared predicted T_d and R_d values (A5) that were based on choices of $\rho\sigma_a$, $\rho\sigma_s$, and g, with experimental T_d and R_d values, that were calculated from T_t, R_t, and T_c by rearrangement of (A6). The algorithm efficiently converged on a unique set of intrinsic optical properties for each tissue sample.

APPENDIX II. One-Dimensional Thermal Diffusion

The process of thermal diffusion obeys the relation [Carslaw and Jaeger, 1973; Birngruber, 1980]:

$$\rho C dT/dt = q + \alpha \nabla^2 T \quad \text{(A7)}$$

where ρ is the tissue density (g/cc), C is the specific heat (J/g-°C), α is the thermal diffusivity (J/cm-s-°C), q is the rate of deposition of photon energy (J/cc-s), T is temperature, and t is time (s). This relation neglects the influence of blood flow, metabolic heat generation, surface water evaporation, and convection, which are important for CW laser irradiation but not for laser pulses of only a few seconds in duration. The one-dimensional impulse response solution to equation 7 for an impulse of heat, Q in joules, deposited at time t' and position x', is given:

$$T_0(x,t) = \frac{Q}{2\rho C[\pi\alpha(t - t')]^{1/2}} e^{-(x-x')^2/4\alpha(t-t')} \quad \text{(A8)}$$

The convolution of this impulse response over both the spatial and temporal distribution of the photon energy deposition yields the temperature at a given position, x, and time, t:

$$T(x,t) = [1/\rho C(\pi\alpha)^{1/2}]$$
$$\int_0^{t} \int_{-\infty}^{+\infty} [q(x',t')/(t-t')^{1/2}]e^{-(x-x')^2/4\alpha(t-t')} \, dx' dt' \quad \text{(9)}$$

where $q(x',t')$ represents the rate of photon energy deposition as a function of time and depth within the tissue and can specify any temporal history of irradiation and spatial distribution of photon absorption by the tissue. The optical model (Appendix I) specified the photon deposition, $\rho\sigma_a I_{total}$, which yielded a $q(x')$ for a unity (1 J/cm^2) incident flux, independent of time. In our experiments, the laser output was a step function of magnitude 55 J/cm^2-s; therefore $q(x't')$ was given by the product $55q(x')$ in J/cm^2-s.

Equation A9 is a general description of the 1-D heat flow process, based on the impulse response to a Dirac delta function. During implementation on the computer, a square pulse function of arbitrarily small width replaced the delta function, to yield a "square pulse" response efficiently evaluated [Abramowitz and Stegun, 1972]:

$$T_0(x,t) = (Q/2\rho C)(\pi/a)^{1/2}[erf(a^{1/2}r) - erf(a^{1/2}r)] \quad (A10)$$

where a equals $(4\alpha t)^{-1/2}$, and r is the radius of the square pulse, which was set to 0.5 μm in this case since the tissue model was composed of 1-μm-wide elements for calculations. The erf function was evaluated by reference to a table held in the computer.

The continuous laser irradiation was treated as a series of impulses spaced at 1-ms intervals, each having an energy $Q(x)$ equal to (55 J/cm^2-s)(1 ms), or 55 mJ/cm^2, and calculations were made in time steps of 1 ms. The choice of interval was arbitrary, based on the resolution desired, and can be as short as required in other problems. At each time step, the square pulse response (eq. A10) was evaluated for time t and for all distances, $x - x'$, from a source, and the results were stored in an array for efficient access. Then, the contributions of heat to a given element from all other elements were calculated:

$$\text{heat contribution} = \sum_x Q(x',t)T_0(|x-x'|,t) \quad (A11)$$

As t increased with each time step, the contribution from heat flow finally arriving at time t at a given element was added to the accumulated heat content of that element. This accumulation constituted the time integral of equation A9, and equation A11 constituted the spatial integral of equation A9. Once laser irradiation was halted, the time-consuming time steps on the computer were no longer necessary. Equation A11 could yield the heat distribution at any later time by a single calculation.

The air/skin interface constituted an insulating boundary, and any heat flow to the surface was reflected back into the tissue. The mirror image of the heat source term $q(x')$ was extended into the air space above the skin, and heat was considered to flow from this image tissue. This mirror image technique properly solved the insulating boundary problem.

ERRATA for Jacques, Prahl (1987), Lasers Surg. Med. 6:494-503.

p. 496, ¶ 3:   after "... in the following propagation model."
add   " ($r_i = 0.3$)."

p. 502, 3:   after "The definitions of these fluxes are given: .... where"
add a final term to the equation for B:

$$B = h(-\rho\sigma_t A \exp(-\rho\sigma_t z) + \kappa_d[C_1\exp(\kappa_d z) - C_2\exp(-\kappa_d z)])/2$$
$$- F_o \rho\sigma_s g \exp(-\rho\sigma_t z)/(4\pi\rho\sigma_{tr})$$

p. 502, Eq. A9:   relabel equation as Eq. A9 and rewrite as:

$$T(x,t) = \left[\frac{1}{2\rho C(\pi\alpha)^{1/2}}\right] \int_0^t \int_{-\infty}^{\infty} [q(x',t')/(t-t')^{1/2}] \exp[-(x-x')^2/4\alpha(t-t')] \, dx' \, dt' \quad (A9)$$

p. 503, Eq. A10:   rewrite equation as:

$$T_o(x,t) = (Q/2\rho C)[erf(a^{1/2}(x+r)) - erf(a^{1/2}(x-r))] \quad (A10)$$

where a equals $(4\alpha t)^{-1}$, ...

Reprinted with permission from *Lasers in Surgery and Medicine*, Vol. 9, pp. 405-421 (1989). ©1989 Wiley-Liss division of John Wiley & Sons, Inc.

Time Constants in Thermal Laser Medicine

Martin J.C. van Gemert, PhD, and **A.J. Welch**, PhD

The University of Texas at Austin, Austin, Texas 78712

Temperature rise of laser-irradiated tissue due to direct absorption of laser light is related to laser parameters (power, spot size, irradiation time, and repetition rate) and tissue parameters (absorption and scattering coefficients, density, heat capacity, and thermal conductivity). Solutions to the bio-heat equation are approximated by introducing axial *(z)* and radial *(r)* time constants for heat conduction that represent two parallel channels for heat conduction. These axial (τ_z) and radial (τ_r) time constants are found proportional to squared distances (z_0^2, r_0^2) that represent the extent of axial and radial temperatures respectively. For convenience, z_0 and r_0 are approximated to the axial and radial extent of laser light in the tissue. The resulting solution of the bio-heat equation, expressed as temperature rise as function of time and position, is obviously exact for irradiation times short compared to τ_z, τ_r (adiabatic heating), but is also a quite reasonable approximation up to irradiation times three times the overall time constant. Comparison with (exact) numerical computations show that this holds for all ratios of (light) penetration depth to laser-beam radius; for strongly scattering materials, smaller laser beams give better predictions than do larger laser beams. Several examples of clinical relevance are discussed, such as multiple-laser-pulse irradiation of high- and low-absorbing tissues and laser treatment of port-wine stains, with some unexpected results that also show potential clinical relevance.

Key words: thermal time constants, temperature response, port-wine stain, penetration depth, multiple laser pulses

INTRODUCTION

Most of the clinical procedures with lasers use the so-called thermal mode of laser-tissue interaction [1]; that is, tissue is heated and irreversibly damaged by direct absorption of the laser light. The degree and extent of tissue damage depends strongly on the rate of heat generation (so-called heat-source term) in laser-irradiated tissue that is dependent on both laser and tissue parameters. Important laser parameters are wavelength, power, spot size, irradiation time, and repetition rate; and important tissue parameters are the optical properties that describe absorption and scattering and the thermal properties that describe the storage and transfer of heat. The temperature response is typically modeled by the heat-conduction equation [2]. For irradiation times less than about 5 sec, the influence of blood perfusion plays a minor role [3] and will be neglected here.

Accepted for publication April 7, 1989.

Address reprint requests to A.J. Welch, Biomedical Engineering Program, The University of Texas at Austin, Austin, TX 78712.

Martin J.C. van Gemert was on leave during 1984–85 from the St. Joseph Hospital, Eindhoven, The Netherlands, sponsored by the hospital, the Netherlands America Commission for Educational Exchange, and the Dutch Organization for the Advancement of Pure Research (ZWO). Present address: Laser Center, Academic Medical Center, Amsterdam, The Netherlands.

A.J. Welch is Marion E. Forsman Centennial Professor of Electrical and Computer Engineering and Biomedical Engineering.

This work was supported in part by the Free Electron Laser Biomedical/Materials Science Program: ONR Contract Number N-14-86-K-0875.

It is the purpose of this paper to discuss a simple model that approximates tissue temperature rise after laser irradiation in terms of the above-mentioned laser and tissue parameters. To this end, time constants for heat conduction are introduced in a cylindrical symmetric geometry. Several cases of relevance for clinical laser treatments are discussed, such as multiple-laser-pulse treatments of laser wavelengths that have high- and low-tissue absorbing properties and laser treatment of port-wine stains.

Typically, time-constant analysis for describing the thermal response of tissue to laser irradiation has considered either penetration depth (1/attenuation coefficient) or image size (spot diameter) but not these combined effects. Priebe and Welch [4] noted that for a nonscattering medium, the heat-conduction equation could be transformed to a dimensionless equation with a single parameter $\mu_a w_L$, where μ_a is the absorption coefficient and w_L is the $1/e^2$ diameter of the laser beam. Numerical solutions indicated that when $\mu_a w_L$ is much greater than one (i.e., the laser-beam size is much greater than the light-penetration depth), the heat-conduction equation is approximately a one-dimensional (axial) problem until the axial gradients become small with respect to the radial gradients. Then, the radial gradient becomes significant and the conduction is essentially in the radial direction. For values of the parameter $\mu_a w_L$ less than one, the axial gradient is de-emphasized and conduction is primarily in the radial direction. This concept was employed by Furzikov [5] in defining a single-characteristic thermal diffusion time, τ, $\tau = \pounds^2/(4\nu)$, where $\pounds$ is a characteristic length (m) and ν is thermal diffusivity (m^2/s). For short penetration depths (axial conduction), Furzikov used $\pounds = 1/\mu_a$, whereas for large penetration depths (radial conduction), Furzikov used $\pounds = w_L$ that is, he assumed either dominant axial conduction or radial conduction. The purpose of this paper is to consider the relative importance of these components and advantages and limitations associated with a time constant model.

THE MODEL
Introduction

A slab of tissue in air irradiated with a Gaussian-shaped laser beam is illustrated in Figure 1. The resulting temperature rise $\Delta T(t,z,r)$ at time t after onset of the laser, at depth z and radial co-

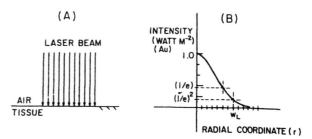

Fig. 1. **A**: A slab of tissue in air irradiated with a laser beam. **B**: Intensity profile of the laser beam, assumed to be Gaussian, with an "exp(-2)" radius of w_L.

ordinate r follows from the solution of the bio-heat equation in cylindrical geometry

$$\frac{\partial \Delta T(t,z,r)}{\partial t} = \frac{\mu_a \phi(z,r)}{\rho c} + \frac{k}{\rho c}\left[\frac{\partial^2 \Delta T}{\partial z^2} + \frac{\partial^2 \Delta T}{\partial r^2} + \frac{1}{r}\frac{\partial \Delta T}{\partial r}\right], \quad (1)$$

where μ_a is the tissue-absorption coefficient (m^{-1}), $\phi(z,r)$ is the (local) fluence rate of the laser light (Watt [W] m^{-2}), k is the thermal conductivity (W m^{-1} °C^{-1}), ρ is the tissue density (kg m^{-3}), and c is the heat capacity (Joule [J] kg^{-1} °C^{-1}). As was stated in the introduction section, convective heat losses by blood perfusion (and other possible heat losses) are neglected, indicating that long irradiation times (longer than a few seconds) are disregarded. Equation (1) does not include tissue removal (ablation). The first term on the right hand side of Equation (1) represents the rate of temperature increase caused by direct absorption of light; the second term is the rate of temperature increase due to heat conduction (this term is negative for a Gaussian radial heat source, so, in fact, it represents the rate of temperature *decrease*). The solution to Equation (1), assuming appropriate boundary and initial value conditions and assuming the optical and thermal parameters to be independent of temperature, has been obtained both analytically [6,7] and numerically [4,8,9].

These solutions to Equation (1) are not obvious, and it is difficult to predict intuitively changes in $\Delta T(t,z,r)$ caused by changes in laser or tissue parameters. In addition, when determination of fluence rate $\phi(z,r)$ requires solution of the so-called transport equation of radiative transfer, intuitive solutions become even more difficult. This integro-differential equation [10], for which there are mainly approximate solutions, does not provide obvious relations between the fluence rate and optical parameters. In a real situation, a temperature increase in tissue can result in dehydration, denaturation, carbonization, and vaporization of tissue. All of these conditions change the values of the optical and thermal properties of tissue. Moreover, whether all these processes take place after each other or not depends on the rate of change of the temperature. In other words, the optical and thermal parameters of Equation (1) depend on the actual temperature and on the rate of change of the temperature. These mathematical difficulties suggest that the resulting temperature distribution in tissue after laser irradiation is not an obvious function of the laser and tissue parameters involved.

In this paper, a simplified treatment of the heat-conduction differential operator of Equation (1) will be discussed. This leads to a simple analytical solution of ΔT in terms of optical- and thermal-tissue parameters. The price to pay is that this solution is not exact. Nevertheless, applied to situations of clinical importance in laser surgery, this solution can lead to identification of important conceptual knowledge that otherwise could have been hidden in the full mathematical solution. So, despite inaccuracies of the quantitative solution, our model may provide more accuracy in the physical concepts of the thermal response to laser radiation.

In the next section, relations for the time constants of heat conduction are derived. The time constants relate to axial (z_0) and radial (r_0) penetration depths of the temperature and fluence rate. Following sections give the assessment of z_0 and r_0 in terms of the optical properties of the tissue and laser-beam size, respectively; summarize all assumptions used in the derivation; and assess the range of validity of the model by comparing its predictions with those from exact numerical computations.

Time Constants for Heat Conduction

Introducing the concept of time constants to represent the heat conduction Laplacian differential operator in Equation (1) requires several assumptions. In this section, assumptions are introduced so heat conduction can be represented exactly by time constants. The first is to assume that the spatial part of $\Delta T(t,z,r)$ is proportional to $\phi(z,r)$ for all times;

$$\Delta T(t,z,r) = \theta(t)\phi(z,r) \text{ for } t \geq 0 \quad (2a)$$

where $\theta(t)$ is the time-dependent proportionality factor. Second, we assume that $\phi(z,r)$ can be written as a product of a z-dependent part, $Z(z)$, and a r-dependent part, $R(r)$:

$$\phi(z,r) = I_L f_s Z(z) R(r) = I_L \psi(z,r), \quad (2b)$$

where I_L (W m^{-2}) denotes the peak laser incident irradiance:

$$I_L = P_L / (\pi w_L^2 / 2). \quad (2c)$$

P_L denotes the incident laser power (W); $f_s \geq 1$ is a positive factor representing the ratio of the fluence rate just inside the medium that depends on the tissue optical properties and the laser-beam spot size to the incident irradiance (see [11]); and $\psi(z,r)$ denotes the normalized fluence rate in response to a unit peak laser incident irradiance $I_L = 1$ W m^{-2} (used later on in this paper). Third, we assume that the spatial behavior of $\Delta T(t,z,r)$ is such that the differential operators on $Z(z)$ and $R(r)$ create z- and r-dependent functions that are proportional to $Z(z)$ and $R(r)$, respectively. Thus, $Z(z)$ and $R(r)$ are chosen to be eigenfunctions of their respective differential operators:

$$\frac{k}{\rho c} \frac{\mathrm{d}^2 Z(z)}{\mathrm{d}z^2} = -\frac{1}{\tau_z} Z(z) \quad (3a)$$

$$\frac{k}{\rho c} \left\{ \frac{\mathrm{d}^2 R(r)}{\mathrm{d}r^2} + \frac{1}{r} \frac{\mathrm{d}R(r)}{\mathrm{d}r} \right\} = -\frac{1}{\tau_r} R(r), \quad (3b)$$

where $-1/\tau_z$ and $-1/\tau_r$, which are called "eigenvalues," are the proportionality factors [chosen to be negative because the heat conduction term in Equation (1) is negative]. These assumptions permit solutions of $Z(z)$ and $R(r)$ and the values of τ_z and τ_r, respectively.

Assuming irradiation at an air-tissue interface with a circular symmetric beam, the reasonable boundary conditions are

$$\frac{\mathrm{d}Z(z)}{\mathrm{d}z} = 0 \text{ for } z = 0 \quad (4a)$$

$$\frac{\mathrm{d}R(r)}{\mathrm{d}r} = 0 \text{ for } r = 0 \quad (4b)$$

Solutions of Equation (3) with the above boundary conditions typically involve a series of cosine terms for axial temperatures and zero-order bessel functions for radial temperatures [6]. Two possible terms that fit the boundary conditions are

$$Z(z) = \cos\left(\frac{\pi}{2}\frac{z}{z_0}\right) \qquad (5a)$$

$$R(r) = J_0(2.40\, r/r_0), \qquad (5b)$$

where z_0, r_0 are imposed limits of temperature rise and light distribution in the axial and radial directions, respectively; that is, $\Delta T(t,z,r) = \phi(z,r) = 0$ whenever $z \geq z_0$ or $r \geq r_0$. The constant 2.40 is the first zero of the zeroth-order bessel function $J_0(x)$. Substitution of Equations (5) into Equations (3) leads to values for τ_z and τ_r:

$$\frac{1}{\tau_z} = \frac{k}{\rho c}\left(\frac{\pi}{2z_0}\right)^2 \qquad (6a)$$

$$\frac{1}{\tau_r} = \frac{k}{\rho c}\left(\frac{2.4}{r_0}\right).^2 \qquad (6b)$$

Equations (6) demonstrate that the time constants for heat conduction are indeed proportional to penetration depth squared divided by the thermal diffusivity ($\nu = k/\rho c$). Note that the proportionality constants differ from the constant used by Furzikov [5] (viz. 0.173 in τ_r and 0.405 in τ_z vs. 0.250).

Substitution of Equations (3) in Equation (1) leads to

$$\frac{d}{dt}\Delta T(t,z,r) = \frac{\mu_a \phi(z,r)}{\rho c} - \frac{\Delta T(t,z,r)}{\tau}, \qquad (7a)$$

with solution

$$\Delta T(t,z,r) = \frac{\tau \mu_a \phi(z,r)}{\rho c}(1 - e^{-t/\tau}). \qquad (1.0)$$

Notice that the steady-state solution for $t\to\infty$, ΔT_{ss} is

$$\Delta T_{ss}(z,r) = \frac{\tau \mu_a \phi(z,r)}{\rho c}. \qquad (7c)$$

τ is the time constant for heat conduction representing a parallel circuit of axial and radial heat conduction with corresponding time constants τ_z, τ_r, respectively,

$$\frac{1}{\tau} = \frac{1}{\tau_z} + \frac{1}{\tau_r} \qquad (8a)$$

According to Equation (8a), the time constant τ is smaller than the smallest individual time constant τ_z or τ_r. Slight rearrangement of Equation (6) in Equation (8a) and noting the product $(2.4) * (2/\pi) = 1.53 \approx 1.5$ finally gives

$$\tau = \frac{\rho c}{k(2.40)^2}\left[\frac{r_0^2}{1 + r_0^2/(1.5z_0)^2}\right]. \qquad (8b)$$

Using the thermal properties of water, that is, $\rho \sim 10^3$ (kg m^{-3}); $c \sim 3.5 \times 10^3$ (J kg^{-1} °C^{-1}); $k \sim 0.62$ (W m^{-1} °C^{-1}) yields that the time constants are approximately

$$\tau_z = 5.64\left(\frac{2z_0}{\pi}\right)^2 \sim (1.5z_0)^2 \quad (\tau \text{ in } s; z_0 \text{ in mm}) \quad (8c)$$

$$\tau_r = 5.64\left(\frac{r_0}{2.4}\right)^2 \sim r_0^2 \quad (\tau \text{ in } s; r_0 \text{ in mm}) \quad (8d)$$

$$\tau \sim \frac{r_0^2}{1 + r_0^2/(1.5z_0)^2} \quad (\tau \text{ in } s; z_0, r_0 \text{ in mm}) \quad (8e)$$

where τ_z, τ_r, and τ remain expressed in seconds, but r_0, z_0 are expressed in *millimeters*.

Equation (7b) is an exact solution to the bioheat equation (1) when the spatial light and temperature distributions can be represented by Equations (2) and (3). In reality, however, Equations (2) and (3) are usually not fulfilled, implying that Equations (7) can only be an approximation. For irradiation times much shorter than τ, Equation (7b) is obviously again the exact solution to Equation (1) (adiabatic heating).

Fig. 2. A: Axial distribution of the laser light fluence rate $\phi(r,z)$ at $r = 0$ as a function of tissue depth z (____), and the approximations

$$\cos(\frac{\pi}{2}\frac{z}{z_0})$$

where $z_0 = 2/\mu_{tr} = 0.4623$ mm and exp $[-\mu_{tr}z]$ (----). The exact result, from [11], refers to Monte Carlo computations using $\mu_a = 0.6$/mm, $\mu_s = 41.4$/mm, $g = 0.91$, a delta-Eddington scattering phase function [12], refractive index of tissue = 1.37, and $\mu_{tr} = 4.326$/mm. The factor of 2 is the factor f_s (from Monte Carlo computations) occurring in Equation (2b). Input was a Gaussian beam, $w_L = 0.5$ mm with a power of 7.85 mW, with a peak irradiance, I_L, of 2.0 W/cm^2. Two values of z (0.164 and 0.279 mm), used in B are indicated. B: Radial distribution of the laser light fluence rate $\phi(r,z)$ (from [11]) and the approximation $2I_L J_0(2.4\, r/r_0)$. Cos $(\pi z \mu_{tr}/4)$ with $r_0 = 0.5$ mm equal to beam radius w_L, for three values of z ($z = 0, 0.164$ and 0.279 mm). Exact results (____); approximate results (----).

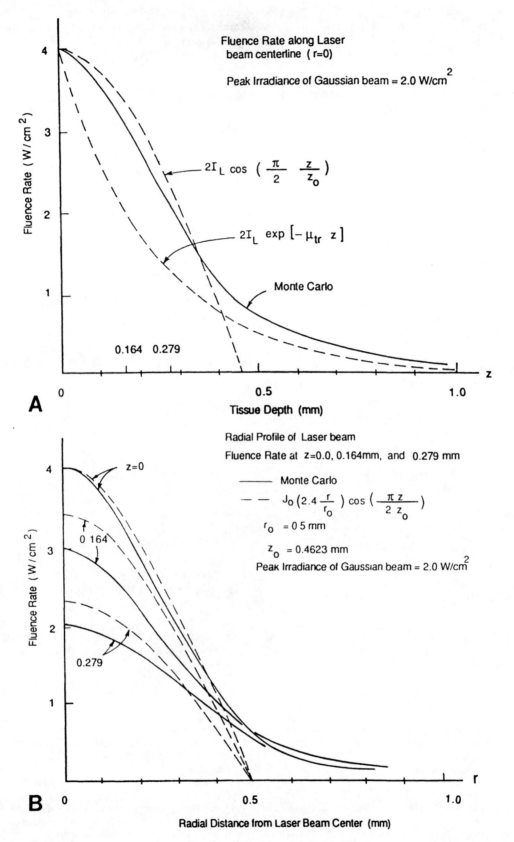

Fluence Rate along Laser
beam centerline (r=0)

Peak Irradiance of Gaussian beam = 2.0 W/cm^2

$2I_L \cos \left(\dfrac{\pi}{2} \dfrac{z}{z_0} \right)$

$2I_L \exp \left[-\mu_{tr} z \right]$

Monte Carlo

0.164 0.279

A

Tissue Depth (mm)

Radial Profile of Laser beam

Fluence Rate at z=0.0, 0.164mm, and 0.279 mm

——— Monte Carlo

— — $J_0 \left(2.4 \dfrac{r}{r_0} \right) \cos \left(\dfrac{\pi z}{2 z_0} \right)$

$r_0 = 0.5$ mm

$z_0 = 0.4623$ mm

Peak Irradiance of Gaussian beam = 2.0 W/cm^2

z=0

0.164

0.279

B

Radial Distance from Laser Beam Center (mm)

Figure 2.

Assessment of $\phi(z,r)$ and z_0, r_0

Assume a Gaussian-shaped laser beam is incident on an air-tissue interface with power P_L and $1/e^2$ radius w_L. The fluence rate in the tissue $\phi(z,r)$ follows from the solution to the equation of radiative transfer. This solution is unknown analytically. For simplicity, we assume the fluence rate is represented by Equations (2)–(4), so the radial dependence of $\phi(z,r)$ is represented by a zeroth-order bessel function, Equation (5b) and the axial dependence by a cosine, Equation (5a). Relations selected for z_0, r_0 are

$$z_0 = 2/\mu_{tr} \qquad (9a)$$

$$r_0 = w_L, \qquad (9b)$$

where the transport attenuation coefficient, μ_{tr}, is defined as

$$\mu_{tr} = \mu_a + (1 - g)\mu_s \qquad (9c)$$

and where μ_s is the scattering coefficient, and g, the anisotropy factor of scattering. The assumed solutions $R(r)$ and $Z(z)$ and the form of an actual light fluence rate computed by Keijzer et al. [11] using a Monte Carlo model are compared in Figure 2. Calculations were based on $\mu_a = 0.6$ mm^{-1}, $\mu_s = 41.4$ mm^{-1}, and $g = 0.91$. The agreement between exact and approximate results are encouraging.

The subsequent relations for τ_z, τ_r, and τ are

$$\tau_z = \frac{\rho c}{k}\left(\frac{4}{\pi\mu_{tr}}\right)^2 \qquad (10a)$$

$$\tau_z \sim (3/\mu_{tr})^2 \qquad (\mu_{tr} \text{ in mm}^{-1}; \tau_z \text{ in s}) \quad (10b)$$

$$\tau_r = \frac{\rho c}{k}\left(\frac{w_L}{2.40}\right)^2 \qquad (10c)$$

$$\tau_r \sim w_L^2 \qquad (w_L \text{ in mm}; \tau_r \text{ in s}) \quad (10d)$$

$$\tau = \frac{\rho c}{k(2.40)^2}\left[\frac{w_L^2}{1 + (w_L\mu_{tr}/3)^2}\right] \qquad (10e)$$

$$\tau \sim \frac{w_L^2}{1 + (w_L\mu_{tr}/3)^2}$$

$$(w_L, 1/\mu_{tr} \text{ in mm}; \tau \text{ in s}). \quad (10f)$$

Substitution of Equation (10e) in Equation (7b) and using the notation of Equation (2b) finally gives

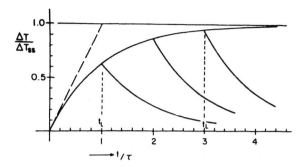

Fig. 3. Model prediction, according to Equation (7b). Note that ΔT_{ss} is virtually reached after three times τ. Switching off the laser after irradiation time t_L leads to a decay with time constant τ, given by $\Delta T/\Delta T_{ss} = [1 - \exp(-t_L/\tau)] \exp[(-t + t_L)/\tau]$.

$$\Delta T = \frac{\mu_a I_L \Psi(z,r)}{k(2.40)^2}\left[\frac{w_L^2}{1 + (w_L\mu_{tr}/3)^2}\right](1 - e^{-t/\tau}). \quad (11)$$

Predictions of temperature rise based on Equation (11) during laser irradiation (with irradiation time t_L) indicate that after $t_L \sim 3\tau$ the maximum temperature has been reached (see Figure 3). When the laser power is switched off, the temperature rise decreases with time constant τ. Three examples for the laser being turned off at τ, 2τ, and 3τ are illustrated in Figure 3. Interestingly, ρ and c canceled out the final results of Equation (11); but the time constant is proportional to ρc. Typically, nondimensional solutions of the heat conduction Equation (1) are independent of ρc; however, "nondimensional time," defined in [4] as

$$\frac{4kt}{\rho c\, w_L^2}$$

is inversely proportional to ρc [4].

Discussion of Time Constant Model

Equation (11) relates temperature behavior in response to a laser pulse to optical and thermal properties of the tissue and to the laser-beam parameters. It requires choosing a (simple approximate) relation for the reduced fluence rate $\psi(z,r)$ defined in Equation (2b). In many situations, reduced scattering is less than or approximately equal to absorption. A realistic form of the normalized fluence rate as a function of r and z is then

$$\Psi(z,r) = e^{-2(r/w_L)^2}e^{-\mu_{tr}z}. \qquad (12a)$$

1. Fluence rate distribution is proportional to the spatial distribution of the temperature increase for all irradiation times

2. The *radial* distribution of the fluence rate is represented by a zero-order bessel function. The *axial* distribution by a cosine function

3. There is zero temperature rise and zero fluence rate distribution for z larger than $z_0 = 2/\mu_{tr}$ and r larger than $r_0 = w_L$

4. Optical and thermal properties of the tissue and thus the time constants for heat conduction are constants, irrespective of the temperature rise and (irradiation) time

For strongly scattering tissues, Figure 2a confirms that a reasonable guess may be

$$\Psi(z,r) = f_s e^{-2(r/w_L)^2} \cos\left(\frac{\pi}{2}\frac{z}{2}\mu_{tr}\right)$$

$$\sim f_s J_0(2.40 r / w_L) \cos\left(\frac{\pi}{2}\frac{z}{2}\mu_{tr}\right). \quad (12b)$$

In deriving Equation (11), several approximations were made that are summarized in Table 1. Based on these assumptions, and in view of the fact that these are seldomly obeyed in a real situation during the full laser irradiation period, the time constants analysis can have only approximate validity. In particular, as time progresses during laser irradiation, the temperature spatial distribution expands, implying that the radial and axial time constants will increase in value. This is not accounted for in the analysis. So the model will tend to be of limited value when the laser irradiation time becomes much larger than a few τ. In any case, the better the radial and axial initial light distributions can be represented by zeroth-order bessel and cosine functions, the better the model will tend to predict the temperature-increase distribution. Also, the τ developed in this paper and used by other authors [5] is simply a device for describing the short-time temperature response. It is not an indicator of time to the steady-state temperature. Also, the steady-state temperature ΔT_{ss} of Equation (7c) cannot repre-

sent the true steady-state temperature, but is a lower boundary that permits estimation of the short-time response (see the next paragraph).

Questions that need to be addressed are the following: 1) Does the time constant model do any better than a simple solution assuming no heat conduction?

$$\Delta T(t,r,z) = \frac{\mu_a \phi(r,z)}{\rho c} t. \quad (13)$$

2) Can the model approximate the steady-state solution? These questions and the usefulness of the model for understanding the thermal response of tissue to laser irradiation is described in the following sections.

Comparison With Numerical Results

The complete temperature response computed with a finite difference model of the heat-conduction equation [2] is compared to temperature estimated by the time constant analysis for three important cases:

1. Penetration depth > beam radius.
2. Penetration depth = beam radius.
3. Penetration depth < beam radius.

In the first case, conduction is initially in the radial direction, whereas in the third case, the initial conduction is in the axial direction. The second case provides an example of initial conduction in both directions. In addition, temperature responses assuming no conduction, Equation (13), are computed so the time constant model can be compared to the "no conduction" model.

Case 1. The temperature behavior for $w_L = 0.1$ mm, $\mu_a = 1$ mm^{-1}, and $\mu_s = g = 0$, so $\mu_{tr} = \mu_a$, is shown in Figure 4A. Here, $z_0 = 2/\mu_{tr} = 2$ mm is much larger than w_L. The heat-conduction process starts at about $t \sim 0.001$ s. The time constant model appears to represent the exact (numerical) results extremely well up until $t \sim 3\tau$, where it is only 16% lower than the exact temperature. At $t = 3\tau$, the "no conduction" model predicts a temperature that is 2.6 times larger than the numerical solution of the full heat-conduction equation. The predicted steady-state value is a factor of 2.7 lower than the exact result. It is important to note that the time constant, τ_N, for heat conduction in the full numerical situation can be substantially larger than τ. τ_N is defined by as-

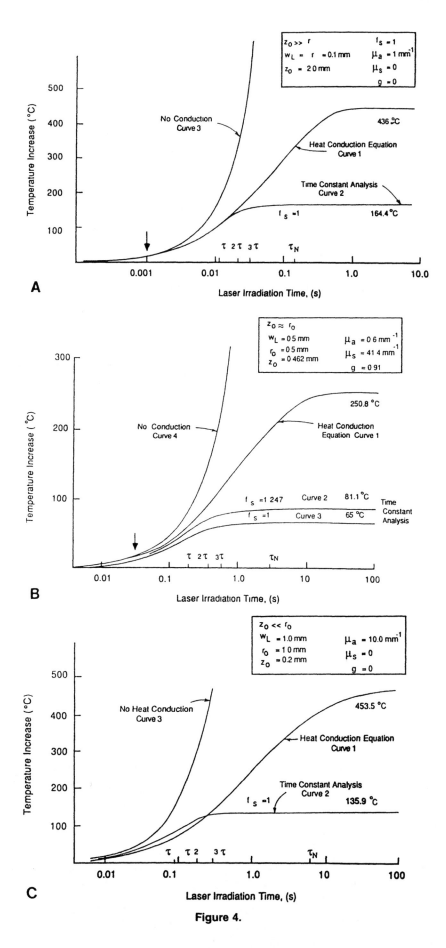

Figure 4.

suming that at three times τ_N the temperature rise would be within 95% of the final value; that is, for the computed temperature response in Figure 4A $[1 - \exp(-3)]\, 436 = 414°C$ so (from Figure 4A), $3\tau_N \sim 0.44$ s or $\tau_N \sim 0.15$ s (the steady state temperature of 436 was obtained from Figure 4A). Thus, τ_N is about 14 times longer than the τ of Equation (10e). The time of the first noticeable heat conduction is over *one hundred* times shorter than τ_N. This is due to the fact that the radial and axial extensions of the temperature profile at (close to) steady state are larger than those at the start of laser irradiation. Note that the definition for τ_N is arbitrary as the exact temperature time behavior is not exponential for large values of t.

An important conclusion from Figure 4A is that for penetration depth $>>$ beam radius, and $f_s = 1$, the time-constant model works well for $t_L \leq 3\tau$, τ given by Equation (10e), but should not be used quantitatively for longer irradiation times.

Case 2. The temperature behavior for $w_L = 0.5$ mm and a set of optical properties suggested for arterial tissue at 476 nm [11] $\mu_a = 0.6$ mm^{-1}, $\mu_s = 41.4$ mm^{-1}, and $g = 0.91$ is shown in Figure 4B. For these optical parameters, $\mu_{tr} = 4.326$ mm^{-1}, and, hence, $z_0 = 2/\mu_{tr} = 0.46$ mm, which is roughly equal to w_L, with a δ-Eddington scattering phase function [12]. The heat-conduction process starts at about $t \approx 0.03$ s. The time constant model, with $f_s = 1$, is about 55–75% lower than the exact (numerical) results until $t \approx 3\tau$. However, using $f_s = 1.247$ (which follows from the numerical results), the time constant model is only 30% lower at $t \approx 3\tau$. Without additional information, it is virtually impossible to estimate the value for f_s in a real clinical situation. For very strongly scattering and very weakly absorbing media, f_s can be as large as about 4 for a very large radial beam size. This factor drops to much smaller values, close to one, for small radial beam sizes. So the time constant model is also limited to

smaller beam sizes when strongly scattering media are involved. Here, $\tau_N \approx 2.7$ s, about 15 times larger than the $\tau = 0.17848$ s of Equation (10e). The time of the first noticeable heat conduction is 90 times shorter than τ_N. The other aspects of comparison between the time constant model and exact results are the same as those shown in Figure 4A.

Case 3. This case refers to $w_L = 1$ mm, $\mu_a = 10$ mm^{-1}, $\mu_s = g = 0$, and, hence, $z_0 = 2/\mu_a = 0.2$ mm is much smaller than w_L. Here, $f_s = 1$. Figure 4C shows that the time constant model gives slightly larger temperatures than the exact numerical results (up to about 25%), but levels off for large values of t/τ in the same way as before. Here, $\tau_N \approx 6.3$ s.

Overall, Figure 4 shows quite reasonable agreement between the time constant model and exact behavior for $t \leq 3\tau$, for all ratios of penetration depth to beam radius, provided that f_s is close to 1 (that is, for small radial laser beams when the tissue is strongly scattering).

EXAMPLES
Beam Size Much Larger or Smaller Than Penetration Depth

Consider first that beam radius w_L is much larger than the thermal penetration depth z_0, which is equal to $2/\mu_{tr}$. This situation usually occurs when using CO_2, excimer and Er:YAG lasers. When

$$w_L^2(\mu_{tr}/3)^2 >> 1 \qquad (14a)$$

or $\tau \sim \tau_z$, Equation (10b), Equation (11) reduces to

$$\Delta T(t,z,r) = \frac{I_L \mu_a}{k(2.4)^2}\left(\frac{3}{\mu_{tr}}\right)^2 \Psi(z,r)(1 - e^{-t/\tau}). \qquad (14b)$$

Equations (14) are a reasonable approximation when the beam radius w_L is larger than four or

---

Fig. 4. A: Curve 1 is the computed temperature rise according to [8] vs. laser irradiation time for the situation $z_0 >> r_0$. Parameters are $w_L = 0.1$ mm $= r_0$, $\mu_a = 1/$mm, $\mu_s = g = 0$ and $f_s = 1$; $z_0 = 2$ mm. The time constant analysis (curve 2), with $\tau = 0.01084$ s shows good agreement until $t < 3\tau$. The "no conduction" model (curve 3) deviates from the numerical model at $t \geq 0.001$ s (arrow). Values of τ, 2τ, 3τ, and τ_N are indicated on the horizontal axis. **B:** Computed temperature rise (curve 1) vs. laser irradiation time for the situation $z_0 \approx r_0$. Parameters are $w_L = 0.5$ mm $= r_0$, $\mu_a = 0.6$ mm^{-1}, $\mu_s = 41.4$ mm^{-1}, $g = 0.91$, and a delta-Eddington scattering-phase function [12], $\mu_{tr} = 4.326$ mm^{-1}, $z_0 = 2/\mu_{tr} = 0.462$ mm. The light distribution is calculated with the diffusion approximation assuming index of refraction matching; the temperature distribution is calculated according to [8]. The time-constant analysis, with $\tau = 0.17848$ s and with $f_s = 1.247$ (curve 2) is in reasonable agreement with the solution to the heat-conduction equation for $t \leq 3\tau$. Note that the f_s used here (from diffusion theory) differs from the value used in Figure 2A (from exact Monte Carlo computations). The agreement decreases when $f_s = 1$ (curve 3). The "no conduction" model (curve 4) deviates from the numerical model at $t \geq 0.03$ s (arrow). Values of τ, 2τ, 3τ, and $\tau_N = 2.7$ are indicated on the horizontal axis. **C:** As in A and B for the situation that $z_0 << r_0$. Parameters are $w_L = r_0 = 1$ mm, $\mu_a = 10$ mm^{-1}, $\mu_s = g = 0$, $f_s = 1$, $z_0 = 2/\mu_a = 0.2$ mm. Curve 1; exact results: curve 2; time-constant model: curve 3; no conduction model: $\tau_N \sim 6.33$ s, $\tau = 0.0896$ s.

five times the penetration depth z_0; that is, eight to ten times the $1/e$ optical penetration depth $1/\mu_{tr}$. According to Equation (14b), temperature increase and steady-state temperature rise is proportional to the *laser irradiance* I_L. This holds for all values of t/τ.

Consider next that w_L is much smaller than z_0, a situation representative of Nd:YAG laser surgery or small image argon irradiations in uncolored tissue. When

$$w_L^2(\mu_{tr}/3)^2 << 1, \qquad (15a)$$

$\tau \cdot \tau_r$ and Equation (11) reduces to, using Equation (2c)

$$\Delta T(t,z,r) = P_L \frac{\mu_a}{k(2.4)^2 \pi/2} \Psi(z,r)(1 - e^{-t/\tau}). \quad (15b)$$

For this condition, the beam radius w_L should be smaller than half of the penetration depth z_0, that is, $w_L \lesssim 1/\mu_{tr}$. Under these circumstances, our model predicts that the steady-state temperature rise is proportional to the *laser power,* independent of the laser-beam size. As $\tau \sim w_L^2$ (w_L in mm) in this case and

$$1 - e^{-t/\tau} \sim t/\tau \sim t/w_L^2, \quad t << \tau, \quad (15c)$$

the initial temperature rise will again be proportional to the incident irradiance (W/m^2). Although our model really does not apply for very large values of t/τ, and, hence, the conclusion that ΔT_{ss} is proportional to laser power P_L should be interpreted with caution, there have nevertheless been experimental observations [13] that indeed seem to confirm this sort of behavior. Hopefully, the above analysis will stimulate further studies in this direction.

Repetition Rate for Pulsed Lasers

Introduction. Clinically, a series of laser pulses is often used for coagulation or ablation. A large number of pulse lasers are available with wavelengths from the ultraviolet to the infrared with repetition rates from a few pulses per second to thousands of pulses per second. In certain cases, the repetition rate should be chosen such that accumulation of temperature rise is avoided; that is, the temperature rise due to one pulse should return to normal before the next laser pulse arrives. In other situations, it is desirable to create an average temperature due to the summation of overlaying temperature responses due to the individual laser pulses. The present model provides simple relations for the temperature rise of the tissue in response to multiple laser pulses.

In view of the limitations of the model, discussed above (comparison with Numerical Results), the laser pulse length, t_L, is limited to 3τ. So,

$$t_L < 3\tau. \qquad (16)$$

With this constraint, our model temperature predictions (Fig. 3) are expected to be virtually identical to those of the bio-heat equation (1). Hence, model calculations for multiple-pulse laser irradiations are expected to provide valuable predictions for temperature behavior in the tissue. However, it is also tacitly assumed that only thermal laser tissue interaction occurs.

Relations for the steady-state temperature rise. The steady-state temperature response for a sequence of laser pulses that started very long ago is illustrated in Figure 5A. Consider the resulting steady-state temporal behavior of temperature between time $t = 0$ and time $t = F$, where F is the time between pulses; $1/f = F$, where f is the repetition rate of the pulses. Assume the duration of the laser pulse is t_L seconds; thus, the time between the end of a pulse and the beginning of the next pulse is $(F - t_L)$. We use "t" to denote the time coordinate starting from the beginning of the laser pulse, and "$(t - t_L)$," the time coordinate starting at the end of the laser pulse (Fig. 5A). The resulting steady-state temperature rise, $0 \leq t \leq F$, consists of the sum of individual temperature responses in that particular time window due to laser pulses in the "past."

Consider first $0 \leq t \leq t_L$, and let ΔT_{ss}, Equation (7c), represent the steady-state due to cw irradiation as illustrated in Figure 5B. The first contribution to $\Delta T(t)$ due to direct absorption and heat conduction of the laser power density between $t = 0$ and $t = t_L$, is given by

$$\Delta T(t) = \Delta T_{ss} (1 - e^{-t/\tau}) \text{ for } (0 \leq t \leq t_L). \qquad (17a)$$

The second contribution is from the previous laser pulse, and according to Figure 5B, is given by

$$T_0 e^{-(t - t_L + F)/\tau} \text{ where } T_0 = \Delta T_{SS}(1 - e^{-t_L/\tau}). \quad (17b)$$

The first part, T_0, of Equation (17b) is the final temperature rise after t_L seconds of laser irradiation, and the second part is the exponential tem-

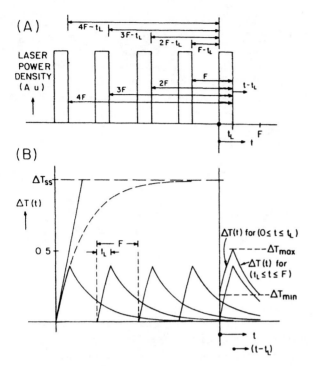

Fig. 5. A: Cartoon of a sequence of laser pulses of pulse duration t_L (seconds) and repetition rate f(Hz); time between pulses F(seconds) $= 1/f$. Time t starts at the beginning of the shaded pulse. **B:** Temperature responses $\Delta T(t)$ for each laser pulse. The steady-state periodic temperature for $0 \leq t \leq F$ is indicated in two parts as $\Delta T(t)$ for $(0 \leq t \leq t_L)$ and $\Delta T(t)$ for $(t_L \leq t \leq F)$; see Equations (17c) and (18) respectively. The maximum and minimum temperature responses are indicated as ΔT_{max} and ΔT_{min} given by Equations (19b) and (21b) respectively.

poral decay after a time interval of $(t - t_L + F)$ seconds. In a similar way, the contributions from all other previous pulses can be written down. Adding all contributions yields

$$\Delta T(t) = \Delta T_{ss}(1 - e^{-t/\tau}) + T_0 e^{-(t - t_L + F)/\tau}$$

$$+ T_0 e^{-(t - t_L + 2F)/\tau} + \cdots$$

$$= \Delta T_{ss}(1 - e^{-t/\tau}) + T_0 e^{-(t - t_L)/\tau}\left[\frac{e^{-F/\tau}}{1 - e^{-F/\tau}}\right],$$

$$\text{for } (0 \leq t \leq t_L). \quad (17c)$$

The term between [ ], in Equation (17c) represents the influence of all previous pulses on the steady-state temperature increase $\Delta T(t)$.

Consider next $t_L \leq t \leq F$. In a similar way as explained under Equation (17b) and illustrated in Figure 5B, $\Delta T(t)$ follows as

$$\Delta T(t) = T_0 e^{-(t - t_L)/\tau} + T_0 e^{-(t - t_L + F)/\tau}$$

$$+ T_0 e^{-(t - t_L + 2F)/\tau} + \cdots$$

$$= T_0 e^{-(t - t_L)}\left(\frac{e^{F/\tau}}{e^{F/\tau} - 1}\right) \text{ for } (t_L \leq t < F). \quad (18)$$

Here, the term $\exp(F/t)/[\exp(F/\tau) - 1]$ represents the contribution of all previous pulses to $\Delta T(t)$ for $t_L \leq t \leq F(t)$. Figure (5B) shows $\Delta T(t)$ for the example $t_L/\tau = 0.5$ and $F/\tau = 1.5$. The maximum temperature rise, ΔT_{max}, follows from

$$\Delta T_{max} = \Delta T(t = t_L), \quad (19a)$$

and by using $T_0 = \Delta T_{ss}(1 - e^{-t_L/\tau})$

$$\Delta T_{max} = \Delta T_{ss}[1 - \exp(-t_L/\tau)]$$

$$\times \left(\frac{\exp(F/\tau)}{\exp(F/\tau) - 1}\right). \quad (19b)$$

Noting that ΔT_{max} for $F \to \infty$ is

$$\Delta T_{max}(F \to \infty) = \Delta T_{ss}(1 - e^{-t_L/\tau}) \quad (20a)$$

yields for Equation (19b)

$$\frac{\Delta T_{max}}{\Delta T_{max}(F \to \infty)} = \frac{e^{F/\tau}}{e^{F/\tau} - 1}. \quad (20b)$$

The curve of Equation (20b) is presented in Figure 6.

The minimum temperature rise, ΔT_{min}, follows from

$$\Delta T_{min} = \Delta T(t = 0) \quad (21a)$$

or

$$\Delta T_{min} = \frac{\Delta T_{ss}(e^{t_L/\tau} - 1)}{e^{F/\tau} - 1}, \quad (21b)$$

which is shown in Figure 7. Interestingly, when t_L/τ is very small, it is only possible to realize a substantial ΔT_{min}-value for F/τ (almost) equally small. Note that F cannot be smaller than t_L ($F = t_L$ indicates a zero time difference between consecutive pulses). Figure 8 shows F/τ-values versus t_L/τ for $\Delta T_{min}/\Delta T_{ss} = 0.1$.

In conclusion, Figure 6 shows that ΔT_{max} is only 5% larger than ΔT_{max} $(F \to \infty)$ or the single-pulse maximum, when $F/\tau \geq 3$. Also, from Figure 7, a ΔT_{min} less than, say, 5% with respect to $\Delta T =$

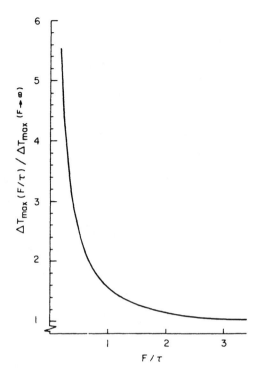

Fig. 6. Plot of $\Delta T_{max}(F/\tau)/\Delta T_{max}$ $(F = \infty)$ vs. F/τ, according to Equation (20b).

ΔT_{max}, requires $F/\tau \geq 3$ and $t_L/\tau < 1$. So, as a rule of thumb, an $F/\tau > 3$ will usually be sufficient for preventing temperature accumulation, except when t_L/τ is close to or exceeds one. So, defining a critical repetition rate f_c that virtually always avoids temperature accumulation yields

$$f_c < (3\tau)^{-1} \text{ for } t_L < \tau. \quad (22)$$

Very large absorption (excimer, Er-YAG, superpulsed CO₂ lasers). Consider the case of very large absorption and $r_0 = w_L >> z_0 = 2/\mu_a$, as would be expected when using the UV excimer, the IR Er:YAG or superpulsed CO_2 lasers. Then, Equation (10e) with $\mu_{tr} = \mu_a$

$$\tau = \frac{\rho c}{k(2.4)^2}\left(\frac{3}{\mu_a}\right)^2. \quad (23a)$$

Since $\rho c/[k(2.4)^2]$ is approximately unity when τ is in seconds and μ_a is in mm^{-1}, we have

$$\tau \sim (3/\mu_a)^2 \quad (\tau \text{ in s}; \mu_a \text{ in mm}^{-1}), \quad (23b)$$

and repetition rate f_c that avoids temperature accumulation is characterized by, Equation (22),

$$f_c < \mu_a^2/27 \quad \text{for } t_L < \tau \ (\mu_a \text{ in mm}^{-1}). \quad (24)$$

TABLE 2. Estimate of the Maximum Frequency f_c.*

Wavelength (nm)	Estimated absorption coefficient (mm^{-1})	f_{cmax} (Hz)
193	1,000	37,037
248	65	156
308	20	15
2,940	500	9,259
10,600	50	93

*According to Equation (24), where f_c is the critical repetition frequency of laser pulses that (just) avoids temperature accumulation for high-absorption materials, the possible occurrence of tissue bond breaking and/or shock-wave generation is neglected.

So f_c depends only on the absorption coefficient (μ_a) of the tissue when conduction is primarily in the axial direction. Table 2 gives estimated values for f_c for some of the lasers used clinically, recalling that thermal heating is the only allowed cause for temperature increase (thus neglecting the possibilities of tissue bond breaking and/or shock-wave generation).

Very small absorption (superpulsed Nd-YAG laser).

Consider now the opposite case that $r_0 << z_0$, or very small axial attenuation with respect to w_L that occurs when using the superpulsed Nd-YAG laser [14]. Then, Equation (10e) reduces to

$$\tau = \frac{\rho c}{k(2.4)^2} w_L^2 \quad (25a)$$

or

$$\tau \approx w_L^2 \ (\tau \text{ in s}, w_L \text{ in mm}). \quad (25b)$$

Here, the repetition rate to avoid temperature accumulation should obey, Equation (22),

$$f_c < 1/(3w_L^2) \quad \text{for } t_L < \tau \ (w_L \text{ in mm}) \quad (26)$$

and, hence, depends on the radial dimensions of the laser-beam profile. This relation suggests that reducing the beam size will increase f_c (see Table 3).

Discussion of periodic laser pulses.

The limiting repetition rate to avoid temperature accumulation is inversely proportional to the 1) penetration depth squared for highly absorbing wavelengths and 2) the laser-beam radius squared for highly penetrating wavelengths. Val-

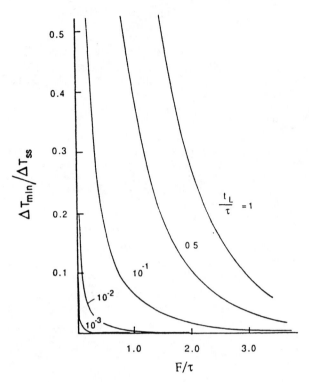

Fig. 7. Plot of $\Delta T_{min}/\Delta T_{ss}$ vs. F/τ for various values of t_L/τ, according to Equations (21b).

TABLE 3. Estimate of the Maximum Repetition Frequency f_{cmax} That Just Avoids Temperature Accumulation for Low-Absorption Materials

Beam radius w_l (mm)	f_{cmax} (Hz)
0.1	33.3
0.2	8.33
0.5	1.33

ues for limiting repetition rates for normal aorta at various wavelengths of interest are presented in Table 4 using the penetration depths presented by Furzikov [5]. The above method of analysis and results are similar to those of Furzikov [5] for highly penetrating wavelengths (425–2,000 nm), but differences in the definition of the axial time constant produce rather large differences between our results and Furzikov's for highly absorbing wavelengths.

Laser Treatment of Port-Wine Stains

Introduction. Port-wine stain (PWS) is a vascular skin abnormality caused by dilated blood vessels in the superficial dermis. The result is a bluish-red-colored stain on the skin that has been treated by laser coagulation of the enlarged

TABLE 4. Normal Aorta Penetration Depths and Limiting Repetition Rates for a Beam Radius of 0.2 mm, Using the Penetration Depths of Furzikov [5]*

Laser	Wavelength (nm)	Penetration depth (μm)	Limiting repetition rate (Hz)
ArF	193	1	37,000
KrF	248	15	156
XeCl	308	50	15
Dye	465	384	8.3[a]
Ar	514.5	313	8.3[a]
Nd:YAG	1,064	1,400	8.3[a]
Er:YAG	2,940	2	9,260
CO_2	10,600	20	93

*Pulse width (t_L) is assumed to be (much) less than three times the relaxation time, Equation (16). Again, the possible occurrence of tissue bond breaking and/or shock-wave generation is neglected.
[a]Limiting repetition rate governed by beam radius.

blood vessels. Curiously, seven different laser wavelengths have been considered suitable for this treatment [15], but the yellow 577 nm, millisecond-pulsed dye-laser is now generally assumed to be the best choice [16].

Analysis. A model for PWS, consisting of an epidermis, a dermis, and one ectatic blood vessel located at (an average dermal) depth $z_{bl} \approx 0.4$ mm [17] is shown in Figure 9. Ideal treatment of PWS is defined here as selective destruction of the blood vessel without irreversible damage to either the dermis or the epidermis. The primary absorbers in this system are the hemoglobin of the blood plexus and the black melanin pigment in the epidermis. There is substantial variation in epidermal pigmentation among Caucasians and Orientals. Nevertheless, only one (model) pigmentation (from [15]) is assumed in this paper, as the analysis intends only to demonstrate the use of time constants for practical purposes. Dermal absorption will be neglected; that is, only laser wavelengths that have a substantial absorption for blood and melanin but a much smaller absorption for dermal tissue will be considered. Thus, an ideal treatment would have the blood vessel temperature much larger than the epidermal temperature. At least the ratio of temperature increase at the top of the blood vessel, ΔT_{bl} at $z = z_{bl}$, and at the air-epidermis junction at $z = 0$, should be as large as possible to minimize thermal damage to the epidermis; that is,

$$\frac{\Delta T_{bl}(t,z_{bl},0)}{\Delta T_e(t,0,0)} = \text{as large as possible.} \quad (27)$$

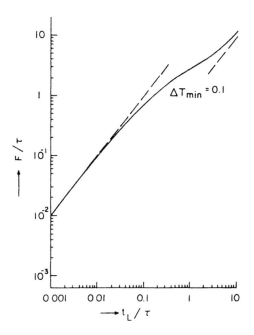

Fig. 8. Plot of F/τ vs. t_L/τ for which $\Delta T_{\min}/\Delta T_{ss} = 0.1$, from Equation (21b). The dashed line at the left-hand side represents $\Delta T_{\min}/\Delta T_{ss} = 0.1$ for $t_L/\tau \ll 1$; the dashed line at the right-hand side represents $\Delta T_{\min}/\Delta T_{ss} = 0.1$ for $t_L/\tau \gg 1$. Note that our model is invalid for $t_L \geq 3\tau$.

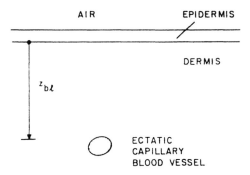

Fig. 9. Model used to represent a port-wine stain. The ectatic capillary blood vessel is located at dermal depth $z_{bl} \approx 0.4$ mm.

Using Equation (7b), and assuming that the blood vessel is located at $r = 0$, and $\rho c(\text{blood}) = \rho c(\text{tissue})$ yields

$$\frac{\Delta T_{bl}}{\Delta T_e} = \frac{\tau_{bl}}{\tau_e} \frac{\mu_a(bl)}{\mu_a(e)} \frac{\phi(z_{bl})}{\phi(0)} \frac{(1 - e^{-t/\tau_{bl}})}{(1 - e^{-t/\tau_e})} \quad (28)$$

Where $\mu_a(bl)$, $\mu_a(e)$ are the absorption coefficients of the blood and epidermis, respectively, and $\phi(z_{bl})$ is the attenuated fluence rate at skin depth z_{bl}. Even though the epidermis and dermis are in series for heat conduction, for most visible and

near infrared wavelengths, the rate of heat generation in the dermis is small and the effect of the dermis on the time constants has been neglected. Let the r_{bl} represent the average radius of the enlarged blood vessels that are assumed to be small cylinders in the blood plexus. Then,

$$\tau_e \approx \left[\frac{\rho c}{k(2.4)^2}\right]\left[\frac{w_L^2}{1 + (w_L\mu_{tr}(e)/3)^2}\right]. \quad (29a)$$

Also,

$$\tau_{bl} \approx \left[\frac{\rho c}{k(2.4)^2}\right]\left[\frac{r_{bl}^2}{1 + (r_{bl}\mu_{tr}(bl)/3)^2}\right]. \quad (29b)$$

Usually, $\tau_{bl} \ll \tau_e$ because $r_{bl} \ll w_L$ and (usually) $\mu_{tr}(bl) \geq \mu_{tr}(e)$.

As a result, $[1 - \exp(-t/\tau_{bl})] > [1 - \exp(-t/\tau_e)]$ and the largest difference occurs when t is small. When $t \ll \tau_{bl}$ and τ_e, the exponential terms can be expanded and Equation (28) reduces to

$$\frac{\Delta T_{bl}(t)}{\Delta T_e(t)} = \frac{\mu_a(bl)\phi(z_{bl})}{\mu_a(e)\phi(0)} \equiv R_{\max}, \quad (30)$$

which is the maximum possible ratio between ΔT_{bl} and ΔT_e. Ideally, this ratio would be maintained while applying sufficient energy to coagulate the blood vessels. Curves of τ_{bl} and τ_e as a function of wavelength are given in Figure 10, based on previously published absorption and scattering coefficients of skin tissues (fig. 1 of van Gemert et al. [15]).

Equations (29) will be used to evaluate and maximize the ratio $\Delta T_{bl}/\Delta T_e$ of Equation (28) for various laser pulse times, t_L, as a function of wavelength and/or laser-beam radius (w_L). We consider three categories of laser pulses: (A) $t_L \ll \tau_{bl}$; (B) $t_L \approx \tau_{bl}$, and (C) $\tau_{bl} \ll t_L < \tau_e$. The cases where t_L is about equal to, or much larger than, τ_e are not considered because of the limitations of the time constant model.

Case (A): $t_L \ll \tau_{bl} \ll \tau_e$

By approximating $[1 - \exp(-t_L/\tau)] \approx t_L/\tau$, Equation (28) reduces to Equation (30). It describes the maximal possible temperature selectivity ratio when there is no heat-conduction. Wavelength dependence according to Equation (30) is shown in Figure 11. Based on the data used, it indicates that ideal treatment can be realized only in the region of 415, 540, 560, and

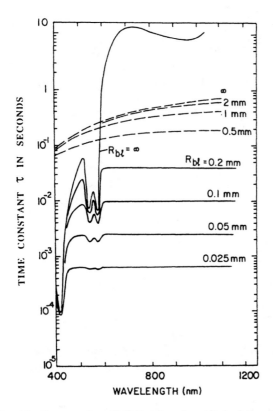

Fig. 10. Curves of τ_{bl} (full lines) and τ_e (dashed lines) as a function of wavelength, for various values of, respectively, r_{bl} (for τ_{bl}) and w_L (for τ_e). The curves are based on figure 1 of [15] and Equations (29).

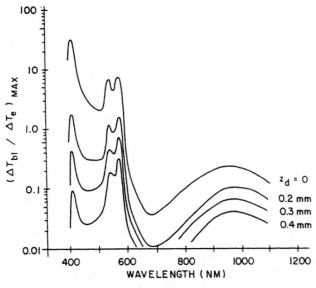

Fig. 11. $(\Delta T_{bl}/\Delta T_e)_{\max} = R_{\max}$ vs. wavelength. Absorption and scattering coefficients are from figure 1 of [15].

577 nm. For all other wavelength regions, including those of the argon laser, the epidermis always heats up faster than does the blood vessel. Equa-

tion (30) is independent of w_L, indicating that for such short pulses any laser-beam radius will do as long as $w_L > r_{bl}$. Previous clinical work [18] using a microsecond-pulsed yellow dye-laser at 577 nm indeed showed that selective vessel coagulation is possible. However, the PWS did not bleach with time most likely because these short pulses caused cavitation within the blood, which tears the vessel wall because of the pressure shock wave. Uniform coagulation of the vessel and wall has not been achieved by microsecond pulses. The wall heals subsequently without forming a new net of (normal) capillaries. It seems, therefore, that category (A) is not suitable for clinical PWS treatment. However, if the laser irradiation time is about equal to τ_{bl}, there would be sufficient time for heat to be conducted to the vessel wall and the capillary wall could be "cooked."

Case (B) $\tau_{bl} \approx t_L \ll \tau_e$

Using once again that $[1 - \exp(-t_L/\tau_e)] \approx t_L/\tau_e$, Equation (28) reduces to

$$\frac{\Delta T_{bl}(t_L)}{\Delta T_e(t_L)} \sim R_{\max}\left(\frac{1 - e^{-t_L/\tau_{bl}}}{t_L/\tau_{bl}}\right), \qquad (31a)$$

where $R_{\max}$ is given by Equation (30). For $\tau_{bl} = t_L$, this reduces to

$$\frac{\Delta T_{bl}(t_L)}{\Delta T_e(t_L)} = 0.63 R_{\max}. \qquad (31b)$$

Clinically, Equation (31) represents the optimal situation for ideal PWS treatment. Again, this prediction is independent of laser-beam size w_L. Figure 11 still applies concerning the wavelengths that can be used for ideal treatment.

Case (C) $\tau_{bl} \ll t_L < \tau_e$

This category leads to

$$\frac{\Delta T_{bl}(t_L)}{\Delta T_e(t_L)} \approx R_{\max}\frac{1}{t_L/\tau_{bl}}, \qquad (32)$$

where $[1 - \exp(-t_L/\tau_{bl})] \approx 1$ was used. To maximize Equation (32) further, consider making τ_{bl} as large as possible. This requires, for a given r_{bl}, making

$$r_{bl}^2\left(\mu_{tr}(bl)/3\right)^2 \ll 1. \qquad (33a)$$

In the same way as described under Equation (15a), this leads to the relation

$$2r_{bl} < 2/\mu_{tr}(bl), \qquad (33b)$$

that is, a wavelength is needed so that the penetration depth of the laser beam in the blood is larger than the diameter of the blood vessel. For $r_{bl} \approx 0.03-0.05$ mm [17] and noting that $\mu_{tr}(bl) \approx \mu_a(bl)$ for most of the wavelengths of interest (see fig. 1 of van Gemert et al. [15]), Equation (33b) suggests that

$$\mu_a(bl) < 20-30 \text{ mm}^{-1}. \qquad (33c)$$

This implies, for example, that the violet laser at about 413 nm with an absorption coefficient of $\mu_a(bl) \sim 300$ mm^{-1} is unsuitable for PWS treatment for these laser pulses $(10^{-3}$ s $< t_L < 0.1$ s), which is in agreement with previous numerical computations [19]. The explanation is that the penetration of light in the blood vessel is small: the light is absorbed at the top of the vessel, a large temperature gradient results, and the lumen of the vessel is heated by conduction. To provide sufficient energy to heat the entire vessel, laser power must be increased leading to increased epidermal damage. The 540, 560, and 577 nm wavelengths, with $\mu_a(bl) \sim 34$, 24, and 36 mm^{-1}, respectively, marginally meet the condition of Equation (33c).

Discussion of port-wine stain analysis

For all cases that predict $\Delta T_{bl}/\Delta T_e > 2.5$ $(\Delta T_{bl} \sim 40°\text{C}, \Delta T_e < 16°\text{C})$, selective destruction of the capillaries seems feasible. Category (B) above $(t_L \approx \tau_{bl})$ seems the best (clinical) choice for PWS treatment. For the violet 413 nm wavelength, this means $t_L \approx 0.1$ ms and for the green (540 nm) and yellow (577 nm) lines $t_L \approx 1.5$ ms. These results correlate well with numerical computations [19] and clinical results by Tan and Stafford [16].

DISCUSSION

Heat-conduction losses in the bio-heat equation have been approximated by time constants, assuming cylindrical symmetry and axial and radial channels for heat conduction occurring in parallel. Hence, the overall time constant for heat conduction (τ) has a reciprocal relation with the radial and axial components (τ_r, τ_z, respectively). The extent of the temperature field has been limited to the extent of radial and axial light distributions, thereby relating τ_r, τ_z to laser-beam radius and optical tissue penetration, respectively. In this way, a simple model (and relation) for temperature increase due to laser irradiation could be obtained, involving all laser and tissue determinants of interest. The model gives a quite reasonable picture for laser irradiation times smaller than three times the time constant for heat conduction and small laser-beam spot sizes (for strongly scattering tissues).

The model has been applied to various cases of clinical relevance, representing for example, laser wavelengths of high- and low-tissue absorption, critical repetition rates for pulsed lasers, and port-wine stain treatment. In general, the model provides a good picture of gross *concepts* occurring in thermal laser medicine. Obviously, the model is unsuitable for explaining subtle events at irradiation times much longer than 3τ.

Time constants for heat conduction have been discussed before. Anderson and Parrish [20] discussed *radial* heat conduction only whereas Boulnois [1] discussed *axial* effects only. Furzikov [5] discussed both, albeit in a separate way. The present model shows clearly that considering both effects in a parallel geometry leads to interesting predictions and explanation of observed clinical behavior. It is worth mentioning that τ_r derived by Anderson and Parrish [20] is virtually identical to our τ_r (proportionality with the radial dimension squared). Also, the τ_z quoted by Boulnois [1] is virtually identical to ours (proportional to penetration depth squared). The relations used by Furzikov [5] are given in the introduction section. The fact that the numerical factors occurring in their and our results may slightly differ is unimportant because they concern only the choice of the axial penetration or radial extension of the temperature. This choice is obviously arbitrary to a certain extent until experimental data is generated to help in the selection of constants.

ACKNOWLEDGMENTS

The authors gratefully acknowledge processing of the manuscript by Rian Becker in Eindhoven and Molly Moonwind in Austin and the performance of the numerical computations by Dr. Gilwon Yoon in Austin.

REFERENCES

1. Boulnois JL. Photophysical processes in recent medical laser developments: A review. Lasers Med Sci 1986; 1:47–67.

2. Welch AJ. Laser irradiation of tissue. In Shitzer A, Eberhart RC (eds.): "Heat Transfer in Medicine and Biology," Vol. 2. New York: Plenum Press, 1985, pp 135–184.

3. Welch AJ, Wissler EH, Priebe LA. Significance of blood flow in calculations of temperature in laser irradiated tissue. IEEE Trans Biomed Eng 1980; BME-27:164–166.

4. Priebe LA, Welch AJ. A dimensionless model for the calculation of temperature increase in biologic tissues exposed to nonionizing radiation. IEEE Trans Biomed Eng 1979; BME-26:244–250.

5. Furzikov NP. Different lasers for angioplasty: Thermo-optical comparison. IEEE J Quantum Electron 1987; QE-23:1751–1755.

6. Wissler EH. An analysis of choroid-retinal thermal response to intense light exposure. IEEE Trans Biomed Engr 1976; BME-23:207–215.

7. Birngruber R. Thermal modeling in biological tissues. In Hillenkamp F, Pratesi R, Sacchi CA (eds): "Lasers in Biology and Medicine." New York: Plenum Publishing Co., 1980, pp 77–97.

8. Takata AN. Development of criterion for skin burns. Aerospace Med 1974; 45:634–637.

9. van Gemert MJC, deKleijn WJ, Hulsbergen Henning JP. Temperature behaviour of a model portwine stain during argon laser coagulation. Phys Med Biol 1982;27:1089–1104.

10. Ishimaru A. "Wave Propagation and Scattering in Random Media." New York: Academic Press, 1978.

11. Keijzer M, Jacques SL, Prahl SA, Welch AJ. Light distributions in artery tissue: Monte Carlo simulations for finite-diameter laser beams. Submitted.

12. Joseph JH, Wiscombe WJ, Weinman JA. The delta-Eddington approximation for radiative flux transfer. J Atmospheric Sci 1976; 33:2452–2459.

13. Motamedi M. Private communication.

14. Cross FW, Bowker TJ, Bown SG. Arterial healing in the dog after intraluminal delivery of pulsed Nd-YAG laser energy. Br J Surg 1987; 74:430–435.

15. van Gemert MJC, Welch AJ, Amin AP. Is there an optimal laser treatment for portwine stains? Lasers Surg Med 1986; 6:76–83. Tan OT, Stafford TJ: Treatment of port-wine stains at 577nm: Clinical results. Med Instrum 1987; 21:218–221.

16. Barsky SH, Rosen S, Geer DE, Noe JM. The nature and evolution of portwine stains: A computer-assisted study. J Invest Dermatol 1980; 74:154–157.

17. Hulsbergen Henning JP, van Gemert MJC, Lahaye CTW. Clinical and histological evaluation of port-wine stains with a microsecond pulsed dye laser at 577nm. Lasers Surg Med 1984; 4:375–380.

18. Lahaye CTW, van Gemert MJC. Optimal laser parameters for portwine stain therapy: A theoretical approach. Phys Med Biol 1984; 30:573–589.

19. Anderson RR, Parrish JA. Microvasculature can be selectively damaged using dye lasers: A basic theory and experimental evidence in human skin. Lasers Surg Med 1981; 1:263–276.

Reprinted from *Optical Engineering*, Vol. 31(7), pp. 1417-1424 (July 1992).
©1992 SPIE.

Heating of biological tissue by laser irradiation: theoretical model

Aharon Sagi
Tel Aviv University
School of Physics and Astronomy
Raymond and Beverly Sackler Faculty of
  Exact Sciences
Tel Aviv, Israel 69978

Avraham Shitzer
Technion–Israel Institute of Technology
Department of Mechanical Engineering
Haifa, Israel 32000

Abraham Katzir, FELLOW SPIE
Solange Akselrod
Tel Aviv University
School of Physics and Astronomy
Raymond and Beverly Sackler Faculty of
  Exact Sciences
Tel Aviv, Israel 69978

Abstract. A mathematical model has been developed for calculating the heating effects of a laser beam on biological tissue. The model may be used for calculating the temperature rise and the extent of damage in tissue exposed to laser irradiation. It can be applied in conjunction with laser coagulation, laser surgery, laser hyperthermia, etc. We briefly describe the model and discuss its use for calculating temperature fields in lased tissue. Experimentally, we measured the temperature profiles in soft and hard tissue under nonablating conditions. The experimental results are in good agreement with the theoretical ones.

Subject terms: biomedical optics; laser irradiation; tissue damage.

Optical Engineering 31(7), 1417–1424 (July 1992).

1 Introduction

Lasers have been widely used in medicine for almost three decades. Some laser applications, such as the use of luminescence for diagnostics or the use of specific wavelengths for triggering chemical reactions, do not involve thermal effects. However, the majority of laser applications in medicine do involve thermal effects. The laser beam is absorbed by the tissue and the heat generated is used for therapy. In the early days, the laser beam was simply focused on tissue so that the generated heat could be used for coagulation or for ablation of tissue. The operating conditions such as laser wavelength, irradiance, etc., were determined by trial and error processes. With the development of the laser field, a better understanding of laser-tissue interaction has been obtained. A need for a better understanding of the thermal effects of laser beams on tissue thus emerged.

Let us briefly mention some of the applications of lasers in medicine:

1. *Coagulation:* Laser beams achieve direct coagulation during surgery. They can also be transmitted through optical fibers and used endoscopically to stop bleeding in the case of bleeding ulcers.[1]

2. *Welding:* Laser beams are used for welding of tissue, such as in the case of the anastomosis of blood vessels.[2,3]

3. *Laser hyperthermia:* The laser beam heats a localized tumor area[4] with the hope that the heat treatment may cause remission. Alternatively, photodynamic therapy is used and the laser heating is used in conjunction with the photochemotherapy.[5]

4. *Ablation:* Focused laser beams heat tissue to temperatures above the ablation temperature, thus causing tissue removal. This is widely used for laser surgery[6] and angioplasty.[7]

In all of these applications, the operating conditions must be carefully chosen. When heating without evaporation, it may sometimes be preferable to use laser wavelengths that are not highly absorbed in tissue, so that they can generate heat deep inside the tissue. However, the irradiance must be within certain limits to cause minimal thermal damage in neighboring areas. In the case of laser surgery, the situation becomes even more difficult. In such cases, it is desirable to remove tissue in one area, i.e., the temperature in this area must exceed the vaporization temperature, while the heat transferred to neighboring areas must be low enough to limit thermal damage.

The theoretical problem of calculating the temperature distribution and the resulting thermal effects in laser irradiated tissue is not an easy one. Normally, its solution requires simplifying assumptions and the use of numerical methods. Such methods were used in the past by various authors for calculating the temperature distribution in tissue exposed to laser radiation.

A review of works and models that were developed to study the thermal processes in laser irradiated tissues is presented by McKenzie.[8] Most of the studies were very

Paper BM-009 received Jan. 14, 1992; revised manuscript received April 22, 1992; accepted for publication April 22, 1992.
© 1992 Society of Photo-Optical Instrumentation Engineers. 0091-3286/92/$2.00.

specific and aimed at investigating thermal processes in certain parts of the body and under limited physical conditions. For example, Takata[9] suggested a model to calculate temperatures in eye tissues that were exposed to a laser beam. Halldorsson and Langerholc[10] calculated the temperatures at a bladder wall and a number of other examples are cited in Ref. 8 including studies of gastrointestinal, cardiac, and coronary tissue. Other studies were conducted by Sagi, Segal, and Dagan[11] to calculate temperature profiles and thermal damage in teeth exposed to CO_2 laser irradiation and by Anderson and Parrish[12] to selectively destroy dermatological tissues. Furzikov[13] introduced simple and efficient rules of thumb to evaluate the ablation during laser angioplasty. These studies, however, were usually able to give only a rough estimate of the threshold parameters for thermal processes. Among other studies, a model for the calculation of tissue removal rate was presented by Walsh and Deutsch[14]. However, this model is limited to short laser pulses, where thermal diffusion processes have little effect.

In this paper we describe a model that we have developed for calculating the thermal response of tissue to laser irradiation. The model is similar, in essence, to some of the previously described models, but it is more flexible and allows for easier modification for various geometries and different irradiation conditions. The model may be easily modified and used for various specific applications. Here, we describe the model, its basic characteristics, and some possible applications; we compare the theoretical results to experimental measurements; and illustrate the use of the model with the computation of temperature distribution in tissue where the resulting temperature remains below the vaporization temperature. This model is relevant for treatments such as laser hyperthermia, coagulation, and welding. In a companion paper,[15] we expand the model to include ablation, such as that required for laser surgery; we calculate the temperature distribution, the thermal damage, and the tissue removal; and the results obtained by the expanded model are compared to experimental measurements.

2 Model

In the general case, a tissue sample is exposed to a laser pulse of specific duration and spatial distribution. The mathematical model developed in this study was designed to:

1. calculate the temperature field inside a body and on its surface as a result of its exposure to laser irradiation

2. incorporate various irradiation conditions, such as spatial distribution or temporal behavior

3. be readily adaptable to various conditions and to specific applications.

Laser beams usually have a cylindrical symmetry around their axis. This feature of the laser beam and the obvious advantage of reducing a 3-D problem into a 2-D problem led us to the choice of an axisymmetric cylindrical model, in which the axis of symmetry of the irradiated body coincides with the optical axis of the laser beam.

To accommodate different laser irradiation conditions, it is essential to design a model that can take all of the important thermal processes into account. These processes include heat conduction inside the body and heat convection and thermal radiation at the analyzed body surfaces. In our

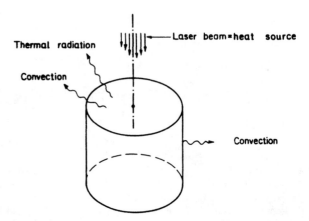

Fig. 1 Schematic description of the thermal processes considered in the theoretical model.

model, the heat source is the laser radiation absorbed by the irradiated body. The surface processes are described schematically in Fig. 1, where the irradiated body is assumed to be a cylinder.

The numerical method is based on dividing the irradiated sample into a large number of volume elements. The elements are not necessarily of equal volume, and each is treated separately.

The heat transfer mechanisms are incorporated into Fourier's law and the energy conservation equation. Let us consider a small volume element ΔV, exposed to laser irradiation to yield the temperature increase ΔT, during a time interval Δt. We may use the expression:

$$\Delta V \rho c \frac{\Delta T}{\Delta t} = \sum Q_c + Q_h + Q_r + Q_l \ . \tag{1}$$

In Eq. (1), ρ is the density, c is the specific heat, Q_h is the heat convection flow, and Q_r is the heat radiation flow from the element. The term Q_l is the laser beam power absorbed by the volume element and Q_c is the conducted heat flow from or into a neighboring volume element. The term ΣQ_c is the sum of the contributions of the heat flow conducted between the element and its neighbors. This equation is applied to a very fine numerical grid using very small time iteration steps Δt. These time steps are automatically varied according to the physical conditions and the accuracy required. When fast temperature changes occur, the time steps are automatically shortened.

In general, $Q_i = q_i \Delta S_i$, where Q_i is any of the thermal heat flows, q_i is the corresponding heat flux, and ΔS_i is the area of the relevant interface. The conducted heat flux, q_c, between the element and one of its surrounding elements, can be approximated by

$$q_c = -k \frac{\Delta T}{\Delta x} \ . \tag{2}$$

In Eq. (2), k is the thermal conductivity and ΔT and Δx are the temperature difference and the distance between the centers of the volume elements involved, respectively.

It is obvious that for all the inner volume elements of the analyzed body $q_h = q_r = 0$. However, for other elements

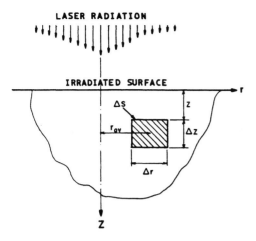

Fig. 2 Cross section of a ring-shaped grid element in the axisymmetrical case.

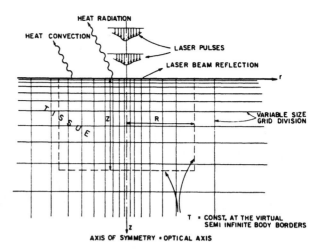

Fig. 3 Schematic description of the semi-infinite body approximation, the boundary processes, and the variable grid.

where surface thermal processes take place, the heat convection flux is given by:

$$q_h = H(T - T_\infty) \ . \tag{3}$$

In Eq. (3), H is the convection coefficient, T is the temperature of the relevant element, and T_∞ is the temperature in the surroundings. The heat radiation flux term is given by:

$$q_r = \varepsilon\sigma(T^4 - T_\infty^4) \ , \tag{4}$$

where ε is the emissivity and σ is the Stephan-Boltzmann coefficient.

The Q_1 term in Eq. (1) is the part of the laser beam power that is absorbed by the body element. Most commercial laser beams have a Gaussian-shaped profile, given by:

$$I(r) = I_0 \exp(-2r^2/a^2) \ . \tag{5}$$

In Eq. (5), $I(r)$ is the irradiance at the body surface and at a distance r from the beam center, I_0 is the irradiance at the center of the beam ($r = 0$), and a is the $1/e^2$ radius of the beam. The attenuation of a laser beam in a material is mainly due to two processes: direct absorption and scattering. When a laser beam is highly absorbed in material, such as for CO_2 or excimer laser radiation, the scattering process may be neglected. In such cases, it can be assumed that the laser irradiation is attenuated only by direct absorption according to Beer's law:

$$I(r,z) = I(r) \exp(-\beta z) \ . \tag{6}$$

In Eq. (6), β is the absorption coefficient and z is the distance from the irradiated surface of the sample. Here, the laser fluence rate at any point in the body is given by:

$$I(r,z) = I_0 \exp(-2r^2/2a^2 - \beta z) \ . \tag{7}$$

A typical grid element in the axisymmetrical numerical model is ring-shaped. Consider a small element of average

radius r_{av} at a depth z relative to the irradiated surface, as depicted in Fig. 2. The laser heat flux into the element is approximated by:

$$Q_l = \Delta S I_0 \exp[-2r_{av}^2/a^2 - \beta z)(1 - \exp(-\Delta z)] \ , \tag{8}$$

where Δz is the "height" of the element and ΔS is the area of the upper and lower surfaces of the element. This approximation is good when the "width" of the element Δr is much smaller then the laser beam radius a.

This description is adequate for the case of the cw laser beam. Whenever the pulsed laser is used, the laser heat source is time dependent and can be described as:

$$Q_l(t) = U(t) \, Q_l \ , \tag{9}$$

where

$$U(t) = \begin{cases} 1 & \text{when the laser beam is ``ON''} \\ 0 & \text{when the laser beam is ``OFF''} \end{cases} \tag{10}$$

In many practical cases, even when the irradiated body is notably different from a cylinder, it is possible to use the semi-infinite body approximation. In these cases, the existence of virtual borders, kept at a constant temperature, is assumed. The additional boundary conditions imposed are $\partial T/\partial z = 0$ at the bottom surface, $\partial T/\partial r = 0$ at the lateral surfaces, but at the upper surface, radiation and convection terms may be included to account for these processes resulting from the temperature gradient there. A schematic description of the semi-infinite body approximation is given in Fig. 3. Some limitations are imposed on the use of this approximation to obtain meaningful results, as discussed later.

The grid subdivision in the numerical model can be varied in different ways. A variable grid was adopted (see Fig. 3) to account for the very large temperature gradients usually generated near the laser irradiation site and the decrease of these gradients as z and r increase. In this grid, the element size is very small close to the irradiated surface and to the axis of symmetry, and it increases gradually along r and z.

The model utilizes the Continuous System Modeling Program (CSMP) software package[16] for the heavy task of

351

solving the heat equations for each of the numerical elements. A simultaneous temporal integration of the heat equations for each element is performed. The integration step varies automatically according to accuracy criteria determined utilizing the fourth-order Runge-Kutta method, or the fifth-order Milne method, depending on the accuracy required.

The analyzed body is considered to be homogeneous with regard to its thermal parameters. However, when the body is composed of a few layers with different thermal parameters, it is easy to define the spatial dependence of these parameters. Also, the temperature dependence of the thermal parameters, if known, can be easily taken into account. The numerical method assesses the temperature of each body element at the end of every time iteration step. Consequently, a continuous updating of the thermal parameters is possible throughout the calculating process, at any iteration step.

3 Results

The model was applied to calculate the temperature fields in several test cases. The calculated results were evaluated in comparison to analytical results or in comparison to temperature measurements in soft biological material and in hard biological tissue.

Case 1. Comparison of results obtained by the model and analytical solutions. Carslaw and Jaeger[17] give a 1-D analytical solution for an insulated semi-infinite body with a heat source of the form:

$$S(z) = I_0 \exp(-\beta z) . \tag{11}$$

This problem is analogous to the case in which an imaginary laser beam with infinite radius and an irradiance of I_0 is absorbed in the infinite body according to Beer's law with an attenuation coefficient β. This case can be simulated by our model if we assume that the surface of the body is exposed to a laser beam of a very large radius and an irradiance I_0 at the center of the beam, while the thermal surface processes are neglected (the convection and emissivity coefficients were set equal to zero). For points at $r = 0$ on the surface of the irradiated body or at very small depths (compared to the laser beam radius), this simulation is very good. A description of this configuration is given in Fig. 4(a).

Let us consider, for example, the absorption of a CO_2 laser beam in hard tissue. The thermal parameters chosen for the analytical and the numerical calculations are similar to those of hard dental tissue: $k = 6.28 \times 10^{-3}$ W/cm °C, $C = 1.17$ J/g °C, and $\rho = 1.5$ g/cm². We chose $I_0 = 2210$ W/cm², $\beta = 1200$ cm^{-1}, and the beam radius $a = 20$ cm. The radius and depth of the virtual semi-infinite body are 0.3 cm and 0.6 cm, respectively.

Figure 4(b) shows the temperature profiles at points A (on the surface) and B (at a small depth). Because of the size of the absorbing elements and the semi-infinite body approximation, some limitations are imposed on the numerical solutions obtained for very short or after very long periods of time. Those limitations will be discussed later. However, in the time range shown in Fig. 4(b), the agreement between the results obtained from our model and the analytical solution is very good.

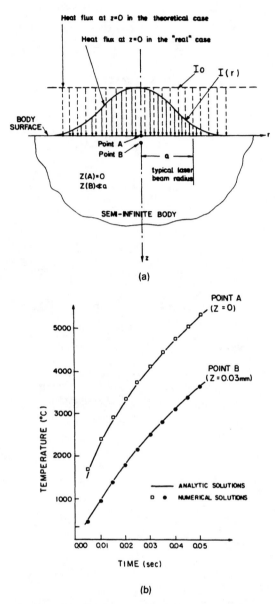

Fig. 4 (a) A uniform theoretical heat source I_0 for the analytical case (represented by the dashed lines), and its simulation by a very wide laser beam $I(r) = I_0 \exp(-r^2/a^2)$ in our model (the solid line). Both are attenuated inside the semi-infinite body as $I(z) = I_0 \exp(-\beta z)$. (b) Comparison of the results obtained by the numerical model and the analytical solution for points A and B. "Numerical solution" symbols refer to the numerical method for the very broad but finite Gaussian beam as depicted in (a). Lines refer to the analytical solution by Carslaw and Jaeger[17] for an infinitely uniform beam.

Case 2. Soft biological material. Experiments were performed to measure the temperature field in egg albumin (egg white) at room temperature exposed to a CO_2 laser pulse. Egg albumin was chosen primarily for its well-known thermal characteristics[19] and its ease of handling.

To avoid burning or evaporation, the egg albumin was exposed to laser pulses with relatively low irradiances. A Sharplan 743 CO_2 laser was utilized for this purpose. A 0.005-in. (125-μm) chromel-alumel thermocouple was mounted on an *x-y-z* manipulator, and its tip was inserted

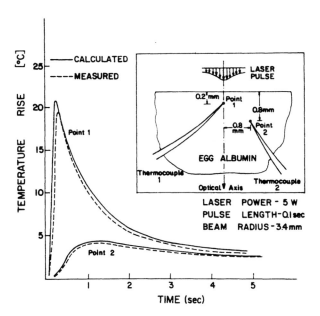

Fig. 5 Comparison of the calculated and experimental results obtained at two points in egg albumin under CO_2 laser irradiation. The geometry is illustrated by the insert.

inside the egg albumin and positioned at the desired location. Figure 5 presents a comparison of the temperature pulses measured at two different locations and the temperature pulses calculated numerically by the model.

The exposure parameters were as follows: laser peak power = 5 W, pulse length = 0.1s, and beam radius = 3.4 mm. The thermal parameters for egg albumin chosen[18] for the numerical calculations were $k = 5.56 \times 10^{-3}$ W/cm°C, $C = 3.36$ J/g°C, and $\rho = 1.036$ g/cm^3. The approximated value for the absorption coefficient β was 767 cm^{-1}, similar to the CO_2 absorption coefficient of water.

The comparison of the experimental measurements and the theoretical calculations is shown in Fig. 5, which indicates a very good fit.

Case 3. Hard biological material. Experiments were carried out to measure the temperature pulses developed in extracted human teeth exposed to irradiation from a Sharplan 743 CO_2 laser. The temperature was measured by a 0.005-in. chromel-alumel thermocouple, which was inserted inside a hole drilled through the back surface of the tooth, as shown in Fig. 6(a). The thermocouple was secured by filling the hole with zinc-phosphate cement. An x-ray photograph was taken to study the exact location of the thermocouple junction and to verify the homogeneity of the cement filling. The same photograph was used for the measurement of the size and geometry of the different inner tissues and cement regions. The tooth was exposed to one laser pulse of 6.3 J with a 0.2-s duration, and the beam was focused onto a spot radius of 1 mm. The measured temperature pulse is shown by the dashed line in Fig. 6(c).

The theoretical model was used to simulate this experiment and to calculate the temperature pulse at the point where it was measured. The tooth was approximated by a cylinder with concentric inner layers as shown in Fig. 6(b). The thermal parameters chosen for the different regions in the tooth are shown in Table 1.[19,20] The heat convection

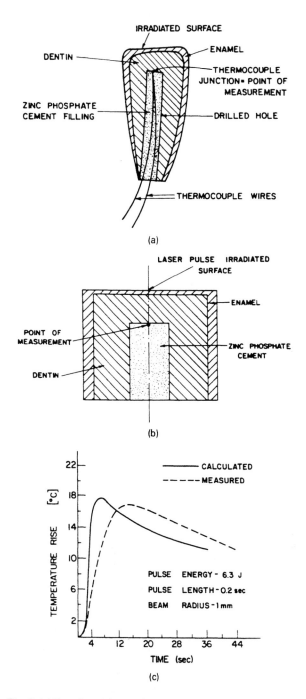

Fig. 6 (a) Experimental setup for temperature measurement inside a tooth; (b) cylindrical approximation to (a), as used in the numerical calculations; and (c) comparison of the calculated and the experimental results for the temperature pulse at a point on the optical axis of the laser beam at a depth of 2.5 mm inside an extracted human tooth (the location of the thermocouple).

parameter used[21] was $H = 0.031$ W/cm^2 °C and the emissivity was assumed to be $\varepsilon = 1$, by comparing emissivities of similar materials.[22] Note, however, that the results obtained for temperature fields in the relevant experiments discussed in this work are hardly sensitive to variation in ε.

The theoretical result is represented by the solid line in Fig. 6(c). The agreement between the measured and theoretical results is satisfactory. The comparison proves the

Table 1 Thermal parameters of the hard dental tissue and the cement used in the numerical calculations.[19,20]

Thermal Parameter / Tissue	Thermal Conductivity k (W/cm °C)	Heat Capacity C (J/g °C)	Density ρ (g/cm³)
Enamel	9.34×10^{-3}	0.71	2.8
Dentin	5.69×10^{-3}	1.59	1.96
Zinc Phosphate Cement	11.72×10^{-3}	0.963	2.4

power of the model to calculate the thermal processes in a complex structure composed of different materials.

4 Discussion

The model described in this study is adaptable and easy to use. It can be applied to a variety of materials, body geometries, and laser exposure parameters. The theoretical results obtained by the model were compared to analytical and experimental results to test its effectiveness.

The model used the semi-infinite body approximation in the simulations described in the first two cases in the previous section. Note that this approximation is valid when certain conditions are met: (1) r and z, the "radius" and the "depth" of the virtual semi-infinite body (Fig. 3), are much larger than the laser beam radius; (2) the laser pulse length is much shorter than the diffusion time from the laser irradiation site to these virtual boundaries; and (3) in exceptional cases where it is important to assess the temperature fields during long time intervals, it is essential to verify that the total absorbed laser energy is not so high as to cause a significant temperature rise at the virtual boundaries (after the energy has diffused throughout the virtual volume).

In case 1, in the comparison to the analytical calculation, the model simulated an isolated semi-infinite body. Surface processes of heat radiation and convection were not considered to fit the conditions (i.e., insulated body) of the analytical case. As shown in Fig. 4(b), good agreement was obtained between our numerical results and the analytical computations. These results were obtained even though the theoretical conditions in case 1 did not comply with requirements (1) and (3). However, the relatively long diffusion time (more than 6 s) from the points of interest to the virtual borders will ensure the accuracy of the results during the time interval considered in Fig. 4(b) (and even during much larger time intervals).

In the egg albumin experiment (case 2), we assumed the semi-infinite body approximation as well. The processes of heat radiation and convection from the surface were ne-

glected in this case, considering the relatively low laser power densities applied and, consequently, the small rises in temperature. In the simulation of the egg albumin experiment, the virtual boundaries were chosen to be $R = 0.5$ cm and $Z = 1$ cm. The thermal diffusivity of the egg albumin (corresponding to the thermal properties cited before) is 1.6×10^{-3} cm²/s. Accordingly, the heat diffusion time to the virtual borders is of the order of tens of seconds. Moreover, if the pulse energy diffuses throughout the virtual volume, the temperature rise of this volume will be of the order of 0.1°C. Therefore, conditions (1) and (3) mentioned previously are met. The value $R = 0.5$ cm is not large enough to comply with condition (1), however, the distance of the virtual boundaries from the analyzed points ensures that the results for these points will not be significantly altered during the time period shown in Fig. 5. It should be noted that, in principle, all the conditions can be easily met by placing the virtual boundaries as far as necessary from the analyzed area. However, this might result in a heavy penalty in computing efforts.

The human tooth used in case 3 was approximated by a multilayered cylinder. Although the agreement between the experimental and the numerical results was satisfactory, some discrepancy was found between the two sets of results. The reason is primarily the uncertainty in the values of the thermal parameter for the dental tissues. Different studies have shown a very wide range for these parameters. Furthermore, significant experimental errors are caused by the imperfect thermal contact between the thermocouple junction and the hard tissue. Such errors are extremely difficult to eliminate or to assess, particularly during fast transient temperature measurements inside hard materials.

Although heat radiation and convection from the surface may be neglected in many cases, situations exist where these processes must be considered to obtain accurate results. This is true, in particular, for cases where materials are being heated to high temperatures (e.g., dental enamel treatments) or for long periods of time (e.g., hyperthermia heating treatments). As mentioned previously, higher power densities and energies were used in the case of the tooth irradiation. Subsequently, the temperature of the enamel surface was much higher than the temperature of the egg albumin. Heat radiation and convection were thus taken into account. This is particularly important because they are the only processes that allow cooling during and after the absorption and diffusion of the laser energy. The extracted human tooth was simulated by a multilayered cylinder with a radius of 3.5 mm and a height of 10 mm. Neglecting surface processes in this case would eventually cause a final temperature rise in the tooth of more than 5°C. As shown in Fig. 6(c), good agreement was obtained between the theoretical results and the experimental ones for hard tissue and higher irradiation energies.

In our studies, which involve mostly tissue exposures to CO_2 laser beams, the scattering mechanism has been neglected. Moreover, when dealing with the highly absorbed CO_2 laser radiation, the model may be simplified by defining a "surface" heat source. In this case, the laser power is considered to be absorbed in the irradiated surface elements only. This simplification imposes some limitations in very short time intervals. The numerical results for the temperature calculations will be meaningful only after the heat diffusion process becomes dominant. As mentioned before, the absorption coefficient of the CO_2 laser beam in tissue is similar to that of water (767 cm^{-1}). A choice of surface elements of a 0.003- to 0.005-cm thickness causes the absorption of 90 to 98% of the laser power in the surface layer. A thermal diffusion time of $\tau = 1.4 \times 10^{-3}$ to 3.9×10^{-3} s is typical for the egg albumin surface elements of this thickness (corresponding to thermal diffusivity coefficients of 1.6×10^{-3} cm^2/s). A value of $\tau \simeq 6 \times 10^{-4}$ s is representative of the thermal diffusion time throughout an enamel element with a 0.003-cm thickness. If we then consider the results to be meaningful after time intervals that are larger than approximately 10τ, then the results for cases 1 and 3 are meaningful after a time span of 6×10^{-3} s and the results for case 2 are meaningful after 3.9×10^{-2} s, which are compatible with the range of results shown in this study.

For most cases where tissue is exposed to short laser pulses, heat convection by blood can be neglected in the vicinity of the irradiation point, because of the fast temperature changes in that region. Therefore, the model can deal adequately with short and local laser treatments. However, when continuous heating in living tissue is required, the model should include the effect of convection by blood flow or use "modified" values for the thermal parameters of the tissue that incorporate the effects of blood perfusion.

The model proved to be very powerful and accurate in assessing the temperature profile $T(t)$ at any point in the irradiated body at any practical time interval. The temperature profile obtained is the basis for the calculations of the thermal damage in tissue. In fact, the results of this model are sufficient for calculation of the thermal damage at any point in the irradiated body according to the damage model by Henriques and Moritz[23,24] or to other models. The ability to predict the desirable and undesirable thermal damage is of great importance for the evaluation and optimization of different laser treatments.

5 Summary

In this work we presented a numerical model for the calculation of heat transfer and temperature fields in bodies exposed to laser irradiation. The model was developed to accept a wide range of physical conditions and laser parameters. The power of the model to calculate accurately the temperature profiles in a body was tested by comparing its computed results against both analytical and experimental results.

The model is versatile and flexible and can easily be modified for a variety of specific applications. The heat source, i.e., the absorbed laser beam power, may have different forms of distribution depending on the attenuation mechanisms and the different material characteristics. Any of the existing models describing the attenuation of laser beams in tissue can be utilized to determine the heat source distribution and can be easily incorporated into the model. Having an accurate assessment of the temperature profiles $T(t)$ at any point in the body allows for the evaluation of the thermal damage at each point.

The model presented in this study was examined in calculating temperature fields in soft biological materials exposed to low-power laser beams. Such laser exposures occur in hyperthermia, tissue destruction, and tissue welding. The model was also tested extensively for evaluating the temperature rise in teeth, such as may be used in dental treatments. Usually these treatments call for very high temperatures on the tooth surface, while the vitality of the adjacent pulp is endangered by even a small temperature rise.

All of the above-mentioned features make the model an important and effective tool that can be used to evaluate different laser treatments. The capability of the model to describe physical processes such as heating, as well as its ability to assess secondary thermal damage, will allow the determination of the most suitable exposure parameters. Optimization of various laser treatments will be possible when ablation processes are required, as described in our companion paper.[15]

Acknowledgments

The authors would like to express their gratitude to R. Wallach-Kapon and M. Gerstmann for their considerable help and to N. Corcos for the figures.

References

1. D. Flischer, "Lasers and gastroenterology," *Am. J. Gastroenterol.* **79**, 406–415 (1984).
2. G. Kopchok, R. A. White, R. Fujitani, G. H. White, L. Dayhovsky, W. S. Grunfest, and J. Blasak, "Laser vascular welding: a comparison of thermal properties of argon and CO_2 energy," *Proc. SPIE* **907**, 71–74 (1988).
3. R. Schober, F. Ulrich, T. Sandor, H. Durselan, and S. Hessal, "Laser induced alteration of collagen substructure allows microsurgical tissue welding," *Science* **232**, 1421–1422 (1986).
4. N. Daikizano, S. Suzuki, H. Tajiri, H. Tsumekawa, M. Ohyama, and S. M. Joffe, "Laserthermia: a computer-controlled contact Nd:Yag system for interstitial local hyperthermia," *Lasers Surg. Med.* **8**, 254–258 (1988).
5. B. W. Henderson, S. M. Waldow, W. R. Potter, and T. J. Dougherty, "Interaction of photodynamic therapy and hyperthermia," *Cancer Res.* **45**, 6071–6077 (1985).
6. J. A. Dixon, "Lasers in surgery," *Curr. Prob. Surg.* **12**, 1–65 (1984).
7. W. S. Grundfest, F. Litvack, A. Hickey, L. Doyle, D. Glik, M. Lee, A. Chaux, R. Treiman, L. Cohen, R. Foran, P. Levin, R. Carroll, L. Morgenstern, and J. Forrester, "The current status of angiosopy and laser angioplasty," *J. Vasc. Surg.* **5**, 667–673 (1987).
8. A. L. McKenzie, "Physics of thermal processes in laser-tissue interaction," *Phys. Med. Biol.* **35**, 1175–1209 (1990).
9. A. J. Welch and G. Polhamus, "Measurement and prediction of thermal damage in the retina of the rhesus monkey," *IEEE Trans. Biomed. Eng.* **BME-31**, 623–644 (1984).
10. T. Halldorsson and J. Langerholc, "Thermodynamic analysis of laser irradiation of biological tissue," *Appl. Opt.* **17**, 3948–3958 (1978).
11. A. Sagi, T. Segal, and J. Dagan, "A numerical model for temperature distribution and thermal damage calculations in teeth exposed to a CO_2 laser," *Math. Biosci.* **70**, 1–17 (1984).
12. R. R. Anderson and J. A. Parrish, "Selective photothermolysis precise microsurgery by selective absorption of pulsed radiation," *Science* **220**, 524–527 (1983).
13. N. P. Furzikov, "Different lasers for angioplasty: thermooptical comparison," *IEEE J. Quantum Electron.* **QE-23**, 1751–1755 (1987).
14. J. T. Walsh and T. F. Deutsch, "Pulsed CO_2 laser tissue ablation: measurement of the ablation rate," *Lasers Surg. Med.* **8**, 264–275 (1988).
15. A. Sagi, A. Avidor-Zehavi, A. Shitzer, M. Gerstmann, S. Akselrod, and A. Katzir, "Heating of biological tissue by laser irradiation: temperature distribution during laser ablation," *Opt. Eng.* **31**(7), pp TK (1992).
16. F. H. Speckhart and W. L. Green, *CSMP—The Continuous System Modeling Program*, Prentice-Hall, New Jersey (1976).
17. H. S. Carslaw and J. C. Jaeger, *Conduction of Heat in Solids*, 2nd ed., p. 80, Oxford University Press, London (1959).
18. H. F. Bowman, E. G. Cravalho, and M. Woods, "Thermal properties of biomaterials," *Ann. Rev. Biophys. Bioeng.* **4**, 43–80 (1975).
19. W. S. Brown, W. A. Dewey, and H. R. Jacobs, "Thermal properties of teeth," *J. Dent. Res.* **49**, 752–755 (1970).
20. R. G. Craig and F. A. Peyton, *Restorative Dental Materials*, 5th ed., pp. 44–45, Mosby, St. Louis (1975).
21. R. F. Boehm, "Thermal environment of teeth during open mouth respiration," *J. Dent. Res.* **51**, 75–78 (1972).

22. G. G. Gubarelf, J. E. Jansen, and R. H. Turborg, "Thermal radiation properties survey," pp. 195–200, Honeywell Research Center, Minneapolis (1960).
23. F. S. Henriques and A. R. Moritz, "Studies of thermal injury, I," *Am. J. Pathol.* **23,** 531–549 (1947).
24. F. S. Henriques, "Studies of thermal injuries, V," *Am. J. Pathol.* **48,** 489–502 (1947).

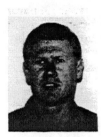

Aharon Sagi received the BSc and MSc degrees in physics from Bar-Ilan, Ramat-Gan, Israel, in 1976 and 1980, respectively, and the PhD in biomedical engineering from Tel Aviv University, in 1988. His major research interests are in the field of heat transfer and laser-tissue interaction.

Avraham Shitzer received BSc and MSc degrees in mechanical engineering from the Technion—Israel Institute of Technology in 1965 and 1968, respectively, and a PhD degree in mechanical and industrial engineering from the University of Illinois at Urbana-Champaign in 1971. From 1971 to 1972 he was a National Research Council research associate with NASA Ames Research Center, Moffett Field, California. In 1972 he joined the Department of Mechanical Engineering at the Technion and was appointed professor in 1984. He is currently the dean of the department and holds the James H. Belfer Chair in mechanical engineering. His research activities include thermal modeling and behavior of biological media, applications of heat transfer in medicine and biology, human thermal comfort and protective garments, computer-aided design and optimization of energy and solar energy systems, and air conditioning and refrigeration systems.

Abraham Katzir: Biography and photograph appear with the special section guest editorial.

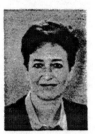

Solange Akselrod received a BSc in physics-mathematics in 1971, an MSc degree in solid state physics in 1974, and a PhD in electrophysiology in 1979, all from Tel Aviv University (TAU). From 1979 to 1981, she was a post-doctoral research associate with the Health Science and Technology Department at MIT, Cambridge, Mass., and since then has spent most of her summers there as a visiting professor. In 1981 she joined the Department of Physics at TAU and started a medical physics research group. She was appointed associate professor at TAU in 1989. Her research activities include the study of autonomic and cardiovascular control, analysis of fluctuations in biological systems, cardiovascular physiology, arrhythmia detection and fetal ECG detection, as well as laser tissue interaction and measurement of tissue blood perfusion by contrast echo-cardiography.

RADIATION PROPAGATION IN TISSUES AND LIQUIDS WITH CLOSE PARTICLE PACKING

A. P. Ivanov, S. A. Makarevich,   UDC 535.36
and A. Ya. Khairullina

Many studies have been made [1-4] on the transmission spectra in the visible and near-IR ranges for various tissues and biological liquids: muscle, heart, bone, blood, plasma, etc. Particular interest attaches to laser beams (440-1115 nm) for therapeutic and diagnostic purposes. The transmission increases rapidly at 600-814 nm, which shows that hemoglobin is mainly responsible for the spectrum. However, sometimes the interpretations, particularly on tissue compression in [5], are crudely qualitative.

We have examined the effective parameters governing light transport in biological media by reference to blood. Scattering components constitute the basic mass of tissue, while cooperative phenomena determine the elementary-volume parameters [6]: attenuation index ε, absorption coefficient k, proton survival probability $\Lambda = (\varepsilon - k/\varepsilon)$, and scattering indicatrix $x(\varphi)$, or integral parameters of this. One can interpret the regularities for biological media from the primary characteristics of blood layers at various packing densities C_v (volume proportion occupied by particles) or from the secondary characteristics (reflection and transmission coefficients). The dilute case occurs for $C_v < 0.1$, where cooperative effects do not occur for all the parameters, apart from the angular distribution in $x(\varphi)$ at small angles [7], where the elementary-volume parameters and the particle ones ε_0, k_0, Λ_0, and so on coincide. The effective absorption parameter k_{ef} and attenuation parameter ε_{ef} can be used for the close-packed case in examining transmission for thin layers [8] and thick ones [9] of soft particles ($n_{rel} \to 1$, the refractive index of the particle relative to the reflecting medium). The transmission coefficient for directly transmitted light is [9] as follows in a close-packed medium:

$$T(0) = \exp(-\varepsilon_{ef} l) \tag{1}$$

Translated from Zhurnal Prikladnoi Spektroskopii, Vol. 47, No. 4, pp. 662-668, October, 1987. Original article submitted June 20, 1986.

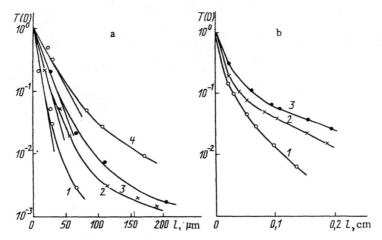

Fig. 1. Transmission coefficient as a function of blood layer thickness for various packing densities C_V and wavelength λ: a) 450 (1), 600 (2), and 805 nm (3, 4) for C_V = 0.5 (1-3) and 0.39 (4); b) C_V = 0.6 (1), 0.27 (2), and 0.19 (3) at 805 nm.

for single scattering or

$$T_{\text{M}} = B \exp(-\gamma_{ef}\varepsilon_{ef}l) \tag{2}$$

with multiple scattering, where l is thickness, B a constant dependent on the illumination and collection conditions, and γ_{ef} the effective depth-attenuation parameter. By analogy with ε_{ef} and k_{ef}, we introduce the effective photon survival probability $\Lambda_{ef} = (\varepsilon_{ef} - k_{ef})/\varepsilon_{ef}$ and examine how this varies for weak and strong absorption. See [8-10] for the methods of measuring ε_{ef} and k_{ef} at 400-800 nm.

Figure 1 shows transmission coefficients for blood layers with weak and strong absorption in the range 400-805 nm. Table 1 gives the erythrocyte optical constants and some elementary-volume characteristics, as the erythrocytes represent the main scattering component, which are taken as having the average diffraction parameter $\rho_{32} = (2\pi r_{32}n/\lambda)$ (n is refractive index for the medium, while the particles are characterized by the radius

$$r_{32} = \frac{\int_0^\infty r^3 f(r)\,dr}{\int_0^\infty r^2 f(r)\,dr}$$

where f(r) is the size distribution). It is evident that the applicability of (1) and (2) is largely determined by the absorption. Strong absorption ($\varkappa = 2.5\cdot10^{-3}$ at 400 nm) leads to the transmission following Bouguer's law down to T(0) = 0.01 (curve 1), while with weak absorption, $\varkappa = 2.3\cdot10^{-5}$ (805 nm), the relation applies only down to T(0) = 0.1 (curve 3). Multiple-scattering conditions at 805 nm ($\varkappa = 2.5\cdot10^{-5}$) set in for $l > 0.1$ cm, as Fig. 1b shows.

Figure 2 shows C_V plots for k_{ef}, ε_{ef}, and $l - \Lambda_{ef}$. The formulas give the dashed lines, while the solid lines are from experiment.

TABLE 1. Wavelength Dependence of Erythrocyte Optical Parameters

λ. nm	n_{rel}	$\varkappa_{rel}$	Λ_0	ρ_0
400	1,0410	$2,5\cdot10^{-3}$	0,574	60
440	1,0410	$6,6\cdot10^{-4}$	0,824	54
500	1,0418	$5,2\cdot10^{-4}$	0,960	47
580	1,0412	$4,2\cdot10^{-4}$	0,924	41
660	1,0414	$8,5\cdot10^{-5}$	0,997	36
700	1,0420	$9,5\cdot10^{-6}$	0,998	34
805	1,0413	$2,3\cdot10^{-5}$	0,9976	30

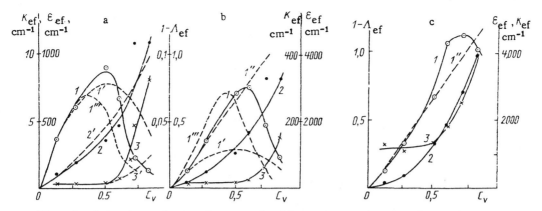

Fig. 2. Behavior of ε_{ef} (1 and 1'-1''') and k_{ef} (2 and 2'); 1) Λ_{ef} (3 and 3') for λ = 805 nm (a), 500 nm (b), and 400 nm (c); 1-3) experiment; 1', 1'', 1''', 2' and 3' calculations of the approximations described correspondingly by (3), (11), (13), (4), and (10).

Various approximations were tested:

1) equal scattering probabilities for the weakly absorbing soft large particles, refractive index n_r, and gaps between them ($2\rho(n_r - n_{rel}) < 1$) [11];

2) an approximation based only on the differences in particle distribution at small and large C_v [12]; and

3) with allowance for the interference beween the fields scattered by the particles for various real and imaginary parts n_{rel} and $\varkappa$ for the particle-material refractive index [13].

The relationship and published data lead to the following conclusions.

The effective attenuation parameter is [8] closely described by the following for weak absorption:

$$\varepsilon_{ef} = \frac{\varepsilon_0}{C_{v0}} C_v (1 - C_v) \tag{3}$$

for the range $0.1 \leqslant C_v \leqslant 0.6$. At higher values, the particles are no longer randomly distributed, which was the condition for deriving (3).

An empirical formula applies for k_{ef}:

$$k_{ef} = \frac{k_0}{C_{v0}} C_v f(C_v), \tag{4}$$

as derived in [10], where $f(C_v)$ = 1.0-1.5 for 650-1000 nm.

Here $f(C_v)$ can be determined from the diffuse-reflection coefficients for two planar optically thick layers R_{ef} and R_0, one having $C_v > 0.1$ and the other $C_v < 0.1$ (these are obtained by diluting the same blood specimen). The erythrocytes can be considered as scattering independently for $C_v < 0.1$.

The diffuse-reflection coefficient for a planar optically thick layer is [14]

$$R = \frac{R_c(1 - A)(1 - A_c)}{1 - AR_d} \quad \text{for } R \geqslant 0.06, \tag{5}$$

where $A_c \approx 0.04$ is the reflection coefficient at the air-glass-blood boundary, $A \approx 0.48$ is the same for the blood-glass-air one, and $R_d = \exp(-4q\gamma)$, $R_c = \exp(-5.2q\gamma)$ are the diffuse-reflection coefficients of blood on diffuse and collimated illumination at 0°, with

$$q = \frac{1}{3 - 3\langle X_1 \rangle} \; ; \; \langle X_1 \rangle = \frac{\int_{-\pi}^{\pi} X(\varphi) \cos \varphi d\varphi}{\int_{-\pi}^{\pi} X(\varphi) d\varphi}$$

359

the mean cosine of the scattering indicatrix $X(\varphi)$.

From R_{ef} and R_0, one can calculate $(q\gamma)_{ef}$ and $(g\gamma)_0$, which can be used on the basis that $k = q\gamma\gamma\epsilon$ for weak absorption [10], while the indicatrix-elongation parameter is

$$q_{ef} = q_0(1.1 - C_v) \quad [15],\tag{6}$$

and then simple steps from (3) and (6) give

$$f(C_v) = \left[\frac{(q\gamma)_{ef}}{(q\gamma)_0}\right]^2 \frac{f(C_v)}{1.1 - C_v}.\tag{7}$$

The effective photon survival probability is

$$1 - \Lambda_{ef} = (1 - \Lambda_0)\frac{f(C_v)}{1 - C_v},\tag{8}$$

which can be used over the same range as (3).

One measures γ_{ef} from the transmission-coefficient ratio $T_M(l_1)/T_M(l_2)$ for thick layers. For weak absorption, we can approximate γ_{ef} as follows by analogy with γ_0:

$$\gamma_{ef} = \sqrt{\frac{1 - \Lambda_{ef}}{q_{ef}}}\tag{9}$$

and on the basis of (3), (4), and (7)

$$\gamma_{ef} = \gamma_0\sqrt{\frac{f(C_v)}{(1 - C_v)(1.1 - C_v)}}, \text{where} \gamma_0 = \sqrt{\frac{1 - \Lambda_0}{q_0}}\tag{10}$$

Figure 3 shows C_v curves for γ_{ef} as measured and as calculated from (9) and (10). The derivations in the measured γ_{ef} from (9) and (10) are largest for $C_v > 0.6$, where the particle distribution is not random.

For strong absorption, the formulas for ϵ_{ef} and k_{ef} are

$$\epsilon_{ef} = \frac{1}{2r_{32}}\ln(1 + 1.5C_v\exp 1.5C_v) \quad [12],\tag{11}$$

$$k_{ef} = \frac{2\pi n}{\lambda}C_v\exp[b(\varkappa)C_v + a(\varkappa)] \quad [8].\tag{12}$$

As $k_{ef}(C_v, \varkappa)$ is complicated and it is difficult to attain the multiple-scattering case (Fig. 1b) because of the strong absorption, one cannot compare the observed curves properly with the theoretical ones. The range in which (3) for ϵ_{ef} applies is dependent on the refractive index (Fig. 2b and c).

Figure 2a compares the measurements and calculations on ϵ_{ef} for strong absorption, the latter being from the formula of [13], which incorporates interference:

where

$$\epsilon_{ef} = \frac{1}{2r_{32}}\ln\left\{1 - Q \cdot 1.5C_v + (1.5C_v)^2\frac{4\pi x(0)Q\Lambda}{\rho^2}\right\},$$

$$Q = 2 - 4e^{-\delta \, tg\, \beta}\frac{\cos\beta}{\delta}\sin(\delta - \beta) - 4e^{-\delta \, tg\, \beta}\left(\frac{\cos\beta}{\delta}\right)^2 \cos(\delta - 2\beta) + 4\left(\frac{\cos\beta}{\delta}\right)^2\cos 2\beta;$$

$$\frac{4\pi x(0)Q\Lambda}{\rho^2} = Q - 1 + \frac{2Q}{\delta^2};$$

$$\delta = 2\rho_0(n_{rel} - 1); \quad tg\,\beta = \frac{\varkappa_{rel}}{n_{rel} - 1}; \quad \rho_0 = \frac{2\pi r_0 n_{rel}}{\lambda};$$

(13)

and r_0 is the modal radius. However, this is restricted to $C_v < 0.4$ for weak absorption. With strong absorption, it is necessary to incorporate at least pair particle-field interactions rather than the interference between fields scattered by independent particles [13]. A better approximation is that of [12] (Fig. 2c), which incorporates the change in particle distribution as C_v increases.

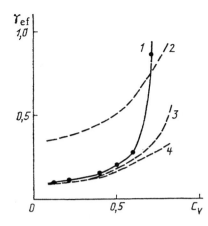

Fig. 3. Dependence of γ_{ef} on C_V at $\lambda = 805$ nm (1, 3, and 4) and 400 nm (2): 1) experiment; 2-4) calculated from (14), (9), and (10) correspondingly. The data for curves 1, 3, and 4 should be multiplied by 10^{-1}.

For strong absorption, it is difficult to attain the multiple-scattering condition, so we have not performed direct γ_{ef} measurements but instead examined the trend with C_V on the basis of the relation [16] for γ_0:

$$\gamma_{ef} = (1 - \Lambda_{ef}) + \sqrt{\frac{(1 - \Lambda_{ef})\Lambda_{ef}}{q_{ef}}} \tag{14}$$

We have calculated q_{ef} for 400 nm from (6) on the basis that $\dfrac{q_0(\lambda)}{q_0(\lambda_1)} = \dfrac{\lambda_1}{\lambda}$ and $q_0 = 40$ ($\lambda_1 = 800$ nm) [15]. As $(1 - \Lambda_{ef}) \to 1$ for $C_V = 0.8$ (Fig. 2c), $\gamma_{ef} \to 1$. Then γ_{ef} (Fig. 3) reproduces almost exactly the course of $1 - \Lambda_{ef}$, with the term under the root in (14) making a negligible contribution.

When a tissue is compressed (C_V increased), $1 - \Lambda_{ef} = k_{ef}/\varepsilon_{ef}$ increases by a substantial factor, no matter what the original Λ_0 (Table 1), and the increase in C_V may cause absorption to exceed scattering considerably (Figs. 2 and 3). For strong absorption and high C_V, $1 - \Lambda_{ef} \to 1$, and the medium produces hardly any scattering, with the attenuation following Bouguer's law no matter what the thickness, since $\gamma \sim 1$, $1 - \Lambda_{ef} \to 1$, with ε_{ef} very large and the attenuation heavy.

For weak absorption, ε_{ef} is much reduced for $C_V > 0.6$, and the radiation is attenuated slowly under multiple-scattering conditions, where γ_{ef} is increased by about a factor 10 for $C_V \approx 0.8$, but one still has $\gamma_{ef} \ll 1$, and the attenuation in thick layers is slower than in thin ones. These trends in ε_{ef} and k_{ef} mean that tissues transmit well at 600-800 nm. One can thus increase radiation penetration substantially, particularly for weak absorption, by diffuse illumination. For strong absorption and large C_V ($k_{ef} \approx \varepsilon_{ef}$), there is less effect from the illumination conditions on the transmission coefficient.

Sensitizers can be used [17] to increase absorption by living tissues in order to increase laser therapy effects, but this can be replaced by transfer to another spectral region, in particular, a shorter-wave one for blood.

LITERATURE CITED

1. V. G. Pinchuk, V. L. Isakov, V. A. Shuklinov, and L. I. Isakova, Dokl. Akad. Nauk Ukr. SSR, No. 3, 73-76 (1980).
2. W. S. Parrish, A. John, and R. R. Anderson, Photochem. Photobiol., 34, No. 6, 679-681 (1981).
3. K. V. Timofeev, V. V. Ryl'kov, A. L. Shurygin, and V. E. Kholmogorov, Dokl. Akad. Nauk SSSR, 255, No. 3, 751-755 (1980).
4. G. S. Dubova, A. Ya. Khairullina, and S. F. Shumilina, Zh. Prikl. Spektrosk., 27, No. 5, 871-878 (1977).
5. G. A. Askar'yan, Pis'ma Zh. Tekh. Fiz., 9, No. 5, 311-313 (1983).
6. G. V. Rozenberg, Theoretical and Applied Light-Scattering Topics [in Russian], Minsk (1971), pp. 159-170.
7. A. P. Ivanov, A. Ya. Khairullina, and T. N. Khar'kova, Opt. Spektrosk., 28, No. 2, 380-385 (1970).
8. A. Ya. Khairullina, Opt. Spektrosk., 53, No. 6, 1043-1048 (1982).
9. G. S. Dubova and A. Ya. Khairullina, Zh. Prikl. Spektrosk., 37, No. 5, 832-836 (1982).

10. G. S. Dubova, A. Ya. Khairullina, and S. F. Shumilina, Zh. Prikl. Spektrosk., 34, No. 6, 1058-1064 (1981).
11. V. Twersky, J. Opt. Soc. Am., 60, No. 6, 1084-1083 (1970).
12. A. N. Ponyavina and V. G. Vereshchagin, Zh. Prikl. Spektrosk., 22, No. 3, 518-524 (1975).
13. A. N. Ponyavina and V. G. Vereshchagin, Zh. Prikl. Spektrosk., 40, No. 2, 302-308 (1984).
14. E. P. Zege and I. L. Katsev, Zh. Prikl. Spektrosk., 31, No. 2, 327-332 (1979).
15. A. Ya. Khairullina, Abstracts for the Third All-Union Conference on Laser Radiation Propagation in Scattering Media [in Russian], Obninsk (1985), pp. 116-119.
16. E. P. Zege, Some Results in the Asymptotic Theory of Radiation Transport in Absorbing Anisotropically Scattering Media [in Russian], Minsk (1982) (Preprint No. 274, IF AN BSSR).
17. V. D. Pinchuk and V. L. Isakov, Dokl. Akad. Nauk SSSR, 279, No. 5, 1257-1260 (1984).

Reprinted from *Optical Engineering*, Vol. 31(7), pp. 1436-1440 (July 1992).
©1992 SPIE.

Optical density of vascular tissue before and after 308-nm excimer laser irradiation

Hans-Joachim Schwarzmaier, MEMBER SPIE
Heinrich-Heine University
Department of Laser Medicine
Moorenstrasse 5
D-W-4000 Düsseldorf 1, Germany

Matthias P. Heintzen
Heinrich-Heine University
Department of Cardiology
Moorenstrasse 5
D-W-4000 Düsseldorf 1, Germany

Wolfram Müller
Heinrich-Heine University
Department of Pathology
Moorenstrasse 5
D-W-4000 Düsseldorf 1, Germany

Raimund Kaufmann
Heinrich-Heine University
Department of Laser Medicine
Moorenstrasse 5
D-W-4000 Düsseldorf 1, Germany

Myron Lee Wolbarsht, MEMBER SPIE
Duke University
Department of Biomedical Engineering
Durham, North Carolina 27706

Abstract. Eleven autopsy specimens of healthy human abdominal aorta were irradiated under normal saline at room temperature ($21.5 \pm 1.5°C$) using an excimer laser (308 nm, 40 Hz, 115 ns, 57 mJ/mm^2, 900-μm fused silica fiber). After irradiation, transmission spectra from untreated areas and from the damage zone next to the ablation area were obtained by microspectrophotometry (250- to 800-nm spectral range, 25-μm cryosections, 6.3-μm-diam measured area). The optical density (OD) of the damage zone was significantly increased over that of untreated areas in the near ultraviolet and parts of the visible spectral range. The OD of the irradiated tissue was higher, up to a factor of 2.4 for intima, a factor of 3.7 for media, and a factor of 2.3 for adventitia. At 308 nm, OD increased from 0.094 ± 0.019 to 0.237 ± 0.041 for intima ($p < 0.001$), from 0.165 ± 0.053 to 0.501 ± 0.034 for media ($p < 0.001$), and from 0.119 ± 0.017 to 0.276 ± 0.026 for adventitia ($p < 0.001$). We show that excimer laser irradiation using a high repetition rate in combination with a high energy density changes significantly the optical properties of a human vessel wall.

Subject terms: biomedical optics; blood vessels; optical properties, optical changes; lasers; laser-tissue interaction.

Optical Engineering 31(7), 1436–1440 (July 1992).

1 Introduction

In 1978 transluminal balloon angioplasty was introduced to the clinical therapy of cardiovascular stenosis.[1] Conventional balloon dilatation techniques, however, are still limited by the occurrence of a restenosis in one third of the treated lesions.[2] Low success rates are also reported in calcified plaques and chronic occlusions.[3]

Since 1980, the laser has been suggested as an alternative approach to angioplasty.[4] At the present time, the 308-nm excimer laser represents the most common system for vascular and cardiovascular applications in patients.[5-7] However, little is known so far about the impact of pulsed excimer laser radiation on the optical properties of vascular tissue.

Our goal in this study was to determine the optical density (OD) in a normal arterial wall before and after 308-nm excimer laser irradiation.

2 Materials and Methods

2.1 Materials

Healthy abdominal aorta was obtained during the autopsy of six patients. Eleven specimens were selected and rinsed

in normal saline to remove blood. The tissue samples were positioned in an appropriate vessel and immersed under normal saline.

2.2 Laser Irradiation

Laser irradiation was performed at room temperature using a pulsed excimer laser ($\lambda = 308$ nm, 115-ns pulse width, model Max 10, Technolas). Irradiation time was 45 s at a repetition rate of 40 Hz and an energy density of 57 ± 2.9 mJ/mm^2 (36-mJ laser energy, 900-μm fused silica fiber, contact mode). Irradiation parameters were chosen according to the upper limit of excimer laser irradiation used in patients. Energy densities above 60 mJ/mm^2 have been reported to deteriorate the clinical outcome of excimer laser angioplasty.

Because heating has been shown to change optical tissue properties,[8] the temperature was measured during the irradiation procedure.

Temperature monitoring was performed using a NiCr-Ni thermocouple [model EB 01, Ebro; 0.2-s response time (τ_{99} water)]. The sensing tip was attached to the distal end of the quartz fiber to control the temperature next to the area of ablation. The amplified and digitized signal of the thermocouple was stored in a computer (see Fig. 1). The applied force during irradiation was kept constant at 10 ± 2 g by a digital balance positioned below the vessel.

The laser energy was monitored before and after laser irradiation with a separate energy meter (model 365; detector

Paper BM-016 received Jan. 14, 1992; revised manuscript received May 4, 1992; accepted for publication May 4, 1992.
© 1992 Society of Photo-Optical Instrumentation Engineers. 0091-3286/92/$2.00.

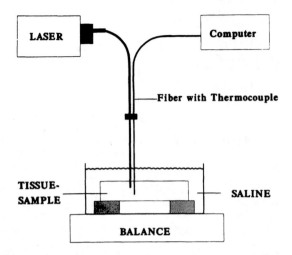

Fig. 1 Temperature monitoring during laser ablation. Note the thermocouple directly attached to the silica fiber.

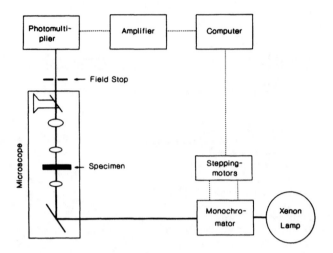

Fig. 2 Experimental configuration for microspectrophotometry. Note the field stop to limit the area measured.

head, model 380107; Scientech). After laser irradiation, specimens were cut into small pieces, each containing irradiated and untreated areas, and were stored at $-196°C$ until further analysis. This quick-freezing technique also used in electron microscopy[9] did not affect the optical tissue properties in this study.

2.3 Microscopy

For spectroscopic analysis, 25-μm cross sections were cut from the tissue samples using a microtome. The sections were immersed in normal saline and positioned between a quartz microscope slide and a quartz coverslip. Stained sections from the same specimen (Elastic van Gieson) were examined microscopically to identify unexposed tissue and the irradiated areas next to the ablation lesion. In addition, the damage zone was measured by micrometry. Ninety-six areas (46 irradiated) were selected for transmission spectroscopy. Twenty-five spectra (11 irradiated) were taken from intima, 47 spectra (23 irradiated) from media, and 24 spectra (12 irradiated) from adventitia.

2.4 Microspectrophotometry

Transmission spectroscopy was performed as reported previously.[10] In short, an ultraviolet transmission microscope (Zeiss Universal) was employed in combination with a xenon high-pressure light source and a prism monochromator. The light from the monochromator was projected onto the tissue section on the object stage of the microscope by a 32/0.3 condensor (Zeiss, Ultrafluar).

The transmitted light was collected by a 100/1.25 glycerol immersion objective (Zeiss, Ultrafluar) and measured using a photomultiplier tube (R446, Hamamatsu). The diameter of the area analyzed was restricted to 6.3 μm by a field diaphragm.

The amplified signal of the photomultiplier was digitized and stored in a personal computer that also controlled the monochromator settings by stepping motors (see Fig. 2).

Transmission spectra were recorded by first scanning a blank area for reference (I_0) and then the area of interest (I). In addition, the dark current of the system (I_D) was recorded and, in order to calculate the transmission (T), was subtracted from the spectroscopic data [$T = (I - I_D)/$

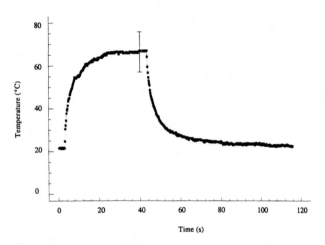

Fig. 3 Time-resolved temperature rise during pulsed excimer laser irradiation.

$(I_0 - I_D)$]. Optical density was defined as $OD = -\log(T)$. The spectral range investigated extended from 250 to 800 nm with a spectral resolution of 10 nm (spectral bandwidth < 10 nm).

At 308 nm, transmission data were obtained separately using the same experimental design with the reduced spectral bandwidth of 0.7 nm (see Fig. 2).

2.5 Statistics

A Student's t-test was performed for each wavelength to evaluate differences in OD.

3 Results

The tissue temperature at the fiber tip increased from $21.5 \pm 1.5°C$ to $68.8 \pm 8.5°C$. The time-resolved temperature increase during excimer laser irradiation is presented in Fig. 3. The damage zone was measured by micrometry. This area extended over 14 ± 5 μm next to the ablation canal. A typical example of this damage zone is presented in Fig. 4.

The digitized and averaged spectra of untreated versus irradiated tissue structures are presented in Figs. 5, 6, and

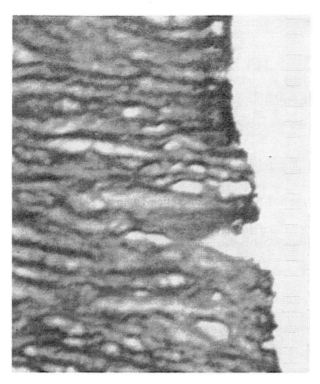

Fig. 4 Light microscopic examination of the ablation canal. Note the small damage zone at the tissue edge (Elastic van Gieson, 50 ×, 308-nm excimer laser, 40 Hz, 57 mJ/mm²).

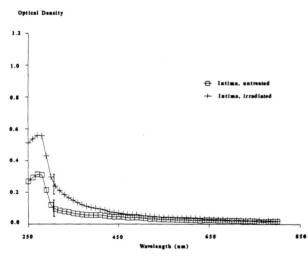

Fig. 5 Optical density of intima before (lower curve) and after (upper curve) 308-nm excimer laser irradiation.

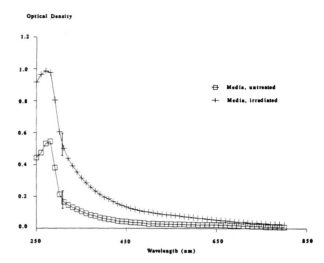

Fig. 6 Optical density of media before (lower curve) and after (upper curve) 308-nm excimer laser irradiation.

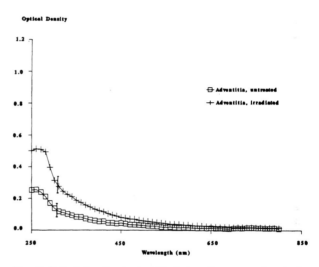

Fig. 7 Optical density of adventitia before (lower curve) and after (upper curve) 308-nm excimer laser irradiation.

7. The OD at 308 nm of unexposed versus irradiated tissue areas is compared in Table 1.

Transmission spectra of normal intima exhibited a maximal absorption at 270 nm, mainly on account of the absorption by aromatic amino acids and nucleic acids (see Fig. 5). Over the remaining spectral range investigated, the curves of OD decreased smoothly and steadily with no other relevant chromophores present between 300 and 800 nm.

After laser irradiation, the OD of the intima was up to 2.4 times higher than that of untreated tissue samples in the ultraviolet and parts of the blue spectral range (all data, 250 to 440 nm; $p < 0.05$). The ratios in OD then decreased steadily and were no longer significant above 440 nm.

Similar results were obtained for media (see Fig. 6). In the ultraviolet spectral range, the OD of the irradiated tissue areas were up to three times higher compared to that of untreated tissue structures. In the blue and partly in the green spectral range, ratios in OD of irradiated over untreated tissue areas increased up to a factor of 3.7 (all data, 250 to 640 nm; $p < 0.05$). Over the remaining green and red spectral range, ratios in OD decreased steadily and were no longer statistically significant.

In adventitia, the OD of irradiated tissue was up to 2.3 times higher than that of untreated areas in the ultraviolet and parts of the visible spectral range (all data, 250 to 510 nm; $p < 0.05$) (see Fig. 7). Over the remaining visible spectral range, the ratios that formed between irradiated and untreated areas decreased and were no longer significant above 510 nm. At 308 nm, the OD of irradiated over un-

Table 1 Optical density of untreated versus irradiated vascular tissue at 308 nm.

	O D untreated (u)	O D irradiated (i)	ratio i/u	significance
Intima	0.094 ± 0.019	0.237 ± 0.041	2.4	p < 0.001
Media	0.165 ± 0.053	0.501 ± 0.034	3.0	p < 0.001
Adventitia	0.119 ± 0.017	0.276 ± 0.026	2.3	p < 0.001

treated tissue was increased by a factor of 2.4 for intima, 3.0 for media, and 2.3 for adventitia (see Table 1).

4 Discussion

Since interest developed in the use of lasers in angioplasty, vascular tissue has been investigated spectroscopically to find suitable wavelengths.[11,12] These studies, however, were based on untreated tissue samples. Little is known thus far about the consequences of laser irradiation on the optical properties of vascular tissues.

Some studies demonstrated substantial changes in the optical properties in biological tissue because of heating as well as continuous wave laser irradiation. After heating a slice of canine myocardium to 65 to 70°C, Thomsen, Jacques, and Flock[8] found a 7-fold increased scattering and a 1.5- and 2-fold increased absorption at 594 and 634 nm, respectively. Derbyshire, Bogen, and Unger[13] documented an irreversible heat-related decrease in light transmittance (45%) at 1.06 μm in porcine myocardial tissue. Agah et al.[10] demonstrated a wavelength-dependent change in the optical tissue properties after thermal alteration (68 to 74°C) of vascular tissue. They found an increased absorption and scattering coefficient at 512 and 633 nm, respectively, but not at 1064 nm.

In former investigations, we demonstrated a wavelength-dependent 2- to 10-fold increase of the OD (250 to 800 nm) in vascular tissue caused by continuous wave Nd:YAG laser irradiation.[10] However, there is no information available thus far about the induction of optical changes in vascular tissue caused by pulsed laser irradiation.

In histological investigations, a small damage zone was seen in excimer laser irradiated vascular tissue.[6] We also confirmed this finding in our studies. The damage zone extended over 14 ± 5 μm beneath the ablation canal. We performed transmission measurements in this area to determine the OD before and after laser irradiation.

Two major findings emerged in our study. First, the OD of irradiated tissue samples was significantly higher compared to unexposed tissue. This increase was wavelength dependent. In the absence of any indication for the *de novo* formation of chromophores, the increase of the OD must be caused by changes of the scattering properties probably in combination with enrichment of pre-existing tissue absorbers.

Second, the transmission properties in excimer irradiated areas were substantially different from the data obtained in continuous wave Nd:YAG lasers. The OD of Nd:YAG irradiated tissues increased three to seven times compared to untreated areas over the entire spectral range investigated. In contrast, excimer laser irradiated tissue areas exhibited an increased OD over unexposed tissue zones only in the ultraviolet and parts of the visible spectral range. In addition,

these increases were limited to a factor of 3.7. The light absorption by proteins in the ultraviolet spectral range remained, while this absorption hump at 270 nm tended to disappear after continuous wave laser irradiation.[14]

These findings suggest that the mechanism underlying the optical tissue changes caused by excimer laser irradiation may be different from the coagulation process seen in heated tissues or in continuous wave laser irradiation.

Nevertheless, the above-mentioned studies demonstrated heating to change optical tissue properties. To investigate whether heating is also related to the optical changes in pulsed laser irradiation, we measured the temperature during the ablation process next to the area of ablation. Temperature increases have already been reported with excimer laser applications. Wolgin et al.[15] found temperatures up to 47.2°C during 308-nm excimer laser disintegration (20 Hz, 55 mJ/mm², 120 ns) of human intervertebral disks using thermography. We confirmed the heat generation by pulsed excimer lasers in this study. The tissue temperature increased during excimer laser irradiation from 21.5 ± 1.5°C to 66.8 ± 8.5°C.

Thus, we demonstrated that a temperature increase was involved also in pulsed laser-tissue interaction. These temperatures, however, were substantially lower than those usually seen in continuous wave laser irradiation and may have a different impact on the optical tissue properties. With regard to this finding, the optical changes seen in this study may also be temperature related. However, this cannot be derived with certainty from this study.

In unstained sections, the identification of relevant tissue zones in the damage area can sometimes be difficult. Occasionally, partly normal areas might have been contributed to analysis. Thus, the extent of optical changes might have been underestimated. Nevertheless, we demonstrated that 308-nm excimer laser radiation changes the optical properties of the vessel wall significantly even with short pulses (115 ns) at least when using a high energy density (57 mJ/mm²) in combination with a high repetition rate (40 Hz).

5 Conclusion

Pulsed excimer laser radiation using a high repetition rate in combination with a high energy density changes significantly the optical properties of a human vessel wall.

References

1. A. Gruentzig, "Transluminal treatment of atherosclerotic obstructions," *Lancet* 1, 263 (1978).
2. D. R. Holmes, R. S. Schwartz, and M. W. I. Webster, "Coronary restenosis: What have we learned from angiography?" *J. Am. Coll. Cardiol.* 17(6), 14B–22B (1991).
3. P. Melchior, B. Meier, P. Urban, L. Fince, G. Steffenino, J. Nobel, and W. Ruitshouser, "Percutaneous transluminal coronary angioplasty for total chronic occlusions," *Am. J. Cardiol.* 59, 535–538 (1987).

4. R. Macruz, J. R. M. Martins, A. da Silveira Tupinamba, E. A. Lopes, H. Vargas, A. F. Pena, V. B. de Carvalho, E. Armelin, and L. V. Decourt, "Possibilidades terapeuticas do raio laser em anteromas," *Arq. Bras. Cardiol.* **34**(1), 9–12 (1980).
5. M. D. Chutorian, P. M. Selzer, J. Kosek, S. C. Quay, D. Profitt, and R. Ginsburg, "The interaction between excimer-laser energy and vascular tissue," *Am. Heart J.* **112**(56), 739–745 (1986).
6. W. S. Grundfest, F. Litvack, J. S. Forrester, T. Goldenberg, H. J. C. Swan, L. Morgenstern, M. Fishbein, S. McDermid, D. M. Rider, T. J. Pacala, and J. B. Laudenslager, "Laser ablation of human atherosclerotic plaque without adjacent tissue injury," *J. Am. Coll. Cardiol.* **5**, 929 (1985).
7. K. R. Karsch, K. K. Haase, W. Voelker, A. Baumbach, M. Mauser, and L. Seipel, "Percutaneous coronary excimer-laser angioplasty in patients with stable and unstable angina pectoris. acute results and incidence of restenosis during 6-month follow up," *Circulation* **81**(6), 1849–1859 (1990).
8. S. Thomsen, S. Jacques, and S. Flock, "Microscopic correlates of macroscopic optical property changes during thermal coagulation of myocardium," *Proc. SPIE* **1202**, 2–10 (1990).
9. T. E. Phillips and A. F. Boyne, "Liquid nitrogen based quick freezing: experiences with bounce-free delivery of cholinerc nerve terminals in a metal surface," *J. Electron. Microsc. Technique* **1**, 9–29 (1984).
10. H.-J. Schwarzmaier, M. Heintzen, M. Zumdick, R. Kaufmann, and M. L. Wolbarsht, "Changes in optical density of normal vessel wall and lipid atheromatous plaque after Nd:YAG laser irradiation," *Proc. SPIE* **1427**, 120–133 (1991).
11. M. R. Prince, T. F. Deutsch, M. M. Mathews-Roth, R. Margolis, J. A. Parrish, and A. R. Osseroff, "Preferential light absorption in atheromas in vitro," *J. Clin. Invest.* **78**, 295–302 (1986).
12. M. J. C. van Germert, R. Verdaasdonk, E. G. Stassen, G. A. C. M. Schets, G. H. M. Gijsbers, and J. J. Bonnier, "Optical properties of human blood vessel wall and plaque," *Las. Surg. Med.* **5**, 235–237 (1985).
13. G. J. Derbyshire, D. K. Bogen, and M. Unger, "Thermally induced optical property changes in myocardium at 1.06 μm," *Las. Surg. Med.* **10**, 23–34 (1990).
14. R. Agah, M. Motamedi, P. Dalmia, E. Ettedgui, L. Song, and J. R. Spears, "Potential role of collagen in optical behavior of arterial tissue during laser irradiation," *Proc. SPIE* **1202**, 246–252 (1990).
15. M. Wolgin, J. Finkenberg, T. Papaioannou, C. Segil, C. Soma, and W. Grundfest, "Excimer ablation of human intervertebral disc at 308 nanometers," *Las. Surg. Med.* **9**, 124–131 (1989).

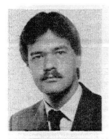

Hans-Joachim Schwarzmaier received his MD from the Heinrich-Heine University of Düsseldorf in 1984. He joined the Department of Cardiology there and worked in ablation techniques for ventricular arrhythmias and laser angioplasty. In 1988, he switched to the Department of Laser Medicine. His current research interests are laser angioplasty and laser-tissue interaction.

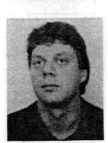

Matthias P. Heintzen received his MD at the University of Kiel in 1985. He started his clinical training at the cardiology department of the Marburg University and continued his education in cardiology and angiology at the Heinrich-Heine University of Düsseldorf in 1987. His interests include basic mechanisms of laser-tissue interaction and interventional cardiovascular therapy, especially the clinical laser application in peripheral and coronary angioplasty.

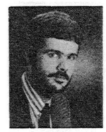

Wolfram Müller works at the Department of Pathology, Heinrich-Heine University of Düsseldorf. His research interests include cardiovascular pathology and tumor pathology of the gastrointestinal tract.

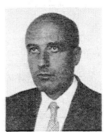

Raimund Kaufmann is the chairman of the Department of Laser Medicine at the Heinrich-Heine University of Düsseldorf. He has been a professor of clinical physiology at the University of Düsseldorf Medical School. Kaufmann has a long record in cardiac electrophysiology and muscle cell biology research. One of his major interests relates to modern physical methods, especially laser optical techniques as applied to biomedical research. He was a codeveloper of the laser microprobe mass analysis technique and was one of the early pioneers in exploring the potential of dynamic light scattering on mobile biological systems. He has published more than 150 papers. Kaufmann serves on numerous governmental advisory and peer review boards and is the chair of a governmental working group on unconventional methods in cancer therapy.

Myron Lee Wolbarsht studied zoology and chemistry at the University of Maryland, College Park, and chemical engineering at Johns Hopkins University, Baltimore, Maryland. He received the AB degree in philosophy and mathematics from St. John's College, Annapolis, Maryland, and the PhD degree in biophysics and biology from Johns Hopkins University. He served in the U.S. Army Air Corps in bombsight and automatic flight equipment development. He was a physicist and the head of the physical biology branch and the biophysics division of the Naval Medical Research Institute, Bethesda, Maryland. He is now a professor of ophthalmology and biomedical engineering, an associate professor of physiology, a lecturer in psychology, and assistant director for the laboratory for interventional cardiac catheterization at Duke University, Durham, North Carolina. In addition to his publications on various research, Wolbarsht is the editor of the book series *Laser Applications in Biology and Medicine* and coauthor of the book *Safety with Lasers and Other Optical Sources*. He holds patents on camera focusing and various machines for vision testing and screening.

Reprinted with permission from *Applied Optics,* Vol. 32(4), pp. 477-487
(February 1, 1993). ©1993 Optical Society of America.

Light dosimetry: effects of dehydration and thermal damage on the optical properties of the human aorta

Inci F. Çilesiz and Ashley J. Welch

The influences of dehydration and thermal damage on *in vitro* optical properties of human aorta were studied. The absorption coefficient increased by 20–50%, especially in the visible range when at least 40% of total tissue weight was lost as a result of dehydration. The reduced scattering coefficient increased by 10–45% in the visible and 30% to over 150% in the near IR after the tissue samples were heated in a constant temperature water bath at 100°C for 300 ± 10 s. This study implies that dehydration and protein coagulation during photothermal treatment of tissue are important factors altering optical properties of tissue.

Key words: Dosimetry, hydration, optical properties, protein coagulation, spectrophotometer.

Introduction and Background

The choice of lasers and exposure parameters in general has been based on clinical results rather than on an understanding of (1) the mechanisms involved in laser treatment, (2) the optical and thermal properties of tissue, and (3) a rational theoretical approach to maximize therapeutic benefits. Previous studies on laser–tissue interaction have shown that the appearance of tissues changes considerably during photothermal processes.[1–3] A number of authors have observed that the clinical levels of laser irradiations vaporize water in the near-surface tissue causing sharp increases in temperature.[4–6] Increasing the tissue temperature above 50°C may also cause denaturation of molecules, dehydration, coagulation, and eventually ablation.[7]

Previous investigations showed that tissue thickness and volume shrink as a result of dehydration during thermal insult to the human aorta. Significant changes in transmittance and reflectance started between 45° and 70°C where transmission decreased and reflectance increased. At higher temperatures (80–100°C) dehydration was the dominating factor increasing transmittance and decreasing reflectance. Beyond 110°C reflectance increased, whereas trans-

mittance decreased.[8] More recently, studies on thermally induced optical property changes in myocardium emphasized irreversible changes between 60° and 75°C, the temperature range in which extracellular protein and collagen denaturation are known to occur. Derbyshire et al.[9] and Splinter et al.[10] speculated that protein macromolecules that are responsible for light scattering had little effect on absorption, because they observed a twofold to threefold increase in the reduced scattering coefficient as a result of thermal insult, whereas the absorption coefficient remained relatively constant.

Hence the deposition of thermal energy in tissue is not only a function of laser irradiation parameters, but it also depends on the physical properties of tissue including the optical properties. Thus the photothermal response of tissue depends on temperature, water content, and tissue condition. An understanding of the influence of these parameters on optical properties will enhance our ability to predict the photothermal response of tissue to laser irradiation.

Most of the recent advances describing laser–tissue interactions are based on transport theory. Tissue is considered to be a medium of dense distributions of random scatterers.[11] Although analytic models have been developed to solve Maxwell equations for scattering particles, transport theory is preferred in studies of tissue optics involving optically thick biological media. Yet implicit assumptions must be made if transport theory is used to describe laser–tissue interaction: (1) The biological medium under investigation is homogeneous. (2) Each particle in the

I. F. Çilesiz and A. J. Welch are with the Biomedical Engineering Program, University of Texas at Austin, Austin, Texas 78712-1084.

Received 6 December 1991.
0003-6935/93/040477-11$05.00/0.
© 1993 Optical Society of America.

biological medium is sufficiently isolated that its scattering pattern is independent of all other particles. (3) Scattering by all particles may be described by a single phase function. (4) Polarization effects are neglected. (5) Radiation is transverse with only small changes in electrical permittivity at boundaries. A description of transport theory applied to tissue can be found in Ishimaru's book.[11]

The optical properties of tissue are obtained by converting measurements of observable quantities into parameters that characterize light propagation in tissue. The fundamental optical properties of tissue related to the radiative transfer theory[12] are the absorption coefficient μ_a (1/cm), the scattering coefficient μ_s (1/cm), and the average cosine of the scattering angle associated with the single-scattering phase function g. The products of each of the former two parameters with path length Δs give the probabilities that a photon will be absorbed or conservatively scattered in Δs as $\Delta s \to 0$. The phase function describes the angular distribution for a single-scattering event, i.e., the probability per unit solid angle that a photon will be scattered from an angle Θ' into an angle Θ''. When the average cosine of the phase function g is equal to 1, scattering is purely forward; when $g = 0$ the scattering is isotropic.

For an *in vitro* tissue sample the computation of μ_a, μ_s, and g requires the measurement of thickness of a uniform sample and three optical measurements such as total reflection, total or diffuse transmission, and collimated transmission. Assuming a preset g value, the similarity relations permit the determination of an absorption coefficient μ_a and a reduced scattering coefficient $\mu_s' = \mu_s(1 - g)$ from two optical measurements: typically diffuse reflection R_d and total transmission T_t, which are measured by using an integrating sphere system.[13]

Unfortunately there is no direct relation between permitting the calculation of μ_a and μ_s' from reflection and transmission measurements. If R_d and T_t are measured, it is necessary to form an iterative computation that varies μ_a and μ_s' until the measured values of R_d and T_t are computed within a preselected error criteria. A one-dimensional diffusion approximation model with a δ-Eddington phase function[14] has been used for this purpose.

Materials and Methods

A Varian 2300 UV–visible–near-IR spectrophotometer was used to measure diffuse reflection and total transmission. The experiments within the context of this study covered a spectrum ranging from 300 to 1800 nm.

Data were taken at 5-nm intervals, and a two-point calibration was performed by using experimental and standard data from two stimulated Raman scattering series reflectance standards (2% and 99%) manufactured by LabSphere Inc. The diffusion approximation with a δ-Eddington phase function, which assigns forward-scattered light into a δ function, was used in an iterative program developed by S. Prahl to compute diffuse reflection and total transmission for an assumed pair of values for absorption and reduced scattering coefficients.[14] This program considered multiple reflections that occurred at air–slide–tissue–slide–air interfaces. New values of μ_a and μ_s' were automatically computed until reflection and transmission matched measured values. An outline of the experimental protocol is shown in Fig. 1.

Tissue Preparation

Aorta segments were harvested from human cadavers within 24 h postmortem and delivered in an airtight container. To remove residual blood, we soaked the segments in 0.9% isotonic saline solution for at least 1 h. Although the cleaning did not alter the *in vitro* hydration levels, placing tissue in fluid may have slightly increased the *in vitro* hydration level relative to the *in vivo* level. Segments were checked for any visible plaque and fatty streaks. Those with clean tunica intima were prepared for experiments. The outer part of the adventitia with most blood vessels was removed.

Squares of ~1 cm × 1 cm were cut. Some samples were stripped to a thickness of 500–700 μm leaving mostly intimal and medial layers. A microtome was used for most samples, and thicknesses down to 250 μm were obtained without freezing the samples. Microtome cuts were more uniform both in thickness and in surface quality. The thin samples were moistened with saline and carefully sandwiched between two slides so that no air bubbles were trapped between the tissue and each slide. Finally this assembly was mounted in a custom-made frame for spectrophotometric measurements as shown in Fig. 2. Quartz slides (GM Associates Inc., part 7525-02) were used to minimize losses in the UV spectrum. Prepared but not immediately used samples were wrapped in saline-moistened gauze, sealed, and refrigerated at 4°C. Except for dehydration studies, samples were not kept longer than 24 h. The maximum time of refrigeration was limited to 72 h.[15]

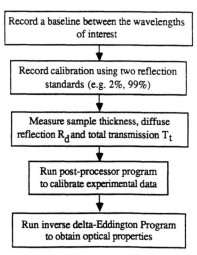

Fig. 1. Experimental protocol.

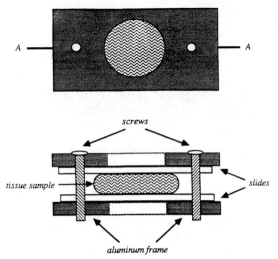

Fig. 2. Tissue preparation for spectrophotometric measurements. Top: view of the assembled sample from the top; bottom: view at the AA cross section.

To determine the effects of hydration levels, we scanned and weighed the samples. Then they were subjected to slow dehydration in a refrigerator for at least 20 h. To isolate the influence of dehydration from that of thermal damage, we induced dehydration in a refrigerator instead of in a low-temperature oven. A weight loss of at least 40% was achieved within 2–3 days without any visible sign of tissue decay. The samples were maintained between the sandwiching slides but with the seals loosened to provide dehydration and to maintain smooth surfaces. The samples were weighed, and the thicknesses were measured after each scan. A Mettler PE 360 digital scale ($\pm$1 mg) and a Hommel Schnelltaster caliper ($\pm$25 μm) were used to weigh and measure the thicknesses of the samples, respectively.[15]

Thermal damage, as characterized primarily by protein coagulation, was induced by bathing aorta samples in a constant-temperature isotonic saline bath (Nesleb RTE-190 constant-temperature bath). The evaporation of water in the bath was minimized by covering the bath. Saline levels at the start and finish of the experiment were approximately the same. Samples were either exposed directly to heat or wrapped in aluminum foil at temperatures of 60°, 70°, and 100°C for 300 $\pm$ 10 s.[15] Since the thermal diffusion time for a 1.0-mm sample is ~1.0 s,[16] the 300-s heating time ensured that the temperature at the center of a 1-mm-thick tissue sample approximated the surface temperature. For thermal damage tests at 60° and 70°C aorta segments were placed in the constant-temperature water bath. Following immersion cooling, to avoid further thermal damage, we prepared thin samples as described before. Different samples from the same specimen were used for the control and thermal damage experiments. Two groups of experiments were conducted at 100°C. In one group samples were processed in the same manner as discussed above, whereas in the other

group prepared thin samples were heated in a constant-temperature water bath after control measurements. The samples in this second group were wrapped in aluminum foil before being placed in a constant-temperature water bath. The aluminum foil was employed to prevent diffusion of saline into tissue and diffusion of chromophores into the bath[17] and thus to investigate the influence of such diffusion on optical properties. After immersion cooling at room temperature (~22°C) for 5 min, the optical measurements were repeated.

Since the scattering is known to decrease as a power of wavelength, we assumed that

$$\mu_s' \propto \lambda^{-n}, \qquad (1a)$$

$$\ln \mu_s' = C - n \ln \lambda, \qquad (1b)$$

where C is a constant. Least-squares values of n were computed for normal, dehydrated, and damaged tissue samples in the 500–1200-nm range, where the slope of the reduced scattering spectra is the most linear in the logarithmic scale. A t-test was used to compare the significance between paired conditions. The hypothesis that samples from two sets of data could come from the same population, i.e., the expected value of one set is equal to the expected value of another set, is tested.

Results

A total of 22 tissue segments was used in the experimentation. In the experiments involving the direct heating of tissue, these segments were cut in two or more pieces; one or two samples were used for control measurements, and the other(s) was placed in the temperature bath. Typical curves for transmission, reflection, and the corresponding optical properties are shown in Figs. 3 and 5 for dehydrated and heated samples, respectively.

Effects of Dehydration

Nine sets of experiments were carried out. Typical transmission and reflection curves are presented in Figs. 3(a) and 3(b). The corresponding absorption and reduced scattering spectra are shown in Figs. 3(c) and 3(d). It was observed that the absorption coefficient of the human aorta increased, particularly in the 400–1300-nm range, when at least 40% of the total weight of tissue was lost because of dehydration. The average weight loss of 46.4 $\pm$ 7.6% was accompanied with an average thickness shrinkage of 19.5 $\pm$ 4.8%. The loss of water decreased the sample thickness. Primarily because of shrinkage the absorption coefficient was increased by 20–50% in this range. Even though data points in the water absorption band were occasionally lost because of low levels of detected signals, there was an increase in the transmission of dehydrated samples between 1400 and 1550 nm as seen in Fig. 3(a). Yet the absorption coefficient was not affected by water loss. The fraction of

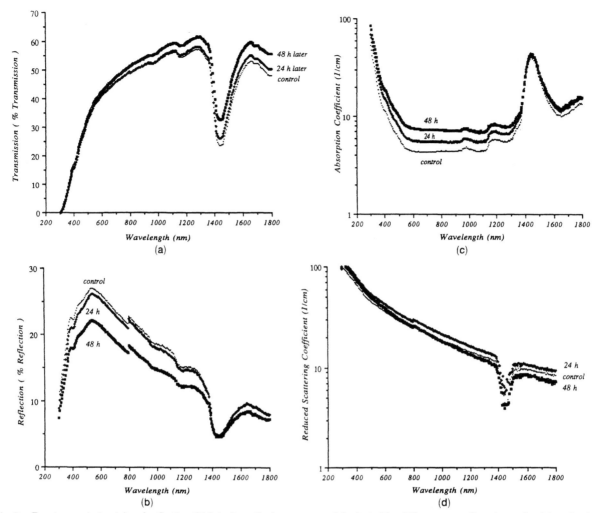

Fig. 3. Raw transmission (a) and reflection (b) data from the human aorta dehydrated for 48 h, corresponding absorption (c), and reduced scattering spectra (d). In control measurements the thickness was 300 μm, the weight was 162 mg. The 24-h-dehydrated sample was 250 μm thick and weighed 98 mg. Following the 48-h dehydration the sample was 225 μm thick and weighed 74 mg. Note that the discontinuity at 800 nm is an instrument artifact caused by detector change. The dips in the reduced scattering spectra are artifacts caused by the δ-Eddington approximation that cannot give accurate properties for regions of very high absorption, such as the water absorption band.[14,18]

light absorbed at near-IR wavelengths beyond 1550 nm decreased by 10–20%.

By assuming that the aorta is composed of 60–80% water, an average weight loss of 46% corresponded to 58–77% dehydration. The optical properties of normal and 50–90% dehydrated human aorta at selected wavelengths are summarized in Table 1. The changes in the reduced scattering coefficient of human aorta were not as consistent and as pronounced as the changes in the absorption coefficient as seen in Fig. 4. Yet there was a slight increase of 2–15% in the visible range.

It became more and more difficult to prepare tissue samples for measurements for dehydration levels beyond 90% (i.e., a weight loss over 60%) since surfaces were no longer smooth and air bubbles were trapped between slides and tissue samples.

Effects of Thermal Damage

Fourteen sets of experiments were carried out. They were divided into three groups according to the temperature of the isotonic saline bath. Samples were heated at 60°C (three sets), 70°C (two sets), or 100°C (nine sets) for 300 ± 10 s. Typical curves for transmission, reflection, the absorption coefficient, and the reduced scattering coefficient for thermal damage studies at 100°C are shown in Fig. 4.

In our initial experiments on the influence of thermal damage at 60° and 70°C on the optical properties of the human aorta, we obtained results with large standard deviations as seen in Tables 2 and 3. Therefore experiments were continued on the effects of thermal damage at 100°C.[15]

When a human aorta was exposed to a temperature of 100°C for 300 ± 10 s, a slight decrease was

Table 1. Optical Properties of Normal and Dehydrated Human Aorta at Selected Wavelengths: $n_{normal} = n_{dehydrated} = 9$ [a]

λ (nm)	μ_a Normal (cm^{-1})	μ_a Dehydrated (cm^{-1})	Change in μ_a (%)	λ (nm)	μ_s' Normal (cm^{-1})	μ_s' Dehydrated (cm^{-1})	Change in μ_s' (%)
350	20.5 ± 2.8	25.7 ± 4.1	+25.9	350	53.0 ± 13.9	60.3 ± 12.9	+15.7
490	4.7 ± 0.8	6.5 ± 1.8	+35.1	490	35.8 ± 4.9	39.1 ± 5.7	+9.3
515	3.7 ± 0.8	5.2 ± 1.7	+35.3	515	33.3 ± 4.8	36.4 ± 5.3	+9.4
630	2.5 ± 0.7	3.6 ± 1.4	+42.2	630	25.4 ± 3.9	27.6 ± 3.9	+9.1
1065	3.2 ± 0.7	4.4 ± 1.1	+35.8	1065	14.2 ± 2.2	14.8 ± 2.0	+5.4
1320	5.4 ± 0.6	6.5 ± 1.0	+19.1	1320	10.7 ± 1.7	10.9 ± 1.6	+3.0
1400	26.7 ± 3.5[b]	26.5 ± 2.7[b]	+11.7[c]	1400	6.2 ± 3.2[c]	6.2 ± 2.9[b]	−35.3[c]
1450	43.1 ± 4.1[d]	42.0 ± 0.7[d]	+5.9[e]	1450	4.1 ± 1.4[d]	3.1 ± 1.3[d]	−20.4[e]
1500	28.6 ± 3.2[f]	29.5 ± 3.2[f]	+12.4[g]	1500	4.1 ± 3.3[f]	5.7 ± 2.5[f]	−14.2[g]
1550	16.7 ± 1.9	17.5 ± 1.7	+5.5	1550	6.8 ± 1.8	6.6 ± 1.8	+5.5
1650	9.4 ± 0.8	10.2 ± 1.0	+8.8	1650	7.8 ± 1.3	7.7 ± 1.2	+0.9
1750	12.2 ± 1.1	13.3 ± 1.3	+9.8	1750	6.7 ± 1.3	6.4 ± 1.4	−0.4

[a] The values are given as a mean ± standard deviation. The corresponding tissue thicknesses for normal and dehydrated samples were 575 ± 138 and 464 ± 116 μm, respectively. The percentage weight loss and thickness shrinkage caused by dehydration were 46.4 ± 7.6% and 19.5 ± 4.8%, respectively. % change = {[μ (dehydrated)/μ (control)] − 1}100.
[b] From only five control and five dehydrated samples, which are not necessarily the same samples.
[c] From scans of only two samples, which did not miss data points in the water absorption band.
[d] From only two control and two dehydrated samples, which are not necessarily the same samples.
[e] From scans of only one sample, which did not miss data points in the water absorption band.
[f] From only five control and four dehydrated samples, which are not necessarily the same samples.
[g] From scans of only two samples, which did not miss data points in the water absorption band.

observed in the absorption coefficient in the visible spectrum above 500 nm. However, the reduced scattering coefficient increased at all wavelengths as seen in Tables 4 and 5. Representative spectra of changes in the optical properties are shown in Figs. 4(c) and 4(d).

It was observed that direct and indirect (i.e., as wrapped in aluminum foil) exposure to a hot saline bath had similar results qualitatively as seen in Figs. 5 and 6, respectively. Yet the changes in the optical properties were less pronounced when tissue samples were first wrapped in aluminum foil and then bathed in an isotonic saline bath. It was also observed that the thickness of the samples wrapped in aluminum foil increased by 16% on average. Microscopic studies revealed increased tissue thickness accompanied by a reduced surface area. It was found that the reduced scattering coefficient of human aorta changed by 10–40% in the range from 400 to 800 nm and by 30 to over 90% above 800 nm when it was bathed in a hot saline solution wrapped in aluminum foil, whereas the reduced scattering coefficient of a human aorta changed by 15–45% in the range from 300 to 800 nm and by 30% to over 150% above 800 nm when it was in direct contact to the hot saline.

Reduced Scattering Coefficient as a Function of Wavelength

The average value of n [for Eq. (1)] and the corresponding standard deviation for normal, dehydrated, and heated samples is given in Table 6. The significance of dehydrated and heated samples relative to the control data is also shown in the table. Typically, if the significance is <5%, we reject the hypothesis that both sets of data come from the same population. According to this criterion, there is a significant increase in the reduced scattering coefficient for 70° and 100°C heated specimens. Another t-test per-

formed for 100°C heated samples revealed that there is no significant difference in the reduced scattering coefficient for directly and wrapped heated samples.

Discussion

In this study we analyzed the effects of dehydration and protein coagulation on the optical properties of the human aorta *in vitro*. It was found that when the average weight loss resulting from dehydration was 46%, the absorption coefficient of the human aorta increased by 20–50% in the 500–1100-nm range and somewhat less in the 300–500- and 1100–1350-nm ranges. The relatively large increase in the absorption coefficient is basically a result of denser packing of cells owing to shrinkage of the tissue samples while the number of chromophores remained constant. However, at 1350–1550 nm (a water absorption band) and up to 1730 nm, the absorption coefficient remained largely unaffected by water loss. Although water is the primary chromophore in this band, the decrease in water content is balanced by tissue shrinkage yielding approximately the same absorption coefficient at the levels of dehydration that we tested.

Since dehydration did not significantly change the reduced scattering coefficient, the authors assumed that the observed optical property changes were attributed only to water loss; actually dehydration may also change collagen cross linking. Indeed it was reported that water is intimately involved in the collagen structure.[19] Electron micrographs of the replicas of wet collagen showed relatively smooth cylindrical fibrils in contrast to the corrugated appearance of dry collagen.[20] Furthermore, in our analysis of the power relationship the value of n for normal and dehydrated samples was 1.15 ± 0.10 and 1.22 ± 0.13, respectively. Since the significance level was

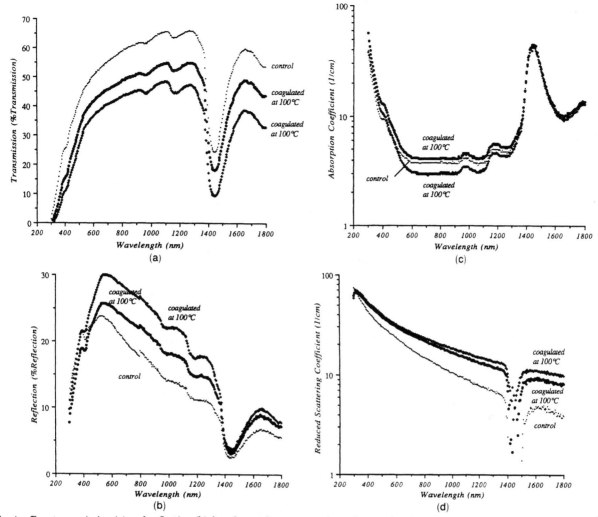

Fig. 4. Raw transmission (a) and reflection (b) data from a human aorta heated in a saline bath at 100°C for 300 ± 10 s, corresponding absorption (c), and reduced scattering spectra (d). There are two different damaged samples. The control sample was 325 μm thick, whereas the damaged samples were 350 (O) and 450 (+) μm thick. Note that the discontinuity at 800 nm is an instrument artifact caused by the detector change. The dips in the reduced scattering spectra are artifacts caused by the δ-Eddington approximation that cannot give accurate properties for regions of high absorption such as the water-absorption band.[14,18]

~ 15%, dehydration did not affect the power-law relation between the wavelength and the reduced scattering coefficient.

We observed that exposure to a temperature of 60–70°C for 300 ± 10 s did not result in predictable and distinct changes in the optical properties as seen in Fig. 5.[15] Our findings are consistent with the fact that collagen denaturation starts dominating tissue behavior between 55° and 70°C.[2] Tissue progresses from normal to denatured states between 60° and 75°C.[21–23] Thus heterogeneous tissue samples such as the aorta may have reached different end points at the end of the 300-s heating period. Although heating tissue to temperatures of ~ 60°C for more than 10 s leads to protein denaturation in cells,[24] it has been reported that some changes in the optical properties caused by thermal damage are still reversible even though the thermal threshold for protein coagulation is exceeded.[25,26]

Although coagulation was first suspected of increasing both the absorption and the reduced scattering coefficients of the human aorta,[25] exposure to hot saline at 100°C for 300 ± 10 s resulted in a slight decrease in the absorption coefficient in the visible spectrum and up to 1400 nm and no dramatic changes over 1400 nm. Only when tissue samples were wrapped in aluminum foil before they were bathed was there a distinct increase in the absorption coefficient at wavelengths of <400 nm. Yet when we compared the curves representing the average change in the absorption coefficient as a result of thermal damage at 70° and 100°C, they were similar, as seen in Fig. 5(a). We believe that a slight decrease from 500 to 1300 nm may be due to denaturation of tissue chromophores. We have also observed that the influence of saline and chromophore diffusion on the absorption coefficient for 100°C heated samples was negligible above 500 nm. On the other hand the

Table 2. Optical Properties of Normal and Thermally Damaged (at 60°C for 300 ± 10 s) Human Aorta at Selected Wavelengths: $n_{normal} = 4, n_{damaged} = 4$[a]

λ (nm)	μ_a Normal (cm^{-1})	μ_a Damaged (cm^{-1})	Change in μ_a (%)	λ (nm)	μ_s' Normal (cm^{-1})	μ_s' Damaged (cm^{-1})	Change in μ_s' (%)
350	22.7 ± 1.8	24.6 ± 3.6	+11.7	350	46.3 ± 3.5	58.2 ± 12.9	+16.2
490	5.4 ± 0.5	6.4 ± 1.0	+14.6	490	31.7 ± 2.1	36.5 ± 7.3	+16.0
515	4.3 ± 0.6	5.2 ± 1.0	+14.9	515	29.3 ± 2.2	33.7 ± 6.8	+16.8
630	2.7 ± 0.8	3.6 ± 0.8	+28.0	630	21.9 ± 2.0	25.0 ± 4.9	+18.1
1065	3.3 ± 0.6	4.1 ± 0.8	+23.7	1065	11.9 ± 1.8	13.1 ± 2.7	+19.0
1320	5.5 ± 0.7	5.9 ± 0.8	+9.8	1320	9.0 ± 1.5	9.8 ± 2.2	+16.2
1400	27.1 ± 4.8[b]	22.9 ± 3.7[b]	−4.9[e]	1400	4.3 ± 2.1[b]	8.5 ± 1.0[b]	+185.0[e]
1450	37.6 ± 0.0[c]	37.8 ± 7.8[c]	+15.2[f]	1450	1.2 ± 0.0[c]	4.4 ± 1.5[c]	+179.2[f]
1500	29.1 ± 4.6[d]	23.5 ± 4.2[d]	−6.5[g]	1500	3.1 ± 1.8[d]	7.7 ± 0.6[d]	+392.9[g]
1550	15.6 ± 1.3	14.9 ± 2.2	+0.3	1550	6.2 ± 1.3	7.3 ± 2.1	+15.0
1650	9.0 ± 0.6	9.0 ± 1.3	+1.6	1650	6.9 ± 1.3	7.6 ± 1.8	+14.9
1750	11.7 ± 0.8	11.5 ± 1.8	+0.9	1750	5.9 ± 1.2	6.8 ± 1.7	+17.3

[a]The samples were directly exposed to hot saline. The values are given as mean ± standard deviation. The corresponding tissue thicknesses for normal and thermally damaged samples were 575 ± 115 and 425 ± 75 μm, respectively. Note that normal and damaged samples were different samples from the same specimen. % change = {[μ (damaged)/μ (control)] − 1}100.
[b]From only three control and three damaged samples, which are not necessarily from the same specimen.
[c]From only one control and three damaged samples, which are not necessarily from the same specimen.
[d]From only three control and three damaged samples, which are not necessarily from the same specimen.
[e]From scans of only two specimens, which did not miss data points in the water absorption band.
[f]From scans of only one specimen, which did not miss data points in the water absorption band.
[g]From scans of only two specimens, which did not miss data points in the water absorption band.

reduced scattering coefficient of the human aorta increased by 10–45% from 400 to 1300 nm and 30% to over 100% above 1500 nm and considerably less in the 300–400-nm range. Assuming that other experimental conditions remained the same, saline and chromophore diffusion resulted in an increased reduced scattering coefficient for 100°C directly heated samples, especially above 1300 nm, even though our analysis of the power relationship between the wavelength and reduced scattering coefficient as given in Eq. (1) revealed no statistical difference in n for 100°C heated samples. There was a consistent decrease in n with thermal damage at 70° and 100°C as can be seen in Table 6. Since a t-test showed a significance level of $<5\%$ between n values for the control and 70° and 100°C heated samples, this decrease in n would represent a change in the shape factor for scatterers and scattering anisotropy in Mie theory. Our hypothesis is supported by the observations of another study on optical-property changes during the thermal coagulation of myocardium. In this study the analyses based on Mie theory suggested that the appearance of coarse and small thermally coagulated granular cellular proteins could be responsible for the increase in the reduced scattering coefficient.[27] Recently Essenpreis et al.[28,29] pointed to changes in the scattering phase function in coagulated rat liver. Essenpreis et al. observed a nearly 35% decrease in the anisotropy

Table 3. Optical Properties of Normal and Thermally Damaged (at 70°C for 300 ± 10 s) Human Aorta at Selected Wavelengths: $n_{normal} = 2, n_{damaged} = 3$[a]

λ (nm)	μ_a Normal (cm^{-1})	μ_a Damaged (cm^{-1})	Change in μ_a (%)	λ (nm)	μ_s' Normal (cm^{-1})	μ_s' Damaged (cm^{-1})	Change in μ_s' (%)
350	21.0 ± 0.3	17.0 ± 1.8	−18.8	350	65.6 ± 17.1	68.5 ± 6.1	+1.1
490	5.6 ± 0.8	4.7 ± 0.4	−16.3	490	38.9 ± 7.8	41.5 ± 5.4	+1.7
515	4.8 ± 0.8	4.0 ± 0.3	−18.1	515	36.3 ± 7.6	38.4 ± 4.9	+0.8
630	3.5 ± 0.8	2.9 ± 0.1	−18.8	630	27.7 ± 6.2	29.2 ± 3.6	+0.6
1065	3.6 ± 0.8	2.9 ± 0.1	−21.9	1065	14.1 ± 3.2	16.9 ± 3.1	+13.7
1320	5.7 ± 0.8	4.9 ± 0.2	−15.7	1320	10.3 ± 2.2	13.7 ± 3.0	+24.8
1400	24.1 ± 1.2	22.6 ± 2.8	−5.1	1400	7.1 ± 3.0	11.2 ± 4.7	+38.5
1450	39.0 ± 0.0[b]	34.0 ± 0.1[b]	−12.8[c]	1450	5.4 ± 0.0[b]	10.9 ± 3.7[b]	+101.0[c]
1500	26.1 ± 1.0	23.0 ± 2.7	−11.1	1500	5.7 ± 2.9	10.2 ± 4.4	+57.9
1550	15.4 ± 0.2	13.6 ± 1.1	−11.8	1550	7.3 ± 2.2	11.3 ± 3.4	+41.0
1650	9.4 ± 0.6	8.4 ± 0.6	−11.5	1650	7.7 ± 1.8	11.0 ± 3.0	+33.4
1750	11.8 ± 0.7	10.7 ± 0.8	−9.7	1750	6.9 ± 1.6	10.4 ± 3.2	+37.6

[a]The samples were directly exposed to hot saline. The values are given as mean ± standard deviation. The corresponding tissue thicknesses for normal and thermally damaged samples were 388 ± 88 μm and 458 ± 12 μm, respectively. Note that normal and damaged samples were different samples from the same specimen. % change = {[μ (damaged)/μ (control)] − 1}100.
[b]From only one control and two damaged samples, which are not necessarily from the same specimen.
[c]From scans of only one specimen, which did not miss data points in the water absorption band.

Table 4. Optical Properties of Normal and Thermally Damaged (at 100°C for 300 ± 10 s) Human Aorta at Selected Wavelengths: $n_{normal} = 6$, $n_{damaged} = 9$[a]

λ (nm)	μ_a Normal (cm^{-1})	μ_a Damaged (cm^{-1})	Change in μ_a (%)	λ (nm)	μ_s' Normal (cm^{-1})	μ_s' Damaged (cm^{-1})	Change in μ_s' (%)
350	18.9 ± 2.8	20.3 ± 2.5	+7.6	350	56.1 ± 7.9	66.3 ± 7.0	+22.2
490	6.2 ± 0.9	5.9 ± 0.9	−5.8	490	33.7 ± 3.6	41.4 ± 3.1	+28.9
515	5.4 ± 0.7	4.6 ± 0.6	−14.0	515	30.1 ± 3.1	38.4 ± 2.8	+29.6
630	4.3 ± 0.6	3.4 ± 0.6	−21.4	630	22.1 ± 2.1	29.9 ± 2.3	+36.7
1065	4.0 ± 0.4	3.4 ± 0.5	−15.1	1065	11.0 ± 1.4	17.5 ± 1.7	+62.0
1320	5.5 ± 0.4	5.2 ± 0.7	−8.1	1320	8.2 ± 1.6	13.8 ± 1.8	+76.5
1400	16.3 ± 5.1	17.4 ± 6.2	−2.0	1400	7.1 ± 3.4	12.4 ± 3.5	+127.0
1450	34.9 ± 4.3[b]	35.9 ± 8.4[b]	−0.9[d]	1450	7.5 ± 5.6[b]	10.1 ± 8.6[b]	+21.5[d]
1500	26.2 ± 3.3[c]	26.4 ± 5.7[c]	+1.3[e]	1500	5.9 ± 4.7[c]	10.6 ± 6.3[c]	+426.6[e]
1550	16.2 ± 2.2	15.4 ± 2.2	−3.5	1550	6.3 ± 3.0	11.7 ± 3.4	+148.6
1650	9.6 ± 0.8	9.3 ± 1.0	−2.9	1650	6.3 ± 2.0	11.2 ± 2.2	+97.7
1750	11.1 ± 0.9	11.1 ± 1.4	−1.5	1750	5.8 ± 2.3	10.6 ± 2.5	+112.1

[a]The samples were directly exposed to hot saline. The values are given as mean ± standard deviation. The corresponding tissue thicknesses for normal and thermally damaged samples were 305 ± 37 μm and 420 ± 59 μm, respectively. Note that normal and damaged samples were different samples from the same specimen. % change = {[μ (damaged)/μ (control)] −1}100.
[b]From only three control and seven damaged samples, which are not necessarily from the same specimen.
[c]From only five control and nine damaged samples, which are not necessarily from the same specimen.
[d]From scans of only two specimens, which did not miss data points in the water absorption band.
[e]From scans of only five specimens, which did not miss data points in the water absorption band.

factor when rat liver was coagulated. His results may well be applicable to the human aorta.

The thermal response of biological tissues to laser light can be predicted by using an optical model such as a δ-Eddington diffusion approximation to determine the fluence rate of light in combination with the heat-conduction equation. However, none of the published models so far incorporates dynamic changes in the optical behavior of tissue during laser irradiation. The photothermal response of laser-irradiated tissue is given by the so-called heat diffusion equation[4] with the heat source term given by

$$Q = \mu_a \phi(z, r), \tag{2}$$

where μ_a is the absorption coefficient of the tissue (cm^{-1}) and $\phi(z, r)$ is the local fluence rate of the laser light (W cm^{-2}).

Since the thermal response of tissue is directly proportional to its absorption characteristics and the local fluence rates, changes in the optical properties will affect the source term. Therefore the local heating patterns will be changed as a function of hydration and protein denaturation. Since the reduced attenuation coefficient is given by

$$\mu_t' = \mu_a + \mu_s', \tag{3}$$

an increase in either of the optical properties will

Table 5. Optical Properties of Normal and Thermally Damaged (at 100°C for 300 ± 10 s) Human Aorta at Selected Wavelengths: $n_{normal} = n_{damaged} = 5$[a]

λ (nm)	μ_a Normal (cm^{-1})	μ_a Damaged (cm^{-1})	Change in μ_a (%)	λ (nm)	μ_s' Normal (cm^{-1})	μ_s' Damaged (cm^{-1})	Change in μ_s' (%)
350	15.4 ± 2.3	17.0 ± 1.5	+11.7	350	62.3 ± 7.6	70.9 ± 7.6	+14.7
490	4.3 ± 1.1	4.1 ± 0.7	−3.0	490	37.0 ± 4.5	45.0 ± 2.2	+23.0
515	3.9 ± 1.0	3.4 ± 0.6	−9.8	515	34.3 ± 4.3	41.9 ± 2.0	+23.3
630	3.1 ± 1.0	2.5 ± 0.6	−17.5	630	25.9 ± 3.4	32.5 ± 1.4	+26.6
1065	3.2 ± 0.9	2.6 ± 0.7	−18.7	1065	13.6 ± 1.6	19.2 ± 0.9	+42.4
1320	4.6 ± 0.9	4.2 ± 0.8	−8.6	1320	10.2 ± 1.2	15.5 ± 1.0	+53.6
1400	11.7 ± 1.3	11.7 ± 0.6	+0.2	1400	9.0 ± 1.0	14.2 ± 1.2	+58.7
1450	38.1 ± 4.2[b]	42.1 ± 5.3[b]	+3.3[d]	1450	1.6 ± 2.0[b]	5.7 ± 3.8[b]	+65.0[d]
1500	28.6 ± 3.3[c]	30.2 ± 2.6[c]	+4.3[e]	1500	4.0 ± 2.7[c]	9.6 ± 2.4[c]	+130.5[e]
1550	16.3 ± 1.9	16.8 ± 1.0	+3.9	1550	7.2 ± 0.8	12.1 ± 1.3	+69.5
1650	9.9 ± 1.1	9.2 ± 0.7	+3.2	1650	7.5 ± 0.9	12.2 ± 1.1	+64.0
1750	10.0 ± 1.2	10.4 ± 0.7	+5.6	1750	7.0 ± 0.8	11.5 ± 1.1	+64.9

[a]The samples were wrapped in aluminum foil before being immersed in a hot saline bath. The values are given as the mean ± standard deviation. The corresponding tissue thicknesses before and after the hot saline bath were 460 ± 116 and 530 ± 124 μm, respectively. The percentage thickness increase caused by thermal damage was 16 ± 5.5%. % change = {[μ (damaged)/μ (control)] − 1}100.
[b]From only three control and five damaged samples.
[c]From only four control and five damaged samples.
[d]From scans of only three specimens, which did not miss the data points in the water absorption band.
[e]From scans of only four specimens, which did not miss the data points in the water absorption band.

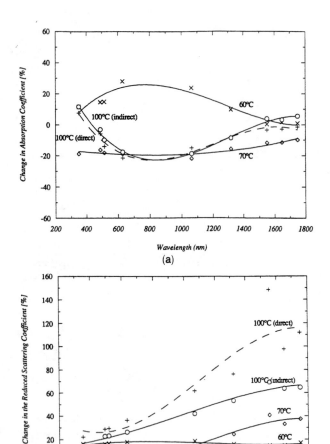

(a)

(b)

Fig. 5. Effects of thermal damage on the (a) absorption and (b) reduced scattering coefficients of the human aorta at selected wavelengths. The average change in optical properties was curve fit with a third-order polynomial.

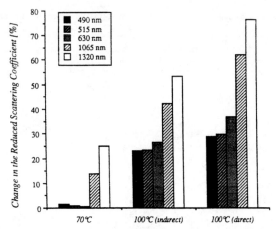

Fig. 6. Effects of thermal damage at 70° and 100°C on the reduced scattering coefficient at frequently used laser wavelengths.

and Nd:YAG laser wavelengths reported by van Gemert *et al.*[33] and Lozano are significantly lower than the values reported in this study. Whereas the absorption coefficient at 632.8 nm reported by Keijzer *et al.*[31] is somehow close to the values found in this study, the absorption coefficient reported by Yoon[35] is close to the values reported by van Gemert *et al.*

The reduced scattering coefficient at 476, 580, and 600 nm reported by Keijzer *et al.*[31] is significantly higher than the values reported in this study. Even though there is reasonable agreement between the values of the reduced scattering coefficient found by Oraevski *et al.*[32] and in our study at 488 nm, the value at 514.5 nm obtained in our study almost doubles the values reported by van Gemert *et al.*[33] The values for the reduced scattering coefficient at 515 and 633 nm found by Lozano[35] are close to the values in this study. Values for the reduced scattering coefficient at 632.8 nm as reported by van Gemert *et al.*[33] are significantly lower than the values found in our study, whereas Yoon[36] and Keijzer *et al.*[31] found higher reduced scattering values at this wavelength. At Nd:YAG laser wavelength of 1064 nm, the values found in this study doubled the reduced scattering coefficient reported by van Gemert *et al.*,[33] but they are lower than the value reported by Lozano.[35]

Why is there such a variation in the value of the optical properties reported by various laboratories? Undoubtedly differences in the measurement tech-

result in a reduced penetration depth, increased attenuation, and thus higher temperatures closer to the tissue surface. By incorporating dynamic changes during laser irradiation in tissue optical behavior, it is possible to estimate the required dosimetry more precisely.

In Table 7 optical properties of normal aorta samples are compared with published values from other research groups. The absorption coefficient at 470 nm reported by Prince *et al.*[30] (as converted from Kubelka–Munk optical properties) and at 476 and 580 nm as reported by Keijzer *et al.*[31] are significantly higher than the absorption coefficient found in this study. Yet the absorption coefficient at 600 nm reported by Keijzer *et al.* is in close agreement with the value found in this study. At argon laser wavelengths, 488 and 514.5 nm, there is reasonable agreement between values of the absorption coefficient found in this study and those reported by Oraevski *et al.*[32] and van Gemert *et al.*,[33] respectively, who used Kubelka–Munk theory. Yet the absorption coefficient at 515 nm reported by Lozano,[35] and at He–Ne

Table 6. Power Relationship Between the Wavelength and the Reduced Scattering Coefficient and the Significance of *n* Values for Control and Experimental Reduced Scattering Spectra as Obtained from a *t*-Test

Description	$n_{control}$	$n_{experimental}$	Significance (%)
Dehydration	1.15 ± 0.10	1.22 ± 0.13	~15
Heating at 60°C	1.21 ± 0.12	1.28 ± 0.04	~25
Heating at 70°C	1.30 ± 0.01	1.10 ± 0.10	<5
Heating at 100°C (Direct heating)	1.38 ± 0.11	1.06 ± 0.07	<5
Heating at 100°C (Wrapped heating)	1.26 ± 0.08	1.03 ± 0.05	<5

Table 7. Published Optical Properties of Normal Human Aorta at Selected Wavelengths Compared with Values Obtained in This Study

λ (nm)	μ_a (cm^{-1})	μ_s' (cm^{-1})	Methods and Reference[a]
470	13 ± 2	—	KM[30]
	5.9 ± 1.2^b	37.8 ± 6.1^b	DA
476	7.5	39.20	DA ($d = 250$ μm)[31]
	26.1	58.76	DA ($d = 233$ μm)[31]
	10.8	38.56	DA ($d = 375$ μm)[31]
	5.7 ± 1.2^b	36.8 ± 6.4^b	DA
488	3.9	30.23	KM[31]
	5.2 ± 2.1^b	35.9 ± 5.8^b	DA
514.5	7.0	16.67	KM ($d = 1.4$ mm)[33]
	6.25	16.75	KM ($d = 1.88$ mm)[38]
	5.0	17.67	KM ($d = 1.23$ mm)[33]
	4.3 ± 1.0^b	33.0 ± 5.4^b	DA
515	2.7	32.6	DA[33]
580	6.6	27.75	DA ($d = 250$ μm)[31]
	9.2	45.75	DA ($d = 233$ μm)[31]
	11.0	28.96	DA ($d = 375$ μm)[31]
	3.5 ± 1.1^b	27.9 ± 4.9^b	DA
600	4.1	28.48	DA ($d = 250$ μm)[31]
	4.7	28.32	DA ($d = 233$ μm)[31]
	3.3	26.85	DA ($d = 375$ μm)[31]
	3.4 ± 1.1^b	26.6 ± 4.6^b	DA
632.8	0.75	10.12	KM ($d = 1.4$ mm)[33]
	0.70	9.17	KM ($d = 1.88$ mm)[33]
	0.55	9.25	KM ($d = 1.23$ mm)[33]
	2.3	40.95	DA[30]
	0.52	31.0	ADT[34]
	3.3 ± 1.1^b	24.6 ± 4.4^b	DA
633	1.4	26.0	DA[33]
1060	1.17	17.0	DA[33]
1064	0.30	6.77	KM ($d = 1.28$ mm)[33]
	0.30	6.77	KM ($d = 1.47$ mm)[33]
	0.45	4.15	KM ($d = 2.87$ mm)[33]
	3.5 ± 0.8^b	13.2 ± 2.6^b	DA

[a]KM, Kubelka–Munk properties converted by using[34] $A_{KM} = 2\mu_a$, $S_{KM} = (3\mu_s' - \mu_a)/4$; DA, diffusion approximation; ADT, asymptotic diffuse transmission.

[b]Mean ± standard deviation from 22 samples.

nique and the difficulty in performing an experiment that matches the mathematical theory are a major source of error. Although little information has been published on the sensitivity of μ_a and μ_s' to errors in the measurement of R and T, adding doubling computation by Prahl[14] suggests that a 5–10% change in total reflection can change the calculated total attenuation coefficient, $\mu_t = \mu_a + \mu_s$, by a factor of 2 for $g = 0.875$, $a = 0.9$, $a = \mu_s/(\mu_s + \mu_a)$. Thus a small error in the measurement of reflection can produce a factor-of-2 change in the albedo a. In this situation it appears that the scattering coefficient is extremely sensitive to errors in the measurement of reflection.

During this study we have noted that measurements with a spectrophotometer system predict greater values of the absorption coefficient than an equivalent laser-based integrating sphere system. Furthermore there is considerable variability in the measurement of the absorption coefficient below 3 cm^{-1} as a function of tissue thickness and unaccounted losses associated with the integrating sphere

measurements.[13,35,37] The data of Keijzer et al.[31] and van Gemert et al.[33] as presented in Table 7 and measurements in our laser laboratory support the observation that the calculated values of the absorption coefficient decrease as the sample thickness increases.[13,15,37] Undoubtedly, the variability in these results is partly due to the nonhomogeneity of the tissue. Yet we can improve the results by minimizing the effects of other sources of error. With tunable laser sources the beam divergence associated with spectrophotometer systems can be reduced. Integrating sphere measurements can also be improved with a double integrating sphere system. Measurements should be corrected for various losses as described by Cheong[37] and Pickering et al.[38] Tissue samples must be fresh and uniform, and dehydration must be avoided, as noted above.

Conclusion

The optical properties of the human aorta are a function of hydration levels and previous thermal damage. A water loss of ~50% increases the absorption coefficient by 20–50% in the visible spectrum, whereas thermal damage induced at 100°C increases the reduced scattering coefficient by 10% to over 150%. Neither the power of the wavelength dependency of the reduced scattering coefficient [see Eq. (1)] nor the reduced scattering coefficient is significantly altered by dehydration or heating at 60°C. However, the value of n decreased by 16–24% as a result of heating at 70° and 100°C, and this change was accompanied by a significant increase in the reduced scattering coefficient.

The authors thank Roberto Bayardo and his assistants at the Travis County Medical Examiner's Office for providing the tissue samples.

This work was supported in part by the U.S. Office of Naval Research under grant N00014-91-J-4065 and in part by the Albert and Clemmie Caster Foundation.

References

1. S. Rastegar and M. Motamedi, "A theoretical analysis of dynamic variation of temperature dependent optical properties in the response of laser irradiated tissue," in *Laser–Tissue Interaction*, S. L. Jacques, ed., Proc. Soc. Photo-Opt. Instrum. Eng. **1202**, 253–259 (1990).
2. R. Agah, M. Motamedi, D. Praveen, E. Ettedgui, L. Song, and J. R. Spears, "Potential role of collagen in optical behavior of arterial tissue during laser irradiation," in *Laser–Tissue Interaction*, S. L. Jacques, ed., Proc. Soc. Photo-Opt. Instrum. Eng. **1202**, 246–252 (1990).
3. E. Ettedgui, L. Song, R. Agah, and M. Motamedi, "Optical behavior of tissue at elevated temperatures," Lasers Surg. Med. Suppl. **2**, 5 (1990).
4. A. J. Welch, "The thermal response of laser irradiated tissue," IEEE J. Quantum Electron. **QE-20**, 1471–1481 (1984).
5. A. J. Welch, J. W. Valvano, J. A. Pearce, L. J. Hayes, and M. Motamedi, "Effects of laser irradiation on tissue during laser angioplasty," Lasers Surg. Med. **5**, 251–264 (1985).
6. S. Thomsen, W.-F. Cheong, and J. A. Pearce, "Histopathologic assessment of water dominated photothermal effects produced with laser irradiation," in *Lasers in Dermatology and Tissue*

Welding, O. T. Tan, J. V. White, and R. A. White, eds., Proc. Soc. Photo-Opt. Instrum. Eng. **1422**, 14–18 (1991).

7. S. A. Prahl, W.-F. Cheong, G. Yoon, and A. J. Welch, "Optical properties of human aorta during low power argon laser irradiation," in *Laser Interaction with Tissue*, M. W. Berns, ed., Proc. Soc. Photo-Opt. Instrum. Eng. **908**, 29–33 (1988).

8. Z. F. Gourgouliatos, "Behavior of optical properties of tissue as a function of temperature," M.S. thesis, Biomedical Engineering Program (University of Texas at Austin, Austin, Tex., 1986).

9. G. J. Derbyshire, D. K. Bogen, and M. Unger. "Thermally induced optical property changes in myocardium at 1064 nm," Lasers Surg. Med. **10**, 28–34 (1990).

10. R. Splinter, R. H. Stevenson, L. Littmann, J. R. Tuntelder, C. H. Chuang, G. P. Tatsis, and M. Thompson, "Optical properties of normal, diseased, and laser photocoagulated myocardium at the Nd:YAG wavelength," Lasers Surg. Med. **11**, 117–124 (1991).

11. A. Ishimaru, *Wave Propagation and Scattering in Random Media* (Academic, New York, 1987), Vols. 1, 2.

12. S. Chandrasekhar, *Radiative Transfer* (Oxford U. Press, London, 1960).

13. W.-F. Cheong, S. A. Prahl, and A. J. Welch, "A review of the optical properties of biological tissues," IEEE Quantum Electron. **26**, 2166–2185 (1990).

14. S. A. Prahl, "Light transport in tissue," Ph.D. dissertation, Biomedical Engineering Program (University of Texas at Austin, Austin, Tex., 1988).

15. I. F. Çilesiz, "The effects of dehydration and thermal damage on the optical properties of biological tissues," M.S. thesis, Biomedical Engineering Program (University of Texas at Austin, Austin, Tex., 1990).

16. M. J. C. van Gemert and A. J. Welch, "Time constants in thermal laser medicine," Lasers Surg. Med. **9**, 405–421 (1989).

17. S. Thomsen and S. L. Jacques, Laser Biology Research Laboratory, University of Texas M.D. Anderson Cancer Center, Houston, Tex. 77030 (personal communication, 1991).

18. G. Yoon, S. A. Prahl, and A. J. Welch, "Accuracies of the diffusion approximation and its similarity relations for laser irradiated biological media," Appl. Opt. **28**, 2250–2255 (1989).

19. M. Luescher, "Effect of hydration upon the thermal stability of tropocollagen and its dependence on the presence of neutral salts," Biopolymers **13**, 2489–2503 (1974).

20. W. Traub and K. A. Piez, "The chemistry and structure of collagen," Adv. Protein Chem. **25**, 320–325 (1971).

21. G. Müller and B. Schaldach, "Basic laser–tissue interaction," in *Advances in Laser Medicine II: Safety and Laser–Tissue Interaction*, G. J. Müller and H.-P. Berlien, eds., Proc. Soc. Photo-Opt. Instrum. Eng. **1143**, 17–25 (1989).

22. F. Chambettaz, X. Clivaz, F. Marquis, and R. P. Salathé, "Temperature variations of reflection, transmission, and fluorescence of the arterial wall," in *Laser–Tissue Interaction II*, S. L. Jacques, ed., Proc. Soc. Photo-Opt. Instrum. Eng. **1427**, 134–140 (1991).

23. S. Rastegar and T. Glenn, "An analysis of kinetic rate modeling of thermal damage in laser irradiated tissue," in *Laser–Tissue Interaction II*, S. L. Jacques, ed., Proc. Soc. Photo-Opt. Instrum. Eng. **1427**, 300–306 (1991).

24. K. Dörschel and T. Brodzinski, "Proposal for dosimetry of nonionizing radiation," in *Advances in Laser Medicine II: Safety and Laser–Tissue Interaction*, G. J. Müller and H.-P. Berlien, eds., Proc. Soc. Photo-Opt. Instrum. Eng. **1143**, 346–357 (1989).

25. G. Yoon, P. S. Sriram, R. C. Straight, and A. J. Welch, "Thermal response during tissue coagulation by successive laser exposures," Lasers Surg. Med. Suppl. **3**, 4 (1991).

26. G. Yoon, Laser Institute, University of Utah, Salt Lake City, Utah 84108 (personal communication, 1991).

27. S. Thomsen, S. Jacques, and S. Flock, "Microscopic correlates of macroscopic optical property changes during thermal coagulation of myocardium," in *Laser–Tissue Interaction*, S. L. Jacques, ed., Proc. Soc. Photo-Opt. Instrum. Eng. **1202**, 2–11 (1990).

28. M. Essenpreis, P. van der Zee, P. S. Jones, P. Gewehr, and T. N. Mills, "Changes in scattering phase function of rat liver at 1.064 μm and 1.32 μm following coagulation," Lasers Surg. Med. Suppl. **3**, 5 (1991).

29. M. Essenpreis, Department of Medical Physics and Engineering, University College, London WC1E 6JA, Great Britain [personal communication during *Laser Coagulation of Superficial and Deep Lesions: A Workshop for Basic Scientists and Clinicians*, at University of Texas M.D. Anderson Cancer Center, Houston, Tex. 77030 (May 1991)].

30. M. R. Prince, T. F. Deutsch, M. M. Mathews-Roth, R. Margolis, J. A. Parrish, and A. R. Oseroff, "Preferential light absorption in atheromas *in vitro*—implications for laser angioplasty," J. Clin. Invest. **78**, 295–302 (1986).

31. M. Keijzer, R. R. Richards-Kortum, S. L. Jacques, and M. S. Feld, "Fluorescence spectroscopy of turbid media: autofluorescence of the human aorta," Appl. Opt. **28**, 4286–4292 (1989).

32. A. A. Oraevsky, V. S. Lethokov, S. E. Ragimov, V. G. Omel'Yanenko, A. A. Belyaev, B. V. Shekhonin, and R. S. Akchurin, "Spectral properties of human atherosclerotic blood vessel walls," Lasers Life Sci. **2**, 275–288 (1988).

33. M. J. C. van Gemert, R. Verdaasdonk, E. G. Stassen, G. A. C. M. Schets, G. H. M. Gijsbers, and J. J. Bonnier, "Optical properties of human blood vessel wall and plaque," Lasers Surg. Med. **5**, 235–237 (1985).

34. W. M. Star, J. P. A. Marijnissen, and M. J. C. van Gemert, "Light dosimetry in optical phantoms and tissues," Phys. Med. Biol. **33**, 437–454 (1988).

35. R. A. Lozano, "Spectrophotometric measurement of optical properties of biological tissues," M.S. thesis, Biomedical Engineering Program (University of Texas at Austin, Austin, Tex., 1989).

36. G. Yoon, "Absorption and scattering of laser light in biological media-mathematical modeling and methods for determining optical properties," Ph.D. dissertation, Biomedical Engineering Program (University of Texas at Austin, Austin, Tex., 1988).

37. W.-F. Cheong, "Photothermodynamics of tissue irradiated by Nd:YAG laser (1064 nm, 1320 nm)," Ph.D. dissertation, Biomedical Engineering Program (University of Texas at Austin, Austin, Tex., 1990).

38. J. W. Pickering, S. A. Prahl, N. van Wieringen, J. F. Beek, H. J. C. M. Sterenborg, and M. J. C. van Gemert, "A double integrating sphere system to measure optical properties of tissue," submitted to J. Opt. Soc. Am.

Errata

Light dosimetry: effects of dehydration and thermal damage on the optical properties of the human aorta

I. Çilesiz and A. J. Welch

The program used to compute the optical properties of tissue was based on measurements of total reflection R_t and total transmission T_t.[1] Diffuse reflection R_d was not converted to total reflection R_t during the execution of the program as the authors assumed. This wrong assumption affected calculations of the reduced scattering coefficient μ_s' when diffuse reflection R_d was small in the 300–400-nm band and the water absorption band at greater than 1300 nm. Recomputed values of the reduced scattering coefficient μ_s' were slightly higher in these wavelength bands. The artifact about the 1450-nm water absorption band noted in Figs. 3(d) and 4(d) was eliminated. Overall trends of change in the optical properties were not affected although individual values in Tables 1–5 were modified. Corrected tables and figures can be obtained from the authors.

Several reference numbers in Table 7 are wrong. A corrected version of this table is given here.

The authors regret the errors.

Reference

1. I. Çilesiz and A. J. Welch, "Light dosimetry: effects of dehydration and thermal damage on the optical properties of the human aorta," Appl. Opt. **32**, 477–487 (1993).

The authors are with the Biomedical Engineering Program, The University of Texas at Austin, 639 Engineering Science Building, Austin, Texas 78712-1084.

Received 3 January 1994.
0003-6935/94/163571-01$06.00/0.
© 1994 Optical Society of America.

Table 7. Published Optical Properties of Normal Human Aorta at Selected Wavelengths Compared with Values Obtained in This Study

λ (nm)	μ_a (cm^{-1})	μ_s' (cm^{-1})	Method and Reference[a]
470	13 ± 2	—	KM[30]
	5.3 ± 0.9	42.6 ± 6.0	DA
476	7.5	39.20	DA (d = 250 μm)[31]
	26.1	58.76	DA (d = 233 μm)[31]
	10.8	38.56	DA (d = 375 μm)[31]
	5.1 ± 0.9	41.9 ± 5.9	DA
488	3.9	30.23	KM[32]
	4.5 ± 0.9	39.9 ± 5.6	DA
514.5	7.0	16.67	KM (d = 1.4 mm)[33]
	6.25	16.75	KM (d = 1.88 mm)[33]
	5.0	17.67	KM (d = 1.23 mm)[33]
	3.7 ± 0.9	36.9 ± 5.4	DA
515	2.7	32.6	DA[35]
580	6.6	27.75	DA (d = 250 μm)[31]
	9.2	45.75	DA (d = 233 μm)[31]
	11.0	28.96	DA (d = 375 μm)[31]
	2.8 ± 0.9	31.1 ± 4.9	DA
600	4.1	28.48	DA (d = 250 μm)[31]
	4.7	28.32	DA (d = 233 μm)[31]
	3.3	26.85	DA (d = 375 μm)[31]
	2.6 ± 0.9	29.6 ± 4.7	DA
632.8	0.75	10.12	KM (d = 1.4 mm)[33]
	0.70	9.17	KM (d = 1.88 mm)[33]
	0.55	9.25	KM (d = 1.23 mm)[33]
	2.3	40.95	DA[31]
	0.52	31.0	ADT[36]
	2.6 ± 0.9	27.4 ± 4.4	DA
633	1.4	26.0	DA[35]
1060	1.17	17.0	DA[35]
1064	0.30	6.77	KM (d = 1.28 mm)[33]
	0.30	6.77	KM (d = 1.47 mm)[33]
	0.45	4.15	KM (d = 2.87 mm)[33]
	2.7 ± 0.5	15.5 ± 2.8	DA

[a]KM, Kubelka–Munk properties converted by using[34] $A_{KM} = 2\mu_a$, $S_{KM} = (3\mu_s' - \mu_a)/4$; DA, diffusion approximation; ADT, asymptotic diffuse transmission.

Reprinted from *Applied Optics*, Vol. 15(9), pp. 2059-2067 (September 1976).

Diffuse reflectance from a finite blood medium: applications to the modeling of fiber optic catheters

Larry Reynolds, C. Johnson, and A. Ishimaru

The scattering and absorption of light by randomly oriented, discretely scattering, red blood cells imbedded in a homogeneous plasma medium can be described by the P1 approximation to the one-speed transport equation, where the cells have the dual role of anisotropic sources for first scattering events and of scattering and absorption sites for subsequent scattering events. Equations for diffuse reflectance defined for a finite size receiver in the plane of a normally incident cylindrical photon beam are derived and compared with experimental data to fundamentally justify the basic sending–receiving charactreristics of a fiber optic catheter model. A model of the fiber optic catheter used for the spectrophotometric measurement of oxygen content in blood is developed from the theory and compared with experimental results to further substantiate the theoretical approach.

Introduction

Diffusion theory as an approach to the solution of photon propagation in a whole blood medium where photons are absorbed and scattered by scattering sites within the medium has been suggested by several sources.[1-3] Substantial experimental evidence indicates that optical propagation in blood may be described by a diffusion theory approach,[1,2,4–6] and further substantiation will be presented.

Conventional theories of light propagation in blood[7,8] based upon the continuously coupled, oppositely traveling photon fluxes due to the backscattering properties of blood are not easily extrapolated to include three-dimensional effects. A more fundamental statistical multiple scattering field theory approach[9,10] is also limited by being easily applied to only one-dimensional configurations. A principal advantage of diffusion theory is that analytical solutions for reflectance and transmittance calculations are readily obtained in three dimensions. The P1 approximation, the zeroth and first order Legendre polynomial approximations to the one-speed transport equation, represents a diffusion theory approach that can be applied to a high albedo medium containing particles such as red blood cells.

There is a great need for an analytical tool useful for the design of optical sensors in biological materials. One application, that of determining oxygen saturation in blood or muscle by optical spectroscopy,[11-13] whether by *in vitro* or *in vivo* techniques, requires measurements by an optical system that is governed to a great extent by three-dimensional effects. Thus a three-dimensional diffusion theory could be of great importance in interpreting experimental results, as well as evolving design criteria for optimum instrumentation and transducer configurations.

Diffusion Analysis (P1 Approximation)

The propagation of scattered light described by the Helmholtz equation

$$[\nabla^2 - (\Sigma_a/D)]\rho_s(r,\theta,z) = -(1/D)S(r,\theta,z) \qquad (1)$$

has been derived heuristically for the case of optical diffusion in a blood medium that assumes light to be isotropically scattered[3] and in the general case for anisotropic sources and scatterers using the P1 approximation to the one-speed transport equation.[14] For the case of isotropic scattering the P1 approximation is equivalent to the diffusion approximation. ρ_s is the scattered photon flux, and Σ_a is the macroscopic absorption cross section. D is the transport diffusion constant for anisotropic scattering and is proportional to the reciprocal of the total transport cross section. S, the generalized source term, defines the injection of photons within the medium, where first scattering events are considered as a volume source distribution. This source distribution is spa-

C. Johnson is with the University of Utah, Department of Biophysics & Bioengineering, Salt Lake City, Utah 84112. The other authors are with the University of Washington, Bioengineering Center & Department of Electrical Engineering, Seattle, Washington 98195.

Received 30 September 1974; revised manuscript received 19 September 1975.

tially defined by the unscattered photon beam within the medium and is proportional to the density of scatterers. For the case of anisotropic scatterers the source term is derived from the coupled $P1$ approximation equation[14] and has the form

$$S(r,\theta,z) = Q_0(r,\theta,z) - 3D\nabla\cdot\mathbf{Q}_1(r,\theta,z), \qquad (2)$$

where the isotropic photon source contribution Q_0 and the anisotropic photon source contribution $\mathbf{Q}_1$ are derived from the coherent source term Q:

$$Q(r,\theta,z,\mu) = q_0\Sigma_d(\mu)\exp(-\Sigma z)R(r),$$

which is closely related to the incident beam radiation. Here Σ is the total macroscopic cross section and is functionally related to the microscopic absorption and scattering cross sections (σ_a and σ_s), thusly,

$$\Sigma = \frac{H}{v}[(1 - H)\sigma_s + \sigma_a] = \Sigma_s + \Sigma_a.$$

The $(1 - H)$ dependence is based on the work of Twersky,[9] where H is the hematocrit of blood, v is the volume of a single erythrocyte, and μ is the cosine of the angle between photon direction before and after scattering. Σ_d is the macroscopic differential scattering cross section, $R(r)$ is the radial source geometry characteristics, q_0 is the source photon flux at $r = z = 0$, and $\hat{z}$ is a unit vector in the z direction.

By taking the first two terms of a Legendre polynomial expansion of the coherent source Q, consistent with the $P1$ approximation,

$$Q_m = 2\pi \int_{-1}^{1} Q(r,\theta,z,\hat{\mu})P_m(\hat{\mu})d\hat{\mu}$$

the isotropic source term is

$$Q_0 = 2\pi \int_{-1}^{1} Q(r,\theta,z,\hat{\mu})d\hat{\mu} = q_0\Sigma_s \exp(-\Sigma z)R(r),$$

and the anisotropic source term is

$$\mathbf{Q}_1 = 2\pi \int_{-1}^{1} Q(r,\theta,z,\hat{\mu})\hat{\mu}d\hat{\mu} = q_0\Sigma_s\bar{\mu} \exp(-\Sigma z)R(r)\hat{z},$$

$\bar{\mu}$ is the average value of the cosine of the scattering angle ($-1 \leq \bar{\mu} \leq 1$), where -1 is purely backscattering, $+1$ is purely forward scattering, and 0 represents isotropic scattering.

The solution to Eq. (1) for the mixed homogeneous boundary condition

$$\rho_s + gn\cdot\nabla\rho_s = 0, \qquad (3)$$

where $\hat{n}$ is a positive unit vector in the outward normal direction from the interface boundaries, and g is a function of the medium, is

$$\rho_s(r,\theta,z) = \frac{1}{D}\int_{v'} S(r',\theta',z')G(r,\theta,z\,|\,r',\theta',z')dv'. \qquad (4)$$

G is the Green's function obtained by solving the inhomogeneous auxiliary Green's function equation,

$$\left(\nabla^2 - \frac{\Sigma_a}{D}\right)G(r,\theta,z\,|\,r',\theta',z')$$
$$= -\frac{\delta(r - r')}{2\pi r}\delta(z - z')\delta(\theta - \theta'), \qquad (5)$$

for a point source in cylindrical coordinates. Equation (4) defines the scattered photon flux at a point (r,θ,z) in terms of an integral over the volume v' that includes all the diffuse photon sources $S(r',\theta',z')$, those scatterers contained within the illuminated unscattered portion of the incident photon intensity that contribute to first scattering events.

Reflectance equations will be obtained from Eq. (4) under the following premises and boundary conditions:

(1) A cylindrical photon beam of radius **b** is normally incident on a slab medium of thickness **d** in the $+z$ direction.

(2) A collimated cylindrical beam of incident photons attenuates as $\exp(-\Sigma z)$ within the medium.[15]

(3) Single anisotropic scattering of the incident photons, described functionally by $S(r,\theta,z)$, occurs within the incident beam, and once an incident photon is scattered it becomes a ρ_s photon.

(4) Reflectance at the interface boundaries $z = 0$ and $z = \mathbf{d}$ due to a mismatch in indices of refraction is neglected.

(5) Mixed homogeneous boundary conditions of the type, Eq. (3), at $z = 0$ and $z = \mathbf{d}$ are used.

Scattered Photon Flux

For a slab of finite thickness **d**, the Green's function defined by Eq. (5) for a ring source where the source function is independent of θ and subject to mixed homogeneous boundary conditions

$$G - g\hat{n}\cdot\nabla G = 0$$

is[6]

$$G(r,z\,|\,r'z') = \frac{2}{\pi}\sum_{n=1}^{\infty}\Gamma_n\rho_n(z)\rho_n(z')G_n(r\,|\,r').$$

$\rho_n(z)$, the eigenfunction, is

$$\rho_n(z) = \sin(k_n z + \gamma_n),$$

and Γ_n, the eigenfunction normalization factor, is given by

$$\Gamma_n = \frac{k_n}{2k_n d + \sin2\gamma_n - \sin[2(k_n d + \gamma_n)]}.$$

$G_n(r\,|\,r')$, the radial component of the Green's function, is

$$G_n(r\,|\,r') = \begin{cases} I_0(\lambda_n r)K_0(\lambda_n r'), & r' > r, \\ K_0(\lambda_n r)I_0(\lambda_n r'), & r' < r, \end{cases}$$

where r' is the radius where scattering occurs, r is the observation radius, and I_0 and K_0 are modified Bessel functions. The eigenvalues k_n are defined by

$$\tan k_n d = \frac{2gk_n}{g^2 k_n^2 - 1},$$

the phase function γ_n is

$$\gamma_n = \tan^{-1}(gk_n)$$

and

381

$$\lambda_n^2 = k_n^2 + \frac{\Sigma_a}{D}.$$

For high albedo media,

$$\left| 1 - \frac{\Sigma_s}{\Sigma_a + \Sigma_s} \right| \ll 1,$$

and plane surface interfaces, the medium dependent constant g, is given by[14]

$$g = (0.7104)/\Sigma_t,$$

where Σ_t is the total transport corrected cross section

$$\Sigma_t = \Sigma_s(1 - \bar{u}) + \Sigma_a.$$

Inserting the Green's function and source function into Eq. (4), the integral form of the scattered photon flux becomes

$$\rho_s(r,z) = \frac{2\Sigma_s}{\pi}\left(\frac{1}{D} + 3\bar{\mu}\Sigma\right)q_0\sum_{n=1}^{\infty}\Gamma_n\rho_n(z)\int_0^{2\pi}d\theta'\int_0^d$$
$$\times \exp(-\Sigma z')\sin(k_n z' + \gamma_n)dz'$$
$$\int_0^b R(r')\begin{bmatrix} I_0(\lambda_n r)K_0(\lambda_n r') \\ K_0(\lambda_n r)I_0(\lambda_n r') \end{bmatrix}r'dr', \quad (6)$$

where the radial functional dependence of the normally incident photon beam of radius **b** is defined as

$$R(r') = U(r') - U(r' - b),$$

and **U** is the unit step function. Integrating the z' dependence gives

$$\int_0^d \exp(-\Sigma z')\sin(k_n z' + \gamma_n)dz' = \frac{z_n}{(k_n^2 + \Sigma^2)}, \quad (7)$$

with

$$z_n = \left\{ \Sigma \sin\gamma_n\left[1 + \exp(-\Sigma d)\left(\frac{k_n}{\Sigma}\sin k_n d - \cos k_n d\right)\right]\right.$$
$$\left. + k_n\cos\gamma_n\left[1 - \exp(-\Sigma d)\left(\frac{\Sigma}{k_n}\sin k_n d + \cos k_n d\right)\right]\right\}.$$

The radial integration in Eq. (6) depends on whether $r < b$ or $r > b$. For $r < b$ the integral consists of two parts:

$$\int_0^r K_0(\lambda_n r)I_0(\lambda_n r')r'dr' = \frac{r}{\lambda_n}K_0(\lambda_n r)I_1(\lambda_n r), \quad (8)$$

and

$$\int_r^b I_0(\lambda_n r)K_0(\lambda_n r')r'dr' = \frac{r}{\lambda_n}I_0(\lambda_n r)K_1(\lambda_n r)$$
$$- \frac{b}{\lambda_n}I_0(\lambda_n r)K_1(\lambda_n b). \quad (9)$$

For $r > b$ the integral gives

$$\int_0^b K_0(\lambda_n r)I_0(\lambda_n r')r'dr' = \frac{b}{\lambda_n}K_0(\lambda_n r)I_1(\lambda_n b). \quad (10)$$

Combining Eqs. (7), (8), (9), and (10), ρ_s becomes

$$\rho_s(r,z) = 4\Sigma_s\left(\frac{1}{D} + 3\bar{\mu}\Sigma\right)q_0\sum_{n=1}^{\infty}\frac{\Gamma_n\rho_n(z)z_nR_n(\lambda_n r)}{(k_n^2 + \Sigma^2)}, \quad (11)$$

where

$$R_n(\lambda_n r) = \begin{cases} \dfrac{1}{\lambda_n^2}[1 - \lambda_n b I_0(\lambda_n r)K_1(\lambda_n b)], & r < b, \\[2mm] \dfrac{b}{\lambda_n}[K_0(\lambda_n r)I_1(\lambda_n b)], & r > b. \end{cases}$$

Diffuse Reflectance

Diffuse reflectance can be calculated by separating the scattered photon flux into two components, the forward and backward traveling partial currents. The total scattered photon current defined by the partial currents Γ_{z+} and Γ_{z-} is given by

$$\Gamma_{sz} = \Gamma_{z+} - \Gamma_{z-},$$

which is just the net current traveling in the positive z direction. These partial currents can be formulated by integrating the z component of Γ_{sz} over the region $0 \le \theta \le \pi$ to obtain Γ_{z+} and $\pi \le \theta \le 2\pi$ to obtain Γ_{z-}.

$$\Gamma_{z-} = \frac{1}{2}\left(\frac{1}{2}\rho_s + \frac{1}{3\Sigma_t}\frac{\partial\rho_s}{\partial z} - \frac{1}{\Sigma_t}\hat{z}\cdot\mathbf{Q}_1\right) \quad (12)$$

and

$$\Gamma_{z+} = \frac{1}{2}\left(\frac{1}{2}\rho_s - \frac{1}{3\Sigma_t}\frac{\partial\rho_s}{\partial z} + \frac{1}{\Sigma_t}\hat{z}\cdot\mathbf{Q}_1\right), \quad (13)$$

when subtracted from the total current,

$$\Gamma_{sz} = -\frac{1}{3\Sigma_t}\frac{\partial\rho_s}{\partial z} + \frac{1}{\Sigma_t}\hat{z}\cdot\mathbf{Q}_1, \quad (14)$$

which contains the diffusion term $-D\nabla_z\rho_s$, where $D = 1/(3\Sigma_t)$ and a term due to the anisotropy of the medium. For isotropic media Eq. (14) reduces to Fick's law with the appropriate definition of Σ_t as the total macroscopic cross section. It may also be noted that the boundary conditions, Eq. (3), may be formulated by requiring that the partial current Γ_{z+} be zero at the $z = 0$ interface, that Γ_{z-} be zero at the $z = $ **d** interface, and that the anisotropic surface contribution due to the finite size scatterer–source characteristics be neglected.

The diffuse reflectance as seen by a finite size receiving aperture of radius **a**, concentric with the incident beam of radius **b**, can be calculated by taking the ratio of the integral of the partial current Γ_{z-} over the receiving aperture to the incident flux at $z = 0$,

$$R_{\text{diff}} = \left.\frac{\int_0^{2\pi}\int_0^a \Gamma_{z-}rdrd\theta}{\int_0^{2\pi}\int_0^b q_0 rdrd\theta}\right|_{z=0} \quad (15)$$

Inserting the partial current Γ_{z-} from Eq. (12) into Eq. (15) and neglecting the anisotropic source contribution at $z = 0$, consistent with the assumptions on the boundary conditions of Eq. (3), the diffuse reflectance is

$$R_{\text{diff}} = \frac{8\Sigma_s}{b^2}\left(\frac{1}{D} + 3\bar{\mu}\Sigma\right)\sum_{n=1}^{\infty}\frac{\Gamma_n z_n}{(k_n^2 + \Sigma^2)}$$
$$\left(\frac{1}{2}\sin\gamma_n + Dk_n\cos\gamma_n\right)R_a, \quad (16)$$

where

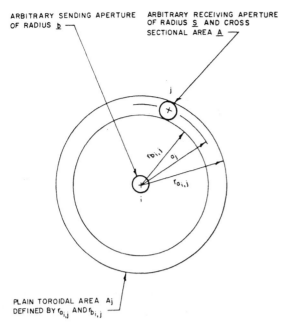

ARBITRARY SENDING APERTURE OF RADIUS b

ARBITRARY RECEIVING APERTURE OF RADIUS S AND CROSS SECTIONAL AREA A

PLAIN TOROIDAL AREA A_j DEFINED BY $r_{o_{i,j}}$ AND $r_{b_{i,j}}$

Fig. 1. Diagrammatic representation of the receiving aperture weighting function for reflectance calculations.

$$R_a = \begin{cases} \frac{1}{\lambda_n^2}\left[\frac{a^2}{2} - ab I_1(\lambda_n a) K_1(\lambda_n b)\right], & a \leq b, \\ \frac{1}{\lambda_n^2}\left[\frac{b^2}{2} - ab K_1(\lambda_n a) I_1(\lambda_n b)\right], & a \geq b. \end{cases}$$

Reflectance at an arbitrary location in the interface plane can be calculated by weighting the reflectance obtained from Eq. (16) by the ratio of the areas A/A_1, where A is the area of the receiving aperture, and A_1 is the plane toroidal area described by r_a, r_b (see Fig. 1).

$$R = [R_{\text{diff}}(r_a) - R_{\text{diff}}(r_b)]\frac{A}{A_1} . \tag{17}$$

It is assumed that there is no collimated beam reflectance at the interface boundaries, thus Eq. (16) and (17) give the diffuse reflectance for a finite receiving aperture. In practice, specular reflection occurs at the $z = 0$ interface and must be accounted for in interpreting experimental results.

Experimental Determination of σ_s and σ_a and Comparison with Mie Scattering

An independent measurement of σ_s, σ_a and $\bar{\mu}$ of the red blood cell was desired to compare diffuse reflectance calculated from Eqs. (16) and (17) with experiment. Since the angular scattering characteristics of the red blood cell $\sigma_d(\mu)$,

$$\sigma_d(\mu) = \frac{v}{H(1-H)}\Sigma_d(\mu)$$

could not be obtained from experimental setups available at our laboratory; the calculation of $\bar{\mu}$ must come from assumptions based on the forward and backward microscopic scattering cross sections σ_s^+ and σ_s^-.

$$\sigma_s = \sigma_s^+ + \sigma_s^-,$$

where

$$\sigma_s^+ = 2\pi \int_0^1 \sigma_d(\mu)d\mu$$

and

$$\sigma_s^- = 2\pi \int_{-1}^0 \sigma_d(\mu)d\mu$$

Experimental procedures for the generation of the cross-section data of Table I have been described previously[16] and duplicated in the 0.63–0.8-μm wavelength range.[17] The data are obtained by measuring optical density for a very low hematocrit ($0.05\% \leq H \leq 0.1\%$), single scattering blood medium. A simulated delta function receiver (cone of reception 1.3°) was used to measure total loss in the incident power due to absorption, forwardscattering, and backscattering; and the total forward directed power from a narrow incident beam was measured by a receiver with a cone of reception of 100° to determine losses due to backscattering and absorption. By performing optical density measurements as a function of cuvette thickness with each receiver at different oxygen saturation levels, wavelengths, and hematocrits the forwardscattering, backscattering, and absorption microscopic cross sections can be obtained. A modified Mie scattering program[18] for which the average value of the radius 2.79 μm, volume 91.3 μm³, and indices of refraction of an erythrocyte were used to simulate the scattering and absorption properties of the red blood cell. Values obtained with the Mie scattering program for the scattering and absorption cross sections approximate the experimentally determined cross-sectional values. Therefore, the calculated values of $\bar{\mu}$, σ_s, and σ_a from the Mie scattering program were used in the two fiber and catheter model comparisons to follow.

Calculations comparing the theoretical and experimental values of σ_s^+, σ_s^-, and σ_a in a transport derived reflectance equation,[19] where $\sigma_s^+ \gg \sigma_s^-$ have shown that the reflectance data used in these comparisons are not sufficiently sensitive to changes in

Table I. Comparison of Mie Scattering Calculation for a Sphere of 2.79-μm Radius and Experimentally Derived Cross Sections for the Red Blood Cell at 100% Oxygen Saturation[a]

		Mie scattering		
$\lambda(\mu)$	0.63	0.66	0.685	0.8
σ_s^+	60.98	57.73	55.09	44.28
σ_s^-	0.01	0.01	0.01	0.01
σ_a	0.10	0.066	0.059	0.131
		Experiment		
σ_s^+	56.13	53.96	53.3	42.03
σ_s^-	0.241	0.235	0.233	0.210
σ_a	0.099	0.066	0.063	0.131

[a] Cross sections in μ^2, STD of data: $\sigma_s^+ \leq 2\%$, σ_s^- and $\sigma_a \leq 5.3\%$.

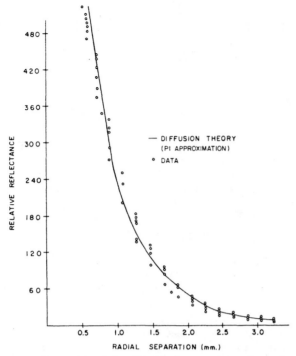

Fig. 2. Comparison of the diffusion theory and experimental results for reflectance from whole human blood vs radial separation distance between two optical fibers at a wavelength of 0.685 µm, 100% oxygen saturation, and a hematocrit of $H = 0.41$.

σ_s^- to warrant the use of the experimental values of the backscattering cross section.

Two Fiber Reflectance

A two fiber cuvette was constructed to measure relative reflectance from a homogeneous medium of discrete scatterers to generate a fundamental set of reflectance data to verify Eq. (17) as a basis for the fiber optic catheter model. The cuvette consists of two parallel optical fibers: a 0.508-mm diam emitter fiber that is normal to, in contact with, and fixed in relation to the scattering medium and a 0.127-mm diam receiving fiber that is also in contact with the scattering medium and continuously adjustable to ±5 mm in the radial direction about the center of the emitting fiber. Both emitting and receiving apertures remain in the same plane during measurements.

The input signal to the emitting fiber is from a Bausch & Lomb (B&L) tungsten light source model (33-86-39-01) connected to a monochromator (B&L, 33-86-25-03) with a visible grating (B&L, 33-86-25-02). The signal was chopped by a mechanical chopper operating at 540 Hz and then focused on the cuvette emitter fiber. The output signal from the receiving fiber is optically coupled to a photomultiplier tube (RCA 7265) and then fed to a lockin amplifier (PAR model 128) to produce an amplified voltage that is recorded.

For the data as shown in Figs. 2 and 3, both fibers are in contact with a controlled blood medium.

Blood is continuously pumped through the cuvette into a disk oxygenator in which N_2 and O_2 are introduced in amounts necessary to control oxygen saturation at a given level, and CO_2 is introduced to maintain the pH at 7.4 ± 0.01. HbO_2, HbCO, and hemoglobin are periodically monitored by an International Laboratories model 182 CO oximeter, and the PH is determined by a Beckman gas analyzer (model 160). Free plasma–hemoglobin solutions were obtained from samples of blood that were periodically removed from the cuvette system to colorimetrically measure hemolysis. Sedimentation was reduced by continuous pumping of the blood and monitored by frequent hematocrit test. Outdated whole human cells were used, and the change in hematocrit was accomplished by dilution of the cells with a sodium heparinized Ringer's solution.

Figure 2 is a plot of relative reflectance vs radial separation between emitting fiber and receiving fiber where the solid line is a computer generated theoretical reflectance curve using Eq. (17) and the data shown in Table II. The blood is at 100% oxygen saturation and a normal hemoglobin level of 14.7 and hematocrit of 0.41. The data are characterized by the exponential like decay of received intensity vs radial separation for a constant density medium as has been shown for the case of scattered photon density from a finite cylindrical beam normally incident upon an infinite half-space, blood medium.[3]

Figure 3 is a plot of relative reflectance from a whole blood medium vs change of hematocrit where the solid line is a computer generated theoretical reflectance curve using the data of Table II. The change of hematocrit is obtained by reducing outdated cells at an initial hematocrit of 0.6–0.2 by addition

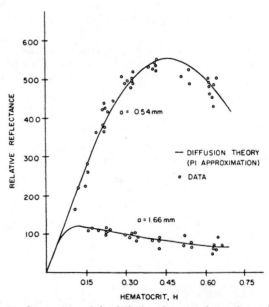

Fig. 3. Comparison of the diffusion theory and experimental results for reflectance from whole human blood vs hematocrit for two different fiber separation distances at a wavelength of 0.685 µm and 100% oxygen saturation.

Table II. Simulation of the Scattering and Absorption Characteristics of a Red Blood Cell by Mie Scattering (Relative Index of Refraction $\eta = \eta_r + j\eta_i$)

$\lambda(\mu)$	η_r	η_i ($\times 10^4$)	$\sigma_s{}^a$ (u^2)	σ_a (u^2)	$\bar{\mu}$	$\sigma_s(1-\bar{u})$ (u^2)	Σ_t (mm^{-1})
			100% Oxygen saturation				
0.665	1.036	0.240	57.20	0.060	0.9951	0.283	0.747
0.675	1.036	0.244	56.14	0.060	0.9950	0.281	0.744
0.685	1.036	0.248	55.09	0.059	0.9949	0.281	0.739
0.955	1.036	0.111	33.47	0.191	0.9925	0.251	0.666
0.960	1.036	0.109	33.18	0.187	0.9924	0.251	0.666
0.965	1.036	0.109	32.90	0.185	0.9924	0.251	0.665
			0% Oxygen saturation				
0.665	1.036	2.203	56.58	0.542	0.9951	0.279	0.738
0.675	1.036	2.207	55.53	0.535	0.9950	0.278	0.735
0.685	1.036	2.023	54.56	0.484	0.9949	0.278	0.731
0.955	1.036	0.052	33.54	0.090	0.9925	0.252	0.668
0.960	1.036	0.049	33.27	0.085	0.9924	0.252	0.667
0.965	1.036	0.047	32.98	0.080	0.9924	0.252	0.666

^{a} Differences in σ_s due to oxygen saturation variations had negligible effect on the computational results.

of normal heparinized Ringer's solution. The curves are for radial separation distances of 0.54 mm and 1.66 mm and 100% oxygen saturation. For small fiber separation distances the reflectance curve has a parabolic shape previously reported for the case of a solid core cylindrical 5 French catheter containing approximately 100–0.127-mm diam fibers.[12,20] It can be seen from Fig. 2 that the closely spaced sending–receiving fiber pairs account for a large percentage of the backscattering intensity, thus considering the catheter as a summation of closely grouped two fiber pairs, the two fiber experiment agrees qualitatively with published results. The parabolic shape of the 0.54-mm fiber separation reflectance curve is characterized by the second order functional dependence of the macroscopic scattering cross section on the density.[9] Higher order multiple scattering effects that have been experimentally investigated[19,21] dominate the 1.66-mm fiber separation distance reflectance curve, which shows an exponential like reflectance vs density relationship that is independent of the individual erythrocyte differential scattering cross section.

Since the measurements made with the two fiber cuvette are of relative reflectance, absolute reflectance values were not obtained. Therefore, the theoretical results were normalized to the experimental relative reflectance data at one point (the value of relative reflectance at 0.90 mm in Fig. 2) and the theoretical curves of Fig. 3 use this normalization factor and follow accordingly. The theoretical–experimental correlation for the ranges of radial separation distances and hematocrit values shown indicate that for a high albedo blood medium, Eq. (17) can be used as a basis for a fiber optic catheter model for oximetry.

Fiber Optic Oximeter Catheter

The fiber optic catheter illuminates blood by conveying light to the tip, or distal end, of the cathe-

ter by means of optical fibers. Light is backscattered by blood cells in the vicinity of the tip and transmitted by a second bundle of fibers to the proximal end for evaluation by an oximeter[12,13,22–24] to determine the oxygen saturation in blood. A catheter fiber configuration such as the ring catheter shown in Fig. 4 consists of a consecutively interspaced set of optical fibers, one quarter of which transmits light at 0.96 μm, another quarter that transmits light at 0.685 μm, and the remaining one-half that is used as receiving fibers. Measuring the ratio of the backscattered intensity at two wavelengths, one of which is most sensitive to oxygen saturation, 0.6–0.7 μm, and the other that is relatively insensitive to oxygen saturation, 0.8–0.9 μm, cancels out reflectance variations due to PH changes and blood velocity pulsations that affect the reflectance at both wavelengths in approximately an equal manner. An analytical model of the catheter can be constructed using the previous general description and reflectance Eqs. (16) and (17) for **a > b**.

By summing the light collected from each detector fiber at each wavelength over the receiving apertures the oxygen saturation can be calculated. Reflectance at an arbitrary receiving fiber can be calculated from Eq. (17), where the area A is that of a single optical fiber, and A_j is the plane toroidal area previously described. Thus the reflectance R_T for an arbitrary set of sending and receiving fibers, neglecting diffraction effects, is

$$R_T = \sum_{i=1}^{m} \sum_{j=1}^{n} [R_{\text{diff}}(r_{a_{i,j}}) - R_{\text{diff}}(r_{b_{i,j}})]\frac{A}{A_j}, \quad (18)$$

where m is the total number of sending fibers, and n is the total number of receiving fibers.

Various fiber optic geometries other than the ring

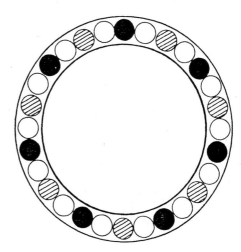

CATHETER Z-13

● SENDING FIBER AT 0.685μ

◐ SENDING FIBER AT 0.960μ

○ RECEIVING FIBER

Fig. 4. Schematic representation of a twenty-eight fiber ring catheter configuration (Z-13).

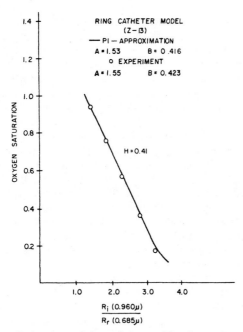

Fig. 5. Comparison of the catheter model and experimental results for oxygen saturation vs reflectance ratio from whole human blood (catheter Z-13).

can be tried using Eq. (18) optimizing the configuration, the number, and the diameter of internal fibers[5,25] for sensitivity and linearity for oximetry.

Comparative Results from the Catheter Model and Related Experimental Data

The motivation for constructing a fiber optic catheter model is to develop a theoretical criterion for the design of the fiber configuration in the distal tip of a catheter to ultimately be used for the measurement of oxygen saturation in blood. Oxygen saturation OS is defined by the ratio of oxyhemoglobin to total hemoglobin. An empirically established relation for oxygen saturation in terms of the ir reflectance R_i and the red reflectance R_r is given by

$$OS = A - B(R_i/R_r),$$

where R_i and R_r are the backscattered intensities at 0.96 μm and 0.685 μm, respectively; and the constants A and B (functions of the geometry of the fiber bundle and blood parameters) can be empirically determined. Thus for different fiber configurations the constants A and B will differ, and a calibration curve for each configuration is necessary for an accurate clinical verification of the *in vivo* operation of the fiber optic oximeter. This calibration curve was in part the object of study of various researchers,[12,22,23] and their experimental procedures have been duplicated as a basis of comparison and as a standard of determining the validity of the fiber optic catheter model. The A constant has been determined empirically and sustantiated theoretically to be relatively independent of the details of the individual fiber optic emitter–receiver positions for a

given over-all catheter tip shape, while the B constant is proportional to the ratio of the emitted intensities.

Figures 5, 6, and 7 show plots of calibration curves for various fiber geometries (data points) and the theoretically derived catheter model curves (solid lines) where the data of Table II were used in the computer simulation of the catheter model. Catheter (Z-13) is a twenty-eight fiber ring catheter of the configuration in Fig. 4, having a minimum average separation between fiber centers of 0.156 mm, an over-all average maximum separation of 1.25 mm, seven sending fibers in the red (0.685 μm), seven sending fibers in the ir (0.96 μm), and fourteen receiving fibers. Catheter (Z-2) is a thirty-five fiber ring catheter of the configuration in Fig. 8, having a minimum average separation between fiber centers of 0.145 mm, an over-all average maximum separation of 1.7 mm, four sending fibers in the red (0.665 μm), fifteen sending fibers in the ir (0.955 μm), and sixteen receiving fibers. Catheter (V-10) is an eighteen-fiber 2-lm configuration (Fig. 9), having a minimum average separation between fiber centers of 0.132 mm, an over-all maximum separation of 0.87 mm, four sending fibers in the red (0.675 μm), five sending fibers in the ir (0.965 μm), and nine receiving fibers. All catheters have an average fiber diameter of 0.127 mm.

Since it is assumed in the catheter model that equal intensities are emitted into the blood medium at each wavelength, the relative backscattered intensity from milk and the attenuation losses in the fibers are measured at both wavelengths and then normalized to unity. Spectral characteristics of the emitter

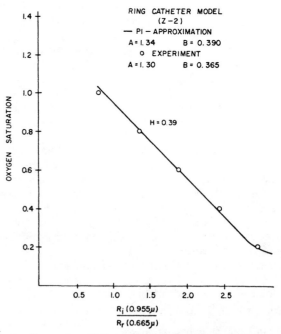

Fig. 6. Comparison of the catheter model and experimental results for oxygen saturation vs reflectance ratio from whole human blood (catheter Z-2).

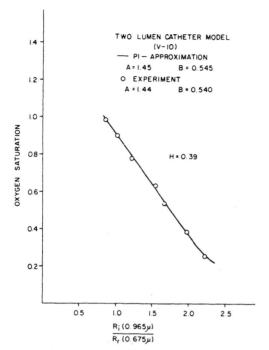

Fig. 7. Comparison of the catheter model and experimental results for oxygen saturation vs reflectance ratio from whole human blood (catheter V-10).

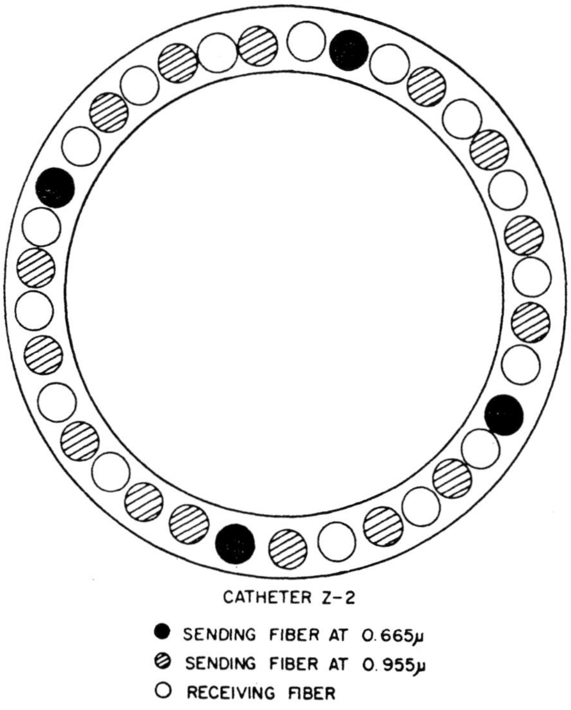

for the experimental procedure used to be of only a negligible effect and thus omitted.

All experimental and theoretical curves show the linear oxygen saturation, reflectance ratio correlation previously reported, and discrepancies between the model and experiment can be explained due to minor inaccuracies in the theoretical data, specular reflectance at the fiber–blood interface, and nonideal single wavelength light sources (LED's having a finite bandwidth rather than a single frequency output).

Conclusion

Despite the obvious limitation of calibrating the catheter input intensities to match the intensities used theoretically, the close correlation between experiments and catheter model plus the excellent agreement shown in Figs. 2 and 3 establish the validity of the theoretical approach, the approximations used, and the potential usefulness in optical instrumentation design. These equations represent a distinct advantage over previously derived one-dimensional models where fine interface detail may be needed. More extensive modeling for various fiber geometries and more fundamental two-fiber type experiments are being performed by the authors over a wide range of physiological parameters to define rigidly the limits of validity of the derivations.

A special thanks is extended to Jonathan Molcho of the University of Washington for many helpful comments and to Peter Cheung of Case Western University for his measurements of reflectance from blood from the fiber optic catheters V-10 and Z-2.

CATHETER Z-2

● SENDING FIBER AT 0.665μ

⊘ SENDING FIBER AT 0.955μ

○ RECEIVING FIBER

Fig. 8. Schematic representation of a thirty-five fiber ring catheter configuration (Z-2).

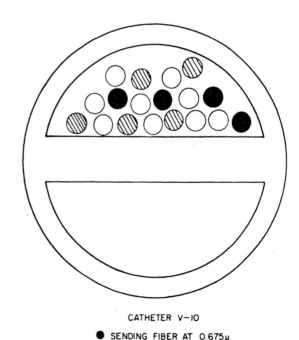

CATHETER V−10

● SENDING FIBER AT 0.675μ

⊘ SENDING FIBER AT 0.965μ

○ RECEIVING FIBER

Fig. 9. Schematic representation of an eighteen-fiber 2-lm catheter configuration (V-10).

and receiver are not compensated for in the experimental results shown, but by comparison with data in which the spectral characteristics of the emitter, receiver, and fibers are considered, it has been found

References

1. R. Longini and R. Zdrojkowski, IEEE Trans. Biomed. Eng. **BME-15**, 4 (January 1968).
2. R. Zdrojkowski and N. Pisharoty, IEEE Trans. Biomed. Eng. **BME-17**, 122 (April 1970).
3. C. Johnson, IEEE Trans. Biomed. Eng. **BME-17**, 129 (April 1970).
4. F. Janssen, Med. Biol. Eng. **10**, 231 (1972).
5. L. Reynolds, "Three Dimensional Reflection and Transmission Equations for Optical Diffusion in Blood," M.S. Thesis, Electrical Engineering Department, University of Washington (1970).
6. L. Reynolds, "Optical Diffuse Reflectance and Transmittance from an Anisotropically Finite Blood Medium," Ph.D. Thesis, Electrical Engineering Department, University of Washington (1975).
7. A. Shuster, Astrophysics **21**, 1 (January 1905).
8. P. Kubelka, J. Opt. Soc. of Am. **38**, 448 (May 1948).
9. V. Twersky, Opt. Soc. Am. **60**, 1084 (1970).
10. M. Moaveni, "A Multiple Scattering Field Theory Applied to Whole Blood," Ph.D. Thesis, Electrical Engineering Department, University of Washington (1970).
11. A. Cohen and R. Longini, Med. Biol. Eng. **9**, 61 (January 1971).
12. C. Johnson, R. Palm, and D. Stewart, Assoc. Adv. Med. Instrum. **5**, No. 2 (March–April 1971).
13. M. Polanyi and R. Hehir, Rev. Sci. Instrum. **33**, 1050 (1962).
14. K. Case and P. Zweifel, *Linear Transport Theory* (Addison-Wesley, Reading, Mass., 1967), Chap. 8.
15. V. Twersky, J. Math. Phys. **3**, No. 4, 724 (1962).
16. R. Pierce, "An Experimental Determination of the Average Scattering and Absorption Cross Sections of Human Red Blood Cells for Near Infrared Light," M.S. Thesis, Electrical Engineering Department, University of Washington (1972).
17. L. Reynolds, J. Molcho, C. Johnson, and A. Ishimaru, "Optical Cross Sections of Human Erythrocytes," *Proc. of the 27th Annual Conf. on Eng. in Med. and Biol. (1974)*, Vol. 16.
18. J. Dave, "Stokes Parameters of the Radiation Scattered by a Homogeneous Sphere," IBM Prog. 360D-17.4.002, IBM Scientific Center, Palo Alto, Calif. (1968).
19. G. Petersen, N. McCormick, and L. Reynolds, "Transport Calculations for Light Scattering in Blood," Biophys. J. (in press).
20. N. Anderson and P. Sekelj, Phys. Med. Biol. **12**, 185 (1967).
21. F. Janssen, Med. Biol. Eng. **10**, 9 (1972).
22. J. Cole, W. Martin, P. Cheung, and C. Johnson, Am. J. Cardiol. **29**, 383 (1972).
23. E. Woodroof and S. Koorajian, J. Assoc. Adv. Med. Instrum. **7**, No. 5, 287 (December 1973).
24. W. Blom and V. H. deVilleneuve, Med. Biol. Eng. 537 (July 1974).
25. L. Reynolds and C. Johnson, "Three-Dimensional Optical Diffusion Theory for Spectrophotometric Instrumentation Design," *Proc. of the 24th Annual Conf. on Eng. in Med. and Biol. (1971)*, Vol. 13.

Reprinted with permission from *Journal of the Optical Society of America A,* Vol. 5(6), pp. 813-822 (June 1988). ©1988 Optical Society of America.

Diffusion model of the optical absorbance of whole blood

J. M. Steinke and A. P. Shepherd

Department of Physiology, University of Texas Health Science Center, San Antonio, Texas 78284

Received August 20, 1987; accepted January 26, 1988

Photon-diffusion theory has had limited success in modeling the optical transmittance of whole blood. Therefore we have developed a new photon-diffusion model of the optical absorbance of blood. The model has benefited from experiments designed to test its fundamental assumptions, and it has been compared extensively with transmittance data from whole blood. The model is consistent with both experimental and theoretical notions. Furthermore, when all parameters associated with a given optical geometry are known, the model needs no variational parameters to predict the absolute transmittance of whole blood. However, even if the exact value of the incident light intensity is unknown (which is the case in many situations), only a single additive constant is required to scale experiment to theory. Finally, the model is shown to be useful for simulating scattering effects and for delineating the relative contributions of the diffuse transmittance and the collimated transmittance to the total optical density of whole blood. Applications of the model include oximetry and measurements of the arteriovenous oxygen difference in whole, undiluted blood.

1. INTRODUCTION

Many different theories have been proposed to account for the complex optical properties of turbid media[1–3] such as whole blood.[4–10] Models that attempt to predict the amount of incident light that blood reflects or transmits have primarily employed two different approaches: wave-scattering theory and photon-diffusion theory. Although the equations from Twersky's wave-scattering theory[4,5] agree reasonably well with measured optical density (O.D.) data,[11–13] researchers have had to resort to curve-fitting techniques to evaluate the parameters in Twersky's equations. Furthermore, unlike the photon-diffusion approach of Reynolds[6] and Reynolds *et al.*[14] and Schmitt and co-workers,[7,15] Twersky's theory does not describe the spatial distribution of the reflected and transmitted light. Finally, Twersky's model does not lend itself to simulating the optical effects of fundamental hematological variables such as mean corpuscular hemoglobin concentration and red blood cell (RBC) volume, nor does it accommodate light detectors and sources that do not share a common optical axis.

By contrast, photon-diffusion theory not only agrees well with experimental data[14,16] but also needs no variational parameters. In addition, it predicts the radial-intensity distribution from the axis of the light source. The radial intensity is useful for simulating practical light sources such as light-emitting diodes (LED's), which emit a diverging beam.[17] Furthermore, photon-diffusion theory is useful for modeling the performance of fiber-optic catheters in which the light-emitting and light-detecting fibers lie side by side.[14] Unfortunately, the success of diffusion theory has been restricted primarily to reflectance data. When its predictions have been compared with transmittance data, they have been applied either to O.D.-versus-sample thickness data[9,18] or to qualitative determinations of O.D. versus hematocrit.[8,18] Consequently, the literature lacks detailed comparisons of photon-diffusion theory with the optical absorbance of blood as a function of hematocrit. Furthermore, we believe that previous treatments[8] have overlooked some important ideas in explaining the failure of photon-diffusion theory to account for the optical transmittance of whole blood.

Therefore we have tested the assumptions of photon-diffusion theory by making careful measurements of fundamental optical properties of blood, and we have developed a new photon-diffusion model of optical absorbance by whole blood. Finally, by making detailed comparisons of our model with experimental data, we have identified the limits of our model's validity.

2. THEORY AND NEW MODEL

The diffusion equation, which is a special case of the general transport equation, has been used successfully by Reynolds and co-workers[6,14] to describe light propagation in whole blood. Schmitt and co-workers[7,15] have solved the transport approximation of the diffusion equation under special boundary conditions for an optical geometry with a collimated light source. In this section we specify certain boundary conditions and otherwise follow the work of Schmitt[7] to derive a transmittance equation to describe the optical absorbance of blood.

To begin we need to define certain cross sections for the RBC (the primary scatterer in whole blood): σ_s and σ_a are the scattering and absorption cross sections of an arbitrary scatterer, defined as the total scattered or absorbed power, respectively, divided by the incident power flux density. Similarly, σ_{ao} and σ_{ar} are the absorption cross sections for RBC's when they contain completely oxygenated or deoxygenated hemoglobin, respectively. The macroscopic scattering and absorption coefficients, Σ_s and Σ_a, respectively, describe the actual optical properties of whole blood. They are defined to represent the scattering and absorption (fractional changes in light flux per unit length) in a volume of whole blood. The relations among the coefficients and cross sections have been assumed[7] to be approximately as follows:

$$\Sigma_a = H[\sigma_{ao}SO_2 + \sigma_{ar}(1 - SO_2)]/V,$$

$$\Sigma_s = H\sigma_s(1 - H)/V \qquad \text{(incorrect, explained below)},$$

$$\Sigma_{st} = \Sigma_s(1 - \bar{\mu}),$$

$$\Sigma_t = \Sigma_a + \Sigma_{st}, \qquad (1)$$

where H is the hematocrit ($0 \leq H \leq 1$), V is the volume of a single RBC ($\sim$90 μm^3), SO_2 is the fractional oxyhemoglobin saturation, and $\bar{\mu}$ is the average value of the cosine of the scattering angles for an isolated scatterer. Σ_{st} is the modified macroscopic scattering coefficient, and Σ_t is the sum of the macroscopic absorption and modified scattering coefficients.

The diffusion equation for the average diffuse intensity Ψ of light in the blood medium takes the form

$$-D\nabla^2\Psi(\bar{\rho}) + \Sigma_a\Psi(\bar{\rho}) = S(\bar{\rho}), \qquad (2)$$

where D is the modified diffusion constant, $D = 1/(3\Sigma_t)$, and S is the source or driving function describing, at any point $\bar{\rho}$, the photon distribution established in the medium by the incident light.

Figure 1 shows the model geometry assumed in the derivation of our transmittance equation. The source is assumed to be a collimated, monochromatic beam of light normally incident upon a slab of blood of thickness z_0. The blood medium is assumed to extend to $\pm\infty$ in the x and y directions. The detector is assumed to have radius b and to be located at or beyond $z = z_0$ along the same axis as the source aperture (of radius a).

The boundary conditions that we use are those derived by Reynolds[6] for the $z = z_0$ and $z = 0$ planes:

$$\Psi(\bar{\rho}) + 3KD\partial\Psi(\bar{\rho})/\partial z = 0 \qquad \text{at } z = z_0, \qquad (3)$$

$$\Psi(\bar{\rho}) - 3KD\partial\Psi(\bar{\rho})/\partial z = 0 \qquad \text{at } z = 0, \qquad (4)$$

where K is the extrapolation distance of the asymptotic flux; $K = 0.7104$ from the solution of the Milne problem.[19] According to Reynolds,[6] these boundary conditions result from neglecting the anisotropic source contribution on the interface boundaries while permitting the medium anisotropy to remain.

The diffusion equation (2) is solved by means of Green's function techniques. According to this method of solution, we obtain

$$\Psi(\bar{\rho}) = (1/D) \int_{v'} S(\bar{\rho}')G(\bar{\rho}; \bar{\rho}')dv', \qquad (5)$$

where S is the source function already mentioned and G is the Green's function, which is the solution of Eq. (2) with $S = -D\delta(\bar{\rho} - \bar{\rho}')$, i.e.,

$$\nabla^2 G(\bar{\rho}; \bar{\rho}') - (\Sigma_a/D)G(\bar{\rho}; \bar{\rho}') = \delta(\bar{\rho} - \bar{\rho}'). \qquad (6)$$

The same boundary conditions [Eqs. (3) and (4)] apply to Eq. (6), and $\delta(\bar{\rho} - \bar{\rho}')$ is the three-dimensional Dirac delta function representing a point source in the volume. The θ-independent Green's function solution for Eq. (5), according to Schmitt and co-workers,[7,15] is

$$G(r, z; r', z') = \sum_{n=1}^{\infty} (1/2\pi N_n)\sin(k_n z + \gamma_n)\sin(k_n z' + \gamma_n)$$

$$\times \begin{cases} I_0(\lambda_n r')K_0(\lambda_n r), & r' < r, \\ I_0(\lambda_n r)K_0(\lambda_n r'), & r' > r, \end{cases} \qquad (7)$$

where r', z' and r, z are the coordinates of the source point and observation point, respectively. The parameters in this equation are as follows:

k_n are the eigenvalues defined implicitly by

$$\tan(k_n z_0) = 2gk_n/[(gk_n)^2 - 1],$$

$$g = 0.7104/\Sigma_t,$$

N_n is the eigenvalue normalization constant

$$(=\{2k_n z_0 + \sin(2\gamma_n) - \sin[2(k_n z_0 + \gamma_n)]\}/k_n),$$

$$\lambda_n^2 = k_n^2 + \Sigma_a/D,$$

γ_n is the phase function [$=\tan^{-1}(gk_n)$],

and I_0 and K_0 are zeroth-order modified Bessel functions of the first and second kind, respectively.[20]

The equation defining the eigenvalues k_n follows from the boundary conditions (3) and (4) and from the form of the

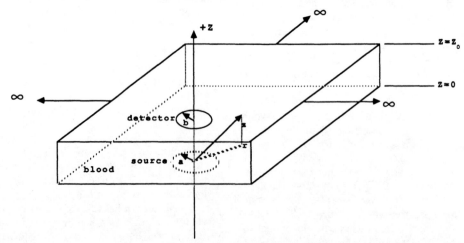

Fig. 1. Optical geometry of the photon-diffusion model [see Eq. (21)]. Assumptions are a collimated source of radius a normally incident upon a blood medium of thickness z_0. Detector aperture is circular, of radius b, and coaxial with the source aperture.

Green's function in Eqs. (7). The source function is the last element necessary to evaluate Eq. (5). The interested reader is again referred to Schmitt's derivation[7] for the source function, which for a collimated source is

$$S(\bar{\rho}) = \Psi_0 \Sigma_{st} \exp(-\Sigma_t z) R(r), \qquad (8)$$

where $R(r)$ describes the radial-intensity distribution of the source and Ψ_0 is the incident light flux. The source is assumed to have a circular aperture of radius a over which the flux is uniform (Fig. 1). Thus, in terms of the unit step function U, $R(r) = U(r) - U(r - a)$. Finally, we may simply substitute Eqs. (7) and (8) into Eq. (5) to obtain the average diffuse intensity $\Psi(\bar{\rho})$:

$$\Psi(r, z) = \sum_{n=1}^{\infty} (\Psi_0 \Sigma_{st}/DN_n) \int_0^{z_0} \exp(-\Sigma_t z')\sin(k_n z + \gamma_n)$$

$$\times \sin(k_n z' + \gamma_n)\mathrm{d}z'$$

$$\times \int_0^a R(r') \begin{cases} I_0(\lambda_n r')K_0(\lambda_n r)r'\mathrm{d}r', & r' < r \\ I_0(\lambda_n r)K_0(\lambda_n r')r'\mathrm{d}r', & r' > r \end{cases}. \quad (9)$$

The integrations are greatly facilitated by the fact that the radial and z' dependencies of the integral are separable, as seen in Eqs. (9). The z' integration is straightforward, but for the radial integral we need the following relations for modified Bessel functions:

$$\int s I_0(s)\mathrm{d}s = s I_1(s) + C_1,$$

$$\int s K_0(s)\mathrm{d}s = -s K_1(s) + C_2,$$

$$I_0(s)K_1(s) + K_0(s)I_1(s) = 1/s. \qquad (10)$$

Here I_1 and K_1 are first-order modified Bessel functions of the first and second kind, respectively.[20,21] Thus, for $a < r$, we simply obtain $(a/\lambda_n)I_1(\lambda_n a)K_0(\lambda_n r)$ for the radial integral. For $a > r$, however, we get two terms:

$$(r/\lambda_n)I_1(\lambda_n r)K_0(\lambda_n r) + \{-(1/\lambda_n)[aK_1(\lambda_n a) - rK_1(\lambda_n r)]I_0(\lambda_n r)\};$$

then, using the third of the relations in Eqs. (10), we obtain $(1/\lambda_n^2) - (a/\lambda_n)K_1(\lambda_n a)I_0(\lambda_n r)$. Performing the z' integral and putting everything together, we obtain

$$\Psi(r, z) = \sum_{n=1}^{\infty} (\Psi_0 \Sigma_{st}/[DN_n \lambda_n (k_n^2 + \Sigma_t^2)])z_n$$

$$\times \sin(k_n z + \gamma_n) \begin{cases} a I_1(\lambda_n a)K_0(\lambda_n r), & a < r \\ (1/\lambda_n) - a I_0(\lambda_n r)K_1(\lambda_n a), & a > r \end{cases}, \quad$$

$$(11)$$

where

$$z_n = k_n \cos(\gamma_n) + \Sigma_t \sin(\gamma_n) - [k_n \cos(k_n z_0 + \gamma_n)$$

$$+ \Sigma_t \sin(k_n z_0 + \gamma_n)]\exp(-\Sigma_t z_0). \qquad (12)$$

The diffusely scattered light flux received in the detector aperture of Fig. 1 can be computed by integrating the partial light current directed in the $+z$ direction over the circular area of the detector aperture. Because at $z = z_0$ the current arising from anisotropic scattering at the interface can be neglected, the positive z-directed partial current can be obtained as

$$|J(r)|_{+z} = -D\partial\Psi/\partial z|_{z=z_0}. \qquad (13)$$

For a circular aperture of radius b, concentric with the source aperture but displaced along z, the transmitted intensity $I(b)$ may be integrated as

$$I(b) = \int_0^b |J(r)|_{+z}\, r\mathrm{d}r. \qquad (14)$$

Substituting Eq. (13) into Eq. (14) and integrating, again using the relations (10), we obtain

$$I(b) = \sum_{n=1}^{\infty} \{-\Psi_0 \Sigma_{st}/[N_n \lambda_n^2 (k_n^2 + \Sigma_t^2)]\}z_n k_n \cos(k_n z_0 + \gamma_n)$$

$$\times \begin{cases} (a^2/2) - baI_1(\lambda_n a)K_1(\lambda_n b), & a < b \\ (b^2/2) - baI_1(\lambda_n b)K_1(\lambda_n a), & a > b \end{cases}. \quad (15)$$

Finally, the diffuse transmittance T_{diff} can be obtained by normalizing $I(b)$ with respect to the incident flux:

$$T_{\text{diff}} = I(b)\left[\int_0^a \Psi_0 r\mathrm{d}r\right]^{-1} = 2I(b)/[\Psi_0 a^2]. \qquad (16)$$

This completes the derivation of the diffuse transmittance T_{diff}. Now we need to determine the collimated transmittance T_c. To remain consistent with the assumptions of the transport approximation, Reynolds et al.[14] express T_c as

$$T_c = \exp(-\Sigma_t d) \qquad \text{(incorrect)} \qquad (17)$$

since Σ_t is assumed to describe the on-axis attenuation of the incident collimated beam. This expression results because of the assumption in the transport approximation that anisotropic scattering is approximated by a small isotropic component (a fraction $1 - \bar{\mu}$) plus a purely forward-scattered component (a fraction $\bar{\mu}$). This expression for T_c turns out to be invalid and will be replaced by a more accurate expression (see Section 4). For now, however, we obtain

$$T_{\text{tot}} = T_{\text{diff}} + T_c = T_{\text{diff}} + \exp(-\Sigma_t d) \qquad \text{(incorrect).} \quad (18)$$

This equation, with the modification of T_c described in Section 4, will be compared with experimental data.

3. MATERIALS AND METHODS

A. Analysis of Blood

To obtain blood for study, we exsanguinated pentobarbital-anesthetized dogs to which 10,000 units of heparin had previously been administered. We then placed the blood in 250-ml buckets and centrifuged it for 20 min at 3000 rpm (1700 g). The packed RBC's were then resuspended in either isotonic saline or Krebs buffer and recentrifuged. After the final centrifugation, the measured hematocrit of the washed, packed RBC's was usually between 80 and 95%.

Aliquots (75–125 ml) of these RBC suspensions were then diluted, placed in revolving drum tonometers, and gassed with 5% CO_2–95% N_2 or 5% CO_2–balance air. In experiments in which transmittance was measured for oxygenated RBC suspensions, the drum tonometer was often not necessary to oxygenate the suspensions completely. Aliquots of low-hematocrit suspensions of RBC's in saline contained few RBC aggregations, but high-hematocrit samples were too concentrated to examine microscopically.

For both optical geometries of our experiments (see Subsection 3.B), we measured transmittance as a function of both hematocrit and oxyhemoglobin saturation (SO_2). To measure transmittance at widely varying oxyhemoglobin saturations, we first completely deoxygenated the RBC suspensions in the drum tonometer and then slowly introduced room air into the sample to oxygenate the suspensions in steps until the cells reached 100% oxygen saturation. The oxygen content of the RBC suspensions was measured on a Lex-O_2-Con (Hospex, Box 353, Boston, Massachusetts 02167), and percentage saturation was computed for each sample by comparing its oxygen content with that of fully oxygenated blood. In other experiments hematocrit was changed by diluting the RBC suspension with saline or Krebs buffer gassed at the same partial pressure of oxygen. Hematocrits were determined by capillary-tube centrifugation (3.5 min) without correction for trapped plasma.

B. Optical Apparatus

To examine the applicability of our new photon-diffusion model to optical absorbance, we reanalyzed data from an earlier study,[13] and we obtained new data by using the optical geometry of a commercial oximeter (Waters Instruments, OSC-80). The first apparatus (illustrated in our earlier study[13]) consisted of a rectangular flow-through cuvette with a blood sample depth of 1.6 mm (Avox Systems, Inc., 15315 Grey Fox, San Antonio, Texas 78255). The geometry of the Waters oximeter was similar to the first apparatus, having a flush-through cuvette (sample depth, 1.27 mm). LED and detector configurations were also similar to our previous geometry.[13] A common feature of both optical geometries was the use of a red (660-nm) and an infrared (800- or 813-nm) LED as light sources. The detector was a United Detector Technology PIN-3DP (with rectangular active area of 3 mm²). The light sources that we used were a red General Instruments MV 5054-3 (660 nm), a Waters Instruments LED (800 nm), and a Motorola MFOE 1200 (813 nm), LED's for which spectral properties were previously reported.[22]

C. Analysis of Data

To produce theoretical curves from Eq. (21), we wrote BASIC programs on a MacIntosh computer and used algorithms from Schmitt[7] to solve for the eigenvalues k_n in Eqs. (7). The parameter values that we used are given in Table 1, and the approximations for the modified Bessel functions[20,21] and the numerical methods that we used were described previously.[17]

To compare our data with the relationships predicted by Eq. (21), we used appropriate values for the particular optical geometry and computed the predicted transmittance for each hematocrit or oxyhemoglobin saturation for which we measured the transmittance of the RBC suspensions.

Table 1. Parameters for Model of Optical Absorbance by Whole Blood As Measured by the Authors

λ (nm)	ϵ_0 (10^6 cm²/ equivalent)	ϵ_r (10^6 cm²/ equivalent)	σ_{ao} (μm²)	σ_{ar} (μm²)	σ_s (μm²)	$\bar{\mu}$
632.8	0.347	1.07[a]	0.155	0.473[a]	63.77[a]	0.9845
660	0.147	0.717	0.0656	0.318	60.65[a]	0.984
800	0.266	0.328	0.1186	0.1462	45.59[a]	0.980
813	0.245	0.315	0.1092	0.1404	45.59[a]	0.980

[a] Value is from Ref. 4.

D. Experiments

Experiment 1

To determine the dependence of the collimated transmittance on hematocrit, we passed a 10-mW He–Ne laser beam (Hughes Aircraft Company, Model 3235H-PC, beam diameter, 1.37 mm at $1/e^2$) through an ultrathin cuvette (37 μm) of fully oxygenated blood. By measuring only the fraction of the incident beam that was neither scattered nor absorbed in samples with various hematocrits, we were able to measure collimated transmittance directly. This measurement was possible because the detector was placed 2 m from the sample, at which point none of the diffuse background would be received by the detector yet the remaining collimated beam could be clearly distinguished by eye from the diffuse background. To avoid RBC sedimentation problems, measurements were made within 2 min of placing the sample in the cuvette. Aliquots of the same samples were centrifuged to measure hematocrit.

Experiment 2

To measure the optical absorbance of blood as accurately as possible, it was necessary to measure the incident intensity exactly. We were unable to fulfill this requirement with LED's because of the marked divergence of their emissions, so we used a narrow He–Ne laser beam that could be captured completely by our detector. Thus we measured the total O.D. exactly as we varied the hematocrit of the sample. Cuvettes with path lengths of 1.27 and 1.6 mm were used.

Experiment 3

To demonstrate the applicability of our new model at wavelengths of interest in oximetry and arteriovenous oxygen difference measurements, we performed experiments in which we measured the O.D. as a function of hematocrit and oxyhemoglobin saturation in the optical geometries and at the LED wavelengths commonly used for such applications. These optical geometries and LED wavelengths were described in Subsection 3.B and in previous reports.[13]

Experiment 4

To study the ability of RBC's to scatter light at various angles, we constructed a simple goniometer in which an American Optical refractometer cuvette was mounted. Dilute RBC suspensions ($H < 1\%$) were placed in the cuvette and illuminated with the previously described He–Ne laser. The detector mentioned earlier was rotated to various angles with respect to the laser beam, and the intensity of the scattered light was measured.

4. INITIAL COMPARISONS OF EXPERIMENT AND THEORY: NEW EXPRESSIONS FOR T_c AND Σ_s

Comparisons of O.D.-versus-hematocrit data with the transmittance equation from the transport approximation, Eq. (18), revealed to us the same two problems that we noticed in the theoretical O.D. curves of Zdrojkowski and Pisharoty.[8] These problems were (1) that their theoretical O.D. was much smaller than experimental values (as Zdrojkowski and Pisharoty also noted) and (2) that the theoretical curves were essentially parabolic in shape. An explanation for the parabolic shape of their theoretical curves may be seen in the following: In Eq. (18) if T_c is large compared with T_{diff}, then Eq. (18) becomes

$$T_{\text{tot}} \cong \exp(-\Sigma_t d).$$

Because the O.D. is simply $-\log_{10}(T_{\text{tot}})$, it follows that

$$\text{O.D.} \cong 0.4343\,\Sigma_t d.$$

Finally, from the equation of Eqs. (1) for $\Sigma_t(1)$ in Section 2, O.D. is seen to become an essentially parabolic function of hematocrit (H). On evaluating T_c and T_{diff} of Eq. (18) in our initial comparisons, we have found that T_c was indeed large compared with T_{diff}. Thus this explanation applies. Similarly, we are convinced that Zdrojkowski and Pisharoty were experiencing the same problem in their comparison of data with theory. In effect, T_c was obscuring the T_{diff} term. This explanation also applies to the first problem, i.e., why their theoretical O.D. predictions were much smaller than their experimental values. Because T_c overestimates experimental values, the theoretical O.D. is much lower than the observed value.

To understand what is causing this sharp disagreement between theory and data, we must review the assumptions used in the transport approximation from which Eq. (18) was derived. First, recall that $\bar{\mu}$ is defined as the mean cosine of the scattering angle of the RBC. Second, Eq. (18) assumes that anisotropic scattering by RBC's can be approximated by a small isotropic component (a fraction $1 - \bar{\mu}$) plus a purely forward-scattered component (a fraction $\bar{\mu}$). Although this assumption seems to be a useful approximation for calculating the diffuse light intensity in the blood, the assumption is not justified for computing the collimated component of transmittance. In our view the correct expression for the collimated component, T_c, should simply be an exponential attenuation due to both absorption and total scattering:

$$T_c = \exp(-\Sigma d) \qquad \text{(correct)}, \qquad (19)$$

where $\Sigma = \Sigma_a + \Sigma_s$ and d = sample depth.

To verify this expression for T_c, we performed Experiment 1, in which a He–Ne laser beam (radius, 0.7 mm) was passed through an ultrathin cuvette (37 μm) of fully oxygenated blood. The results are shown in Fig. 2. By varying hematocrit and measuring only the fraction of the incident beam that was neither scattered nor absorbed 2 m away from the sample, we found that Eq. (19) predicted the collimated transmittance fairly well. Although the magnitude of $\log$-(T_c) is roughly as large as Eq. (19) predicts, the dependence

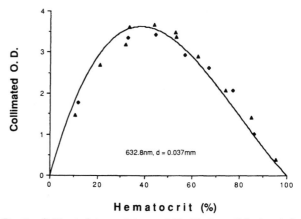

Fig. 2. Collimated transmittance of He–Ne laser light in whole blood. O.D. data are from experiments with RBC suspensions from two different dogs. Solid curve is a graph of O.D. = $15.1H(1 - H)(1.4 - H)$. Functional dependence on H in this figure determines the dependence of Σ_s on H [Eq. (20)].

of $\log(T_c)$ or $(\Sigma_s + \Sigma_a)d$ on H is not so simple as the expression $\sigma_s H(1 - H) + \sigma_a H$. Because σ_s is much larger than σ_a at the wavelengths that we are considering (see values in Table 1), we may set $\log_{10}(T_c) = -0.4343\Sigma_s d$ with little error. In fact, Pisharoty[23] attempted to determine the dependence of Σ_s on H experimentally (although by a different method from the one described here). Pisharoty also found that Σ_s was not simply proportional to $H(1 - H)$, and he fitted his scattering function to a cubic expression in order to describe the relationship better. Pisharoty's scattering function (ignoring his scale factor) is given by

$$H^3 - 2.388H^2 + 1.385H - 0.00390$$
$$= (H - 0.00283)(0.983 - H)(1.402 - H)$$

and is approximately wavelength independent in the range 660–800 nm. Subsequently, Hirko $et\ al.$[24] used a simplified form of Pisharoty's scattering function, which passes through 0 at $H = 0$ and $H = 1$. The results of the collimated transmittance measurements (Experiment 1) are compared in Fig. 2 with a cubic equation that passes through 0 at $H = 0$ and $H = 1$. The expression in Fig. 2 is a scale factor times the polynomial,

$$H(1 - H)(1.4 - H).$$

This expression fits our data and is nearly identical to the factorization of Pisharoty's expression. The maximum of the expression $H(1 - H)(1.4 - H)$ is 0.240, whereas the maximum of $H(1 - H)$ is 0.250. Because 0.240 and 0.250 are quite close to each other, $H(1 - H)(1.4 - H)$ does not need any additional normalization for use in the expression for Σ_s. Therefore, because $H(1 - H)(1.4 - H)$ fits the data shown in Fig. 2 and because it is practically the same as Pisharoty's, we now write the equation for Σ_s in our model as

$$\Sigma_s = \sigma_s H(1 - H)(1.4 - H)/V \qquad \text{(correct)}. \qquad (20)$$

As we show in Section 5, the clarification of this ambiguity about the collimated transmittance permits a more accurate comparison of theory and experiment.

5. FURTHER COMPARISON OF EXPERIMENT AND THEORY: NEW VALUES FOR $\bar{\mu}$ AND THE I_0 PROBLEM

We now rewrite Eq. (18) with the new expressions for T_c and Σ_s:

$$T_{\text{tot}} = T_{\text{diff}} + \exp(-\Sigma d) \qquad \text{(correct)}, \qquad (21)$$

$$\Sigma_s = \sigma_s H(1-H)(1.4-H)/V \qquad \text{(correct)}. \qquad (20)$$

Note here that $\Sigma = \Sigma_a + \Sigma_s$, where Σ_s is now given by Eq. (20). To compare Eq. (21) with O.D. data, the parameters necessary for evaluating T_{diff} and Σ must be determined. Some of these parameters, such as the radius of the light beam incident upon the blood surface, the radius of the detector, and the wavelength of the source, are fairly easy to measure. However, the scattering and absorption cross sections σ_a and σ_s and the mean cosine of the scattering angle $\bar{\mu}$ are more difficult to obtain. Consequently many investigators have used Mie scattering theory[25] to obtain these values by assuming a spherical scatterer with a volume equal to that of a RBC. Although experimental values for σ_a and σ_s have agreed with Mie theory,[14,26,27] similar calculations for $\bar{\mu}$ have not. In particular, from experimental cross-section data at 685 nm, Pedersen et al.[28] obtained $\bar{\mu}$ values that were smaller than those from Mie theory. Using two different scattering models, they determined $\bar{\mu}$ from experiment to be 0.979 or 0.991, whereas Mie scattering theory gave a value of 0.9947. These differences are significant because the modified macroscopic scattering coefficient Σ_{st} is proportional to $1 - \bar{\mu}$, which varies by a factor of 4 from $\bar{\mu} = 0.9947$ to $\bar{\mu} = 0.979$.

Because of this confusion over the value of $\bar{\mu}$, we performed goniometric measurements with a He–Ne laser (Experiment 4) and calculated $\bar{\mu}$ from its definition. By fitting our angular scattering data to the two-parameter scattering phase function of Reynolds and McCormick,[29] we obtained a value of 0.9845 for $\bar{\mu}$. This value falls approximately halfway between the experimental values just cited. Because this value is obviously restricted to 632.8 nm, we could not simply use it for calculations at 660 and 800–813 nm. However, because theory predicts that Σ_{st} is nearly independent of wavelength in the region 630–950 nm, for 660 and 800–813 nm, we chose $\bar{\mu}$ values that preserved the relative magnitudes of Σ_{st} that were predicted by Mie theory at the wavelengths 632.8, 660, and 800–813 nm. As shown in Table 1, this method yielded 0.984 and 0.980 for $\bar{\mu}$ at 660 and 800–813 nm, respectively.

When we first applied Eq. (21) to our own O.D. data by using the values in Table 1, which include the new values for $\bar{\mu}$ and the new expressions for T_c and Σ_s, it became apparent that theory and experiment still differed at least by an additive constant. Because a constant additive offset in O.D. corresponds to a multiplicative constant in transmittance, we suspected a problem in our measurement of I_0. As explained in Section 3, the optical geometry from which the measurements were taken consisted of LED light sources, an optical cuvette, and a P–I–N diode detector. What we discovered was that our measurement of I_0 with a saline-filled cuvette detected only a small fraction of the total incident intensity. This effect was due to the small active area of the detector and to the size and divergence of the beam emitted by the LED's.

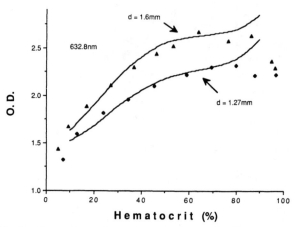

Fig. 3. Comparison of new transmittance model, Eq. (21), with experimental data. Data shown are absolute O.D. versus hematocrit for oxygenated RBC suspensions with a He–Ne laser in cuvette geometry. I_0 is known exactly for these data since the whole incident laser beam can be captured by detector. Agreement between experiment (data points) and model (curve) shows that the model predicts absolute transmittance accurately. For the lower curve, a = 0.685 mm, b = 1.0 mm; for the upper curve, a = 0.685 mm, b = 1.0 mm.

To obtain data in which I_0 would be known accurately, we measured the O.D. as a function of hematocrit in cuvettes with path lengths of 1.27 and 1.6 mm illuminated by a He–Ne laser (Experiment 2). The beam radius was 0.7 mm, and the effective detector radius was approximately 1.0 mm. In this manner we were able to capture essentially the whole incident beam with our detector and thus measure I_0 accurately. We also measured the extinction coefficient of oxyhemoglobin for the laser light (with a 1-cm path-length cuvette) rather than using values in the literature that were obtained with light less monochromatic than the laser. The O.D. data for whole blood are shown in Fig. 3. The RBC suspensions were 100% saturated with oxygen. Also shown in Fig. 3 are the theoretical predictions of Eq. (21). Because of the agreement between our model and the laser data in Fig. 3, we gained confidence in the model's ability to predict absolute transmittance, i.e., no additive constant was needed to fit the laser data to the theory. However, in experiments at LED wavelengths, we could not assess I_0 accurately. Therefore in the rest of this paper, if I_0 was not known exactly, we have allowed ourselves the convenience of adding an arbitrary constant to the data to account for the low I_0 measurements in the experiments at LED wavelengths.

6. DATA FOR LIGHT-EMITTING-DIODE WAVELENGTHS USED IN OXIMETRY

The laser O.D. data of Fig. 3 serve to illustrate the applicability of our transmittance model [Eq. (21)] to the wavelength region used for oximetry. However, practical oximeters typically use inexpensive LED's as light sources and detectors that do not capture all the incident light. In this section we present O.D. data for LED wavelengths of 660, 800, and 813 nm and for optical depths of 1.27 and 1.6 mm (see Subsection 3.B). Each set of data will be compared with Eq. (21). In each case, an additive constant that corrects for I_0 has been added to the data. As in the case of the laser experiments, we preferred to measure the extinction

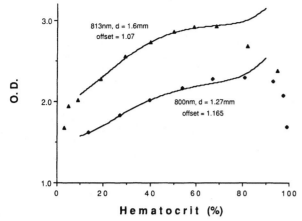

Fig. 4. O.D. versus hematocrit at LED wavelengths. Data shown are measured O.D. for cuvette geometries at 800- and 813-nm LED wavelengths. An additive constant (denoted offset) has been added to the data to account for inability to measure I_0 accurately with LED's. For the lower curve, $a = 2.0$ mm, $b = 1.5$ mm; for the upper curve, $a = 2.5$ mm, $b = 1.0$ mm.

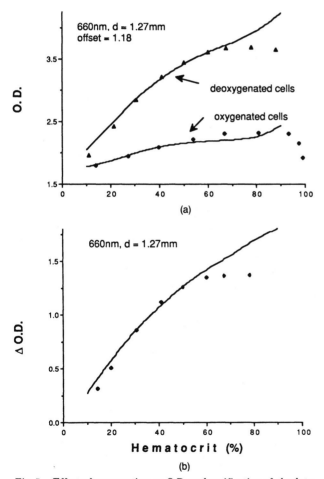

Fig. 5. Effect of oxygenation on O.D. and verification of absolute transmittance predicted by model. (a) Data are from completely oxygenated and deoxygenated red-cell suspensions. A single additive offset has been added to both sets of data. (b) Difference of two sets of data in (a). Data points are the differences in raw data values, and the curve is the difference of the theoretical curves of upper panel. The agreement of data and theory in (b) verifies that absolute transmittance is correctly predicted by new model. For all curves, $a = 3.0$ mm, $b = 1.5$ mm.

coefficients for oxyhemoglobin and deoxyhemoglobin at the LED wavelengths rather than to use the values in the literature. In the LED case we did so because the spectral half-bandwidth of an LED is much wider than that of the spectrophotometers with which the extinction coefficients in the literature were measured. The values that we obtained are shown in Table 1.

Figure 4 shows data at the LED wavelengths 800 and 813 nm from cuvettes of 1.27- and 1.6-mm optical depth. The state of oxygenation of the red-cell suspensions for both curves was 100%. The agreement of the theory with the data appears quite good through a range from 10 to 75% hematocrit.

In Fig. 5(a) we have plotted data at the LED wavelength of 660 nm. The two curves show results for oxygenated and deoxygenated red-cell suspensions. Because the measurements for Fig. 5 were made in the same optical geometry with the same LED, detector, cuvette, etc., one should expect the ratio between the true I_0 and the measured I_0 to be the same for both sets of data. The additive offset values that we used to scale data to theory were the same for the two sets of data. To evaluate further whether the additive constants are indeed the same, we have plotted the difference of the two theoretical curves in Fig. 5(b). The difference in the O.D. between two samples known to have the same incident intensity (I_0) is independent of that intensity since $\log(I_0/I_1) - \log(I_0/I_2) = \log(I_2/I_1)$. Thus, if we plot, without an additive offset, the difference in the raw data from oxygenated and deoxygenated cells [Fig. 5(a)] versus the predicted difference, we should expect agreement. Figure 5(b) confirms this expectation.

In Fig. 6 we have plotted O.D. data as a function of oxyhemoglobin saturation (SO_2) for a fixed hematocrit ($H = 36.5\%$) at the 660-nm LED wavelength. For consistency with the data shown in Fig. 5(a), the same additive constant (1.18) was added to this set of data as was added to the data in Fig. 5(a). Note that the agreement of theory and experiment is good for $SO_2 > 25\%$ and that this agreement breaks down somewhat for lower SO_2 values. We also note here that the data are significantly linear ($r = 0.999$) and that the

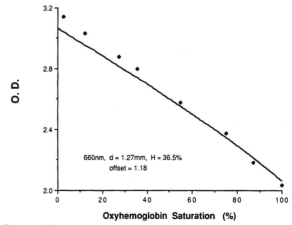

Fig. 6. O.D. versus oxyhemoglobin saturation at fixed hematocrit. Additive offset is same as used for both curves in Fig. 5(a). Data are highly linear in oxyhemoglobin saturation ($r = 0.999$), and the theoretical curve is itself significantly linear, although theory falls below data at low oxyhemoglobin saturation. For this curve, $a = 3.0$ mm, $b = 1.5$ mm.

theoretical curve shown is also an approximately linear function of SO_2. We shall amplify these observations in Section 8.

7. JUSTIFICATION OF THE MODEL

Our model of the diffuse transmittance of whole blood is based primarily on the work of Schmitt and co-workers[7,15] and Reynolds and co-workers.[6,14] However, we have introduced several innovations that need to be justified. They are (1) the use of Σ in place of Σ_t for the collimated attenuation of the incident beam and the redefinition of Σ_s, (2) Eq. (3) for the second boundary condition at $z = z_0$, (3) the experimental measurements of $\bar{\mu}$ and the extinction coefficients for both hemoglobin species with the same detectors and light sources as in the experiments, and (4) for the LED data only, the use of an arbitrary additive constant to scale the O.D. data to theory.

Let us consider each of these aspects of the new model. First, the use of Σ in place of Σ_t means that the total collimated attenuation of an incident beam is due to both absorption and total scattering. We verified in the laser experiments (Experiment 1) that Σ represents the proper collimated attenuation, provided that Σ_s is taken from Eq. (20). When photon-diffusion theory has been applied to the P1 approximation of Reynolds,[6] Σ has been assumed to describe the collimated attenuation. Thus there is a precedent for this use of Σ. Furthermore, the use of Σ_t and the previous expression for Σ_s causes the theoretical O.D. to be too small in magnitude and to be parabolic versus the hematocrit (see Section 4). Second, Eq. (3) merely applies the appropriate boundary condition to the $z = z_0$ plane. This boundary condition was often used by Reynolds[6] throughout his original work on diffuse reflectance and transmittance, and it is necessary to evaluate the light flux at $z = z_0$, whereas the boundary condition used by Schmitt and co-workers[7,15] is a simplification that sets $\Psi = 0$ at $z = z_0$. Third, our measuring the extinction coefficients for both hemoglobin species in our own apparatus rather than using literature values was necessary because it is well known that the spectral bandwidth of a source affects the value obtained for the effective extinction coefficients.[30] Furthermore, the sensitivity of light detectors varies with wavelength. Thus the apparent spectral distribution of the source depends on the particular detector employed. Similarly, our measuring $\bar{\mu}$ from experiment was necessary because the results from Mie theory are for a spherical scatterer, whereas the RBC is actually a biconcave disk. We shall return to $\bar{\mu}$ in Section 8. Finally, the introduction of an arbitrary additive constant to scale the O.D. data to theory is simply a way to account for the actual incident intensity. We used such a scaling constant in the LED experiments in which I_0 was unknown because only a small fraction of I_0 was received by the detector. However, as the laser experiments show (Fig. 3), the model accurately predicts absolute transmittance ($T = I/I_0$) when I_0 can be measured accurately.

8. INSIGHTS AND APPLICATIONS OF THE MODEL

As an example of insights that the model provides, we first consider the variation of $\bar{\mu}$, the mean cosine of the scattering

angle of the RBC. The values for $\bar{\mu}$ computed from Mie theory for the scattering characteristics of a sphere with a volume equal to that of a RBC[14,15] are probably incorrect since the RBC is actually a biconcave disk. As we mentioned earlier, the values for $\bar{\mu}$ from experimental evaluations are smaller than those from Mie theory (see Section 5). Figure 7 shows the effects of changing $\bar{\mu}$ while the other parameters in the model are held fixed. For the sake of comparison, all parameters except $\bar{\mu}$ are the same as those used to generate the theoretical curve of Fig. 3 (lower curve). Figure 7 shows that as $\bar{\mu}$ decreases the theoretical curves take on more closely the shape of the data in Fig. 3 (lower curve). Furthermore, simulations at other wavelengths and sample depths (not shown) indicate trends similar to those in Fig. 7. Thus the theoretical results (from our model) indicate that the appropriate values for $\bar{\mu}$ are indeed smaller than those predicted by Mie theory. Therefore the simulations of Fig. 7 and the experimental values obtained by Pedersen et al.[28] corroborate the value that we obtained in our goniometric measurements of $\bar{\mu}$.

Another example of insights provided by the model is the relative contributions of T_c and T_{diff} to T_{tot} in Eq. (21). For the same theoretical curve shown in Fig. 3 (lower curve), we have plotted in Fig. 8 the components T_c, T_{diff}, and their sum T_{tot}. The T or transmittance axis is on a log scale so that we are essentially plotting O.D. since O.D. $= -\log(T)$. The important feature of Fig. 8 is that between hematocrits of 3 and 97%, T_{tot} is essentially just T_{diff}, and the collimated component T_c is completely negligible. We have also plotted in Fig. 8 the T_c curve corresponding to Eq. (18). As we pointed out above, T_c of Eq. (18) obscures T_{diff}, so that the O.D. from Eq. (18) is approximately equal to the parabola shown in Fig. 8 and labeled T_c from Eq. (18). This is a graphical analysis of what we described in Section 4.

As a first application of our model we consider oximetry, a technique for measuring oxyhemoglobin saturation (SO_2) in whole blood. Recall that in Fig. 6 we plotted O.D. versus SO_2 at a fixed hematocrit in the physiological range. Experimentally, the O.D. at 660 nm has been found to be an approximately linear function of SO_2 at a fixed hemato-

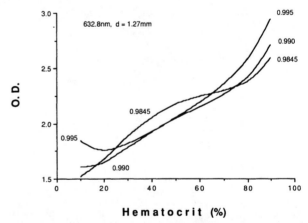

Fig. 7. Effect of $\bar{\mu}$, mean cosine of scattering angle, on predictions of new model [Eq. (21)]. Simulation parameters are the same as those used to generate the theoretical curve of Fig. 3 (lower curve). Note that as $\bar{\mu}$ decreases, the theoretical curve conforms more closely to the shape of the data in Fig. 3 (lower curve). This trend indicates that values of $\bar{\mu}$ from Mie theory are too high.

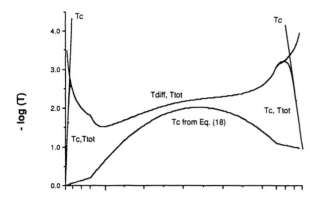

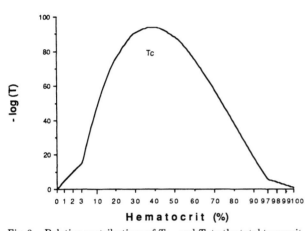

Fig. 8. Relative contributions of T_{diff} and T_c to the total transmittance of whole blood [Eq. (21)]. For comparison, parameters used in this figure are the same as those used to generate the lower, theoretical curve of Fig. 3. Note that between $H = 3\%$ and $H = 97\%$, T_{tot} is essentially just T_{diff}. When an incorrect expression [Eqs. (17) and (18)] is used for T_c, T_c obscures T_{diff} so that T_{tot} would be approximately T_c.

crit.[31,32] This observation has been the basis of whole-blood oximetry.[33] Not until recently, however, has such a linear relationship been justified on a theoretical basis.[13] Therefore, inasmuch as the theoretical curve in Fig. 6 may be approximated by a straight line, we now have further verification of this experimental result. Finally, although we do not discuss it here, our model may be used to predict the hematocrit dependence of the whole-blood oximeter curve, a phenomenon that we reported previously.[13]

Our second application of the model is the spectrophotometric measurement of the difference in oxygen content between arterial and venous blood ($a - v\, O_2$). We recently delineated the role that light scattering plays in such measurements of $a - v\, O_2$. In that study[12] with 1.6-mm cuvettes, we found that (1) the difference in the O.D. between fully oxygenated and fully deoxygenated blood at 660 nm is proportional to hematocrit and (2) that the O.D. at 660 nm is an approximately linear function of SO_2 at a fixed hematocrit. These two observations imply that the difference in O.D. between two samples of whole blood is directly proportional to their difference in oxyhemoglobin concentration, i.e., to $a - v\, O_2$. The predictions of our model shown in Figs. 5(b) and 6 indicate that these two observations also hold at a

different optical depth (1.27 mm). Thus it may be expected that the difference in the O.D. between two samples of whole blood in 1.27-mm cuvettes would also be directly proportional to the difference in their oxyhemoglobin concentrations. However, with this path length, the range of hematocrits for which this technique would work is limited to the range for which the theory and the data in Fig. 5(b) are approximately proportional to hematocrit (e.g., up through approximately 50% hematocrit).

9. ADVANTAGES AND LIMITATIONS OF THE MODEL

Comparisons of data and theory (Figs. 3–6) have demonstrated the validity of our model. Fundamental to photon-diffusion theory, however, is the assumption that scattering dominates absorption.[7] Therefore we shall assess the limitations that this assumption imposes on our model. A convenient measure of the ratio of scattering to absorbance is the quantity $\Sigma_{st}/\Sigma_a = \sigma_s(1 - \bar{\mu})(1 - H)(1.4 - H)/\sigma_a$. For the wavelengths that we have considered, $\sigma_s(1 - \bar{\mu})$ stays between 0.85 and 0.95 μm^2, and σ_a varies from 0.066 to 0.318 μm^2 for oxygenated and deoxygenated RBC's at 660 nm. This expression for Σ_{st}/Σ_a reveals that if $\sigma_a/[(1 - H)(1.4 - H)]$ becomes comparable with $\sigma_s(1 - \bar{\mu})$, scattering will no longer dominate absorption. Because $\sigma_a/[(1 - H)(1.4 - H)]$ becomes large if H approaches 1 or if σ_a is large, these limiting values constitute the range in which photon-diffusion theory may no longer be valid. In fact, all but one of the theoretical curves shown in Figs. 3–5 diverge from the data at high hematocrits (i.e., as $H \rightarrow 1$).

The only exception is the theoretical O.D. curve for oxygenated RBC's at 660 nm. However, of all the data presented here, this set represents the smallest value for σ_a. Thus, at 660 nm, H must be close to 1 before Σ_{st}/Σ_a falls significantly. Finally, in Fig. 6, which shows data for a constant hematocrit ($H = 36.5\%$), the absorption cross section σ_a varies linearly from 0.066 to 0.318 μm^2 as oxyhemoglobin saturation (SO_2) varies from 100 to 0%. Note that the model deviates from the data as σ_a increases, i.e., as SO_2 decreases. In summary, we see from our comparisons of theory with data that as H approaches 1 and as σ_a becomes large, our model loses its validity. Fortunately, in most biomedical applications, hematocrit will be less than 60% and oxyhemoglobin saturation will be greater than 25%. Therefore our model remains valid in these regions.

Comparisons of experiment and theory have pointed out several advantages of our model over other transmittance models. First, because the model includes emitter and detector radii, it can easily simulate various practical optical geometries that might be evaluated for possible instrument designs. Second, by incorporating the detector radius, the model automatically determines what fraction of the total transmitted diffuse light will be detected, an ability that eliminates the considerable guesswork that other models[4,5,9,18] require. In fact, Moaveni and Razani[18] stressed the importance of knowing the fraction of the transmitted light that is detected, a quantity that other models assume is fixed. Unfortunately, the fraction of the total transmitted diffuse light reaching a given detector aperture is actually a function of hematocrit and other parameters and thus cannot be specified by a single value even for a fixed optical geometry. Such considerations underscore this second advantage of our model. Third, when all apertures are known and I_0 is measured correctly, our model needs no variational parameters to predict absolute transmittance accurately (Fig. 3). Thus our model is superior to previous treatments, most of which require curve-fitting techniques and variation of unknown parameters to obtain realistic theoretical predictions.

REFERENCES

1. A. Ishimaru, Y. Kuga, R. L. T. Cheung, and K. Shimizu, "Scattering and diffusion of a beam wave in randomly distributed scatterers," J. Opt. Soc. Am. **73**, 131–136 (1983).
2. W. G. Tam and A. Zardecki, "Off-axis propagation of a laser beam in low visibility weather conditions," Appl. Opt. **19**, 2822–2827 (1980).
3. S. A. W. Gerstl, A. Zardecki, W. P. Unruh, D. M. Stupin, G. H. Stokes, and N. E. Elliott, "Off-axis multiple scattering of a laser beam in turbid media: comparison of theory and experiment," Appl. Opt. **26**, 779–785 (1987).
4. V. Twersky, "Absorption and multiple scattering by biological suspensions," J. Opt. Soc. Am. **60**, 1084–1093 (1970).
5. V. Twersky, "Interface effects in multiple scattering by large, low-refracting, absorbing particles," J. Opt. Soc. Am. **60**, 908–914 (1970).
6. L. O. Reynolds, "Optical diffuse reflectance and transmittance from an anisotropically scattering finite blood medium," Ph.D. dissertation (University of Washington, Seattle, Wash., 1975).
7. J. M. Schmitt, "Optical measurement of blood oxygen by implantable telemetry," Ph.D. dissertation (Stanford University, Stanford, Calif., 1986).
8. R. J. Zdrojkowski and N. R. Pisharoty, "Optical transmission and reflection by blood," IEEE Trans. Biomed. Eng. **BME-17**, 122–128 (1970).
9. M. K. Moaveni, "A multiple scattering field theory applied to whole blood," Ph.D. dissertation (University of Washington, Seattle, Wash., 1970).
10. P. Kubelka, "New contributions to the optics of intensely light-scattering materials. Part I," J. Opt. Soc. Am. **38**, 448–457 (1948).
11. H. H. Lipowsky, S. Usami, S. Chien, and R. N. Pittman, "Hematocrit determination in small bore tubes from optical density measurements under white light illumination," Microvasc. Res. **20**, 51–70 (1980).
12. J. M. Steinke and A. P. Shepherd, "Role of light scattering in spectrophotometric measurements of arteriovenous oxygen difference," IEEE Trans. Biomed. Eng. **BME-33**, 729–734 (1986).
13. J. M. Steinke and A. P. Shepherd, "Role of light scattering in whole blood oximetry," IEEE Trans. Biomed. Eng. **BME-33**, 294–301 (1986).
14. L. Reynolds, C. Johnson, and A. Ishimaru, "Diffuse reflectance from a finite blood medium: applications to the modeling of fiber optic catheters," Appl. Opt. **15**, 2059–2067 (1976).
15. J. M. Schmitt, J. D. Meindl, and F. G. Mihm, "An integrated circuit-based optical sensor for in *vivo* measurement of blood oxygenation," IEEE Trans. Biomed. Eng. **BME-33**, 98–107 (1986).
16. J. M. Steinke and A. P. Shepherd, "Reflectance measurements of hematocrit and oxyhemoglobin saturation," Am. J. Physiol. **253**, H147–H153 (1987).
17. J. M. Steinke and A. P. Shepherd, "Diffuse reflectance of whole blood: model for a diverging light beam," IEEE Trans. Biomed. Eng. **BME-34**, 826–834 (1987).
18. M. K. Moaveni and A. Razani, "Application of invariant imbedding for the study of optical transmission and reflection by blood: Part II—Application," Indian J. Biochem. Biophys. **11**, 30–35 (1974).
19. G. Bell and S. Glasstone, *Nuclear Reactor Theory* (Van Nostrand Reinhold, New York, 1970), pp. 93–97.
20. M. Abramowitz and I. A. Stegun, *Handbook of Mathematical Functions with Formulas, Graphs, and Mathematical Tables* (Wiley, New York, 1972), pp. 375, 378–379.
21. I. S. Gradshteyn and I. M. Ryzhik, *Tables of Integrals, Series, and Products* (Academic, New York, 1965), p. 970.
22. A. P. Shepherd, J. W. Kiel, and G. L. Riedel, "Evaluation of light-emitting diodes for whole blood oximetry," IEEE Trans. Biomed. Eng. **BME-31**, 723–725 (1984).
23. N. R. Pisharoty, "Optical scattering in blood," Ph.D. dissertation (Carnegie-Mellon University, Pittsburgh, Pa., 1971).
24. R. J. Hirko, R. J. Fretterd, and R. L. Longini, "Application of the diffusion dipole to modelling the optical characteristics of blood," Med. Biol. Eng. **13**, 192–195 (1975).
25. C. F. Bohren and D. R. Huffman, *Absorption and Scattering of Light by Small Particles* (Wiley, New York, 1983), pp. 82–129.
26. L. Reynolds, J. Molocho, C. Johnson, and A. Ishimaru, "Optical cross-sections of human erythrocytes," in *Proceedings of the 27th Annual Conference on Engineering in Medicine and Biology* (Alliance for Engineering in Medicine and Biology, Chevy Chase, Md., 1974), Vol. 16, p. 58.
27. R. Pierce, "An experimental determination of the average scattering and absorption cross sections of human red blood cells for near infrared light," M.S. thesis (Department of Electrical Engineering, University of Washington, Seattle, Wash., 1972).
28. G. D. Pedersen, N. J. McCormick, and L. O. Reynolds, "Transport calculations for light scattering in blood," Biophys. J. **16**, 199–207 (1976).
29. L. O. Reynolds and N. J. McCormick, "Approximate two-parameter phase function for light scattering," J. Opt. Soc. Am. **70**, 1206–1212 (1980).
30. Varian Instrument Division, *Optimum Parameters for Spectrophotometry* (Varian, Palo Alto, Calif., 1975).
31. K. Kramer, J. O. Elam, G. A. Saxton, and W. N. Elam, Jr., "Influence of oxygen saturation, erythrocyte concentration and optical depth upon the red and near-infrared light transmittance of whole blood," Am. J. Physiol. **165**, 229–246 (1951).
32. N. M. Anderson and P. Sekelj, "Studies on the light transmission of nonhemolyzed whole blood. Determination of oxygen saturation," J. Lab. Clin. Med. **65**, 153–166 (1965).
33. J. W. Kiel and A. P. Shepherd, "A microcomputer oximeter for whole blood," Am. J. Physiol. **244**, H722–H725 (1983).

Summary of paper from *Akademiya Navuk Belarusskai SSSR Vestsi—Seryya Fizika-Matematychnykh Navuk*, Vol. 1, pp. 79-84 (1984).

Dispersion of the real and imaginary part of the complex refractive index of hemoglobin in the range 450-820 nm

S.F. Shumilina

Summary

The problem of determinating the real and imaginary parts of the hemoglobin refractive index by using the Kramers-Kronig relation is considered. The absorption spectra of oxy- and deoxyhemoglobin and the dispersion n in the spectral range 450-820 nm are given.

Reprinted from *Optical Engineering*, Vol. 32(2), pp. 253-257 (February 1993).
©1993 SPIE.

Optical properties of blood in motion

Lars-Göran Lindberg
Per Åke Öberg, MEMBER SPIE
Linköping University
Department of Biomedical Engineering
S-581 85 Linköping, Sweden

Abstract. An *in vitro* model is developed for application in studies of the optical and physical characteristics of flowing blood in rigid and flexible tubes (artificial vessels). The results indicate that both transmission and reflection of light are dependent on blood volume changes and orientation as well as the deformability of the red blood cells. Light transmission and reflection in human blood shows a parabolic behavior at hematocrit levels greater than 40%, when plotted against blood flow. At both low and high flow rates, the light transmission increases when compared to an intermediate flow where the transmission shows a minimum. The optical wavelength used also affects the light transmission and reflection in moving blood. The results of studies of blood in flow-through models are important for the understanding of the optical mechanisms behind the signal generation in photometrical measurement techniques.

Subject terms: biomedical optics; transmission and reflection; rigid and flexible flow-through models; steady flow.

Optical Engineering 32(2), 253–257 (February 1993).

1 Introduction

A number of medical diagnostic methods utilize the absorption, reflection, and scattering of light in whole blood and tissue. Light is brought to illuminate human tissue or a sample of blood in a cuvette. The reflected or transmitted light is modulated in some way by the parameter studied, e.g., blood flow, oxyhemoglobin saturation, hematocrit, hemoglobin concentration, arteriovenous oxygen difference, etc.

Noninvasive optical instruments have increased in popularity over the last decade. These methods monitor steady or pulsatile perfusion levels and have been applied in clinical work, for example, for (1) the assessment of wound and burn healing, the viability of skin flaps after plastic surgery, and skin perfusion using photoplethysmography[1]; (2) the monitoring of the respiratory rate[2]; (3) laser blood flow measurements using the laser Doppler technique[3]; and (4) the measurement of arterial oxygen saturation using pulse oximetry.[4] Pulse oximetry is a relatively new method that has progressed from its first technical appearance to commercial production in less than 10 yr.

A thorough understanding of the processes of light absorption and scattering in tissue and blood is of great importance in the design of practical diagnostic instruments. It is not surprising that many different theories have been proposed to describe the complex propagation of light in blood and tissue. However, although good agreement has often been found between theoretical predictions and experimental data, there are often certain conditions under which the theories either fail or lack generality. Simplifying assumptions, such as homogenously distributed blood in tissue and isotropic scattering, are often made when the photon pathways in tissue are simulated. Another limitation of these theories is that they often assume a stationary blood volume. In biological tissue, however, the blood is always in steady and/or pulsatile movement in vessels of different size. Motion of course affects the optical properties of red blood cells.

The aim of this work is to study how light is transmitted and scattered in blood in motion.

2 Methods and Materials

2.1 Experimental Setup

The developed *in vitro* setup (Fig. 1) consists of three main parts: a pressure controlled roller pump, a cylindrical blood

Paper BM-011 received Feb. 1, 1992; revised manuscript received July 31, 1992; accepted for publication July 31, 1992.
© 1993 Society of Photo-Optical Instrumentation Engineers. 0091-3286/93/$2.00.

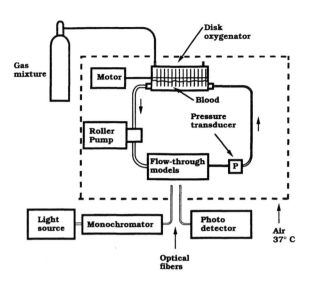

Fig. 1 The flow-through model setup.

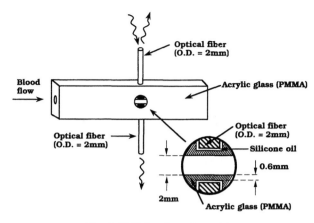

Fig. 2 Rigid flow-through model.

reservoir (and disk oxygenator), and rigid and flexible flow-through models (artificial blood vessels). Fresh blood (20 ml) from healthy blood donors was put into the reservoir. A gas mixture (19% oxygen and 5.6% carbon dioxide in nitrogen) was lead into the reservoir and mixed with the blood by the disk oxygenator. A roller pump, specially designed to circulate blood, transported the blood through different types of flexible and rigid flow-through models. The roller pump and the connections of the tubing system were designed so as to minimize the damage to the red blood cells. The pump was controlled by a waveform generator to accurately (within 2%) maintain the steady pressures that were preset.

The light was guided to and from the circulating blood by optical plastic fibers, placed outside the flow-through models. A pressure transducer was placed at the outlet of the flow-through model. The blood temperature was maintained at $37 \pm 0.1°C$ by circulating warm air. The optical illuminating and detecting system consisted of a Quartz Halogen lamp (250 W), a monochromator (model 77250, Oriel Co., U.S.A.), a photodetector (model 835, silicon, 818-SL, Newport Co., U.S.A.), and optical plastic fibers (Super Eska, Mitsubishi Rayon Co., Japan).

The steady blood flow was varied between 0.5 and 18 ml/min, and the shear rate was never below 10 s^{-1} to avoid blood sedimentation.[5]

2.2 Handling of the Blood

Venous blood (20 ml) from healthy blood donors was put into the reservoir within 20 min after being taken. Glucose, 0.1 ml (50 mg/ml), and 0.5 ml of heparin (5000 IE/ml) were added to the blood. To ensure that the blood parameters were maintained at normal physiological values, each experiment included measurement of hematocrit (micro-centrifugation); mean cell volume (MCV; flow cell cytometry, Technicon*1, U.S.A.); osmolality (freezing point method, model 3L, Advanced Instruments, Inc., U.S.A.); and pCO_2, pO_2, and pH (ABL 3, Radiometer, Copenhagen). MCV and osmolality were measured to check that isotonic conditions were maintained. In addition, the amount of hem-

olysis was visually checked (microcentrifugation) after each experiment.

Several experiments were performed on plasma containing no red blood cells or on blood that had been diluted by adding plasma. Frozen plasma (blood group = AB) was thawed in water at 35°C for approximately 10 min before use. Each experiment was performed within 2 h after the blood was taken to ascertain normal physiological blood conditions.

2.3 Light Transmission and Reflection from a Rigid Flow-Through Model

Figure 2 shows the rigid flow-through model. A flow-through hole (i.d. = 2 mm) was drilled in an acrylic block [poly-methyl methacrylate (PMMA)]. During transmission experiments, two optical fibers (o.d. = 2 mm, numerical aperture = 0.5, Super Eska, Mitsubishi Rayon Co., Japan) were placed in holes in the acrylic block facing each other and placed perpendicular to the longitudinal axis of the flow-through hole. The distance between the end of the fibers and the blood was 0.6 mm. In the reflection experiments, the light was transmitted and picked up by the same optical fiber (numerical aperture = 0.5, Super Eska, Mitsubishi Rayon Co., Japan). Viscous silicone oil was placed between the fiber ends and the bottom of the holes.

The refraction indices of the optical fibers ($n = 1.495$), the silicone oil ($n = 1.530$), and the acrylic block (1.491) were chosen to allow the maximum amount of light to reach the flowing blood. Measurements were performed using three optical wavelengths, namely, 560, 660, and 940 nm.

2.4 Light Transmission from a Flexible Flow-Through Model

These experiments actually used two models—an elastic flow-through model and a rigid one—so that the two models at the same blood flow and at similar optical conditions could be compared. A silicone flexible tube (i.d. = 1.9 mm, length = 15 mm, wall thickness = 0.05 mm) was inserted into a circular hole (i.d. = 3 mm) in a rod made of acrylic glass (PMMA), see Fig. 3.

The ends of the silicone tube were connected to the circulating system and fixed to the inside of the circular hole with silicone glue. To measure the blood volume changes in the flexible tube, a water column was incorporated in the tubing system (Fig. 3). The total blood volume change was

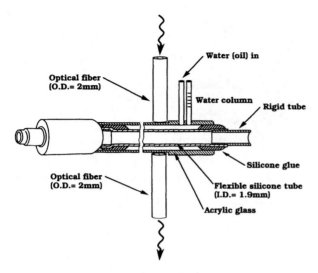

Fig. 3 Flexible flow-through model.

8.5%, corresponding to a pressure change of 80 mm Hg and a blood flow change from 0.5 to 18 ml/min. In the rigid flow-through model, a glass tube (i.d. = 1.9 mm, wall thickness = 0.1 mm) was coated with a flexible silicone tube. The glass tube was inserted into the hole and the optical fibers used were the same as described in Sec. 2.3.

3 Results

3.1 Light Transmission and Reflection from a Rigid Flow-Through Model

Figure 4 shows relative changes in light transmission and reflection versus blood flow at different optical wavelengths. The light transmission decreased with increasing blood flow [Fig. 4(a)] until it reached a minimum value. The light transmission then rose with a further increase in blood flow (parabolic behavior). At 560 nm, the changes in light transmission with flow were small at a high hematocrit.

The light reflection [Fig. 4(b)] showed similar responses to blood flow changes in the sense that a decrease in light transmission was accompanied by an increase in light reflection. In both transmission and reflection modes, the maximal relative change in detected light relative to a minimum flow increased with the wavelength at normal hematocrits. The total relative change in light transmission increased with decreasing hematocrit (Fig. 5). At a hematocrit (HCT) of below approximately 40%, the parabolic behavior in light transmission was not observed. Instead, the light transmission continued to decrease with increasing blood flow toward an asymptotic value. This also occurred at 560 and 940 nm.

3.2 Light Transmission from a Flexible Flow-Through Model

Figure 6 shows relative changes in light transmission versus blood flow in a rigid and flexible tube using a wavelength of 660 nm. The greatest change in light transmission within the flow range was observed in the flexible tube. The blood volume increased 6.6% within the flow range 0.5 to 14ml/min, and the blood volume changed linearly with the pressure change.

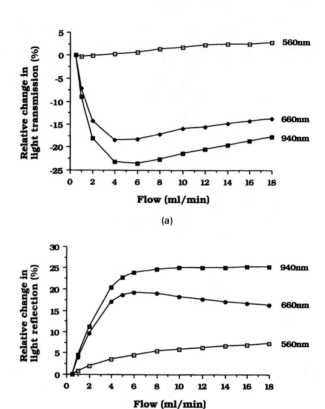

Fig. 4 Relative changes in light transmission (a) and reflection (b) plotted as a function of blood flow.

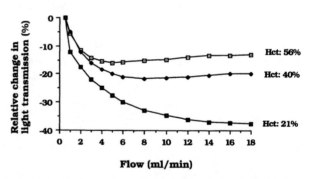

Fig. 5 Changes in light transmission (660 nm) plotted against blood flow at different hematocrits.

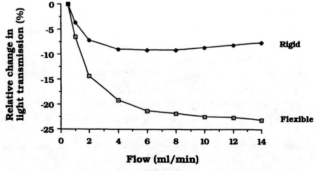

Fig. 6 Light transmission versus blood flow for rigid and flexible flow-through models: wavelength = 660 nm and HCT = 40%.

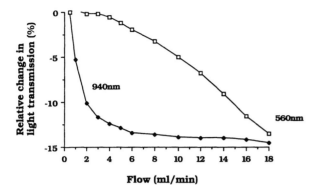

Fig. 7 Light transmission as a function of blood flow in a flexible tube at 560 and 940 nm (HCT = 43%).

Table 1 Blood flow, velocity, and shear rate for a 2-mm-diam tube.

Q (ml/min)	v (cm/s)	shear rate (s^{-1})
18	9.6	382
16	8.5	340
14	7.4	297
12	6.4	255
10	5.3	212
8	4.2	170
6	3.2	127
5	2.7	106
4	2.1	85
3	1.6	64
2	1.1	42
1	0.53	21
0.5	0.27	11

In Fig. 7 relative changes in light transmission is plotted against blood flow at 560 and 940 nm. The light transmission using 560 nm decreased approximately linearly with blood flow, whereas at 940 nm the light transmission decreased exponentially before reaching an asymptotic value.

4 Discussion

To put the mean velocity v and shear rate in physiological perspective it is useful to calculate the values (Table 1). The shear rate (at the wall) was calculated using the equation[6] $4Q/\pi R^3$, where Q is the volume flow and R the radius of the tube.

The Reynolds number was calculated to be maximally 100, which is far from the critical number of 2000. Therefore, the steady blood flow was regarded strictly as laminar flow. In addition, the measuring point (including the tube connection) was designed to establish a steady viscous flow with a parabolic velocity profile.

It is known that the arrangement of the flow tubes in horizontal or vertical position is important to the physical behavior of blood because of sedimentation and/or aggregation of red cells at lower shear rates.[5] In all experiments, the flow-through models and the optical fibers were arranged in horizontal positions. For control reasons, all experiments were, however, performed once or twice, with the tubes in vertical position. There were no differences in results comparing horizontally and vertically oriented flow-through models.

4.1 Transmission and Reflection from a Rigid Flow-Through Model

When plotting the light transmission of human blood as a function of blood flow, parabolic behavior was observed for hematocrits greater than 40% [Fig. 4(a)]. It is possible to identify three blood flow levels that correspond to different rheological and optical mechanisms in moving blood:

1. At a low shear rate (high viscosity) the red blood cells are aggregated into rouleaux and other networks, which leave clear plasma gaps.[7] This makes it possible for the light to propagate through the plasma, which is accompanied by high light transmission.

2. At ''intermediate'' shear rates the aggregates are dispersed and the red blood cells perform as separate cells. Many cells are randomly oriented and exhibit angular rotation, but they also start to align with the major axis parallel to the flow direction and migrate toward the axis of the tube.[8] This increases the total absorption area in the tube model, which in turn reduces the light transmission.

3. At a high shear rate and at a high hematocrit (above approximately 40%) the following two important mechanisms must be considered.

   a. The red cells are deformed into long ellipsoids and the time intervals during which the cells are aligned with flow increases.[9] The deformation is a result of the shear stress acting on the surface of the blood cell.[7] This deformation of the red cells may be accompanied by an increase in light transmission.

   b. The axial accumulation of red blood cells[10] may increase the hematocrit in the middle of the tube, which may favor the formation of aggregates. Light is passed through the plasma gaps, which causes an increase in light transmission.

The results obtained in the reflection mode [Fig. 4(b)] can be explained in a similar way if we consider that higher reflection corresponds to less transmission.

These three rheological states may provide an explanation for the parabolic behavior of light transmission and reflection seen in human blood.

At a high hematocrit, the changes in light transmission and reflection versus blood flow are dependent on the wavelength used (Fig. 4). The penetration depth of light in the blood increases with the wavelength. Light of 940 nm has been scattered in many red blood cells before it escapes from the tube, whereas light of 560 nm is strongly absorbed. The light detected at 940 nm will therefore reflect transmission/reflection changes from a greater volume of blood.

The change in light transmission always decreased toward an asymptotic value for diluted blood (Fig. 5). The total relative change in light transmission (and reflection) is also greater for diluted blood (Fig. 5). This may be explained as follows: At a low hematocrit, the degree of alignment with flow decreases and the red blood cells become more randomly oriented. Angular rotation and changes in orientation without deformation[9] continue at higher blood flows. Additionally, the migration of red cells toward the axis of the tube is favored at a low hematocrit.[10] This means that rotation and tumbling, changes in red cell orientation, and the degree of cell migration toward the tube axis is not limited as in the case of higher hematocrits.

4.2 Transmission from a Flexible Flow-Through Model

Figure 6 shows differences in light transmission when rigid and flexible flow-through models are compared. In a rigid tube, the changes in light transmission primarily depend on the orientation of red blood cells. In a flexible tube, both changes in red cell orientation and blood volume changes due to increased lumen of the tube must be considered.

In a flexible tube, the light transmission at 560 nm changes approximately proportionally to blood flow changes in contrast to infrared light at 940 nm (Fig. 7). For green light, absorption in whole blood is approximately 10 times scattering, whereas for infrared light, scattering dominates absorption.[11] The different results obtained at the two wavelengths may primarily result from the light absorption properties, which dominate in blood in flexible tubes and especially for shorter wavelengths.

To be able to understand the light distribution in tissue it is important to study the interaction between light and blood in more detail, especially with regard to the fact that the blood is enclosed in conduits of different sizes and is always, more or less, in a permanent state of motion. Such studies can be performed in physical models that permit a variety of controlled parameters and conditions.

Acknowledgments

The authors would like to thank P. Sveider for his skillful technical assistance. This work was supported by grants from the National Swedish Board for Technical Development (project 90-00469).

References

1. A. A. R. Kamal, J. B. Harness, G. Irving, and A. J. Mearns, "Skin photoplethysmography—a review," *Comp. Meth. Progr. Biomed.* **28,** 257–269 (1989).
2. L.-G. Lindberg, H. Ugnell, and P. Å. Öberg, "Monitoring of respiratory and heart rates using a fibre optic sensor," *Med. Biol. Eng. Comput.* **30,** 533–537 (1992).
3. A. P. Shepherd and P. Å. Öberg, Eds., *Laser Doppler Flowmetry,* Kluwer Academic Publishers, Boston (1991).
4. K. Tremper and S. Barker, "Pulse oximetry," *Anesthesiology* **70,** 98–100 (1989).
5. W. Reinke, P. Gaehtens, and P. C. Johnson, "Blood viscosity in small tubes: effect of shear rate, aggregation and sedimentation," *Am. J. Physiol.* **253,** H540–H547 (1987).
6. D. A. McDonald, *Blood Flow in Arteries,* The Camelot Press Ltd., Southampton, Great Britain (1974).
7. H. J. Klose, E. Volger, H. Brechtelsbauer, L. Heinich, and H. Schmid-Schönbein, "Microrheology and light transmission of blood. 1. The photometric effects of red cell aggregation and red cell orientation," *Pflugers Arch.* **333,** 126–139 (1972).
8. U. Dinnar, *Cardiovascular Fluid Dynamics,* pp. 23–55, CRC Press, Boca Raton, La. (1981).
9. S. Chien, "Biophysical behavior of red cells in suspensions," in *The Red Blood Cell,* Vol. II, D. M. N. Surgenor, Ed., pp. 1031–1133, Academic Press, New York (1975).
10. Y. C. Fung, *Biomechanics. Mechanical Properties of Living Tissues.* Springer-Verlag, New York (1981).
11. R. N. Pittman, "In vivo photometric analysis of hemoglobin," *Ann. Biomed. Eng.* **14,** 119–137 (1986).

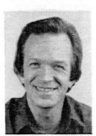

Lars-Göran Lindberg received the MS degree in applied physics and electrical engineering in 1983 and the PhD in biomedical engineering in 1991, both from Linköping University, Sweden. He is currently working as a research associate at the Department of Biomedical Engineering, Linköping University. His research interests include the interaction between optical radiation and tissue and blood and biomedical optical instrumentation.

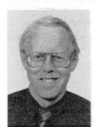

Per Åke Öberg received the MSEE degree from Chalmers University of Technology, Göteborg, Sweden, in 1964, and the PhD in biomedical engineering from Uppsala University in 1971. From 1963 to 1972 he worked at the Department of Physiology and Medical Biophysics, Uppsala University. In 1972 he joined Linköping University, where he is currently a professor of biomedical engineering and director of the Department of Clinical Engineering, University Hospital. His research interests include biomedical instrumentation, transducers, and clinical engineering. Dr. Öberg is a past president of the Swedish Society of Medical Physics and Medical Engineering, a board member of the IFMBE's Division of Clinical Engineering, and a fellow of the Swedish Academy of Engineering Sciences (1980) and the Royal Swedish Academy of Sciences (1987).

Reprinted with permission from *Optics and Spectroscopy [USSR],* Vol. 68(2), pp. 236-239 (February 1990). ©1990 Optical Society of America.

Scattering matrix of a monolayer of optically soft close-packed particles

A. N. Korolevich, A. Ya. Khairullina, and L. P. Shubochkin

(Received 29 November 1988; in revised form, 3 June 1989)

Opt. Spektrosk. **68**, 403–409 (February 1990)

We have studied the angular distribution of the elements of a scattered-light matrix of a monolayer of optically soft disk-shaped and spherical particles during a change in their packing density $c_v = 0.06$–0.6 (c_v being the relative fraction of the volume occupied by the particles). The measurements were conducted on disk-shaped and spherulized erythrocytes. The influence of packing density on the angular variation of element a_{11} at $\gamma = 15$–$16°$ for disks as well as spheres has been determined. The factor determining the angular variation of elements $a_{11}, a_{22}, a_{33}, a_{21}$ in the range of angles $\gamma = 110$–$160°$ is the shape of the particles, not their packing density. The possibility of determining the refractive index of optically soft particles ($n_{rel} \leqslant 1.055$) from the magnitude of element a_{12} at angles $\gamma = 140$–$160°$ from the direction of the incident flux is indicated.

In problems of radiation propagation in biological media and their diagnostics, there arises the question of determining the parameters of a volume element in media with close-packed particles. While the question of radiation scattering in the scalar case in a monolayer has been discussed in an appreciable number of papers,[2-7] we do not know of any studies of the polarization characteristics of a monolayer of close-packed particles. Therefore, the purpose of the present work was an experimental study of the angular distribution of the scattering matrix (SM) elements of a monolayer of particles as their packing density (relative fraction of the volume occupied by the particles) changes. Also discussed is the question of the effect of nonsphericity of close-packed particles in the layer on the SM, since many biological objects can have a shape other than spherical. The asphericity parameter is $p = a/b$, where a and b are, respectively, the maximum and minimum dimensions of the particle (the average value of the asphericity parameter of an erythrocyte is $p = 3.5$–4).

Since the packing density c_v of the scattering particles was measured experimentally over a considerable range ($c_v = 0.06$–0.6), the condition of quasisingleness of scattering was achieved by using a thin cell ($l = 7 \mu$m). The cell thickness was determined by the size of the scattering particles chosen for the experiment, i.e., human erythrocytes. In their natural state, erythrocytes are biconcave disks of radi-

us $r = 3.5$–4μm with an edge thickness of 2.4μm.[8]

It should be noted that disk-shaped erythrocytes, in contrast to spherulized ones, can be highly deformed owing to their shape. In spherulized erythrocytes, the membrane is in a stressed state, and therefore, they exhibit practically no change in shape.[8] The real part of the relative index of refraction of erythrocytes is $n_{rel} = 1.037$–1.055, the imaginary part is $\varkappa = 10^{-5}$–10^{-4},[4,9] and the most probable diffraction parameter is $\rho_0 = 2\pi rn/\lambda = 24$–$36$, where n is the refractive index of the medium in which the particles are located. The relative halfwidth of the distribution of erythrocytes is $\Delta = 0.4$–1.0.[4] The indicated optical parameters of the erythrocytes are given for radiation wavelength $\lambda = 0.63 \mu$m, used in the measurements. The shape of the erythrocytes (spherical or aspherical) is checked visually under the microscope. The maximum packing density c_v was obtained by centrifuging whole blood. The packing density values were obtained by successive dilution of the erythrocyte mass in saline solution.

Erythrocytes were chosen as the model medium for several reasons: first, because the object itself is of interest (in their natural state in whole blood, erythrocytes are close-packed), and second, because of the ability of erythrocytes to change shape at constant volume.[10] In addition, it is easy to obtain different packing densities of the erythrocyte mass, and finally, despite a low refractive index, because of the

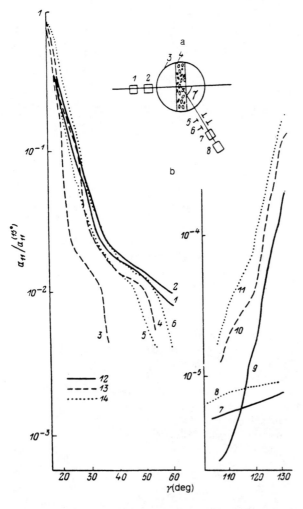

FIG. 1. (a) Optical line diagram of a device for measuring SM elements; (b) scattering functions of disk-shaped (1,3,5,9,10,11) and spherulized (2,4,5,7,8) erythrocytes as their density c_r changes: 0.6(12), 0.3(13), 0.1(14).

larization unit 2, spherical cell 3 with scattering volume 4, limiting diaphragms 5 and 6, and polarization unit 7, and enters radiation detector 8. The spherical surface of cell 3 (radius of curvature $R = 50$ mm) focuses the erythrocyte-scattered light on diaphragm 6. Microdiaphragms 5 and 6 form a point volume on the planar surface of two hemispheres. Because of the finite angular sizes of the source and receiver, and constructive conditions of formation of the scattering volume, the 0–15°, 70–110°, and 160–180° angular intervals were dead zones for measuring the SM elements and are not shown in the figures.

In general, for randomly oriented anisotropic spheres and for isotropic ellipsoids, the scattered-light matrix is[10,11]

$$\begin{pmatrix} a_{11} & a_{12} & 0 & 0 \\ a_{21} & a_{22} & 0 & 0 \\ 0 & 0 & a_{33} & a_{34} \\ 0 & 0 & a_{43} & a_{44} \end{pmatrix}. \tag{1}$$

For spherical isotropic scatterers $a_{12} = a_{21}$, $a_{34} = -a_{43}$, $a_{11} = a_{22} = 1$. $a_{33} = a_{44}$.[11] The complex measurements performed on all the SM elements of disk-shaped and spherulized erythrocytes, as their packing density changed, showed, first, that the general structure of the SM changed (the zero elements were considered to be those whose values were < 0.1). Second, for spherulized erythrocytes in comparison to matrix (1), the additional elements a_{41} and a_{42} ($a_{41} = a_{42}$) appeared, although they were small compared to the 0.1 level (Fig. 2).

$$\begin{pmatrix} a_{11} & a_{12} & 0 & 0 \\ a_{21} & a_{22} & 0 & 0 \\ 0 & 0 & a_{33} & a_{34} \\ a_{41} & a_{42} & a_{43} & a_{44} \end{pmatrix}. \tag{2}$$

The appearance in the SM of still another element a_{32} for disk-shaped erythrocytes can be explained by the presence of partial orientation of the particles in the monolayer[11]

large size of the particles studied, a dependence of the angular variation of the SM elements on their shape exists.[11]

The measurements were carried out with an automated polarization nephelometer, described in detail in Ref. 12, and permitting measurement of the angular dependence of all sixteen elements of the scattered-light matrix.

To estimate the measurement errors of the elements of the scattered-light matrix, verification measurements were made on model media with well-known properties. For this purpose, it was convenient to use polystyrene latexes embedded in agar, whose refractive index is well known, and the absorption coefficient in the visible region of the spectrum is negligible and does not affect the values being measured. The measurement errors were estimated from the deviations of the normalized elements of the scattered-light matrix of monodisperse latexes from the values calculated theoretically from Mie equations. It is shown that the error of determination of the SM elements (for latex diameters of 180 and 500 nm) does not exceed 10%.[12]

The optical layout of the apparatus is shown in Fig. 1(a). The beam of a He–Ne laser (LGN-207) traverses po-

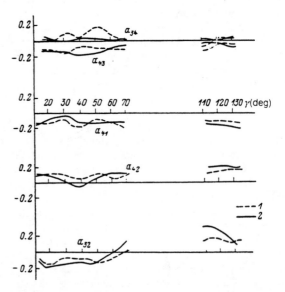

FIG. 2. Angular distributions of SM elements for disk-shaped (1) and spherulized (2) erythrocytes.

$$\begin{pmatrix} a_{11} & a_{12} & 0 & 0 \\ a_{21} & a_{22} & 0 & 0 \\ 0 & a_{32} & a_{33} & a_{34} \\ a_{41} & a_{42} & a_{43} & a_{44} \end{pmatrix}. \qquad (3)$$

It should be noted that the indicated elements a_{41}, a_{42}, a_{32} are much smaller than the remaining nonzero SM elements (Figs. 2 and 3). The small difference from zero of elements a_{41}, a_{42}, but larger than the measurement errors, is apparently due to the presence of a slight anisotropy of the optical properties of erythrocytes,[11] and the appearance of element a_{32} in the matrix (2) is due to the orientation of aspherical particles,[11,13] which will be manifested in our case, since the density of the preferred orientation of the disk-shaped particles is perpendicular to the scattering plane.[11]

We shall examine in more detail the angular dependence of the remaining nonzero SM elements of disk-shaped and spherulized erythrocytes as their packing density changes.

Element a_{11} characterizes the angular distribution of scattered light (scattering function), provided that unpolarized radiation is incident on the sample.

For clarity, the scattering functions [Fig. 1(b)] are represented as small angles ($\gamma \leqslant 70°$), where the dependence on the packing density c_v is visible, and at large angles ($\gamma \geqslant 110°$), where differences are observed in the variation of the scattering function for disk-shaped (curves 1,3,6,9,10,11) and spherulized (curves 2,4,5,7,8) erythrocytes.

Analysis of the experimental data showed that at small scattering angles ($\gamma \leqslant 60°$), as the packing density changes both for disks and for spheres, the slope of the scattering function $a_{11}(\gamma)$ changes [Fig. 1(b)], and not continuously, but with a minimum at $c_v \approx 0.25$ (curves 3 and 4). At low packing densities ($c_v < 0.1$), the scattering function for spheres (curve 5) is elongated more than for disks (curve 6), similarly to the data cited in Ref. 14. Conversely, at large c_v for spheres, the fall of $a_{11}(\gamma)$ (curve 2) has a milder slope as angle γ increases (curves 2 and 1).

The nonmonotonicity of the shift of the diffraction maxima for disk-shaped particles is manifested more strongly [Fig. 1(b), curves 1, 3, and 6]; this may be due to the fact that the intervals between the disks will, as c_v increases, be smaller than they are for spheres. It may be assumed that at significant packing densities, mainly the intervals between particles do the scattering, not the particles themselves, in accordance with the approximation discussed in Ref. 2. Small intervals between the particles make the indicatrix of the monolayer for disks more diffuse at large c_v.

As noted in Refs. 13 and 14, at observation angles $\gamma > 110°$, the angular variation of the scattering function for disk-shaped and spherulized erythrocytes may differ considerably. The measurements performed indicate that this pattern is preserved for higher packing densities [Fig. 1(b), curves 7–11], and the asphericity of erythrocytes exerts a stronger influence on the absolute value of scattering intensity than does the packing density. Summarizing the results of the measurements, calculations using Mie equations, as well as the results of Refs. 13 and 14, one can distinguish two groups of factors which differently affect the variation of the scattering function at large angles γ. The relative index of refraction and the asphericity and crenation (i.e., the presence of a microstructure on the surface of erythrocytes) have a greater effect on the scattering function. The influence of the absorption coefficient $\varkappa$ (10^{-6}–10^{-3}) and of polydispersity of the particles, characterized by modal dimension ρ, and distribution halfwidth Δ, is appreciably weaker.

Elements a_{12}, a_{21}. The measurements showed that in the range of measurement error, for spherulized erythrocytes, irrespective of the change in packing density, $a_{12} = a_{21}$ (Table I). For disk-shaped erythrocytes at angles $50 < \gamma < 140°$, the element $|a_{21}|$ is greater than $|a_{12}|$, and their difference, related to the partial orientation of erythrocytes in the monolayer, increases with the observation angle. In the remaining cases, $|a_{21}| = |a_{12}|$. A discrepancy of 0.1 between the values of a_{21} of spherulized erythrocytes (and correspondingly, disk-shaped ones) and the theoretical calculations of Ref. 15 is due to the fact that in our experiment, the observation angle γ is indicated without allowing for the refraction at the monolayer—cell glass boundary.

Our theoretical calculations using Mie equations[15] showed that a change in the diffraction parameter ρ for particles with $n_{rel} = 1.02$–1.05 at $\gamma > 130°$ has practically no effect on the magnitude of element a_{12} (Table II for the possible values of the erythrocyte parameters ($\rho_0 = 24$–36, $n_{rel} = 1.0$–1.05). The only parameter on which a_{12} substan-

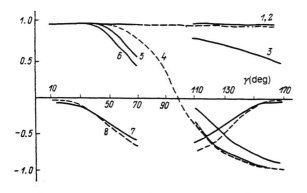

FIG. 3. Angular distributions of SM elements: $a_{12}(7)$, $a_{21}(8)$, $a_{33}(4,5,6)$, $a_{22}(1,2,3)$ for disk-shaped (3,4,7,8) and spherulized (2,6) erythrocytes. Dashed curves—theoretical calculation using Mie equations.

TABLE I. Matrix elements a_{12} (I) and a_{21} (II) of spherulized and disk-shaped erythrocytes for different packing densities c_v and scattering angles γ (γ in air).

c_v	Type of erythrocyte		40°	50°	120°	130°	140°
0.6	Sphere	I	0.22	0.3	0.48	0.31	0.24
		II	0.22	0.3	0.48	0.32	0.28
	Disk	I	0.14	0.42	0.4	0.33	0.22
		II	0.18	0.54	0.61	0.49	0.27
0.3	Sphere	I	0.19	0.35	0.45	0.30	0.30
		II	0.18	0.35	0.47	0.32	0.31
	Disk	I	0.17	0.24	0.55	0.31	0.24
		II	0.18	0.27	0.7	0.44	0.21
0.1	Sphere	I	0.28	0.41	0.46	0.29	0.23
		II	0.28	0.41	0.46	0.30	0.22
	Disk	I	0.2	0.29	0.54	0.35	0.24
		II	0.18	0.31	0.61	0.44	0.23

TABLE II. Values of matrix elements a_{12} calculated for different diffraction parameters ρ_0 and refractive indices n of the medium ($\Delta\rho/\rho_0 \lesssim 1$).

n	γ(deg)	ρ_0		
		24	36	48
1.036	110	0.805	0.803	0.799
	130	0.428	0.428	0.428
	140	0.269	0.268	0.268
1.05	110	0.709	0.654	0.526
	130	0.465	0.461	0.411
	140	0.320	0.319	0.285

tially depends at $\gamma > 140°$ was found to be the relative index of refraction n_{rel} (Table II).

Thus, since at $\gamma > 140°$ a_{12} substantially depends on the relative index of refraction n_{rel} of the particles and much less on the packing density c_v or particle size, it becomes possible in this range of γ to determine n_{rel} from the magnitude of a_{12}.

Element a_{22}. As is evident from Fig. 3, for disk-shaped erythrocytes, the magnitude of element a_{22} decreases as the observation angle γ increases (although the deviation from unity is not as large as for low packing densities,[13] where the value of a_{22} decreases as γ increases from 1 to 0.5). Apparently, this dependence is due to the appreciable contribution of multiple scattering at large scattering angles.[16] It is well known[11] that the deviation of a_{22} from unity increases with asphericity p. This most likely accounts for the decrease in a_{22} for disks.

Within experimental error, the change in packing density c_v did not affect the angular variation of element a_{22} for either disks or spheres. Therefore, these relationships are not shown in the figures.

Element a_{33}. It follows from the experimental data that at high packing densities c_v, just as in the case of low ones,[14] the asphericity of erythrocytes does not violate the relation $a_{33} = a_{44}$. The variation of element a_{33} does not differ from that of elements a_{44} in the entire range of observation angles and packing densities. A study of the effect of the shape of the behavior of element a_{33} found that the angular variation of element $a_{33}(\gamma)$ for disks and spheres differs quantitatively, while the general form of the curves remains unchanged over the entire range of observation angles (Fig. 3). The same dependence was observed at low packing densities c_v.[14] For all practical purposes, the effect of packing density on

the angular variation of a_{33} is not manifested, and lies in the range of measurement errors.

Thus, experimental studies of the angular variation of nonzero SM elements for disk-shaped and spherulized human erythrocytes have shown that as their packing density changes ($c_v = 0.06$–0.6): with the exception of element a_{11}, the angular variation of nonzero SM elements for disks and spheres remains practically unchanged at both low and high packing densities of erythrocytes; the asphericity of the scattering particles is manifested most strongly in the angular variation of a_{11} (particularly at $\gamma > 110°$), and to a lesser extent for elements a_{22} and a_{33}, irrespective of packing density; the difference between elements a_{12} and a_{21} can serve as a measure of the asphericity of the particles in the presence of their orientation relative to the observation plane.[4] Determination of the refractive index is possible from the value of a_{12} ($\gamma = 140$–$160°$) for an arbitrary shape of the erythrocytes and their packing density.

[1]Yu. M. Barabanenkov, Izv. Akad. Nauk SSSR Fiz. Atm. Okeana **18**, 720 (198).

[2]V. Twersky, J. Opt. Soc. Am. **60**, 1084 (1970).

[3]A. N. Ponyavina and V. G. Vereshchagin, Zh. Prikl. Spektrosk. **22**, 518 (1975).

[4]A. Ya. Khairullina, Opt. Spektrosk. **53**, 1043 (1982) [Opt. Spectrosc. (USSR) **53**, 623 (1982)].

[5]A. N. Ponyavina and V. G. Vereshchagin, Zh. Prikl. Spektrosk. **40**, 302 (1984).

[6]A. G. Borovoi, Opt. Spektrosk. **54**, 757 (1983) [Opt. Spectrosc. (USSR) **54**, 449 (1983)].

[7]V. A. Loiko, A. P. Ivanov, and V. P. Dik, Zh. Prikl. Spektrosk. **42**, 828 (1985).

[8]V. A. Levtov, *Rheology of the Blood* (Moscow, 1982).

[9]A. P. Ivanov, S. A. Makarevich, and A. Ya. Khairullina, Zh. Prikl. Spektrosk. **47**, 662 (1987).

[10]E. Ponder, J. Exp. Biol. **13**, 298 (1963).

[11]C. F. Bohren and D. R. Hufman, *Absorption and Scattering of Light by Small Particles* (Wiley, New York, 1983; Moscow, 1987).

[12]L. P. Shubochkin, *Author's abstract of candidate's dissertation* (Saratov), 1987.

[13]I. N. Plakhina, *Author's abstract of candidate's dissertation* (Moscow, 1975).

[14]G. S. Dubova, A. N. Korolevich, and A. Ya. Khairullina, Zh. Prikl. Spektrosk. **40**, 630 (1984).

[15]K. S. Shifrin and I. N. Salganik, *Tables on Light Scattering* (Leningrad, 1973).

[16]L. I. Chaikovskaya, *Author's abstract of candidate's dissertation* (Minsk, 1985).

Reprinted with permission from *Cytometry,* Vol. 8, pp. 539-544 (1987).
©1987 Wiley-Liss division of John Wiley & Sons, Inc.

Light-Scattering Polarization Measurements as a New Parameter in Flow Cytometry

B.G. de Grooth, L.W.M.M. Terstappen, G.J. Puppels, and J. Greve

Department of Applied Physics, Cell Characterization Group, University of Twente, 7500 AE Enschede,
The Netherlands

Received for publication August 8, 1986; accepted June 8, 1987

Polarization measurement of orthogonal light scattering is introduced as a new optical parameter in flow cytometry.

In the experimental setup, the electrical field of the incident laser beam is polarized in the direction of the sample flow. The intensity of the orthogonal light scattering polarized along the direction of the incoming laser beam is called depolarized orthogonal light scattering. Theoretical analysis shows that for small values of the detection aperture, the measured depolarization is caused by anisotropic cell structures and multiple scattering processes inside the cell.

Measurements of the orthogonal depolarized light scattering in combination with the normal orthogonal light scattering of human leucocytes revealed two populations of granulocytes. By means of cell sorting it was shown that the granulocytes with a relatively high depolarization are eosinophilic granulocytes. Similar experiments with human lymphocytes revealed a minor subpopulation of yet-unidentified lymphocytes with a relative large orthogonal light-scattering depolarization. The results were obtained with an argon ion laser tuned at different wavelengths as well as with a 630-nm helium neon laser.

These results show that measurement of depolarized orthogonal light scattering is a useful new parameter for flow-cytometric cell differentiation.

Key terms: Eosinophilic granulocytes, neutrophilic granulocytes, depolarization, blood cell differentiation

Light-scattering measurements are routinely used in flow cytometry (FCM). Most frequently, the forward or small angle light scattering (0.5° to 3°) is detected from which the cell size can be estimated (5). Since the forward light scattering is strongly dependent on the refraction index difference between cells and the external medium, cells with a damaged membrane show a decreased forward light scattering. This phenomena is used to discriminate vital from dead cells (3).

Another useful light-scattering parameter is obtained when scattered light within a cone at 90° with respect to the incoming laser beam is collected. This so-called orthogonal light scattering provides additional information on the structureness of the cells (1). Salzman et al. (6) have shown that human lymphocytes, monocytes, and granulocytes can be distinguished in unstained blood cells by light-scattering measurements, mainly due to differences in orthogonal light scattering. Similar measurements of mouse bone marrow cells, performed by Visser et al., revealed at least four subpopulations (9). Recently we have shown that human lymphocytes can be divided into two subpopulations on the basis of orthogonal light-scattering measurements (7,8). Cytotoxic lymphocytes, including natural killer cells, show an orthogonal light scattering which is about 70% larger than that of B-lymphocytes and regulatory T-cells.

Up to now, no efforts have been reported to obtain information on cell morphology by measuring the polarization of light scattering. In this paper we demonstrate that by using this technique a further discrimination between human blood cells can be obtained.

MATERIALS AND METHODS

Human blood was obtained by venipuncture from healthy individuals. Heparine was used as anticoagulant (150 USP U sodium heparine/10 ml Venoject Terumo Europe NV). Purified lymphocytes and granulocytes were obtained by density separation as described in detail elsewhere (7). Human leucocyte preparations were obtained by adding 190 ml of lysing buffer (8.29 g/liter NH_4Cl, 0.0037 g/liter Na_2EDTA, 1.00 g/liter $KHCO_3$) to 10 ml of whole blood and incubating for 20 min at 4°C. The lysed blood suspension was washed three times in phosphate-buffered saline (PBS). Cell suspensions were

---

Address reprint requests to B.G. de Grooth, University of Twente, Dept. of Applied Physics, Cell Characterization Group, P.O. Box 217, 7500 AE Enschede, The Netherlands.

adjusted to a concentration of 1×10^6/ml in PBS containing 0.005% sodium azide and 1% bovine serum albumin (BSA). Measurements were performed the same day to preserve cell viability.

Monodisperse polystyrene microspheres with a diameter of 1.6 μm and standard deviation of 0.05 μm were purchased from Polysciences (Polysciences Inc., Warrington, PA; cat. No. 7310).

Flow cytometric experiments were done with a homemade FCM equipped with a 3-W argon ion laser tuned to 488 nm, unless otherwise indicated (Coherent Radiation, Palo Alto, CA: model CR3) or when indicated with a 5mW helium neon laser (Spectra Physics, San Jose, CA; model 120 S). The optical measurements were performed in a quartz flow cell with a 250 μm $\times$ 250 μm square flow channel designed by us and produced by Hellma (Hellma GmbH & Co, Mullheim/Baden, W. Germany); additional experiments were done with a jet in air, using a FACS flow cell (Becton Dickinson, Sun Valley, CA). The argon laser was focused on the cell stream by means of two cylindrical lenses (focal length 200 and 20 mm) and the helium neon laser by means of a single spherical lens (focus length 70 mm). The forward light scatter was detected with a photodiode (model Pin 10-D, United Detector Technology) at angles between 2 and 17°. Orthogonal light scattering was collected with a Leitz microscope objective (H32, NA 0.6 collecting angles between 115° and 65°) and imaged on a diaphragm. With a normal glass plate placed at 45° toward the light beam, a small portion of the scattered light was directed to the first photomultiplier (Hamamatsu R928), which measured the total orthogonal light scattering. The transmitted portion of the light was led to the second photomultiplier (Hamamatsu R928), provided with a polaroid filter (HN7, Melles Griot, Irvine, CA). The filter was placed so as to absorb the scattered light polarized in the direction along the sample stream. The scattered light detected with this photomultiplier is referred to as depolarized orthogonal light scattering.

In order to obtain the absolute values of the depolarization ratio (D), we have calibrated the photomultipliers with respect to each other for both polarization directions. This was done by measuring $I_\perp$ and $I_\parallel$ (see theoretical considerations) of monodisperse polystyrene microspheres in two subsequent measurements with one photomultiplier. For these measurements the beam splitter was removed and the polarization filter was placed to transmit $I_\perp$ and $I_\parallel$, respectively. The value of D thus obtained was used to calibrate the signals, measured with the two photomultipliers, with respect to each other in the presence of the beam splitter. In this way the polarization effects of the beam splitter are also included.

Data were analyzed with a LSI 11/23 microcomputer and displayed as two-parameter density maps.

THEORETICAL CONSIDERATIONS

Figure 1 illustrates the optical arrangement of the orthogonal light-scattering experiments described here

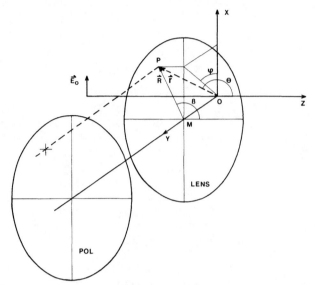

FIG. 1. Schematic drawing of the orthogonal light-scattering experiments defining the geometrical parameters involved. The incident light propagating along the z-axis is polarized along the x-direction. The light is scattered by a particle at the origin 0. The propagation direction of the scattered light is described by polar coordinates r, θ, and ϕ. The light is collected with a lens placed at the focal distance from the origin and analyzed with a polarizer (P). See Appendix for derivations of formal equations.

and defines the geometrical parameters used. An incoming laser beam propagates along the z-axis and is linearly polarized with incident electrical field E_0 along the x-axis. At the origin of our coordinate system the laser beam intersects the particles of the flow cytometer moving along the x-axis. The direction of the scattered light is described in spherical coordinates r, θ, and ϕ.

In general the amplitudes of the scattered light polarized in the θ and ϕ direction can now be described as (2)

$$E_\phi = (S_4 \cos\phi - S_1 \sin\phi) \, f \, E_0 \quad (1)$$
$$E_\theta = (S_2 \cos\phi - S_3 \sin\phi) \, f \, E_0 \quad (2)$$

where f is a complex expression for a spherical wave, inversely proportional to r, the distance between the scatterer and the detector, and S_1, S_2, S_3, and S_4 are the so-called amplitude functions (2), dependent on ϕ, θ, and the geometry and physical composition of the scatterer. The measurable light-scattering intensities I_ϕ and I_θ are related to these fields by

$$I_\phi = |E_\phi|^2 \quad (3)$$
$$I_\theta = |E_\phi|^2 \quad (4)$$

The light intensities measured using ideal polarizers transmitting only the x polarized or the z polarized fields are called $I_\parallel$ and $I_\perp$, respectively. $I_\perp$ is called the depolarized light-scattering intensity and the depolarization ratio is defined here as

$$D = \frac{I_\perp}{I_\perp + I_\parallel} \qquad (5)$$

For light scattered in the yz plane, i.e., orthogonal with respect to the polarization direction of the incident light, we have $\phi = 90°$ and we can write for $I_\parallel$ and $I_\perp$:

$$I_\parallel = \mid S_1 \, f \, E_0 \mid^2$$
$$I_\perp = \mid S_3 \, f \, E_0 \mid^2 \qquad (6)$$

Thus, whereas $I_\parallel$ is determined by S_1, measurement of the depolarized light-scattering intensity in this geometry yields information on the term S_3. The importance of this term will be illustrated briefly.

Mie theory shows that for homogeneous spheres, spherical shells, etc., the term S_3 is zero (2). S_3 becomes important for particles which are optically anisotropic (due to shape and/or composition) and for particles containing structures, so that multiple scattering becomes important. A simple but striking example of the latter is illustrated in Figure 2. We imagine a cell containing two intracellular spheres located on the x-axis. A particular incoming ray, traveling along the z-axis, is reflected along the x-axis by the first sphere and along the y-axis by the second sphere. Applying the laws of reflection we find that the polarization direction of this ray changes from along the x-axis to along the z-axis. Thus we see how multiple reflections can lead to depolarization and thus to contributions to the term S_3. The reader can easily verify this example with two mirrors and two polarizer sheets. In a similar way it can be shown that multiple scattering due to diffraction and refraction can also lead to depolarization (Puppels, unpublished results).

In a practical flow cytometer, the optical configuration is such that the detector, which collects orthogonally scattered light, gathers light from a conus around the y-axis. In that case depolarization is not only caused by S_3 but also by the other amplitude functions S_1, S_2, and S_4.

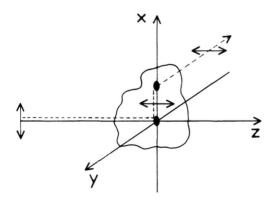

FIG. 2. Depolarization of orthogonal light scattering by multiple-scattering processes. An incident light ray is traced as it is reflected by two intracellular particles. The final scattered ray propagating along the negative y-axis is completely polarized in the z-direction.

This extra depolarization is due to the geometry of the measuring system and is called cross depolarization. It is closely related to the term "aperture polarization" used when describing fluorescence polarization experiments. In order to determine the origin of a measured depolarization signal we can analyze the dependence of the depolarization ratio on the angle ϕ. We place a rectangular diaphragm in front of the collection lens, limiting the angles of the collected light between $\phi = 90° \pm \Delta\phi$ and $\theta = 90° \pm \Delta\theta$. As is shown in the appendix, depolarization due to pure cross depolarization drops to zero proportional to $\Delta\phi^2$. The polarization ratio due to the S_3 term, however, reaches a constant nonzero value for small values of $\Delta\phi$.

RESULTS

We have investigated the orthogonally depolarized light scattering of human blood cells measured with a flow cytometer. Lymphocytes, granulocytes, and monocytes were selected by gating on forward and orthogonal light scattering of lysed peripheral blood cell preparations obtained from healthy donors. Erythrocytes were taken from whole blood diluted in PBS.

In Figure 3 two-parameter density maps of the depolarized orthogonal light scattering vs. the total orthogonal light scattering are plotted for the different cell populations. Figure 3a clearly reveals two populations of granulocytes. From Figure 3b it appears that the large majority of the lymphocytes and all monocytes have about the same polarization ratio (depolarized light scattering divided by the total orthogonal light scattering) but that a minor subpopulation of lymphocytes exists with a relatively large depolarization. The monocytes with a relatively larger orthogonal light scattering show no heterogenity (Fig. 3b). The results of Figure 3a and b could be reproduced with granulocytes and lymphocytes purified with density separation. Erythrocytes show no heterogenity (Fig. 3c).

The granulocyte subpopulations have been sorted and examined under the light microscope after May-Grünwald staining. The cells with a relatively high depolarization of orthogonal light scattering were identified as eosinophylic granulocytes (99% purity) whereas the other population consists of neutrophilic granulocytes (99% purity). The identification of the minor lymphocyte subpopulation of Figure 3b is still under investigation.

Whether the measured depolarization signals are due to cross depolarization or due to cellular structures was examined according to the method outlined in the theoretical considerations given above. The measured depolarization ratio was plotted vs. the acceptance angle $\Delta\phi$ of the collection objective for the different cell populations (Fig. 4). The curves were normalized at the maximum angle of 14.5°. Also included are the values measured with polystyrene microspheres with a diameter of 1.16 μm and a theoretical curve for perfect homogeneous spheres.

The absolute values of the depolarization ratios of the different particles are given in Table 1 for a small and a

411

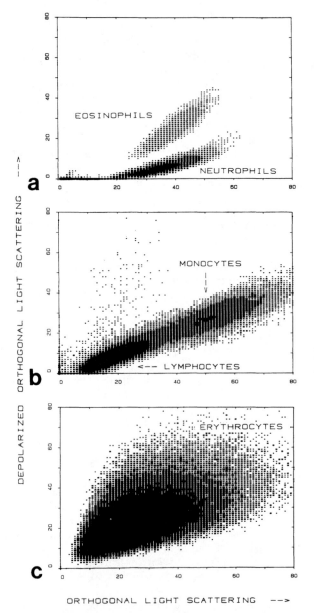

FIG. 3. Flow cytometric density map of orthogonal light scattering vs. depolarized orthogonal light scattering of different human blood cells. a) Lysed peripheral blood revealing neutrophilic and eosinophilic granulocytes. b) The same sample as Figure 3a but at different amplifications showing lymphocytes and monocytes. c) Erythrocytes.

large value of the angle of acceptance $\Delta\phi$.

Since the intensity of the depolarized orthogonal light scattering is not very high we verified that the measured light is indeed only due to elastic light scattering and not caused by autofluorescence. This was done by inserting a 500-nm shortwave pass filter in the detection optic; it did not affect the results. In addition, the illumination wavelength of the argon ion laser used was

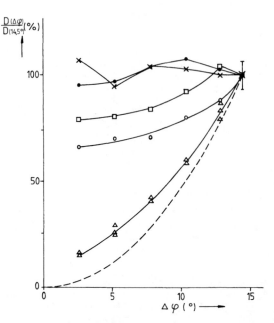

FIG. 4. Normalized depolarization ratio measured as function of the acceptance angle $\Delta\phi$ for neutrophils ($\bullet$), eosinophils ($\times$), lymphocytes ($\bigcirc$), monocytes ($\square$), and microspheres with a diameter of 1.16 μm ($\triangle$). The dashed line represents the theoretical curve for ideal spheres. The curves were normalized at a value for $\Delta\phi$ of 14.5°.

changed from 488 to 509 and 514 nm, and a helium neon laser of 630 nm was used. In all cases, the results obtained were the same.

Many flow cytometers, in particular flow sorters, make use of a jet in air configuration. In these systems a small obscuration bar is placed in front of the orthogonal light detection objective in order to block the laser light scattered by the cylindrical liquid jet. With such an obscuration bar, the relative contribution of the cross depolarization to the total depolarization is increased. We have used such a system with an obscuration bar effectively blocking the orthogonal light scattering with an angle ϕ between 87° and 92°. With this system using a 5 mW helium neon laser as light source, a clear discrimination between neutrophilic and eosinophilic granulocytes still was obtained (Fig. 5).

Table 1
Absolute Values of the Depolarization Ratios (D)[a]

	$\Delta\phi = 2.5°$	$\Delta\phi = 14.5°$
Eosinophilic granulocytes	0.047	0.044
Neutrophilic granulocytes	0.013	0.013
Monocytes	0.005	0.007
Lymphocytes	0.005	0.008
Microspheres	0.0062	0.039

[a]$D = I_\perp/(I_\perp + I_\parallel)$ is given for a small ($\Delta\phi = 2.5°$) and a large ($\Delta\phi = 14.5°$) value of the angle of acceptance $\Delta\phi$ of eosinophilic, neutrophilic granulocytes, monocytes, lymphocytes, and polystyrene microspheres with a diameter of 1.16 μm.

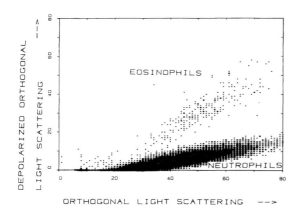

FIG. 5. Density map of orthogonal light scattering vs. the depolarized orthogonal light scattering of lysed whole blood measured with a 5 mW helium neon laser and a stream in air flow system. A clear discrimination between eosinophilic and neutrophilic granulocytes is obtained.

DISCUSSION

We have shown that measurement of the depolarized orthogonal light scattering adds to existing flow cytometers a new parameter which can provide useful information not available by other means. The observation that, with this parameter, eosinophylic granulocytes can be distinguished from neutrophylic granulocytes, is of practical as well as of theoretical importance. It is now feasible to construct a simple flow cytometer, provided with a low-power helium neon laser, which can perform white blood cell differentiation with unstained cells. The cells can be differentiated into cytotoxic lymphocytes (8), noncytotoxic lymphocytes (8), monocytes (6), neutrophilic granulocytes, and eosinophilic granulocytes (this study). Up to now, additional staining procedures had to be applied, or the weak autofluorescence had to be measured with an expensive argon ion laser (10). From a theoretical point of view, it is interesting to note that the eosinophils, with a large number of small intracellular particles (granulae), show a relative high depolarization ratio. This is in agreement with theoretical considerations that multiple-scattering processes result in depolarization. In Figure 4 we have investigated the nature of the measured depolarization signal. As discussed in the theoretical section, the cross-depolarization contributions vanish proportional to $\Delta\phi^2$. From the figure we may conclude that the observed depolarization of both granulocyte populations is mainly due to true cellular depolarization effects. For lymphocytes and monocytes about 25% of the depolarization measured with the full aperture (na = 0.6) might be due to cross depolarization.

The observed angle dependency of the depolarization ratio found with microspheres does not completely follow the theoretically expected behaviour for ideal spheres. For small values of $\Delta\phi$ a constant depolariza-

tion ratio is reached. This can either be caused by imperfect optical components or geometry used in the measurements or by imperfections in the spheres. The minor subpopulation of Figure 3b with a large depolarization could be cytotoxic cells in view of the relatively large orthogonal light scattering.

Weil and Chused (10) have shown that eosinophilic granulocytes show a larger autofluorescence than neutrophilic granulocytes. By changing the illumination and detection wavelengths we have excluded that autofluorescence contributes significantly to our depolarization measurements.

The frequently used jet in air flow cytometers are not particularly well suited for depolarization experiments since the angular region with minimal contributions from cross depolarization is blocked. However, even with such a system we could clearly resolve the two granulocyte subpopulations. This is in agreement with the results given in Figure 4 which show that cross depolarization, even for large apertures, is small for granulocytes.

We have shown that the explicit use of the polarization of the orthogonal light scattering extends the ability of flow cytometric cell differentiation. Measurement of depolarized light scattering can also be applied to other angles, e.g., forward and/or backward light scattering. We are currently investigating in our laboratory whether such measurements give additional information.

LITERATURE CITED

1. Benson MC, McDougal DC, Coffey DS: The applications of perpendicular and forward light scatter to assess nuclear and cellular morphology. Cytometry 5:515–522, 1984.
2. Hulst van de HC: Light scattering by small particles. Dover Publications, Inc., New York, 1981, Chapter 4, pp 28–39.
3. Julius MH, Sweet RG, Fatham CG: Fluorescence-activated cell sorting and its applications. In: Mammalian Cells: Probes and Problems, ERDA Symposium Series CONF-731007, Richmond CR, Petersen DF, Mullaney PF, et al. (eds). Technical Information Center, Oak Ridge, Tenn., 1975, p 107.
4. Marston PL: Uniform Mie theoretic analysis of polarized and crow-polarized optical glories. J Opt Soc Am 73:1816–1819, 1983.
5. Mullaney PF, Dean PN: The small angle light scattering of biological cells. Biophys J 10:764–772, 1970.
6. Salzman GC, Growell JM, Martin JC: Cell classification by laser light scattering: Identification and separation of unstained leukocytes. Acta Cytol (Baltimore) 19:374–377, 1975.
7. Terstappen LWMM, de Grooth BG, Nolten GMJ, ten Napel CHH, van Berkel W, Greve J: Physical discrimination between human T-lymphocyte subpopulations by means of light scattering, revealing two populations of T8-positive cells. Cytometry 7:178–183, 1986.
8. Terstappen LWMM, de Grooth BG, ten Napel CHH, van Berkel W, Greve J: Discrimination of human cytotoxic lymphocytes from regulatory and B-lymphocytes by orthogonal light scattering. J Immunol Methods 95:211–216, 1986.
9. Visser JW, Van den Engh GJ, van Bekkum DW: Light scattering properties of murine hematopoietic cells. Blood Cells 6:391–407, 1980.
10. Weil GJ, Chused TM: Eosinophil autofluorescence and its use in isolation and analysis of human eosinophils using flow microfluorometry. Blood 57:1099, 1981.

APPENDIX

In this appendix we will derive the formal equations for the amplitudes of the scattered electrical fields, as collected with an ideal lens and analyzed with a polaroid sheet. We will use the notation of Marston (4). Figure 1 shows the basic geometry. The lens is centered around the y-axis at point M and placed parallel to the xz plane at the focal distance from the origin 0. When the scattered wave reaches the lens it can be described by

$$\vec{E}_{sca} = E_\theta \vec{e}_\theta + E_\phi \vec{e}_\phi$$

with E_θ and E_ϕ given by eq. 1 and 2.

The scattered wave enters the lens at point P. We define the vector R from M to P and the angle between R and the z-axis β. The unit vector $\vec{e}_\beta$, defined in the usual way, is perpendicular to e_r and thus lies in the plane through $\vec{e}_\phi$ and $\vec{e}_\theta$. Therefore we can rewrite the previous equation as

$$\vec{E}_{sca} = E_\beta \vec{e}_\beta + E_\rho \vec{e}_\rho$$

where $\vec{e}_\rho$ is in the plane through $\vec{e}_\phi$ and $\vec{e}_\theta$ and is orthogonal to $\vec{e}_\beta$. E_β and E_ρ can be obtained by calculating

$$E_\beta = (\vec{e}_\theta \cdot \vec{e}_\beta) E_\theta + (\vec{e}_\phi \cdot \vec{e}_\beta) E_\phi$$
$$E_\rho = (\vec{e}_\theta \cdot \vec{e}_\rho) E_\theta + (\vec{e}_\phi \cdot \vec{e}_\rho) E_\phi$$

After the scattered field has passed the lens, the propagation direction is parallel toward the y-axis and the amplitude can be expressed in the polar coordinates $\vec{e}_R$ and $\vec{e}_\beta$

$$\vec{E}_{sca} = E_R \vec{e}_R + E_\beta \vec{e}_\beta$$

By passing through the lens, the amplitude in the direction of e_β remains unchanged, whereas $E_R = E_\rho$. If we now analyze the scattered wave in the direction parallel and perpendicular to the polarization direction of the incident field, with $e_\parallel = e_x$ and $e_\perp = e_z$, we obtain:

$$\vec{E}_{sca} = E_\parallel \vec{e}_\parallel + E_\perp \vec{e}_\perp$$

with

$$E_\parallel = [E_\theta(\vec{e}_\theta \cdot \vec{e}_\rho) + E_\phi(\vec{e}_\phi \cdot \vec{e}_\rho)] (\vec{e}_R \cdot \vec{e}_x)$$
$$+ [E_\theta(\vec{e}_\theta \cdot \vec{e}_\beta) + E_\rho(\vec{e}_\phi \cdot \vec{e}_\beta)] (\vec{e}_\beta \cdot \vec{e}_x)$$

$$E_\perp = [E_\theta(\vec{e}_\theta \cdot \vec{e}_\rho) + E_\phi(\vec{e}_\phi \cdot \vec{e}_\rho)] (\vec{e}_R \cdot \vec{e}_z)$$
$$+ [E_\theta(\vec{e}_\theta \cdot \vec{e}_\beta) + E_\phi(\vec{e}_\phi \cdot \vec{e}_\beta)] (\vec{e}_\beta \cdot \vec{e}_z)$$

By geometrical analysis the values of the scalar products can be obtained and in combination with 1 and 2 we get

$$E_\parallel = \frac{(\sin\phi + \sin\theta)(S_4\cos\phi - S_1\sin\phi) - \cos\phi\cos\theta(S_2\cos\phi - S_3\sin\phi)}{1 + \sin\phi \sin\theta} \cdot f E_0$$

$$E_\perp = \frac{(\sin\phi + \sin\theta)(S_2\cos\phi - S_3\sin\phi) - \cos\phi\cos\theta(S_4\cos\phi - S_1\sin\phi)}{1 + \sin\phi \sin\theta} \cdot f E_0$$

We see that for a practical situation E is not only dependent on S_3 but also on the other amplitude functions S_1, S_2, and S_4. These latter contributions are called cross or aperture depolarization.

We take $\phi = 90° + \Delta\phi$ and $\theta = 90° + \Delta\theta$. For small values of $\Delta\phi$ and $\Delta\theta$ we get

$$E_\perp = [-S_3 + \Delta\phi \, S_2 + O(\Delta\phi^2, \Delta\theta^2, \Delta\phi\Delta\theta)] \cdot f E_0$$

where $O(\Delta\phi^2, \Delta\theta^2, \Delta\phi\Delta\theta)$ stands for higher orders than $\Delta\phi$ and $\Delta\theta$. Thus, the depolarized orthogonal light scattering is determined by S_3 and the cross depolarization is in first-order approximation dependent on $\Delta\phi S_2$. To analyze the $\Delta\phi$ dependency we maintain a fixed value for $\Delta\theta$ and vary $\Delta\phi$. If the depolarization is entirely due to cross depolarization we have $S_3 = S_4 = 0$ (as for ideal spheres) and we obtain

$$R = \frac{I_\perp}{I_\parallel + I_\perp}$$

$$= \frac{\int_{90-\Delta\theta}^{90+\Delta\theta} \int_{90-\Delta\phi}^{90+\Delta\phi} |E_\perp|^2 \, d\theta d\phi}{\int_{90-\Delta\theta}^{90+\Delta\theta} \int_{90-\Delta\phi}^{90+\Delta\phi} |E_\parallel|^2 + |E_\perp|^2 \, d\theta d\phi}$$

$$= \frac{1}{3} \Delta\phi^2 \cdot k$$

where k is independent on $\Delta\phi$. The polarization term due to S_3, is independent of $\Delta\phi$.

Section Three
Eye Tissue Optics

Reprinted from *Applied Optics*, Vol. 10(3), pp. 459-473 (March 1971).

Theory of Transparency of the Eye

G. B. Benedek

The present work relates the turbidity of the eye to microscopic spatial fluctuations in its index of refraction. Such fluctuations are indicated in electron microscope photographs. By examining the superposition of phases of waves scattered from each point in the medium, we provide a mathematical demonstration of the Bragg reflection principle which we have recently used in the interpretation of experimental investigations: namely, that the scattering of light is produced only by those fluctuations whose fourier components have a wavelength equal to or larger than one half the wavelength of light in the medium. This consideration is applied first to the scattering of light from collagen fibers in the normal cornea. We demonstrate physically and quantitatively that a limited correlation in the position of near neighbor collagen fibers leads to corneal transparency. Next, the theory is extended to predict the turbidity of swollen, pathologic corneas, wherein the normal distribution of collagen fibers is disturbed by the presence of numerous *lakes*—regions where collagen is absent. A quantitative expression for the turbidity of the swollen cornea is given in terms of the size and density of such lakes. Finally, the theory is applied to the case of the cataractous lens. We assume that the cataracts are produced by aggregation of the normal lens proteins into an albuminoid fraction and provide a formula for the lens turbidity in terms of the molecular weight and index of refraction of the individual albuminoid macromolecules. We provide a crude estimate of the mean albuminoid molecular weight required for lens opacity.

I. Introduction

In 1957, Maurice produced a pioneering analysis of the transparency of the corneal stroma.[1] Electron microscope photographs[2,3] had shown that the stroma consists of long fibers of collagen in a mucopolysaccharide ground substance. Maurice calculated the scattering of light produced by each collagen fiber. He was able to show that, if each fiber radiated *independently* of the others, a little more than 90% of the incident light would be scattered. Such a cornea would be opaque. Maurice rightly concluded that to understand the transparency it was necessary to take into account the correlation in the phases of the waves scattered from each fiber.

Perhaps the simplest and most striking demonstration of the effects of phase correlation in scattering is found in the diffraction of light and x rays from perfectly regular gratings or lattices. In such arrays the position of each scatterer is known exactly relative to all the others, and it is simple to calculate the summation of the phases of the scattered waves.

Calculation shows that the light scattered from a perfectly regular lattice is essentially zero in all directions except those few which correspond to Bragg reflections. It was therefore natural for Maurice to suggest that a similar perfect regularity existed in the corneal stroma: "For a tissue to be transparent it is necessary that its fibrils are parallel, equal in diameter and have their axes disposed in a lattice."[1]

Despite the mathematical appeal of the perfect lattice, it is not necessary that the stromal fibers be arranged in a lattice to obtain transparency. Lattice regularity neither is required theoretically nor is it found experimentally. The Bowman's zone of the shark is a striking experimental case in point. Here the collagen fibers are arranged in apparently complete disorder, their axes being randomly oriented in every direction. Goldman and Benedek observed that the thickness of this zone in the shark is so great that if these fibers were treated as independent scatterers the shark cornea would be opaque.[4] Clearly, even in this disordered array, the phase relations between the waves scattered from each fiber reduces substantially the intensity of the scattered light. To understand this theoretically, Goldman and Benedek pointed out that the collagen fibers in both human and shark stroma are spaced by distances small compared to the wavelength of light. As a result there is considerable correlation between the phases of light waves scattered by neighboring fibers, and this will produce the required reduction in the scattered intensity. They went on to point

The author is with the Department of Physics and Center for Materials Science and Engineering, Massachusetts Institute of Technology, Cambridge, Massachusetts 02139.

Received 28 July 1970.

out that the theory of the scattering of light from random arrays shows that large scattering and consequent opacity results only if there are substantial fluctuations in the index of refraction which take place over distances comparable to or larger than the wavelength of light.[4] In a later experimental investigation they showed that opaque corneas did in fact contain irregularities in the density of the collagen fibers and so-called lakes where there was no collagen. The dimensions of those irregularities and lakes were indeed comparable to or larger than the light wavelength.[5] Our assertion that lattice structure is not essential for transparency has been investigated in detail in two recent papers by Feuk[6] and by Hart and Farrell.[7] The former author observed that the arrangement of stromal fibers was pictorially consistent with random displacements of the fibers around perfect lattice positions. The rms displacement found to be qualitatively consistent with the electron micrographs was about one tenth of the average interfiber spacing. Feuk then used the Debye-Waller theory of thermal diffuse x-ray scattering to calculate the scattering of light from this arrangement of fibers and found that the theoretical magnitude of the scattering was consistent with the observed scattering from normal stroma. While this approach provides a useful semiquantitative analysis of the scattering, it suffers from the defect of not properly including the effects of correlation in position between pairs of neighboring fibers. It is important to include this correlation to calculate correctly the wavelength dependence of the scattering.

Hart and Farrell alternatively computed the detailed probability distribution function for the relative position of fibers from photographs of corneal stroma. This distribution function showed that the position of pairs of collagen fibers remained correlated only over two near neighbors at most. This is very different from a perfect lattice. They were able to show, by a precise mathematical summation of the phases of the waves scattered by such a partially ordered array, that both the magnitude and the wavelength dependence of the scattered light was in good agreement with that found experimentally.

In this paper we present:

1. A simple rigorous proof of the principle that light is scattered only by those fluctuations in the index of refraction whose wavelengths are larger than one-half of the wavelength of light in the medium. This principle was used without proof as the theoretical basis of our previous papers,[4,5] which originally demonstrated that a perfect lattice of collagen fibers was not necessary for transparency.

2. A physical explanation of the complex mathematical analysis of Hart and Farrell[7] which shows how their main numerical results can be obtained approximately in a simple way.

3. The first theoretical computation of the turbidity of a swollen pathologic cornea. The calculation numerically supports our view[5] that the lakes present in

the electron micrographs are responsible for the opacity of these edematous corneas.

4. Finally, we present a calculation of the turbidity of the cataractous lens under the assumption that the opacity is produced by high molecular weight protein aggregates whose index of refraction differs from that of the background proteins. This calculation provides a quantitative relationship between the turbidity of the lens and the molecular weight, index of refraction, and concentration of such aggregates. It is hoped that this calculation will stimulate biochemical efforts to establish (or disprove) the existence of such aggregates.

As this subject is of great interest to the research ophthalmologist, we have endeavored to present the theory in its simplest mathematical form. We hope by this means and by careful presentation of the concepts involved to bring out clearly the subtle physical considerations that lead to transparency or opacity.

II. Scattering of Light from a Two-Dimensional Array

A. Normal Corneal Stroma

Electron microscope photographs show that the corneal stroma consists of lamellae within which collagen fibers are laid down approximately parallel to each other in a mucopolysaccharide ground substance. We shall consider the scattering of light from a single lamella. The scattering effect of many lamella follows simply from that of a single one. Let the fibers be arranged so that their axes are parallel to the z direction, as shown in Fig. 1. In Fig. 1, 0 is the arbitrary origin of the xyz coordinate system. Then the vector $\mathbf{R}_j$ from this origin to the intersection of each fiber with the xy plane will specify the position of each fiber. In general, regardless of the orientation of the fibers, or the location of the field point, the fiber positions can be specified completely in terms of the two-dimensional position vectors $\mathbf{R}_j$ which specify the points of intersection of the fibers in that plane which includes the observation point and is normal to the fiber axis.

The incident light wave has the form $E_0 e^{i(\mathbf{k}_0 \cdot \mathbf{r} - \omega_0 t)}$;

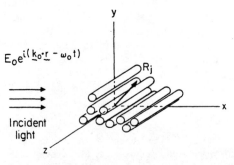

Fig. 1. Schematic diagram of arrangement of collagen fibers in a lamella. The incident light is shown propagating along the x direction.

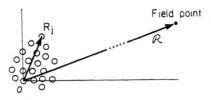

Fig. 2. Schematic diagram showing the positions of the observation point (or field point) ℛ and the source point $\mathbf{R}_j$ for fibers in a lamella.

$\mathbf{k}_0$ is the wave vector of the incident wave in the medium. The magnitude of $\mathbf{k}_0$ is $2\pi/(\lambda/n)$, where λ is the wavelength of the light in vacuum and n is the mean index of refraction. $\omega_0 = 2\pi\nu_0$ is the angular frequency of the light wave. We use here the complex exponential as a mathematically convenient means of expressing the sinusoidal traveling light wave. As this light wave falls on the fiber–ground substance combination, the oscillating electric field in the light wave induces at each point in the medium an oscillating electric dipole moment whose size depends on the square of the index of refraction at that point. These oscillating dipoles then each reradiate a new electric field in all directions in space. All these radiated wavelets add together to produce both the transmitted light beam and the sideways scattered light. The scattered light removes energy from the incident beam and thereby decreases the intensity of the transmitted beam. Thus, because of the sideways scattering, the transmitted beam is weaker than the incident beam. Consequently, we find that the scattering medium is not perfectly transparent. The calculation of the turbidity of a medium therefore requires an evaluation of the amount of light it scatters.

If the stromal collagen fibers had an index of refraction (n_c) that was the same as that of the ground substance (n_t) there would be no net scattered field. The sum of all the fields radiated from each point in the medium would add up to zero in all directions except in the direction of the transmitted beam. The scattering of light can occur only if there is a difference between the index of refraction of the collagen and the ground substance. Insofar as the scattering of light is concerned, we may regard the corneal stroma as being made up of fibers each of which produces a scattered field proportional to $(n_c{}^2 - n_t{}^2)$.

1. The Field Scattered by Each Collagen Fiber

The electric field radiated from a single collagen fiber located at the position $\mathbf{R}_j$ contains two parts: an amplitude part and a phase part. The amplitude part gives the size of the radiated field. The phase part tells precisely where this scattered field is in its oscillation cycle. This phase factor crucially determines the scattering process, because, as we add together the effect of many scatterers, the net result depends in detail on the summation of phases of the waves scattered from each fiber.

If a collagen fiber is at the point $\mathbf{R}_j$, the electric field

that it scatters to the field point at the position ℛ (see Fig. 2) is given by

$$E_j(\mathcal{R},t) = E'_{0j} e^{i(k_0\mathcal{R} - \omega_0 t)} e^{i(\mathbf{k}_0 - \mathbf{k}) \cdot \mathbf{R}_j}. \tag{1}$$

In the succeeding paragraphs we shall discuss and define each of the factors that enters into Eq. (1).

We assume that $\mathcal{R} \gg R_j$. The amplitude factor is E'_{0j}, and the phase factor is $e^{i(\mathbf{k}_0 - \mathbf{k}) \cdot \mathbf{R}_j}$. The factor $e^{i(k_0\mathcal{R} - \omega_0 t)}$ is the same for all the fibers since ℛ is the distance from the origin to the field point. This factor represents the fact that the radiated field is an electromagnetic disturbance with the same wavelength and frequency as that of the exciting field.

In subsequent analysis the amplitude factor $\mathbf{E}'_0$ will not be consequential. Nevertheless for the sake of completeness we write below the magnitude and direction of $\mathbf{E}'_{0j}$ if the incident field $\mathbf{E}_0$ is polarized as shown in Fig. 3. The scattered field is a function of the distance r in the xy plane and the angle θ between the x axis and the direction of r. As indicated in Fig. 3, r is the distance in the xy plane from the axis of the fiber to the observation or field point. We break $\mathbf{E}'_0$ into a component in the z direction and a component in the xy plane in terms of the unit vectors $\hat{1}_z$ and $\hat{1}_\theta$. In the case that the radius of the fiber r_0 is small compared to the wavelength of light λ in the medium outside the fiber, and if all the fibers are within a region small compared to the distance ℛ to the field point, then E'_{0j} is independent of the position $\mathbf{R}_j$ of fiber and is given by

$$E'_0 = \frac{E_0}{4} \left(\frac{\lambda}{r}\right)^{\frac{1}{2}} \left(\frac{2\pi r_0}{\lambda}\right)^2 (m^2 - 1)\left[\hat{1}_z \cos\gamma \right.$$
$$\left. + \hat{1}_\theta \left(\frac{2}{m^2 + 1}\right) \sin\gamma \, \cos\theta \right], \tag{2}$$

where $m = n_c/n_i$. This result[7,8] states that when the incident field is polarized along z, the scattered field is polarized entirely along the z direction and is independent of θ. However, when the incident field is polarized along y, the field is in the xy plane in the di-

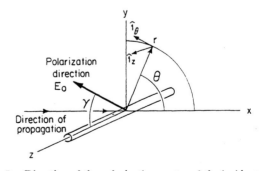

Fig. 3. Direction of the polarization vector of the incident light field (E_0) and incident propagation direction (x). Also shown are the unit vectors $\hat{1}_z$ and $\hat{1}_\theta$ that are used to specify the polarization of the scattered field as observed a distance r from the axis of a single scattering collagen.

419

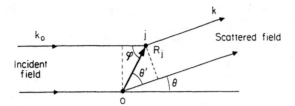

Fig. 4. Geometric representation of the difference in optical path between scattering from a fiber situated at the origin O, and one situated at the source point $\mathbf{R}_j$. The scattered direction is specified by the scattering angle θ.

rection of $\hat{1}_\theta$ and its amplitude varies as $\cos\theta$ in accordance with dipole radiation. The amplitude of the scattering from each fiber is proportional to the square of the fiber radius and is inversely proportional to $r^{\frac{1}{2}}$ because each fiber is regarded as an infinite cylinder. Because of the cylindrical symmetry the radiated field propagates only in the plane of the vector $\mathbf{R}_j$. In Figs. 1–3 this plane is the xy plane.

The factor $e^{i(\mathbf{k}_0-\mathbf{k})\cdot\mathbf{R}_j}$ in Eq. (1) merits careful consideration. Here, $\mathbf{k}_0$ is the wave vector of the incident light, and $\mathbf{k}$ is the wave vector of the scattered light wave. This exponential represents the effect on the scattered field of the difference in path between rays scattered from the fiber at $\mathbf{R}_j$ and a fiber at O. We can see this in Fig. 4. The ray emanating from O and moving in the scattered direction θ travels a distance $R_j \cos\theta'$ further in its path to the observer of the scattered field than the ray scattered from j. In units of the optical phase this difference is $[2\pi/(\lambda/n)](R_j \cos\theta')$, where λ/n is the wavelength of light in the stroma. It must be observed, however, that the oscillation induced by the incident field at the point $\mathbf{R}_j$ took place at a time later than that at O. This introduces a factor $(2\pi/\lambda/n)R_j \cos\varphi$ to describe this retardation. The net difference in optical phase between rays scattered from O and j then is

$$\Delta\Phi = [2\pi/(\lambda/n)]R_j(\cos\theta' - \cos\varphi). \quad (3)$$

It is convenient to express this in terms of the wave vectors $\mathbf{k}_0$ and $\mathbf{k}$. $\mathbf{k}_0$ is a vector pointing in the propagation direction of the incident light and having length $2\pi(\lambda/n)$, whereas $\mathbf{k}$ is a vector of the same length but pointing in the direction of the scattered wave. Using the dot product notation, viz.,

$$\mathbf{k}_0\cdot\mathbf{R}_j = [2\pi/(\lambda/n)]R_j \cos\varphi, \quad (4)$$

$$\mathbf{k}\cdot\mathbf{R}_j = [2\pi/(\lambda/n)]R_j \cos\theta', \quad (5)$$

we see that we may write the phase difference $\Delta\Phi$ in terms of the difference vector $\mathbf{k} - \mathbf{k}_0 = \mathbf{K}$. Here $\mathbf{K}$ is called the scattering vector:

$$\Delta\Phi = (\mathbf{k} - \mathbf{k}_0)\cdot\mathbf{R}_j = \mathbf{K}\cdot\mathbf{R}_j. \quad (6)$$

The scattering vector $\mathbf{K}$ will enter our discussion continually, so let us examine its properties at this point. Since $\mathbf{K}$ is the difference between $\mathbf{k}_0$ and $\mathbf{k}$, we see from Fig. 5 that its magnitude is

$$K = 2k_0 \sin\theta/2 = [4\pi/(\lambda/n)] \sin(\theta/2). \quad (7)$$

This figure also shows clearly that the direction of $\mathbf{K}$ is perpendicular to the plane bisecting $\mathbf{k}_0$ and $\mathbf{k}$.

2. The Field and the Intensity of Light Scattered from Many Fibers

We now calculate the total electric field and the total power scattered by all the fibers. The total electric field as observed at some field point is the sum of the electric fields radiated by each fiber. If the observation distance $\mathfrak{R}$ is large compared to the corneal thickness then E'_{0_j} is independent of fiber position (j), so that if there are a total of N illuminated fibers we have the following expression for the total scattered field $E_{\text{tot}}(\mathfrak{R}, t)$:

$$\mathbf{E}_{\text{tot}}(\mathfrak{R}, t) = \sum_{j=1}^{N} \mathbf{E}_j(\mathfrak{R}, t) = \sum_{j=1}^{N} \mathbf{E}'_0 e^{i\mathbf{K}\cdot\mathbf{R}_j} e^{ik_0\mathfrak{R} - \omega t}, \quad (8)$$

or

$$\mathbf{E}_{\text{tot}}(\mathfrak{R}, t) = \mathbf{E}'_0 e^{ik_0\mathfrak{R} - \omega t} \sum_{j=1}^{N} e^{i\mathbf{K}\cdot\mathbf{R}_j}. \quad (9)$$

The last term, which is the sum of the phase factors of each of the scattered fields can be called the interference function I:

$$I \equiv \sum_{j=1}^{N} e^{i\mathbf{K}\cdot\mathbf{R}_j}. \quad (10)$$

Since, as we have pointed out earlier, the $\mathbf{R}_j$ vectors are in a plane, the interference function is a sum over positions in a plane. Equation (9) shows very clearly that the total scattered field is determined by the summation of many waves at a particular point in space. Each of the constituent waves has a different phase from the others. The summation of waves is illustrated schematically in Fig. 6. The interference function I describes the total sum of all the waves adding together, some with positive values, some with negative values. It is an interference function because the net result of all the waves is determined by the total effect of many constructive and destructive interferences between the constituent waves. The scattering of light waves from collagen fibers is perfectly analogous to the superposition of many waves on the surface of a ripple tank. In such a tank, surface waves are generated at one side of the tank by two or more ripple generators. At every point in the tank the net displacement of the

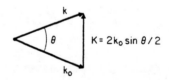

Fig. 5. Geometry of the scattering process. The wave vector of the incident light is $\mathbf{k}_0$, the wave vector of the scattered light is $\mathbf{k}$. The scattering vector is the difference vector. Its length is $2k_0 \sin\theta/2$.

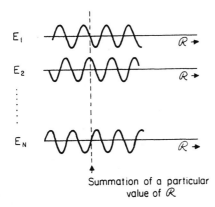

Fig. 6. The total scattered electric field at some particular field point ($\mathcal{R}$) is the sum of the fields radiated from each fiber. The value of the sum depends on the phases of each of the constituent waves, as is indicated above.

surface is fixed by the superposition of the surface waves. In some regions at a particular moment the waves interfere constructively to produce a large amplitude disturbance. At other points the waves destructing interfere and give no net displacement. The light waves superpose in a similar way. The result at any point in space is determined by the superposition of the phases of all the waves that exist at that point. The interference function therefore is at the very heart of the calculation of the scattered field. In the discussion that follows we show how a careful consideration of this function leads to an understanding of the transparency and the opacity of the cornea.

Let us write the interference function of Eq. (10) in an alternative form. For convenience we introduce the well known delta function $\delta(R - R_j)$ which has the property that its integral

$$\int_A d^2R\delta(R - R_j)$$

is zero if the area of integration does not include $\mathbf{R}_j$, and the integral is unity if the area does include the point $\mathbf{R}_j$. In terms of these delta functions, which in effect locate the positions of the fibers, we may write I as an integral over a sum of delta functions, viz.,

$$I = \int_A d^2R e^{i\mathbf{K}\cdot\mathbf{R}}\left(\sum_{j=1}^{N}\delta(\mathbf{R} - \mathbf{R}_j)\right). \quad (11)$$

Here A is the total illuminated area of the lamella and N is the total number of fibers in the illuminated area.

Now, if the number of fibers in the scattering region is sufficiently large that there are many such particles in each area of dimension $(1/K) \times (1/K)$, then, since the factor $e^{i\mathbf{K}\cdot\mathbf{R}}$ is constant in each such small area, we may describe the sum of delta functions as a local number density $\rho(R)$. Thus we write

$$\sum_{j=1}^{N}\delta(\mathbf{R} - \mathbf{R}_j) = \rho(\mathbf{R}). \quad (12)$$

This density ρ has some average value $\langle\rho\rangle$ which is

the same at all points in space. However, as one moves from one region to another the density of fibers will fluctuate around this average value, so that we should write

$$\rho(\mathbf{R}) = \langle\rho\rangle + \Delta\rho(\mathbf{R}), \quad (13)$$

where $\Delta\rho(\mathbf{R})$ is the deviation of the density in the region around $\mathbf{R}$ from the average density $\langle\rho\rangle = (N/A)$. If we put Eq. (13) into Eq. (11) we obtain

$$I = \int_A d^2\mathbf{R}e^{i\mathbf{K}\cdot\mathbf{R}}\langle\rho\rangle + \int d^2\mathbf{R}e^{i\mathbf{K}\cdot\mathbf{R}}\Delta\rho(\mathbf{R}). \quad (14)$$

The first integral has the property that it is equal to zero, if A is large compared to the wavelength of light, for all values of $\mathbf{K}$ except for $\mathbf{K} = 0$. Thus the uniform part of the density produces no scattering of light to the side. The scattering light is produced entirely by fluctuations in the density, and the magnitude of the scattering grows larger as the fluctuations in density grow larger. We may carry this observation further by recognizing that the final term in Eq. (14) is in fact just the fourier component of the density fluctuation whose wave vector is equal to the scattering vector $\mathbf{K}$. The meaning of this remark may be understood in the following way. In Fig. 7 is plotted schematically the fluctuation in the density as one moves in some direction in the scattering medium. This random fluctuation in the density can be looked upon as being made up of many perfectly sinusoidal waves of wave vector $\mathbf{q}$, each of which has some amplitude $\Delta\rho(\mathbf{q})$ in the following way:

$$\Delta\rho(\mathbf{R}) = \frac{1}{2\pi}\int_A d^2\mathbf{q}e^{i\mathbf{q}\cdot\mathbf{R}}\Delta\rho(\mathbf{q}). \quad (15)$$

This is the mathematical statement that $\Delta\rho(\mathbf{R})$ is a sum of sinusoidal waves $e^{i\mathbf{q}\cdot\mathbf{R}}$ each of which has amplitude $\Delta\rho(\mathbf{q})$. This amplitude $\Delta\rho(\mathbf{q})$ is determined by $\Delta\rho(\mathbf{R})$ by inverting Eq. (15), namely

$$\Delta\rho(\mathbf{q}') = \frac{1}{2\pi}\int_A d^2\mathbf{R}e^{i\mathbf{q}'\cdot\mathbf{R}}\Delta\rho(\mathbf{R}). \quad (16)$$

This equation is very similar to Eq. (14). In fact the final term in Eq. (14) is exactly equal to $\Delta\rho(\mathbf{q}')$ when $\mathbf{q}' = \mathbf{K}$. Thus, of all the fourier components present in a sinusoidal decomposition of the density fluctuations only that which has a periodicity or a wavelength (λ_f) equal to $2\pi/K$ is responsible for the scattering of light in the direction θ. Since

$$2\pi/\lambda_f = K = [4\pi/(\lambda/n)]\sin\tfrac{1}{2}\theta, \quad (17)$$

we may write

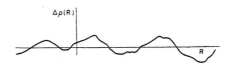

Fig. 7. Representation of the random spatial fluctuation in the fiber density $\Delta\rho(R)$ as a function of position (R) inside the cornea.

421

$$\lambda_f = \frac{(\lambda/n)}{2 \sin(\theta/2)}. \tag{18}$$

This equation is nothing other than the famous Bragg reflection condition. In the present context it can be understood to mean that light is scattered an angle θ if there exists in the scattering medium a fluctuation in density or index of refraction whose wavelength is given by $[\lambda/2n \sin(\theta/2)]$. The smallest such wavelength is one-half of the wavelength of light in the medium. It is on the basis of this very general consideration (which also applies in three dimensions) that we have suggested previously[4,5] that the scattering of light is produced by those fluctuations in density whose spatial dimensions are comparable to or larger than one half of the wavelength of light. Electron microscope photographs resolve much smaller structures, of course. In examining such photographs for the source of the transparency or opacity of ocular media, one must search for those structural features that contain fourier components whose wavelengths are comparable to or larger than the wavelength of light.

In the discussion which follows, I shall show why the fourier amplitude $\Delta\rho(\mathbf{K})$ is small in normal corneal stroma. The discussion given above shows that

$$I = \int d^2 R e^{i\mathbf{K}\cdot\mathbf{R}} \Delta\rho(\mathbf{R}) = 2\pi\Delta\rho(\mathbf{K}). \tag{19}$$

The intensity of the scattered light is proportional to the square of the scattered electric field. Using Eqs. (9) and (10) the squared electric field is

$$E^2_{tot}(\mathfrak{R}, t) = |E'_0|^2 |I|^2 = 4\pi^2 |E'_0|^2 |\Delta\rho(\mathbf{K})|^2. \tag{20}$$

To calculate $|I|^2$ it would appear that we would need to know in detail the precise distribution of fibers in the lamella. This we do not know. The difficulty can be circumvented as follows. Suppose we imagine that we scatter light not from a single lamella but from a succession or an ensemble of many lamella. The intensity of the light scattered from each lamella will be different, but all the scattered intensities will fluctuate around an average value. Similarly, the square of the interference function will fluctuate around some average $\langle |I|^2 \rangle$. It is this ensemble average, denoted by $\langle \rangle$, which measures the magnitude of the scattered intensity, and it is this average that we will calculate. It should be realized that in the corneal stroma such an average occurs as the light is scattered from many lamellae. Thus the scattered light intensity is proportional to the product $\langle |E'_0|^2 \rangle \langle |I|^2 \rangle$. The first average is taken over all orientations of fibers relative to the incident light polarization. The second average is taken over the distribution of fiber positions. The great advantage of the ensemble average is that it does not require knowledge of the detailed microscopic properties of a particular lamella but depends only on a statistical or probabilistic description of the fiber arrangements.

We can now calculate $\langle |I|^2 \rangle$ in the following way. From Eq. (10) we have

$$\langle |I|^2 \rangle = \left\langle \sum_j \sum_k e^{i\mathbf{K}\cdot(\mathbf{R}_j - \mathbf{R}_k)} \right\rangle. \tag{21}$$

Introducing the delta function representation again, this can be expressed as

$$\langle |I|^2 \rangle = \int_A d^2\mathbf{R} \int d^2\mathbf{R}' e^{i\mathbf{K}\cdot(\mathbf{R}-\mathbf{R}')}$$
$$\times \left\langle \sum_j \sum_k \delta(\mathbf{R} - \mathbf{R}_j)\delta(\mathbf{R}' - \mathbf{R}_k) \right\rangle. \tag{22}$$

The ensemble average of the double sum can be decomposed as follows:

$$\left\langle \sum_j \sum_k \delta(\mathbf{R} - \mathbf{R}_j)\delta(\mathbf{R}' - \mathbf{R}_k) \right\rangle$$
$$= \left\langle \sum_{l=1}^{N} \delta(\mathbf{R} - \mathbf{R}_l)\delta(\mathbf{R}' - \mathbf{R}_l) \right\rangle$$
$$+ \left\langle \sum_{\substack{j \neq k \\ j,k}} \delta(\mathbf{R} - \mathbf{R}_j)\delta(\mathbf{R}' - \mathbf{R}_k) \right\rangle. \tag{23}$$

N is the total number of fibers illuminated. The first term on the right-hand side of Eq. (23) comes from the $j = k$ term, the second from the $j \neq k$ term. The second term in Eq. (23) is an ensemble average over N rows of $(N - 1)$ terms. The terms in the row with $j = 1$ are $\delta(\mathbf{R} - \mathbf{R}_1)\delta(\mathbf{R}' - \mathbf{R}_2) + \delta(\mathbf{R} - \mathbf{R}_1)\delta(\mathbf{R}' - \mathbf{R}_3) + \ldots \delta(\mathbf{R} - \mathbf{R}_1)\delta(\mathbf{R}' - \mathbf{R}_N)$. The ensemble average over each row gives the same result, so that the sum is N times as big as the sum over a single row. The ensemble average over a single row with $j = 1$ is $\delta(\mathbf{R} - \mathbf{R}_1) [\rho(\mathbf{R}'|\mathbf{R}_1)]$. Here $\rho(\mathbf{R}'|\mathbf{R}_1)$ may be called the conditional number density distribution. $\rho(R'|R_1)d^2R'$ is the average number of particles within area d^2R' around R', under the condition that there is certainly a particle at the position $\mathbf{R}_1$. Thus we may write

$$\left\langle \sum_j \sum_k \delta(\mathbf{R} - \mathbf{R}_j)\delta(\mathbf{R} - \mathbf{R}_k) \right\rangle$$
$$= \left\langle \sum_{l=1}^{N} \delta(\mathbf{R} - \mathbf{R}_l)\delta(\mathbf{R}' - \mathbf{R}_l) \right\rangle$$
$$+ N\rho(\mathbf{R}'|\mathbf{R}_1)\delta(\mathbf{R} - \mathbf{R}_1). \tag{24}$$

On putting this into Eq. (22) we find using the properties of the delta function that

$$\langle |I|^2 \rangle = N + N \int_A d^2\mathbf{R} \int_A d^2\mathbf{R}' e^{i\mathbf{K}\cdot(\mathbf{R}-\mathbf{R}')}$$
$$\times \delta(\mathbf{R} - \mathbf{R}_1)\rho(\mathbf{R}'|\mathbf{R}_1) \tag{25}$$

or

$$\langle |I|^2 \rangle = N + N \int_A d^2R e^{i\mathbf{K}\cdot(\mathbf{R}_1-\mathbf{R}')} \rho(R'|R_1). \tag{26}$$

Since the conditional number density $\rho(R'|R_1)$ is a function only of the distance $|R' - R_1|$ we can define a new variable $R'' = R_1 - R'$ in terms of which Eq. (26) takes the form

$$\langle |I|^2 \rangle = N + N \int d^2R'' e^{i\mathbf{K}\cdot R''} \rho(R''|0). \tag{27}$$

In Maurice's analyses of the scattering of light he first considered the scattering assuming that each fiber scattered *independently* of the others. In terms of the present analysis this means that the second term on the right side of Eq. (27) is assumed equal to zero. Maurice found that under such an assumption the total scattered intensity would be so great that the cornea would certainly be opaque. It is not opaque because the second term in Eq. (27) which describes the correlation between the phases of waves scattered from nearby pairs of particles nearly cancels the N term. Maurice's thesis was that for such a cancellation to take place, the distribution of neighboring fibers had to be that of a perfect lattice. While such a distribution can indeed produce the required cancellation, it is by no means *necessary* that such an extreme correlation occur. We now show that even with the relatively poor correlation that exists in the position of pairs of fibers in the cornea that the second term in Eq. (27) can nearly cancel the first. To do this, let us examine the properties of $\rho(R''|0)$. For small values of R'', $\rho(R''|0)$ must go to zero because a second fiber cannot be closer to the fiber at 0 than a distance equal to the fiber diameter. In fact, in the cornea $\rho(R''|0)$ is zero for larger values of R'' than the fiber diameter. For values of R'' substantially greater than some correlation range R_c the number of particles in d^2R'' will be completely unaffected by the presence of the particle at the origin and $\rho(R''|0)$ will become equal to the average density $\langle\rho\rangle = (N/A)$. In Fig. 8 we plot the general form of $\rho(R''|0)$. *Wiggles* occur in $\rho(R''|0)$ above and below the value of $\langle\rho\rangle$ if the neighbors are located in fairly well-defined positions relative to a particle at the origin. The first positive bump in Fig. 8 corresponds to the location of near neighbors, the small negative bump is the space before the next position of second nearest neighbors. In the schematic diagram shown below there is no correlation over more than, say, the distance to second nearest neighbors. The actual form of $\rho(R''|0)$ has been constructed by Hart and Farrell[7] from electron microscope photographs of fiber position in normal corneas. Their function has the form shown in Fig. 8 and demonstrates clearly that after about two near neighbors there is no correlation in the position of particles. Nonetheless the required reduction in scattering takes place. We can see why this occurs. Because of the

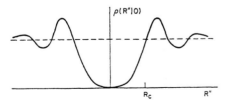

Fig. 8. General form for the conditional number density $\rho(R''|0)$. When R'' becomes appreciably larger than the correlation range R_c, the conditional probability becomes equal to the mean density $\langle\rho\rangle$. For values substantially less than the correlation range $\rho(R''|0)$ is zero.

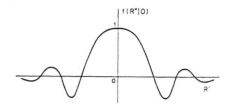

Fig. 9. General form for the function $f(R'') = 1 - \rho(R''|0)/\langle\rho\rangle$.

form of $\rho(\mathbf{R}''|0)$ we can write it as

$$\rho(\mathbf{R}''|0) = \langle\rho\rangle[1 - f(\mathbf{R}'')]. \qquad (28)$$

Here

$$f(\mathbf{R}'') = 0, \qquad R \gg R_c,$$
$$f(\mathbf{R}'') = 1, \qquad R \ll R_c.$$

This function $f(\mathbf{R}'')$ is plotted schematically in Fig. 9. Putting Eq. (28) into Eq. (27) we find

$$\langle|I|^2\rangle = N - N\int_A \langle\rho\rangle f(\mathbf{R}'')e^{i\mathbf{K}\cdot\mathbf{R}''}d^2\mathbf{R}''$$
$$+ N\langle\rho\rangle\int_A e^{i\mathbf{K}\cdot\mathbf{R}''}d^2\mathbf{R}''. \qquad (29)$$

The last term is identically zero if the illuminated area A is much larger than the wavelength of light unless $K = 0$. Thus for scattering in any direction other than the forward direction we have

$$\langle|I|^2\rangle = N(1 - \langle\rho\rangle\int_A f(\mathbf{R}'')e^{i\mathbf{K}\cdot\mathbf{R}''}d^2\mathbf{R}''). \qquad (30)$$

This equation tells us precisely how the correlation in the relative position of particles, as expressed in the function $f(\mathbf{R}'')$, reduces the scattering depending on the size of the second term in the brackets in Eq. (30) compared to unity. It is possible at the outset to make an estimate of the size of this term. Let us suppose for convenience that $f(\mathbf{R}'')$ goes to zero for values of R'' so much smaller than the wavelength of light that the integral can be evaluated assuming that $e^{i\mathbf{K}\cdot\mathbf{R}}$ changes very little from unity. If this condition applies, then we can write

$$\langle|I|^2\rangle \simeq N(1 - \langle\rho\rangle\int_A f(\mathbf{R}'')d^2\mathbf{R}''). \qquad (31)$$

The integral $\int f(R'')dR''$ is an effective correlation area A_c. Since $f(R'') \sim 1$ up to the correlation distance R_c, the integral is equal approximately to the correlation area (A_c) over which there exists substantial correlation in the position of particles. Thus we may write Eq. (31) simply as

$$\langle|I|^2\rangle \cong N(1 - \langle\rho\rangle A_c). \qquad (32)$$

Now, we must recognize that $\langle\rho\rangle$ is the number of particles per unit area

$$\langle\rho\rangle = N/A \equiv 1/A_0. \qquad (33)$$

Calling (A/N) the average *available* area per particle

(A_0) we see that

$$\langle |I|^2 \rangle \cong N[1 - (A_c/A_0)]. \qquad (34)$$

Clearly, if the scattering particles have a small area of correlation (this is of the same order as the size of the particle itself) in comparison to the area, on average, available to the particle, the factor A_c/A_0 will be small compared to unity and the scattering proportional to the total number of particles N. On the other hand, when the correlation area is about equal to the area *available* to the particle, i.e., when the particles become closely packed, A_c/A_0 becomes close to unity and as a result $|I|^2$ is reduced very markedly below N.

In three-dimensional systems the factor A_c/A_0 is replaced by V_c/V_0, the ratio of the correlation volume to the available volume. For gases at low density $V_c/V_0 \sim 1/1000$ and the scattered light intensity is N times the scattering produced by a single particle. However, in a liquid V_c/V_0 is of the order of unity and the scattering per particle is much smaller than that produced by an isolated particle.

In the cornea the correlation effect represented by the factor A_c/A_0 is very important. This can be seen at the very outset since A_c and A_0 can be estimated from electron microscope photographs of normal stroma. $A_0 = 1/\langle \rho \rangle$ is approximately $0.3 \times 10^6 (\text{Å}^2)$.[1] We may estimate A_c by noting that the average spacing of collagen fibers is 550 Å and that the centers of two fibers are never closer than about 300 Å. Taking the correlation range R_c as about 400 Å, we see that $\pi R_c^2 \sim A_c$ estimated in this crude manner is $0.5 \times 10^6 (\text{Å}^2)$. Thus we crudely estimate from the outset that $A_c/A_0 \simeq 1.7$. This number is of the order of unity so that it is immediately obvious that the correlation in positions of fibers plays a very important role in the determination of the transparency. To establish more accurately the effect of this correlation we must return to Eq. (31) and evaluate more accurately the correlation area A_c by computing the integral $\int f(R'')dR''$.

Hart and Farrell have constructed the form of the correlation function $\rho(R''|0)$ by making a statistical computation of the density of fibers around any given starting fiber. These authors have kindly informed me that the integral $\langle \rho \rangle \int f(R'')dr''$ has a value between 0.8 and 0.95.[9] Thus the actual scattering from the cornea is between 0.2 and 0.05 times smaller than the estimate of $\sim 90\%$ computed by Maurice on the basis of independent scatterers. It is important to point out that this reduction takes place even though the particles are correlated by distances no greater than the spacing of two neighbors.

Hart and Farrell have also computed[9] the quantity

$$\langle \rho \rangle \int f(\mathbf{R}'')e^{i\mathbf{K} \cdot \mathbf{R}''}d^2\mathbf{R}'',$$

which appears in the accurate expression for $\langle |I|^2 \rangle$ in Eq. (30) and includes the phase factor $e^{i\mathbf{K} \cdot \mathbf{R}''}$. In the cornea R_c is large enough so that for backward scattering $KR_c \sim 0.5$. Thus the exponential factor $e^{iK \cdot R''}$ does change somewhat during the integration. Their calcu-

lations take this into account. They have kindly informed me that, when this factor is included, for a light wavelength of 6000 Å this integral has the value 0.87.[9] It is to be observed that this accurate result is quite consistent with the cruder estimate given above. The scattering in effect is reduced to a value eight times smaller than that produced by independent scatterers because of the correlation between the position of the fibers.

There is yet another way to understand the marked reduction in the intensity of scattering below that which obtains when the particles are treated as independent scatterers. This is to observe that the mean square fluctuation $\langle \delta N^2_\Omega \rangle$ in the number of particles in some area Ω, which is arbitrary (but must be large compared with the correlation area $A_c \simeq \pi R_c^2$) can be written as

$$\langle \delta N^2_\Omega \rangle = \langle (N_\Omega - \langle N_\Omega \rangle)^2 \rangle = \langle N^2_\Omega \rangle - \langle N^2_\Omega \rangle \qquad (35)$$

$$= \langle N_\Omega \rangle \left(1 - \langle \rho \rangle \int_\Omega f(\mathbf{R}'')d^2\mathbf{R}'' \right). \qquad (36)$$

This last equation is of the same form as Eq. (31). That is, if Ω is equal to the illuminated area, and if the range of the correlation R_c is small compared to 2π divided by the wavelength of light, then $e^{iK \cdot R''}$ can be replaced by unity in Eq. (30), and Eq. (31) results. Under these conditions $\langle |I|^2 \rangle$, the mean square value of the interference function, is equal to the mean square fluctuation in the number of particles in the area of illumination:

$$\langle |I|^2 \rangle = \langle \delta N^2_\Omega \rangle. \qquad (37)$$

Equation (36) states that the mean square fluctuation in the number of particles in any chosen area Ω is proportional to the average number of particles $\langle N_\Omega \rangle$ in that area. The constant of proportionality $(1 - A_c/A_0)$ is much smaller than unity, however, when the particles are densely packed in the sense that the correlation area A_c is about as large as the available area A_0. This is the case in the cornea. There appears to be an interaction between collagen fibers which keeps them from coming very close to one another. This raises A_c to such a value that $A_c/A_0 \sim 1$. In terms of fluctuation in the number of fibers, the collagen fibers act as if they were nearly close-paced. Under these conditions, of course, the fluctuation in the number of fibers in any area will be small because a considerable expenditure of energy would be required to change the number in that area. The reduction in the scattering thus can be interpreted as resulting from the fact that the collagen is effectively densely packed, and as a result fluctuations in the density of these fibers are suppressed to values much smaller than that appropriate to a random arrangement of point particles.

B. Swollen, Opaque Corneas

Having now discussed the delicate conditions required for the transparency of the corneal stroma, let us give an analysis of the scattering of light produced by the microstructural alterations observed in swollen corneas. Electron microscope photographs, like that shown in Fig. 10, show that swollen corneal stroma contains

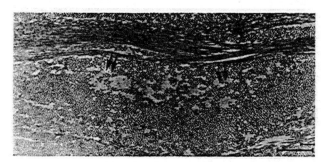

Fig. 10. Electron microscope photograph of swollen pathologic corneal stroma from paper in Ref. 5. The arrows point to some of the lakes where the collagen fibers are not present. The short scale marker has the length of 2000 Å.

irregular regions or lakes in which there is no collagen present at all. These lakes are irregular in cross section and are taken to have the form of long cylinders. Such regions represent places where there is a large fluctuation in the density of collagen. As we have seen in the previous discussion, the scattering of light is produced by fluctuations in the fiber density or, equivalently, by fluctuations in the index of refraction. Hence we can expect such lakes to scatter light.

In Fig. 11(a) we plot how the index of refraction of the stroma varies as one moves along some particular direction in a swollen cornea containing lakes. The index of refraction (n) shows sharp bumps at the position of the fibers by an amount equal to the difference between the index of the fibers (n_c) and the index (n_i) of the mucopolysaccharide ground substance.[10] The spatial variation in index of refraction shown in Fig. 11(a) produces a scattered field which can be regarded as originating as the sum of two arrangements of scattering sources. In Fig. 11, we show the scattering amplitudes which correspond to the two arrangements. The first arrangement, (b) in Fig. 11, is the distribution of fibers which would have occurred had the lakes not been present. The second arrangement (c) consists of fibers, each of which has a negative scattering amplitude, located at positions in the lakes where the fibers in arrangement (b) were placed. The scattered field from (b) plus (c) will be the same as that from that of Fig. 11(a), the stroma with lakes. Using the decomposition indicated in Figs. 11(b) and 11(c) we can now estimate simply the scattering produced by the swollen stroma.

1. Elementary Analysis of the Scattering from Small Lakes

The mean intensity of the light scattered by (b) and (c) is the sum of the mean intensity of light scattered by configuration (b) plus that scattered by (c). That is,

$$\langle |E_{\text{tot}}|^2 \rangle = \langle |E_b|^2 \rangle + \langle |E_c|^2 \rangle. \tag{38}$$

(We shall see in 2, below, the reason why $\langle E_b E_c \rangle$ can be neglected.) We calculated previously the value of $\langle E_a{}^2 \rangle$ in Eq. (30) and found

$$\langle |E_b|^2 \rangle = NE'_0{}^2[1 - \langle \rho \rangle \int f(\mathbf{R}'') e^{i\mathbf{K}\cdot\mathbf{R}''} d^2\mathbf{R}'']. \tag{39}$$

$\langle E_c{}^2 \rangle$ can be estimated in the following simple way. Each fiber in configuration (c) scatters a field whose amplitude is $(-E'_0)$. If the size of each lake is smaller than, or of the same order as the light wavelength, each fiber radiates a field coherently with all the others. That is, the factor $e^{i\mathbf{K}\cdot\mathbf{R}}$ is about the same for all the fibers in a lake. As a result the fields scattered from each are in phase, and the total scattered field from each lake is $(-N_\alpha E'_0)$, where N_α is the number of fibers missing in the lake labeled with the index α. Since we assume that the positions of the lakes are completely uncorrelated with one another, each lake radiates independently and the total scattered intensity is the sum of the intensities scattered by each lake. Thus

$$\langle |E_c|^2 \rangle = \sum_{\alpha=1}^{p} N_\alpha{}^2 E'_0{}^2. \tag{40}$$

Here, p is the total number of lakes in the illuminated region. We may conveniently define the mean square value of the number of particles per lake as $\langle N_\alpha{}^2 \rangle$, where

$$\langle N_\alpha{}^2 \rangle = \frac{1}{p} \sum_{\alpha=1}^{p} N_\alpha{}^2. \tag{41}$$

Thus

$$\langle |E_c|^2 \rangle = p\langle N_\alpha{}^2 \rangle E'_0{}^2. \tag{42}$$

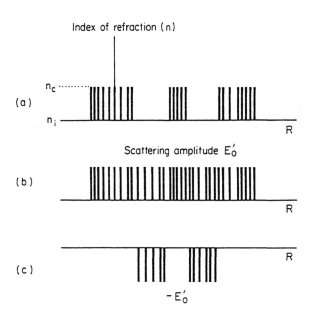

Fig. 11. Characterization of the scattering from lakes. In (a) we represent the fluctuation in index of refraction as a function of position in a lamella containing lakes. Each line represents a collagen fiber and the gaps represent the lakes. In (b) and (c) we represent an arrangement of scattering amplitudes which will radiate the same field as would be radiated from the fiber arrangement in (a). In (b) the missing fibers are randomly replaced with the average fiber density in the region of the lakes. In (c) fibers with negative scattering amplitudes cancel the field radiated by the replaced fibers. The field radiated by the sum of the configuration (b) plus (c) is the same as that radiated by the original swollen cornea represented in (a).

Thus the intensity scattered by configuration (b) is proportional to the number of lakes and to the mean *square* number of missing particles per lake. This scattering can be very effective in reducing transparency, as we now demonstrate. Adding Eqs. (42) and (39) together we find using Eq. (38) that

$$\langle E^2_{\text{tot}} \rangle = NE'^2_0 \left(1 - \langle \rho \rangle \int f(\mathbf{R}'') e^{i\mathbf{K} \cdot \mathbf{R}''} d^2\mathbf{R}'' \right.$$
$$\left. + \frac{p}{N} \langle N_\alpha^2 \rangle \right). \quad (43)$$

It is clear that if the factor $(p/N)\langle N_\alpha^2 \rangle$ is unity or larger, the cornea will be opaque. For in this case $\langle E^2_{\text{tot}} \rangle \simeq NE'^2_0$, which we know from Maurice's calculation leads to about 93% loss of light intensity. We thus have a convenient criterion for effectiveness of the scattering from the lakes, i.e., if we define the quantity ϵ as

$$\epsilon \equiv (p/N)\langle N_\alpha^2 \rangle. \quad (44)$$

Then if ϵ is about unity or larger, the cornea will be opaque. On the other hand, if $(p/N)\langle N_\alpha^2 \rangle$ is small compared to unity, the lakes will not scatter much light. It is possible to estimate ϵ by means of an analysis of the electron microscope photographs. Writing

$$\epsilon = (p\langle N_\alpha \rangle/N)(\langle N_\alpha^2 \rangle/\langle N_\alpha \rangle), \quad (45)$$

we recognize that the first factor in Eq. (45) is the fractional number of collagen fibers that are missing in the stroma. Alternatively, this first bracket $(p\langle N_\alpha \rangle/N)$ is equal to the ratio of the area of the lakes to the area of the stroma in the illuminated area. Cursory examination of Fig. 10 suggests that for this cornea $p\langle N_\alpha \rangle/N \sim 0.1$. The quantity $\langle N_\alpha^2 \rangle/\langle N_\alpha \rangle$ is crudely equal to the mean number of fibers missing in the average lake. This is easily twenty to forty for the lakes in Fig. 10. Thus ϵ is indeed of the order of or greater than unity for that cornea.

The analysis we have just given also can be used to show why lakes whose characteristic dimension is small compared to the wavelength of light are ineffective scatterers compared with those whose size is comparable to the light wavelength. This conclusion flows from the fact that the scattering is proportional to N_α^2, the square of the number of particles in the lake. This is proportional to the square of the area of the lake or to the *fourth power* of the linear size of the lake. Thus, the light scattered from a lake of diameter say one fourth of the wavelength of light is sixteen times smaller than the scattering from a lake of diameter equal to one half of the wavelength of light. This analysis demonstrates the action of the principle which we have expressed earlier in this paper and have emphasized in earlier experimental work,[5] namely that irregularities in the ocular media whose linear dimensions are comparable to or larger than the wavelength of light are most effective in scattering light incident upon them.

As the size of the lakes grows large in comparison to the light wavelength the scattering from the lakes will continue to grow, but not so strongly as the square of

the number of fibers in each lake. This occurs because the waves scattered from each of the fibers in the lakes in arrangement (b) are not in phase with one another. Hence there is a cancellation between the radiated fields within a lake, and the scattered *field* no longer is proportional to the number $\langle N_\alpha \rangle$ of fibers in each lake. Of course, if the size of the lakes becomes very large compared to the wavelength of light one may use geometrical optics to determine the reflection and refraction from the irregularities.

2. Quantitative Analysis of Scattering from Lakes

We now give a quantitative analysis of the scattering from the lakes which permits a more rigorous determination of the scattered intensity even for lakes large compared to the light wavelength. To calculate E_c we return to the basic equation, Eq. (9), for the field scattered by a distribution of fibers. In the present case the distribution is that given in Fig. 11(c), and the scattered field amplitude E'_0 is the negative of that given in Eq. (2). Let the vector $\mathbf{R}_\alpha$ represent a position at or near the *center* of that lake which is labeled by index α. $\alpha = 1, 2 \ldots p$, where p is the total number of lakes in the illuminated area. Let $\mathbf{R}_{\alpha j}$ represent the position of the jth fiber in the αth lake relative to the origin $\mathbf{R}_\alpha$, i.e.,

$$\mathbf{R}_j = \mathbf{R}_\alpha + \mathbf{R}_{\alpha j}. \quad (46)$$

Using Eq. (9) we find

$$E_c = (-E'_0) e^{i(k_0 R - \omega t)} \sum_{\alpha=1}^{p} e^{i\mathbf{K} \cdot \mathbf{R}_\alpha} \left(\sum_{j=1}^{N_\alpha} e^{i\mathbf{K} \cdot \mathbf{R}_{\alpha j}} \right). \quad (47)$$

N_α is the number of fibers missing from the αth lake. Using the delta function representation for the position of the fibers we see that

$$\sum_{j=1}^{N_\alpha} e^{i\mathbf{K} \cdot \mathbf{R}_{\alpha j}} = \int_{A_\alpha} d^2 R e^{i\mathbf{K} \cdot \mathbf{R}} \left(\sum_{j=1}^{N_\alpha} \delta(\mathbf{R} - \mathbf{R}_{\alpha j}) \right), \quad (48)$$

where A_α is the area of the αth lake. It is this area over which the integral is to be evaluated. If, on the average, the number of fibers missing in each lake is sufficiently large (say greater than ~ 10), we may replace the sum $\Sigma \delta(\mathbf{R} - \mathbf{R}_\alpha)$ by the average number density of fibers $\langle \rho \rangle = (N/A)$. We may then define the quantity $\mathcal{I}_\alpha(K)$ as

$$\mathcal{I}_\alpha(K) = \sum_{j=1}^{N_\alpha} e^{i\mathbf{K} \cdot \mathbf{R}_{\alpha j}} = \int_{A_\alpha} \langle \rho \rangle e^{i\mathbf{K} \cdot \mathbf{R}} d^2 R. \quad (49)$$

$\mathcal{I}_\alpha(K)$ is the Kth fourier component in a two-dimensional sinusoidal decomposition of a step function which is equal to $\langle p \rangle$ inside the lake area and zero outside it. If the αth lake is taken for convenience to be a circle of diameter $2a_\alpha$, then we see that if $Ka_\alpha \ll 1$, $\mathcal{I}_\alpha(K)$ is independent of $\mathbf{K}$ and equal to

$$\mathcal{I}_\alpha(K) = \langle \rho \rangle \pi a_\alpha^2 = N_\alpha. \quad (50)$$

Using Eq. (49) in Eq. (47) we see that

$$E_c = (-E'_0) e^{ikR - \omega t} \left(\sum_{\alpha=1}^{p} \mathcal{I}_\alpha(K) e^{i\mathbf{K} \cdot \mathbf{R}_\alpha} \right). \quad (51)$$

E_b is the field scattered by configuration (b) in Fig. 11. The total scattered field (E) is the sum of E_b and E_c. The scattered intensity is, as we mentioned previously, proportional to the square of the total scattered field. We may calculate the mean square total scattered field by making use of the ensemble average. On carrying out the squaring process and ensemble averaging over all possible locations of lakes and arrangements of fibers the cross term $\langle E_a E_b \rangle$ in the ensemble average of the square may be neglected. We can understand why the $\langle E_b E_c \rangle$ term is negligible in the following way: E_b, the field scattered by the full array of collagen fibers, is proportional to the fourier transform of the fluctuation in the density $\Delta\rho(R)$. The mean density makes no contribution to E_b because, as we observed earlier, the integration is carried out over the entire illuminated region which is very large compared to the light wavelength. On the other hand E_c, the field scattered by the substituted negative fibers in each lake, is proportional to the fourier transform of the sum of the mean density $\langle\rho\rangle$ and the fluctuation $\Delta\rho(R)$ in fiber density. In the case of the lakes, the contribution to the fourier transform from the average density $\langle\rho\rangle$ far outweighs that from the fluctuations because the fourier transform integral is computed over a region which is not very large compared to the light wavelength. Thus, when the cross term $\langle E_b E_c \rangle$ is computed we see that the term $E_b E_c$ which is proportional to $\Delta\rho\langle\rho\rangle$ will give zero when the ensemble average is carried out. The term proportional to $[\Delta\rho(R)]^2$ will not be zero, but it will be very small compared to the $\langle E_c^2 \rangle$ term which is proportional to the square of the fourier transform of $\langle\rho\rangle$. We therefore may neglect the cross term $\langle E_b E_c \rangle$.

Thus

$$\langle |E_{\text{tot}}|^2 \rangle = \langle |E_b|^2 \rangle + \langle |E_c|^2 \rangle. \tag{52}$$

Now,

$$\langle |E_b|^2 \rangle = E'_0{}^2 \langle |I|^2 \rangle, \tag{53}$$

where $\langle |I^2| \rangle$ is given by Eq. (30). $\langle |E_c|^2 \rangle$ is given by

$$\langle |E_c|^2 \rangle = E'_0{}^2 \left\langle \sum_{\alpha=1}^{p} \sum_{\alpha=1}^{p} \vartheta_\alpha(K) \vartheta_{\alpha}{}'(K) e^{i\mathbf{K}\cdot(\mathbf{R}_\alpha - \mathbf{R}_\alpha')} \right\rangle. \tag{54}$$

If the position of the various lakes R_α and R_α' are completely uncorrelated, as appears from the electron microscope photographs, only the $\alpha = \alpha'$ terms contribute to the ensemble average and we find

$$\langle |E_c|^2 \rangle = E'_0{}^2 \sum_{\alpha=1}^{p} |\vartheta_\alpha(K)|^2. \tag{55}$$

Thus, the total scattered intensity is proportional to

$$\langle |E_{\text{tot}}|^2 \rangle = N E_0{}^2 \left[1 - \langle\rho\rangle \int f(R'') e^{iK\cdot R''} d^2 R'' \right.$$

$$\left. + \frac{1}{N} \sum_{\alpha=1}^{p} |\vartheta_\alpha(K)|^2 \right]. \tag{56}$$

This is of the same form as Eq. (43), except that now we have $|\vartheta_\alpha(K)|^2$ instead of $N_\alpha{}^2$.

We saw in Eq. (50) that $\vartheta_\alpha(K) = N_\alpha$ if the lake is small compared to the wavelength of light. We now calculate the magnitude of $\vartheta_\alpha(K)$ even when this is not the case. The evaluation of $\vartheta_\alpha(K)$ is quite straightforward as it is mathematically identical to the well-known problem of the diffraction of light from a circular aperture. If we regard the lake as being a circle of radius a_α, the dimensional area differential d^2R is equal to $RdRd\varphi$, where φ is the angle in the plane of integration between R and the direction of K. Thus

$$\vartheta_\alpha(K) = \langle\rho\rangle \int_{R=0}^{R=a_\alpha} RdR \int_0^{2\pi} d\varphi e^{iKR\cos\varphi}. \tag{57}$$

The integral over φ is the integral representation of the Bessel function or order zero $[J_0(KR)]$. Thus

$$\vartheta_\alpha(K) = 2\pi\langle\rho\rangle \int_0^{a_\alpha} RdR J_0(KR). \tag{58}$$

The radial integral is also readily evaluated,[11] and we find that

$$\vartheta_\alpha(K) = \langle\rho\rangle \pi a_\alpha{}^2 \left[\frac{2J_1(Ka_\alpha)}{Ka_\alpha} \right]. \tag{59}$$

Here $J_1(Ka_\alpha)$ is the Bessel function of order one. Since $\langle\rho\rangle\pi a_\alpha{}^2 = N_\alpha$ we see that the intensity of the scattering from each lake is given by

$$\vartheta_\alpha{}^2(K) = N_\alpha{}^2 \left[\frac{2J_1(Ka_\alpha)}{Ka_\alpha} \right]^2. \tag{60}$$

We plot in Fig. 12 the quantity $[2J_1(Ka_\alpha)/Ka_\alpha]^2$ as a function of Ka_α.

We can draw a number of useful conclusions by considering Eq. (60) and Fig. 12. First we examine how $\vartheta_\alpha{}^2(K)$ varies with the size of the lake. From the asymptotic form of the Bessel functions[11] we see that for $Ka_\alpha < 3$

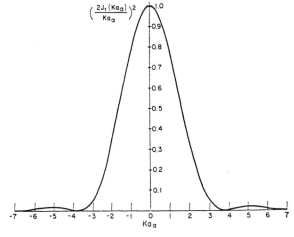

Fig. 12. A plot of the function $[2J_1(Ka_\alpha)/(Ka_\alpha)]^2$ vs Ka_α.

$$\mathcal{G}_\alpha{}^2(K) \simeq \langle\rho\rangle^2 (\pi a_\alpha{}^2)^2 \left[1 - 1.12\left(\frac{Ka_\alpha}{3}\right)^2 \right.$$
$$\left. + 0.422\left(\frac{Ka_\alpha}{3}\right)^4 \cdots \right]^2. \quad (61)$$

This shows that for $Ka_\alpha < 1$, $\mathcal{G}_\alpha{}^2(K)$ will be accurately proportional to the fourth power of the radius of the lake. On the other hand, for large size lakes, i.e., for $Ka_\alpha > 3$

$$\mathcal{G}_\alpha{}^2(K) = \langle\rho\rangle^2 (\pi a_\alpha{}^2)^2 \frac{8}{\pi} \frac{\cos^2[Ka_\alpha - (3\pi/4)]}{(Ka_\alpha)^3}. \quad (62)$$

If we replace the cosine squared factor in this equation by one half to obtain the mean value of $\mathcal{G}_\alpha{}^2$ we find

$$\mathcal{G}_\alpha{}^2(K) \rightarrow \langle\rho\rangle^2 (\pi a_\alpha{}^2)^2 \frac{4}{\pi} \frac{1}{(Ka_\alpha)^3}. \quad (63)$$

Thus for a_α large enough so that $Ka_\alpha > 3$ the scattering per lake increases linearly with the radius of the lake.

We may express these results in a somewhat simpler form. For small lakes ($Ka < 1$), $\mathcal{G}_\alpha{}^2(K)$ is equal to $\langle\rho\rangle^2 (\pi a_\alpha{}^2)^2 = N_\alpha{}^2$, the square of the number of fibers missing from the lake. On the other hand, if the lake is large ($Ka > 3$), $\mathcal{G}_\alpha{}^2(K)$ is equal to $(4/\pi)N_0{}^2(Ka_\alpha)$. Here $N_0 = \langle\rho\rangle(\pi/K^2)$. If we chose the K value appropriate for backward scattering, i.e., $K = 4\pi/(\lambda/n)$, N_0 is the number of fibers missing from a lake of radius $(\lambda/4\pi n)$.

The intensity of the light scattered from each lake is a continuously increasing function of the size of the lake. In the size range $1 < Ka_\alpha < 3$, however, the dependence on size changes from a fourth power dependence on the lake radius to a linear dependence on the lake radius. Since $Ka_\alpha = [4\pi/(\lambda/n)] \sin\frac{1}{2}\theta$, we see that this crossover region occurs (for backward scattering $\theta = 180°$) when the diameter of the lake $d_\alpha = 2a_\alpha$ falls in the range

$$\left(\frac{1}{2\pi}\right) < \frac{d_\alpha}{(\lambda/n)} < \left(\frac{3}{2\pi}\right). \quad (64)$$

The crossover region in diameter occurs when d is between one half and one sixth the light wavelength (λ/n) in the cornea. Those lakes that have diameters large compared to this crossover size (d_α) scatter more effectively than those smaller because the scattering from the smaller lakes falls as the fourth power of the size of the lake. Goldman's photographs (see Fig. 12, Ref. 5) show that lakes in opaque corneal stroma have size $\sim$2333 Å and will therefore be very effective scatterers.

Equation (56) permits us to generalize the opacification factor (ϵ) first defined in Eq. (44) for lakes whose radius is small compared to the light wavelength. For lakes whose radius is either large or small compared to the light wavelength we may define the quantity ϵ' as

$$\epsilon' = \frac{1}{N} \sum_{\alpha=1}^{p} |\mathcal{G}_\alpha(K)|^2. \quad (65)$$

If ϵ' is of the order of unity or even larger the cornea will be opaque, but if ϵ is less than, say, 0.1 it will be

transparent. To compute ϵ' from an electron microscope photograph covering some large area A of the cornea one should first make a statistical measurement of the number of lakes $[\mathfrak{N}(a)da]$ whose radii fall between a and $a + \mathfrak{N}$. $\mathfrak{N}(a)$ is the number distribution for lake sizes. From such a distribution one may find ϵ' by integrating over all the lake sizes in accordance with the formula

$$\epsilon' = \frac{1}{N} \int da \mathfrak{N}(a) \pi a^2 \langle\rho\rangle \left[\frac{2J_1(Ka)}{Ka}\right]^2, \quad (66)$$

which is the representation of Eq. (65) for a continuum of lake sizes. Equation (63) has also been used here for $\mathcal{G}_\alpha(K)$. The subscript α has been dropped in the argument of the Bessel function since the lake radius is now regarded as a continuous variable. The quantity N is the total number of collagen fibers which would be on average in the area A of the electron micrograph:

$$N = \langle\rho\rangle A. \quad (67)$$

3. Turbidity of the Cornea

Our discussion so far has established the condition under which light is or is not transmitted by the cornea. It is now appropriate to describe the turbidity of the cornea more precisely in terms of the numerical fraction of the incident light transmitted by the cornea. It is well known that the attenuation of a beam of light, which is being scattered as it traverses the medium, follows an exponential law, namely,

$$P(z) = P_0 e^{-\tau z}. \quad (68)$$

Here $P(z)$ is the power in the light beam after it has passed through a distance z in the medium. P_0 is the power in the incident beam. τ is the turbidity of the medium. A large value of τ implies great attenuation, while a small value implies little attenuation. Maurice[1] has expressed the turbidity of the cornea (τ) in terms of the size, density, and index of refraction of the collagen fibers under the assumption that each fiber scatters independently of the others. We can easily adapt his result so that it includes the effect of the correlation in fiber position and the presence of lakes. This can be done simply by recognizing that whenever the number density of fibers appears in his formula we must multiply it by the factor in brackets in Eq. (56), namely, $1 - \langle\rho\rangle \int f(R'') e^{iK \cdot R''} d^2R'' + (1/N)\Sigma|\mathcal{G}_\alpha(K)|^2$. If we use for convenience the definition of ϵ' given in Eq. (65) we see that[1,7]

$$\tau = \frac{\pi^2}{8} r_0{}^4 \left(\frac{2\pi}{\lambda}\right)^3 (m^2 - 1)^2 \left[1 + \frac{2}{(m^2 + 1)^2}\right]$$
$$\times \langle\rho\rangle[1 - \langle\rho\rangle \int f(R'') e^{i\mathbf{K} \cdot \mathbf{R}''} d^2R'' + \epsilon'], \quad (69)$$

where $m = n_c/n_i$, λ is the wavelength of light in the ground substance, r_0 is the radius of the collagen, and the incident light is unpolarized. On using the corneal thickness as 0.046 cm, $\lambda = 5000$ Å, and Maurice's values[1] for the various parameters in Eq. (69), one finds from Eqs. (68) and (69) that the power transmitted by the cornea (P_{tr}) is numerically related to the incident power by

$$P_{tr} \simeq P_0 \exp - \{2.5[1 - \langle \rho \rangle \int f(R'')e^{i\mathbf{K}\cdot\mathbf{R}''}d^2R'' + \epsilon']\}. \quad (70)$$

This formula for the scattered intensity is numerically not so exact as the more complex results of Hart and Farrell,[7] because it does not include certain small effects such as the coupling between the angular dependence in the scattered field and the angular dependence of the factor $e^{i\mathbf{K}\cdot\mathbf{R}}$. It also does not include small corrections of the order of $(k_0r_0)^2$ in the scattering from individual fibers. Nevertheless, this formula gives results at 5000 Å which compare quite favorably with the numerical values obtained by Hart and Farrell. Equation (70) shows that in the case where there is no correlation in position of collagen fibers and no lakes [the integral in Eq. (70) is zero and ϵ' is zero], the transmitted power is $\exp(-2.5) \simeq 0.08$ times smaller than the incident power. The correlation in fiber positions measured by Hart and Farrell reduces the exponent in Eq. (70) to the value $\exp 2.5(1 - 0.87) = 0.73$. If the additional small but mathematically complicated effects mentioned above are included, the theoretical power transmitted by the cornea will be about 83% of the incident power. In view of experimental uncertainties about the actual turbidity of the cornea, and the accuracy of existing estimates of the collagen and mucopolysaccharide indices of refraction,[1] this must be considered in satisfactory agreement with experimental data.[7]

If the cornea undergoes swelling, ϵ' grows from zero, and the factor in braces in Eq. (70) grows large. Thus, for example, when ϵ' is 1.0, the exponent has the value $\exp - [2.5(1 - 0.87 + 1)] = 0.06$, and only 6% of the incident light will penetrate the cornea in this case. As ϵ' grows larger with swelling to values larger than unity, the exponent describes an even greater loss in transmission. Of course, if ϵ' becomes quite large compared to unity, multiple scattering will occur and the simple exponential decrease of intensity given in Eqs. (68) and (70) will not apply.

On concluding this discussion of the scattering of light by the corneal collagen fibers it is worthwhile noting that in the sclera the collagen fibers are quite large. In fact their diameters and spacings are of the same size as the wavelength of light. This produces large fourier amplitudes at wavelengths appropriate for the scattering of light, thus the sclera is opaque.

III. Theory of the Opacity of the Cataractous Lens

It is natural to inquire as to whether the theory of the scattering of light which we have presented earlier in this paper can help us to relate microscopic alterations in the structure of the lens to the loss of transparency which occurs in the cataractous lens. Of course, loss of transparency can be produced either by absorption of light or by scattering of light. In a recent review of experimental and theoretical investigations on cataracts, Phillipson[12] has pointed out that no peaks have been found in the visible absorption spectra of cataractous lens substances. We must therefore look to in-

creased light scattering as the origin of the turbidity of the cataractous lens.

The theory we have presented above indicates that the scattering of light is produced by microscopic fluctuations in the index of refraction. These fluctuations must be of such a size that their spatial fourier components have a wavelength comparable with or larger than the wavelength of light. In the case of the lens, the absence of electron microscope photographs forces us to turn to biochemical analyses for evidence as to the microscopic fluctuations that produce scattering in the cataractous lens.

Biochemical analyses show that cataractous lenses contain in addition to the normal α, β, and γ crystalline lens proteins,[13] an elevated percentage of insoluble protein material called the albuminoid fraction. The physical properties of this fraction are not established, but they are apparently proteins of large molecular weight, and they are formed presumably by a process of aggregation or polymerization of the α, β, or γ proteins.

In the normal lens, light is of course scattered by each of the proteins in the lens. It is essential, however, to realize that, as we found in the cornea, each protein does not scatter independently of its neighbors. The correlation in the position of pairs of proteins reduces the scattering in the lens just as the correlation between the positions of pairs of collagen fibers reduced the scattering in the cornea. In the normal lens, the fluctuation in the number of protein molecules over a dimension comparable to the light wavelength is small because the proteins are densely packed, and transparency therefore results. It is to be emphasized that a "paracrystalline order"[14] of the constituent proteins is not required for transparency of the normal lens.

The presence of substantial numbers of large protein aggregates randomly distributed within the background of the α, β, and γ protein constituents of the lens can have an important effect on the transparency as has been pointed out by Trokel.[14] Using microradiography, Phillipson[12] has demonstrated that the opaque cortical region of lenses having galactose-induced cataracts has marked spatial fluctuations in the protein density. If the aggregated units have an index of refraction different from that of the average refractive index of the lens, and if the aggregated proteins are distributed at random throughout the lens, then they will scatter light proportionately to their number. We can expect that the aggregates can play a role in the lens, like that played by the lakes in the cornea. They produce regions within which the index of refraction is disturbed from the average value appropriate to the lens as a whole.

We may make a quantitative calculation of the effectiveness of such aggregates if we imagine them as being spheres of index of refraction n_a imbedded in a uniform background whose index of refraction is n_l. For convenience we shall assume that the radii of such spheres is smaller than the wavelength of light. (The analysis can easily be extended to spheres comparable to or larger than the wavelength of light just as we extended our treatment to the case of large cylindrical lakes in the previous section.) The problem at hand is essentially the same as the calculation of the turbidity of an aqueous solution of protein macromolecules. We may therefore use the result, well established in that field,[15] to express the turbidity τ for unpolarized light as:

$$\tau = 24\pi^3\xi^2 N_a V_a^2/\lambda^4. \qquad (71)$$

Here

$$\xi = \frac{n_a^2 - n_l^2}{n_a^2 + 2n_l^2}, \qquad (72)$$

N_a is the number of aggregate macromolecules per cubic centimeter, V_a is the volume of each aggregate macromolecule, and λ is the light wavelength. We can make a crude numerical estimate of the size of the turbidity in the following way. First we observe that both N_a and V_a can be expressed in terms of the average molecular weight of the aggregated or albuminoid macromolecules.

Each cubic centimeter of the lens contains about 330 mg of lens protein[16]: of this, a fraction which we denote as ζ is made up of the aggregated proteins. Thus the mass density of albuminoid fraction is $0.3\,\zeta$ g/cc. In the normal lens $\zeta \sim 0.01$, whereas in the cataractous lens ζ can become as large as 0.20.[16] If M_a is the mean molecular weight of the albuminoid macromolecules, and N_0 is Avogadro's number, it follows that

$$N_a = (0.3N_0/M_a)\zeta. \qquad (73)$$

We may also relate V_a to the albuminoid molecular weight by using the partial specific volume $\bar{v}$ for proteins. The quantity $(\bar{v})$ represents the volume of solvent excluded per gram of dispersed solute macromolecules. For most proteins $\bar{v}$ is between 0.6 cc/g and 0.7 cc/g. We may then estimate that

$$V_a = \bar{v}M_a/N_0. \qquad (74)$$

On inserting Eqs. (73) and (74) into Eq. (71) we find that the turbidity is given by

$$\tau = \frac{24\pi^3}{\lambda^4}\frac{(0.3)\bar{v}^2}{N_0}\xi^2 M_a\zeta. \qquad (75)$$

Here we see that the turbidity is directly proportional to the molecular weight of the albuminoid particles. This direct proportionality between turbidity and molecular weight is the basis of the light scattering determination of molecular weight of macromolecules.[13] The scattering also is proportional, of course, to the fraction ζ of albuminoid present and to the difference between index of refraction between the albuminoid and the rest of the lens, as is indicated by the factor ξ^2 in Eqs. (75) and (72).

To calculate the turbidity exactly we must know both ξ^2 and M_a. At present these numbers are not well-established. We can nevertheless crudely estimate the turbidity using reasonable values of these quantities to examine whether the present suggestion for lens opacity is tenable. If we use for n_a and n_l the values that apply to the collagen and ground substance in the cornea we find that $\xi = 0.1$. These values for n_a and n_l are similar to those obtained in microradiographic studies of

the distribution of proteins in galactose cataracts.[17] We shall also use the value $\xi = 0.2$, which is appropriate to the cataractous lens. With these choices for ζ and ξ and $\lambda = 5000$ Å and $\bar{v} = 0.6$ cc/g, we find that Eq. (75) can be expressed numerically as

$$\tau = 0.4 \times 10^{-7}M_a \text{ cm}^{-1}. \qquad (76)$$

Since the thickness of the lens is about 0.5 cm, $\tau z_0 \sim 2 \times 10^{-8}M_a$. The power transmitted by the lens is reduced below the incident power by the factor $\exp(-\tau z_0)$. The lens will certainly appear turbid if τz_0 is about equal to unity or larger. Such a value will be obtained if the albuminoid macromolecules in the lens have a molecular weight of about 50×10^6 g/mole. This may not be an unreasonably large value for the molecular weight of the albuminoid aggregates.

This crude estimate of the turbidity produced by a random distribution of protein aggregates in the lens indicates clearly the desirability of more measurement of the physical properties of these aggregates. In particular it would be very valuable to obtain reliable values of the index of refraction and the molecular weight of these protein aggregates. These data will permit a more accurate estimation of the lens turbidity.

Finally, if these protein aggregates should prove to be the microscopic origin of the lens cataracts, biochemical inhibition of the aggregation process would be effective in preventing cataracts.

The author acknowledges numerous stimulating discussions with Jerome N. Goldman at the Retina Foundation, Boston. Those discussions led to the present theory of corneal transparency and opacity. I am grateful to J. Kinoshita of the Harvard Medical School who pointed out to me the remarkable increase in albuminoid fraction in cataracts and its possible connection with lens opacity. R. W. Hart and R. A. Farrell of the Johns Hopkins Applied Physics Laboratory generously made available numerical results of their calculations. The author expresses his gratitude to C. Dohlman for making possible the collaborative relationship between the Retina Foundation and the Massachusetts Institute of Technology. Finally, the author acknowledges with thanks the support of the Sarah Reed Fund for Research on Diseases of the Eye at the Massachusetts Institute of Technology.

This research was supported in part by the Cornea Research Unit of the Retina Foundation, Boston, Mass., and by the Sarah Reed Fund for Research on Diseases of the Eye at the Massachusetts Institute of Technology.

References

1. D. M. Maurice, J. Physiol. (London) **136**, 263 (1957).
2. W. Schwarz, Z. Zellforsch. **38**, 26 (1953).
3. M. A. Jakus, "The Fine Structure of the Human Cornea," in *The Structure of the Eye*, G. K. Smelser, Ed. (Academic, New York, 1961).
4. J. N. Goldman and G. B. Benedek, Invest. Ophthalmol. **6**, 574 (1967).
5. J. N. Goldman, G. B. Benedek, C. H. Dohlman, and B. Kravitt, Invest. Ophthalmol. **7**, 501 (1968).

6. T. Feuk, IEEE Trans. Biomed. Eng. (in press) (1970) and private communication.

7. R. W. Hart and R. A. Farrell, J. Opt. Soc. Amer. **59**, 766 (1969).

8. H. C. Van de Hulst, *Light Scattering by Small Particles* (Wiley New York, 1957).

9. R. W. Hart and R. A. Farrell, Appl. Phys. Lab., Johns Hopkins Univ., private communication.

10. In Fig. 10 we indicate that in the region of the lakes the index of refraction is the same as that of the ground substance. This is probably not quite correct as there is likely to be water in these lakes. This would tend to lower the index of refraction of the lake to a value closer to that of water. The discussion we give above can be very simply extended to include this effect. We shall neglect this effect as it does not alter substantially the line of argument presented above.

11. M. Abramowitz and I. Stegun, Eds. *Handbook of Mathematical Functions* (Dover, New York, 1965), p. 364, Eq. 9.2.1; p. 370, Eq. 9.4.4.

12. B. Phillipson, Acta Ophthalmol. (Stockholm) Suppl. 103 (1969); see also Acta Ophthalmol. **47**, 1089 (1969).

13. A. Spector, Invest. Ophthalmol. **4**, 579 (1965).

14. S. Trokel, Invest. Ophthalmol. **1**, 493 (1962).

15. D. McIntyre and F. Gornick, Eds., *Light Scattering from Dilute Polymer Solutions* (Gordon and Breach, New York, 1964) (see, for example, article by W. Heller, p. 41).

16. J. Kinoshita, Howe Laboratory, Harvard Medical School, private communication.

17. B. Phillipson, Invest. Ophthalmol. **8**, 281 (1969) (especially p. 288); see also **8**, 271 (1969).

Reprinted with permission from *Experimental Eye Research,* Vol. 41, pp. 1-9 (1985).
©1985 Academic Press Inc. (London) Ltd.

Light Scattering of Normal Human Lens III. Relationship Between Forward and Back Scatter of Whole Excised Lenses

F. A. BETTELHEIM AND S. ALI

Chemistry Department, Adelphi University, Garden City, New York, NY 11530, U.S.A.

(*Received 6 April 1984 and accepted 24 January 1985, New York*)

Twenty-three human lenses from age 3–76 years were studied. Lenses obtained 24–36 post-mortem were exposed to monochromatic light (435·8 and 546·1 nm) in the $I_\parallel$ and I_+ modes and to white (tungsten lamp) unpolarized radiation. The light scattering intensities were obtained as a function of scattering angles from 0 to 135°. The scattering intensities in the forward directions are greater than in the back scatter in all modes of illuminations. The age dependence of a number of light scattering parameters such as percent transmission; I_θ/I_0; dissymmetry and depolarization were obtained using regression analysis. These parameters may serve as standards of normal lenses to which similar parameters of cataractous lenses can be compared.

Relationships between back scatter and forward scatter have been established using the regression coefficients. Thus, the light scattering intensity observed in the slit lamp (at 135° back scatter) can be quantitatively related to the light reaching the retina at different angular displacements.

Key words: age dependence; back scatter; forward scatter; depolarization; dissymmetry; light scattering; whole human lenses.

1. Introduction

In cataract formation, an increase in the light scattering produces a degradation of the image. This degradation is due to the forward scattering of the light. However, for a clinician using the slit lamp only the back scatter of light is available to diagnose the severity of the cataract. A tacit assumption is made that the back scatter of the light by the lens can be used as an index of image degradation (Siegelman, Trokel and Spector, 1974).

In a clinical examination with the slit lamp, the ophthalmologist scans the lens using multiple adjustments of the apparatus and thus forms a three-dimensional picture in his mind. Slit lamp photography preserves the record, but the two-dimensional photograph documents only a limited part of the original examination (Brown, 1969). Although this may be typical yet it is difficult to reproduce. Scanning such photographs gives a semi-quantitative interpretation of the turbidities in the lens (Siegelman et al., 1974). Photographing by the principle of Scheimpflug (1906) has been developed by Hockwin and his associates (Dragomirescu, Hockwin and Koch, 1980; Dragomirescu, Hockwin, Koch and Sasaki, 1978; Hockwin, Weigelin, Hendrickson and Koch, 1975) and this technique yields a three-dimensional reconstruction of turbidity in the lens (with the aid of densitometry).

However, all these techniques deal with back scattering and the angle between the slit lamp illumination and the back scatter is generally 45°. Densitometric scans of back scatter photographs have shown that the intensity of back scatter increases with age (Lerman, 1982; Siegelman et al., 1974). Slit lamp examination discovers turbidity, sometimes even in young lenses, without any apparent impairment of visual acuity. At the same time acuity assessment has been criticized as an insufficient measure in cases where intraocular scattering occurs, and additional measurements have been proposed such as glare recovery (Miller, Jernigan, Molnar, Wolf and Newman, 1972) and contrast thresholds measurement as a function of frequency (Hess and Woo, 1978).

In order to understand the impairment caused by cataract, it is necessary to know the angular distribution of the forward scattered light that reaches the retina and its relationship to the back scatter (diagnosis by slit lamp). Correct understanding of impairment caused by cataract can be assessed only if the relationship between forward and back scatter in normal human lenses is already known. Therefore, it was

Table I

Reproducibility of the light scattering envelope of lenses (tungsten lamp)

Scattering angle (θ)	Eye (72-yr-old)		
	First run	Second run	Third run
		(between two glass plates)	
0	4·75	4·80	4·72
10	4·00	3·95	3·92
20	3·02	3·02	3·05
30	2·06	2·01	2·10
40	1·30	1·32	1·38
45	1·10	1·12	1·12
50	0·92	0·88	0·89
60	0·75	0·75	0·75
65	0·65	0·60	0·61
115	0·41	0·40	0·46
120	0·45	0·46	0·47
125	0·48	0·49	0·49
130	0·50	0·49	0·52
135	0·55	0·60	0·62

Light scattering intensities are reported in volts; in the output of the photomultiplier tube.

decided to obtain the backward and forward scattering envelope of normal human lenses as a function of the age of the lens and also as a function of the wavelength and mode of the illuminating light source.

2. Materials and Methods

Human lenses were obtained from the New York Eye Bank via the Ophthalmological Research Department of College of Physicians and Surgeons, Columbia University. The names of the donors, and cause and time of death were recorded. Most of the lenses were obtained 24–36 h post-mortem. The lenses were kept at 4° in a moist chamber in which a wet filter paper kept the atmosphere saturated with water-vapor.

The light scattering intensities of the lenses were obtained in a universal light scattering photometer (C. N. Wood Manufacturing of Newton, PA, Model 3000). The lenses were positioned slightly flattened between a microscopic slide and a cover glass. The net scattering envelope was obtained by subtracting the blank from the scattering envelop of the lens plus the holder thus minimizing artifacts from reflections.

Light scattering envelopes were obtained with white unpolarized light (tungsten lamp) and with a mercury lamp (blue line 435·8 nm and green line 546·1 nm) both in the $I_\parallel$ and I_+ modes, i.e. when the polarizer and analyzer were aligned parallel or perpendicular to each other. Thus, five scattering envelopes were obtained on each lens. This usually took less than 10 min. The shape of the primary beam in all cases was rectangular (3×5 mm), sufficient to illuminate that portion of the lens which is in the visual axis.

In order to prove that a lens held between two glass plates and placed in the water-vapor-saturated light scattering apparatus does not alter its light scattering properties during a 10-min run, the light scattering envelope of the same lens was measured three times: 0, 5 and 10 min after positioning it in the light scattering apparatus.

As Table I shows, the slight amount of dehydration that may take place during the 10-min run does not change appreciably the light scattering envelope.

Selected light scattering parameters (percent transmission, $(I_{20}/I_0)_\parallel$, etc.) were evaluated from the light scattering envelopes. Their age dependence was studied by regression analysis using the Minitab II program in a Prime Computer. The statistical significance of each regression analysis was established by the standard Student's t-test (Bancroft, 1965).

3. Results

The scattering envelope of whole excised normal human lenses is not symmetrical around 90°. The intensities of the forward scattering are greater than the backward scattering (Table I) in all modes ($I_\parallel$ and I_+) and with the different light sources.

Selected light scattering parameters were evaluated and their age dependence was studied by regression analysis. The slope and the intercept of the regression lines together with the standard deviation and correlation coefficient, r, are given in Table II for a number of light scattering parameters.

Table II

Regression analysis of light scattering parameters (y) *as a function of age of the normal human lens* (x)

y		b (Intercept)	m (Slope)	S.D. of y about the regression line	$r^2\%$
% Transmission	W	101·0	−0·18	3·5	57·4*
	G‖	84·4	−0·26	6·7	42·5*
	B‖	72·6	−0·30	8·9	35·7*
(I_{20}/I_0)	W	0·579	+0·001	0·114	4·6
	G‖	0·336	+0·003	0·126	25·2*
	B‖	0·366	+0·001	0·113	7·3
(I_{45}/I_0)	W	0·121	+0·002	0·091	14·3†
	G‖	0·027	+0·001	0·074	23·0*
	B‖	0·046	+0·001	0·036	29·2*
(I_{115}/I_0)	W	0·044	0·000	0·021	9·3‡
	G‖	0·016	+0·004	0·010	38·0*
	B‖	0·013	0·000	0·008	43·2*
(I_{135}/I_0)	W	0·070	0·000	0·029	6·9
	G‖	0·026	0·000	0·016	28·0*
	B‖	0·021	0·000	0·015	26·9*
(I_{135}/I_{45})	W	0·554	−0·002	0·199	4·1
	G‖	0·784	−0·006	0·175	37·5*
	B‖	0·497	−0·001	0·209	1·8
$(I_{20}/I_0)_+$	G	0·024	0·000	0·020	7·5
	B	0·020	0·000	0·021	16·5†
$(I_{45}/I_0)_+$	G	0·011	0·000	0·009	2·8
	B	0·029	0·000	0·017	1·3
$(I_{115}/I_0)_+$	G	0·011	0·000	0·000	0·6
	B	0·015	0·000	0·011	0·0
$(I_{135}/I_0)_+$	G	0·016	0·000	0·007	8·0
	B	0·010	0·000	0·008	8·0
$(I_{135}/I_{45})_+$	G	0·879	−0·004	0·170	19·3*
	B	0·958	−0·004	0·174	24·0*
$(I_{45}/I_0)_+/(I_{45}/I_0)_‖$	G	0·207	−0·002	0·054	29·4*
	B	0·187	0·000	0·100	0·0
$(I_{115}/I_0)_+/(I_{115}/I_0)_‖$	G	0·491	−0·004	0·111	35·3*
	B	0·477	0·000	0·166	0·2
$(I_{135}/I_0)_+/(I_{135}/I_0)_‖$	G	0·456	−0·004	0·143	32·1*
	B	0·485	−0·002	0·174	6·9

Statistically significant at the: 99*, 95(†) and 90%(‡) levels.

W, G and B denote white, green and blue light, respectively.

The age dependence of the percent of transmission is statistically highly significant (99% confidence level) for all three light sources. The negative slopes (Fig. 1) imply that the percentage of light transmitted to the fovea decreases with age. This decrease is the steepest with the 435·8 nm Hg line followed by the 546·1 nm Hg line, both in the $I_‖$ mode, and the least is with the non-monochromatic white line. The regression analysis also implies that while a newborn infant's lens would have 100% transmission of white light, it would transmit only 84·4% of the green and 72·6% of the blue light of the Hg lamp. The non-transmitted light must be accounted for by scattering and absorption.

The relative amount of light scattered in the forward directions (I_{20}/I_0) and (I_{45}/I_0) increases with the age of the lens. The scattering is stronger with white light than with

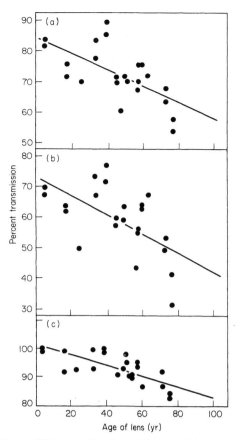

FIG. 1. Percent transmission of light as a function of the age of the lens. (a) $I_{\parallel}$ mode with green (546·1 nm), (b) $I_{\parallel}$ mode with blue (435·8 nm) and (c) white light.

monochromatic radiation. The age dependence of the scattering is greater with the green line of Hg than with the blue line.

A similar trend is found with the back scatter (I_{115}/I_0 and I_{135}/I_0). The relative back scatter is less than the relative forward scatter considering complementary angles $(90+\theta)$ vs. $(90-\theta)$ of scatter (see the respective b value in Table II). The age dependence of the scattered light intensity is also smaller in the back scatter than in the forward scattering (see the respective values of the regression slope m in Table II). The relative scattering intensities in the I_+ modes have little age dependence in either the forward $(I_{20}/I_0$ and $I_{45}/I_0)_+$ or backward scattering $(I_{115}/I_0$ and $I_{135}/I_0)_+$, although the forward scattering has greater intensities than the back scatter, especially with the 435·8 nm blue Hg line.

The dissymmetry ratios (I_{135}/I_{45}) have negative slopes in both the $I_{\parallel}$ and I_+ (Table II). This means that the relative back scatter compared to the forward scatter decreases with age.

A number of depolarization indexes were evaluated in which the relative scattering in the I_+ mode was compared to that in the $I_{\parallel}$ mode at different angles and with different light sources. All the depolarization indices showed a negative slope, implying that the density fluctuation was more important in aging than the orientation fluctuations.

4. Discussion

One purpose of the present investigation was to establish age-dependent light scattering parameters of normal excised whole human lenses. Since the present work is concerned with whole lenses, the simultaneous multiple scattering and the absorption of the light prevents the feasibility of structural analysis in the manner possible on thin sections (Bettelheim and Paunovic, 1979; Siew, Opalecky and Bettelheim, 1981). Therefore, the data obtained here are intended to be used in a phenomenological sense to serve as a comparison with whole excised cataractous human lenses (reported in the succeeding article).

It can be seen that the percent transmission of the incident light is strongly age-dependent (Fig. 1). This is expected, since many studies (Lerman, 1982; Siegelman et al., 1974; Siew et al., 1981) have indicated that light scattering increases with age and, consequently, the percent transmission of light must diminish with age. Therefore, the negative slopes in Fig. 1 came as no surprise. The fact that the percent transmission is less with the blue line of Hg (435·8 nm) than with the green line (546·1 nm) is accounted for by the coloration of the human lens and also by basic light scattering principles. The chromophores in the human lens absorb more light in the blue than in the green region of the visible spectrum (Lerman, 1980). Similarly, the light scattering intensity is inversely related to the wavelength of the light source (Kerker, 1969).

The percent light transmitted with non-monochromatic white light (tungsten lamp) is greater than with monochromatic radiations. Not only do the magnitudes of light intensities reaching the fovea follow this relationship, but the aging of the lens also provides a greater decrease in transmittance with blue light than with green or white.

The correlation between percent transmission and age is statistically (highly) significant (> 99 % level). Using the regression lines of Fig. 1, a useful age-dependent index of the average normal human lenses may be obtained which will serve to compare with cataractous lenses. This is especially important due to the variability of the individual lenses. (An individual's right and left lenses may show a greater difference in percent transmission than the difference between average lenses 10 yr apart in age.) Aging, of the average, would decrease the percent transmission of a lens over a period of 50 yr by 9 % with white light, by 13 % with green and by 15 % with blue light.

In looking at scattered light intensities it can be noted that forward scattering is always stronger than backward scattering, i.e. the scattering intensities are not symmetrical around 90°. This is true with the different light sources and in different modes ($I_\parallel$ and I_+) This is to be expected if the scattering elements in the lens (density and orientation fluctuations) have dimensions comparable to the wavelength of the light (Kerker, 1969).

The scattering intensities rapidly decrease with scattering angle (Table I) in normal lenses. The rapid decrease in angular dependence of the scattering intensities is important to normal vision because even though there may be a high percent transmission of light, the image on the retina will be blurred if the scattering intensities are high at wide scattering angles.

From Table II it can be calculated that an average 50-yr-old lens will have a scattering intensity at a 20° angle of 63, 50 and 44 % of the intensity at zero scattering angle with white, blue and green light, respectively. At 45° scattering angle, these intensities would decrease to 21, 11 and 9 %, respectively.

The positive slopes of the relative scattering intensities (I_θ/I_0) in Table II show that scattering increases with age at every angle with white unpolarized light and in the $I_\parallel$ modes with monochromatic radiations. In contrast, the I_+ modes demonstrate very little variation with the age of the lens.

The values of the regression lines (b and m) in Table II indicate that relative scattering intensities are not only greater at complementary angles in the forward direction (I_{45}/I_0) than in the backward direction (I_{135}/I_0), but also that aging causes a greater increase in scattering intensities in the forward direction than in the back scatter.

This is especially important to note because the second purpose of this investigation was to relate the observations of a clinician in a slit lamp to what actually occurs on the retina.

The back scatter of the slit lamp corresponds to the intensities at 135°. It is seen that in general the back scattering of an average 50-yr-old lens at 135° is 9, 5 and 4 % of that of the transmitted light intensity using unpolarized white and polarized green and blue lights in the $I_\parallel$ mode, respectively. The assumption a clinician makes is that as the back scatter increases so does the forward scattering that reaches the retina. This is a reasonable qualitative assumption.

A quantitative prediction regarding the forward scattering intensities can also be made using the regression analysis values in Table II once the back scatter intensities are available (as in Dragomirescu et al., 1978, 1980; Siegelman et al., 1974). Using the regression equations, the following expression is obtained:

$$(I_f/I_0) - (I_b/I_0) = (b_f - b_b) + (m_f - m_b)x, \tag{1}$$

where I are the intensities at 0, 45 and 135° scattering angles represented by the 0, f(orward) and b(ackward) subscripts; b stands for the intercepts of the regression lines and m for their slopes and x is the age of the lens.

From equation (1),

$$I_f = \frac{(b_f - b_b) + (m_f - m_b)x}{b_b + m_b x} I_b + I_b. \tag{2}$$

Thus, for white tungsten light, if the back scatter intensity (I_b) is known from slit lamp densitometric reading (135°), the forward scattering intensity at 45° can be calculated. For a 50-yr-old average human lens, 128 % more light is scattered forward than backward since

$$I_{45} = 1 \cdot 281\, I_{135} + I_{135}.$$

Scattering intensities at other (scattering) angles can also be predicted using regression coefficients for a particular angle, such as those given in Table II.

Similar predictions can be made for scattering intensities with monochromatic radiations.

It obviously must be kept in mind that data obtained in the present study are on excised whole human lenses and the in vivo relationship between forward and back scattering intensities may be modified by the passage of the light through the cornea and aqueous humor, on the one hand, and the vitreous, on the other. However, under normal conditions, there should be only minor alterations in the scattering intensities going from the in vitro to the in vivo condition. It also should be noted that while the correlations between the relative forward and back scatter and the age of the lens are statistically highly significant with the blue and green lights, the correlation is not as good with the white light.

Even with these precautionary notes, the present study is important because it provides, for the first time, some quantitative relationships between the forward and back scatter of normal human lenses.

Another useful light scattering parameter is the dissymmetry ratio, given here as I_{135}/I_{45}, etc., as this ratio increases the size of the scattering particle decreases (Stacey, 1956). The regression lines of the dissymmetry ratios given here have a negative slope both in the $I_\parallel$ and I_+ modes (Table II). This would imply that the size of the scattering particles on the average in the normal whole lens increases with aging. Such an increase implies an age-related aggregation (Bettelheim and Siew, 1982).

As a phenomenological parameter, it may be noted that calculations using the regression coefficients indicate that an average 50-yr-old human lens scatters twice as much light in the forward direction as in the backward direction. The actual factors are 2·2, 2·1 and 2·3 for white, green and blue light, respectively, in the $I_\parallel$ mode. For the I_+ modes, the corresponding factors are 1·5 and 1·3 for green and blue lights, respectively.

Finally, the relative depolarization ratios, $(I_{45}/I_0)_+/(I_{45}/I_0)_\parallel$, etc., are an important measure of the optical anisotropy of the lens (Bettelheim, 1978; Bettelheim and Bettelheim, 1978). Depolarization ratios at 45 and 135° show negative slopes in their regression lines indicating that the optical anisotropy decreases with age and implying a randomization or disorganization process. The depolarization is greater in the backward than in the forward direction.

In conclusion, the present study provides a number of age-dependent light scattering parameters that can quantitatively describe the optical behavior of an average human lens. These phenomenological parameters can serve as a standard by which turbidities and similar light scattering parameters of cataractous lenses can be compared. Such a comparison can decribe the severity of cataracts in quantitative optical terms.

437

More importantly, however, the data supplied here provide a bridge between the observations of a clinician using a slit lamp ophthalmoscope and the actual amount of light reaching the retina in the fovea as well as at a certain angular displacement from the fovea. Thus, the slit lamp examinations may be correlated to actual image focusing on the retina in normal lenses.

ACKNOWLEDGMENTS

We thank the National Eye Institute for the support of our research with grant EY 02571. We would like to express our gratitude to the Cooperative Cataract Research Group and especially to Dr A. Spector of Columbia University, New York, for providing human lenses.

REFERENCES

Bancroft, H. (1965). *Introduction to Biostatistics*. P. 174. Hoeber Medical Division, Harper and Row, New York.

Bettelheim, F. A. (1978). Induced optical anisotropy fluctuations in the lens of the eye. *J. Colloid Interface Sci.* **63**, 251–8.

Bettelheim, F. A. and Bettelheim, A. A. (1978). Small angle light scattering studies on xylose cataract formation in bovine lenses. *Invest. Ophthalmol.* **17**, 896–902.

Bettelheim, F. A. and Pauvonic, M. (1979). Light scattering of normal human lens. I. Application of random density and orientation theory. *Biophys. J.* **26**, 85–100.

Bettelheim, F. A. and Siew, E. L. (1982). Biological and physical basis of lens transparency. In *Cell Biology of the Eye* (Ed. McDevitt, D.). Ch. 6. Academic Press, New York.

Brown, N. (1969). Slit image photography. *Trans. Ophthalmol. Soc. U.K.* **89**, 397–408.

Dragomirescu, V., Hockwin, O. and Koch, H.-R. (1980). Photo-cell device for slit-beam adjustment to the optical axis of the eye in Scheimpflug photography. *Ophthalmic Res.* **12**, 78–86.

Dragomirescu, V., Hockwin, O., Koch, H.-R. and Sasaki, K. (1978). Development of a new equipment for rotating slit image photography according to Scheimpflug's principle. *Interdiscip. Top. Gerontol.* **13**, 118–30 (Karger, Basel).

Hess, R. and Woo, G. (1978). Vision through cataracts. *Invest. Ophthalmol.* **17**, 428–35.

Hockwin, O., Weigelin, E., Hendrickson, P. and Koch, H.-R. (1975). Kontrolle des Trübungsverlaufs bei der Cataracta senilis durch Linsenphotographie im regredienten Licht. *Klin. Mbl. Augenheilk.* **166**, 498–505.

Kerker, M. (1969). *The Scattering of Light and Other Electromagnetic Radiation*. Pp. 30–40. Academic Press, New York.

Lerman, S. (1980). *Radiant Energy and the Eye*. MacMillan, New York.

Lerman, S. (1982). Densitographie von Spaltlampen–Aufnahmen menschlicher Linsen mit UV-Licht. Ein Hilfsmittel bei zukünftigen Untersuchungen über Veränderungen der Linsentransparenz. *Symposium über die Augenlinse, Strasbourg* (Ed. Hockwin, O.). Pp. 139–54. Integra GmbH. Puchheim, Germany.

Miller, D., Jernigan, M. E., Molnar, S., Wolf, E. and Newman, J. (1972). Laboratory evaluation of a clinical glare tester. *Arch. Ophthalmol.* **87**, 324–32.

Scheimpflug, T. (1906). Der Photoperspektograph und seine Anwendung. *Photogr. Korr.* **43**, 516–31.

Siegelman, J., Trokel, S. L. and Spector, A. (1974). Quantitative biomicroscopy of lens light back scatter. Changes in aging and opacification. *Arch. Ophthalmol.* **92**, 437–42.

Siew, E. L., Opalecky, D. and Bettelheim, F. A. (1981). Light scattering of normal human lens. II. Age dependence of light scattering parameters. *Exp. Eye Res.* **33**, 603–14.

Stacey, K. A. (1956). *Light Scattering in Physical Chemistry*. P. 31. Academic Press, New York.

Reprinted with permission from *Johns Hopkins APL Technical Digest*, Vol. 11(1,2), pp. 191-199 (1990). ©1990 John Hopkins University, Applied Physics Laboratory.

RESEARCH ON CORNEAL STRUCTURE

RICHARD A. FARRELL, DAVID E. FREUND, and RUSSELL L. McCALLY

A strong interplay between theory and experiment is a key feature in our continuing development of light scattering as a probe of corneal structure. A general theory for predicting scattering from the structures depicted in electron micrographs of abnormal corneas is reviewed, and an experimental test verifying that collagen fibrils are the primary scattering elements in the cornea is presented.

INTRODUCTION

The Milton S. Eisenhower Research Center has a long-standing interest in understanding the properties of the cornea. Earlier investigations were reviewed in two previous *Technical Digest* articles.[1,2] The initial work[1] demonstrated that the order in the spatial arrangements of the fibrillar ultrastructure depicted in electron micrographs could produce the interference effects needed to explain transparency, and that macromolecular models in which fibrils are linked by mucoprotein bridges were consistent with the electron micrographs. In a subsequent study,[2] a strong interplay between theory and experiment was used to develop light scattering as a probe of the ultrastructure in fresh corneal tissue and to explain infrared damage to corneal cells. In what follows, we review briefly a general theory that we developed to predict light scattering using electron micrographs of abnormal corneas[3] and an experimental verification that fibrils are the primary scattering elements.[4] The theory applies to arbitrary inhomogeneous distributions of parallel fibrils having an arbitrary distribution of fibril diameters. The experimental test is based on the prediction that the differential scattering cross section, normalized appropriately, should follow a universal curve that depends on wavelength λ and scattering angle θ_s, only through the combination $\lambda/\sin(\theta_s/2)$.

BACKGROUND

The cornea is the transparent part of the eye's outer sheath (Fig. 1) and the primary refractive element in the optical system of the eye. Indeed, its curved interface with the air provides three-fourths of the eye's focusing power (the remainder being provided by the lens). Maintenance of its curvature and clarity is therefore essential for good vision. The structural elements that give the cornea the strength to preserve its proper curvature while withstanding the intraocular pressure (typically 14 to 18 mm Hg) are located within its stromal region, which constitutes 90% of the cornea's thickness.[5] The stroma comprises many layers of stacked sheets called lamellae, which average $\approx 2\ \mu m$ in thickness. A few flat cells (keratocytes) are dispersed between the lamellae, and these occupy 3% to 5% of the stromal volume. Each lamella is composed of a parallel array of collagen fibrils surrounded by an optically homogeneous solution consisting of water, mucoproteins, and various salts[5] (see

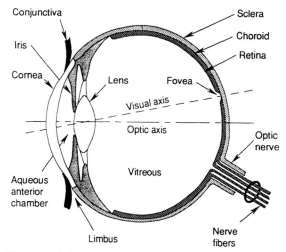

Figure 1. A diagram of the eye showing the location of the curved, transparent cornea.

Figs. 2 and 3). The fibrils have nearly uniform diameters, averaging ≈ 30 nm in man, and extend entirely across the cornea (lying essentially parallel to its surface), where they enlarge and blend into the white sclera at the limbus. The fibril axes in adjacent lamellae tend to make large angles with one another. This fibrillar structure gives the cornea its required strength.

The refractive index of the fibrils differs from that of their surroundings; most estimates of the relative index m range from 1.05 to 1.10.[1,2,5-7] Because of this difference and because the fibrils are so numerous, it was recognized long ago that if they acted as independent scattering elements, they would scatter so much light that the cornea would be opaque.[8] Thus, modern theories predict that the cornea's transparency results from an ordered spatial arrangement of the fibrils that creates essentially complete destructive interference among the waves scattered in all but the forward direction.[1,5-14]

The visibility of the cornea in the ophthalmologist's slit lamp demonstrates that it is not perfectly transparent. In fact, the cornea actually scatters about 2% of the red light and about 10% of the blue light incident on it.[15] The characteristics of this small amount of scattered light contain information about the structural ele-

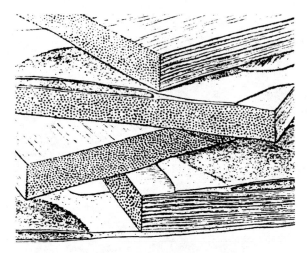

Figure 2. A schematic illustration of several lamellae from a normal cornea. The collagen fibrils are of uniform diameter and, within a given lamella, are all parallel to each other and run the entire breadth of the cornea. The lamellae are oriented at various angles with respect to each other. Three keratocytes are also shown between the lamellae. (Reprinted, with permission, from Hogan, M. J., Alvarado, J. A., and Weddell, J. E., *Histology of the Human Eye*, p. 93, Philadelphia, 1971; © 1971 by W. B. Saunders.)

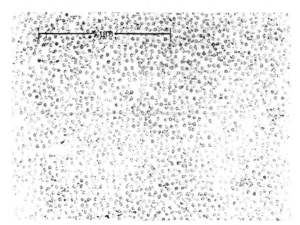

Figure 3. Electron micrograph showing the fibrils within the stroma of a normal rabbit cornea.

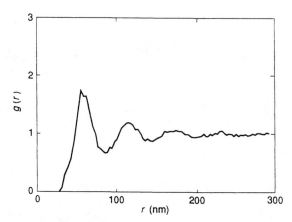

Figure 4. The radial distribution function, $g(r)$, for the fibrils shown in Figure 6. This function is the ratio of the local number density of fibrils at a distance r from an arbitrary fibril to the overall bulk number density; it represents the probability of finding a fibril a distance r from any given fibril and goes to unity at large distances.

ments from which the light is scattered, thereby permitting us to combine theory and experiment to develop light scattering as a tool for probing the stroma's ultrastructure.[2,4,12-16] The general approach, which has been quite successful, is to characterize corneas through measurement and analysis of their light scattering properties. By comparing experimental scattering data and theoretical predictions based on structures depicted in electron micrographs, model structures, or both, we can test the validity of the structures.

Previously we devised methods to calculate the scattering expected from the distributions of collagen fibrils depicted in electron micrographs of the normal cornea, such as that shown in Figure 3.[1,6,7] We showed that the fibril positions could be described by a radial distribu-

tion function, $g(r)$, an example of which is presented in Figure 4. Thus, the theory developed for X-ray scattering in liquids[17,18] could be applied. In swollen or damaged corneas, however, we cannot describe fibril distributions in this way, and consequently the earlier theory is not valid. The following section describes our efforts to devise a calculation procedure based on a direct summation of fields from the measured positions of fibril centers in electron micrographs.[3] This procedure would be applicable to swollen or damaged corneas as well as normal corneas, and would also enable one to account explicitly in the calculations for the wide variability of fibril diameters that has been reported in certain types of scars.[19]

The various models developed to explain corneal transparency, as well as our development of light scattering as a probe of fibrillar structure, rest on the fundamental assumption that the collagen fibrils are the primary source of scattering in the stroma. On the basis of this assumption, models to explain corneal transparency and its loss when the cornea swells have been analyzed and tests devised to discern among them, especially on the basis of the predicted wavelength dependencies of scattering.[2,12,15] Although experiments continue to support the theories that are based on the structures revealed by electron microscopy, we must remember that stromal structure is complex, and other potential sources of scattering, such as cells, are present. Such an important hypothesis, therefore, should be subjected to whatever tests can be devised. In a subsequent section of this article, we examine the experimental conditions for which the hypothesis is valid (and those for which it is not, *viz.*, specular scattering), and describe an experimental test of a theoretical prediction of how angular scattering scales with light wavelength and scattering angle.[4] Experiments confirm the predicted scaling relationship, which provides additional strong support for the idea that the collagen fibrils are the principal scatterers, except at specular scattering angles.[4]

DIRECT SUMMATION–OF–FIELDS METHOD

The underlying problem is to calculate the field that would be scattered by L stacked sheets composed of fibrils embedded in a ground substance. In general, the total scattered field $\mathbf{E}_s$ can be written as

$$\mathbf{E}_s = \sum_{l=1}^{L} \mathbf{E}_s(l) , \tag{1}$$

where $\mathbf{E}_s(l)$ is the field scattered by the fibrils in the lth lamella. The scattered intensity equals the absolute square of the scattered field, so that

$$I = \sum_{l=1}^{L} |\mathbf{E}_s(l)|^2 + \sum_{l=1}^{L} \sum_{\substack{m=1 \\ m \neq l}}^{L} \mathbf{E}_s(l) \cdot \mathbf{E}_s^*(m) , \tag{2}$$

where * denotes complex conjugation.

As with the Zernike–Prins-type analysis developed in Ref. 6, we evaluate the average intensity for an ensemble of corneas of a given type. We assume that the lth lamella of the corneas in the ensemble all have the same bulk number density of fibril axes and the fibril positions and diameters are distributed similarly, but that the specific position of fibrils, in general, differs throughout the ensemble. The field scattered from the lth lamella can depend on that from the mth lamella in two ways, namely, if the positions of their fibrils are correlated or if multiple scattering is important. For the cornea, fibril positions in different lamellae are uncorrelated, and we are primarily interested in semitransparent tissues for which multiple scattering can be neglected. Thus, the Born approximation in which the field experienced by the fibrils is replaced by the incident field can be used, and one finds

$$\langle I \rangle = \sum_{l=1}^{l} \langle |\delta \mathbf{E}_s(l)|^2 \rangle + |\langle \sum_{l=1}^{l} \mathbf{E}_s(l) \rangle|^2 , \tag{3a}$$

where $\langle \ \rangle$ denotes the ensemble average, and

$$\delta \mathbf{E}_s(l) \equiv \mathbf{E}_s(l) - \langle \mathbf{E}_s(l) \rangle . \tag{3b}$$

Although the members of the ensemble have similar spatial distributions of fibrils, the actual positions in different members of the ensemble are uncorrelated. Thus, $\langle \sum_{l=1}^{L} \mathbf{E}_s(l) \rangle$ is the field that would be scattered by a perfectly homogeneous cornea. Its absolute square represents the diffraction that would arise from the finite-sized illuminated region. This diffraction term depends only on the overall size and shape of the illuminated region and is negligible (except in the forward direction) for typical profiles of the incident beam intensity.

We obtain the scattering from fibrils by neglecting the second term in Equation 3a, so that

$$\langle I \rangle = \sum_{l=1}^{L} Q(l) , \tag{4a}$$

with

$$Q(l) \equiv \langle |\delta \mathbf{E}_l|^2 \rangle . \tag{4b}$$

In principle, we could evaluate $Q(l)$ by averaging over many corneas; however, we devised a method for approximating it from an electron micrograph of a single lamella. We first place a grid consisting of $M(l)$ rectangular boxes over the lth lamella (cf. Fig. 5) and write $\delta \mathbf{E}_l$ as

$$\delta \mathbf{E}_l = \sum_{j=1}^{M(l)} \delta \mathbf{E}_l^{(j)} , \tag{5}$$

where, analogous with Equation 3b, $\delta \mathbf{E}_l^{(j)}$ is the field scattered by the fibrils in the jth box minus the ensemble average field that would be scattered by fibrils within such a box. If the boxes are made large compared with the correlation length, then correlations among fibrils in different boxes can be neglected, and Equation 4b can be written as

$$Q(l) = \sum_{j=1}^{M(l)} \langle |\delta \mathbf{E}_l^{(j)}|^2 \rangle \tag{6a}$$

$$= M(l) \left[\langle |\mathbf{E}_l^{(r)}|^2 \rangle - |\langle E_l^{(r)} \rangle|^2 \right] , \tag{6b}$$

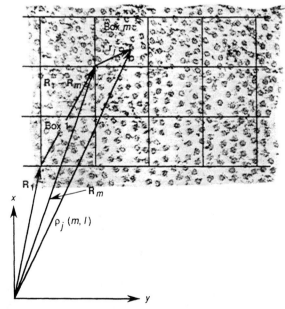

Figure 5. Hypothetical grid placed over a lamella. The fixed, arbitrary coordinate system is used to locate fibril centers ρ_j and boxes $\mathbf{R}_m$. An illustrative translation is shown for box 1 and box m; box 1 corresponds to the reference box.

where we have used the facts that the ensemble average of $|\delta\mathbf{E}_l^{(j)}|^2$ is independent of the particular box, j, and $\langle|\delta\mathbf{E}_l^{(j)}|^2\rangle = \langle|\mathbf{E}_l^{(j)}|^2\rangle - |\langle\mathbf{E}_l^{(j)}\rangle|^2$. The superscript r in Equation 6b denotes a generic or reference rectangular box.

We can approximate the ensemble average in Equation 6 from the fibril distributions in the K boxes of that portion of the grid covering the fibrils depicted in an electron micrograph. Specifically, we choose one box as the reference rectangle and treat the other $(K-1)$ boxes as if they were the reference box from other corneas in the ensemble. This identification requires that the other boxes be translated so that they overlap the reference box. In the Born approximation, the field scattered by a fibril located at a position $\mathbf{r}_j$ is of the form

$$\mathbf{E}_{sc} = \mathbf{E}_{sc}^{(0)} \exp(i\mathbf{q} \cdot \mathbf{r}_j) , \qquad (7)$$

where $\mathbf{E}_{sc}^{(0)}$ is the field that would be scattered from the fibril if its axis were at the origin, $\mathbf{q} = \mathbf{k}_i - \mathbf{k}_s$ ($\mathbf{k}_i$ and $\mathbf{k}_s$ being the wave vectors of the incident and scattered waves), and we have assumed that the detector is not in the near field of the scatterer. From the form of Equation 7, one can show that the effect of the above translation is to introduce a phase factor $\exp\{i\mathbf{q} \cdot [\mathbf{R}_r - \mathbf{R}_m]\}$ in the scattered field, where $\mathbf{R}_r$ and $\mathbf{R}_m$ locate a reference point (e.g., the lower left-hand corner) in the reference and mth box, respectively (cf. Fig. 5). Thus, an unbiased estimate for $Q(l)$ can be obtained from

$$Q(l) = \frac{M(l)K}{(K-1)} \left[\overline{\mathbf{E}_r^2} - \overline{\mathbf{E}}_r^2 \right] , \qquad (8a)$$

where the bars denote sample average, specifically,

$$\overline{\mathbf{E}_r^2} = \frac{1}{K} \sum_{m=1}^{K} |e^{i\mathbf{q} \cdot (\mathbf{R}_r - \mathbf{R}_m)} \mathbf{E}_m|^2 , \qquad (8b)$$

and

$$\overline{\mathbf{E}}_r = \frac{1}{K} \sum_{m=1}^{K} e^{i\mathbf{q} \cdot (\mathbf{R}_r - \mathbf{R}_m)} \mathbf{E}_m . \qquad (8c)$$

The phase factor $e^{i\mathbf{q} \cdot (\mathbf{R}_r - \mathbf{R}_m)}$ is included in Equation 8b to emphasize the translation, and the factor $K/(K-1)$ in Equation 8a arises because the sample average field $\overline{\mathbf{E}}_r$ differs from the ensemble average field $\langle\mathbf{E}_r\rangle$.

The field scattered by the fibrils within the mth box, $\mathbf{E}_m$, is the sum of the fields scattered by the individual fibrils within it. The latter fields depend on fibril positions through the phase factor in Equation 7, and their dependence on the fibril diameter and refractive index is contained in $\mathbf{E}_{sc}^{(0)}$ (of that equation), which can be calculated from the series solution. For the normal and swollen corneas discussed here, all fibrils have essentially the same diameter and refractive index, and the field $\mathbf{E}_m$ is given by

$$\mathbf{E}_m = \mathbf{E}_{sc}^{(0)} \sum_{j=1}^{N(m)} e^{i\mathbf{q} \cdot \mathbf{r}_j} \equiv \mathbf{E}_{sc}^{(0)} S_m(\lambda, \theta_s) , \qquad (9)$$

where the summation is over the $N(m)$ fibrils in the mth box, and $S_m(\lambda, \theta_s)$ is the phase sum, which depends on scattering angle θ_s and light wavelength λ.

The application of Equation 4a to calculate transmission through normal and swollen corneas can be simplified by noting that, for total scattering, the layered nature of the cornea can be ignored since, for unpolarized light, the *total* scattering from each fibril is independent of its azimuthal orientation. As we will emphasize in the following section, the azimuthal orientations profoundly affect angular scattering and must be considered in analyzing measurements of angular scattering. For transmission, however, the cornea can be treated as a single lamella whose thickness is that of the entire cornea. The total cross section is obtained by integrating the differential (or angular) cross section over scattering angles. With these assumptions, the differential scattering cross section per fibril becomes

$$\sigma_s(\lambda, \theta_s) = \frac{\sigma_0(\lambda, \theta_s)K}{(K-1)\bar{N}_r} \{ \overline{|S_r(\lambda, \theta_s)^2|}$$
$$- \overline{|S_r(\lambda, \theta_s)|^2} \} , \qquad (10)$$

where

$\sigma_0(\theta_s) \equiv |\mathbf{E}_{sc}^{(0)}|^2/|E_0|^2$ is the differential scattering cross section for an isolated fibril,
$|E_0|^2$ is the intensity of the incident beam,
the barred quantities within the brackets are sample average values of the phase sums defined in analogy to Equations 8b and 8c, and
$\bar{N}_r$ is the sample average number of fibrils within the reference box.

The calculation is performed by first recording the coordinates of the fibril centers from a micrograph of a region in a single lamella. The sample average of the phase sums in Equation 10 is evaluated over a series of angles θ_s between 0 and 2π for various wavelengths, and then $\sigma_s(\lambda, \theta_s)$ is integrated numerically between 0 and 2π to obtain the total scattering cross section per fibril per unit length, σ_{tot}. The fraction of light transmitted through the cornea is then found from the relation

$$F_T = \exp(-\rho\Delta\sigma_{\text{tot}}) , \qquad (11)$$

where ρ is the number density of fibril centers in the lamella, and Δ is the thickness of the cornea.[2,6-7] In Ref. 3, we performed this calculation for the large region indicated in Figure 6 and compared the results with those obtained using the earlier formulation based on the radial distribution function.[6,7] The results, plotted in Figure 7, show excellent agreement between the two

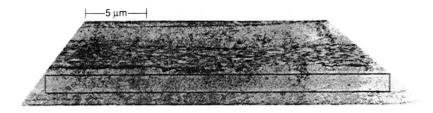

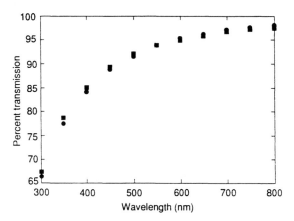

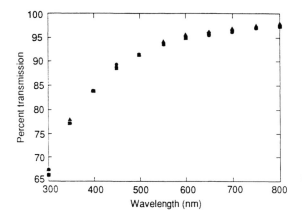

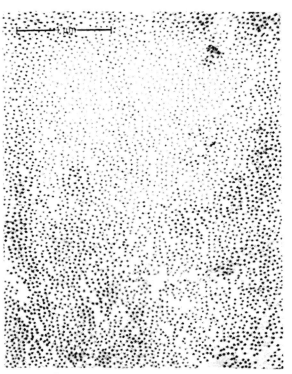

Figure 6. Electron micrograph of a region in the central stroma of a normal rabbit cornea that was fixed while applying a transcorneal pressure of 18 mm Hg. The large rectangle indicates the area of the lamella used for analysis.

Figure 7. Calculated light transmission plotted as a function of wavelength. The circles were computed by the direct summation of fields for a grid with 157 fibrils per box. The squares were computed using the radial distribution function.

Figure 8. Calculated light transmission plotted as a function of wavelength. The squares were computed from the entire region using a grid with 157 fibrils per box. The circles were computed from the entire region using a grid with 1262 fibrils per box. The triangles were computed from a subregion using a grid with 10 boxes containing 162 fibrils per box. The results are virtually identical for all three computations.

methods. (Previously we showed that the calculations based on the radial distribution function agreed closely with experimental determinations of the fraction transmitted.[6,7,15]) Figure 8 shows that the calculations are independent of grid size, thus supporting our assumption that correlations between boxes could be ignored if the box size was larger than the correlation length. In addition, Figure 8 shows that accurate results can be obtained from a subregion that is closer in size to typical micrographs (cf. Fig. 3).

We have also used the method to calculate scattering from a micrograph (Fig. 9) of a cornea that was swollen to 1.25 times its initial thickness.[20] Again, the fibril positions in swollen corneas cannot be described by a radial distribution function, and, therefore, scattering from such micrographs could not be calculated before now. The predicted transmission closely agrees with measured values (taken from Ref. 15); but, more importantly, Figure 10 shows that the wavelength dependence of the total scattering cross section agrees with the measured value. The figure shows that σ_{tot} contains a term that varies as λ^{-2}, which agrees with our extension of Benedek's lake theory.[2,9,12-15] This agreement between the calculated and measured values suggests that the small voids (or lakes) noted in the micrograph (Fig. 9) are not artifacts of the preparation method.

STROMAL SCATTERING

Specular Versus Nonspecular Scattering

In addition to the matrix of collagen fibrils, other possible sources of scattering in the stroma are cells and un-

Figure 9. Electron micrograph of the stroma from the posterior region of a 25% swollen rabbit cornea.

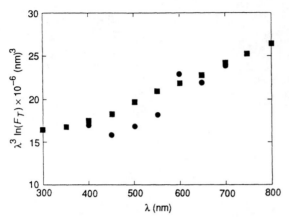

Figure 10. Comparison of calculated (■) and measured (●) values of $\lambda^3 \ln|F_T|$ as a function of wavelength for a 25% swollen rabbit cornea. Multiplication by the cube of the wavelength removes the inverse cubic dependence that characterizes the individual fibril cross section. The straight line of positive slope indicates the increased effect of scattering by lakes in swollen corneas, which, according to our extension of Benedek's theory,[15] contributes a term proportional to λ^{-2}.

dulations in the lamellae that exist at low intraocular pressures when the tension in the fibrils is relaxed. These undulations are the source of the small angle scattering patterns that we discussed in a previous *Technical Digest* article and elsewhere.[2,16,21] To understand the relative importance of these possible sources of scattering, it is instructive to view the cornea in the scattering apparatus (shown in Fig. 11) under different conditions of illumination. In Figure 12A the incident light is normal to the central cornea, and the scattering angle θ_s is 120°. The bands at the front and back surfaces are caused by scattering from the epithelial and endothelial cell layers, respectively. The stromal region contains a few bright "flecks," which presumably are scattering from cells, on a diffuse background, which presumably represents the scattering from the fibrillar matrix. This appearance is typical at all scattering angles for this setup. Figure 12B shows the same cornea shifted laterally to produce specular scattering at $\theta_s = 144°$. (Here, the incident light is no longer normal to the corneal surface.) In this photograph, which received 13 times less exposure than the one in Figure 12A, the cells in the stroma shine intensely against a darker background. Scattering from the cellular layers at the front and back of the cornea also is much more intense in Figure 12B.

We obtain a similar result when we view the stroma with a scanning-slit specular microscope. This instrument, lent to us by David Maurice of Stanford University, operates using the same principles now employed in confocal microscopes and, as configured here, isolates a thin optical section of the stroma (≈ 2 μm thick).[22] Figure 12C shows a representative view in the stroma in which the bright ovals are keratocytes, and the complex background pattern arises from the lamellar undulations found at low intraocular pressures. Similar patterns have been observed and reported by Gallagher and Maurice.[23] We see from Figures 12B and 12C that the flat keratocytes, which have lateral dimensions of several wavelengths, act like tiny mirrors under the condition of specular reflection and dominate the scattering. The specular condition must therefore be avoided in scattering experiments designed to probe fibrillar structures.

Tests for Fibrillar Scattering–Nonspecular Scattering

The idea for a test to determine whether stromal scattering derives primarily from fibrils comes directly from

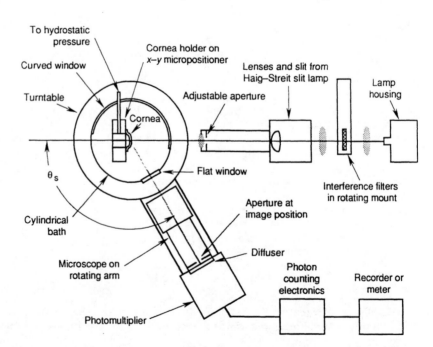

Figure 11. Schematic diagram of the experimental scattering apparatus.

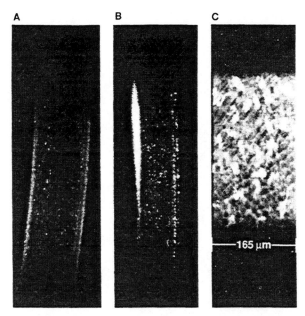

Figure 12. Three different views of a cornea. **A.** Scattering at $\theta_s = 120°$ from a rabbit cornea, with the incident light normal to the surface as viewed in the scattering apparatus shown in Figure 11. **B.** Scattering at $\theta_s = 144°$ from the same rabbit cornea, except that it has been shifted laterally; the incident light is no longer normal to the cornea's surface. Scattering from stromal cells and the front and back cellular layers of the cornea is much more intense. This photograph received 13 times less exposure than the one in Figure 12A. **C.** The cornea viewed with a scanning-slit specular microscope. The bright ovals are keratocytes, and the background pattern is caused by lamellar undulations.

our earlier theory based on the radial distribution function. As discussed in the previous section, this theory treated the stroma as a single lamella of parallel, infinitely long fibrils, which for this discussion we take to be aligned perpendicular to the scattering plane defined by the incident beam and the axis of the collection optics (cf. Fig. 11). We defined the azimuthal angle of this plane measured from the vertical to be $\varphi_s = \pi/2$. We then showed that, if the fibril diameters were small compared with the wavelength, the scattering intensity (per unit length) could be expressed as[6]

$$I_s(\theta_s, \pi/2) = \frac{AI_0}{r_s} \left(\frac{1 + B\cos^2\theta_s}{\lambda^3} \right) \left\{ 1 - 2\pi\rho \right.$$

$$\left. \times \int_0^{R_c} r\,dr[1 - g(r)]J_0[2kr\sin(\theta_s/2)] \right\}, \quad (12)$$

where

I_0 is the intensity of the incident light,
r_s is the distance to the field point,
A is a constant having dimensions (length),[4] which depends on the diameter and dielectric properties of the fibrils,
B is a dimensionless constant, which depends on the relative refractive index of the fibrils and their surroundings,

R_c is the distance over which fibril positions are correlated,
ρ is the number density of fibrils in the lamella,
k is the magnitude of the incident wave vector, and
J_0 is the 0th-order Bessel function of the first kind.

From Equation 12 we clearly see that if the scattering were primarily from a single lamella of parallel fibrils, the quantity

$$S(\lambda, \theta_s) \equiv \frac{\lambda^3[I_s(\theta_s, \pi/2)/I_0]}{1 + B\cos^2\theta_s} \quad (13)$$

should scale with wavelength and scattering angle via an effective wave number

$$k_{\text{eff}} \equiv k\sin(\theta_s/2) . \quad (14)$$

In a real cornea, however, the nature of scattering from long cylinders requires that the azimuthal orientations of the fibrils in the different layers of the stroma be considered in deriving an expression for angular scattering. Scattering from an infinitely long cylinder is a cylindrically outgoing wave, with the wave vector of the scattered wave orthogonal to the cylinder axis at all points along its (infinite) length. For finite cylinders, the situation is similar at intermediate distances, where the scattering is also a cylindrically outgoing wave confined to the narrow band, which is defined by the height of the illuminated region of the cylinder (assumed here to be much smaller than the size of the detector). In the far field, the scattering peaks sharply about the plane that is perpendicular to the cylinder axis and passes through its center. When using the apparatus shown in Figure 11 to measure angular scattering, therefore, only those lamellae whose fibrils are oriented to within a certain tilt angle from the scattering plane (defined by the incident beam and the optic axis of collection optics) will contribute to the measured scattering. We see this schematically in Figure 13, which also shows that the number of these lamellae varies with the scattering angle θ_s. In Ref. 4, we used these considerations to derive the proper form of Equation 12, which accounts for the azimuthal orientations of the stromal lamellae, the net result being that the form of the constant A is slightly different, and an additional factor of $\sin\theta_s$ appears in the denominator. Thus, the quantity that should scale with k_{eff} is $\sin\theta_s S(\lambda, \theta_s)$ and not simply $S(\lambda, \theta_s)$.

We used the scattering apparatus in Figure 11 to test this relationship. For the measurements, the corneas were bathed in normal saline solution (0.154 molar concentration of NaCl) and maintained at an intraocular pressure of 18 mm Hg. Measurements were made at scattering angles of 35°, 40°, 50°, 60°, 115°, 120°, 130°, 140°, and 150° and at the four strong lines in the mercury arc's visible spectrum, 404.7, 435.8, 546.1, and 577.7 nm. Full experimental details can be found in Ref. 4. The results are plotted in Figure 14, where we used a value of 1.09

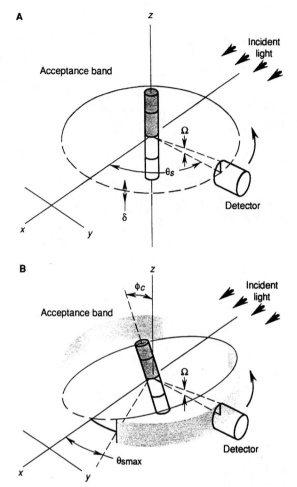

Figure 13. A schematic representation of scattering from a cylindrical fibril. **A.** This geometry shows the finite acceptance band δ resulting from the angular acceptance of the detection optics. The scattering from the fibril, which is oriented perpendicular to the x-y plane, is confined to directions very near that plane, whose intersection with the acceptance band is indicated by the solid and dashed line (the angular spread of the scattering out of the plane is much less than the detector acceptance angle Ω). Scattering from such a fibril would be detected at all scattering angles θ_s. **B.** Scattering from a fibril lying in the y-z plane, but tilted at an angle ϕ_c with respect to the z axis, is essentially confined to the plane through its center, which makes an angle ϕ_c with the x-y plane. The intersection of this plane with the top of the acceptance band defines the maximum scattering angle in the forward direction θ_{smax} for which a fibril tilted at an angle ϕ_c would contribute to the measured signal. Similarly, the intersection also defines the minimum scattering angle in the backward direction $\pi - \theta_{smax}$ for which such a fibril would contribute (scattering angles θ_s are measured between 0 and π). For scattering angles $\theta_{smax} \leq \theta_s \leq \pi - \theta_{smax}$, the scattering misses the acceptance band. From these considerations, it is obvious that all fibrils (or lamellae) would contribute to the measured scattering at $\theta_s = 0$ or π, whereas at $\theta_s = \pi/2$, the number of contributing lamellae diminishes to those having tilt angles $< \Omega$.

for the relative refractive index m to determine the constant $B = 4/(m^2 + 1)$ in Equation 13. All of the values collapse to a single curve, indicating that the predicted scaling is observed.

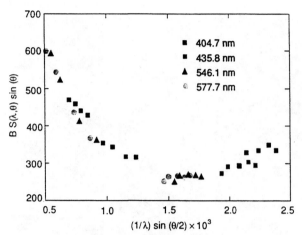

Figure 14. Experimental measurements of the function $\sin \theta_s \, S(\lambda, \theta_s)$, defined in Equation 13, plotted as a function of k_{eff}. These data are the average values from four normal rabbit corneas. The observed scaling agrees with the hypothesis that fibrils are the primary source of nonspecular light scattering in the cornea.

This confirmation of the scaling provides additional, strong evidence that the matrix of collagen fibrils is the primary source of scattering in the corneal stroma. Thus, transparency theories, which are all based on this assumption, remain on firm ground. Further, our continued use of light scattering to probe fibrillar structures in the stroma is justified.

REFERENCES

[1] Hart, R. W., Farrell, R. A., and Langham, M. E., "Theory of Corneal Structure," *APL Tech. Dig.* **8**, 2-11 (1969).

[2] Farrell, R. A., Bargeron, C. B., Green, W. R., and McCally, R. L., "Collaborative Biomedical Research on Corneal Structure," *Johns Hopkins APL Tech. Dig.* **4**, 65-79 (1983).

[3] Freund, D. E., McCally, R. L., and Farrell, R. A., "Direct Summation of Fields for Light Scattering by Fibrils with Applications to Normal Corneas," *Appl. Opt.* **25**, 2739-2746 (1986).

[4] Freund, D. E., McCally, R. L., and Farrell, R. A., "Effects of Fibril Orientations on Light Scattering in the Cornea," *J. Opt. Soc. Am. A* **3**, 1970-1982 (1986).

[5] Maurice, D. M., "The Cornea and Sclera," in *The Eye*, Vol. 1B, Davson, H., ed., Academic Press, Orlando (1984).

[6] Hart, R. W., and Farrell, R. A., "Light Scattering in the Cornea," *J. Opt. Soc. Am.* **59**, 766-774 (1969).

[7] Cox, J. L., Farrell, R. A., Hart, R. W., and Langham, M. E., "The Transparency of the Mammalian Cornea," *J. Physiol. (Lond.)* **210**, 601-616 (1970).

[8] Maurice, D. M., "The Structure and Transparency of the Corneal Stroma," *J. Physiol. (Lond.)* **136**, 263-286 (1957).

[9] Benedek, G. B., "The Theory of Transparency of the Eye," *Appl. Opt.* **10**, 459-473 (1971).

[10] Feuk, T., "On the Transparency of the Stroma in the Mammalian Cornea," *IEEE Trans. Biomed. Eng.* **BME-17**, 186-190 (1970).

[11] Twersky, V., "Transparency of Pair-Related, Random Distributions of Small Scatterers, with Applications to the Cornea," *J. Opt. Soc. Am.* **65**, 524-530 (1975).

[12] Farrell, R. A., and McCally, R. L., "On Corneal Transparency and Its Loss with Swelling," *J. Opt. Soc. Am.* **66**, 342-345 (1976).

[13] McCally, R. L., and Farrell, R. A., "Interaction of Light and the Cornea: Light Scattering versus Transparency," in *The Cornea: Transactions of the World Congress on the Cornea III*, Cavanagh, H. D., ed., Raven Press, New York (1988).

[14] McCally, R. L., and Farrell, R. A., "Light Scattering from Cornea and Corneal Transparency," in *New Developments in Noninvasive Studies to Evaluate Ocular Function*, Masters, B., ed., Springer-Verlag, New York (in press, 1990).

[15]Farrell, R. A., McCally, R. L., and Tatham, P. E. R., "Wavelength Dependencies of Light Scattering in Normal and Cold Swollen Rabbit Corneas and Their Structural Implications," *J. Physiol. (Lond.)* **233**, 589–612 (1973).

[16]McCally, R. L., and Farrell, R. A., "Structural Implications of Small-Angle Light Scattering from Cornea," *Exp. Eye Res.* **34**, 99–111 (1982).

[17]Zernike, F., and Prins, J. A., "Die Beugung von Röntgenstrahlen in Flüssigkeiten als Effekt der Molekülanordnung," *Z. Phys.* **41**, 184 (1927).

[18]Debye, P., and Menke, H., "Bestimmung der Inneren Struktur von Flüssigkeiten mit Röntgenstrahlen," *Phys. Z* **31**, 797 (1930).

[19]Schwarz, W., and Graf Keyserlingk, D., "Electron Microscopy of Normal and Opaque Human Cornea," in *The Cornea*, Langham, M. E., ed., The Johns Hopkins Press, Baltimore (1969).

[20]McCally, R. L., Freund, D. E., and Farrell, R. A., "Calculations of Light Scattering from EM of Swollen Corneas by Direct Summation of Fields," *Invest. Ophthalmol. Vis. Sci.* (Supplement) **27**, 350 (1986).

[21]Andreo, R. H., and Farrell, R. A., "Corneal Small-Angle Light Scattering Patterns: Wavy Fibril Models," *J. Opt. Soc. Am.* **72**, 1479–1492 (1982).

[22]Maurice, D. M., "A Scanning Slit Optical Microscope," *Invest. Ophthalmol.* **13**, 1033–1037 (1974).

[23]Gallagher, B., and Maurice, D. M., "Striations of Light Scattering in the Corneal Stroma," *J. Ultrastruct. Res.* **61**, 100–114 (1977).

ACKNOWLEDGMENTS: This work was supported in part by the National Eye Institute (Grant EY01019), by the U.S. Army Medical Research and Development Command, and by the U.S. Navy under Contract N00039-89-C-5301. We thank James Cox (Wilmer Institute of the Johns Hopkins Medical Institutions), who did the electron microscopy; Ray Wisecarver (McClure Computing Center), who digitized the fibril locations in Figure 6; and Ujjal Ghoshtagore, who, as a summer apprentice, digitized and helped analyze the results from the micrograph in Figure 9. Special thanks are due to Stanley Favin (Mathematics and Information Science, APL), who aided in the development of the computer programs for the direct summations method, and to Robert W. Hart, who gave valuable insights on the effects of fibril orientations.

THE AUTHORS

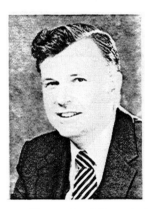

RICHARD A. FARRELL is a principal staff physicist and supervisor of the Theoretical Problems Group in APL's Milton S. Eisenhower Research Center. Born in Providence, Rhode Island, he obtained a B.S. degree from Providence College in 1960, an M.S. degree from the University of Massachusetts in 1962, and a Ph.D. degree from The Catholic University of America in 1965. Dr. Farrell's research interests include relating the cornea's structure to its function, developing theoretical methods for calculating wave scattering in random media, analyzing the statistical mechanics of phase transitions, and modeling ocular blood flow. He has been involved in collaborative efforts with the Johns Hopkins Medical School since joining APL in 1965. Dr. Farrell is the principal investigator on a grant from the National Eye Institute and recently served on their steering committee for a workshop on corneal biophysics. He is a member of the American Physical Society, the Optical Society of America, the Association for Research in Vision and Ophthalmology, the International Society for Eye Research, and the New York Academy of Sciences. He recently received an Alcon Research Institute recognition award for outstanding research in ophthalmology.

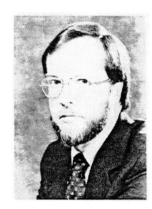

RUSSELL L. McCALLY was born in Marion, Ohio. He received a B.Sc. degree in physics from Ohio State University in 1964 and shortly thereafter joined APL's Aeronautics Division, where he was involved in research on explosives initiation. In 1969, he joined the Theoretical Problems Group in APL's Milton S. Eisenhower Research Center. He received M.S. (1973) and M.A. (1983) degrees in physics from The Johns Hopkins University, and in 1979–80 was the William S. Parsons Fellow in the Physics Department. Mr. McCally's research interests include the application of light scattering methods to the study of corneal structure, the physics of laser-tissue interactions, and magnetism in amorphous alloys. He is co-principal investigator on a grant from the National Eye Institute that supports corneal light scattering research. His professional memberships include the American Physical Society and the Association for Research in Vision and Ophthalmology.

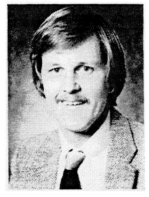

DAVID E. FREUND is a physicist in the Theoretical Problems Group. He joined APL's Milton S. Eisenhower Research Center in 1983. Born in Hamilton, Ohio, he received a B.A. degree from Lycoming College in 1972, an M.S. degree from Purdue University in 1974, and a Ph.D. degree from the University of Delaware in 1982. Dr. Freund's research interests include developing theoretical methods for calculating acoustic and electromagnetic wave scattering in random media and the use of light scattering for probing the ultrastructure of the cornea.

Light-scattering matrices of the crystalline lens

I. L. Maksimova, V. V. Tuchin, and L. P. Shubochkin

(Received 14 August 1987)

Opt. Spektrosk. **65**, 615–620 (September 1988)

Experimental studies have been carried out on the polarized light scattering characteristics of the crystalline lens. The experimental setup and the technique for measuring the elements of the scattering matrix are described.

INTRODUCTION

It is known that certain general illnesses, eye diseases, old age, traumas, and electromagnetic radiation may cause irreversible opacity in the crystalline lens—various forms of cataract.[1] For most forms of cataract, the injured tissues of the crystalline lens do not possess intense spectral absorption peaks in the visible range, and therefore the fundamental reason for the loss of transparency in the crystalline lens, one would suppose, is significant light scattering.[2] Light scattering is the result of local inhomogeneities in the index of refraction of the lens tissue, which is brought about by conglomerates of proteins with different refractive indices.[3] The main fraction of the albumin of the transparent crystal-

line lens is conglomerates of proteins, homogeneous in size ($\sim 0.5 \, \mu$m); however, the scattering by them is small because of their regular distribution. Opacity of the crystalline lens is accompanied by an increase in the size of the protein conglomerates and the appearance of significant inhomogeneities in their sizes.

At present, noninvasive analysis of the opacities in the crystalline lens is usually based on biomicroscopic investigative methods. However, the practical limits for resolving the microstructure using optical microscopes do not exceed 7–10 μm, whereas the formations of conglomerates with small molecular weight amount to hundreds of nanometers.[4] Therefore, for a better understanding of the pathogenesis of opacities in the optical media of the eye, it is necessary to use noninvasive methods with submicron resolution. To study the ultrastructure of the crystalline lens we use various physical diagnostic methods, for example: the spectroscopic method of optical mixing,[5] laser picosecond spectroscopy,[6] Raman spectroscopy.[7] However, all these methods possess a series of significant shortcomings. They either require long observation times, or provide low accuracy given polydispersion of scattering particles, or require comparatively high power levels for the laser radiation. All this complicates the use of the indicated methods on subjects in vivo. Along with this the most complete information on the optical properties of the scattering medium can be obtained, by studying the angular and spectral dependences of the nonzero components of the light scattering matrix (LSM) of the medium.[8] Knowledge of the LSM allows us to solve the problem of light propagation and the structure of the light field in the medium by using matrix transposition theory, and to obtain information on the properties of the particles, suspended in the scattering medium: their form, size, symmetry etc.

The goal of the present work is to experimentally determine the structure of the LSM of transparent and turbid crystalline lenses, to study the angular dependences of its nonzero components during blurring of the lens and analyze certain optical properties of the scattering particles of the objects under study.

MEASUREMENT TECHNIQUE

To conduct our investigations we developed a polarization nephelometer, whose fundamental principle is the modulation of a light beam by rotating the polarization elements with subsequent photoelectric detection of the signal, analog-to-digital conversion and calculation, using the obtained data, of the optical characteristics of the object using a microcomputer coupled to the nephelometer. A scheme was realized with a rotating compensator, which possesses a comparatively simple working algorithm and low electrical requirements.[9,10]

The measurement setup contains a fixed polarizer P, analyzer A, and two rotating phase plates F and F', positioned before and after the object under study (Fig. 1). The polarizer and analyzer were oriented parallel to one another, and their transmission planes perpendicular to the scattering plane; the fast axes of the phase plates F and F' make angles of φ and φ' with the scattering plane, and the phase differences induced by them are equal to δ and δ', respectively. Then, if $S_0\{I_0, Q_0, U_0, V_0\}$ is the Stokes parameter vector at the entrance to the system, and $S\{I, Q, U, V\}$ is the Stokes parameter vector at the exit of the system, then the matrix equation, which relates these vectors, has the form[8]

$$S = A \times F' \times M \times F \times P \times S_0. \tag{1}$$

where P and A are the matrices of the polarizer and analyzer, F and F' are the matrices of the phase plates, M is the matrix of the object under study. The ratio of the rotation rates of the phase plates F and F' was chosen equal to 1/5, i.e., $\varphi' = 5\varphi$. Such a choice for the rate relation allows us to obtain the optimal resulting system of linear equations for the unknown elements of the LSM of the object under study.[11]

Multiplying the matrices in Eq. (1) and carrying out the appropriate trignometric transformations, one can show

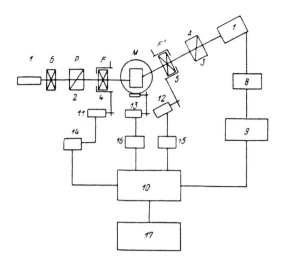

FIG. 1. Block diagram of a polarization nephelometer.

that the intensity I at the output of the system is represented by a Fourier series of the form[11]

$$I = a_0 + \sum_{k=1}^{12} (a_{2k} \cos 2k\varphi + b_{2k} \sin 2k\varphi). \tag{2}$$

The coefficients of the Fourier series (2) may be calculated based on the experimental data using the discrete Fourier transform

$$a_{2k} = \sum_{i=1}^{N} I(\varphi_i) \cos 2k\varphi_i, \qquad b_{2k} = \sum_{i=1}^{N} I(\varphi_i) \sin 2k\varphi_i, \tag{3}$$

where $I(\varphi_i)$ is the radiation intensity recorded by the photodetector by orienting the fast axis of the phase plate F at an angle φ_i to the scattering plane.

The values of the Fourier coefficients a_{2k} and b_{2k} are unambiguously associated with the parameters of the object and the polarization setup used. Their explicit expressions have a simple form if $\delta = \delta' = \pi/2$; however in practice accurate preparation of such plates is quite complicated and deviation of the actually obtained values of δ from $\pi/2$ cannot be considered negligible. Therefore in what follows we will use the general expressions for the coefficients a_{2k} and b_{2k}, obtained for arbitrary δ and δ'. It is easy to show that in this case the matrix elements of the object under study are expressed via the Fourier coefficients a_{2k} and b_{2k} in the following form:

$$\left.
\begin{aligned}
M_{11} &= a_0 - (1+\beta)\beta_1 a_{24} - (1+\beta')\beta_1' a_{20} \\
&\quad + (1+\beta)(1+\beta')\beta_1\beta_1'(a_{24} + a_{16}), \\
M_{12} &= -2\beta_1 a_4 + 2(1+\beta')\beta_1\beta_1'(a_{24} + a_{16}), \\
M_{14} &= -\mu b_2 + (1+\beta')\beta_1'\mu(b_{22} - b_{18}), \\
M_{21} &= -2\beta_1 a_{20} + 2(1+\beta)\beta_1\beta_1'(a_{24} + a_{16}), \\
M_{22} &= 4\beta_1\beta_1'(a_{24} + a_{16}), \\
M_{33} &= 4\beta_1\beta_1'(a_{16} - a_{24}), \\
M_{34} &= 2\beta_1'\mu(a_{18} - a_{22}), \\
M_{41} &= \mu b_{10} + (1+\beta)\beta_1'\mu'(b_{14} + b_6), \\
M_{43} &= 2\beta_1\mu'(a_{14} - a_6), \\
M_{44} &= \mu\mu'(a_{12} - a_8),
\end{aligned}
\right\} \tag{4}$$

where $\beta = \cos\delta$, $\beta' = \cos\delta'$, $\mu = 1/\sin\delta$, $\mu' = 1/\sin\delta'$.

$\beta_1 = 1/(1 - \beta)$, $\beta'_1 = 1/(1 - \beta')$, and the expressions for the matrix elements M_{13}, M_{31}, M_{23}, M_{32}, M_{24}, M_{42}, are obtained from the expressions for M_{12}, M_{21}, M_{22}, M_{33}, M_{14}, M_{41}, respectively, by replacing a_{2k} by b_{2k}.

Thus, to determine all 16 elements of the LSM, it is necessary to measure the light intensity I at the output of the system for N different angular positions of the phase plates F and F' for a period during which, as has been indicated, the rotation rate of the phase plate F' is 5 times greater than the rotation rate of plate F. Then having determined the coefficients a_{2k} and b_{2k} using Eqs. (3), where N for efficient realization of the fast Fourier transform was chosen equal to 256, one can determine the elements M_{ij} of the LSM according to Eqs. (4).

THE EXPERIMENTAL SETUP

The setup is a polarizing nephelometer with rotating phase plates, automated using a microcomputer, which allows us to determine all 16 elements of the LSM in no more than 100 sec.[12] The possibility of conducting accurate angular measurements is ensured by positioning the main terminals of the polarimeter on the G-5 goniometer to an accuracy of no worse than 5″. As light source 1 we used an LHN-207 ($\lambda = 0.63 \mu$m) helium–neon laser, which possesses high stability in the energy characteristics of the output radiation. On the arms of the goniometer, in place of the collimator and the eyepiece, are mounted optical angle-measuring devices with an accuracy for measuring rotation angle of 1′, with which one can visually control the rotation angles of the polarizer 2, analyzer 3, and compensators 4 and 5. Rotation of the angle-measuring devices of the polarizing elements is accomplished using the stepper motors 11 and 12. The controlling pulses to the stepper motors is fed through power amplifiers 14 and 15 by the junction 10 under control of an Electronika DZ-28 microcomputer 17. In front of the angle-measuring devices of the polarizer one can place a quarter-wave plate 6, which transforms the linearly polarized radiation of the laser into circularly polarized radiation.

As is known the highest accuracy and sensitivity when measuring weak light signals can be attained by using the photon-counting method. Therefore for the photodetector 7, we used an FEU-79 photomultiplier, which possesses satisfactory single-electron characteristics.[13] The signal from the PM enters the amplitude discriminator 8—a cut-off device with an amplifier. The discriminator partially cuts off the noise pulses of the PM, and also amplifies an calibrates the signal pulses. The cut-off device of the discriminator passes only those pulses from the PM whose amplitudes are greater than 1 mV, whereupon the amplitude of the amplified pulses does not depend on the amplitude of the initial pulse transmitted by the cut-off device.

The microcomputer puts out a series of pulses which enter the stepper motors through the junction, and on rotation of the optical devices of the polarized elements by a given angle the measured signal from the PM is recorded by the frequency meter 9. The digital values of the light intensity for given angular positions of the polarized elements undergo Fourier analysis to determine the polarization parameters of the radiation under consideration.

Angular scanning with a 4′ step of the analyzer arm is accomplished using stepper motor 13 under control of a microcomputer.

To estimate the measurement accuracy by the indicated method, the LSM were determined in suspensions of polystyrene latex with known parameters. As a result it turned out that the greatest deviations in the values of the elements of the experimental matrix from those calculated according to Mie theory did not exceed 5%.

RESULTS AND DISCUSSION

The studies were carried out on native material. In accordance with the technique illustrated in Ref. 14, crystalline lenses with various degrees of opacity were obtained from rabbits which underwent daily inoculations of naphthalene. As the studies indicated, good measurement results are observed when conducted for an interval of no more than 2 hours; in this case the error in determining any matrix element does not exceed the instrumental error. Individual differences in the transparent crystalline lens were found within the limits of 5–10%, while the variations in the properties of the turbid lenses were more noticeably delineated, which explains the different degrees of maturity of the cataracts.

Measurements of the angular dependences of the LSM elements of transparent and turbid crystalline lenses were carried out in the 20–140° range. In Figs. 2 and 3 we present the results of the measurements, with the values of all matrix elements normalized to the value of element M_{11}.

An analysis of all components of the LSM of various lenses indicates that, to an accuracy of the measurement error, the LSM have the following structure:

$$\begin{bmatrix} M_{11} & M_{12} & M_{13} & 0 \\ M_{12} & M_{22} & M_{23} & 0 \\ M_{13} & M_{23} & M_{33} & M_{34} \\ 0 & 0 & -M_{34} & M_{44} \end{bmatrix}$$

In this case the differences in the M_{33} and M_{34} elements does not exceed 10%. The presence of nonzero values for elements M_{13} and M_{23} suggests that the scattering particles of the crystalline lens are characterized by a coefficient of cross-polarization which is different from zero.[8] A possible explanation of this may be the optical activity of the material of the crystalline lens or, more likely, scattering in structures of the lens whose axis of symmetry is inclined to the scattering plane. The smooth character of all the obtained curves is explained by the polydispersion of the scattering particles of the lens.

Elements M_{12} and M_{21} are equal, within the limits of experimental accuracy, and satisfy the inequality $M_{12} \leqslant 0$ over the whole range of scattering angles, i.e., the degree of polarization $P = -M_{12}/M_{11}$ is positive,[8] which is characteristic of scattering by particles which are significantly smaller than the light wavelength. As is obvious from Fig. 2, the maximum degree of linear polarization P in the case of a transparent crystalline lens is attained for 90°, however, even for this scattering angle the degree of linear polarization is less than unity.

The zero point of the angular distribution of the M_{33} element for all transparent lenses we studied was located at an angle of 90° or shifted by 2–3° to the side of larger scattering angles. Element M_{22} is essentially constant over all the region under study, with an increase in the scattering angle its value decreases somewhat. The values of the elements M_{34} and M_{43} for a transparent lens are opposite in sign, how-

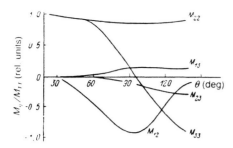

FIG. 2. Characteristic curves of the LSM elements of a normal crystalline lens.

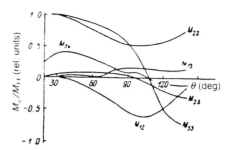

FIG. 3. Characteristic curves of the LSM elements of a cataractous crystalline lens.

ever, their value is so small that it is comparable to the experimental error, and they are not presented in Fig. 2. One should note that in the whole range of angles that were measured the elements of the LSM of a transparent crystalline lens satisfy the inequality

$$M_{11}^2 > M_{12}^2 + M_{33}^2 + M_{34}^2, \tag{5}$$

which is valid for an accumulation of spherical particles that are inhomogeneous in size or composition.[15]

As is evident from Fig. 3, the angular characteristics of the LSM for a turbid crystalline lens varies considerably. The values of the elements M_{12} and M_{21}, while remaining negative, decrease in absolute value, and the extremum point shifts to the side of larger scattering angles. The angular dependence of the element M_{22} indicates the presence in the medium of large nonspherical scattering particles. Large-scale particles are also responsible for shifting the intersection point of the M_{33} curve along the x axis to the direction of angles > 100°. At the same time, inasmuch as the value of P is positive over the whole region of scattering angles, taking into account the calculations of Ref. 16, one can conclude that the most likely particle size determining the behavior of this characteristic does not exceed 0.5 μm. One should note that for a turbid crystalline lens, an increase in the absolute value of the elements M_{34} and M_{43} in the region of scattering angles 30–40° is observed. The behavior of the components M_{23} and M_{32} of transparent and turbid crystalline lenses is identical, their values are less than zero for scattering angle greater than 80°, and close to zero for small scattering angles. One should note that for small scattering angles the matrix elements of a turbid lens do not satisfy inequality (5).

Thus the study indicates that the elements of the LSM of transparent and cataractous crystalline lenses possess clearly pronounced differences in absolute value and angular dependences. This is promising for conducting experiments in the dynamics of variation in the LSM elements of crystalline lenses during the process of developing opacity, with the goal of developing methods of quantitative diagnostics of the pathological processes of crystalline lens tissue.

The authors wish to thank P. I. Saprykin for his useful consultations, and also V. V. Bakutkin and A. G. Safaryan for help in conducting the experiments on the biological subjects.

[1]V. V. Shmeleva, *Cataracts* (Moscow, 1981).

[2]G. B. Benedek, Appl. Opt. **10**, 459 (1971).

[3]J. A. Jedziniak, D. F. Nicoli, H. Baram, and G. B. Benedek, Invest. Ophthalm. Visual Sci. **17**, 51 (1978).

[4]A. Spector and S. Li, Invest. Ophthalm. **13**, 795 (1975).

[5]T. Tanaka and G. B. Benedek, Invest. Ophthalm. **14**, 449 (1975).

[6]A. B. Bruckner, Appl. Opt. **17**, 3177 (1978).

[7]Y. Ozaki and K. Iriyuma, in *Laser Scattering Spectroscopy of Biological Objects* (Prague, 1986), p. 56.

[8]C. F. Bohren and D. R. Huffman, *Absorption and Scattering of Light by Small Particles* (Wiley, New York, 1973; Moscow, 1986).

[9]V. V. Tuchin, L. P. Shubochkin, I. L. Maksimova, and Yu. P. Volkov, in *XII All-Union Conference on Coherent and Non-Linear Optics: Lecture Summaries* (1985), p. 171.

[10]M. L. Aleksandrov, L. I. Asinovskii, A. L. Meltsin, and V. A. Tolokonnikov, Zh. Prikl. Spektrosk. **44**, 887 (1986).

[11]P. S. Hauge, Surf. Sci. **96**, 108 (1980).

[12]Yu. P. Volkov, I. L. Maksimova, V. V. Tuchin, and L. P. Shubochkin, in *Electronics Industry*, No. 1 (1987), p. 48.

[13]S. S. Vetokhin, I. R. Gulakov, A. N. Pertsev, and I. V. Reznikov, *Single Electron Photodetectors* (Moscow, 1986).

[14]L. A. Linnik, N. I. Usov, P. P. Chechin, and O. S. Pelepchuk, Oftalm. Zh. **4**, 193 (1982).

[15]E. S. Fry and G. W. Kattawar, Appl. Opt. **20**, 2811 (1981).

[16]K. S. Shifrin and I. L. Zeldovich, *Light Scattering Tables, Vol. 2* (Leningrad, 1968).

Reprinted with permission from *Journal of Molecular Biology,* Vol. 205,
pp. 713-728 (1989). ©1989 Academic Press Inc. (London) Ltd.

Molecular Basis of Eye Lens Transparency

Osmotic Pressure and X-ray Analysis of α-Crystallin Solutions

Françoise Vérétout[1], Mireille Delaye[2]† and Annette Tardieu[1]

[1] *Centre de Génétique Moléculaire*
CNRS, 91190 Gif sur Yvette, France

[2] *Laboratoire de Physique des Solides*
Université Paris-Sud, 91405 Orsay, France

Short range, liquid-like order of the crystallin proteins accounts for eye lens transparency. The relationship between structural and thermodynamic properties of eye lens was further investigated using osmotic pressure and small-angle X-ray scattering measurements of calf lens α-crystallins. The consistency of both data sets confirms that the macroscopic thermodynamic properties are determined by the structural properties accessible to X-ray scattering. In addition, the experimental data were correctly accounted for using a model developed in liquid-state physics: the rescaled mean spherical approximation combined with a Verwey–Overbeek potential. This model provides as best fit parameters the excluded volume, the charge and the diameter of an "equivalent" particle that compare well with the corresponding values found in the literature for α-crystallins. As a result, transparency may now be expressed as a function of a few structural parameters, the role of which is discussed. The approach presented here may be extended to studies of the thermodynamic–structural relationships of other protein solutions.

1. Introduction

Eye lens offers an example of a biological function, i.e. light focusing on the retina, which is linked to macroscopic physical properties such as refractive index and light transmission. For several years we have been interested in relating these global properties to local structure and composition.

Mammalian lens fibre cells enclose, as a major component, high concentrations (20 to 40%, w/w) of lens-specific proteins, the crystallins. In the normal state, eye lens transparency is limited mainly by light-scattering owing to these proteins. In a previous paper (Delaye & Tardieu, 1983), we discussed the relationships between lens transparency and the protein spatial organization. A short-range, liquid-like order of the crystallins was shown to account for lens transparency. The aim of this work is to go a step further, i.e. to relate such spatial organization to crystallin structure and interactions (or interaction potentials).

Among crystallins, the most efficient light-scatterers are the largest, the α-crystallins. The use in this study of purified α-crystallins instead of lens

cytoplasmic extracts (Delaye & Tardieu, 1983), was therefore justified and has greatly simplified the analysis. Calf lens α-crystallins are polydisperse globular particles made of a large number of two types of subunit (Harding & Dilley, 1976; Siezen *et al.*, 1978; Bloemendal, 1981), for which we have proposed a quaternary structure model (Tardieu *et al.*, 1986).

The coupling of approaches sensitive either to macroscopic or to structural properties was essential. In this paper we develop an approach that associates osmotic pressure (Prouty *et al.*, 1985) and solution X-ray scattering (Tardieu *et al.*, 1987) measurements, while data analysis relies on models developed in liquid-state physics (Hayter & Penfold, 1981; Hansen & Hayter, 1982).

All of the results obtained allowed us to sort out a few structural parameters particularly relevant for transparency and to express transparency as a function of them. At the same time, these results open the way to the study of other lens properties. The approach presented here could be applied to a variety of protein solutions.

2. Theory

Two major physical phenomena limit lens transparency, absorption and scattering of visible

---

† Deceased.

light. In the normal state, absorption is negligible, since the lens components contain few visible chromophores. Light-scattering arises from short-range fluctuations of refractive index, essentially owing to the lens-specific proteins, the crystallins. At the high concentration of protein prevailing in the lens fibre cells (up to about 400 mg/cm³), the level of scattering is determined by the spatial organization, or local order, of the crystallin proteins (Trokel, 1962; Benedek, 1971; Delaye & Tardieu, 1983; see also Tardieu & Delaye (1988) for a more detailed account of the theoretical background).

Transparency is usually quantified by the extinction coefficient τ, which allows us to calculate the transmitted intensity, I_t, for an incident intensity I_0, through a sample of thickness l:

$$I_t = I_0 \exp(-\tau l). \qquad (1)$$

The extinction coefficient is related to the integral of scattered light in all directions, which for isotropic light-scattering may be written:

$$\tau = (16\pi/3) R^2 I_s / I_0, \qquad (2)$$

where I_s is the scattered intensity measured at a distance R from the sample. This scattered intensity may be expressed in terms of macroscopic parameters according to the thermodynamic approach, or in terms of structural parameters according to the particle approach.

(a) The thermodynamic approach

Whenever the wavelength, λ, is large compared to particle sizes, the scattered intensity is invariant with the scattering angle and is conveniently expressed with macroscopic, thermodynamic parameters. This is the case for lens proteins studied by light-scattering.

Whenever the solution can be considered ideal, the following scattering expression, for unpolarized radiation and for polydisperse particles, may be considered as a reasonable approximation (Kerker, 1969; Eisenberg, 1976):

$$R^2 I/I_s/I_0 = (2\pi^2/\lambda^4)n_0^2(\partial n/\partial c)^2 M_w c/N_a, \qquad (3)$$

where n_0 is the refractive index of the solvent, $(\partial n/\partial c)$ is the refractive index increment due to the presence of solute, M_w is the weight average molecular weight ($M_w = \Sigma c_i M_i / \Sigma c_i$), c is the protein concentration in g/cm³, and N_a is Avagadro's number.

Departure from ideality, which is usually observed in concentrated solutions, corresponds to departure from 1 of an interference term introduced as a multiplying factor, $cRT\beta/M_n$. R is the gas constant, T is absolute temperature, M_n is the number average molecular weight ($M_n = \Sigma c_i / \Sigma(c_i/M_i)$) and β the compressibility of the solution. The compressibility is related to fluctuations in the number N of particles around the average value. It may be expressed in terms of

osmotic pressure, Π, by (Guinier & Fournet, 1955; Eisenberg, 1976):

$$\beta = (-1/V)(\partial\Pi/\partial V)^{-1} = (1/c)(\partial\Pi/\partial c)^{-1}, \qquad (4)$$

therefore:

$$R^2 I_s/I_0 = (2\pi^2/\lambda^4)n_0^2(\partial n/\partial c)^2 (M_w c/N_a) \\ \times (RT/M_n)(\partial\Pi/\partial c)^{-1}. \qquad (5)$$

Note that we distinguish here the weight average, M_w, and the number average, M_n, molecular weight since, usually, the values do not coincide with polydisperse particles.

In the thermodynamic approach, the osmotic pressure is often expanded as a series of virial coefficients:

$$\Pi = cRT((1/M_n) + A_2 c + A_3 c^2 + \ldots). \qquad (6)$$

The interference term in equation (5) is then expressed as a function of these coefficients. Another possibility is to relate the osmotic pressure to the partition function $Z(c)$ of the system:

$$\Pi = (RT/M_n)Z(c). \qquad (7)$$

In the case of hard spheres, i.e. of impenetrable spheres without any other interaction neither repulsive nor attractive, Carnahan & Starling (1969) have developed a closed analytical expression of the partition function as a function of one parameter, ϕ, which is the excluded volume fraction associated with the particles:

$$Z(c) = c(1 + \phi + \phi^2 - \phi^3)/(1-\phi)^3. \qquad (8)$$

The interference term in equation (5) is then obtained from derivatives of $Z(c)$.

(b) The particle approach

Whenever λ is small compared to particle sizes, the scattering varies with the scattering angle. This is the case for lens proteins studied with X-ray scattering. The particle approach is then particularly rewarding, since it provides a structural expression for the scattering.

The intensity scattered by one particle as a function of s (where $s = 2\sin\theta/\lambda$, and 2θ is the scattering angle), usually called the particle form factor, is the Fourier transform of the spherically averaged auto-correlation function of the electron density contrast associated with the particle. When the solution is ideal, the total scattering, $I(0,s)$, is the sum of the scattering of the individual particles. When normalized to one electron of solute particle, and assuming particles of identical chemical composition and partial specific volumes, the forward scattered intensity, or intensity at the origin, $I(0,0)$, becomes (Luzzati & Tardieu, 1980):

$$I(0,0) = m_w(1 - \rho_0\psi)^2, \qquad (9)$$

where m_w is the average number of electrons of one particle ($m_w = \Sigma c_i m_i / \Sigma c_i$), ρ_0 is the electron density of the solvent ($e/\text{Å}^3$) and ψ is the partial electronic volume of the particle ($\text{Å}^3/e$) (1 Å = 0·1 nm).

With concentrated solutions of monodisperse, spherical particles, departure from ideality may be accounted for simply by a multiplying factor or interference term, $S(c,s)$, which is a function of the scattering angle:

$$I(c,s) = I(0,s)S(c,s). \qquad (10)$$

$S(c,s)$ is usually called the solution structure factor. Since the solution can be described mathematically as the convolution product of a particle shape and a particle distribution (i.e. a set of delta functions placed at the particle centres), $S(c,s)$ is the Fourier transform of the spherically averaged auto-correlation function $g(r)$ of the particle distribution:

$$S(c,s) = 1 + (N/V) \int_0^\infty 4\pi r^2 (g(r) - 1) \\ \times (\sin 2\pi rs / 2\pi rs) \, \mathrm{d}r, \qquad (11)$$

where (N/V) is the number of particles per unit volume. Equation (10) can still be considered valid, yet in a smaller s range, with quasi-spherical particles and/or polydisperse particles.

(c) Relationships between thermodynamic and structural parameters

Since the value at zero angle of the interference term (or X-ray structure factor) in equation (10) must coincide with the light interference term of equation (5), one obtains the following relationships between macroscopic thermodynamic and microscopic structural parameters:

$$(RT/M_n)(\partial\Pi/\partial c)^{-1} = S(c,0) \qquad (12)$$

or

$$\Pi = (RT/M_n) \int_0^c (1/S(c,0)) \, \mathrm{d}c. \qquad (13)$$

One aim of this paper is to show that such relationships are indeed valid for α-crystallin solutions (and for protein solutions in general).

τ may now be written as a function of either thermodynamic or structural variables:

$$\tau = (32\pi^3/3\lambda^4)n_0^2(\partial n/\partial c)^2(cRT/N_a)(M_w/M_n)(\partial\Pi/\partial c)^{-1}, \qquad (14)$$

$$\tau = (32\pi^3/3\lambda^4)n_0^2(\partial n/\partial c)^2(M_w c/N_a)S(c,0). \qquad (15)$$

In the case of hard spheres, equations (8) and (12) provide a simple expression for $S(c,0)$:

$$S(c,0) = (1-\phi)^4/(1+4\phi+4\phi^2-4\phi^3+\phi^4). \qquad (16)$$

(d) Modelling the structure factors and the osmotic pressure

Since the solution structure factor $S(c,s)$ is related to particle distribution, $S(c,s)$ can be calculated from the interactions or interaction potentials between neighbouring particles that govern such distributions. Through a model, the interactions and thus $S(c,s)$, are usually expressed

as a function of a few macromolecular structural parameters. Once $S(c,s)$ is known, the osmotic pressure Π may be calculated from the $S(c,0)$ variation as a function of c by equation (13). Reciprocally, model-fitting provides us with the relevant structural parameters. Finally, the extinction coefficient (eqns (14) and (15)) and therefore the transparency (eqn (1)) may be expressed as a function of these parameters.

A particularly convenient analytical procedure has been developed in liquid-state physics to calculate the case of repulsive screened coulombic interactions; the rescaled mean spherical approximation (RMSA†) coupled to a Verwey–Overbeek (VO) potential (Verwey & Overbeek, 1948; Hayter & Penfold, 1981; Hansen & Hayter, 1982). The validity of the hypotheses involved in modelling structure factors of α-crystallin solutions has been discussed (Tardieu et al., 1987), using two protein concentrations and two ionic strengths.

The model depends upon three structural parameters; the excluded volume fraction ϕ, the charge Ze and the particle diameter σ. (When the charge is small, or screened at high ionic strength, this model is essentially equivalent to a hard sphere model and the $S(c,0)$ values are similar to those calculated from eqn (16).)

The screened Coulomb potential between spherical particles, in the MKS system is described by:

$$v(r) = (\pi\varepsilon_0\varepsilon\sigma^2\psi_0^2/r)\exp((-k(r-\sigma)) \quad \text{for } r > \sigma, \qquad (17)$$

where r is the interparticle centre to centre distance, ε is the dielectric constant of the solvent medium, ε_0 is the permittivity of free space and k is the Debye–Hückel inverse screening length:

$$k = 1/\lambda_d = (2e^2 10^3 N_a I/\varepsilon_0\varepsilon k_B T)^{1/2}, \qquad (18)$$

where e is the electronic charge, k_B is the Boltzmann constant and I is the ionic strength of the solvent (in mol). Typically, in an aqueous solution at 25°C one finds:

$$\lambda_d(\text{Å}) = 3/\sqrt{I}. \qquad (19)$$

ψ_0 is the surface potential related, in the Debye–Hückel approximation, to an "effective" particle charge Ze through:

$$\psi_0 = Ze/\pi\varepsilon_0\varepsilon\sigma(2+k\sigma). \qquad (20)$$

Typically for aqueous solutions, one has, σ being expressed in ångström units:

$$\psi_0(mV) = 720Z/\sigma(2+k\sigma). \qquad (21)$$

The model usually assumes impenetrable spheres, i.e. ϕ and σ linked by the following relationship:

$$\phi = (cN_a/6M_w)\pi\sigma^3. \qquad (22)$$

---

† Abbreviations used: RMSA, rescaled mean spherical approximation; VO, Verwey–Overbeek; HPLC, high-pressure liquid chromatography; MKS, metre-kilogram-second.

Tardieu *et al.* (1987) assumed this relationship to be fulfilled. In this work it was not, as explained in Results.

3. Materials and Methods

(a) α-Crystallin preparation

α-Crystallins were prepared as described by Tardieu *et al.* (1986). Briefly, α-crystallins were extracted from the cortex (i.e. periphery) of fresh calf lenses. The cortex was first homogenized in 4 vol. physiological buffer B1 (B1 is a phosphate buffer (pH 6·8), ionic strength $I = 150$ mM adjusted with KCl, supplemented with NaN_3, dithiothreitol and phenylmethylsulphonyl fluoride). The solution was centrifuged for 30 min at $10,000 g$ to separate the membrane fragments. α-Crystallins were prepared from the centrifuged solution by gel filtration, using a Fractogel (TSK-HW55S) column (volume 600 ml) eluted with buffer B1. Under these conditions, α-crystallins elute as a first broad peak. The top portion of the α-peak was pooled for the experiments, resulting in an α population with about 10 to 15% size polydispersity.

For the X-ray experiments as a function of concentration and ionic strength, a stock solution at high concentration was prepared first. The stock solution was then divided. One part was diluted with buffer B1 to reach various concentrations. The others were dialysed for 2 days against the appropriate low ionic strength buffers ($I = 17$ mM: 10 mM-phosphate (pH 6·8) $I = 35$ and $I = 75$ mM were further adjusted with KCl) before dilution with the corresponding buffer.

To reach α-crystallin concentrations up to about 0·10 g/cm^3, an Amicon ultrafiltration cell with a YM100 membrane was used. For higher concentrations, the solutions were further concentrated by ultrafiltration (180,000 g for 4 h at 20°C) to reach $c = 0·35$ g/cm^3.

HPLC controls were performed with a SW4000 TSK column (30 cm).

(b) Concentration measurements

At low concentrations, α-crystallin concentrations were usually measured by absorbance, using $A_{1cm}^{1\%} = 8·45$. At high concentrations, either dry weight (2 days at 45°C in a Savant Speed Vac concentrator connected to a liquid nitrogen trap) or refractive index measurements were used. The refractive index calibration curve *versus* concentration c (g/cm^3) was itself established using either dry weight or absorbance measurements to yield the following relationships:

$$n = 1·3342 + 0·183\,c \quad \text{at } 150 \text{ mM};$$
$$n = 1·3328 + 0·186\,c \quad \text{at } 17 \text{ mM}.$$

(c) X-ray scattering

Experiments were performed using the small-angle instrument D24 at the Synchrotron Radiation Laboratory LURE (Orsay) (Depautex *et al.*, 1987). The X-ray beam was monochromated ($\lambda = 1·608$ Å, K-edge of Co) and focused with a bent germanium crystal. Point collimation geometry was used. The X-ray beam had a full-width cross-section of about 0·5 mm × 1·0 mm at the detector level. The detector was a linear position-sensitive detector with delay line readout linked to a data-acquisition system designed at the E.M.B.L., Heidelberg and Hamburg (Bordas *et al.*, 1980). A 1 mm slit was

placed in front of the detector to maintain point collimation conditions.

In the 1st series of experiments, the sample to detector distance was 2 m, ds/channel was $0·62 \times 10^{-4}$ Å^{-1} ($s = 2 \sin \theta / \lambda$, with 2θ the scattering angle) and the recorded s range was $0·8 \times 10^{-3} < s < 1·1 \times 10^{-2}$ Å^{-1}. In the 2nd and 3rd series, the sample to detector distance was 1 m. Accordingly the ds/channel was about twice as large: $1·355 \times 10^{-4}$ Å^{-1} and the recorded s range was $1·3 \times 10^{-3} < s < 2·2 \times 10^{-2}$ Å^{-1}.

Samples were contained in calibrated quartz capillary tubes, about 1 mm in diameter. Experiments were performed at room temperature. Average exposure time for samples with $c > 0·10$ g/cm^3 was from 10 to 20 min. The $c < 0·01$ g/cm^3 sample, the scattering curve of which is used as the form factor, and the background were recorded several times during the run, for a total exposure time of about 100 min.

After background subtraction, the experimental intensities $I_{exp}(c,s)$ were put on an absolute scale $I(c,s)$ according to (Luzzati & Tardieu, 1980):

$$I(c,s) = I_{exp}(c,s)/\mu E_0 \phi_c c,$$

where μ takes into account physical constants, E_0 is the photon number of the incident beam measured by reference to a previously calibrated carbon black sample, and ϕ_c is the thickness of the capillary tube, determined by measurement of water absorption.

Since the absolute scale normation is only accurate within about 10%, the scattering curves recorded at different concentrations and plotted on a log scale were found to be parallel, yet not identical, for $s > 0·0095$ Å^{-1}. To render the scattering curves identical in this region, these curves were re-normalized to the same integrated intensity for $s > 0·0095$ Å^{-1}.

(d) Osmotic pressure

The osmotic pressure of the α-crystallin solutions was measured using a "secondary" osmometer, directly copied from that designed and described by Prouty *et al.* (1985). This osmotic stress technique is, in principle, simple and straightforward; the solution of interest is equilibrated against a polymer solution of known osmotic pressure.

For most experiments, we used a "carousel" osmometer, i.e. a simple beaker (volume 250 cm^3) in which 4 bags of protein solution could be equilibrated against the same polymer solution. The dialysis bag was from either Union Carbide, after normal soaking (cutoff 12,000 to 14,000 M_r) or Spectrapor 2. Trials with Spectrapor 6 and a larger cutoff (50,000 M_r) did not lead to reduced dialysis times. Dialysis tubing was 6·4 mm flat-width. Intramedic tubing was made of glass, simply positioned in a rubber stopper regularly spaced on the cover. The sample volume in the bag was from 0·2 to 0·5 cm^3 and the volume of polymer solution was 120 to 180 cm^3. The stressing reservoir solution was therefore in large excess compared to the studied solution, so that the activity of the reservoir components could be regarded as fixed during the experiment. A magnetic stirrer ensured mixing.

The limitation of the osmotic stress technique clearly lies in establishing accurate calibration curves for the stressing polymer solutions. Dextran was chosen for the availability of such curves and for the range of osmotic pressure covered. The osmotic pressure of dextran T250, with number average molecular weight 100,000, was measured as a function of concentration by LeNeveu *et* al. (1976). Prouty *et al.* (1985) and Parsegian *et al.* (1986) showed that, for concentrations above 10% (w/w), dextrans of different number average molecular weight are remarkably alike and that osmotic pressure is well-represented as a function of weight %, w (since dextran solutions are prepared by weighing the components), by the relationship:

$$\log \Pi = 2 \cdot 75 + 1 \cdot 03 \omega^{0 \cdot 383}$$

In this work, dextran T500 (Pharmacia Fine Chemicals), i.e. a fractionated sample of number average molecular weight of about 185,000, was chosen for its high level of purity. The above relationship was used for $w > 0 \cdot 1$ g/g. For $w < 0 \cdot 1$ g/g, the calibration curve of T500 was established using T250. The following relationship was obtained:

$$\log \Pi = 2 \cdot 48 + 1 \cdot 05 \omega^{0 \cdot 416}$$

In the range of dextran concentrations used, the osmotic pressure was found to be virtually independent of the buffer and the ionic strength.

The concentration after equilibration was checked by refractive index measurements using an Abbe refractometer. Calibration was made using freshly weighted dextran solutions at 2 ionic strengths. The regression lines led to:

$$n = 1 \cdot 3338 + 0 \cdot 154 \ w \quad \text{at 150 mM;}$$
$$n = 1 \cdot 3323 + 0 \cdot 152 \ w \quad \text{at 17 mM.}$$

(e) *Model calculations*

Theoretical structure factors $S_{\text{th}}(c, s)$ were calculated using the Fortran package developed by Hayter & Penfold (1981) and as modified by Hansen & Hayter (1982) implemented on an IBM computer at the Centre Inter Régional de Calcul Electronique (CIRCE, Orsay).

4. Results

(a) *X-ray analysis*

(i) *Experimental data*

Three series of experiments were performed, corresponding to three different preparations. In the first series, the protein concentration was from $0 \cdot 01$ to about $0 \cdot 10$ g/cm^3 and the experiments were performed at four ionic strengths, 150, 75, 35 and 17 mM. In the second series, the protein concentration varied from $0 \cdot 01$ to $0 \cdot 34$ g/cm^3 and the experiments were performed at 150 and 17 mM. The normalized scattering curves recorded in this second series are shown in Figure 1. The last series was performed essentially to check the reproducibility of the results from one preparation to another. Four protein concentrations, from $0 \cdot 01$ to $0 \cdot 32$ g/cm^3, were studied at 150 and 17 mM.

In each series of experiments, a low protein concentration ($0 \cdot 005 < c < 0 \cdot 010$ g/cm^3) curve recorded at I $= 150$ mM in the same conditions, yet with a long accumulation time, was used as the form factor. This concentration was chosen as a compromise between the contradictory requirements of sufficient signal yet negligible interactions in the recorded range. The form factor was found to vary slightly from one preparation to the other. The

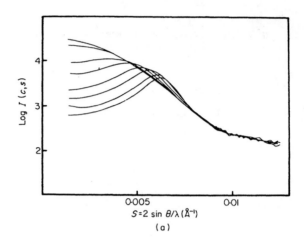

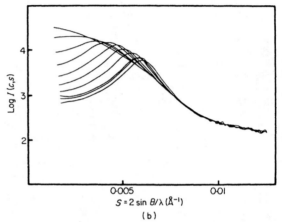

Figure 1. X-ray scattering curves selected within the 2nd series of experiments at (a) 150 and (b) 17 mM. The data are subtracted for background and normalized as indicated in Materials and Methods but otherwise uncorrected. From top to bottom, protein concentration was (a) 10, 25, 84, 147, 205, 273, 308, 343 mg/cm^3; and (b) 10, 36, 66, 107, 147, 184, 215, 272, 284, 308 mg/cm^3.

measured radii of gyration and average molecular weight were found to be, respectively, 65 Å and 1,000,000 in the first preparation, 67 Å and 1,000,000 in the second and 61 Å and 800,000 in the third. In a previous paper (Tardieu *et al.*, 1986), we discussed the fact that α-crystallins are rather sensitive to physico-chemical conditions, temperature and age of the preparation (see also Van den Oetelaar *et al.*, 1985). Differences such as those observed here have been observed between fresh and "aged" preparations, or because of a different pooling of the fractions after gel filtration. On the other hand, no evolution of the form factor was observed during the one or two days necessary to record a series of scattering spectra. After the central peak, the form factor displays one broad shoulder around $s = 0 \cdot 01$ Å^{-1} but no well-defined minimum (Fig. 1). All these features were accounted for by a three-layer model, displaying tetrahedral symmetry (Fig. 9), in which the variation of the average molecular weight from one

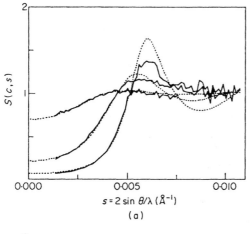

(a)

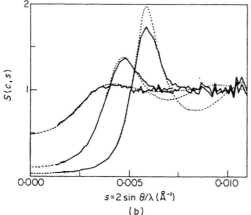

(b)

Figure 2. Continuous lines, examples of experimental structure factors calculated from scattering curves of the 2nd series as described in Materials and Methods. Dotted lines, best fits calculated from the RMSA+VO model. (a) 150 nM; protein concentration, 25, 99 and 205 mg/cm^3; (b) 17 mM; protein concentration, 36, 107 and 215 mg/cm^3.

preparation to the other and/or as a function of time, and the polydispersity around this average value corresponds to a variable filling of the external layers (Tardieu *et al.*, 1986).

As a function of protein concentration, the scattered intensity near the origin decreases, while a more pronounced maximum is observed at medium angles (Fig. 1). In each series, all the curves coincide at high angles. The coincidence indicates that the form factor remains essentially the same whatever the concentration, and it is only a function of the α-crystallin population selected for the experiments. The qualitative behaviour is similar at both ionic strengths yet, when the ionic strength decreases at a given concentration, the height of the maximum increases while its position is shifted towards lower s values. From one series to another, the variation of the scattering spectra with protein concentration and ionic strength was found

to be the same. The peak position, however, at a given concentration, may vary slightly from one preparation to another. Such variation is correlated with the radius of gyration variation; the higher the radius of gyration, the lower the s value of the peak position.

(ii) *Structure factor modelling*

We found it convenient to calculate experimental structure factors $S_{exp}(c, s)$ as described in Materials and Methods, using equation (10), and to model them using the rescaled mean spherical approximation (RMSA) coupled to a Verwey–Overbeek (VO) potential, the adequacy of which has been discussed (Tardieu *et al.*, 1987). Therefore, only the main features of the model are recalled here.

In the whole concentration range, the experimental structure factors start from values lower than 1 near $s = 0$, rise to a maximum (height of the peak higher than 1) and fall to 1. Some examples are shown in Figure 2. Such features, coupled to ionic strength sensitivity, are typical of repulsive electrostatic interactions.

The model depends upon three parameters, the excluded volume fraction ϕ, the particle diameter σ and the charge Ze. In the absence of charges, the amplitude of the minima and maxima of the structure factors is determined only by ϕ and their position essentially by σ. ϕ and σ can thus be determined independently. The charges essentially affect the amplitude of the maxima and minima in such a way that when nothing is known about ϕ and Ze, these amplitudes may be accounted for by a number of coupled ϕ and Ze values. To resolve the ambiguity, experiments may be performed at different ionic strengths to change the screening of the charges and thus their effect on the structure factor amplitudes. ϕ and Ze can then be determined if both parameters are assumed to be independent of ionic strength.

The RMSA+VO potential model cannot take polydispersity into account. Polydispersity, however, essentially results in an experimental first maximum lower than the calculated one, and in the disappearance of subsequent minima and maxima. Neglecting polydispersity, therefore, does not affect the determination of the other parameters significantly, provided the fit is restricted to the low-angle part of the scattering curve, typically out to $s = 0.004$ Å^{-1}.

Tardieu *et al.* (1987) assumed that the fitting parameters were invariant with protein concentration. In addition, ϕ and σ were assumed to be related by equation (22). These hypotheses were found inappropriate when the analysis was carried out over a large range of protein concentrations. A modified fitting procedure had to be designed, which is explained below and summarized in Table 1. Since at high ionic strength the charges are at least partly screened, each of the 150 mM scattering curves is fitted in a first step (S1), with ϕ and σ as the only variables, keeping Ze equal to an

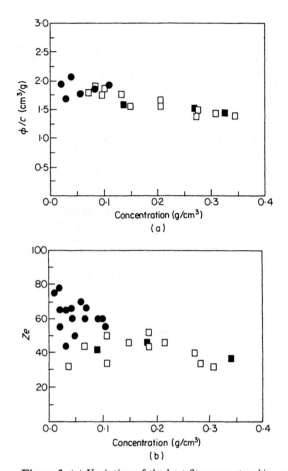

Figure 3. (a) Variation of the best fit parameter ϕ/c as a function of protein concentration. The fit was done on the 150 mM data. (●) 1st, (□) 2nd and (■) 3rd series of experiments. (b) Variation of the best fit parameter Ze, determined from the 17 mM data, as a function of protein concentration. (●) 1st, (□) 2nd and (■) 3rd series of experiments (the data at 35 and 75 mM of the first series are included).

Each of the 17 mM curves is then fitted with Ze and σ as the only variables. An average Ze value is thus determined as well as the variation of σ as a function of c at 17 mM. The average Ze value is then reintroduced at $I = 150$ mM and the process reiterated until convergence. When the charge is totally unknown, it is advisable to start with $Ze = 1$. Using the results from our previous work (Tardieu *et al.*, 1987), this initial value was chosen to be 50.

Examples of typical fits at 150 mM are shown in Figure 2(a). The agreement is excellent out to $s = 0.005$ Å^{-1} and reasonably good around the first maximum, where the difference between experimental and calculated intensity, which can be ascribed to polydispersity, remains less than 20% up to $c = 0.25$ g/cm^3. This difference increases to about 30% at higher concentrations, which could mean that other effects, such as departure from sphericity, begin to play a role. Typical fit examples at 17 mM are shown in Figure 2(b). The agreement between experimental and calculated structure factors is even better than at 150 mM up to $c = 0.25$ g/cm^3. The additional repulsive effect introduced by the unscreening of the charges may partly mask the size polydispersity and/or the charge polydispersity is lower than the size polydispersity. Around $c = 0.30$ g/cm^3, however, the difference between experimental and calculated structure factors become similar to that observed at 150 mM. Figure 2 shows that for a given experiment, a change of a few per cent in the maximum position or in the low angle amplitude is easily detectable, even by eye, and therefore that, within the strategy adopted, the best fit parameters are determined without ambiguity. The uncertainties in the parameters' determination lie elsewhere; namely, in the concentration determination and, especially at low concentration, in the background subtraction.

The resulting Ze values after one fit cycle are shown on Figure 3(b). Ze was found to vary from about 60 at low concentration to about 40 at $c = 0.30$ g/cm^3, with an average value close to 50. We therefore did not find it necessary to reiterate the process. Note that the corresponding surface charge remains small, so that at 150 mM the charge is almost completely screened and barely affects the fits.

initial value. Thus, we derive the variations of ϕ and σ as a function of c. In a second step (S2), this variation of ϕ with c is assumed to be independent of ionic strength and thus to be valid at 17 mM.

Table 1
X-ray data: fitting procedure

Step	I (mM)	Known param.	Fixed param.	Fitting param.	Result
			For the ith experiment		From the series of experiments
S1	150	c_i	$Ze_i = Ze_1$	ϕ_i, σ_i	$\phi(c) = f_1(c)$ $\sigma(c) = g_1(c)$
S2	17	c_i'	$\phi_i' = f_1(c_i')$	$Z'e_i, \sigma_i'$	$Z'e_1 = \Sigma Z'e_i/n'$ $\sigma'(c) = g_1'(c)$

Test: $Z'e_1 = Ze_1$?   No: go to S1 with $Ze_i = Z'e_1$
Yes: stop here

Control: $\sigma(c) = \sigma'(c)$?

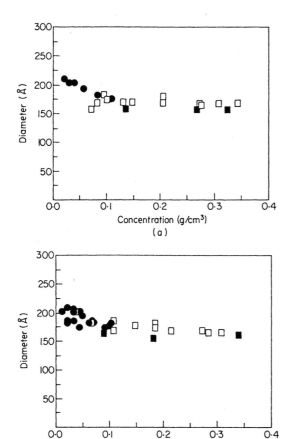

Figure 4. Variation of the best fit parameter σ as a function of protein concentration. (a) 150 mM and (b) 17 (or 35 or 75) mM. (●) 1st, (□) 2nd and (■) 3rd series of experiments.

The resulting ϕ values are plotted in Figure 3(a) in the form $\phi/c = f(c)$. ϕ/c was found particularly convenient, since it is analogous to a specific volume; when the excluded volume fraction is equal to the dry volume fraction, ϕ/c is equal to the partial specific volume of the solute which, for proteins, is close to 0·74 cm³/g. Although there is some scatter in the data of Figure 3(a), ϕ/c can be seen to vary from about 2 at low concentrations up to about 1·4 at $c = 0·35$ g/cm³. The values obtained from the three preparations follow the same variation. ϕ/c thus seems independent of the molecular weight. The ϕ/c data of Figure 3(a) were fitted by a straight line; $\phi/c = 1·953 - 1·72\,c$.

The variation of σ as a function of protein concentration at 150 and 17 mM (qualitatively visible on Fig. 2) is shown in Figure 4. Interestingly, the σ variation observed at 150 mM may be exactly superimposed with the σ variation observed at 17 mM, the two sets of fit parameters having been determined independently. Such an agreement supports the validity of the fitting procedure.

The σ values may be compared to the ϕ/c values. Whenever the particles under study behave as impenetrable spheres, ϕ and σ are related by equation (22). The relationship seems to be valid for $c > 0·10$ g/cm³. For instance, at $c = 0·30$ g/cm³, using ϕ/c of Figure 3(a) and the molecular weight of the appropriate form factor, σ is calculated from equation (22) to be 171 and 154 Å in the second and third series, respectively, in excellent agreement with the data of Figure 4. For $c < 0·10$ g/cm³, the σ values calculated from equation (22), about 185 Å for the first series, are slightly lower than those of Figure 4, close to 200 Å.

All these results show that the solution is well described by a a model of charged spheres interacting through repulsive coulombic interactions. The spheres provided by the model are not invariant with protein concentration. Their size decreases with increasing concentration, while the spheres become more and more impenetrable. At 150 mM, where the charge is screened, and at high protein concentration, the model approaches a hard sphere model.

(iii) *Forward X-ray scattering*

Finally, the fits performed provided us with an extrapolation of the X-ray scattering curves to the origin. These extrapolated $S(c, 0)$ values, which are relevant for comparison to osmotic stress measurements, are shown in Figure 5(a) (150 mM) and (b) (17 mM). These values correspond to the thermodynamic counterpart of the structural model. No difference could be detected between the three preparations, in agreement with a ϕ/c variation essentially independent of the α-crystallin M_w.

(b) *Osmotic pressure analysis*

(i) *Controls*

The validity of the approach to measure the osmotic pressure of protein solutions has been demonstrated and discussed for haemoglobin solutions (Prouty *et al.*, 1985). However, since the approach has not been widely used, and since different proteins might behave differently, we designed a series of experiments to ensure that an equilibrium concentration of the α-crystallin solution was reached that was a function only of the osmotic pressure of the stressing polymer solution.

The osmotic pressure measurements were performed at two ionic strengths, 150 and 17 mM. The samples were found to reach a constant concentration after three or four days and to remain stable at that concentration for about six more days. This equilibrium concentration was checked to be independent of the initial sample concentration. Preset sample concentrations did not seem to speed equilibration. The initial concentrations and volumes were then simply chosen to limit the volume changes during equilibration and to ensure a sufficient surface to volume ratio for rapid equilibrium. From 4 to 25°C, no significant

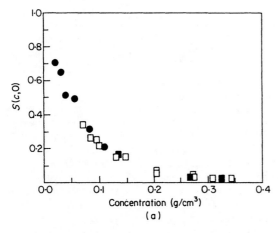

(a)

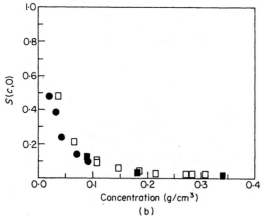

(b)

Figure 5. Variation of the structure factor at the origin $S(c, 0)$, as a function of protein concentration. (a) 150 mM; (b) 17 mM. (●) 1st, (□) 2nd and (■) 3rd series of experiments.

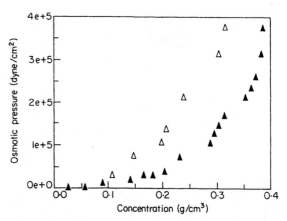

Figure 6. Experimental osmotic pressure data: (▲) 150 mM; (△), 17 mM. ($1e + 5 = 100{,}000$.)

difference in the equilibrium concentration was measurable. For convenience, the experiments were performed at room temperature. No significant difference was observed for α-crystallins obtained from different preparations.

When controlled with HPLC after six days of osmotic stress, the α-crystallin average molecular weight was found to have decreased, to reach at 150 mM values between 600,000 and 700,000, and at 17 mM values around 600,000. The α-crystallin polydispersity, as estimated from the width of the peak, was increased only slightly after the osmotic pressure measurements. In addition, the presence of a tiny amount of low molecular weight compounds could sometimes be detected, especially at low ionic strength, probably corresponding to dissociated α-crystallin subunits. This amount, however, never exceeded 5%. When the osmotic pressure experiment was pursued for longer times, a slow evolution of the α-crystallin concentration was observed as a function of time, probably linked to α-crystallin degradation.

Finally, neither rough calculations (Eisenberg,

1976) nor comparison with the X-ray data, indicated that the Donnan effect had to be taken into account.

(ii) *Osmotic pressure of α-crystallin solutions*

The data obtained for the two ionic strengths are plotted in Figure 6, which shows that, in both cases, the osmotic pressure increases rapidly with protein concentration. This variation significantly departs from what would be expected from "ideal" behaviour, i.e. from a linear variation of the form $\Pi = cRT/M_n$ (Theory, section (a)). Figure 6 shows that, for a given protein concentration, the osmotic pressure measured at 17 mM is always significantly higher than at 150 mM. Such behaviour is indeed expected with unscreening of the charges for particles interacting *via* repulsive electrostatic interactions, as found previously. In addition, it can be seen that increasing the osmotic pressure after $\Pi = 3 \times 10^5$ dyne/cm^2 no longer results in a concentration increase of the α-crystallin solutions. The limiting concentration that can be reached seems to be about 0·38 g/cm^3 at 150 mM and 0·31 g/cm^3 at 17 mM.

When the M_n and M_w values of the solute particles are known, the consistency of osmotic pressure and X-ray measurements may be checked simply by verifying that equations (12) and (13) are satisfied. α-Crystallin M_w relevant for the X-ray experiments was known. In principle, M_n could be obtained from the "solution regime", i.e. from osmotic pressure data recorded at very low concentrations of protein, where ideality of the solution can be assumed. In practice, however, equilibrium was particularly slow and difficult to reach at low final concentrations of protein, probably because of the rather small osmotic pressures and osmotic pressure gradients involved. We therefore operated in a different way. The integral of d$c/S(c, 0)$ (eqn (13)) was calculated from the X-ray data as a function of c and plotted on a log scale with the osmotic stress data. The M_n value

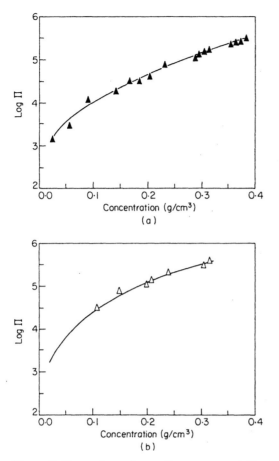

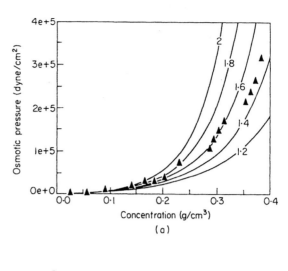

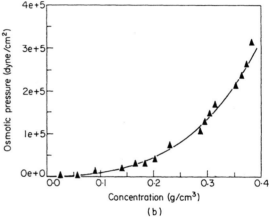

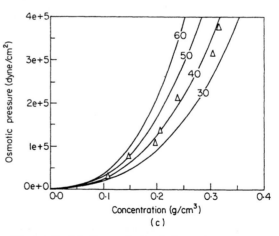

Figure 7. Comparison of osmotic pressure and X-ray data: (a) 150 mM; (b) 17 mM. Continuous line, osmotic pressure calculated using eqn (13) from the $S(c, 0)$ variation as a function of c shown in Fig. 5. Symbols, experimental osmotic pressure data from Fig. 6.

Figure 8. (a) Comparison of the 150 mM osmotic pressure data with the theoretical osmotic pressures calculated using eqns (7) and (8) and the ϕ/c values indicated in the Figure. (b) Best fit of the 150 mM osmotic pressure data using RMSA+VO. ϕ/c was assumed to vary linearly as a function of c. The best fit was obtained for $\phi/c = 1.965 - 1.91\ c$. (c) Comparison of the 17 mM osmotic pressure data with the theoretical osmotic pressures calculated using RMSA+VO, the ϕ/c variation of Fig. 8(b) and the Ze values indicated on the Figure.

allowing the best superimposition of both sets of data was sought. An excellent agreement, as shown in Figure 7, was found in the whole experimental range with M_n equal to 630,000 at I = 150 mM and M_n equal to 500,000 at 17 mM. The 150 mM value is perfectly consistent with the average molecular weight determined by HPLC after the osmotic stress experiments. The lower M_n value at 17 mM may be accounted for entirely by a major component at about 600,000 and a small percentage of low molecular weight compounds as observed with HPLC. In addition, since the X-ray experiments were performed with α-crystallins of larger molecular weight, the agreement of osmotic pressure and X-ray data relevant to α-crystallin solutions indicate that the interactions are essentially independent of the molecular weight between 600,000 and 1,000,000.

(iii) *Osmotic pressure modelling*

It seemed most probable, from the comparison with the X-ray data in Figure 7, that the

461

Table 2
Osmotic pressure data: fitting procedure

			For the series of experiments	
Step	I (mM)	Known param.	Fixed param.	Fitting param.
S1	150	c_i	$Ze_i = Ze_1$	$\phi(c) = f_1(c)$
S2	17	c'_i	$\phi(c') = f_1(c')$	$Z'e_1$

Test: $Z'e_1 = Ze_1$?   No: go to S1 with $Ze_1 = Z'e_1$
Yes: stop here

RMSA + VO potential model would be able to account for the osmotic pressure variation as a function of protein concentration at both 150 and 17 mM. It seemed interesting, however, to test whether simpler models could be discarded on the basis of osmotic pressure measurements alone. Since the charge was previously seen barely to play a role at 150 mM, a fit with a hard sphere model was attempted for the 150 mM data, using equations (7) and (8). This is the simplest model to try, as there exists an analytical expression. The osmotic pressure calculated from equations (7) and (8) depends upon only one parameter, the ϕ/c ratio, which in this model is assumed invariant with protein concentration. As can be seen from Figure 8(a), it is impossible to fit the data with a unique ϕ/c value (in contrast, the haemoglobin osmotic pressure data of Prouty *et al.* (1985) can be accounted for correctly using eqns (7) and (8) and a constant ϕ/c value of about 0·83). Figure 8(a), however, clearly indicates the range of ϕ/c values and of their variation with concentration that would account for the data.

The data were then modelled using the RMSA + VO potential model to calculate $S(c,0)$ as a function of c (by steps of 0·01 g/cm^3), from which osmotic pressure as a function of c was obtained using equation (13). Since $S(c,0)$ is barely dependent upon σ, especially at high ionic strength, there is no way to determine σ from the osmotic pressure data. ϕ/c and σ were assumed to be linked by the equation (22) relationship and the fit was done on only two parameters, ϕ/c and Ze. To find the best fit parameters, we adopted the strategy described in Table 2, which is copied from that of Table 1. Since it had been shown that a constant ϕ/c ratio could not account for the experimental data, ϕ/c was assumed to vary linearly as a function of c. The fit at 150 mM was done with Ze fixed to determine the best linear variation compatible with the data. The fit at 17 mM was done on Ze assuming that the linear ϕ/c variation determined at 150 mM was valid. The process was then reiterated until convergence. Since this approach was applied for the first time to osmotic pressure measurements, the initial Ze value was set equal to 1. Ze was found to converge to about 40 after two iterations, in good agreement with the X-ray data at high concentrations of protein. The best fit for the 150 mM data is shown in Figure 8(b). It corresponds to $\phi/c = 1·965 - 1·91\,c$, again in good agreement with the X-ray data. The osmotic pressure calculated at 17 mM for the same ϕ/c variation and various values of Ze are shown in Figure 8(c) to illustrate the sensitivity of the Ze determination.

The excellent agreement between osmotic pressure and X-ray data indicates that the thermodynamic properties of the α-crystallin solutions are entirely accounted for by the structural properties accessible to X-ray analysis, i.e. by the local properties. In addition, the results obtained show that osmotic pressure measurements are perfectly adequate to determine two interaction parameters, ϕ/c and Ze, in a system where repulsive interactions are predominant.

(c) Relationships between the model parameters and the particle structural parameters

The model used is, of course, an oversimplification. The interest of the model is that it allows us to predict osmotic pressure values and to simulate the scattering curves in a large angular domain with two or three parameters. In the framework of the model, the particles are homogeneous spheres and the three parameters have simple structural meanings. σ, ϕ and Ze are, respectively, the sphere diameter, the excluded volume fraction occupied by these spheres, and the sphere charge. Furthermore, when the spheres are impenetrable, σ and ϕ are related by equation (22). When the particles under study are polydisperse oligomeric proteins, the physical meaning of the three parameters is less direct. The three parameters define an "equivalent" spherical particle. As far as osmotic pressure and X-ray scattering are concerned, a solution made of such equivalent particles of diameter σ and charge Ze, occupying an excluded volume fraction ϕ, behave essentially as the real α-crystallin solution.

The values of the equivalent particle parameters may, however, be compared to the α-crystallin structural parameters that have been determined in other studies. The Ze value, which is an effective charge, is coherent with the evaluation $Ze = 46$ deduced from electrophoretic measurements (Siezen & Owen, 1983). The physico-chemical events underlying the slight Ze variation observed as a function of c remain, however, unclear. (The approximations involved in the approach might become invalid at high concentrations of protein and low ionic strength.)

The excluded volume and the diameter of the equivalent particle were seen to be closely related. The excluded volume per equivalent particle is found to vary from about 2·8 times ($\phi/c = 2$) the dry α-crystallin volume at low protein concentration to about two times ($\phi/c = 1·4$) at high concentrations of protein.

Independently of any α-crystallin quaternary structure model, one may observe that, at high protein concentration, σ coincides with the

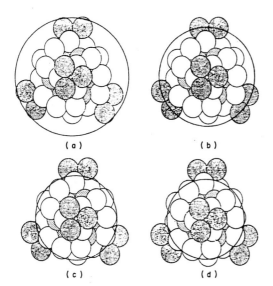

Figure 9. A representation of the α-crystallin quaternary structure model described by Tardieu *et al.* (1986). The model displays tetrahedral symmetry and consists of 3 concentric layers with 12, 24 and 24 sites, respectively. The subunits are modelled by spheres and only 12 equivalent sites were filled in the 3rd layer to yield a 48-subunit particle. Comparison of the model with (a) the equivalent sphere at low protein concentration; (b) the equivalent sphere at high protein concentration, (c) the sphere occupying the α-crystallin hydrated volume; (d) the sphere occupying the α-crystallin dry volume.

The equivalent particle parameters determined by our approach, and their variation with protein concentration, thus appear entirely consistent with α-crystallin structural properties analysed in other studies. In particular, the equivalent particle diameter and excluded volume appear closely related to the external shape. Such a consistency justifies the simulation of α-crystallin interactions with the RMSA + VO potential model. As a consequence, some essential properties of α-crystallin solutions, that may seem at first sight rather complicated, may now be described with only three parameters.

(d) *Physiological relevance*

From the results obtained, the structural parameters that govern transparency *in vivo* may now be analysed. In Theory, the extinction coefficient (eqn (15)) was written as a function of n_0, ∂_n/∂_c, M_w and $S(c,0)$. With proteins in aqueous solutions, n_0 is close to the water refractive index, 1·334, ∂_n/∂_c is almost independent of the protein under study and is close to 0·185 (the choice of this value is not critical). With α-crystallin solutions, $S(c,0)$ was shown to be determined by three parameters, ϕ, σ and Ze, that define an equivalent particle. Therefore, and at least for α-crystallin solutions, four parameters (and possibly their variation with concentration) are relevant to scattering and transparency; M_w, ϕ, σ and Ze.

What is relevant to the situation *in vivo* is even simpler. At the protein concentrations prevailing *in vivo*, the particles may be considered invariant and, in addition, impenetrable since the equation (22) relationship between ϕ and σ is satisfied. The four parameters reduce to three constant parameters. Furthermore, at the ionic strength *in vivo*, about 150 mM (Duncan & Jacob, 1984), the α-crystallin charges are essentially screened and barely affect $S(c,0)$. In other words, in physico-chemical conditions close to the situation *in vivo*, α-crystallins behave essentially as hard spheres. Scattering and transparency are thus mainly determined by two parameters, M_w and the equivalent particle parameter ϕ/c.

The light-scattering and transparency calculated for various values of M_w and ϕ/c are shown in Figure 10, at two different magnifications: (a) and (c), and (b) and (d). Three molecular weights were chosen for the illustration, which cover a large range of protein M_w values, 1,000,000, 500,000 and 50,000, and three ϕ/c values, 1·5 as observed with α-crystallins, 1·0 and 0·75, the last of which corresponds to the dry weight volume. The scattering is represented as the product $M_w c S(c,0)$. For such an illustration, $S(c,0)$ may be calculated quite simply using equation (16). The case of 500,000 M_w particles, the scattering of which would be proportional to concentration, i.e. the case of a solution that would display an "ideal" behaviour is also indicated (this corresponds to set $\phi = 0$ in eqn (16), i.e. $S(c, 0) = 1$). The percentage of

diameter of the sphere having the same radius of gyration as the average α-crystallin; 171 compared to 173 Å for the second series and 154 Å compared to 157 Å for the third series. The diameters of the spheres occupying the same dry volume as an average α-crystallin would be 137 and 123 Å, respectively. At low concentrations of protein, the σ value of about 200 Å compares well with twice the α-crystallin hydrodynamic radius: 96 ($\pm$2) Å (Tardieu *et al.*, 1986).

Within the framework of the α-crystallin quaternary structure model described by Tardieu *et al.* (1986) (and to a large extent the model proposed by Bindels *et al.*, 1979), the variation of ϕ and σ with protein concentration (in the absence of any change in particle quaternary structure) can be rationalized easily, as can be seen from Figure 9. At low concentration, α-crystallins behave as if they were free to rotate, and the equivalent particle diameter is the spherical envelope diameter. At the same time, the large excluded volume fraction associated with α-crystallins is partially penetrable. With increasing concentration, α-crystallins take advantage of their non-sphericity to pack more closely. The equivalent particle diameter is then close to the real envelope average diameter, while the excluded volume fraction so defined becomes impenetrable.

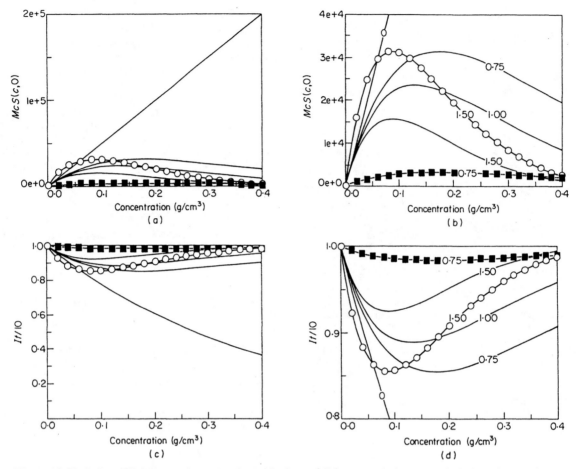

Figure 10. Variation of light-scattering ((a), enlarged in (b)) and light transmission ((c), enlarged in (d)) as a function of protein concentration, calculated with various M_w: (-■-) 5×10^4; (——) 5×10^5; (-○-) 10^6 and with the ϕ/c values indicated in the Figure. The light-scattering is represented by $M_w c S(c, 0)$. The light transmission is calculated from eqn (1), assuming a 1 cm thick sample; τ is calculated from eqn (15) using $\lambda = 5000$ Å. For both light-scattering and light transmission, $S(c, 0)$ is calculated from eqn (16).

transmitted light was calculated using equations (1) and (15) for each curve of Figure 10(a) with $\lambda = 5000$ Å and a 1 cm sample thickness.

Figure 10(a) and (c) illustrates the drastic effect of solution departure from ideality. If the scattering was simply proportional to concentration, only about 50% of the incident light would be transmitted in the physiological concentration range, and the sample would appear turbid. On the other hand, with a fluid of hard spheres and in a large range of protein M_w values and ϕ/c ratios, the scattering first increases with protein concentration, reaches a maximum, and then decreases sufficiently to preserve transparency. The effect of variations of M_w and ϕ/c is better seen in Figure 10(b) and (d). Essentially, the scattering increases with increasing M_w and decreasing ϕ/c ratio. The role of M_w is simple, since it is a multiplying factor. The unexpected result, however, is the importance of the ϕ/c ratio, which significantly affects both the maximum position and the level of scattering, especially at high concentrations. In the physio-

logical range of concentrations, the scattering calculated with $M_w = 500,000$ increases by a factor of about 15 when ϕ/c decreases from 1·50 to 0·75. Accordingly, the percentage of transmitted light would decrease from 99% to 89%. It appears that, for a given molecular weight, ϕ/c variation or, in other words, variation of the compactness of the macromolecule, is a rather efficient way to modify the solution structural properties and, in particular, transparency. α-Crystallins, with $M_w = 1,000,000$ and $\phi/c = 1·5$ are compatible with transparency in the physiological concentration range, while α-crystallins of the same M_w with a compact structure, and thus $\phi/c = 0·75$, would be slightly turbid. The same transparency as observed with α-crystallins could, however, be obtained with compact particles of about 50,000 M_w.

In the same way, theoretical osmotic pressure can be calculated as a function of M_n and ϕ/c. In this case, osmotic pressure increases with decreasing M_n and increasing ϕ/c. Again, for a given M_n, ϕ/c plays a major role, as can be seen in Figure 11. For

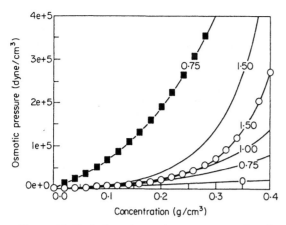

Figure 11. Variation of osmotic pressure as a function of protein concentration calculated from the same series of M_{w}: (—■—) 5×10^4; (——) 5×10^5; (—○—) 10^6 and ϕ/c values as in Fig. 10. The ϕ/c values are also indicated on the Figure. Osmotic pressure is calculated from eqns (7) and (8) using $M_{\mathrm{n}} = M_{\mathrm{w}}$.

instance, in the physiological concentration range, the osmotic pressure decreases by a factor of 10 when ϕ/c decreases from 1·5 to 0·75. Again, at high concentrations of protein, osmotic pressure similar to that obtained with α-crystallins could be achieved with compact proteins, of about 50,000 M_{n}. However, to appreciate the physiological relevance of the osmotic pressure of the α-crystallin solutions better, the calculated values may be converted to mosmol. At 150 mM and $c = 0·350\,\mathrm{g/cm^3}$, the α-crystallin solution osmotic pressure is calculated to be about 10 mosmol, close to the osmolarity of haemoglobin in erythrocytes (Prouty *et al.*, 1985), but well below the lens osmolarity, which is of the order of 300 mosmol (Cotlier *et al.*, 1968; Patterson, 1981; Duncan & Jacob, 1984). Therefore, even at high concentrations of protein, the protein contribution to the osmotic pressure remains limited. In this case, however, increasing the α-crystallin compactness would result in lowering the osmotic pressure, probably without any damage for cells, while 50,000 M_{n} molecules with $\phi/c = 1·5$ would lead to large osmotic pressures, possibly unacceptable for cells.

The analysis of the parameters relevant for α-crystallin solution properties therefore indicates that concomitant variations of M_{w} or M_{n} and ϕ/c may lead to scattering (and thus transparency) and osmotic pressure values practically unchanged at high concentrations of protein. Such a constraint might have played a role in evolution of the lens proteins. In this context, one may note that oligomeric proteins as compared to monomeric proteins seem good candidates for an increased ϕ/c value associated with an increased molecular weight.

The real case of interest is, however, the whole mixture of α, β and γ-crystallins observed in

mammalian lenses. In a previous study (Delaye & Tardieu, 1983), the experimental scattering values obtained with lens cortical cytoplasmic extracts were accounted for by a hard sphere model and equivalent particles of $M_{\mathrm{w}} = 500,000$ and $\phi/c = 1·15$. The present study of α-crystallin solutions justifies, *a posteriori*, the choice of this model and shows that, as far as scattering is concerned, the addition of β and γ-crystallins essentially leads to scattering that may be accounted for by an equivalent particle of lower M_{w} value and ϕ/c ratio. As can be inferred from Figure 10, the light-scattering of such equivalent particles and of α-crystallins is similar at high concentrations. Other properties of cytoplasmic extracts will be discussed in a forthcoming article.

5. Discussion

The approach presented in this paper to study the relationships between thermodynamic and structural parameters, i.e. between eye lens protein interactions and transparency, introduces two novelties. The first is the coupling of the osmotic stress technique developed by Prouty *et al.* (1985) to solution X-ray scattering experiments. The second is to use models developed in liquid-state physics for the study of colloids to account for either the X-ray or the osmotic pressure measurements with a small number of structural parameters relevant to the particle under study.

No model is required to show that the spatial organization viewed by X-ray scattering is responsible for macroscopic transparency and osmotic pressure. It is sufficient to extrapolate the X-ray data one way or another, as was done by Delaye & Tardieu (1983) for instance, and to show the consistency of the thermodynamic and the structural data sets. In this context, measuring light-scattering or osmotic pressure is just a question of convenience. Light-scattering was used by Delaye & Tardieu (1983) and other light-scattering measurements, not reported here, are indeed in agreement with the X-ray data. Our interest in using osmotic stress instead of light-scattering was mainly that these two techniques involve totally different experimental protocols. Also, osmotic stress was found particularly convenient and attractive for its simplicity and provided another physiologically relevant parameter. From a more theoretical standpoint, the relationships between osmotic pressure and forward X-ray scattering were, of course, well known. That they could be relatively easily verified in a large concentration range with protein solutions was less obvious. Such a success owes much to synchrotron radiation facilities for allowing us to measure a large number of unsmeared X-ray scattering curves, with good statistics, in a reasonable time.

The present study confirms that the models developed in liquid-state physics for the study of colloids are adequate to model, in a large angular domain, the scattering of concentrated protein solutions, where departure from ideality is essentially due to excluded volume effects and repulsive electrostatic interactions. The approximations involved and the hypotheses implicit in the fitting procedure have been discussed (Tardieu *et al.*, 1987). Among them, the assumption of spherically symmetric interactions has often been assumed to restrict the analysis to particles also displaying spherical symmetry. The present study demonstrates that α-crystallin solutions behave as if the interaction symmetry and the particle symmetry were uncoupled. Work is in progress on other protein solutions to further substantiate this point (in collaboration with Claude Poyart, Patrick Tauc and Patrice Vachette). One may anticipate that the model also holds in a variety of cases, which is particularly satisfying since concentration effects in X-ray solution scattering were, for years, inadequately described. The present study shows that such effects can now be analysed, even if they cannot yet be predicted accurately. Unfortunately, the case where attractive interactions are predominant has not been solved satisfactorily. Reciprocally, such a study shows that protein solutions could perhaps be helpful for physicists. Protein solutions offer the advantage that the form factor is independent of concentration. The consequences of particle shape and compactness variation may be analysed by the appropriate choice of different proteins.

The RMSA + VO potential model is as useful for analysing the osmotic pressure data as it was for X-ray scattering. The osmotic pressure experiments of Prouty *et al.* (1985) were designed to study a phase transition phenomenon. With the model, interparticle interactions become accessible. In the simple case where the particles in solution behave as hard spheres invariant with concentration, our approach is essentially equivalent to that developed, for instance, by Ross & Minton (1977), on the basis of virial expansion of the osmotic pressure. Our approach is, however, more powerful and more general since, in calculating the osmotic pressure from $S(c; 0)$, charges and excluded volume variations as a function of c may be taken into account easily.

The structural parameters particularly relevant for a description of the properties of concentrated α-crystallin solutions have been specified. There are only three physico-chemical parameters, to a large extent independent of the specificity of the solute. They can be interpreted as defining an equivalent, yet simplified spherical particle with a charge, an excluded volume and a diameter. These equivalent particle parameters compare well with what is known of α-crystallin charge and quaternary structure from other studies.

As far as transparency is concerned, after the early theoretical work of Trokel (1962) and Benedek (1971), after the experimental evidence that short-range order of the crystallin proteins accounts for eye lens transparency (Delaye & Tardieu, 1983), the molecular basis of such a short-range order seems to

be understood. We have learned that α-crystallin solutions behave as a fluid of charged spheres and their properties are correctly described by a model of repulsive screened coulombic interactions between particles. Under physiological conditions, the behaviour of α-crystallin solutions simplifies to that of a fluid of hard spheres, i.e. of a solution of impenetrable spheres, where departure from ideality is essentially due to the excluded volume effect. In such solutions, the position correlations of the particles are only short-range. The scattering, and therefore the transparency, of such solutions is essentially determined by two parameters; the particle M_w and excluded volume, and can be calculated and/or predicted as a function of these two parameters. Calculation of transparency using a large range of values for these two parameters indicate that in the physiological range of protein concentration, transparency is enhanced when M_w decreases and when the excluded volume per particle increases. Yet, the calculations show also that transparency could be achieved in many ways. Comparison of the α-crystallin scattering and of the cytoplasm scattering is a good example; as far as light-scattering is concerned, the major effect of the presence of $β$ and $γ$-crystallins is to lead to lower values of both average M_w and excluded volume. At high concentrations of protein, the light-scattering is similar in both cases. We are reminded that lens proteins are the response to a number of different constraints; for instance, stability with ageing, or tendency to avoid aggregation that could produce opacities. The advantage of a protein mixture, which seems to have been retained in all vertebrate species, also needs to be considered. Work is in progress along these lines.

We gratefully acknowledge the excellent technical assistance of Brigitte Krop. We thank Peter Rand for sending us dextran calibration curves prior to publication. We are indebted to Linda Sperling and Patrice Vachette for constant friendly interest and advice. We thank the operators of the storage ring DCI at LURE. This work is part of the Ph.D. thesis of F.V. This work was supported in part by an MRT grant (Interface Physique-Biologie) and was pursued within the scope of the EC Concerted Action on Cellular Aging and Disease (EURAGE).

References

Benedek, G. B. (1971). *Appl. Opt.* **10**, 459–473.

Bindels, J. G., Siezen, R. J. & Hoenders, H. J. (1979). *Ophthal. Res.* **11**, 441–452.

Bloemendal, H. (1981). In *Molecular and Cellular Biology of the Eye Lens* (Bloemendal, H., ed.), pp. 1-48, Wiley, New York.

Bordas, J., Koch, M. H. J., Clout, P. N., Dorrington, E., Boulin, C. & Gabriel, A. (1980). *J. Phys. Sci. Instrum.* **E13**, 938–944.

Carnahan, N. F. & Starling, K. E. (1969). *J. Chem. Phys.* **51**, 635–636.

Cotlier, E., Kwan, B. & Beaty, C. (1968). *Biochim. Biophys. Acta*, **150**, 705–722.

Delaye, M. & Tardieu, A. (1983). *Nature (London)*, **302**, 415–417.

Depautex, C., Desvignes, C., Feder, P., Lemonnier, M., Bosshard, R., Leboucher, P., Dagneaux, D., Benoit, J. P. & Vachette, P. (1987). *LURE Rapport d'activité pour la période Aout 1985-Avril 1987*, p. 87, doc. CEN Saclay.

Duncan, G. & Jacob, J. C. (1984). *The Eye*, **1**, 159–206.

Eisenberg, H. (1976). *Biological Macromolecules and Polyelectrolytes in Solution*, Clarendon Préss, Oxford.

Guinier, A. & Fournet, G. (1955). *Small-Angle Scattering of X-rays*, Wiley, New York.

Hansen, J. P. & Hayter, J. B. (1982). *Mol. Phys.* **46**, 651–656.

Harding, J. J. & Dilley, K. J. (1976). *Exp. Eye Res.* **22**, 1–73.

Hayter, J. B. & Penfold, J. (1981). *Mol. Phys.* **42**, 109–118.

Kerker, M. (1969). *The Scattering of Light and other Electromagnetic Radiations*, Academic Press, New York.

LeNeveu, D. M., Rand, R. P. & Parsegian, V. A. (1976). *Nature (London)*, **259**, 601–603.

Luzzati, V. & Tardieu, A. (1980). *Annu. Rev. Biophys. Bioeng.* **9**, 1–29.

Parsegian, V. A., Rand, R. P., Fuller, N. L. & Rau, D. C. (1986). *Methods Enzymol.* **127**, 400–416.

Patterson, J. W. (1981). *Exp. Eye. Res.* **32**, 151–162.

Prouty, M. S., Schechter, A. N. & Parsegian, V. A. (1985). *J. Mol. Biol.* **184**, 517–528.

Ross, P. D. & Minton, A. P. (1977). *J. Mol. Biol.* **112**, 437–452.

Siezen, R. J. & Owen, E. A. (1983). *Biophys. Chem.* **18**, 181.

Siezen, J. R., Bindels, J. G. & Hoenders, H. J. (1978). *Eur. J. Biochem.* **91**, 387–396.

Tardieu, A. & Delaye, M. (1988). *Annu. Rev. Biophys. Biophys. Chem.* **17**, 47–70.

Tardieu, A., Laporte, D., Licinio, P., Krop, B. & Delaye, M. (1986). *J. Mol. Biol.* **192**, 711–724.

Tardieu, A., Laporte, D. & Delaye, M. (1987). *J. Phys.* **48**, 1207–1215.

Trokel, S. (1962). *Invest. Ophthalmol.* **1**, 493–501.

Van den Oetelaar, P. J. M., Clauwaert, J., Van Laethem, M. & Hoenders, H. J. (1985). *J. Biol. Chem.* **260**, 14030–14034.

Verwey, E. J. W. & Overbeek, J. T. G. (1948). *Theory of the Stability of Lyophobic Colloids*, Elsevier, Amsterdam.

Edited by M. F. Moody

Section Four
Coherent Light Scattering by Biotissues

Reprinted with permission from *Optics and Laser Technology*, Vol. 20(6), pp. 309-316
(December 1988). ©1988 Butterworth-Heinemann Ltd.

Non-contact blood flow determination using a laser speckle method

B. RUTH

An electro-optical device is described which allows the non-contact determination
of the skin blood flow and its temporal course. As the laser light penetrates the
skin, it is not only scattered from the epidermis but also from the moving red blood
cells in the capillaries. The scattered light is time dependent and can be described
in terms of the dynamic laser speckle effect. Measurements at the skin demonstrate
that there is a so-called 'involuntary body movement' which must be taken into
account when the measurement of the blood flow is determined. Theoretical
considerations show a way to reduce the influence of this movement. Some
measurements demonstrate the response of the device to blood flow variations.

KEYWORDS: speckles, blood flow, flow measurement, biological tissue

Introduction

Micro-circulation is essential for the supply of
biological tissue with oxygen and nutritive substances
and the removal of waste products. It has been shown
that it is possible for the micro-circulation to be
insufficient although the flow in the corresponding
arteries and veins is not impaired[1]. The determination
of the blood flow in the capillaries is, therefore, of great
interest in the diagnosis of diseases such as leg ulcers
and arterial occlusive disease.

Several methods for blood flow determination have
been introduced, for example the evaluation of the
transcutaneous oxygen tension, the vital capillaroscopy
method, and the laser Doppler method[2-5]. The optical
methods are based on the light penetration of the skin.
As scattering and absorption decrease the light
intensity, the mean penetration depth of skin is defined
by that depth where the initial intensity is reduced to
a fraction $1/e$ (37%). For HeNe laser light a value of
about 0.5 mm is found[6]. Since the thickness of the
epidermis ranges from 38 µm to about 370 µm, some
of the light is scattered by the red blood cells in the
dermis[7].

In the vital capillaroscopy method a microscope
objective is placed on the skin and the capillaries are
directly observed[2].

The number of capillaries per unit area and the form
of the capillaries give information about the efficiency
of the micro-circulation. When the microscopic image
is processed by a video camera, a recorder and a

correlator, the velocity of the red blood cells in the
capillaries can be determined, and is found to vary[8]
between 0 and approximately 2 mm s^{-1}. This method
is preferably applied to the nailfold because the thin
epidermis allows the formation of an image with
sufficient quality. However, in medical diagnosis other
positions of the skin are also of great importance, for
example, the skin at the feet and lower legs. It seems
to be difficult to apply vital microscopy to these sites
presumably because the epidermis is too thick.

Blood flow in the skin can also be estimated utilizing
laser light scattering. Since no image formation is
necessary this method should be applicable to skin even
with a thick epidermis. The scattered light is interpreted
and processed as a Doppler signal and the resulting
measurement is shown to be dependent on the blood
flow[4,5,9]. As proved by a theoretical derivation, the
mean signal frequency is proportional to the mean
blood velocity if the following assumptions are valid
1 — the surrounding tissue is stationary, 2 — the
direction of the scattered light in the depth of the
capillaries is randomly distributed, and 3 — the
direction of the blood flow in the capillaries is also
random[10].

Several instruments have been designed utilizing optical
fibres for illumination and detection[5,9,11]. The fibre
ends are mounted close together in a measuring head
which is fastened to the skin by use of double-sided
adhesive tape. Since the fibre ends are positioned
perpendicular to the skin surface the scattered light is
measured with high efficiency.

The method has already been tested in clinical practice,
for example on patients with peripheral vascular

The author is in the Insitut für Angewandte Optik, Gesellshaft für Strahlen-
und Umweltforschung Ingolstädter Landstr.1, D-8042 Newherberg, FRG.
Received 27 April 1988. Revised 27 June 1988.

disease, diabetes, and Raynaud's syndrome and it has been shown that useful results are obtained[12-14].

The main disadvantage of the instruments is that the probe has to be attached to the skin by adhesive tape. In this way, the blood flow itself is considerably influenced because of the pressure on the skin and, more especially, the temperature are affected. Furthermore, the skin of patients suffering from insufficient microcirculation is very sensitive and may easily be injured when the adhesive tape is removed. Measurements in open wounds are also not possible with this method. Consequently, a device for non-contact determination of the blood flow would be of great advantage.

The primary aim of this paper is to present such a device and to show the dependence of the measurement on the tissue blood flow in some examples.

As indicated by the mean penetration depth of 0.5 mm, the light is scattered from different layers of the skin. Since the skin can therefore be considered as a rough object, the scattered light is described by the laser speckle effect. The scattering from the surrounding tissue and from the red blood cells simultaneously determines the speckle pattern.

In a previous paper a laser speckle method has been described for the evaluation of the velocity of an object with an in-plane movement[15]. A laser beam is focused on the object surface and the speckle pattern is measured by an aperture with a diameter somewhat smaller than the mean speckle width. The signal $I(t)$ of the photomultiplier behind the aperture depends on time and the quantity V, derived from $I(t)$, according to

$$V = (\int \dot{I}(t)^2 \, dt)^{1/2} \qquad (1)$$

can be shown to be proportional to the object velocity. A modification of this device is now used to measure the tissue blood flow.

As described in a previous paper, a device based on this measuring principle provides a signal which is empirically shown to be a quantitative measure of the blood flow[24]. With a further device a two-dimensional image can be obtained when a CCD sensor is used for speckle detection[25].

The second aim of the paper is to describe the scattered light in terms of the speckle effect and to explain the dependence of the measuring value on blood velocity, blood volume and surrounding tissue.

Description of the measuring head

The principle of velocity determination with the laser speckle method has been described in a previous paper[15]. The measuring head and the circuit for the signal processing are modified in order to adapt the device to the requirements of tissue blood flow determination.

As shown in Fig. 1, an optical fibre for laser light illumination (HeNe laser 632.8 nm) facilitates the measurements at all locations of the skin. The laser light is focused by a lens with a focal length of 60 mm into an optical fibre 600 μm in diameter. Since the light diverges at the fibre end, it is focused again by a second lens (focal length 16 mm) and forms a laser spot of

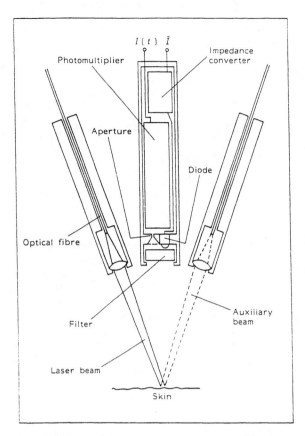

Fig.1 Measuring head for blood flow determination using the laser speckle method

about 1.5 mm in diameter on the skin. In front of the photodetectors an interference filter with a central frequency of 633 nm eliminates most of the stray light. As the diameter of the aperture (30 μm) is smaller than the mean speckle width, the photomultiplier signal (PM-signal) is proportional to the speckle intensity $I(t)$. Close to the aperture a diode is mounted with a sensitive area of 1 mm² for the determination of the speckle pattern mean intensity $\bar{I}$. The signal is fed into an impedance converter which provides an output that is less noisy than the original diode output and is proportional to $\bar{I}$.

For reproducible measurements adjustment of the measuring head at the correct distance of 50 mm to the skin is necessary. An auxiliary beam which is also derived from the laser source indicates the correct distance when its laser spot coincides with that of the measuring beam. An accuracy of ± 5 mm is sufficient for the measurements. The measuring head is mounted on a tripod and can be fixed in all positions above the skin.

Involuntary body movement

The measuring head outlined in Fig. 1 is used for investigations on the hand dorsum. The signals $I(t)$ and $\bar{I}$ are processed to give a value V according to (1). For perfused skin a value V_s is obtained. When the blood supply is suppressed by inflating a cuff around the upper arm, V drops below V_s, but does not reach the value for a stationary object.

In order to investigate these findings the spectra of $I(t)$ are shown for perfused skin (Fig. 2, Curve 1) and skin with suppressed blood supply (Curve 2). Below 50 Hz the amplitudes seem to be unaffected, but above 50 Hz the amplitudes clearly decrease although they do not reach very small values.

The origin of Curve 2 is obtained by the following: skin-coloured adhesive tape is fastened to the perfused skin at the same position on the hand dorsum. Since the tape does not transmit light, the blood flow cannot influence the speckle movement. The spectrum of signal $I(t)$, shown as Curve 3 in Fig. 2, is very similar to Curve 2. The only possible explanation for the nearly identical spectra is that the skin not perfused by blood, and the adhesive tape on the perfused skin move in a similar way. Therfore, it is also not possible to regard the perfused skin to be stationary.

As a control of this interpretation a piece of the same tape was fastened to a stationary object. The resulting spectrum (Curve 4) shows a clear reduction of the amplitudes for all frequencies and proves that the tape on the skin is moving. Further control measurements with the laser source and the photomultiplier show that Curve 4 is due to the noise of these components.

Since movement is present at all sites of the body and cannot consciously be suppressed, it is called 'involuntary body movement'. As a result. the movement of the skin provides a considerable contribution to the dynamics of the speckle pattern. This must be taken into account when assessing the blood velocity.

Superposition of two dynamic speckle patterns

Blood flow and involuntary body movement jointly determine the time-dependent signal $I(t)$ and the spectrum. In order to separate both these motions a speckle pattern (1) is assumed to be formed by the light which is scattered from the tissue. At a given observation point the speckle intensity and mean intensity are denoted as $I_1(t)$ and $\overline{I}_1$, respectively. Speckle pattern (2) with the corresponding

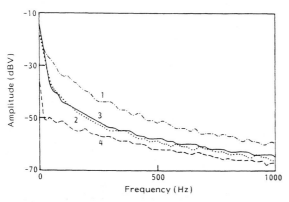

Fig. 2 Spectrum of the speckle intensity $I(t)$ obtained from the skin of the hand dorsum with normal blood flow (Curve 1) and suppressed blood flow (Curve 2). Spectrum from a skin-coloured adhesive tape fastened to the skin of the hand dorsum (Curve 3) and to a stationary object (Curve 4). The difference between Curves 3 and 4 indicates the so-called 'involuntary body movement'

abbreviations $I_2(t)$ and $\overline{I}_2$ originates from the light scattered by the red blood cells. As a simplification. speckle pattern (1) is not assumed to be influenced by the blood flow and vice versa.

The normalized intensity is given by

$$i_j(t) = \frac{I_j(t)}{\overline{I}_j} \quad j = 1, 2 \tag{2}$$

and the corresponding power spectrum is

$$p_j(\omega) = \mathscr{F}(i_j(t) \otimes i_j(t)) \tag{3}$$

$\mathscr{F}$ denotes the Fourier transformation and the $\otimes$ indicates the convolution defined by

$$r_1(t) \otimes r_2(t) = \int r_1(t - t') r_2(t')\, dt' \tag{4}$$

with the example functions $r_1(t)$ and $r_2(t)$.

The corresponding normalized amplitude $a_j(t)$ and mean amplitude $\overline{A}_j$ are related to the intensity by

$$I_j(t) = (\overline{A}_j a_j(t))^* (\overline{A}_j a_j(t)) \tag{5}$$

$$i_j(t) = a_j^*(t)\, a_j(t) \tag{6}$$

where the superscript * indicates the complex conjugate function. The speckle pattern which can be measured is characterized by the mean amplitude $\overline{A}$ and the normalized amplitude $a(t)$, and is formed by the coherent superposition of speckle patterns (1) and (2). This is shown in Refs 16 and 17.

$$\overline{A}\, a(t) = \overline{A}_1\, a_1(t) + \overline{A}_2\, a_2(t) \tag{7}$$

Accordingly the intensity is given by

$$I(t) = (\overline{A}\, a(t))^* (\overline{A}\, a(t)) \tag{8}$$

As described in Appendix 1 the power spectrum of $I(t)$ is

$$P(\omega) = \overline{I}_1^2\, p_1(\omega) + \overline{I}_2^2\, p_2(\omega) + \overline{I}_1\, \overline{I}_2\, p_{1.2}(\omega) \tag{9}$$

with

$$\overline{I}_j = \overline{A}_j^2 \quad (j = 1.2) \tag{10}$$

$p_{12}(\omega)$ is a function and depends on $a_1(t)$ and $a_2(t)$

In order to investigate the influence of the blood velocity on the spectrum $P(\omega)$ let us look at an arbitrary time instant t_E. The positions of all red blood cells determine the speckle pattern and the amplitude $a_2(t_E)$. When the velocity of all blood cells is simultaneously increased by the same factor k this position and the same amplitude are already reached at the time instant t_E/k. Therefore, the amplitude $a_{2.k}(t)$ of the speckle pattern with the increased velocity can be described by

$$a_{2.k}(t) = a_2(kt) \tag{11}$$

Since the blood volume within the range of the laser light, the optical properties of the tissue, and the involuntary body movement are assumed to be constant, the quantities $\overline{I}_2$, $\overline{A}_2$, $\overline{I}_1$, $\overline{A}_1$, $i_1(t)$, and $p_1(\omega)$ do not vary. The time dependent intensity $I_k(t)$ of the speckle pattern is now given by

$$I_k(t) = (\overline{A}_1 a_1(t) + \overline{A}_2 a_2(kt))^* \, (\overline{A}_1 a_1(t) + \overline{A}_2 a_2(kt)) \quad (12)$$

and the corresponding spectrum has the form (see Appendix 2)

$$P_k(\omega) = \overline{I}_1^2 \, p_1(\omega) + \frac{1}{k} \, \overline{I}_2^2 \, p_2 \left(\frac{\omega}{k} \right) + \overline{I}_1 \, \overline{I}_2 \, p_{1,2}(k,\omega) \quad (13)$$

$p_{1,2}(k,\omega)$ depends on the quantities $a_1(t)$, $a_2(t)$ and k. Corresponding to (1), the quantity $L(k)$ is defined by

$$L^2(k) = \int \omega^2 \, P_k(\omega) \, d\omega \quad (14)$$

Substituting (13) in (14) yields

$$L^2(k) = \overline{I}_1^2 \int \omega^2 \, p_1(\omega) \, d\omega + k^2 \, \overline{I}_2^2 \int \omega^2 \, p_2(\omega) \, d\omega$$
$$+ \overline{I}_1 \, \overline{I}_2 \int \omega^2 \, p_{1,2} \, (k,\omega) \, d\omega \quad (15)$$

where the substitution rule is applied to the second term. $L(k)$ is now investigated when the tissue is assumed to be stationary. This means that $i_1(t)$ and $a_1(t)$ are constant:

$$a_1(t) = \alpha_1 \quad (16)$$

Since the spectrum of a constant is a δ-function, the first term of (15) becomes zero because of the factor ω^2 (see Ref. 19.) The integral of the second term is abbreviated by

$$K_2 = \int \omega^2 \, p_2 \, (\omega) \, d\omega \quad (17)$$

and depends on the optical device and the spatial distribution of the blood velocity. The third term of (15) is calculated in Appendix 3. (15) can now be written as

$$L^2(k) = k^2 \overline{I}_2^2 K_2 + k^2 \overline{I}_1 \, \overline{I}_2 \, K_3 \quad (18)$$

$$L(k) = k \, (\overline{I}_2^2 \, K_2 + \overline{I}_1 \, \overline{I}_2 \, K_3)^{\frac{1}{2}} \quad (19)$$

(19) proves that $L(k)$ is proportional to the blood velocity when the surrounding tissue is considered stationary. The proportionality factor depends in the spatial blood flow distribution (K_2, K_3), the blood volume in the range of the laser light ($\overline{I}_2$), and the scattering from the tissue ($\overline{I}_1$).

What is now the influence of the involuntary body movement on quantity $L(k)$?

As can be concluded from the mean penetration depth, the mean intensity of the light scattered from the tissue ($\overline{I}_1$) can be considered to be large compared to the light ($\overline{I}_2$) from the red blood cells ($\overline{I}_1 \gg \overline{I}_2$). From (15) $L(k)$ is a quantitative measure of the blood velocity, but not a proportional one.

In particular, an increased body movement may simulate a high blood velocity. Since there is no clear knowledge about the quantities $\overline{I}_1$, $\overline{I}_2$, p_1 (ω), p_2 (ω),

and $p_{1,2}$ (k, ω), it is not possible to define a quantity which is proportional to the blood flow in all cases. For this reason, an empirical method is chosen in order to find a method to separate the blood flow and the involuntary body movement.

The spectra in Fig. 2 shows that the blood flow mainly affects the frequencies above 50 Hz. In (14) the term ω^2 can be regarded as a weighting function of the spectrum P_k (ω). A quantity M derived with a reduced weighting below 50 Hz and an increased weighting above 50 Hz may allow a reduction of the perturbation due to the involuntary body movement. With new weighting functions $T_n(\omega)$ ($n = 1, 2, \ldots$), M_n is defined by

$$M_n = \frac{1}{\overline{I}} (\int T_n^2 \, (\omega) \, P(\omega) \, d\omega)^{\frac{1}{2}} \quad (20)$$

Several weighting functions $T_n(\omega)$ were tested in order to achieve simultaneously a high sensitivity for the blood flow variations and a reduction in the influence of the involuntary body movement.

The division by $\overline{I}$ compensates for variations of the laser intensity and the scattering conditions at the skin.

Signal processing

The processing of the signals $I(t)$ and $\overline{I}$, corresponding to (20), is performed by the electronic circuit shown in Fig. 3 $T_n(\omega)$, the weighting function in (20), is realized by a series connection of electronic filters. First, signal $I(t)$ passes an active high-pass and low-pass filter with cut-off frequencies of 50 Hz and 800 Hz, respectively. The high-pass filter reduces the influence of the involuntary body movement and the low-pass filter eliminates the high frequencies which contain no information about the blood flow. A further frequency dependent amplifier (FDA) is responsible for the sensitivity due to blood flow variations.

The action of the filter combination is characterized by the transfer function which is given by the spectrum of the output when the input signal is white noise. Since the transfer function is identical to the weighting function, it is denoted by the same symbol: $T_n(\omega)$. Equation (20) is modified in order to explain the further processing. When $S_n(t)$ denotes the output of the FDA characterized by $T_n(\omega)$ (see Fig. 3) the corresponding power spectrum is given by

$$\mathcal{F}(S_n(t) \otimes S_n(t)) = T_n^2 \, (\omega) \, P(\omega) \quad (21)$$

Using the power theorem for Fourier transformations, (20) is transformed to

$$M_n = \frac{1}{\overline{I}} (\int S_n^2(t) \, dt)^{\frac{1}{2}} \quad (22)$$

For this reason, the further processing of $S_n(t)$ is carried out by the rms-dc converter which successively forms square, mean-value, and square-root. The formation of the mean value corresponds to the integral in (22). Finally, the divider takes account of the mean intensity $\overline{I}$.

Since the blood flow may unexpectedly change[20], a

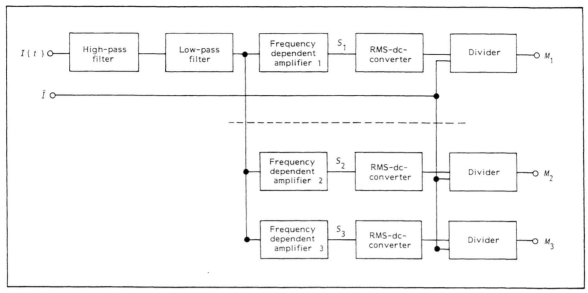

Fig. 3 Electronic circuit for signal processing

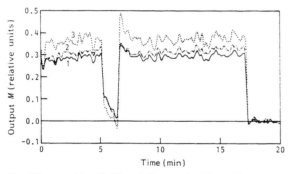

Fig. 4 The quantities M_1, M_2, and M_3 are derived from different frequency dependent amplifiers and are synchronously obtained from the hand dorsum during ischaemia and reactive hyperaemia. The corresponding transfer functions T_n are given in Fig. 5, Curves 1–3

comparison of different FDAs is only possible if the corresponding output signals M_n are derived from the same input signals $I(t)$ and $\bar{I}$. For this reason, the values M_1, M_2, and M_3 are synchronously formed by the different frequency dependent amplifiers in Fig. 3. One example of the measurements obtained from the hand dorsum is shown in Fig. 4.

In the first five minutes the blood flow was relatively constant. After the blood supply was suppressed by inflating a cuff around the upper arm M_n fell to a minimum value within 1 min. When the cuff was released, M_n rapidly increased, passed a maximum, and then fell to a level near the initial value. This effect is called reactive hyperaemia. In the last three minutes a skin coloured adhesive tape was fastened to the skin in the same position. This measurement served as a control and the fluctuations of the measurement indicated the perturbation by involuntary body movements.

The quantities M_1 and M_2 were obtained using a differentiator and a band pass filter respectively, with a centre frequency of $f_c = 170$ Hz, as a frequency

dependent amplifier. A comparison of curves 1 and 2 in Fig. 4 shows that the characteristics of the electronic filters do not necessarily influence the measurements very much. Nevertheless, there are other filters which considerably improve the sensitivity to variations in blood flow. M_3, for example, derived from a band pass filter with $f_c = 370$ Hz, declines rapidly to a minimum value and reveals a high peak value after the opening of the cuff. Hence, the frequency range between 300 Hz and 400 Hz is obviously very important for sensitivity to blood flow variations. The corresponding transfer functions are shown in Fig. 5. The fluctuations of the measurements during the control with the adhesive tape in the last three minutes represent the perturbation by the involuntary body movement and can be considered as the noise of the method. As shown in Fig. 4, the fluctuations of M_3 do not considerably exceed those of M_1 and M_2. Since the sensitivity of M_3 is increased the application of the band pass filter $f_c = 370$ Hz improves the signal-to-noise ratio. M is shown to be a quantitative but not a proportional measure of the blood velocity. In order to indicate this, it is denoted as the blood flow parameter (BFP).

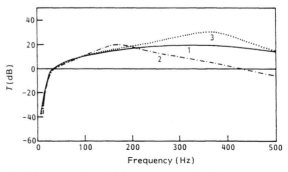

Fig. 5 Transfer function T of the series connection of low and high-pass filters (cut-off frequencies 50 Hz and 800 Hz, respectively) and different frequency dependent amplifiers. Curve 1 — Differentiator, Curves 2 and 3 — Band pass filters with a centre frequency $f_c = 170$ and 370 Hz, respectively

Blood flow measurements

As an example, a synchronous measurement of the blood flow parameter with the transcutaneous oxygen tension obtained from the hand dorsum is shown in Fig. 6.

Since the blood flow is constant for the first nine minutes the transcutaneous oxygen tension is constant and the blood flow parameter fluctuates with a constant mean value. After the blood supply is suppressed by inflating a cuff around the upper arm (downward arrow) both values decline to a minimum. The release of the cuff (upward arrow) causes the blood flow parameter to increase rapidly to a peak value followed by a slow decrease to the initial value. The transcutaneous oxygen tension rises with a time constant of about 1 min to the initial value.

A comparison of the curves in Fig. 6 suggests that the blood flow parameter and the transcutaneous oxygen tension show a similar reaction to rapid changes of the blood flow. However, the response of the blood flow parameter is faster than that of the transcutaneous oxygen tension.

As a second example, the laser speckle method was tested in a simple physiological experiment. After the hand had been held in water of temperature T between 5° C and 45°C for 1 min it was wiped dry and the blood flow parameter was determined at the hand dorsum. Measurements with $T = 5$°C, 15°C, 30°C, and 45°C are shown in Fig. 7. With 5°C and 45°C a high BFP is obvious at the beginning. These findings correspond to the high blood flow which is necessary

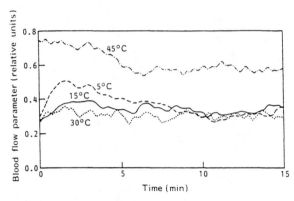

Fig. 7 Blood flow parameter obtained from the hand dorsum after the hand was held in water of different temperatures T

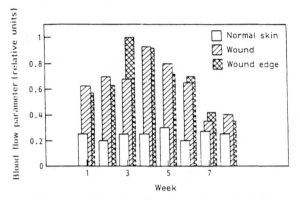

Fig. 8 Development of the blood flow parameter measured on a patient leg ulcers during the healing process. The measurements were obtained from the wound, wound edge and normal skin

to compensate for the difference from the normal skin temperature of about 30°C. For this reason only a small increase is noticeable at 15°C, whereas the blood flow parameter does not considerably change at 30°C.

As a third example, the development of the blood flow parameter was investigated in patients with healing leg ulcers. The measurements were taken from nine patients during their stay in hospital. From measurements at several positions mean values were formed corresponding to the classification into the groups 'wound', 'wound edge', and 'normal skin'. As the positions were marked on photographs the measurements could be repeated every week.

One example is shown in Fig. 8. The initial values for wound and wound edge exceed that for normal skin because there is no epidermis which normally absorbs a large quantity of light scattered from the red blood cells. Subsequently, the values increase, pass a maximum, and decrease to a level near that for normal skin. The increase may be the result of the therapy and the decline is surely due to the formation of new epidermis. In contrast to this pronounced time-dependence, the values for normal skin are comparatively constant.

Discussion

The involuntary body movement represents the main perturbation of blood flow measurements when using

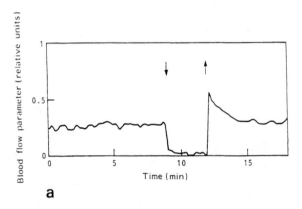

a

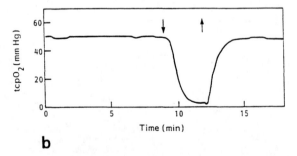

b

Fig. 6 Simultaneous measurement of a — the blood flow parameter; and b — the transcutaneous oxygen tension

the laser speckle method. However, the influence of this movement is reduced by an electronic circuit specially matched to the optical device. Additional measurements with adhesive tape attached to the skin allow the control of the residual influence of the involuntary body movements.

Measurements with the laser Doppler method are also affected by the involuntary body movement[21,22]. Since the probe is fixed to the skin, the relative movement between the optical fibres and the tissue is reduced. However, when the probe and fibres move together with the skin the light transmitted by the moving fibres is shifted in frequency because it is transferred from one optical mode to another[15]. As stated in Ref 10, the laser Doppler method provides a proportional measure of the blood flow if the surrounding tissue can be considered to be stationary. This assumption is clearly not valid and in measurements with the laser Doppler method the involuntary body movement simulates a high blood flow in the same way as in the laser speckle method. However, control measurements are easier to perform with the laser speckle method.

Flow measurements using ultrasound are not affected by the involuntary body movement because they measure the blood flow in large arteries and in these the blood velocity exceeds that of capillaries by two orders of magnitude[23].

It has been found that a measurement at one position can be performed within 2 min. This is advantageous when compared to the determination of blood flow by the method of transcutaneous oxygen tension, as this takes about 20 min. As the skin blood flow in patients with arterial occlusive disease may vary considerably from one position to another[1], several positions must be investigated. With the laser speckle method these measurements can be performed in a reasonable time interval.

The device for the determination of the two-dimensional image of the skin blood flow[25] is based on the same measuring principle. However, in Ref. 25 no relation between the output signal and the blood velocity is given and the influence of the involuntary body movement is not discussed. The spatial resolution of the device described in this paper is given by the diameter of the laser spot (1.5 mm).

As shown by thermography, the skin blood flow may vary within a few centimetres[26]. Therefore, the given resolution is sufficient to investigate this effect. The high resolution of the image, however, can probably not be utilized in medical applications.

The non-contact method allows measurements without affecting the blood flow by the measurement itself. Blood flow determination in wounds is possible and no difficulties arise from the sterilization of the probe. Further work will show whether it is a useful tool in clinical practice.

Appendix 1

The power spectrum of $I(t)$

Substituting (7) into (8) yields

$$I(t) = (\overline{A}_1\, a_1(t) + \overline{A}_2 a_2(t))^* \,(\overline{A}_1 a_1(t) + \overline{A}_2\, a_2(t))\,(23)$$

Corresponding to (3) the power spectrum is given by

$$P(\omega) = \mathcal{F}(I(t) \otimes I(t)) \tag{24}$$

(23) is substituted into (24). Then the commutative property of convolutions and the addition theorem of Fourier transforms are applied. The result is

$$P(\omega) = \overline{A}_1^4 \mathcal{F}(a_1^*(t)\, a_1(t) \otimes a_1^*(t)a_1(t)) + \\ \overline{A}_2^4\, \mathcal{F}(a_2^*(t)a_2(t) \otimes a_2^*(t)a_2(t)) \\ + \overline{A}_1^2\overline{A}_2^2\, \mathcal{F}(2a_1^*(t)a_1(t) \otimes a_2^*(t)a_2(t) \tag{25}$$
$$+ (a_1^*(t)a_2(t) + a_2^*(t)a_1(t)) \otimes (a_1^*(t)a_2(t) + \\ + a_2^*(t)\, a_1(t)))$$

It can be shown that further terms with products of amplitudes like $A_1^3 A_2$ and $A_1 A_2^3$ vanish[18]. Equation (10) is applied for the amplitudes and (6) and (3) for the first and second term.

The third term is abbreviated by

$$p_{12}(\omega) = \mathcal{F}\,[2a_1^*(t)\, a_1(t) \otimes a_2^*(t)\, a_2(t) \\ + (a_1^*(t)\, a_2(t) + a_2^*(t)\, a_1(t)) \otimes (a_1^*(t)a_2\,(t) \\ + a_2^*(t)\, a_1(t))] \tag{26}$$

The result is (9).

Appendix 2

The power spectrum of $I_k(t)$

The calculation is equivalent to Appendix 1. The result, corresponding to (25), is

$$P_k(\omega) = \overline{A}^4{}_1\, \mathcal{F}(a_1^*(t)a_1(t) \otimes a_1^*(t)\, a_1(t)) \\ + \overline{A}_2^4\, \mathcal{F}(a_2^*(kt)\, a_2(kt) \otimes a_2^*(kt)\, a_2(kt)) \\ + \overline{A}_1^2\overline{A}_2^2\, \mathcal{F}(2a_1^*(t)\, a_1(t) \otimes a_2^*(kt)a_2(kt) \tag{27} \\ + (a_1^*(t)a_2(kt) + a_2^*(kt)a_1(t)) \otimes \\ (a_1^*(t)a_2(kt) + a_2^*(kt)a_1(t)))$$

The first term is identical to the first term of (25). For the second term (6) and (3) together with the similiarity theorem are applied with the result

$$\mathcal{F}(a_2^*(kt)\, a_2(kt) \otimes a_2^*(kt)\, a_2(kt)) \\ = \mathcal{F}(i_2(kt) \otimes i_2(kt)) \tag{28} \\ = \frac{1}{k} p_2\!\left(\frac{\omega}{k}\right)$$

The third term is abbreviated by

$$P_{12}(k,\omega) = \mathcal{F}\,[\,2a_1^*(t)a_1(t) \otimes a_2^*(kt)a_2(kt) \\ + (a_1^*(t)\, a_2(kt) + a_2^*(kt)a_1(t)) \otimes (a_1^*(t)a_2(kt) \\ + a_2^*(kt)a_1(t))] \tag{29}$$

and the use of (10). The result is (13).

Appendix 3

Equation (29) is inserted into the integral of the third term of (15) and the addition theorem for Fourier transforms is applied

$$\int \omega^2 \, P_{12}(k,\omega) \, d\omega = \int \omega^2 \mathscr{F}(2a_1^*(t)\, a_1(t) \otimes a_2^*(kt)a_2(kt)) \, d\omega$$

$$+ \int \omega^2 \mathscr{F} \left[(a_1^*(t)a_2(kt) + a_2^*(kt)a_1(t)) \otimes (a_1^*(t)a_2(kt) + a_2^*(kt)a_1(t)) \right] d\omega \qquad (30)$$

$a_1(t)$ is replaced by the constant α_1 (16).

$$\int \omega^2 P_{12}(k,\omega) \, d\omega = \int \omega^2 \mathscr{F}(2\alpha_1^* \, \alpha_1 \otimes a_2^*(kt)a_2(kt)) \, d\omega \qquad (31)$$

$$+ \int \omega^2 \mathscr{F} \left[(\alpha_1^* a_2(kt) + a_2^*(kt)\alpha_1) \otimes (\alpha_1^* a_2(kt) + a_2^*(kt)\alpha_1) \right] d\omega$$

In the first term of (31) a convolution with a constant is performed. As the result is also a constant (see (4)) the Fourier transform is a δ-function and the integration of the first term yields zero because of the factor ω^2.

In the second term of (31) the only time dependency is given by the function $a_2(kt)$.

When the similarity theorem is applied to this term, the integral in the third term of (15) is, in this special case, given by

$$\int \omega^2 \, p_{12}(k,\omega) \, d\omega = \int \omega^2 \frac{1}{k} \, \bar{p}\left(\frac{\omega}{k}\right) d\omega \qquad (32)$$

where $\bar{p}(\omega)$ is defined by

$$\bar{p}(\omega) = \mathscr{F}((\alpha_1^* a_2(t) + a_2^*(t)\alpha_1) \otimes (\alpha_1^* a_2(t) + a_2^*(t)\alpha_1)) \qquad (33)$$

When the substitution rule is used and a further constant K_3 is defined by

$$K_3 = \int \omega^2 \bar{p}(\omega) d\omega \qquad (34)$$

the result is

$$\int \omega^2 \, p_{12}(k_1,\omega) = k^2 K_3 \qquad (35)$$

Similar to K_2, the constant K_3 depends on the optical device and the spatial blood flow distribution.

References

1 **Fagrell, B.** 'Microvascular skin changes in severe arterial insufficiency', *Int J Microcirc Clin Exp* **5** (1986) 178–183
2 **Fagrell, B.** 'Ischemic skin ulcers and gangrene — Mainly a microcirculatory problem?', *Bibl anat* **13** (1975) 360–361
3 **Kessler, M., Höper, J., Kumme, B.A.** 'Monitoring of tissue perfusion and cellular function', *Anesthesiology* **45** (1986) 184–197
4 **Stern, M.D.** '*In vivo* evaluation of microcirculation by coherent light scattering', *Nature* **254** (1975) 56–58
5 **Holloway, G.A. Watkins, D.W.** 'Laser Doppler measurement of cutaneous blood flow', *J Invest Derm* **69** (1977) 306–309
6 **Anderson, R.R., Parrish, J.A.** 'The optics of human skin', *J Invest Dermatol* **77** (1981) 13–19
7 **Whitton, J.T., Everall, J.D.** 'The thickness of the epidermis', *Br J Dermatol* **89** (973) 467–476
8 **Butti, P., Intaglietta, M., Reiman, H., Hollinger, Ch., Bollinger, A., Anliker, M.** 'Capillary red blood cell velocity measurements in human nailfold by videodensitometric method', *Microvasc Res* **10** (1975) 220–227
9 **Nilsson, G.E., Tenland, T., Öberg, P.A.** 'A new instrument for continuous measurement of tissue blood flow by light beating spectroscopy', *IEEE Trans Biomed Eng* **BME–27** (1980) 12–19
10 **Bonner, R., Nossal, R.** 'Model for laser Doppler measurements of blood flow in tissue', *Appl Opt* **20** (1981) 2097–2107
11 **Haumschild, D.J.** 'An overview of laser Doppler flowmetry', *Biomed Sci Instrum* **22** (1986) 35–40
12 **Karanfilian, R.G., Lynch, T.G., Lee, B.C., Long, J.B., Hobson, R.W.** 'The assessment of skin blood flow in peripheral vascular disease by laser Doppler velocimetry', *The Am Surgeon* **50** (1984) 641–644
13 **Rayman, G., Hassan, A., Tooke, J.E.** 'Blood flow in the skin of the foot related to posture in diabetes mellitus', *Br Med J.* **292** (1986) 87–90
14 **Kristensen, J.K., Engelhart, M., Nielsen, T.** 'Laser-Doppler measurement of digital blood flow regulation in normals and in patients with Raynaud's phenomenon', *Acta Dermatovener.* **63** (1983) 43–47
15 **Ruth, B** 'Velocity measurement by the laser speckle method using optical fibres', *Opt Laser Technol* **19** (1987) 83–90
16 **Briers, J.D.** 'The statistics of fluctuating speckle patterns produced by a mixture of moving and stationary scatterers', *Opt Quant Electron* **101** (1978) 364–366
17 **Ohtsubo, J.** 'The time-space cross-correlation of speckle patterns under illumination of double-crossed laser beams', *J Opt* **10** (1979) 169–177
18 **Ruth, B.** 'Superposition of two dynamic speckle patterns — An application to non-contact blood flow measurements', *J Mod Opt* **34** (1987) 257–273
19 **Bracewell, R.** 'The fourier transform and its applications', New York, McGraw-Hill Book Company, (1965)
20 **Bollinger, A., Butti, P., Barras, J.P. Trachsler, H., Siegenthaler, W.** 'Red blood cell velocity in nailfold capillaries of man measured by a television microscopy technique', *Microvasc Res* **7** (1974) 61–72
21 **de Mul, F.F.M., v. Spijker, J., van der Plas, D., Greve, J., Aarnoudse, J.G., Smits, T.M.** 'Mini laser-Doppler (blood) flow monitor with diode laser source and detection integrated in the probe', *Appl Opt* **23** (1984) 2970–2973
22 **Heden, P.G., Hamilton, R., Arnander, C., Jurell, G.** 'Laser Doppler surveillance of the circulation of free flaps and replanted digits', *Microsurgery* **6** (1985) 11–19
23 **Kilpatrick, D., Tyberg, J.V., Parmley, W.W.** 'Blood velocity measurement by fibre optic laser Doppler anemometry', *IEEE Trans Biomed Eng.* **BME 29** (1982) 142–145
24 **Ruth, B., Haina, D., and Waidelich, W.,** 'Determination of a blood flow parameter by the Doppler method', *Optica Acta* **31** (1984) 759–66
25 **Fujii, H., Nohira, K., Yamamoto, Y., Ikawa, H., and Ohura, T.,** 'Evaluation of blood flow by laser speckle image sensing. Part 1 *Appl Opt* **26** (1987) 5321–5
26 **Winsor, T.,** 'Vascular aspects of thermography', *J Cardiovas Surg* **12** (1971) 379–88

Reprinted with permission from *Optics and Laser Technology*, Vol. 23(4),
pp. 205-219 (1991). ©1991 Butterworth-Heinemann Ltd.

Bio-speckle phenomena and their application to the evaluation of blood flow

Y. AIZU, T. ASAKURA

The study of time-varying speckle phenomena observed in light-fields scattered from living objects is reviewed. The laser speckles produced from living objects may be called 'bio-speckles' and fluctuate temporally due to various physiological movements such as blood flow. The time-varying properties of the bio-speckles are experimentally investigated from the analyses of the power spectrum and the autocorrelation function. Based on the knowledge of dynamic bio-speckles, some methods are introduced for evaluating blood flow in the skin surface, internal organs, and ocular fundus. The experimental results show that the degree of blood flow is reflected sensitively by the time-varying properties of the bio-speckles and this can be utilized for monitoring the blood flow.

KEYWORDS: speckles, blood flow, flow measurement, biological tissue

Introduction

When a diffuse object with an optically-rough surface is illuminated by laser light, laser speckle phenomena can be observed in the reflected or transmitted light. If the diffuse object moves with a certain velocity, the individual grains of the speckle pattern also move and change their shape: the moving speckle pattern thus contains information about the object's motion. Therefore, the dynamic properties of the speckles have been extensively studied and are being applied to velocity measurements[1]. However, most of these studies have been carried out for inanimate objects — such as a solid diffuse plate with a simple structure. Except for a few studies[2, 3], the dynamic speckles produced from living objects have not been sufficiently investigated. The speckles observed from living objects generally fluctuate in a space–time random fashion owing to the complicated structure and inconsistent physiological activity of living objects. Therefore, the dynamic behaviour of such speckles is considerably different from that of speckles produced from solid diffuse objects. From this point of view, the speckles from living objects may be called 'bio-speckles'[4, 5].

With the recent increase of laser applications in the medical and physiological fields, bio-speckles are receiving much attention from researchers. This is because the temporal fluctuation of bio-speckles is expected to provide much information about the physiological activity of living objects, such as blood flow and heartbeat. In addition, the dynamic behaviour of bio-speckles is an interesting subject in the field of laser light scattering. This is due to the fact that bio-speckles result from multiple scattering from various complex media of living objects.

On the other hand, a number of studies[6-14] have been performed for the measurement of blood flow using the laser Doppler effect. This Doppler method has been reported to be useful because of its non-invasive and repeatable characteristics. However, it is limited to cases where the blood vessel is exposed to the laser beam or in which the vessel permits insertion of an optical fibre probe. In other cases, such as skin blood flow, some of the studies which are described as laser Doppler velocimetry may, in fact, be distinguished from the original principle of laser Doppler velocimetry: red blood cells are illuminated through a surface tissue, which acts as a diffuser, and the 'Doppler-shifted light' is detected, also through this diffuser. Therefore, the phase distribution of light fields to be detected is fully randomized by the mass scattering of the tissues and blood flows. These scattering processes seem to be more suitably described as dynamic speckle phenomena rather than the Doppler effect and, therefore, may be appropriately reinterpreted from the viewpoint of speckle phenomena. On the basis of

YA is in the Department of Mechanical Systems Engineering, Muroran Institute of Technology, Muroran, Hokkaido 050, Japan. TA is in the Research Institute of Applied Electricity, Hokkaido University, Sapporo, Hokkaido 060, Japan. Received 20 March 1991.

this consideration, some recent articles[15-17] have discussed the relation between the bio-speckle fluctuation and blood flow.

In this paper, the time-varying properties of bio-speckles are experimentally investigated on the basis of the power spectral and autocorrelation analyses. As one of the interesting applications of bio-speckles, several techniques are introduced for non-invasively evaluating the blood flow in the skin surface, internal organs, and ocular fundus. Some other applications of bio-speckle phenomena are also described briefly.

Bio-speckles from the skin surface

Observation of bio-speckles

We first discuss the dynamic properties of bio-speckles observed from the human skin surface[15] as shown in Fig. 1. A HeNe laser beam illuminates a fingertip and is scattered back to an observation plane O_p, where a bio-speckle pattern is formed. The photographs (a) and (b) show bio-speckle patterns taken at the plane O_p with different exposure times of (a) 0.5 s and (b) 1 s. With increasing exposure time, it is found that the bio-speckle pattern is blurred and that its contrast becomes lower. The photograph (c) shows a high-contrast speckle pattern obtained from a static styrene-form plate. These observations imply that the bio-speckle pattern from the skin surface fluctuates spatially and temporally in a random fashion. This is due to dynamic scattering by the blood flow in dermal capillaries. Figure 2 shows the intensity fluctuations of bio-speckles detected by a photomultiplier, through a pinhole placed at the plane O_p. The signals (a) and (b) were recorded for normal flow, and for reduced flow with an inflated cuff on the upper arm, respectively. High frequency components are clearly suppressed in Fig. 2(b) and this seems to reflect the reduction of blood flow. Thus, frequency analysis of the bio-speckle fluctuations may give useful information on the degree of skin blood flow.

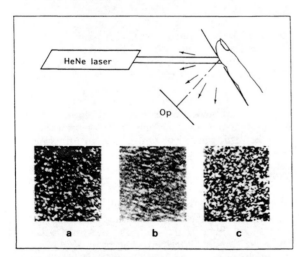

Fig. 1 Bio-speckle patterns produced in (a) 0.5 s; and (b) 1 s; from the skin surface of a fingertip and a usual speckle pattern (c) obtained from a styrene-form plate

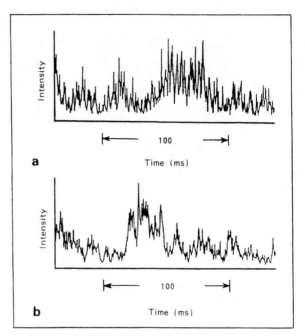

Fig. 2 Bio-speckle fluctuations (a) and (b) obtained from the normal and reduced skin blood flows, respectively

It can be observed that the entire structure of the low-contrast pattern in the photograph Fig. 1(b) is stable with a further increase of exposure time unless the skin surface moves laterally. This means that the bio-speckle pattern produced by the skin tissue consists of two components: (1) the fast fluctuation due to the skin blood flow and (2) the slow movement due to the deformation of the outer skin tissue. The latter slowly-moving component causes the low frequency noise in the output signals. Then, the bio-speckles from the blood flow in the inner skin tissue may be modulated by the movement of the outer skin tissue before detection.

Despite the modulation, the bio-speckle signals in Fig. 2 possibly show the dependence of bio-speckle fluctuations on the skin blood flow. This observation was also confirmed by a simulation study[18] in which the dynamic speckles were produced by two ground-glass plates set in layers with a small separation distance. Static-front ground-glass and the moving-back ground-glass plates were used, respectively, for modelling the static outer skin tissue and the blood flow in the inner skin tissue. The illuminating laser light was firstly transmitted through the static front diffuser, secondly reflected by the moving back diffuser, and thirdly passed through the static front diffuser. Thus, the triply-scattered speckle is detected and its intensity fluctuation is investigated from the autocorrelation function. In spite of the phase modulation by the front ground-glass, the intensity fluctuation of triply-scattered speckles was found to depend linearly on the moving velocity of the back ground-glass plate.

Evaluation of skin blood flow

The time-varying properties of bio-speckles may be applied to measurements of skin blood flow. Figure 3

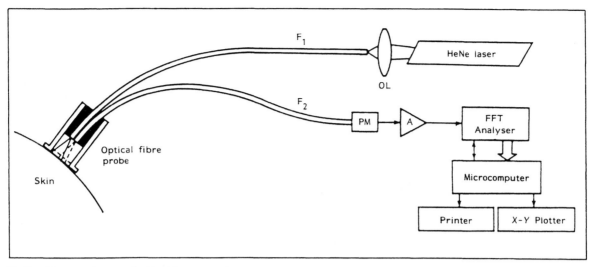

Fig. 3   Schematic diagram of a blood-flow monitoring system using bio-speckle phenomena

shows schematically[15] the measuring system using an optical fibre probe. A HeNe laser beam is radiated onto the skin surface via a multimode optical fibre F_1 with a core diameter of $80\,\mu$m. The scattered light is picked up by a single-mode optical fibre F_2 with a core diameter of $10\,\mu$m installed in parallel to fibre F_1. This pair of multimode and single-mode fibres is effective for achieving high output radiation from the illuminating fibre, high signal-to-noise ratio, and low modal noise from the vibration of the fibre. Bio-speckle fluctuations are detected by a photomultiplier, PM, and are fed into a spectrum analyser where the power spectral distribution is obtained.

Figure 4 shows the typical power spectral distributions obtained from three different regions of the human skin surface. Two interesting features are found in Fig. 4: (1) the power spectral distribution plotted on a log scale decreases monotonically from the low to the high frequency; and (2) the rate of decrease is characterized by the region of human skin being measured as the degree of blood flow may be different. These features indicate that skin blood flow can be characterized by the slope of the power spectral distribution.

To evaluate quantitatively the slope of the power spectral distribution, a simple signal processor was constructed. This has two band-pass filters with central frequencies of 640 Hz and 40 Hz. By measuring the powers $|V_H|^2$ and $|V_L|^2$ of the high and the low frequency components obtained from these filters, a blood flow parameter HLR can be calculated by

$$HLR = \frac{|V_H|^2}{|V_L|^2} \qquad (1)$$

and used to evaluate the skin blood flow. Figure 5 shows the variation of the blood flow parameter HLR according to the skin blood flow in the palm of the hand. Region (a) shows normal flow, while regions (b) and (c) show the flow stopped by an inflated cuff on the upper arm and the enhanced

flow as the cuff is deflated, respectively. The value of HLR is found to indicate sensitively the change of skin blood flow. The separation of the two pass-bands determines the sensitivity of the measuring system. It should be carefully noted that the bio-speckle phenomena observed here reflect the overall characteristics of the blood flows, but do not directly give flow properties, such as velocity.

The depth of the probed volume is generally determined by the depth of the light penetration into the skin. In Fig. 6, HeNe laser light with a wavelength of 632.8 nm penetrates into the dermis, while blue light with a wavelength of nearly 450 nm is mainly absorbed and scattered in the epidermis, under which papillary loops exist. Selection of the wavelength of the illuminating light may provide the discriminative measurements of the total dermal flow and the superficial dermal flow in the papillary loops. In the measuring system of Fig. 3, however, the discrimination of skin-tissue layers to be probed is made easier by adjusting the separation distance d between the illuminating and detecting fibre ends as shown in Fig. 6. Figure 7 shows the power spectral distributions obtained from the palm of a hand by means of the three fibre probes with different separation distances d. With increasing distance d, the low frequency components decrease and the high frequency components increase. With small distance d, the detecting fibre F_2 mainly receives the scattered light propagated in the short path in and near the region of epidermis. This light is modulated by the low degree of blood flow in papillary loops and shows the low frequency fluctuation. With large distance d, the light coming from the deeper dermal region dominantly contributes to the detected bio-speckles, and the high degree of blood flow in the dermis results in the high frequency fluctuation. The relation between the separation distance d and the depth of the probed volume was quantitatively calibrated by the simulation study using a Teflon sheet as a skin model. This study shows that the separation distance of $d = 1$–2 mm is suitable for evaluating the

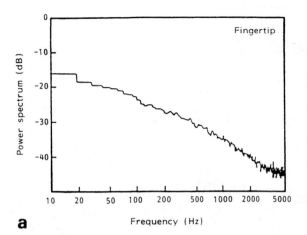

a

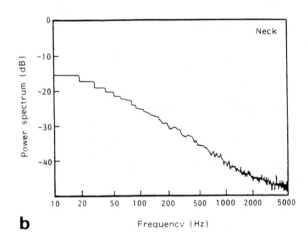

b

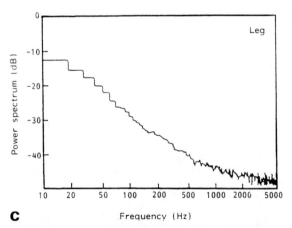

c

Fig. 4   Power spectral distributions obtained from three different skin surfaces

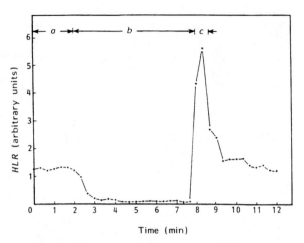

Fig. 5   Variation of the blood flow parameter *HLR* for the different degrees of skin blood flow in the palm of a hand

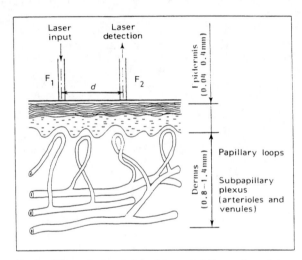

Fig. 6   Schematic description of the optical fibre probe and the vascular structure of skin

blood flow in the dermis, although the simulation is not directly applied to the actual skin tissue.

Two-dimensional blood flow map

The technique of monitoring blood flow using bio-speckles can be extended to the visualization of a two-dimensional microcirculation map[3, 19]. Figure 8

(see Ref. 19) schematically shows an optical system for visualizing a two-dimensional blood-flow map using a CCD linear image sensor. A skin surface is illuminated, via mirror M, with a HeNe laser spot expanded into a line by cylindrical rod lens L_1. The scattered light is reflected by the mirror M and collected by lens L_2 to form an image of the line spot on a CCD linear image sensor (with an array of 256 elements) where a bio-speckle pattern appears. When the intensity pattern of the bio-speckle image is scanned successively by the CCD linear sensor, the profile of the output signals fluctuates temporally due to the blood flow in the dermal tissue layer. The rate of this fluctuation depends on the blood-flow degree.

Figure 9(a) shows two successive scanning outputs of the CCD image sensor. The left and right-hand sides of the scanned position correspond to the areas where the skin blood flow is artificially controlled to be slow and fast, respectively. Considerable difference is found between the two successively scanned signals in the right-hand side. This is due to the rapid

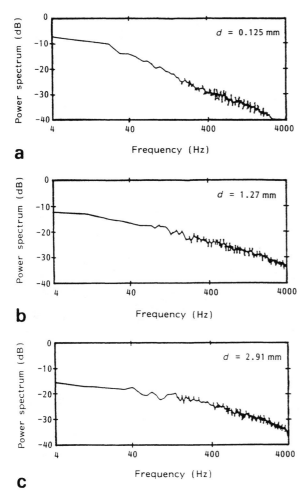

a

b

c

Fig. 7   Power spectral distributions obtained by three fibre probes with the different separation distance d

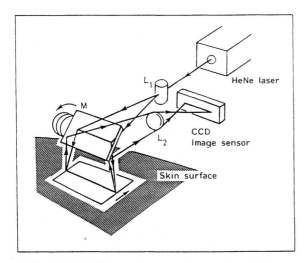

Fig. 8   Schematic diagram of a system for visualizing the two-dimensional blood flow map

fluctuation of bio-speckles resulting from the fast blood flow. The two successive signals in the left-hand side are almost the same because the slow bio-speckles hardly fluctuate in one scanning interval

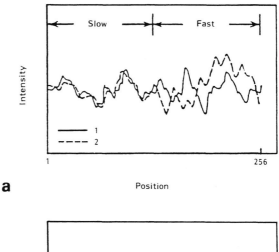

a

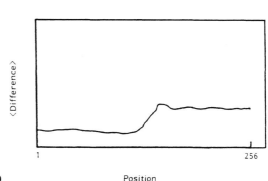

b

Fig. 9   (a) Two successive scanning outputs of a CCD linear image sensor and (b) a one-dimensional blood flow map

owing to the slow blood flow. The difference between a pair of output signals for successive scans, defined as

$$D_{(n)} = \sum_{k=1}^{N} \frac{|I_k(n) - I_{k+1}(n)|}{|I_k(n) + I_{k+1}(n)|} \qquad (2)$$

is measured and integrated for each pixel. In (2), $I_k(n)$ is the amplitude value of the output signal for the nth pixel point of the kth scan in the CCD linear sensor. This process was repeated for more than 100 scans to average the difference data. Figure 9(b) shows the integrated value $D_{(n)}$ of the average difference which provides a one-dimensional blood-flow map. The average difference becomes high for the area where the blood-flow degree is high and vice versa. Figure 10 shows a one-dimensional flow map on the back of a hand where a small scratch scar is left. There was a slightly itchy region in the scar which is represented by a circle in Fig. 10(a). The blood-flow map was measured and plotted along the solid line across the scar. The result, Fig. 10(b), clearly shows that the wound healing process induces a high degree of blood circulation around the scar.

A two-dimensional map of the microcirculation is obtained by scanning the illuminating line spot in a direction perpendicular to the line spot. In Fig. 8, this is done by tilting the mirror M step by step and repeating the same data analysis as in the one-dimensional measurement. The two-dimensional spatial variation of the flow degree is visualized by

483

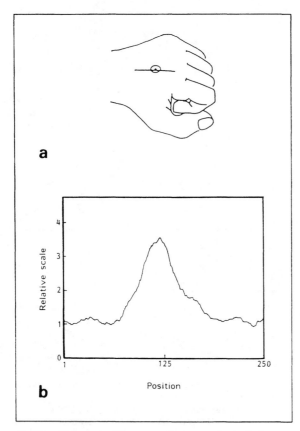

Fig. 10 (a) A scanned line across the scar on the back of a hand and (b) the corresponding one-dimensional blood flow map

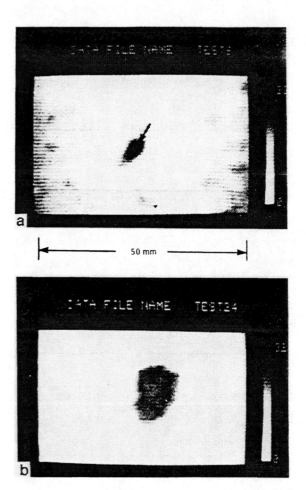

Fig. 11 CRT display of the blood flow map at the skin surface under tuberculin test: (a) 6 h and (b) 24 h after the injection

graphically displaying in colours the integrated values of the average difference. Figure 11 shows black and white photographs of a colour CRT display showing the microcirculation map of human skin under a tuberculin test. The values of the average differences are colour-coded in 32 levels. The results (a) and (b) were obtained 6 h and 24 h after injection of the drug into the skin. As expected, the spot of higher blood-flow degree is small in (a) and is enlarged due to the reaction in (b). Using a two-dimensional area sensor, instead of tilting the mirror mechanically, is more suitable for a practical instrument. However, the scanning rate of commercially available area sensors is not sufficiently high enough to follow the high frequency fluctuation of bio-speckles. Thus, the use of an area sensor is promising for the skin blood flow, but needs to have an improved scanning rate if the more active blood flow in large vessels is to be visualized.

Bio-speckles from internal organs

We next discuss the bio-speckle phenomena observed from internal organs. Figure 12 shows the experimental set-up of the optical fibre probe shown in Fig. 3, which was used for observing the bio-speckle fluctuation from the gastric mucous membrane of an anaesthetized albino rabbit. The optical fibre probe was held by a flexible arm to avoid the effect of body movements. Figure 13 shows the power spectral

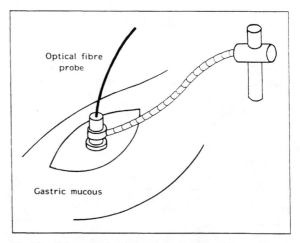

Fig. 12 Schematic illustration of the experimental set-up for evaluating the blood flow in the gastric mucous membrane using bio-speckles

distributions obtained under three different conditions of blood flow in the gastric mucous membrane. The results (I) and (II) were obtained when norepinephrine and prostaglandine E_1 were applied to the mucous membrane as a vasocon-

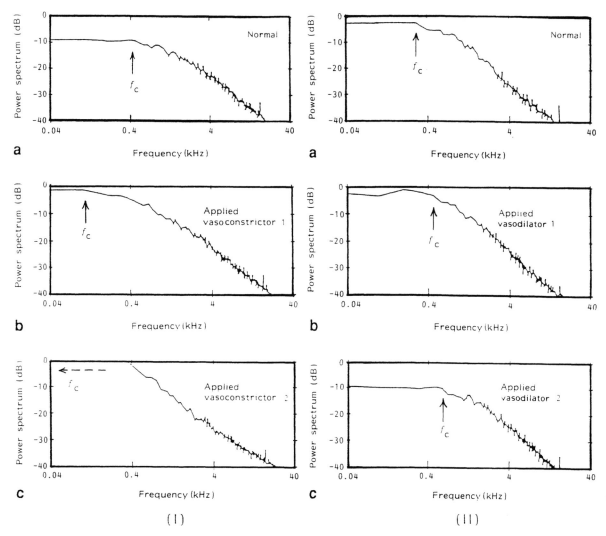

Fig. 13 Power spectral distributions obtained for (I) the normal and the reduced blood flows and (II) the normal and the enhanced blood flows, in a gastric mucous membrane

strictor and a vasodilator, respectively. In addition, the power spectrum (a) is measured for the normal flow, while the power spectra (b) and (c) are measured for single and continuous applications of these drugs, respectively. The blood flow was expected to decrease with the vasoconstrictive effect of norepinephrine and to increase with the vasodilative effect of prostaglandine E_1. The power spectral distribution is nearly flat from the low frequency to a certain frequency f_c which may be regarded as a cut-off frequency and, then, begins to decrease in the higher frequency region. With the application of norepinephrine and prostaglandine E_1, the cut-off frequency f_c is seen to become lower in (I) and higher in (II), respectively, from (a) to (c). This implies a relative increase of lower and higher frequency components in the power spectral distribution corresponding to the reduced and the enhanced blood flows, respectively.

It should be noticed that the form of power spectral distributions shown in Fig. 13 is clearly different from the result for the skin, as shown in Fig. 4. A difference is also found in the variation of the power

spectral distribution according to the change of blood-flow degree. Figure 14 schematically illustrates such a difference in the form of power spectral distributions obtained from the skin surface and the gastric mucous membrane. This difference is probably due to the structure of tissues and vessels. The blood vessels and capillaries in the gastric mucous membrane are directly exposed to the laser light for illumination and detection, and the photomultiplier dominantly receives the high-frequency fluctuation scattered by the blood flow. In the skin, the low-frequency fluctuation due to involuntary movements of the outer skin surface primarily contributes to the photodetector signals. This latter effect results in the relative increase of low frequency components as shown in Fig. 14(a).

The blood flow parameter *HLR* in (1), which is used for evaluating the skin blood flow, is not suitable for analysing the power spectral distributions obtained from the gastric mucous membrane, because of their different decreasing forms. To evaluate appropriately the variation of the power spectral distribution

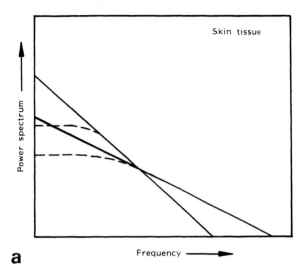

a

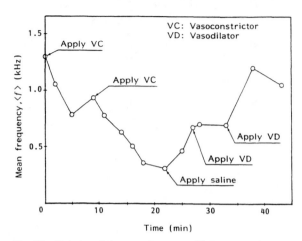

Fig. 15 Variation of the mean frequency $\langle f \rangle$ for the application of vasoconstrictor (VC) and vasodilator (VD)

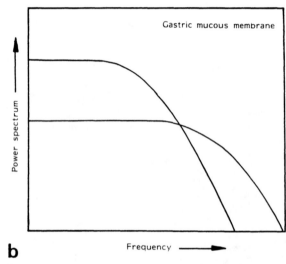

b

Fig. 14 Schematic comparison of the power spectral distributions obtained from (a) the skin tissue and (b) the gastric mucous membrane

according to the change of the blood-flow degree, the mean frequency $\langle f \rangle$ is introduced here and is given by

$$\langle f \rangle = \frac{\sum\limits_i f_i P(f_i)}{\sum\limits_i P(f_i)} \qquad (3)$$

where $P(f_i)$ is the signal power at frequency f_i. Figure 15 shows the variation of the mean frequency $\langle f \rangle$ obtained for the application of norepinephrine as the vasoconstrictor (VC) and prostaglandine E_1 as the vasodilator (VD). As expected, the mean frequency $\langle f \rangle$ decreases with the VC-application and then increases again with the VD-application. Therefore, the mean frequency $\langle f \rangle$ is found to be another useful indicator for the evaluation of blood-flow degree as well as for the blood-flow parameter *HLR*. The experiment was also carried out for the intestinal mucous membrane of an anaesthetized albino rabbit. The blood flow was reduced by the clamping of

arteriole and venule. According to this operation, the power spectral distribution shows a substantial decrease in higher frequency components, and the usefulness of the method is also verified for the blood flow in the intestinal mucous membrane. One of the promising potentials in the clinical application of this method may be the installation of the present measuring system into a fibre endoscope.

Bio-speckles from ocular fundus

Evaluation of fundus blood flow

Bio-speckles are also observed from the ocular fundus tissue in which retinal vessels are directly exposed to the laser light. Fercher and Briers[3, 20–23] showed a method for visualization of the retinal blood-flow map. In their method, the bio-speckle fluctuation from the ocular fundus is recorded on a photographic film as the decorrelation effect and is used for visualizing a blood-flow map using optical filtering or image processing. In this section, we discuss the dynamic properties of bio-speckles obtained from the ocular fundus (including retinal and choroidal tissue layers) and introduce a new method[24, 25] for evaluating the ocular-fundus blood flow. Figure 16 shows two basic optical systems for detecting the bio-speckle fluctuations from the ocular fundus (I) at the diffraction plane and (II) at the image plane. In Fig. 16 (I), laser light illuminates a certain area of the retina with an extended spot and is scattered by ocular fundus tissues and blood flows. The scattered light produces, via lenses L_1, L_2, and L_3, a dynamic bio-speckle pattern at the diffraction plane where a detecting aperture DA is placed. Through the detecting aperture DA, the bio-speckle fluctuation is detected by a photomultiplier, PM. Owing to the extended illuminating spot and the setting of the detecting aperture at the diffraction plane, this aperture DA receives the superposition of whole light fields scattered from every point in the spot. Therefore, this optical system enables us to measure the overall activity of the various blood flows observed in the illuminated spot area, rather than the absolute flow velocity at a certain point on

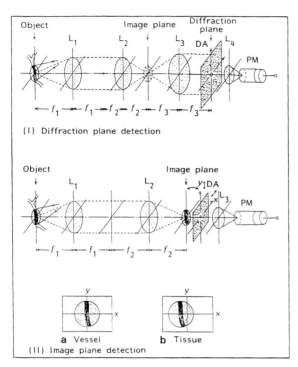

(I) Diffraction plane detection

a Vessel   **b** Tissue

(II) Image plane detection

Fig. 16   Two basic optical systems for detecting bio-speckles from the ocular fundus (I) at the diffraction plane and (II) at the image plane

a blood vessel. In addition, a consistent phase relation between those scattered light fields may not be retained at the detecting point but may be fully randomized. This is due to the rapid fluctuation of the positions of the red blood cells. It is, therefore, noticeable that the bio-speckle fluctuation observed here may be distinguished from the usual Doppler effect.

Figure 17 (see Ref. 25) shows a schematic diagram of the apparatus for detecting the bio-speckle fluctuation from the ocular fundus and for evaluating the ocular-fundus blood flow. A HeNe laser beam with 50–100 μW power illuminates the ocular fundus with an

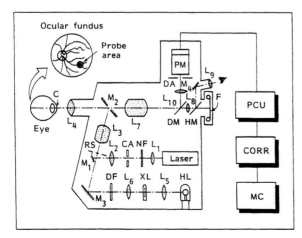

Fig. 17   Schematic diagram of the apparatus for evaluating the blood-flow at the ocular fundus

approximately 1 mm diameter extended spot using the illuminating optical system of a fundus camera. This exposure follows the security conditions for the human retina presented by the WHO[26]. The light scattered from the ocular fundus is received and detected by a photomultiplier PM via a 80 μm diameter detecting aperture, DA, placed at the Fraunhofer diffraction plane. The probe area is easily positioned by a target fixation. The probe volume depth cannot be strictly defined in the present method, but we employ a HeNe laser of 632.8 nm wavelength so that the light penetrates into the choroidal tissue layers. Then, the method may probe both the retinal and choroidal layers.

Figure 18 (see Ref. 24) shows typical power spectral distributions of the bio-speckle fluctuation obtained from the ocular fundus of an anaesthetized albino rabbit. Result (a) was measured when the rabbit was breathing in room air. Results (b) and (c) were measured when the rabbit's mouth was covered with a vinyl bag filled with a gas mixture of CO_2 and O_2 for 2 min and 3 min, respectively. This application was expected to increase the blood flow artificially. With the gas application, the low frequency components of the power spectral distribution are clearly reduced and higher frequency components increase relatively. This variation indicates the substantial increase of the ocular-fundus blood flow. It is interesting to note that the form of the power spectral distribution in Fig. 18 is very similar to the result for the gastric mucous membrane in Fig. 13 but is different from the result for the skin surface in Fig. 4. This is probably due to the fact that the structure of the ocular fundus tissue is closer to that of the gastric mucous membrane than that of the skin tissue. This observation implies that the frequency components of bio-speckle fluctuations are significantly influenced by the structure of the tissues and vessels. Figure 19 shows the temporal variations of the mean frequency $\langle f \rangle$ as the two kinds of gas mixture (a) and (b) were applied to two anaesthetized rabbits. The mean frequency $\langle f \rangle$ increases with the gas mixture (a) after time A and then decreases with room air after time B, but it remains unchanged with gas mixture (b). This difference arises from the effect of CO_2 density on the blood flow. The mean frequency $\langle f \rangle$ reflects favourably the change of the ocular fundus blood flow according to the gas application.

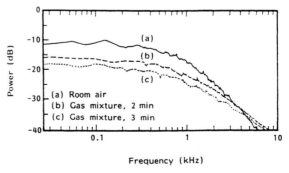

(a) Room air
(b) Gas mixture, 2 min
(c) Gas mixture, 3 min

Fig. 18   Power spectral distributions obtained from the ocular fundus of a rabbit for the three different conditions of breathing

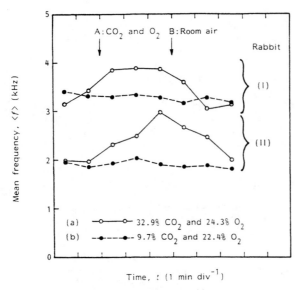

Fig. 19 Variation of the mean frequency $\langle f \rangle$ as the two kinds of the gas mixture (a) and (b) are applied to the two anaesthetized rabbits

Because of the weak-intensity speckles from the ocular fundus, the photon correlation technique is used for analysing effectively output signals. In Fig. 17, photoelectron pulses obtained from the photomultiplier PM are fed into a 256 channel digital correlator, CORR, with which the autocorrelation function of the bio-speckle fluctuation is obtained. Figure 20 shows the fundus photograph of a human

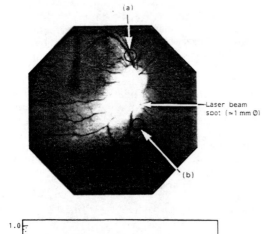

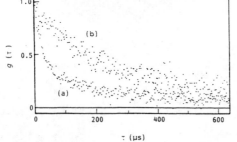

Fig. 20 Fundus photograph of a human volunteer and correlation functions obtained from the two probe points shown in the photograph

volunteer including an illuminated spot, along with typical correlation functions of the bio-speckle fluctuation obtained from the probe positions (a) and (b) indicated in the photograph. The correlation function attenuates rapidly in (a) and slowly in (b). The probe area (a) contains two major retinal vessels (vein and artery), but the area (b) includes no visible vessel. Thus, the blood flow is considered more active in (a) than in (b). The more and less active blood flows in (a) and (b) increase higher and lower frequency components and result in the rapid and slow decays of the correlation functions, respectively.

The attenuation of the correlation function is evaluated by analysing the time-correlation length τ_c which gives half the maximum correlation value of the correlation function. Figure 21 shows the distribution maps of the time-correlation length τ_c obtained from each ocular fundus of three normal volunteers (a), (b) and (c). From the rough estimation of Fig. 21, the smallest or largest values of τ_c are obtained from those probe areas where retinal vessels cross or do not, respectively. In these results, the absolute values of τ_c cannot be directly compared among the three volunteers, because of their individuality with respect to the inhomogeneous structure of tissue and vessels. But the similar dependence of τ_c on the existence or non-existence of blood vessels was observed for the three volunteers. Thus, these results are helpful for investigating the blood circulation at the human ocular fundus. In the present method, the bio-speckle fluctuation mainly reflects blood flows in retinal vessels and capillaries, although the light from capillaries has weak intensity. The light scattered from the underlying choroidal tissue also contributes to the bio-speckle fluctuation, but this is modulated and indirect since the detected light experiences twice the phase modulation due the retinal blood flows and tissues. Therefore, the only possible and useful measurement in the method is to evaluate the overall degree of blood-flow activity in the probed area including both the retinal and choroidal vasculatures.

Retinal blood-flow velocity

As well as the overall degree of blood flow in a finite fundus area, the blood-flow velocity at a point on a retinal vessel also has important information for many diagnostic purposes. Several researchers[6, 8] have extensively studied the laser Doppler method, and recently the usefulness of the method has been reported for the non-invasive assessment of some eye diseases. We shall study a method for measuring the retinal blood-flow velocity using bio-speckle phenomena. In Fig. 16(II), the intensity fluctuation of bio-speckles scattered by red blood cells in a retinal vessel is detected by the aperture DA at the magnified image plane. By positioning the centre of the detecting aperture DA to a measuring point of interest, this optical system enables us to measure the velocity of retinal blood flow at the selected point. Arrangements (a) and (b) in Fig. 16(II) show schematic examples of the measuring point on a vessel and surrounding tissue, respectively. Output pulses are analysed to obtain the autocorrelation

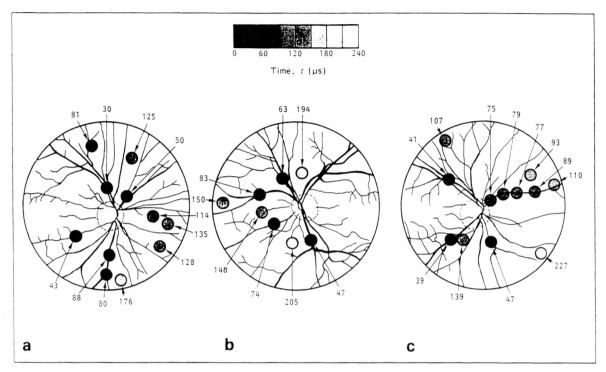

Fig. 21 Distribution maps of τ_c obtained from each ocular fundus of the three normal volunteers

function. The blood-flow velocity is measured in a relative value from the reciprocal of the time-correlation length, $1/\tau_c$. Figure 22 shows the measuring apparatus modified with a microscope

for 22.8× magnification and an *X–Y* micro stage for positioning a measuring point. Nearly 200 μm diameter grains of bio-speckles were detected by a 400 μm diameter detecting aperture. DA, at the mag-

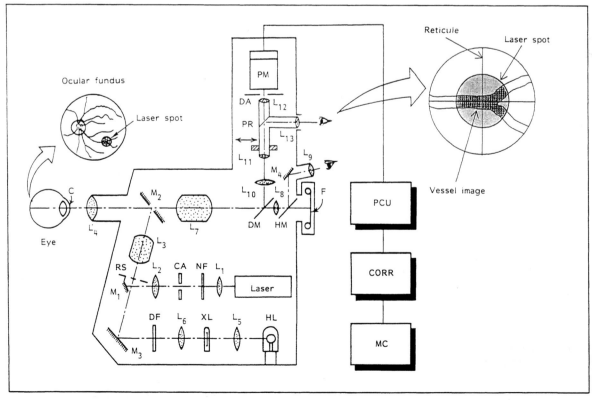

Fig. 22 Schematic diagram of the measuring apparatus modified with a microscope and an *X–Y* micro stage

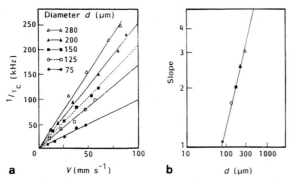

a

Diameter d (μm)
- $\triangle$—$\triangle$ 280
- $\blacktriangle$—$\blacktriangle$ 200
- $\blacksquare$---$\blacksquare$ 150
- $\circ$---$\circ$ 125
- $\bullet$---$\bullet$ 75

b

Fig. 23 (a) Relation between the blood-flow velocity in capillaries and the reciprocal of time-correlation length; (b) Relation between the slope of lines and the capillary diameter obtained from (a)

nified image plane. With this condition, the probe's cross-sectional area was defined to be nearly 20 μm. Thus, more than 50 μm diameter of the vessel is available for blood-flow measurements in this arrangement. By using the reticle of the eyepiece, the position of the detecting aperture can be adjusted to the measuring point of interest.

Before applying the method to human subjects, we performed a preliminary experiment[27, 28] by using blood flow in glass capillaries of various diameters. Figure 23(a) shows the relation between the velocity of the blood flow and the reciprocal of time-correlation length, $1/\tau_c$. Good linearity was obtained for each glass capillary, but the slope of the lines increased with increasing capillary diameters. This means that a certain constant flow velocity was evaluated to be different values of $1/\tau_c$ according to the capillary diameter. We found, however, that the slope of the lines is linearly proportional to the square root of the diameter. Figure 23(b) shows this linearity obtained from the results of Fig. 23(a). Therefore, the diameter dependence of the bio-speckle fluctuations may be compensated for by this experiment, and the velocity of the retinal blood flow can be measured by the present method.

On the basis of the knowledge from the preliminary experiment, we applied the method to human volunteers. Figure 24 shows the fundus photograph of a human volunteer, in which a_1–a_4 indicate the measuring points on the vessel while b_1–b_4 represent the measuring points on the surrounding tissue. Figure 25 shows typical correlation functions obtained from the points a_3 and b_3 of Fig. 24 and τ_c-histograms obtained by repeating the measurements several times at all points of Fig. 24. Each correlation function was measured in 2 s. The correlation function (a) demonstrates an extremely early decay owing to the high blood-flow velocity in the vessel, but the function (b) shows a slow decay owing to the low degree of capillary blood flow and indirect choroidal blood flow. In the histograms, the τ_c-values of (a) and (b) are distributed in shorter and longer time regions, respectively. Therefore, the bio-speckle fluctuation well reflects the retinal blood-flow velocity.

Figures 26 and 27 show the temporal variations of the correlation functions and their $1/\tau_c$ values when

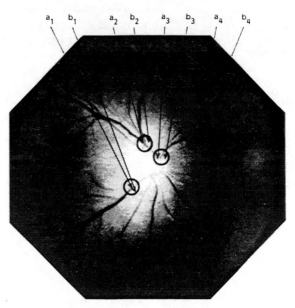

Fig. 24 Fundus photograph of a human volunteer and some measuring points

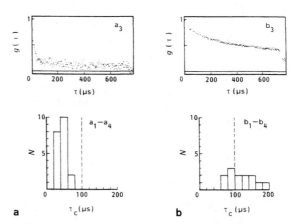

a

b

Fig. 25 Typical correlation functions and τ_c-histograms obtained from the measuring points; (a) a_1–a_4 on retinal vessels; and (b) b_1–b_4 on surrounding tissue areas shown in the photograph of Fig. 24

the measuring point was moving out from (a) the centre of a vessel to (b) the surrounding tissue. We stored the photon count data for about 6 s and then analysed the correlation functions every 52.5 ms. In Fig. 26, the decay of the correlation curve is found to become slower after 4 s because of displacement of the measuring point. This variation is clearly shown by the $1/\tau_c$-value in Fig. 27. This means that the blood flow velocity can be favourably evaluated by the value of $1/\tau_c$. Figure 28 shows the variations of $1/\tau_c$-values and the electrocardiogram (ECG) obtained every 65 ms from the retinal artery (a) and vein (b). In (a), the value of $1/\tau_c$ clearly changes over the same period with the ECG, and the pulsating blood flow is successfully measured. In (b), however, the pulsation of the blood flow is not recognized as expected from the elementary medical knowledge. These experimental results show the usefulness of the present method for measuring the blood-flow

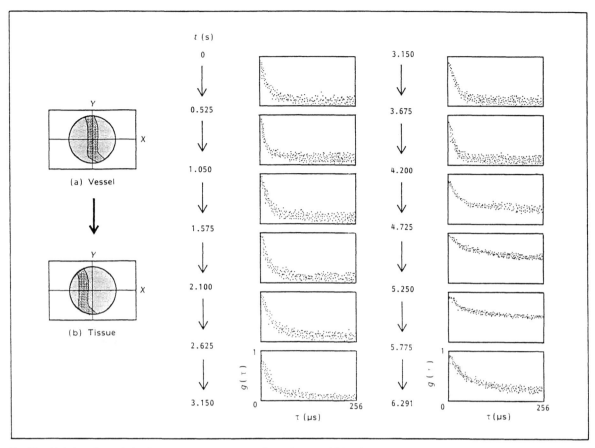

Fig. 26 Variation of correlation functions when the measuring point was shifting from a vessel to a tissue

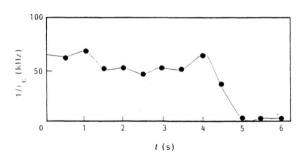

Fig. 27 Variation of $1/\tau_c$-value corresponding to the correlation functions of Fig. 26

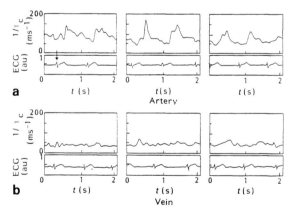

Fig. 28 Variations of $1/\tau_c$ and ECG obtained simultaneously from (a) retinal artery and (b) vein

velocity in retinal vessels. The method detects the temporal fluctuation of bio-speckles but not the Doppler broadening components. Therefore, the present technique is free from the severe scattering geometry conditions.

Other examples of bio-speckles

A few studies[2, 29, 30] have been made on bio-speckles obtained from fruits and eggs. These studies are not directly related to the evaluation of blood flow, but are interesting in other applications of bio-speckle phenomena. Briers[2] investigated the bio-speckle fluctuation obtained from red and green tomatoes, and proposed a method for evaluating the movement

of plastids in the cells with relation to the wavelength of light used. The bio-speckle phenomena observed from some fruits were also studied by Oulamara et al[29] and were applied to the quantitative analysis of the biological activity of the living state of the cells. Another example[30] of bio-speckle was studied for measuring the heart rate of avian embryos in an egg. Figure 29 presents a block diagram of the experiment for measuring minute ballistic movements of the egg using the bio-speckle

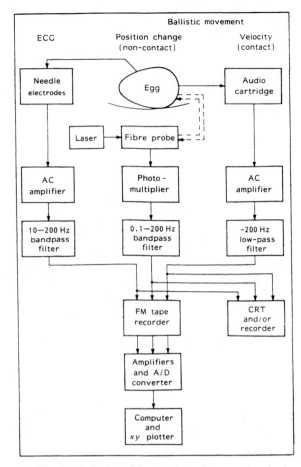

Fig. 29 Block diagram of the experiment for measuring simultaneously minute ballistic movements of the egg using the ECG, audiocartridge, and bio-speckle technique

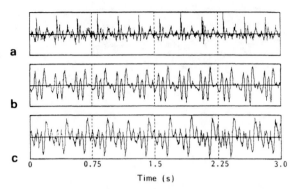

Fig. 30 (a) ECG; (b) audiocartridge signals; and (c) bio-speckle signals simultaneously measured from an embryo 19 days old

phenomena. Two contact methods with the electrocardiogram (ECG) and audiocartridge were also used for comparison purposes. By using the optical fibre probe shown in Fig. 3, a HeNe laser beam illuminates an egg in a non-contact manner and the scattered light is picked up and propagated to the photomultiplier. The intensity fluctuation of biospeckles was measured via a bandpass filter and an amplifier. The bio-speckle signals are compared to the results obtained by the two contact methods. Figure 30 shows typical examples of (a) an electrocardiogram, (b) the output signals of an audiocartridge, and (c) the bio-speckle signals simultaneously measured from an embryo 19 days old. The periodic variation synchronized with the electrocardiogram was clearly obtained in the biospeckle signals (c) with the merit of a non-contact and non-disturbing operation. In addition to heartrate measurements, the bio-speckles from the egg are expected to provide information about other physiological functions and responses of avian embryos within their eggs to altered environments.

Conclusion

This paper reviews the time-varying properties of dynamic bio-speckles obtained from living objects and introduces some methods for measuring the blood flow in the living tissue. The bio-speckle fluctuation has various frequency components according to the probing area of the living objects being measured, but it has now been found to reflect sensitively blood-flow activity such as velocity. This is quite useful for evaluating non-invasively the blood flow. The dynamic behaviour of bio-speckles depends on various factors within the living objects. such as the spatial structures of tissues and vessel network. and their absorption and diffusion characteristics. The theoretical analysis of the relation between these factors and the bio-speckle fluctuation seems to be an interesting but a complicated subject because of the complexity of living objects. However. detailed observation and experimental analysis of bio-speckles are effective for the development of their potential applicability. We hope that dynamic bio-speckle phenomena will be further investigated for various kinds of living objects and will be applied to the measurement of these objects' physiological behaviour.

References

1 Asakura, T., Takai, N. 'Dynamic laser speckles and their application to velocity measurements of the diffuse object'. *Appl Phys* 25 (1981) 179–194

2 Briers, J.D. 'Wavelength dependence of intensity fluctuations in laser speckle patterns from biological specimens'. *Opt Commun* 13 (1975) 324–326

3 Fercher, A.F., Briers, J.D. 'Flow visualization by means of single-exposure speckle photography'. *Opt Commun* 37 (1981) 326–330

4 Asakura, T. 'Dynamic properties of bio-speckles and their application to blood flow measurements'. *Anritsu News* 8 (1988) 4–9

5 Aizu, Y., Asakura, T. 'Bio-speckle phenomena and their applications to blood flow measurements'. *Proc SPIE* 1431 (1991) 239–250

6 Tanaka, T., Riva, C., Ben-Sira, I. 'Blood velocity measurements in human retinal vessels'. *Science* 186 (1974) 830–831

7 Tanaka, T., Benedek, G.B. 'Measurement of velocity of blood flow (in vivo) using a fiber optic catheter and optical mixing spectroscopy'. *Appl Opt* 14 (1975) 189–196

8 Riva, C.E., Grunwald, J.E., Sinclair, S.H., O'Keefe, K. 'Fundus camera based retinal LDV'. *Appl Opt* 20 (1981) 117–120

9 Koyama, T., Horimoto, M., Mishina, H., Asakura, T. 'Measurements of blood flow velocity by means of a laser Doppler microscope'. *Optik* 61 (1982) 411–426

10 Stern, M.D. 'In vivo evaluation of microcirculation by coherent light scattering'. *Nature* 254 (1975) 56–58

11 Stern, M.D., Lappe, D.L., Bowen, P.D., Chimosky, J.E., Holloway Jr., G.A., Keiser, H.R., Bowman, R.L. 'Con-

tinuous measurement of tissue blood flow by laser Doppler spectroscopy', *Am J Physiol* **232** (1977) 441–448

12 **Watkins, D., Holloway, Jr., G.A.** 'An instrument to measure cutaneous blood flow using the Doppler shift of laser light', *IEEE Trans Biomed Eng* **25** (1978) 28–33

13 **Nilsson, G.E., Tenland, T., Öberg, P.A.** 'Evaluation of a laser Doppler flowmeter for measurement of tissue blood flow', *IEEE Trans Biomed Eng* **27** (1980) 597–604

14 **Duteil, L., Bernengo, J.C., Schalla, W.** 'A double wavelength laser Doppler system to investigate skin microcirculation', *IEEE Trans Biomed Eng* **32** (1985) 439–447

15 **Fujii, H., Asakura, T., Nohira, K., Shintomi, Y., Ohura, T.** 'Blood flow observed by time-varying laser speckle', *Opt Lett* **10** (1985) 104–106

16 **Ruth, B.** 'Superposition of two dynamic speckle patterns: an application to non-contact blood flow measurements', *J Mod Opt* **34** (1987) 257–273

17 **Ruth, B.** 'Non-contact blood flow determination using a laser speckle method', *Opt Laser Technol* **20** (1988) 309–316

18 **Iwai, T., Asakura, T.** 'Dynamic properties of speckled speckles with relation to velocity measurements of the diffuse objects', *Opt Laser Technol* **21** (1989) 31–35

19 **Fujii, H., Nohira, K., Yamamoto, Y., Ikawa, H., Ohura, T.** 'Evaluation of blood flow by laser speckle image sensing. Part 1,' *Appl Opt* **26** (1987) 5321–5325

20 **Briers, J.D., Fercher, A.F.** 'Retinal blood-flow visualization by means of laser speckle'. Optics in Biomedical Sciences, eds von Bally, G., Greguss, P. Berlin: Springer-Verlag (1982) 158–161

21 **Briers, J.D., Fercher, A.F.** 'Retinal blood-flow visualization by means of laser speckle photography'. *Invest Ophthalmol Vis Sci* **22** (1982) 255–259

22 **Fercher, A.F., Peukert, M.** 'Retinal blood-flow visualization and measurement by means of laser speckle photography'. *Proc SPIE* **556** (1985) 110–115

23 **Fercher, A.F., Peukert, M., Roth, E.** 'Visualization and measurement of retinal blood flow by means of laser speckle photography', *Opt Eng* **25** (1986) 731–735

24 **Aizu, Y., Ogino, K., Koyama, T., Takai, N., Asakura, T.** 'Evaluation of retinal blood flow using time-varying laser speckle', Laser Anemometry in Fluid Mechanics III, ed. Adrian R.J., Lisbon: Ladoan (1988) 55–68

25 **Aizu, Y., Ogino, K., Sugita, T., Yamamoto, T., Asakura, T.** 'Noninvasive evaluation of the retinal blood circulation using laser speckle phenomena'. *J Clinical Laser Med Surgery* **8** No 5 (1990) 35–45

26 'Optical radiation, with particular reference to lasers'. Regional Office for Europe, World Health Organization, Copenhagen (1977)

27 **Aizu, Y., Ambar, H., Yamamoto, T., Asakura, T.** 'Measurements of flow velocity in a microscopic region using dynamic laser speckles based on the photon correlation'. *Opt Commun* **72** (1989) 269–273

28 **Aizu, Y., Asakura, T., Ogino, K., Sugita, T.** 'Evaluation of flow volume in a capillary using dynamic laser speckles based on the photon correlation', *Opt Commun* **80** (1990) 1–6

29 **Oulamara, A., Tribillon, G., Duvernoy, J.** 'Biological activity measurement on botanical specimen surfaces using a temporal decorrelation effect of laser speckle'. *J Mod Opt* **36** (1989) 165–179

30 **Tazawa, H., Hiraguchi, T., Asakura, T., Fujii, H., Whittow, G.C.** 'Noncontact measurements of avian embryo heart rate by means of the laser speckle: comparison with contact measurements'. *Med Biol Eng Comput* **27** (1989) 580–586

493

Reprinted from *Optical Engineering,* Vol. 32(2), pp. 277-283 (February 1993).
©1993 SPIE.

Speckle fluctuations and biomedical optics: implications and applications

J. David Briers, MEMBER SPIE
Kingston University
School of Applied Physics
Penrhyn Road
Kingston upon Thames, KT1 2EE
United Kingdom

Abstract. Laser speckle limits the resolution that can be achieved in holography. Time-varying speckle, caused by scattering from moving objects, is even more troublesome. It can destroy the correlation needed to obtain fringes in holographic interferometry and even, if the fluctuations are rapid compared with the exposure time needed, the coherence needed to record a hologram. These problems are discussed, with particular reference to biomedical holography, and suggestions are made for minimizing their effect. Some positive aspects of time-varying speckle are also discussed. The fluctuations obey the same statistics as the spatial variations of a stationary speckle pattern. These statistics can be used to measure the movement of the scattering particles, a technique of particular value in biomedical science. Potential applications include monitoring blood flow, motility, and intracellular activity.

Subject terms: biomedical optics; holography; speckle; correlators; light scattering.

Optical Engineering 32(2), 277–283 (February 1993).

1 Introduction

1.1 Laser Speckle

When diffuse objects are illuminated with laser light, a characteristic granular pattern is seen.[1] This effect, today universally referred to as "speckle,"[2] is caused by interference between light scattered from adjacent points on the object. Whether a particular point appears bright or dark depends on whether the amplitudes of the light scattered from within the scattering center around that point sum to a maximum (constructive interference) or to zero (destructive interference). The average size of the scattering centers, and hence of the individual speckles, is equal to the size of the resolution cell of the optics forming the image of the object, and is hence dependent on the aperture of those optics (which may well be the human eye). The effect is illustrated in Fig. 1 and a typical speckle pattern is presented in Fig. 2.

The speckle phenomenon actually occurs with any type of illumination, but with incoherent sources, the overlap of speckle patterns caused by the different wavelengths present greatly reduces the contrast of the pattern; it is possible, however, under certain circumstances, to observe speckle even with sunlight as the light source.[3,4] But it was only with the advent of the laser, with its unique combination of coherence and high intensity, that the effect became readily observable—and troublesome, because it severely restricted the resolution that could be achieved when laser light was used as the illuminating source.

1.2 Speckle Statistics

Laser speckle is a random (stochastic) effect and its properties can only be described statistically. The statistics of speckle have been investigated in great detail, starting with the classic work by Goodman.[5] The statistical properties of speckle can be divided into the first-order statistics, which describe the contrast of the speckle, and the second-order statistics, which describe the size distribution of the speckles.

The main result from the first-order statistics of laser speckle is that in a fully coherent speckle pattern (a "fully developed" speckle pattern, to use the term introduced by Pedersen[6]), the standard deviation of the (spatial) intensity variations is equal to the mean intensity of the pattern. The ratio of the standard deviation to the mean intensity can therefore be used as a measure of the contrast of the speckle pattern; this will, in practice, usually be less than unity. Note, however, that some authors prefer to use the square of this quantity, i.e., the ratio of the variance to the square of the mean intensity, as the parameter for speckle contrast.

The size distribution of the speckles in the pattern can be expressed by the (spatial) autocorrelation function of the intensity, a second-order statistic. As mentioned, the average speckle size is determined only by the limiting aperture of the viewing optics and is, in fact, equal to the size of the Airy disk for that aperture.

Paper BM-042 received July 1, 1992; revised manuscript received Sep. 22, 1992; accepted for publication Sep. 22, 1992. This paper is a revision of papers 1429-08 and 1647-36 presented at the SPIE conferences on Holography, Interferometry, and Optical Pattern Recognition in Biomedicine I, January 1991, Los Angeles, California, and Holography, Interferometry, and Optical Pattern Recognition in Biomedicine II, January 1992, Los Angeles, California, respectively. The papers presented there appear (unrefereed) in SPIE Proceedings Vols. 1429 and 1647.
© 1993 Society of Photo-Optical Instrumentation Engineers. 0091-3286/93/$2.00.

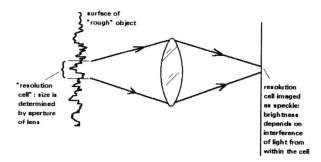

Fig. 1 Origin of the speckle effect.

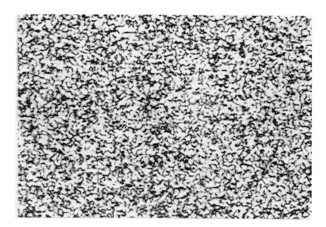

Fig. 2 A typical laser speckle pattern.

1.3 Time-Varying Speckle

Because speckle is an interference effect, it is apparent that any movement of the object producing the speckle pattern gives rise to differences in the relative phases between light scattered from different points on the object and hence causes the intensity distribution in the speckle pattern to change in time. The speckle pattern appears to "twinkle." Under certain circumstances (see below) the temporal statistics of the intensity fluctuations of a single speckle have the same properties as the spatial statistics of a stationary speckle pattern.[7]

Note, however, that the derivation of speckle statistics has traditionally assumed (implicitly) simple scattering of the laser light at a diffusing surface. In the real world, and especially with biological subjects, multiple scattering effects[8-10] should be taken into account. This can lead to some unexpected changes to the statistics of laser speckle,[11] and in particular to the second-order statistics of speckle fluctuations.[12]

2 Speckle Fluctuations and Holography

2.1 Holography and Holographic Interferometry

Conventional photography records only a two-dimensional image of an object because photographic film, in common with most detectors of light, records only the intensity of the light coming from the object. The phase of the light, which carries information about the third dimension, is lost. Holography[13,14] solves this problem by introducing a reference beam that interferes with the light from the object (Fig. 3). Note that this requires coherent light and, in practice, a laser is invariably used. The phase information is then recorded, in coded form, in the resulting interference pattern. The resulting hologram can be decoded simply by illuminating it with the original (or a similar) reference beam (Fig. 4). The interference pattern acts as a complex diffraction grating and the original object beam is "reconstructed" in amplitude and in phase, thus producing a full three-dimensional image of the original object. This occurs because the same mathematics governs the processes of interference and diffraction.

If two almost identical wavefronts are superimposed, they interfere and the resulting fringes provide information about the differences between them. This is the principle of holographic interferometry.[15,16] The reconstructed wavefront from a hologram can be superimposed on the actual wavefront coming from the object itself ("real-time" or "live-fringe" holographic interferometry), or two images

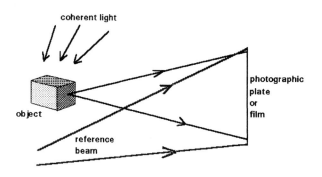

Fig. 3 Recording a hologram.

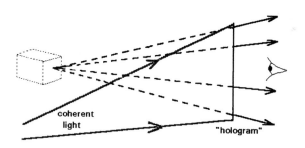

Fig. 4 Reconstructing a hologram.

can be recorded on the same hologram ("double-exposure" or "frozen-fringe" holographic interferometry). If the object is changed slightly, either in real time or between the two exposures, these changes are represented by interference fringes appearing on the reconstructed image. The changes might result from displacement, distortion, strain, or, in the case of biological subjects, growth or elongation. Quantitative evaluation of the fringe patterns is complicated, but can usually be achieved.[17]

2.2 Effect of Speckle Fluctuations on Holographic Recording

It is important to remember that in holography, the speckle pattern itself is effectively the image and must be recorded on the holographic film (or other recording medium), duly coded by interference with the reference beam. If this speckle pattern is destroyed, for example by the fact that it is fluctuating in time and is averaged out over the time of the holographic exposure, no hologram can be recorded. Conversely, in order to record a hologram of an object that is exhibiting time-varying speckle, it is essential to keep the exposure time of the hologram short enough to "freeze" the speckle fluctuations.

2.3 Effect of Speckle Fluctuations on Holographic Interferometry

The image reconstructed from a hologram, then, is essentially a speckle pattern. In holographic interferometry, two such (almost identical) speckle patterns are superimposed. One way of looking at the technique of holographic interferometry is to consider the fringes that are produced as a moiré effect between the two reconstructed speckle patterns.[18] This applies for both double-exposure and real-time holographic interferometry; in the former, both speckle patterns are reconstructed from the same hologram, whereas in the latter the speckle pattern reconstructed from the hologram is superimposed on the speckle pattern observed on the object itself.

It is clear that for these moiré effects to be observed, the two speckle patterns must be correlated. In other words, the two speckle patterns must be essentially identical, except that individual speckles will be slightly displaced where movement has occurred. These speckle displacements give rise to the moiré effect and hence to the fringe patterns of holographic interferometry. Speckle fluctuations tend to destroy this correlation, because the two speckle patterns are no longer identical. If the time interval between the two exposures (or between the recording of the hologram and the viewing of the fringes in the real-time technique) is long enough to allow the speckle pattern to have decorrelated completely, no fringes are observed.

3 Speckle Fluctuations with Biological Subjects

3.1 Holography of Biological Subjects

Anyone who has tried to make holograms of living subjects, and more especially to carry out holographic interferometry on such subjects, knows that it is much more difficult than with inanimate objects. An early experiment to demonstrate this, in which a hologram was taken of a tomato alongside an inanimate object, was reported by the author at an informal meeting of the Institute of Physics in London in 1974 and was later described in a short article by Troup.[19] The fact is that when many biological subjects are illuminated with laser light, the speckle pattern is observed to fluctuate. As discussed, these fluctuations tend to make the fringes of holographic interferometry very difficult to observe and, in extreme cases, may even make the recording of a hologram extremely difficult.

3.2 A Screening Test for Holography

Experiments have shown that there is a very good correlation between the speckle fluctuations observed when botanical objects are illuminated with laser light and the degree of difficulty encountered when such subjects are used for holography and for holographic interferometry. The speckle fluctuations can be characterized by their temporal statistics, and in particular by the ratio of the standard deviation σ of the intensity fluctuations to the mean intensity $\langle I \rangle$ (in the same way that the spatial version of this ratio is used for the contrast of a speckle pattern). These quantities are computed from the variations observed in the intensity of a single speckle. Table 1 shows typical measured values of $\sigma/\langle I \rangle$ for a variety of subjects, together with comments on the difficulties of using the subjects for holography.[20]

The speckle fluctuations were recorded using the experimental arrangement of Fig. 5. Note that far-field speckle[2,5] was used, rather than the image speckle discussed in Sec. 1.1. The statistics of the two versions of speckle are, however, essentially identical and the far-field arrangement was used simply for convenience. An aperture of about one-tenth of the average speckle size was placed in front of the detector to ensure that a single speckle was being monitored. A typical oscilloscope trace is presented in Fig. 6 (the subject in this case is a green tomato, the light source is an argon-ion laser operating at a wavelength of 514 nm, and the time base is 8 s full scale).

Note that the values of σ obtained in these experiments may be limited by the response time of the detector. If the fluctuations are too fast, the detector is not able to follow them and the measured value of σ is too low. In these experiments, the detector was a photomultiplier connected to an oscilloscope. Bearing in mind the proposed cause of the speckle fluctuations (the motion of scattering bodies within the specimens[20]), it is believed that the response time of such a system should be short enough to ensure that the experiment is unlikely to be detector-limited. Further details of these experiments have been published elsewhere.[20]

Results like those outlined in Table 1 were used to propose the use of speckle fluctuations as a screening test in holography with biological subjects[20,21]: subjects exhibiting strong speckle fluctuations would be difficult subjects for holography. By keeping the exposure time short compared with the decorrelation time of the speckle fluctuations, a single-shot hologram is still possible, but if holographic interferometry is the aim, such fluctuations are likely at best to reduce fringe contrast and at worst to make fringes impossible to achieve. (A similar proposal to detect the presence of creep in inanimate objects before taking a hologram was made by Ennos.[22])

3.3 Mixture of Moving and Stationary Scatterers

The highest values of $\sigma/\langle I \rangle$ observed in the fluctuations of speckle patterns from botanical subjects was, as indicated in Table 1, of the order of 0.4. In other words, the fluctuations were never fully developed ($\sigma/\langle I \rangle = 1$). As mentioned, this is unlikely to be caused by the limited response time of the detector. An alternative explanation might be the fact that not only the moving scatterers contribute to the speckle pattern when a biological subject is illuminated with laser light. There is also a contribution to the scattered light, and hence to the speckle pattern, from parts of the object that are not in motion. Thus it should be possible to deduce from the value of $\sigma/\langle I \rangle$ the relative contributions to the speckle pattern of light scattered from moving and from

Table 1 Speckle fluctuations observed with various botanical subjects and their effect on holographic interferometry experiments.

Subject	σ/⟨I⟩ for speckle fluctuations (typical values)	Comments on holographic interferometry
metal and other inanimate objects	0.03 (noise)	no problems with inanimate objects, providing normal precautions taken.
tobacco stem tobacco leaf	0.05 0.11	reasonable fringes obtained with many types of mature plants.
seedlings of pea, bean, etc.	0.20 (base) to 0.40 (tip)	faint fringes near base; more difficult at tip.
coleoptiles of cereals	0.40	very difficult to obtain fringes; often difficult to obtain holograms.

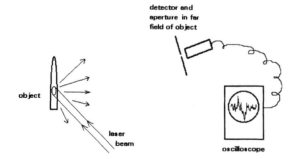

Fig. 5 Experiment to record time-varying speckle.

stationary scatterers.

In fact, it can be shown that[23]:

$$\rho = 1 - \left(1 - \frac{\langle \sigma^2 \rangle_{x,y}}{\langle I \rangle^2} \right)^{1/2} ,$$

where ρ is the ratio of the mean intensity of the light scattered from the moving scatterers to the total mean intensity of the scattered light and $\langle \ \rangle_{x,y}$ indicates spatial averaging (necessary because σ varies from point to point in the speckle pattern).

In practice, because the scattering properties of the moving scatterers are likely to be different from those of the

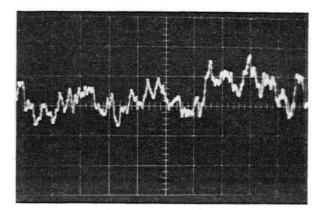

Fig. 6 A typical fluctuating-speckle trace.

stationary scatterers, and because other effects such as vibrations or air currents might also have a contribution, this equation is more likely to be of value for relative rather than for absolute measurements. Nevertheless, it is believed that these first-order statistics of the time variations of a speckle pattern do carry information about the relative contributions from moving and from stationary scatterers.

3.4 Second-Order Statistics of the Speckle Fluctuations

As mentioned, the second-order (spatial) statistics of a stationary speckle pattern carry information about the size distribution of the speckles. The function usually used is the autocorrelation (or autocovariance) function. The second-order (temporal) statistics of a time-varying speckle pattern carry information about the velocity distribution of the scatterers. Again the autocorrelation function is usually used. If the motion of the scatterers is random, the technique is known as intensity fluctuation spectroscopy (also known as light beating spectroscopy or photon correlation spectroscopy) and can be used to measure diffusion constants and cell motility.[24] If the motion is directional, the closely related technique of laser Doppler velocimetry[25] is used. These techniques are now well established and widely used. They are not considered in any detail in this paper and are mentioned mainly to stress the close relationship between the techniques and laser speckle—the mathematics of the two fields are identical.

3.5 Wavelength Dependence of the Speckle Fluctuations

Speckle fluctuations imply that the scattering centers in the illuminated object are in motion. In biomedical subjects, the scattering may well be taking place from discrete bodies within the subject rather than from the surface of the subject. For example, the green color of plants results from chlorophyll and this is largely contained in discrete chloroplasts within the cells of the plants. Microscopic observations on thin-leaved plants such as *Elodea canadensis* show that these chloroplasts move around inside the cells, a process known as cyclosis. Other colorations, for example the red color of a tomato, also result from discrete pigmented bodies (chromoplasts) inside the cells. Similarly, the color of animal tissue is largely caused by the selective scattering of discrete cells such as red blood cells.

Experiments carried out on different colored plant subjects and using different wavelengths of laser radiation showed that there was indeed a correlation between the color, the wavelength, and the degree of speckle fluctuation observed. In general, fluctuations were more pronounced when the color of the laser light was the same as the color of the subject, less so when the colors were complementary. There was also an angular effect, the speckle fluctuations being less pronounced around the specular reflection direction. This led to a model being proposed,[26] which suggested that there were two components to the scattered light, a quasi-specular component giving rise to stationary speckle and a diffuse component from moving (and pigmented) bodies within the subject producing fluctuating speckle. One conclusion to be drawn from this model is that it may be possible to limit the speckle fluctuations, and hence to make holography more practicable, by careful selection of the wavelength of the laser light used for the illumination. Thus if green plants are the subject and the degree of speckle fluctuation in the green light from an argon-ion laser suggests that holography might be difficult, the problem might be solved by changing to the red light from a helium-neon laser. On the other hand, in medical holography better results may be obtained by using an argon laser rather than a helium-neon laser. It has also been suggested[27] that this wavelength dependence of speckle fluctuations could provide a useful additional degree of freedom when studying biological and medical subjects with techniques such as intensity fluctuation spectroscopy.

3.6 Spatial Statistics of Time-Integrated Speckle Patterns

Another way to analyze time-varying speckle patterns is to take a time-exposure photograph of the (fluctuating) speckle pattern and measure the spatial statistics. The second-order statistics, of course, do not yield any additional information. But the first-order statistics, in particular the speckle contrast, depends on the exposure time, the velocity of the moving scatterers, and the proportion of light scattered by the moving scatterers compared with stationary scatterers.

If the time exposure (integration time) is long enough, the speckle pattern from the moving scatterers becomes completely smoothed out and has the effect of adding a uniform (incoherent) background to the speckle pattern produced by the stationary scatterers. It can be shown that[28]

$$\rho = 1 - \frac{\sigma}{\langle I \rangle} \, ,$$

where ρ is again the ratio of the mean intensity of the light scattered from the moving scatterers to the total mean intensity of the scattered light. This time σ is the spatial standard deviation of intensity. For shorter integration times, the degree to which the speckle pattern is blurred out depends on the velocity of the moving scatterers. In other words, the (spatial) speckle contrast depends on the velocity of the moving scatterers (and, of course, on the integration time). Thus, velocity variations in a flow field are mapped as variations in speckle contrast on a time-exposure photograph.[29] This technique has been applied to the visual-

Table 2 Possible applications of speckle statistics in biology and medicine. The techniques of Table 2 have been used to measure: a—flow,[29,30] mobility[26,28] and vibrations;[31] b—velocity;[33] c—mobility;[23] d—intensity fluctuation spectroscopy[24] and laser Doppler velocimetry[25] for diffusion, motility, and flow; e—velocity;[34] f—velocity.[35]

	1st order	2nd order
Spatial statistics of time-integrated speckle	a	
Temporal statistics of time-integrated speckle	b	
Temporal statistics of direct signal	c	d
Temporal statistics of time-differentiated speckle	e	f

ization of blood flow in the retina[30] and to the study of vibrations.[31] In practice, optical filtering techniques may be needed to convert the speckle contrast variations into easier-to-see intensity variations.[32]

3.7 Time-Integrated and Time-Differentiated Speckle

Other variations on the theme of the statistics of fluctuating speckle are possible. In addition to the temporal statistics of what we might call the direct signal and the spatial statistics of the time-integrated speckle, some workers have used the temporal statistics of time-integrated and time-differentiated speckle to measure velocities.[33–35]

4 Applications of Fluctuating Speckle

4.1 Overview of Reported Applications

This discussion indicates a multiplicity of ways in which the fluctuating speckle effect can be used to monitor flow and movement, many of which are applicable to biological and medical subjects. Thus, first- and second-order statistics can be used, and can be applied to the direct signal (the speckle fluctuations themselves), to time-integrated speckle, or to time-differentiated speckle. Table 2 indicates the possibilities available and indicates some applications that have been reported in the literature.

4.2 Examples of Specific Applications

The following examples are in no way a complete list of reported applications of the techniques described in this paper. They do, however, give some idea of the range of applications in the biomedical field that have already been developed.

4.2.1 Blood flow by laser Doppler velocimetry

The well-established technique of laser Doppler velocimetry, which in effect utilizes the second-order statistics of time-varying speckle, has been used to measure blood flow in the retina[36] and in other tissues.[37] In some medical establishments, this technique is now almost a routine tool. The main advantage of the Doppler technique, in addition to the potentially noninvasive nature it shares with all the techniques discussed in this paper, is its precision; its main disadvantage is that it measures the velocity at only one point.

4.2.2 *Blood flow mapping by single-exposure speckle photography*

The mapping of velocity as speckle contrast in a time-exposure photograph, utilizing the spatial statistics of time-integrated speckle, has been used to map retinal blood flow.[30] The technique has the advantage of presenting a global map of the flow field, at the expense of some precision and ease of use. The technique is still under development.

4.2.3 *Blood flow using speckle fluctuations*

The second-order statistics of time-varying speckle are used directly in a method devised to measure blood flow in the skin.[38] A strip of skin is illuminated with laser light and the intensity of individual speckles is monitored repeatedly by means of a linear CCD array. Because each point (speckle) is being monitored separately, this technique has the ability to build up an image of the velocity variations along the illuminated line. Proposals to extend the technique by using two-dimensional arrays, or by scanning the line over the surface of the skin, would allow the mapping of blood flow over areas of the skin surface.

A similar technique has recently been applied to the measurement of blood flow at the ocular fundus.[39]

4.2.4 *Miscellaneous applications of speckle fluctuations*

A review of the use of the second-order statistics of time-varying speckle and its biomedical applications—a field called "bio-speckle" by its authors—was published recently.[40] Applications described included the two-dimensional mapping of the blood velocity in the skin; the measurement of blood flow in internal organs, in the ocular fundus, and in the retina; the analysis of the biological activity of living cells; and the measurement of the heart rate of embryos inside eggs.

5 Conclusions

Many of these techniques have been reported only in terms of the feasibility of the method; it is suggested that there could well be viable applications for some of them in the field of biology and medicine. For example, it may be practicable to study cyclosis and other intracellular motion in plants by one of the noninvasive methods mentioned.[41,42] The potential of the techniques for measuring blood flow has also probably not been exhausted. Of the two gaps in Table 2, the second-order spatial statistics of time-integrated speckle do not, of course, yield any information (other than on the size of the speckle and hence of the aperture of the optics), but there may be possibilities to consider in the second-order temporal statistics. Finally, there may be some advantage in considering the effects of different wave-lengths of laser light on the temporal statistics of time-varying speckle.

References

1. J. D. Rigden and E. I. Gordon, "The granularity of scattered optical maser light," *Proc. IRE* **50**, 2367–2368 (1962).
2. J. C. Dainty, Ed., *Laser Speckle and Related Phenomena* (*Topics in Applied Physics*, Vol. 9), Springer-Verlag, Berlin-Heidelberg-New York (1975).
3. D. A. Palmer, "Speckle patterns in incoherent light and ocular refraction," *Vis. Res.* **16**, 436 (1976).
4. T. S. McKechnie, "Image-plane speckle in partially coherent illumination," *Opt. Quantum. Electron.* **8**, 61–67 (1976).
5. J. W. Goodman, "Statistical properties of laser speckle patterns," Stanford Elec. Lab. Technical Report No. 2303-1 (1963).
6. H. M. Pedersen, "The roughness dependence of partially developed, monochromatic speckle patterns," *Opt. Commun.* **12**, 156–159 (1974).
7. J.-P. Goedgebuer and J.-C. Vienot, "Temporal speckle," *Opt. Commun.* **19**, 229–231 (1976).
8. V. Twersky, "Absorption and multiple scattering by biological suspensions," *J. Opt. Soc. Am.* **60**, 1084–1093 (1970).
9. C. F. Bohren, "Multiple scattering of light and some of its observable consequences," *Am. J. Phys.* **55**, 524–533 (1987).
10. Č. Koňák, J. Jakeš, P. Štěpánek, F. Petráš, M. Kárská, J. Křepelka, and J. Peřina, "Effect of multiple light scattering on transmitted and scattered light," *Appl. Opt.* **30**, 4865–4871 (1991).
11. T. Yoshimura and K. Fujiwara, "Statistical properties of doubly scattered image speckle," *J. Opt. Soc. Am. A* **9**, 91–95 (1992).
12. S. Feng and P. A. Lee, "Mesoscopic conductors and correlations in laser speckle patterns," *Science* **251**, 633–639 (1991).
13. D. Gabor, "A new microscope principle," *Nature* **161**, 777–778 (1948).
14. R. J. Collier, C. B. Burckhardt, and L. H. Lin, *Optical Holography*, Academic Press, New York (1971).
15. R. L. Powell and K. A. Stetson, "Interferometric vibration analysis by wavefront reconstruction," *J. Opt. Soc. Am.* **55**, 1593–1598 (1965).
16. K. A. Haines and B. P. Hildebrand, "Surface deformation measurement using a wavefront reconstruction technique," *Appl. Opt.* **5**, 595–602 (1966).
17. J. D. Briers, "The interpretation of holographic interferograms," *Opt. Quantum. Electron.* **8**, 469–501 (1976).
18. R. J. Collier, E. T. Doherty, and K. S. Pennington, "Application of moiré techniques to holography," *Appl. Phys. Lett.* **7**, 223–225 (1965).
19. G. J. Troup, "Lasers and tomatoes," *Aust. Phys.* **12**, 44 (March 1975).
20. J. D. Briers, "Speckle fluctuations as a screening test in the holographic measurement of plant motion," *J. Exper. Botany* **29**, 395–399 (1978).
21. J. D. Briers, "The measurement of plant elongation rates by means of holographic interferometry: possibilities and limitations," *J. Exper. Botany* **28**, 493–506 (1977).
22. A. E. Ennos, "Speckle interferometry," in *Laser Speckle and Related Phenomena* (*Topics in Applied Physics*, Vol. 9), J. C. Dainty, Ed., pp. 203–253, Springer-Verlag, Berlin-Heidelberg-New York (1975).
23. J. D. Briers, "The statistics of fluctuating speckle patterns produced by a mixture of moving and stationary scatterers," *Opt. Quantum. Electron.* **10**, 364–366 (1978).
24. H. Z. Cummins and E. R. Pike, Eds., *Photon Correlation and Light Beating Spectroscopy, Procs. of NATO Advanced Study Institute, Capri, July 1973*, Plenum Press, New York (1974).
25. J. B. Abbiss, T. W. Chubb, and E. R. Pike, "Laser Doppler anemometry," *Opt. Laser Technol.* **6**, 249–261 (1974).
26. J. D. Briers, "Wavelength dependence of intensity fluctuations in laser speckle patterns from biological specimens," *Opt. Commun.* **13**, 324–326 (1975).
27. J. D. Briers, "Wavelength dependence as an additional degree of freedom in biological applications of intensity fluctuation spectroscopy," in *Recent Advances in Optical Physics* (*Procs. ICO-10*, Prague, 1975), B. Havelka and J. Blabla, Eds., pp. 145–153, Palacky University Olomouc and Society of Czechoslovak Mathematicians and Physicists, Prague (1976).
28. J. D. Briers, "A note on the statistics of laser speckle patterns added to coherent and incoherent uniform background fields, and a possible application for the case of incoherent addition," *Opt. Quantum. Electron.* **7**, 422–424 (1975).
29. A. F. Fercher and J. D. Briers, "Flow visualization by means of single-exposure laser speckle photography," *Opt. Commun.* **37**, 326–330 (1981).
30. J. D. Briers and A. F. Fercher, "Retinal blood-flow visualization by means of laser speckle photography," *Invest. Ophthalmol. Vis. Sci.* **22**, 255–259 (1982).
31. N. Takai, "Contrast of time-averaged image speckle pattern for a vibrating object," *Opt. Commun.* **25**, 31–34 (1978).

32. J. D. Briers, "Optical filtering techniques to enhance speckle contrast variations in single-exposure laser speckle photography," *Optik* **63**, 265–276 (1983).
33. J. Ohtsubo and T. Asakura, "Velocity measurement of a diffuse object by using time-varying speckles," *Opt. Quantum. Electron.* **8**, 523–529 (1976).
34. A. F. Fercher, "Velocity measurement by first-order statistics of time-differentiated laser speckles," *Opt. Commun.* **33**, 129–135 (1980).
35. N. Takai, T. Iwai, T. Ushizaka, and T. Asakura, "Velocity measurement of the diffuse object based on time-differentiated speckle intensity fluctuations," *Opt. Commun.* **30**, 287–292 (1979).
36. T. Tanaka, C. Riva, and I. Ben-Sira, "Blood velocity measurements in human retinal vessels," *Science* **186**, 830–832 (1974).
37. M. D. Stern, D. L. Lappe, P. D. Bowen, J. E. Chinovsky, G. A. Holloway, Jr., H. R. Kaiser, and R. L. Bowman, "Continuous measurement of tissue blood flow by laser Doppler spectroscopy," *Am. J. Physiol.* **232**, 441–448 (1977).
38. H. Fujii, K. Nohira, Y. Yamamoto, H. Ikawa, and T. Ohura, "Evaluation of blood flow by laser speckle image sensing," *Appl. Opt.* **26**, 5321–5325 (1987).
39. Y. Aizu, K. Ogino, and T. Sugita, "Evaluation of blood flow at the ocular fundus by using laser speckle," *Appl. Opt.* **31**, 3020–3029 (1992).
40. Y. Aizu and T. Asakura, "Bio-speckle phenomena and their application to the evaluation of blood flow," *Opt. Laser Technol.* **23**, 205–219 (1991).
41. B. Dance, "Laser-speckle effect monitors intracellular motion," *Laser Focus World* **25**, 32 (September 1989).
42. A. Oulamara, G. Tribillon, and J. Duvernoy, "Biological activity measurement on botanical specimen surfaces using a temporal decorrelation effect of laser speckle," *J. Mod. Opt.* **36**, 165–179 (1989).

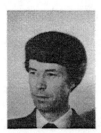

J. David Briers received his MSc and PhD in optics from Imperial College, London. After five years with Pilkington, he moved to New Zealand in 1969 and spent 10 y at the Physics and Engineering Laboratory, New Zealand's national standards laboratory. Three years in Germany, as visiting professor at the University of Essen, were followed by a return to UK industry in 1983, first with Ferranti and later with Omitec Electro-optics. Since June 1990 he has been head of the School of Applied Physics at Kingston University (formerly Kingston Polytechnic), just outside London. Briers is a Fellow of the UK Institute of Physics and Chairman of its Optical Group. He is also a member of SPIE, the Optical Society of America, the European Optical Society, the Biomedical Optics Society, and OWLS (the International Society on Optics Within Life Sciences). Earlier he was the founder Chairman of New Zealand's national Optical Committee.

Reprinted with permission from *Investigative Ophthalmology and Visual Science,*
Vol. 28(1), pp. 175-183 (January 1987). ©1987 J.B. Lippincott Co.

Dynamic Light Scattering in the Intact Rabbit Lens. Its Relation to Protein Concentration

Mark Latina,*† Leo T. Chylack, Jr.,*† Per Fagerholm,§ Isumi Nishio,‡
Toyoichi Tanaka,‡ and Britt M. Palmquist§

The physical-chemical properties of highly concentrated protein systems as seen in the lens are poorly understood. Using the technique of dynamic laser light scattering spectroscopy, the authors have determined changes in the dynamics of lens proteins from the intact rabbit lens as a function of position and age. The authors have identified two heterogeneous populations of mobile scatterers with relaxation times of less than 0.5 msec and greater than 1 msec. A decrease in scattered light intensity at 90°, an increase in protein concentration, and aging are associated with lengthening of the relaxation times of the less mobile population of scatterers. This data provides evidence for the existence of a gel-like structure of the lens proteins. Invest Ophthalmol Vis Sci 28:175–183, 1987

The physical-chemical properties of the crystalline lens cytoplasm are best understood in terms of a protein–water system. Alterations in lens proteins, protein–protein interactions, and protein–water interactions can result in lens opacification. Biochemical studies have provided evidence for the presence of insoluble proteins and high molecular weight aggregates which may be responsible for lens opacification. Experimental results of light scattering,[1-5] Raman spectroscopy,[6] optical anisotropy,[7,8] and x-ray scattering[9,10] of intact lenses and lens cytoplasmic homogenates have furthered our insight into the physical basis of lens transparency and cataract formation. However, our understanding of the relationship between the biochemical and physical properties of the lens is hampered by the complex behavior of its highly concentrated protein system.

Dynamic laser light scattering spectroscopy (DLS), otherwise known as intensity correlation spectroscopy, is a noninvasive technique which can determine protein dynamics of the lens fiber cell cytoplasm. This technique has been used by Benedek and Jedziniak[2] to detect protein aggregation in cataractous lenses, and by

Tanaka and Benedek[1] and Tanaka and Ishimoto[11,12] to measure the susceptibility of the lens cytoplasm to phase separation, the mechanism responsible for lens opacification in cold cataract.

DLS can quantitatively characterize the degree of aggregation of molecules and their approach to phase transition by determining their correlation length. The correlation length represents the range of interaction of protein molecules and is defined as the average distance beyond which thermal random motions of protein molecules become independent. In the case of a dilute solution of noninteracting protein molecules, the correlation length corresponds to the average radius of the protein molecules in solution.[13] Previous DLS studies of the lens have assumed the lens protein–water system to behave as a dilute solution.[2,5,14] However, dynamic light scattering studies of nonideal solutions in which Coulombic interactions, Van der Waals interactions, and excluded volume are no longer negligible, reveal behavior quite different from dilute noninteracting particle solutions.[15]

We report the first study of changes in the DLS properties of the lens cytoplasm in normal intact rabbit lenses in relation to age and protein concentration.

Materials and Methods

Dynamic Light Scattering Methodology—Intact Lenses

Intact lenses from three 4.5-week-, three 8.5-week-, three 15-week-, and two 50-week-old rabbits were studied. The rabbits were killed with air emboli and the lenses carefully extracted via a posterior route from the enucleated eyes. The configuration of the dynamic light scattering apparatus is shown in Figure 1. Each

From the *Howe Laboratory of Ophthalmology, Harvard Medical School, †Massachusetts Eye and Ear Infirmary, and ‡Massachusetts Institute of Technology, Boston, Massachusetts, and the §Karolinska Institute, Stockholm, Sweden.

Supported by the following grants from the National Eye Institute, National Institutes of Health: EY-01276, EY-07063, EY-02433, EY-03247, and the Brigham Surgical Group Foundation.

Data organization and analysis was performed on the PROPHET system, a national computer resource sponsored by the Division of Research Resources, NIH.

Submitted for publication: August 23, 1983.

Reprint requests: Dr. Mark Latina, Massachusetts Eye and Ear Infirmary, 243 Charles Street, Boston, MA 02114.

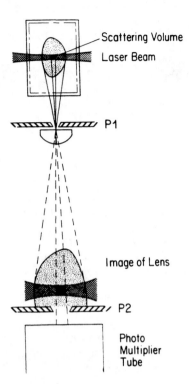

Scattering Volume

Laser Beam

P1

Image of Lens

P2

Photo
Multiplier
Tube

Fig. 1. Experimental setup of dynamic laser light scattering spectroscopy. The laser beam is aligned so that it travels along the optical axis of the lens. Scattered light collected by pinhole 1 (P1) is imaged onto pinhole 2 (P2) resulting in a scattering volume of (100 μm^3).

lens is positioned in an optical cuvette containing Dulbecco's phosphate buffered saline (Gibco; Long Island, NY) with 5.5 mm glucose, 296–300 mOsm. The laser beam traverses the lens along it optical axis in an anterior to posterior direction. A movable, temperature-controlled stage was designed to hold the cuvette. All experiments were controlled at $(37 \pm 0.2)°C$. The incident light is provided by a Spectra Physics model 164 argon ion laser (Mountain View, CA) at 514.5 nm with a power of 60 mW. The optics are arranged so light scattered 90 degrees from the incident direction is collected from small volume (100 μm^3) and imaged onto a photomultiplier tube (RCA type 8850; Harrison, NJ). The output of the photomultiplier tube is amplified, shaped, and discriminated by a pre-amplifier (EG+G, Ortec 9302; Oakridge, TN), and the temporal correlations in the pulse train analysed using either a 56-channel digital autocorrelator (Nicomp model 6864; Santa Barbara, CA) or a 128-channel autocorrelator (Malvern model M-2000; Malvern, England). Correlation functions were obtained using delay times of 20 μsec, 50 μsec, and 100 μsec. Twenty to thirty minutes were required for analysis of each lens.

The average total scattered light intensity at 90°, I_t, was obtained simultaneously with the correlation function at each position. Readings were obtained from

a digital photoncounter connected directly to the pre-amplifier.

Correlation functions were stored on hard disc using a DEC LSI 11/23 (Digital Equipment Corporation; Maynard, MA) computer. Fits of the correlation function were performed using the Marquardt nonlinear least squares gradient expansion algorithm.[16]

Determination of Dry Mass

Immediately after study by DLS, each lens was frozen in isopentane precooled in liquid nitrogen to −140°C. The frozen lenses were shipped on dry ice to Sweden via air freight and processed within 2 days. After freeze sectioning along the optical axis to a thickness of about 20 μm, then freeze drying, the specimens were mounted in close contact with a fine grained photographic emulsion (Kodak AR HI) and exposed to soft x-rays generated at 3 kV. The dry mass was computed from microradiograms separated by 0.1 mm in each lens. The dry mass content corresponds to the protein concentration of the defined volume within 5%.[17]

Data Analysis

The technique of DLS measures temporal fluctuations in the light intensity scattered from protein molecules. The time dependence of the intensity fluctuations is described by the correlation function. An increase in the correlation length, previously defined, results in an increase in the amplitude and relaxation time of the correlation function.

Fluctuations in scattered light intensity are not affected by surface irregularities or by changes in refractive interfaces such as water–glass, glass–air, etc. This is an important advantage of DLS over conventional light scattering techniques.

The correlation function of scattered light intensity can be separated into two components: (1) the function itself, which represents the decay in the fluctuations of the intensity of scattered light; and (2) the baseline to which the function decays. Each correlation function in this study was normalized to the baseline, BASE, using the relation [C(t) − BASE]/[C(o) − BASE]. C(t) is the observed value of the correlation function at delay time, t, and C(o) is the initial value of the correlation function. The baseline of the correlation function is calculated from the average intensity of scattered light during each delay time interval averaged over the elapsed time of the correlation measurement (1000 times the decay time, t).

Light scattered from the lens may arise from cell membranes, free movement of proteins, cytoskeletal structures and organelles. Clark and Benedek[18] and Delaye et al.[5] have shown the phase diagram and correlation function from intact lenses to be qualitatively similar to lens cytoplasmic homogenates where all the cytoskeletal structures and organelles have been removed. The correlation function therefore corresponds only to the protein dynamics of the lens cytoplasm.

The normalized correlation function from the intact rabbit lens has a complex profile. Unlike a monodisperse solution of macromolecules, which produces a single exponential decay function, the correlation function from the intact lens has two major decay components. Delaye et al[5] has called attention to the shape of the correlation function in the bovine lens and applied a double exponential function to fit the observed data. This function was based on dilute solution theory assuming two populations of scattering elements. We have found the double exponential decay function to fit only correlation functions from the lens cortical region and nuclear region of young lenses.

In this study, we are concerned with relative changes in the two components of the correlation function which occur with position and age, but not with absolute values of the amplitudes or relaxation times. We have empirically fitted the correlation functions to the equation below (equation 1), which provides a mode for comparing the two decay components of the correlation function. The correlation coefficient, r, for the fitted curves was 0.98 ± 0.01.

$$C(t) = [Ae^{-t/TAU(1)} + B/\sqrt{t/TAU(2) + 1}]^2$$

(equation 1)

The first term in the function, $Ae^{-t/TAU(1)}$, represents the initial rapid decay in the correlation function. This will be termed the fast decay mode (FDM). The second portion of the correlation function is represented by the term $B/\sqrt{t/TAU(2) + 1}$ and will be termed the slow decay mode (SDM) (Fig. 2). The parameters, A and B, correspond to the amplitude of the fast and slow decay modes, respectively; the ratio B/A is a measure of the relative intensity of light scattered by each component.

Correlation functions using a delay time of 50 μsec are presented in Figure 2. Correlation functions from rabbit lenses older than 15 weeks decayed only 20% of their initial value. A delay time of 100 μsec and a baseline of 100 msec was used to estimate TAU(2) and B/A for these lenses. These estimates do not affect the conclusions of this study but point to the very slow relaxation times in the nuclear region, longer than we have predicted.

Results

Dynamic Light Scattering

Using the technique of DLS spectroscopy, we find scattered light intensity correlations to exist over a very broad time range (20 μsec–10 msec). The biphasic

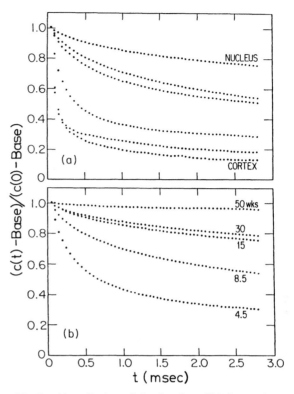

Fig. 2. **a,** Normalized correlation functions, C(t), from an intact 15-week-old rabbit lens as a function of position along the optical axis from cortex to nucleus. Note initial fast decay followed by much slower decay (50 μsec sampling time). **b,** Normalized correlation functions from the central nucleus of intact rabbit lenses ages 4.5- to 50-weeks-old (50 μsec sampling time).

character of the correlation function from intact lens is described by an initial fast decay followed by a much slower decay indicating at least two heterogeneous populations of scatterers can be identified.[5]

Our data demonstrates that relaxation times of protein molecules of the lens fiber cell cytoplasm slow with aging and with position along the optical axis form cortex to nucleus (Figs. 3, 4). TAU(1) increases from 0.05 msec to 0.18 msec in a smooth fashion from cortex to nucleus of 4.5-week-old lenses. In lenses 15 weeks or older, an abrupt increase to TAU(1) occurs approximately 1.3 mm from the capsule and reaches a plateau value in the nuclear region of 0.4 msec. For all lenses, TAU(2) increases in a smooth fashion from cortex to nucleus. TAU(2) of the oldest lens (130 msec) is 15 times greater than that of the youngest lens (9 msec) in the nuclear region.

The ratio B/A which is a measure of the relative intensities of light scattered by each population of molecules increases in a monotonic fashion from cortex to nucleus. As demonstrated in Figure 5, B/A of 50-week-old lenses increases 99-fold over that of 4.5-week-old lenses in the nuclear region. Since the ratio B/A is

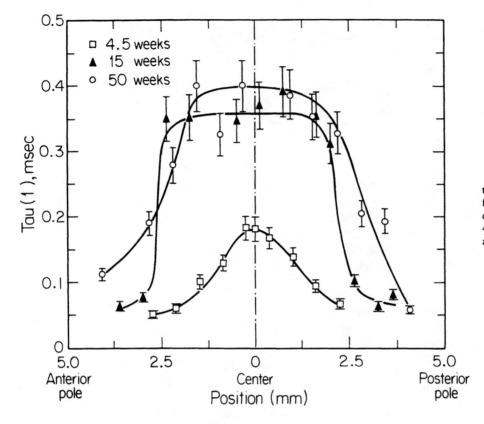

Fig. 3. Tau (1), the relaxation time of the fast decay mode as a function of position along the optical axis of intact lenses ages: 4.5, 15, 50 weeks. Horizontal axis: 0 = lens center.

greater than one, the scattered light is derived predominately from the slow decay mode component.

The average total intensity of scattered light at 90°, I_t, decreases from cortex to nucleus in the lenses stud-

ied. I_t in the nuclear region also decreased slightly with age in lenses from 4.5 to 50 weeks old (Fig. 6). The age and position related decrease in the intensity of scattered light cannot be accounted for by scattering

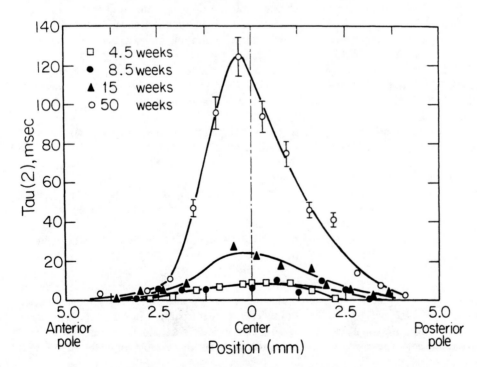

Fig. 4. Tau (2), the relaxation time of the slow decay mode, as a function of position along the optical axis of intact lenses ages: 4.5, 8.5, 15, 50 weeks.

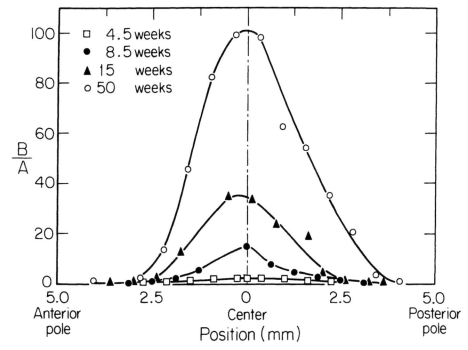

Fig. 5. B/A, the relative intensity of light scattered by the slow and fast decay mode as a function of position along the optical axis of intact lenses ages: 4.5, 8.5, 15, 50 weeks.

through an increase in lens volume which occurs with aging and with position along the optical axis.

Lens Protein Concentration

As shown in Figure 7, the protein concentration immediately beneath the capsule was 0.3 ± 0.02 g/cm^3

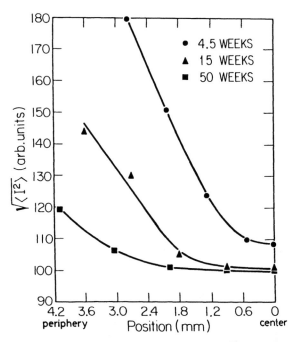

Fig. 6. Mean intensity of scattered light $I_t = \sqrt{\langle I^2 \rangle}$, at 90° with position from lens periphery to nucleus along the optical axis of intact lenses ages: 4.5, 8.5, 15, 50 weeks.

and increased smoothly from cortex to nucleus. The average protein concentration in the nucleus of 4.5-week-old lenses was 0.72 ± 0.02 g/cm^3 and increased to 0.77 ± 0.03 g/cm^3 in 50-week-old lenses. The relationship between the relaxation times TAU(2), or the ratio B/A and protein concentration are not linear (Figs. 8, 9). At high protein concentrations, TAU(2) and B/A increase disproportionately. There was no correlation between TAU(1) and protein concentration.

Discussion

The correlation function of scattered light intensity from intact rabbit lenses was found to have a complex profile similar to that observed by Delaye et al[5] from bovine lenses. In our study, the SDM is the predominant component of the correlation function which changes with age and protein concentration in these noncataractous lenses. The FDM (Fig. 3) shows a radial variation similar to the small scattering elements observed by Delaye et al.[5] As shown in Figures 8 and 9, as the lens ages, the magnitude of TAU(2) and B/A increases at a constant protein concentration and temperature. A change in the degree of protein interaction must occur to account for these observations.

Three mechanisms which can affect a change in the degree of protein interaction and are relevant to the discussion of light scattering are: (1) "steric hindrance" or a change in the degree of molecular packing; (2) the formation of protein aggregates; and (3) the process of gelation.

505

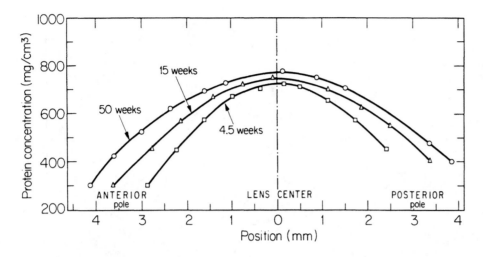

Fig. 7. Protein concentration versus position along the optical axis of intact lenses ages: 4.5, 15, 50 weeks.

By small angle x-ray scattering and light scattering, the spatial correlations of the lens crystallins has recently been investigated.[10] A biphasic change in the transparency of calf lens cytoplasm was observed as the concentration of protein increases. Relatively dilute protein solutions with concentrations less than 175 mg/mL show a decrease in transparency or increase in turbidity as the concentration of protein is increased. Increasing the protein concentration of the lens cytoplasmic preparations above 175 mg/mL resulted in an increase in transparency or decrease in the turbidity of the lens protein preparation. According to the authors,

there is progressively closer packing of the lens proteins with increasing concentration without the formation of a crystallin order. The extent of spatial correlations is consistent with the formation of a short range liquid-like or glass-like order to the crystallins which accounts for lens transparency at high protein concentrations. According to this study, lens proteins cannot act as independent scatterers. Close packing of the lens crystallins decreases refractive index fluctuations reducing scattered light intensity in comparison to that predicted if lens proteins acted as independent scatterers. A diagram of this model is depicted in Figure 10. The

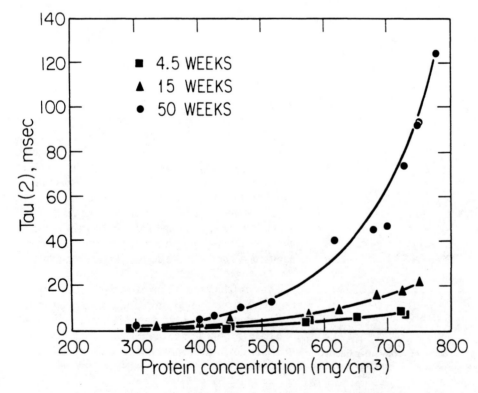

Fig. 8. Tau (2) as a function of protein concentration for lenses ages: 4.5, 15, 50 weeks.

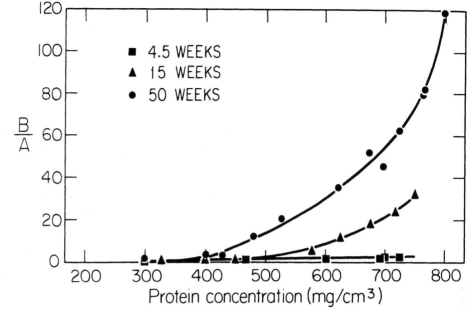

Fig. 9. B/A as a function of protein concentration for lenses ages: 4.5, 15, 50 weeks.

■ 4.5 WEEKS
▲ 15 WEEKS
● 50 WEEKS

changes in TAU(2), B/A, and scattered light intensity with increasing protein concentration supports the authors[10] conclusions that lens proteins cannot act as independent scatterers. However, an increase in the degree of molecular packing due to a concentration effect cannot be the sole factor responsible for the changes in TAU(2), B/A, and scattered light intensity; otherwise, the data would be independent of age.

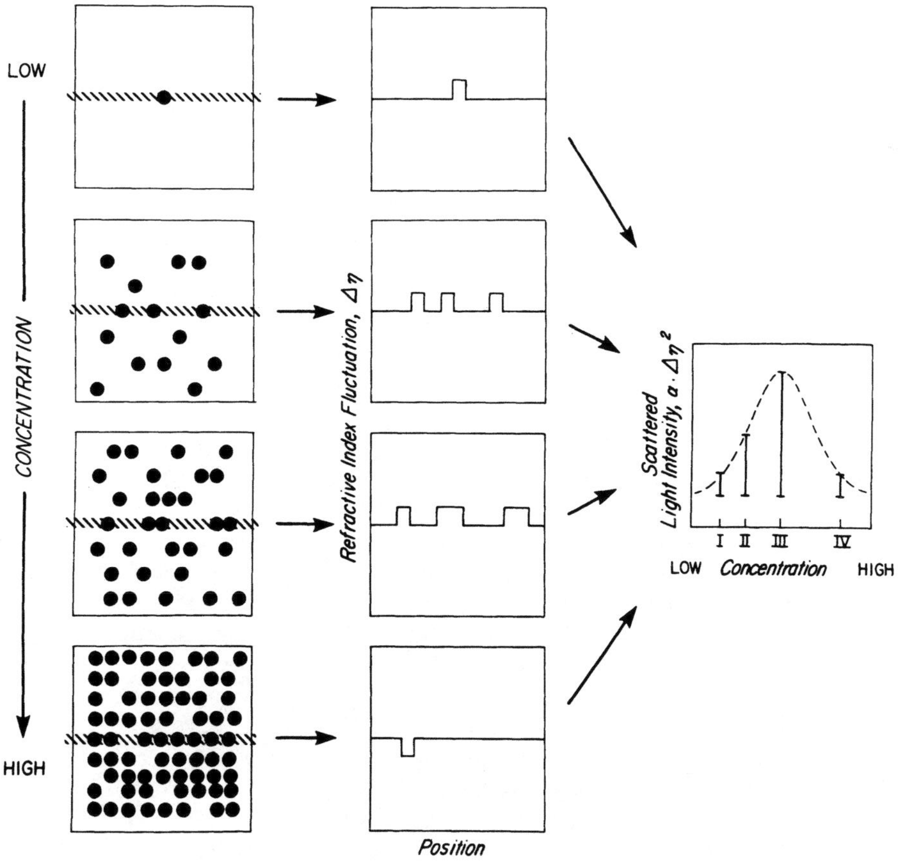

Fig. 10. Diagramatic representation of the relationship between scattered light intensity (turbidity) and the concentration of solute. The first column represents solutions of various concentrations at a given moment. The second column represents the refractive index fluctuation, η, along the line displayed. The scattered light intensity is proportional to the square of the refractive index fluctuation and is shown in the right hand graph. Note the scattered light intensity at low concentration is the same as that at high concentration.

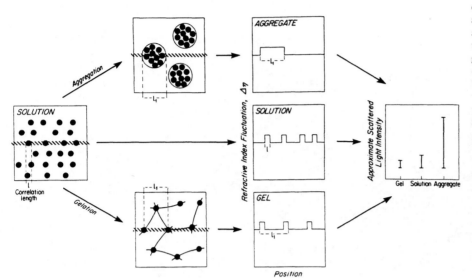

Fig. 11. This figure depicts the differences in correlation length and refractive index properties of a solution of a given concentration undergoing gelation and aggregation. The correlation length of free solute molecules is given by L, and is proportional to particle size. Aggregation and gelation increase the correlation length to L_1, the size of the aggregate and the effective distance between crosslinks, respectively. The correlation length of the aggregate and the gel are the same; therefore, the relaxation times of the two systems are equal. However, the spatial fluctuation of the refractive index is much larger for the aggregate than for either the gel or solution. Therefore, the scattered light intensity of the aggregate is much larger than that of either the gel or the solution.

Various authors[19,20] have suggested the formation of high molecular weight (HMW) protein aggregates may be responsible for visual impairment in cataract. Biochemical studies indicate such aggregates are composed of lens proteins cross linked by disulfide or other covalent bonds. Assuming these aggregates are discrete molecular structures which are distributed at random throughout the lens with the ability to freely diffuse, and have an index of refraction different from the average refractive index of the lens, Benedek[20] has theorized these aggregates can result in an increase in light scattering and decrease in transparency of the lens. As shown in Figure 11, at low to moderate protein concentrations, protein aggregation results in an increase in the correlation length and an increase in scattered light intensity in comparison to the native solution. At high protein concentrations, we have no knowledge of either the concentration of these aggregates or their refractive index in relation to the remaining protein; therefore, it is not clear as to whether these aggregates will increase scattering of light. The fact that we have used young rabbit lenses less than 1 year old argues against a significant degree of protein aggregation.[21,22] We cannot, however, exclude protein aggregation as a mechanism which can account for our results.

Gelation is another mechanism consistent with the results of our study. A gel is a form of matter intermediate between a solid and a liquid. It consists of an entangled protein network formed by covalent bonding between various protein molecules immersed in a liquid medium. Two essential properties of a gel are the elasticity of the protein network and the viscous interaction of the network with the fluid. Elasticity is the ability of the protein network to resist deformation.

Because of its viscoelastic properties, a gel behaves like a solid, that is, it does not flow. Tanaka and coworkers[23-25] have demonstrated that laser light scattering can be used to characterize the viscoelastic properties of gels. The correlation length of a gel increases in comparison to the unlinked proteins in solution (Fig. 11). However, refractive index fluctuations and, therefore, scattered light intensity of a gel are similar to that of the unlinked protein solution. This phenomena has been observed in weakly cross-linked gels in which the gel network underwent a solution to gel phase transition.[24] Again, studies of gelation in highly concentrated protein solutions are sparse. The existence of an entangled gel state for a highly concentrated protein solution of bovine serum albuminoid has recently been confirmed.[26] The entangled proteins in the gel phase form intermolecular bonds and a β-sheet structure.

Because of the biphasic character of the correlation function, it is necessary to conclude that the gel network is not perfect; that is, gel and protein, not incorporated into the gel network, must coexist. Free protein particles not incorporated into the gel network will undergo diffusion within the liquid medium of the gel, resulting in the fast decay mode we have observed. The protein network will greatly restrict molecular movement resulting in the slow decay mode of the correlation function. Based on this model, as the lens ages, one can postulate an increase in the number of covalent cross links between proteins with a resultant increase in the rigidity or decrease in the elasticity of the protein network. Such a change may be related to the loss of accommodative amplitude seen in presbyopia. The phenomenon of gelation does not, we suggest, preclude the existence of short range order of the lens proteins detected by Delaye et al,[10] but points to a longer range order of the lens proteins which cannot be detected by small angle x-ray scattering technique.

In summary, this study excludes a concentration effect as the sole factor responsible for slowing of the correlation functions from these young noncataractous lenses. Until now, such changes in the correlation function have been attributed to protein aggregation. We suggest the formation of a gel-like structure of the lens proteins is another mechanism which can account for these results.

Various authors[21,27] have alluded to the existence of a protein network which deteriorates or collapses to account for the development of cataract. The relation between the gel model we propose in young lenses and the formation of cataract requires further investigation.

Key words: lens, dynamic light scattering, gelation, aggregation, protein concentration

Acknowledgments

The authors thank Dr. John Clark and Dr. George Benedek for their helpful scientific discussions. The authors also thank Gerry Swislow for his implementation of the data acquisition computer programs and Ms. Ann Piccolomini for her secretarial assistance.

References

1. Tanaka T and Benedek G: Observation of protein diffusivity in intact human and bovine lenses with application to cataract. Invest Ophthalmol 14:449, 1975.
2. Jedziniak JA, Nicoli PF, Barun H, and Benedek GB: Quantitative verification of the existence of high molecular weight protein aggretates in the intact normal lens by light scattering spectroscopy. Invest Ophthalmol Vis Sci 17:51, 1978.
3. Bettelheim FA and Bettelheim AA: Small-angle light scattering studies on xylose cataract formation in bovine lenses. Invest Ophthalmol Vis Sci 17:896, 1978.
4. Bettelheim FA and Paunavic M: Light scattering of normal human lens. I. Application of random density and orientation fluctuation theory. Biophysics J 26:38, 1979.
5. Delaye M, Clark JI, and Benedek GB: Identification of the scattering elements responsible for lens opacification in cold cataracts. Biophysics J 37:647, 1982.
6. Schachar R and Solin SA: The microscopic protein structure of the lens with a theory for cataract formation as determined by

7. Raman spectroscopy of intact bovine lenses. Invest Ophthalmol 14:380, 1975.
7. Bettelheim FA: On the optical anisotropy of lens fiber cells. Exp Eye Res 21:231, 1975.
8. Bettelheim FA: Induced optical anisotropy fluctuation in the lens of the eye. J Colloid Interface Sci 63:251, 1978.
9. Bettelheim FA and Wang JJY: X-ray diffraction studies of macromolecular aggregates of bovine lens. Exp Eye Res 25:613, 1977.
10. Delaye M and Tardieu A: Short-range order of crystallin proteins accounts for eye lens transparency. Nature 302:415, 1983.
11. Tanaka T, Ishimoto C, and Chylack LT Jr: Phase separation of a protein–water mixture incold cataract in the young rat lens. Science 197:1010, 1977.
12. Ishimoto C: Phase separation in protein–water mixture and the development of nuclear opacity in cataracts. Dissertation, Massachusetts Institute of Technology, 1978.
13. Pusey PN: The dynamics of interacting brownian particles. J Phys Math 8:1433, 1975.
14. Andries E, Backhavens H, Clauwaest J, DeBlock J, DeVoeght F, and Dhont C: Physical-chemical studies on bovine eye lens proteins. Exp Eye Res 34:239, 1982.
15. Phillies GDJ, Benedek GB, and Mazer NA: Diffusion in protein solutions at high concentrations: A study by quasi-elastic light scattering spectroscopy. J Chem Phys 65:1993, 1976.
16. Bevington PR: Curve fitting. In Data Reduction and Error Analysis for the Physical Sciences, Bevington PR, editor. New York, McGraw Hill, 1972, pp. 134–235.
17. Phillipson G: Distribution of proteins within the normal rat lens. Invest Ophthalmol 8:258, 1969.
18. Clark JI and Benedek GB: Phase diagram for cell cytoplasm from the calf lens. Biochem Biophys Res Commun 95:482, 1980.
19. Trokel S: The physical basis for transparency of the crystalline lens. Invest Ophthalmol 1:493, 1962.
20. Benedek GB: Theory of transparency of the eye. Appl Opt 10:459, 1971.
21. Mostafapour MK and Schwartz CA: Age-related changes in the protein concentration gradient and the crystallin polypeptides of the lens. Invest Ophthalmol Vis Sci 22:606, 1982.
22. Hoenders HJ and Blomendal H: Aging of lens proteins. In Molecular and Cellular Biology of the Eye Lens, Bloemendal H, editor. New York, John Wiley and Sons, 1981, pp. 282–294.
23. Tanaka T, Hocker LO, and Benedek GB: Spectrum of light scattered from a viscoelastic gel. J Chem Phys 59:5151, 1973.
24. Tanaka T, Swislow G, and Ohmine I: Phase separation and gelation in gelatin gels. Physical Rev Lett 42:1556, 1979.
25. Tanaka T: GeLS. Sci Am 244:124, 1981.
26. Kidokoro S and Nagayama K: Ordering of charged particles in solution. Proceedings of Microsymposium, 1981, the Society of Polymer Science, Japan. April 1981. (In Japanese)
27. Siew EL, Opacecky D, and Bettelheim FA: Light scattering of normal human lens. II. Age dependence of the light scattering parameters. Exp Eye Res 33:603, 1981.

Reprinted from *Optical Engineering*, Vol. 32(2), pp. 233-238 (February 1993).
©1993 SPIE.

Coherent fiber optic sensor for early detection of cataractogenesis in a human eye lens

Harbans S. Dhadwal, MEMBER SPIE
State University of New York
Department of Electrical Engineering
Stony Brook, New York 11794

Rafat R. Ansari, MEMBER SPIE
NASA Lewis Research Center/CWRU
21000 Brookpark Road
Cleveland, Ohio 44135

Michael A. DellaVecchia, MEMBER SPIE
Wills Eye Hospital
9th and Walnut
Philadelphia, Pennsylvania 19107

Abstract. A lensless backscatter fiber optic probe is used to measure the size distribution of protein molecules inside an excised, but intact, human eye lens. The fiber optic probe, about 5 mm in diameter, can be positioned arbitrarily close to the anterior surface of the eye; it is a transreceiver, which delivers a Gaussian laser beam into a small region inside the lens and provides a coherent detection of the laser light scattered by the protein molecules in the backward direction. Protein sizes determined from the fast and slow diffusion coefficients show good correlation with the age of the lens and cataractogenesis.

Subject terms: biomedical optics; human lens fibers; light scattering; fiber optic sensors; cataracts; protein aggregates.

Optical Engineering 32(2), 233–238 (February 1993).

1 Introduction

A normal adult eye lens, having an equatorial diameter of 9 mm, is suspended between the vitreous humor and the iris by zonular fibers. It is a continually growing tissue whose transparency is essential for normal vision. The lens comprises a layer of fiber cells enclosing lens-specific proteins known as crystallins, which are subdivided into three types: α (molecular weight = 750,000 to 1,200,000), β (molecular weight = 180,000), and γ (molecular weight = 60,000). The physical and biochemical properties of the lens can be understood in terms of a protein-water system (35% protein by mass and 65% water); α-crystallins, accounting for 47% of the total protein mass, are the predominant scatterers of light. Loss or degradation of the transparency of the lens is referred to as a cataract. The current clinical diagnostic technique, involving visual inspection through a slit-lamp microscope and analysis of a photographic plate, lacks the sensitivity and accuracy to detect small cellular and biochemical changes.[1] Biochemical studies of lens extracts have demonstrated that aging in the normal mammalian lens is accompanied by conversion of the α-crystallin into higher molecular weight species.[2–6] Early detection of changes in the relative concentration and size of the different protein species will permit development of preventive therapy, and possible reversal of cataractogenesis. A reliable, quantitative technique, causing the least trauma to the patient, has been a long-sought goal for the study of cataractogenesis and other ocular disorders.

Mechanisms initiating cataract formation at the molecular level are well understood, and several risk factors have been identified, for example, hyperglycemia and exposure to various types of radiation,[7,8] but the point at which cataractous formation becomes inevitable and irreversible remains to be identified. The most promising clinical technique that has become available is based on quasielastic light scattering (QELS). Early work by Tanaka and Benedek[9] demonstrated the utility of QELS for detection of molecular changes in the lens. A recent clinical QELS study[10] of diabetic and nondiabetic patients has attempted to correlate the QELS results with visual inspection. Early researchers were concerned with solving the mystery of the transparency of a normal adult lens, given the high concentration of proteins in an aqueous solution.[11,12] Based on the assumption of independent scatterers, such a system should have been opaque. Trokel[11] offered the first explanation, which sought an ordering of the protein structure through interprotein interactions. However, Benedek[13] proposed a less stringent ordering requirement, which has been experimentally confirmed by x-ray scattering from an intact lens.[14] Loss of transparency, resulting from the normal aging (senile cataract), attributed to the aggregation of the α-crystallin, has been confirmed by a variety of complementary techniques including biochemical,[15] light scattering,[16–18] QELS,[19–24] and electron microscopy.[25]

This paper focuses on the development of a coherent fiber optic backscatter system for early detection of cataractous changes in human eye lenses. Initial investigations were reported in an earlier publication.[26] The coherent fiber optic probe is about 5 mm in diameter, flexible, can be remotely located, and requires no lenses or apertures. Additionally, conventional QELS systems require fairly dilute concentration to avoid effects caused by multiple light scattering[27] (MLS). The backscatter fiber optic probe has been successfully used in recovering the size of 39-nm polystyrene latex spheres at 10% solids concentration.[28]

2 Theory

QELS, photon correlation spectroscopy (PCS), intensity fluctuation spectroscopy (IFS), and dynamic light scattering (DLS) are synonymous terms used to describe a noninvasive laser light-scattering technique that is used for probing and characterizing the dynamic behavior of fluid systems. For

Paper BM-049 received July 1, 1992; revised manuscript received Oct. 2, 1992; accepted for publication Oct. 15, 1992. This paper is a revision of a paper presented at the SPIE conference on Fiber Optic Medical and Fluorescent Sensors and Applications, January 1992, Los Angeles, California. The paper presented there appears (unrefereed) in SPIE Proceedings Vol. 1648.
© 1993 Society of Photo-Optical Instrumentation Engineers. 0091-3286/93/$2.00.

a historical perspective on the development of the field see Chu's[29] selection of papers on the subject. For understanding the practice of QELS, Chu's[30] text on laser light scattering is excellent.

In this study, Brownian movement of protein molecules in the cytoplasm of the lens fiber cell produce temporal fluctuations in the scattered light, when illuminated by a coherent light source. The scattered intensity from the α-crystallin is about four orders of magnitude stronger than that from the β-crystallin. Consequently β- and γ-crystallins are invisible to probing by QELS. A self-beating QELS experiment involves the self-mixing of the scattered electric field at the detector and gives rise to an intensity-intensity autocorrelation $G^{(2)}(t)$, which for Gaussian statistics is related to the first-order field autocorrelation $g^{(1)}(t)$, through the Siegert relation[31]

$$G^{(2)}(t) = A[1 + \beta|g^{(1)}(t)|^2] \ , \qquad (1)$$

where A is the base line, corresponding to the square of the average value of the scattered intensity, and β is a measure of the self-beating efficiency. The first-order field autocorrelation is a Laplace transform of the characteristic linewidth distribution $G(\Gamma)$,

$$g^{(1)}(t) = \int_a^b G(\Gamma) \exp(-\Gamma t) \, d\Gamma \ , \qquad (2)$$

where $\Gamma = q^2 D$ is a relaxation parameter corresponding to the protein species with a translational diffusion coefficient D. Here Γ is a very useful parameter for investigating trends that result from external factors, when specific information regarding the physical parameters of the system, such as, temperature, viscosity, and index of refraction, are not known. The magnitude of the Bragg wave vector q is dependent on the scattering geometry through the relation,

$$q = \frac{4n\pi}{\lambda_0} \sin\left(\frac{\theta}{2}\right) \ , \qquad (3)$$

where n is the refractive index of the medium, λ_0 is the wavelength of the light source in free space, and θ is the scattering angle. Under the assumption that the α-crystallin molecules are spherical, the Stokes-Einstein relation expresses D_0 as a function of hydrodynamic radius r of the protein,

$$D_0 = \frac{kT}{6\pi\eta r} \ , \qquad (4)$$

where η is the absolute viscosity of the medium, in this case water; k is Boltzmann's constant; T is the absolute temperature; and D_0 is the value D at zero concentration. However, we have previously used a backscatter fiber optic probe to recover D_0 from an aqueous concentration of 10% solids of 39-nm polystyrene latex spheres,[28] without the need to invoke concentration dependence.

The goal of a QELS experiment is to recover $G(\Gamma)$ from a measurement of $G^{(2)}(t)$. For a monodisperse suspension of scatterers, the inversion task of recovering $G(\Gamma)$ is trivial. However, for a polydisperse distribution of scatterers the

inversion procedure is more complex. In the presence of noise, which is unavoidable in the accumulation of experimental data, Eq. (1) represents an ill-posed inversion problem.[32] In recent years, several techniques have been developed to overcome the ill-conditioning, for example, regularization techniques, exponential sampling, and nonnegative least-squares; original papers are collected in Ref. 29. For a dilute concentration, that is, negligible interparticle interactions and multiple light scattering, the Stokes-Einstein relation, together with a knowledge of the scattering strengths from each of the size species leads to a particle size distribution. Suitable commercial software for performing these calculations is usually available from manufacturers of digital correlators.

QELS studies of the protein constituents in a human eye lens has already established the presence of two decay times, which have been attributed to a fast diffusion coefficient D_f arising from the α-crystallin and a slower component D_s caused by the aggregation of the α-crystallins,[21–24] or the mutual diffusion coefficient describing the relaxation of a concentration gradient.[21] Based on these results, we can also postulate a bimodal distribution in diffusion coefficients, giving a first-order autocorrelation

$$g^{(1)}(t) = p_1 \exp(-q^2 D_f t) + p_2 \exp(-q^2 D_s t) \ , \qquad (5)$$

where p_1 and p_2 are proportional to the number concentration and the scattering strengths of the smaller and larger particles, respectively.

3 Experimental Results

3.1 Backscatter Fiber Optic Probe

A generic backscatter fiber optic probe has been described elsewhere.[26,28] Here it suffices to say that the probe comprises two optical fibers, which are positioned in close proximity to each other and mounted into a single stainless steel fiber ferrule. One of the fibers, a monomode optical fiber of the type employed in lightwave communications, is used to transmit a Gaussian beam of coherent radiation from a convenient optical source to the scattering medium; the second, either monomode or multimode, is positioned at some convenient backscatter angle to collect and relay the optical signal to a photon detector. The probe requires no lenses and apertures to control the properties of the transmitting and receiving beams.

Figure 1 shows a schematic of the apparatus used for measuring the intensity autocorrelation from excised human eye lenses. Light from a He-Ne laser operating at a 632.8-nm wavelength was launched into a monomode optical fiber, with about 1 mW emanating from the probe end. The probe tip was positioned so that a point inside the excised lens was illuminated with an expanding Gaussian laser beam, having a diameter of 150 μm. The second optical fiber collects the scattered light at a fixed scattering angle and is connected to a photomultiplier (EMI model 9863B). The photon pulse train after suitable amplification and discrimination was correlated using a digital correlator (Brookhaven Instruments model BI2030 and model BI8000AT). In this study, two types of fiber probes, having scattering angles of 155 deg (probe 1) and 143 deg (probe 2), were used. Figure 2 shows a comparison of the normalized intensity

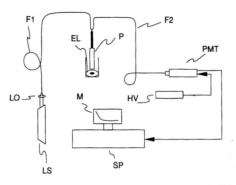

Fig. 1 Schematic of the optical system used for measuring the intensity-intensity autocorrelation of the scattered light from an intact excised human eye lens: F1—monomode transmitting optical fiber, F2—receiving optical fiber, P—probe tip, EL—excised human eye lens, LO—launching optics, LS—He-Ne laser, PMT—photomultiplier, M—monitor, DC—digital correlator, and HV—high voltage power supply for PMT.

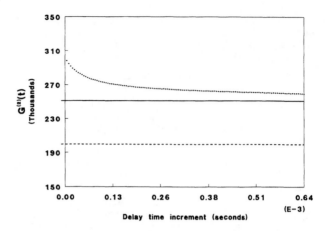

Fig. 3 Typical un-normalized intensity autocorrelation from the excised lens of the 43-yr-old donor. Experimental data was obtained using fiber optic probe 1 and Brookhaven Instruments BI2030 correlator. Solid line is the measured base line, dashed line is the calculated base line.

3.2 Eye Lenses

The cadaver human eye lenses were kindly made available as a gift by the Eye Bank of the Delaware Valley in Philadelphia, Pa. The five pairs of lenses employed in this study belonged to 18-, 43-, 55-, 65-, and 73-year-old donors. The lenses were kept in a biological nutrient solution, which was also provided by the Eye Bank of the Delaware Valley. The nutrient solution was a McCarey-Kaufman solution consisting of dextran media, phenol red, and gentamicin sulfate. On visual inspection by an ophthalmologist (M. A. DellaVecchia), the lenses of the younger patients were found to be transparent, whereas the older lenses had a yellowish tint in them, consistent with senile cataractous changes. Clinically, these older lenses can be classified as having a mild to moderate cataract. None of the lenses was completely opaque.

3.3 Data Analysis

Intensity autocorrelation measurements were performed on the lenses using two different fiber probes, but within 24 h. Figure 3 shows a typical un-normalized intensity-intensity autocorrelation. The calculated base line (dashed line), computed from the total number of samples and the average counts per sample time, and the measured base line (solid line), computed from the average of six delay channels, are superimposed on the same graph. Invariably, all measurements exhibited a similar behavior over a large range of sample times. In a typical QELS experiment, as shown in Fig. 2, the calculated and measured base lines are within 0.5% of each other, indicating a good estimate of the true base line. Errors in the true base line exceeding 0.5% can lead to a distorted normalized first-order autocorrelation, and subsequently produce erroneous estimates of the diffusion coefficient.[33] Previous QELS studies of human eye lenses[19,26] have encountered base-line problems in the measurement of the intensity autocorrelation; their analysis used a floating base line in the fitting procedure. Such an approach is acceptable provided the curve fitting uses the un-normalized intensity autocorrelation data.

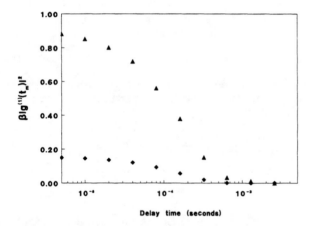

Fig. 2 Normalized first-order autocorrelation function obtained from an aqueous suspension of 85-nm polystyrene latex spheres using a Brookhaven Instruments BI8000AT correlator. The data has been normalized using a measured base line. Self-beating efficiencies are 0.88 and 0.16 for probes 1 (triangles) and 2 (diamonds), respectively. Probe 1 was constructed using monomode optical fibers and for a scattering angle of 155 deg. Probe 2 has a scattering angle of 143 deg and uses a multimode optical fiber for detection and a monomode optical fiber for transmitting.

autocorrelation obtained from a dilute concentration of 85-nm polystyrene latex spheres using the two fiber probes. Probe 1 (triangles) provided the higher self-beating efficiency, as indicated by the value of the normalized first-order autocorrelation at $t = 0$, but a lower count rate. Probe 2 had a much higher count rate but a lower self-beating efficiency. The reduction in the self-beating efficiency is the result of the use of a multimode optical fiber for the detection of the scattered light in probe 2. Choice of a particular probe is dictated by the expected count rate; for example, for weak scattering, the second probe is necessary if the total accumulation time is to be kept short. This consideration may be very important in view of reducing patient exposure to laser radiation.

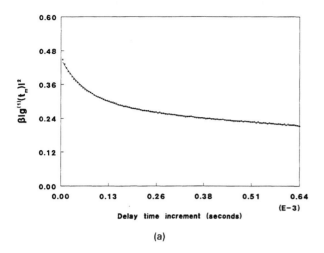

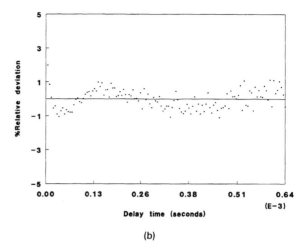

(a)

(b)

Fig. 4 Results of a double-exponential nonlinear least-squares fit to the normalized data shown in Fig. 3: (a) symbols are the data points and the solid line is the fit obtained using Eq. (6) and (b) plot of the percentage relative deviations between data points and fit values computed using Eq. (6).

In this study, we normalized the intensity autocorrelation data using the measured base line to obtain the first-order autocorrelation,

$$\left[\frac{G^{(2)}(t_m)}{A} - 1\right]^{1/2} = p_1 \exp(-p_2 t_m)$$
$$+ p_3 \exp(-p_4 t_m) = \sqrt{\beta}\left|g^{(1)}(t_m)\right| , \quad (6)$$

where A is a measured base line, the p's are the unknowns to be determined from a nonlinear least squares analysis, t_m is the m'th delay channel, $p_2 = q^2 D_f$, and $p_4 = q^2 D_s$. Figure 4(a) shows a typical result of the curve fitting (solid line) and Fig. 4(b) shows a plot of the corresponding percentage relative deviations between the data and fit. The average values of the linewidths P_2 and P_4, and hence diffusion coefficients, were determined from three independent measurements of the intensity-intensity autocorrelation for each of the lenses. The average hydrodynamic diameter, corresponding to the slow and fast diffusion coefficient, was determined using Eq. (4). The results are summarized in Fig. 5, which shows a plot of the average protein size obtained for the two scattering species inside the cytoplasm of lens fibers, as function of the lens age. Triangles and squares are results of measurements made with probes 1 and 2, respectively. Measurements with probe 1 were made within a 24-h period after the measurements with probe 2. Because both eyes, from each donor, were expected to show similar cataractous changes due to aging, no attempt was made to tag either of them. In computing the hydrodynamic diameter from an estimate of the diffusion coefficient, we assumed that the protein molecules of the α-crystallin are spherical and suspended in water, and therefore have used the associated values for the index of refraction and viscosity. The faster component, which results from the smaller particle size, is consistent with values published in the literature for the hydrodynamic diameter of the α-crystallin monomer in a normal adult eye lens.[14,24] Note an increase in the size of the α-crystallin as a function of the age of the lens; the magnitude of this component and the age-dependence

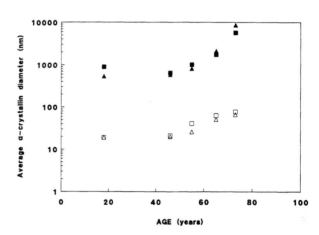

Fig. 5 Summary of the results obtained from the QELS measurements made using two types of coherent fiber probes. Each data point is an average of three independent determinations of the protein size. Average crystallin size is computed from the results of a double-exponential fit to each of the normalized intensity-intensity autocorrelation data. Effective hydrodynamic diameter is computed from the Stokes-Einstein relation by using the viscosity of water, and assuming spherical protein molecules. Triangles and squares represent measurements made with probes 1 and 2, respectively. Hollow symbols correspond to the α-crystallin, and the filled symbols are due to a slower component arising from concentration gradients.

trend are consistent with other published results.[2,4,5,24] Origins of the slower relaxation component are still being debated, but it has been postulated that this may arise from the mutual diffusion describing the relaxation of a concentration gradient.[21]

4 Comments on a Clinical System

Figures 6 and 7 show the incorporation of a backscatter fiber optic into a slit-lamp microscope assembly. The fiber probe, together with a micropositioner, is mounted onto a universal applanation tonometer mounting assembly. This arrangement provides precise positioning and location of the scattering volume in any substantially transparent region of the

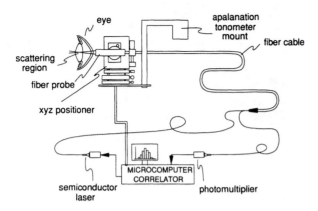

Fig. 6 Slit-lamp microscope with the fiber optic probe mounted on a universal applanation tonometer mounting assembly.

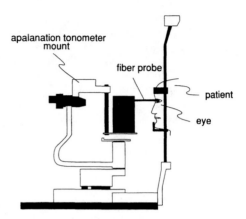

Fig. 7 Schematic of a QELS clinical apparatus using a backscatter fiber optic probe.

anterior segment of the eye. The transmitting monomode optical fiber is pigtailed to a semiconductor laser, and threaded through a ruggedized cable assembly. The receiving optical fiber, also contained within the same cable, is coupled to a miniature photon detection system.

The application of the fiber optic probe for the measurement of cataractogenesis is procedurally similar to techniques familiar to ophthalmologists, most notably applanation tonometry and ultrasonography. The procedure can be easily done at a slit lamp under the installation of topical (drop) anesthesia. The eye movement is negated by having the patient direct vision in the contralateral eye on the fixation light.

Findings from other clinical systems,[34-36] introducing laser beams into patients' eyes, have concluded that a 20-min exposure is the upper limit before patient fatigue becomes a limiting factor. QELS measurements should take less than 2 min per autocorrelation. The maximal retinal irradiance is a function of wavelength, incident power, numerical aperture of the cone of laser light, and exposure time. In our fiber optic system, we expect retinal irradiance to be less than 0.05 mW/mm^2, which is three orders of magnitude below the damage threshold of 2 W/cm^2 for a 10-s exposure.[37,38]

5 Conclusion

In this paper, we have presented results indicating the utility of a coherent backscatter fiber optic sensor in the development of an *in vivo* QELS system for the study of the onset of nucleation, prior to the irreversible cataractous formation. The fiber probe is less than 5 mm in diameter, can be remotely located, and can be incorporated into existing clinical apparatus, as shown in Figs. 6 and 7. The average hydrodynamic diameter of the α-crystallin increased from 20 nm for a normal eye lens to 80 nm for a cataractous lens showing a yellowish tint.

The data analysis presented here represents the currently accepted approach to the recovery of the size distribution from the intensity-intensity autocorrelation data.[24] Improved models, taking into account interprotein interactions, effects resulting from multiple scattering, and causes of the base line fluctuations are needed. However, the subtraction of the base line or the use of a floating base line in the curve-fitting procedures is legitimate and will not give rise

to erroneous conclusions. Note that a 10% solids concentration of 39-nm polystyrene particles is turbid and the light scattered in the forward direction diffuse. However, the 35% by mass of the protein-water system found in the human eye lens is distinctly transparent.

Acknowledgment

Harbans S. Dhadwal would like to thank Brookhaven Instruments Corporation, Holtsville, New York, for the loan of the BI2030 correlator.

References

1. A. Spector, S. Li, and J. Sigelman, "Age-dependent changes in the molecular size of human lens proteins and their relationship to light scatter," *Invest. Ophthalmol. Rep.* **13**(10), 795–798 (1974).
2. H. F. Honders and H. Bloemendal, "Aging of lens proteins," in *Molecular and Cellular Biology of the Eye Lens,* H. Bloemendal, Ed., pp. 229–236, Wiley Interscience, New York (1981).
3. L. J. Takemoto and P. Azari, "Isolation and characterization of covalently linked, high molecular weight proteins from human cataractous lens," *Exp. Eye. Res.* **24**, 63–70 (1977).
4. M. J. McFall-Ngai, L. L. Ding, L. J. Takemoto, and J. Horwitz, "Spatial and temporal mapping of age-related changes in human lens crystallins," *Exp. Eye. Res.* **41**, 745–758 (1985).
5. A. Spector, T. Freund, L. K. Li, and R. C. Augusteyn, "Age-dependent changes in the structure of alpha crystallin," *Invest. Ophthalmol.* **10**(9), 677–686 (1971).
6. J. A. Jedziniak, J. H. Kinoshita, E. M. Yates, and G. B. Benedek, "The concentration and localization of heavy molecular weight aggregates in aging normal and cataractous human lenses," *Exp. Eye. Res.* **20**, 367–369 (1975).
7. J. H. Kinoshita, "Mechanisms initiating cataract formation," Proctor Lecture, *Invest. Ophthalmol.* **13**(10), 713–724 (1974).
8. L. Olson, "Anatomy and embryology of the lens," Chapter 71 in *Clinical Ophthalmology,* Vol. 1, T. Duane, Ed., Harper & Row, Philadelphia (1981).
9. T. Tanaka and G. B. Benedek, "Observation of protein diffusivity intact human and bovine lenses with application to cataract," *Invest. Ophthalmol.* **14**(6), 449–456 (1976).
10. S. Bursell, R. S. Baker, J. N. Weiss, J. H. Haughton, and L. I. Rand, "Clinical photon correlation spectroscopy evaluation of human diabetic lenses," *Exp. Eye. Res.* **49**, 241–258 (1989).
11. S. Trokel, "The physical basis for transparency of crystalline lenses," *Invest. Ophthalmol.* **1**, 493–501 (1962).
12. D. M. Maurice, "The structure and transparency of a cornea," *J. Physiol. (Lond.)* **736**, 263–286 (1957).
13. G. B. Benedek, "Theory of transparency of the eye," *Appl. Opt.* **10**(3), 459–473 (1971).
14. M. Delaye and A. Tardieu, "Short-range order of crystallin proteins accounts for eye lens transparency," *Nature* **302**, 415–417 (1983).
15. J. A. Jedziniak, J. H. Kinoshita, E. M. Yates, L. O. Hocker, and G. B. Benedek, "On the presence and mechanism of formation of heavy molecular weight aggregates in human normal and cataractous lenses," *Exp. Eye. Res.* **15**, 185–189 (1973).

16. J. A. Jedziniak, D. F. Nicoli, H. Baram, and G. B. Benedek, "Quantitative verification of the existence of high molecular weight protein aggregates in the intact normal human lens by light scattering spectroscopy," *Invest. Ophthalmol.* **17**(1), 51–57 (1978).

17. A. P. Bruckner, "Picosecond light scattering measurements of cataract microstructure," *Appl. Opt.* **17**(19), 3177–3183 (1978).

18. F. A. Bettelheim and M. Paunovi, "Light scattering of normal human lens I: Application of random density and orientation fluctuation theory," *Biophys. J.* **26**, 85–100 (1979).

19. C. Andries, W. Guadens, and J. Clauwert, "Photon and fluorescence correlation spectroscopy and light scattering of eye lens proteins," *Biophys. J.* **43**, 345–354 (1983).

20. J. N. Weiss, S. E. Bursell, R. E. Gleason, and B. H. Eichold, "Photon correlation spectroscopy of in vivo human cornea," *Cornea* **5**(1), 19–24 (1986).

21. C. Andries and J. Clauwert, "Photon correlation spectroscopy and light scattering of eye lens proteins at high concentrations," *Biophys. J.* **47**, 591–605 (1985).

22. P. C. Magnante, L. T. Chylack, and G. B. Benedek, "In vivo measurements on human lens using quasielastic light scattering," *Proc. SPIE* **605**, 94–97 (1986).

23. M. Delaye, J. I. Clark, and G. B. Benedek, "Identification of the scattering elements responsible for lens opacification in cold cataracts," *Biophys. J.* **37**, 647–656 (1982).

24. S. E. Bursell, P. C. Magnante, and L. T. Chylack Jr., "In vivo uses of quasielastic light scattering spectroscopy as a molecular probe in the anterior segment of the eye," in *Noninvasive Diagnostic Techniques in Ophthalmology*, Barry R. Masters, Ed., Springer-Verlag, New York (1990).

25. F. A. Bettelheim, E. L. Siew, S. Shyne, P. Farnsworth, and P. Burke, "A comparative study of human lens by light scattering and scanning electron microscopy," *Exp. Eye. Res.* **32**, 125–129 (1981).

26. R. R. Ansari, H. S. Dhadwal, M. C. W. Campbell, and M. A. DellaVecchia, "A fiber optic sensor for ophthalmic refractive diagnostics," in *Fiber Optic Medical and Fluorescent Sensors and Applications*, A. Katzir, Ed., *Proc. SPIE* **1648**, 83–105 (1992).

27. M. Drewel, J. Ahrebs, and K. Schatzel, "Suppression of multiple scattering errors in particle sizing by dynamic light scattering," in *Proc. 2nd Int. Congr. on Particle Sizing*, pp. 130–138, Arizona University Press (1990).

28. H. S. Dhadwal, R. R. Ansari, and W. V. Meyer, "A fiber optic probe for particle sizing in concentrated suspensions," *Rev. Sci. Instrum.* **62**, 2963–2968 (1991).

29. B. Chu, *Selected Papers on Quasielastic Light Scattering by Macromolecular, Supramolecular and Fluid Systems*, SPIE Milestone Series, Vol. MS12, B. J. Thompson, Series Ed., Optical Engineering Press, Bellingham, Wash. (1990).

30. B. Chu, *Laser Light Scattering: Basic Principles and Practice*, Academic Press, New York (1991).

31. A. J. F. Siegert, MIT Radiation Lab. Report No. 465 (1943).

32. A. N. Tikonov and V. Y. Arsenin, *Solutions of Ill-Posed Problems*, W. H. Winstons & Sons, Washington, D.C. (1977).

33. B. Chu, J. R. Ford, and H. S. Dhadwal, "Correlation function profile analysis of polydisperse macromolecular solutions and colloidal suspensions," in *Methods of Enzymology*, Vol. 117, Academic Press, New York (1985).

34. C. E. Riva, G. T. Fake, B. Eberli, and V. Benary, "Bidirectional LDV system for absolute measurement of blood speed in retinal vessels," *Appl. Opt.* **18**, 2301–2306 (1979).

35. B. L. Petrig and C. E. Riva, "Retinal laser Doppler velocimetry: toward its computer-assisted clinical use," *Appl. Opt.* **27**, 1126–1134 (1988).

36. B. L. Petrig and C. E. Riva, "Near-IR retinal laser Doppler velocimetry and flowmetry: new delivery and detection techniques," *Appl. Opt.* **30**, 2073–2078 (1991).

37. W. F. Van Pelt, W. R. Payne, and R. W. Peterson, "A review of selected bioeffects for various spectral ranges of light," DHEW Publication (FDA) 20–24, 74-8010 (June 1973).

38. American National Standards Institute, *Safe Use of Lasers: Z-136.1*, 1436 Broadway, New York, NY 10018 (1986).

Harbans S. Dhadwal obtained his BSc (Hons.) and PhD degrees in electrical engineering from the University of London in 1976 and 1980, respectively. Subsequently, he joined the Royal Aircraft Establishment in Farnborough, England, as a research scientist. In 1984, he joined the faculty in electrical engineering, where he has developed a laboratory facility to study coherent optical processors and develop new fiber optic sensors. His current research interests include development of coherent optical systems for information retrieval, coherent fiber optic sensors, integrated fiber optic systems, development of single photon counting systems, and inverse problems. He is a senior member of the IEEE and a member of SPIE and OSA.

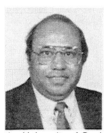

Rafat R. Ansari is a project scientist in the Microgravity Materials Science Division of the NASA Lewis Research Center in Cleveland, Ohio. He earned a BSc (Hons.) and an MSc in physics from the University of Karachi in Pakistan in 1974. He was on the physics faculty of the University of Karachi from 1975 to 1979, where he worked in the area of cryogenics and physical oceanography. He earned an MS and a PhD in physics from the University of Calgary and the University of Guelph in Canada in 1982 and 1985, respectively. Prior to joining NASA, he worked as a researcher at the Department of Energy Mines and Resources Canada in Alberta from 1985 to 1988. Ansari's research interests include colloidal phenomenon, advanced technology development in the area of laser light scattering spectroscopy, and particle sizing. Currently he is involved in the development of a miniaturized, modular and rugged laser light scattering instrument capable of monitoring material processing in a microgravity environment on board the space shuttle orbiter and possibly space station Freedom. He is an active member of the NASA speakers bureau and is a member of SPIE and APS.

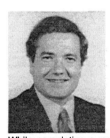

Michael A. DellaVecchia received his BA in physics with a mathematics minor at LaSalle University in Philadelphia, Pennsylvania, in 1970. He earned his MS degree in biomedical engineering from Drexel University. He attended Temple University School of Medicine and received his MD in 1976. He completed full residencies in anatomical pathology and clinical pathology (1977 to 1981) and then served in a fellowship in surgical pathology (1980 to 1981). While completing a residency in ophthalmology (1981 to 1984) he finished his PhD in biomedical engineering (biophysics) at Drexel University (1984). Dr. DellaVecchia is a staff member at Temple University Hospital, University of Pennsylvania Scheie Eye Institute, Wills Eye Hospital, and Drexel University. He belongs to AMA, Sigma Xi, IEEE, and SPIE.

Reprinted with permission from *Optics Letters,* Vol. 14(20), pp. 1098-1100
(October 15, 1989). ©1989 Optical Society of America.

High-resolution imaging of the living human fovea: measurement of the intercenter cone distance by speckle interferometry

Pablo Artal* and Rafael Navarro

Instituto de Optica, Consejo Superior de Investigaciones Científicas, Serrano 121, 28006 Madrid, Spain

A high-resolution method that allows direct measurements of the intercenter cone distance in the living human fovea is proposed. The experimental technique is similar to that used in stellar speckle interferometry. It is based on the recording and posterior processing of coherent short-exposure images of a small area of the central fovea. By using this optical–digital procedure, we have obtained what are to our knowledge the first objective measurements *in vivo* of the cone spacing in the human fovea. The reconstruction of the whole spatial information of the cone mosaic would also be possible by further improvements of the technique by subsequent application of image-reconstruction algorithms.

The sampling of the retinal images by the photoreceptor mosaic plays an important role in the spatial information processing performed by the human visual system. After the low-pass filtering carried out by the optics of the eye, the imaging properties of the mosaic depend directly on the spatial distribution of photoreceptors. However, actual topographic data from the cone mosaic of the living eye, by objective methods, are not yet available. Traditional measurements of the structural parameters of the photoreceptor mosaic in the human fovea and the periphery were obtained by means of histological studies.[1-3] Histological measurements could differ from measurements made in the living human eye owing to tissue distortions during processing, because of the fragility of the photoreceptor mosaic. Williams has proposed an indirect psychophysical method that allows for the estimation of the cone spacing and the packing geometry in the living human retina.[4-6] However, to our knowledge, objective physical measurements on the distribution of cones in the living human fovea have not yet been reported. Such results would clarify important questions, mainly those related to the actual intercenter cone distance and the regularity of the mosaic in the fovea. These are important structural data for evaluating the physical limits of visual resolution and the possible aliasing artifacts that could occur in the sampling of retinal images.

Direct observations of the cone mosaic have been carried out in lower vertebrates,[7] but the application of that method of the living human eye presents many problems. The main reason is that the optical image quality of the eye[8-10] is not good enough to resolve the close separation between cones. Therefore, resolving the human cone mosaic through the optical system of the eye is similar to a high-resolution imaging problem in astronomy. Here we present an objective method to measure directly the spatial distribution of the foveal cone mosaic of the human eye *in vivo*. The method is based on stellar speckle interferometry[11,12] similar to that used in astronomy to resolve binary stars through atmospheric turbulence. We obtain short-exposure speckle images of a small area of the fovea. Then, after selecting the best specklegrams, we compute the averaged power spectrum, which contains spatial frequency information as far as the diffraction limit of the eye.

In our case, for a normal eye with a 7-mm pupil diameter and incident light with a wavelength of 632 nm, the minimum separable size on the retina by diffraction will be approximately 1.8 μm. On the other hand, according to histological studies, the center-to-center spacing between cones in the central fovea is thought to range from 2.1 μm (Ref. 3) to 2.8 μm.[1] Under these conditions, in principle, we will be able to resolve foveal cone details by using this high-resolution technique.

The procedure involves recording a large number of short-exposure images of the central fovea formed with coherent light using the experimental setup shown in Fig. 1. A He–Ne laser beam is expanded by lens L_1 and filtered by a 400-μm pinhole (D) that acts simultaneously as the object and fixation test. The beam collimated by lens L_2 enters the eye after reflection in a pellicle beam splitter (BS) and forms an image of approximately 55-μm diameter on the central foveal mosaic (M). The light reflected from the retina contains information on the spatial distribution of the cone array. It leaves the eye, and after the light is transmitted through the BS and a polarizer (P), lens L_3 forms the aerial foveal image on high-sensitivity photographic film (Kodak Recording 1000 ASA). After development, the aerial foveal images are digitized by using a microdensitometer and stored in a computer. Two examples of typical short-term exposure aerial foveal images are shown in Fig. 2. The exposure time for each image was 4 msec. The corneal irradiance was of the order of 0.3 mW/cm^2, which is more than 1 order below U.S. security standards.

Since the whole imaging process is carried out in

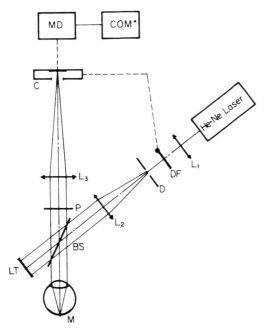

Fig. 1. Experimental setup for the recording of the short-term-exposure foveal images. DF, density filter; LT, light trap; C, camera; MD, digital microdensitometer; COM, computer.

coherent light, the short-exposure aerial images of the central part of the fovea $[i_k(x'', y'')]$ can be expressed by

$$i_k(x'', y'') = |r(x', y') \otimes a_k(x', y')|^2, \quad (1)$$

where $\otimes$ denotes convolution, $r(x', y')$ is the complex reflection factor of the cone mosaic, and $a_k(x', y')$ is the amplitude spread function of the human eye.[8] After the aerial images have been digitized, the power spectrum of each instantaneous image is computed. Since the signal-to-noise ratio is low for a single power spectrum, we have averaged many individual power spectra, as expressed by

$$\langle |\bar{I}|^2 \rangle = \frac{1}{N} \sum_{k=1}^{N} |FT[i_k(x'', y'')]|^2, \quad (2)$$

where FT denotes a Fourier transformation.

A plot of the power spectrum corresponding to the instantaneous image of Fig. 2(a) is presented in Fig. 3. Figure 4 shows the average of 10 two-dimensional power spectra from a normal subject. The mean center-to-center cone distance in the human fovea is directly obtained from the result presented in Fig. 4. The value $1/s$ in the spatial frequency domain is correlated to the local average spacing between rows of cones in the foveola. The ring that appears in this experimental result has the same shape as those obtained by computer simulation and optical transform, using digitized patterns corresponding to excised foveas.[13,14] The cone spacing in the foveola for the same normal subject as above was $0.51' \pm 0.02'$ of arc. This corresponds to 2.45 ± 0.1 μm on the retina using as a conversion factor the focal length of a schematic eye.[15] This result is in the middle of a wide range of data (2–3

μm) obtained from histological studies.[1–3] We have obtained local mean cone spacing for three different normal young subjects. Variations of these results were always lower than the standard deviation of the experimental error. This numerical result can be directly applied to more precise evaluations of the physical limits of visual resolution and to aliasing caused by foveal undersampling. By a method of analysis similar to that used in Ref. 16, we would be able to study the problem of foveal aliasing using our objective data of both the image quality of the eye and cone spacing.

Another important point concerns the regularity of the foveal cone mosaic.[13] To obtain actual high-resolution imaging of the fundus (cone mosaic topogra-

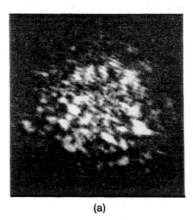

(a)

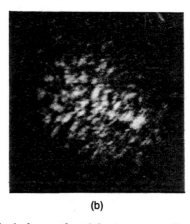

(b)

Fig. 2. Typical examples of short-exposure (4-msec) coherent images from the foveal cone mosaic.

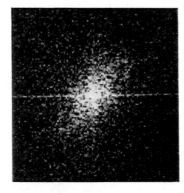

Fig. 3. Two-dimensional power spectrum of the instantaneous image shown in Fig. 2(a).

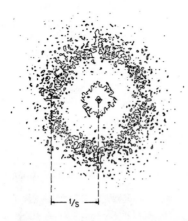

Fig. 4. Average of two-dimensional power spectrum of 10 instantaneous images of the central fovea. $1/s$ is the spatial frequency value corresponding to the mean interdistance between rows of cones.

phy), using the stellar speckle interferometry method presented here, would require the use of algorithms to recover the lost phase information. This is because high resolution is obtained by averaging individual power spectra, with the accompaning loss of phase information and then the ability to reconstruct the image itself. Unfortunately, since the performance of phase-retrieval algorithms on noisy data is poor, further research and higher signal-to-noise ratios will be necessary to obtain high-resolution images of the human retina. Despite this, from the analysis of instantaneous foveal images (Fig. 2) and their two-dimensional power spectra (Fig. 3) we can point out, in a preliminary way, that the distribution of cones at the central fovea is locally a regular triangular array. This is good agreement with previous detailed studies of the primate cone mosaic.[17] The outer ring that appears in Fig. 4 is due to the average of individual power spectra with approximately regular hexagonal structures but in different orientations. The imaged area of the fovea was slightly different for each instantaneous foveal image, and the relative orientation of the mosaic at different areas is also probably different.

In conclusion, we have presented an optical–digital method that is based on stellar speckle interferometry

to obtain diffraction-limited information on the foveal cone mosaic *in vivo* for individual human eyes. The intercenter cone distance has been determined for the first time, to our knowledge, in a completely objective way. These data are useful for evaluating the physical limits of spatial resolution and aliasing artifacts in the sampling of retinal images. Further research to improve this methodology could help to achieve a better understanding of the actual spatial photoreceptor organization.

The authors thank Ana Plaza and Consuelo Gonzalo for their collaboration during the development of this research. This research was supported by the Comision Interministerial de Ciencia y Tecnologia, Spain.

* Present address, Institut d'Optique, Université de Paris-Sud, Bâtiment 503, B.P. 147, 91403 Orsay Cédex, France.

References

1. G. Osterberg, Acta Ophthalmol. Suppl. **6**, 1 (1935).
2. C. A. Curcio, K. R. Sloan, O. Parker, A. E. Hendrickson, and R. E. Kalina, Science **236**, 579 (1987).
3. B. O'Brien, J. Opt. Soc. Am. **41**, 882 (1951).
4. D. R. Williams, Vision Res. **28**, 433 (1988).
5. D. R. Williams, Vision Res. **35**, 195 (1985).
6. D. R. Williams, J. Opt. Soc. Am. A **2**, 1087 (1985).
7. M. F. Land and A. W. Snyder, Vision Res. **25**, 1513 (1985).
8. J. Santamaría, P. Artal, and J. Bescós, J. Opt. Soc. Am. A **4**, 1109 (1987).
9. P. Artal, J. Santamaría, and J. Bescós, J. Opt. Soc. Am. A **5**, 1201 (1988).
10. P. Artal, J. Santamaría, and J. Bescós, Opt. Eng. **28**, 687 (1989).
11. J. C. Dainty, ed., *Laser Speckle and Related Phenomena* (Springer-Verlag, Berlin, 1984).
12. J. W. Goodman, *Statistical Optics* (Wiley, New York, 1985).
13. Y. I. Yellott, Jr., Vision Res. **22**, 1205 (1982).
14. N. J. Colleta and D. R. Williams, J. Opt. Soc. Am. A **4**, 1503 (1987).
15. R. Navarro, J. Santamaría, and R. Bescós, J. Opt. Soc. Am. A **2**, 1273 (1985).
16. P. Artal, "Generation of foveal retinal images: contribution of image quality of the eye and sampling in the photoreceptors," submitted to J. Opt. Soc. Am. A.
17. J. Hirsch and P. Hylton, Vision Res. **24**, 347 (1984).

Reprinted with permission from *Journal of Modern Optics,* Vol. 38(7), pp. 1327-1333 (1991). ©1991 Taylor & Francis Ltd., London.

Measurement of intraocular optical distances using partially coherent laser light

A. F. FERCHER, C. HITZENBERGER

University of Vienna, Institute of Medical Physics,
Währinger Straße 13, A-1090 Wien, Austria

and M. JUCHEM

Department of Ophthalmology, Lainz Hospital,
A-1130 Wien, Austria

(*Received 6 July 1990; revision received 2 November 1990*)

Abstract. The application of partially coherent laser light to measure intraocular optical distances is discussed. In a first step the optical thickness of the retina at the macula and the optical length of the eye has been measured and a precision of ± 0.03 mm has been obtained. The results of a comparison with the acoustically determined eye length and first fundus profile measurements are presented.

1. Introduction

So far optical techniques have mainly been used to measure the depth of the anterior chamber of the eye [1] and the thickness of the cornea [2]. Two basic principles have been used.

(1) A fixed-focus device can be used to scan along the optical axis of the eye [3]. The specific problem here is that the movement of the device does not coincide with the movement of the focus.

(2) A slit lamp can be used and a narrow slit of light can be focused along the optical axis of the eye [4]. The distances seen from a constant angle are to be determined. The specific problem here is that the distances seen do not correspond to intraocular distances.

In addition to the problems already mentioned, these techniques suffer from unavoidable motions of the subject and the accommodation of the eye.

An optical technique which allows an estimation of intraocular axial distances as well as the axial length has been described by Krogsaa *et al.* [5]. They combine the slit lamp and the focusing technique. After the injection of fluorescein intravenously a specially constructed slit-lamp fluorophotometer determines the axial fluorescein concentration profile. A standard deviation of an axial length determination of ± 0.43 mm has been achieved [6].

Recently two closely related laser techniques have been used to measure intraocular axial distances and the axial length of the eye. Fujimoto *et al.* [7] demonstrated the application of the femtosecond optical ranging technique to measure the thickness of the cornea in anaesthetized rabbit eyes. Fercher *et al.* [8] demonstrated the application of an interferometric technique to measure the axial length of the eye of human subjects *in vivo*. The precision of the two techniques depends on the length of the mode-locked light pulses or coherence length Δl of the light used. This length is related by the Fourier uncertainty [9]

$$\Delta l \, \Delta \omega \sim c/2,$$

to the spectral bandwidth $\Delta \omega$ of the radiation used. At present, however, it is much easier to obtain light of short coherence length from multimode semiconductor lasers than to obtain short mode-locked light pulses [8].

If the eye is illuminated by coherent light, several light beams are re-emitted from interfaces of the eye and interfere. First of all there are four reflected beams corresponding to the four Purkinje images [10]. These beams are reflected at the front surface of the cornea, at the rear surface of the cornea, at the front surface of the lens and at the rear surface of the lens. These beams will generate interference fringes. In addition, light is re-emitted from the fundus of the eye, which also produces interference fringes [11]. Furthermore light is back-scattered from the internal structure of the cornea, the lens and the vitreous humour of the normal eye. This is due to geriatric changes in the eye or ocular disorders. These light beams will also interfere and will form a speckle pattern because of the stochastic phases of these beams.

However, the interference phenomena mentioned so far do not provide the absolute distances of the reflecting structures. Only distances to a modulo of the wavelength can be obtained. There is a large variety of interferometric techniques which do provide absolute distances, for example multiple-wavelength techniques [12–15] and wavelength-tuning techniques [15–17]. These techniques might be used in cases with few reflecting surfaces. In the situation here, however, the several reflecting surfaces cause unresolvable ambiguities.

One may, however, use partially coherent light. Then interference will only occur between waves with a path difference less than the coherence length of the light. If the coherence length is less than say 100 µm, the light re-emitted by the eye will not exhibit any interference. In the following section we shall discuss corresponding interferometric techniques.

2. Interferometric length measurement using partially coherent light

Partially coherent light has already been used in interferometry in the past. Brewster fringes or fringes of superposition have been used to measure the spacing between optical surfaces [18, 19]. Channelled spectra have been used to measure the thickness of thin films [20] and for the absolute measurement of small displacements [21]. White-light interferences [22] have been used in an interferometric thickness gauge to monitor continuously the thickness profile of transport layers. We are using partially coherent light together with a Doppler technique to measure intraocular distances. All these techniques are based on the following basic principles.

From standard textbooks [9, 23] it is well known that the power spectrum of a light beam $|E(\omega)|^2$ equals the Fourier transform of the autocorrelation or coherence function $\langle E^*(t)E(t+\tau) \rangle$ of the electric field $E(t)$

$$|E(\omega)|^2 = \frac{1}{(2\pi)^2} \int_{-\infty}^{\infty} \langle E^*(t)E(t+\tau) \rangle \exp(i\omega\tau) \, d\tau. \tag{1}$$

The normalized autocorrelation of the electric field is called the (complex) degree $g_E(\tau)$ of coherence of this beam [9]

$$g_E(\tau) = \frac{\langle E^*(t)E(t+\tau)\rangle}{\langle E^*(t)E(t)\rangle}. \tag{2}$$

Hence the half-width $\Delta\tau$ of the degree $g_E(\tau)$ of coherence and the spectral bandwidth $\Delta\omega$ are related by the Fourier uncertainty

$$\Delta\tau\,\Delta\omega \sim \tfrac{1}{2}. \tag{3}$$

$\Delta\tau$ is the coherence time and $\Delta\tau\,c = \Delta l$ (c is the velocity of light) is the coherence length.

Let this light beam illuminate the structure under investigation and let it be reflected at discontinuities or interfaces 1 and 2 a distance D apart. The electric field $R(t)$ of the reflected beam will contain two components

$$R(t) = E(t) + E(t+T). \tag{4}$$

For simplicity we have assumed equal amplitudes of the reflected beams. A straightforward computation, for example along the lines given on p. 82 of [23] yields the complex degree $g_R(\tau)$ of coherence and the power spectrum $|R(\omega)|^2$ of this field

$$g_R(\tau) = 2g_E(\tau) + g_E(\tau + T) + g_E(\tau - T), \tag{5}$$

$$|R(\omega)|^2 = 2|E(\omega)|^2[1 + \cos(\omega T)]. \tag{6}$$

The degree $g_R(\tau)$ of coherence of the re-emitted light $R(t)$ is composed of three versions of the degree $g_E(\tau)$ of coherence of the illuminating light beam. The time delay between these versions is $T = 2D/V$, where V is the group velocity, because in a medium the coherence function is propagated with the group velocity rather than with the phase velocity [24, 25]. The latter, however, is exclusively used in the classical interferometric techniques, which rely on the measurement of phase differences. The power spectrum of the re-emitted light is a 'channelled' spectrum [20], that is its spectral intensity is modulated by parallel dark and light bands. The spectral distance between adjacent dark channels is $\delta\omega = 2\pi/T$.

Hence we have two basic possibilities to measure the distance D of the re-emitting structures or interfaces. Firstly we can use an interferometer to evaluate the coherence function $g_R(\tau)$ of the re-emitted beam. If the coherence length $\Delta l = \Delta\tau\,c$ of the light beam $E(t)$ is smaller than the distance D, the terms on the right-hand side of equation (5) will be separated and $D = Tc/2$ can be determined. This is the basis of Brewster's fringes and superposition fringe techniques. Secondly we can use a spectrometer to evaluate the spectral modulation given by equation (6). Here D can be obtained from the distance $\delta\omega$ of two dark bands in the channelled spectrum. From equation (6) we have for adjacent bands $\delta\omega\,T = 2\pi$ from which immediately $D = Tc/2 = \pi c N/\Delta\omega$ follows, where N is the number of dark channels in the spectrum $\Delta\omega$.

Let us consider a rough estimate of the precision of both techniques. We shall show that in both techniques the uncertainty ΔD by which D can be determined depends on the coherence length Δl of the beam $E(t)$. In the interferometric technique the distance between adjacent components of the coherence function $g_R(\tau)$ has to be determined. This is possible with an uncertainty equal to the half-width $\Delta\tau$ of these components. Hence ΔD equals the coherence length: $\Delta D = \Delta l$. In the spectrometric technique, however, the number N of dark channels in the spectrum has to be determined. For comparison it is reasonable to assume an uncertainty equal to the width $\delta\omega/2$ of the intensity peaks in the spectrum here, too. Hence the uncertainty when determining N is $\Delta N = \frac{1}{2}$ and the uncertainty in the measurement of D is $\Delta D = \pi c \, \Delta N / \Delta\omega = \pi c / (2 \, \Delta\omega) = \pi \, \Delta l$. This is of the same order of magnitude as in the interferometric technique. In the subsequent section we describe the application of the interferometric technique.

3. Ophthalmic interferometer

Figure 1 shows the basic scheme of the interferometer used in the work described here. The He–Ne laser is used for the adjustment of the subject's eye and the interferometer. If the subject's eye is at the proper position, the examiner will see pulsating interference fringes in the infrared-scope [11]. Subsequently the subject's eye is illuminated by the semiconductor laser. This light beam passes through the Fabry–Pérot interferometer and to a first approximation we can assume the transmitted beam to consist of two components of light according to equation (4) with a delay $T = 2d/c$. Hence the eye is illuminated by a light beam with a complex degree of coherence given by equation (5). The situation here deviates a little from the scheme described in section 2; here the light beam firstly passes through the interferometer and subsquently passes through the structure under investigation. This, however, does not put a different complexion on the results of the analysis given above.

All components of the beam re-emitted from the eye's fundus will have a time delay $T' = 2D/c$ compared with the components reflected at the front surface of the cornea. Here D is the optical length of the eye. In general no interference fringes will be seen in the infrared-scope but, if the time delay $\tau = T'$ caused by the eye equals the time delay T caused by the Fabry–Pérot interferometer, parts of the light beam will interfere again. This can be seen from equation (5)

$$g_R(T') = 2g_E(T') + g_E(T' + T) + g_E(0). \qquad (7)$$

The last term on the right-hand side indicates coherence if $\tau = T'$. Obviously only 25% of the light intensity used will create interference fringes. 75% of the light intensity will form a bright background. Hence it is rather difficult to identify the fringes. Consequently in the first version of this technique it took us approximately 1 h to find these fringes and to measure the optical length of the eye *in vivo*. A

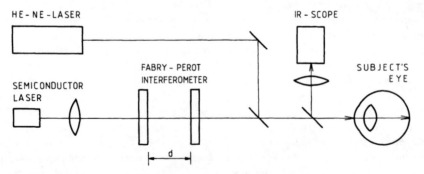

Figure 1.   Optical scheme of the ophthalmic interferometer.

substantial improvement was achieved, however, by using laser Doppler interferometry. One of the Fabry–Pérot plates is moved continuously at a velocity v. Hence the beam reflected at this plate is frequency shifted by the Doppler frequency ω_D

$$\omega_D = \frac{4\pi}{\lambda} v. \tag{8}$$

Instead of the infrared-scope we use a photodetector together with an electronic bandpass filter to detect the Doppler-shifted detector signal. With this technique the time needed to measure the optical length of the eye could be reduced to a few seconds.

4. Results and discussion

The table compares eye lengths obtained by the laser technique on the one hand and the standard ultrasound technique on the other hand. In order to avoid deformations of the cornea by the application of the ultrasound transducer a water bath technique with the subject in supine position was used. In the laser technique the group refractive index [25] has been used to compute the geometrical length. This refractive index is not available for eye media. Because of the high water content of these media we use the dispersion of water to calculate the group refractive index for $\lambda = 780$ nm from the readily available phase refractive index at $\lambda = 550$ nm [26].

As can be seen from the table, the lengths obtained by the two techniques are in good agreement. In spite of this result, one may speculate, however, on whether the acoustic and optic echoes are caused by the same interfaces at the fundus. There is some uncertainty for example about the structure where the acoustical echo is created. Although the same is true for the optical technique, there are first important steps towards clarification of this matter. With some subjects for example an additional Doppler signal can be observed which corresponds to a shorter axial length of the eye compared with the usual Doppler signal. Figure 2 shows a corresponding example obtained from subject M. J. Here the two signals are separated by approximately 280 µm at the centre of the fovea. Perifoveally a separation of approximately 350 µm has been obtained. It is well known in ophthalmology [27] that in young, heavily pigmented subjects some of the incident light is reflected at the vitreoretinal interface. Hence we can assume the usual

Geometric eye length of seven subjects determined optically and acoustically. The standard deviation of the optically determined lengths is ± 25 µm. The standard deviation of the acoustical technique is approximately ± 200 µm.

Subject	Geometric length of the eye (mm)		
	Obtained optically	Obtained acoustically	Difference (mm)
A. F.	24·78	24·64	0·14
G. G.	23·01	22·82	0·19
C. H.	25·50	25·54	−0·04
M. J.	23·55	23·60	−0·05
K. L.	28·42	28·37	0·05
H. S.	24·17	24·36	−0·19
L. S.	25·04	25·04	0·00

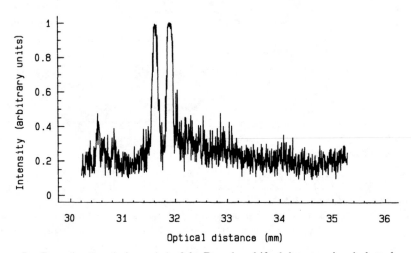

Figure 2. Intensity (in relative units) of the Doppler-shifted detector signal plotted against the separation of the Fabry–Pérot plates. Two peaks separated by approximately 280 μm can be recognized (fovea of subject M. J.).

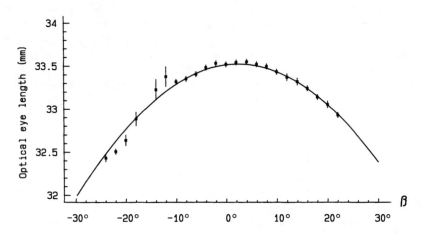

Figure 3. Fundus profile of subject A. F. on a horizontal meridian, showing the optical length of the eye plotted against the azimutal angle β ($\beta < \theta°$, temporal; the fovea is at $\beta = \theta°$): (———), profile of an eye of same optical length with a spherical bulbus and a spherical cornea.

Doppler signal to be caused by an interface at or near the pigment epithelium and the weaker signal to be generated at the concave foveal surface of the inner limiting membrane between the vitreous and the retina. Because of the depression in the centre of the macula the separation of the two signals is smaller there than at the periphery of the fovea, that is at the margin of the macula.

Figure 3 shows the surface profile of the fundus of subject A. F. Light reflected at the pigment epithelium has been used. The position of the fovea is at $\theta°$. The centre of the fovea seems a little elevated, which is in agreement with histological findings. The excavation of the optic disc can be seen between $-10°$ and $-15°$. The margins of the excavation are elevated as is the case in healthy subjects.

5. Conclusion

This preliminary report presents some results and describes some properties of the interferometric length measurement technique. There is a rather significant agreement with the ultrasonic technique. In addition to its high longitudinal and transversal precision, the optical technique gives access to histological structures of the eye media.

Acknowledgments

The work reported here has been supported by the Austrian Fonds zur Förderung der Wissenschaftlichen Forschung (grant No. P 7300 MED). The authors also wish to thank Mr H. Sattmann for his excellent technical assistance.

References

[1] BLEEKER, G. M., 1960, *Archs Ophthalmol.*, **63,** 821.
[2] EHLERS, N., and HANSEN, F. K., 1971, *Acta Ophthalmol.*, **49,** 65.
[3] DONDERS, F. C., 1872, *Klin. Mbl. Augenheilk.*, **10,** 300.
[4] BLEEKER, G. M., 1961, *Archs Ophthalmol.*, **65,** 369.
[5] KROGSAA, B., FLEDELIUS, H., LARSEN, J., and LUND-ANDERSEN, H., 1984, *Acta Ophthalmol.*, **62,** 274.
[6] KROGSAA, B., FLEDELIUS, H., LARSEN, J., and LUND-ANDERSEN, H., 1984, *Acta Ophthalmol.*, **62,** 290.
[7] FUJIMOTO, J. G., DE SILVESTRI, S., IPPEN, E. P., PULIAFITO, C. A., MARGOLIS, R., and OSEROFF, A., 1986, *Optics Lett.*, **11,** 150.
[8] FERCHER, A. F., MENGEDOHT, K., and WERNER, W., 1988, *Optics Lett.*, **13,** 186.
[9] BORN, M., and WOLF, E., 1980, *Principles of Optics* (Oxford: Pergamon).
[10] SAFIR, A., 1980, *Refraction and Clinical Optics* (Hagerstown, Maryland: Harper & Row).
[11] FERCHER, A. F., HU, H. Z., STEEGER, P. F., and BRIERS, J. D., 1982, *Optica Acta*, **29,** 1401.
[12] BIEN, F., CAMAC, M., CAULFIELD, H. J., and EZEKIEL, S., 1981, *Appl. Optics*, **20,** 400.
[13] BOURDET, G. L., and ORSZAG, A. G., 1979, *Appl. Optics*, **18,** 225.
[14] BUHOLZ, N. E., 1981, *Opt. Engng.*, **20,** 325.
[15] FERCHER, A. F., VRY, U., and WERNER, W., 1990, *Proceedings of the International Workshops on Holography and Speckle Phenomena* (Singapore: World Scientific), pp. 353–361.
[16] OLSSON, A., and TANG, C. L., 1981, *Appl. Optics*, **20,** 3503.
[17] SUZUKI, T., SASAKI, O., and MARUYAMA, T., 1989, *Appl. Optics*, **28,** 4407.
[18] STEEL, W. H., 1983, *Interferometry* (Cambridge University Press).
[19] SCHWIDER, J., 1979, *Appl. Optics*, **18,** 2364.
[20] FRANCON, M., 1966, *Optical Interferometry* (New York: Academic Press).
[21] SMITH, L. M., and DOBSON, C. C., 1989, *Appl. Optics*, **28,** 3339.
[22] FLOURNOY, P. A., McCLURE, R. W., and WYNTJES, G., 1972, *Appl. Optics*, **11,** 1907.
[23] LOUDON, R., 1985, *The Quantum Theory of Light* (Oxford University Press).
[24] BERAN, M. J., and PARRENT, G. B., 1964, *Theory of Partial Coherence* (Englewood Cliffs, New Jersey: Prentice-Hall).
[25] PANCHARATNAM, S., 1963, *Proc. Indian Acad. Sci.*, **57,** 231.
[26] OBSTFELD, H., 1982, *Optics in Vision* (London: Butterworths).
[27] VAUGHAN, D., and ASBURY, T., 1983, *General Ophthalmology* (Los Altos, California: Lange Medical Publications).

Reprinted from *Optics Letters,* Vol. 17(1), pp. 4-6 (January 1, 1992).
©1992 Optical Society of America.

High-resolution reflectometry in biological tissues

X. Clivaz, F. Marquis-Weible, and R. P. Salathé

Centre d'Applications Laser, Ecole Polytechnique Fédérale, 1015 Lausanne, Switzerland

R. P. Novàk and H. H. Gilgen

Technical Center, Swiss PTT, 3000 Berne, Switzerland

Optical low-coherence reflectometry is applied for the first time to our knowledge to investigate diffusive biological tissues with a single-mode fiber probe. Samples of fresh arteries are studied, using the backscattered light from the tissue. The probed volume in the vicinity of the fiber tip is estimated to be below 6.7×10^{-10} cm^3. This noninvasive method allows one to determine optical parameters, such as the index of refraction and the transmission properties, and the tissue thickness.

Investigation of the internal structure of biological tissues and membranes generally implies the use of heavy preparation and fixation methods such as freeze drying, freeze fracturing, and microtome slicing. The tissue and its components are then dead and altered to a certain extent, which introduces artifacts that lower the quality of the experimental results. Optical methods often permit noninvasive measurements. For highly diffusive media, however, such techniques are not yet well developed. The thickness of an arterial wall can be evaluated noninvasively with acoustic-wave techniques, however, with a limited resolution.[1] The refractive index of soft diffusive tissue is measured by an invasive technique based on an evanescent field method.[2] In this Letter we report what are to our knowledge the first attempts to apply optical low-coherence reflectometry (OLCR) to measure parameters of diffusive tissue. The OLCR technique was originally developed by Takada *et al.*[3] and Danielson and Whittenberg[4] for reflection measurements in telecommunication devices with micrometer resolution. Fercher *et al.*[5] and Swanson *et al.*[6] used the same technique to investigate corneal tissue. The measurements in this nondiffusive tissue were limited in their experiment to the evaluation of tissue thickness. Without exploiting the full potential of OLCR, we demonstrate here that this technique is well suited to measure optical properties of diffusive biological tissue, such as an arterial wall (e.g., attenuation and refractive index), as well as the thickness of the sample.

OLCR uses a Michelson interferometer with a broadband light source of short coherence time. The technique is based on coherent cross-correlation detection of light reflected from a sample. The apparatus used in the experiment presented here has been described in detail by Novàk *et al.*[7] Briefly, the interferometer is built with single-mode polarization-maintaining fibers with a core diameter of 8.5 μm and a 50:50 Panda coupler (PMC; Fig. 1). A mirror is mounted on a stepper translator at the end of the reference arm (REF). The

scanning of the position of the mirror is recorded. It induces the variation of the propagation time τ. The sample (SAM) is mounted at the end of the measurement arm, either close to or in contact with the fiber. The fiber tip has a radius of curvature of ~4 mm as a result of polishing, which does not significantly alter the geometry of light propagation at the fiber end. An edge-emitting diode (LED) is used as a continuous light source. It delivers 3 μW of power in the fiber at a wavelength of $\lambda = 1300$ nm with a bandwidth $\Delta\lambda = 60$ nm. A phase modulation at ~117 Hz is generated by a 3-cm-long piezoelectric element (MOD) that stresses the fiber on the reference arm. The stress modifies locally the refraction index of the fiber and changes the reference propagation time τ. The modulation amplitude is chosen to induce a phase shift corresponding to one wavelength. The signal is detected by an InGaAs photodiode (PD). The photodiode current, which is proportional to the incident light power, is measured with a lock-in amplifier. Light coming from the reference arm of the Michelson interferometer interferes with light from the sample arm only when their round-trip propagation time difference is smaller than the coherence time of the light source. Homodyne detection with the phase modulation on the reference arm isolates the interference signal from the total photodetected light. A fiber polarizer is placed at the input of the interferometer. It allows one to confine the measurement to one state of polarization. This eliminates the signal degradation due to polarization-dispersion effects in the fiber paths.

The measured physical value is the interference term of the optical power P_i reaching the detector as a function of the round-trip propagation time τ in the reference arm of the interferometer. If we assume a lossless interferometer, the interference signal generated by a single reflection is expressed by[4]

$$P_i(\tau) = 2P_o k(1-k)\beta_i A_i \sqrt{R_i}|\gamma_{12}(\tau - \tau_i)|\cos\theta_i,$$

$$\theta_i = 2\pi\nu(\tau - \tau_i) + \xi. \tag{1}$$

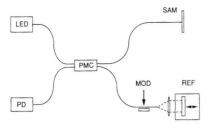

Fig. 1. Schematic of the experimental setup for OLCR measurements.

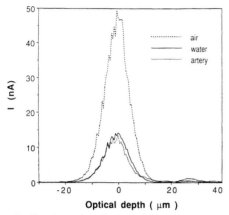

Fig. 2. Reflection signal as a function of the optical depth for three different interfaces: fiber–air, fiber–pure water, and fiber–arterial wall.

Here P_o is the optical power launched into the interferometer, k is the coupling constant of the interferometer, ν is the mean optical frequency of the light source, and β_i is a geometrical factor accounting for the divergence of the light coming out of the fiber, which is not collected on reflection. Each reflection event in the sample, numbered with the index i, is characterized by a round-trip propagation time in the sample arm τ_i, a geometrical factor β_i, a reflection coefficient R_i, and a transmittance A_i. A_i is defined as the ratio of the light power entering the sample to the light power at location of reflection i. γ_{12} is the cross-correlation function for the relative delay $(\tau - \tau_i)$. ξ is a constant phase factor. The theoretical resolution of an OLCR device is determined by the group velocity of the light in the sample v_g and the spectral width $\Delta\nu$ of the light source. The FWHM of a signal generated by a discrete reflection is given approximately by $\Delta z = v_g/2\Delta\nu$, with $\Delta z \approx 15$ μm for LED light sources.[3,4]

Fresh postmortem bovine superior mesenteric arteries are taken at the slaughter house and kept in a Krebs solution at 4°C for a few hours (less than one day), until measurement takes place. Arteries are dissected so that the connective tissue covering the adventitia is removed, then cut longitudinally and slightly stretched on a sample holder so that the sample around the measured spot is in contact with air only. Pieces of the arterial wall $\sim$300 μm thick are placed perpendicular to the beam, with the intima facing the fiber end.

Figure 2 displays the reflection signal probed at the interface between a clean bare fiber and three different media, air, pure water, and arterial wall. An interval of 70 μm is investigated in 0.5-μm steps, and each point is measured during a 1-s period with the scanning stage at rest. The photodiode current is represented in a linear scale as a function of the optical depth. The dashed curve shows the typical interferometric signature of a discrete single reflection. The main peak reaches the intensity $I_{\text{air}} = 49.337$ nA, which is typical of a 4% reflection of light at a glass–air interface. The reflection in pure water, represented by the solid curve, corresponds to a similar peak of lower intensity $I_{\text{water}} = 14.160$ nA, as expected from the larger index of refraction of water. The relative ratio between I_{air} and I_{water} allows one to calculate the index of refraction of the fiber, according to the formula

$$\frac{I_{\text{water}}}{I_{\text{air}}} = \frac{n_{\text{water}} - n_{\text{fiber}}}{n_{\text{water}} + n_{\text{fiber}}} \frac{n_{\text{air}} + n_{\text{fiber}}}{n_{\text{air}} - n_{\text{fiber}}} \quad (2)$$

deduced from Fresnel theory of reflection at an interface. Assuming $n_{\text{water}} = 1.322$,[8] we obtain $n_f = 1.476$. This value represents the effective refraction index of the fiber propagation mode, at the wavelength of the source $\lambda = 1300$ nm. The peak of reflection at the fiber–artery interface, displayed in the lowest curve, reaches the maximum value $I_{\text{artery}} = 13.310$ nA. This value is in the same range as that of I_{water}, which is not surprising since the tissue is composed of $\sim$70% of water.[9] Using for the fiber the index of refraction determined above, we obtain from I_{air} and I_{artery} the value of $n_{\text{artery}} = 1.331$. This is in good agreement with values given in the literature.[2] The FWHM of all these curves is of the order of $\approx$11 μm. In the vicinity of the fiber tip, the mode field radius is $\omega_0 = 4.4$ μm. The corresponding volume is thus $\approx$6.7 $\times$ 10^{-10} cm^3. This estimation constitutes an upper limit for the probed volume in this region and illustrates the fine spatial resolution that can be reached with this technique.

The full dynamic range of the measured curves is shown in Fig. 3, which displays the reflection signal probed in a sample over a depth of 1 mm. Data are represented in decibels relative to a reference current I_0 characteristic of the LED used as the light source. The solid curve displays the reflection signal through the arterial wall, with the artery being in contact with the fiber and exposed to air. It exhibits two peaks corresponding to reflections R_1 and R_2 at the fiber–artery and artery–air interfaces, respectively. The two peaks are separated by a distance $d_2 = 365$ μm. This distance corresponds to the measured displacement of the reference mirror in air. The effective sample thickness is given by $d_2' = d_2/n$, where n is the refraction index of the sample. We neglect the inhomogeneities of n throughout the arterial wall and take in our calculation the value of n_{artery} obtained above for the intima, thus deducing $d_2' = 274$ μm. The maxima of the two reflectivity peaks correspond to the values -26.5 and -49.5 dB for R_1 and R_2, respectively. Based on the measured indices of refraction for the fiber and the artery, we calculate a difference in reflectance of 8.8 dB between the fiber–artery and artery–air interfaces. The total attenuation

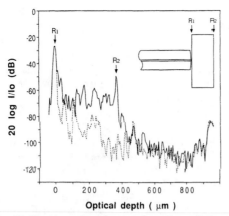

Fig. 3. Reflection signal as a function of the optical depth in a logarithmic representation. Dotted curve, reference curve from the bare fiber in air (normalized); solid curve, arterial wall in contact with the fiber end.

through the arterial wall is thus 31.8 dB. This attenuation includes diffraction, absorption, and diffusion in the tissue and surface scattering at R_2. The dotted curve in Fig. 3 represents the reflection signal without the artery, corresponding to the fiber–air interface. This signal can be used as a reference curve to study the diffusion in the artery. It has been normalized so that the peak at the fiber–air interface has the same size as the peak at the fiber–artery interface. The signal at the interface decreases only slowly with distance. This is due to the Lorentzian shape of the emission profile.[10] On this reference curve, a side peak structure is observed at a depth of $d \approx 470 \ \mu m$, characterized by an intensity at least 40 dB lower than the main reflection peak. This structure, which is reproducible, is characteristic of the spectrum of the source LED in conjunction with a discrete reflection in the setup. Comparing this reference curve with the measurement (solid curve), we notice that the intensity of the solid curve between the peaks at the fiber–artery ($z = 0$) and artery–air ($z = 365$) interfaces is at a level of approximately -65 dB. This level is clearly higher than the intensity of the normalized reference curve at the same position. This is due to the superimposition of a large number of small peaks produced by the retrodiffusion of light in the arterial tissue. Beyond the peak at the artery–air ($z > 365$) interface, the signal in the sample is similar to the signal of the nomalized reference curve at the same position. The maximum dynamic range achieved with this measurement is ~110 dB. This value depends critically on the LED light source and the experimental arrangement. A dynamic range of 130 dB with a spatial resolution of 14 μm has been measured in a previous experiment with a different LED.[7]

The interpretation of reflectometry curves is relatively easy when discrete and distant Fresnel reflections are measured. It is possible to determine the position of the reflecting interface. The reflection coefficient R_i and the transmission factor A_i are two parameters related by Eqs. (1). By taking the geometrical characteristics of the setup into account

and knowing one of these two parameters, it is possible to determine the other one from an OLCR curve. The interpretation becomes much more delicate when reflection events are closer; we then have to consider the interferences of light reflected from interfaces separated by a distance of the same order as the coherence length of the light source. Decorrelation of the measured curve with the curve of a discrete single reflection could be used efficiently for interpreting such measurement. Another solution might be to improve the resolution of the OLCR, by using a light source with a broader frequency bandwidth, to resolve closer reflection events. The precision of the measured curves in Fig. 3 is limited by the number of sampling points and by the 8-bit digital-to-analog converter. This limited precision does not allow us to use deconvolution techniques in order to separate the signatures of two reflection peaks from the arterial wall interfaces. Research in this direction is currently in progress.

Optical low-coherence reflectometry has been applied for the first time to our knowledge to the study of diffusive biological tissues. This technique is noninvasive and allows one to investigate the optical parameters of unprepared biological samples. From measurements on fresh bovine mesenteric superior arteries, we have evaluated the refraction index of the intima surface and the thickness of the arterial wall, and we have estimated the total transmission coefficient for linear polarized light through the sample. The results indicate the usefulness of this technique, which can be refined for a broader use in the study of biological tissues.

The authors thank the Swiss National Fundation for financial support and B. Bolz and G. Bodmer from the Swiss PTT for technical assistance.

References

1. A. Poli, E. Tremoli, A. Colombo, M. Sirtori, P. Pignoli, and R. Paoletti, Atherosclerosis **70**, 253 (1988).
2. F. P. Bolin, L. E. Preuss, R. C. Taylor, and R. J. Ference, Appl. Opt. **28**, 2297 (1989).
3. K. Takada, I. Yokohama, K. Chida, and J. Noda, Appl. Opt. **26**, 1603 (1987).
4. B. L. Danielson and C. D. Whittenberg, Appl. Opt. **26**, 2836 (1987).
5. A. F. Fercher, K. Mengedoht, and W. Werner, Opt. Lett. **13**, 186 (1988).
6. E. Swanson, D. Huang, J. G. Fujimoto, C. P. Lin, and C. A. Puliafito, in *Digest of Conference on Lasers and Electro-Optics* (Optical Society of America, Washington, D.C., 1991), p. 150.
7. R. P. Novàk, H. H. Gilgen, P. Beaud, and W. Hodel, in *Digest of Symposium on Optical Fiber Measurements* (National Institute of Standards and Technology, Boulder, Colo., 1990), p. 35.
8. G. M. Hale and M. R. Querry, Appl. Opt. **12**, 555 (1973).
9. C. G. Carro, T. J. Pedley, R. C. Schroter, and W. A. Seed, *The Mechanics of the Circulation* (Oxford U. Press, London, 1978), p. 91.
10. H. H. Gilgen, R. P. Novàk, R. P. Salathé, W. Hodel, and P. Beaud, IEEE J. Lightwave Technol. **7**, 1225 (1989).

Reprinted from *Holography, Interferometry, and Optical Pattern Recognition in Biomedicine II,* Proc. SPIE Vol. 1647, pp. 9-20 (1992).

Optical Fourier transform analysis of corneal endothelial cell patterns

Barry R. Masters

Department of Anatomy & Cell Biology,
Uniformed Services University of the Health Sciences,
Bethesda, MD 20814-4799,

ABSTRACT

The quantitative analysis of human corneal endothelial cells patterns is analyzed with Fourier transform methods. The optical or digital Fourier transform of the the pattern of endothelial cell borders is analyzed to yield the average cell area and the coefficient of variation of the average cell area. The more difficult problem of cell shape characterization is still under investigation. The advantage of the Fourier transform analysis is the parallel processing of the optical Fourier transform and the potential development of a hybrid digital-optical device for the rapid analysis of large numbers of endothelial specular photomicrographs.

1. INTRODUCTION

The human cornea is about 0.5 mm thick at its center and is an important refractive element in the eye. The corneal endothelium contains active transport systems which transport ions and thus maintain the hydration and the transparency of the cornea. The corneal endothelium consists of about 350,000 to 500,000 polygonal cells about 5 microns thick and 20 microns in diameter. The size and the shape of the cells and the statistical evaluation of these parameters is important for diagnostic evaluation of the state of the layer. The standard method to evaluate these parameters is to manually trace the cell borders and to input their location to a computer for numerical evaluation. This method has been used to analyze only a limited number of cells (50-100) due to the difficulty of the manual operation. The numerical values obtained from these small numbers of cells are often not statistically significant, and may result in false conclusions about endothelial structure. The research described in this paper is aimed at the development of a hybrid optical/digital technique to obtain these statistical perimeters for large numbers of endothelial cells (500-1000) in a short time. Fourier transform methods are widely used in image analysis.

2. METHODS

There are several methods to obtain the images of corneal endothelial cell patters. The standard instrument is the specular microscope which can image the specular reflection of the corneal endothelial cells. The images can be recorded on photographic film or on video tape. An alternative and newer method to obtain images of the posterior surface of corneal endothelial cells is the use of confocal light microscopy.

These images are converted into binary images of the posterior endothelial cell borders with several methods. These methods include: manual tracing of the cell borders from photographs, semi-automatic digital image processing, and optical image processing. The binary images of the cell borders were then converted into two dimensional Fourier transforms of the input images with either digital or optical methods.

The log of the intensity distribution in the two dimensional Fourier transform shows the following characteristics. There is a bright center spot of high intensity light. Around the center spot is a dark ring. Surrounding the dark ring is the first bright annulus of light intensity. The analysis of the position and the width of the first bright ring of light intensity in the two dimensional Fourier transform contains the information on the average endothelial cell area and the coefficient of variation of the average cell area.

3. RESULTS AND DISCUSSION

A typical image of the the posterior surface of the corneal endothelial of a rabbit ex vivo eye is shown in Fig. 1. The sharp polygonal cell borders are the dark lines. Examples of human corneal endothelial cell patterns are shown in Figs. 2, 3. The gray level human corneal endothelial cell patterns have been digitally segmented into binary images and coded with gray levels for identification. Fig. 2 shows a cell pattern with 1000 cells per millimeter squared. Fig. 3 shows an endothelial cell pattern with 3000 cells per millimeter squared.

From observation of Figs 2, 3 the following statements can be made.

(1). The cell patterns are not regular polygons; the lengths of the sides of the polygons differ.

(2) The orientation of the cell polygons differs for all of the endothelial. cells. If all of the cells had the same orientation the problem of cell shape identification and analysis would become a simple problem for pattern recognition.

A typical example of the optical Fourier transform of the binary endothelial cell patterns is shown in Fig. 4. The central bright spot is shown. The first ring of bright intensity is also shown. This ring contains the information on average cell area and the coefficient of variation of average cell area. This Figure should be compared with Fig. 10. The optical method to obtain the optical Fourier transform is shown in Fig. 9.

Figs. 5-8 are examples of digital two dimensional Fourier transform of binary endothelial cell patterns. The central high intensity spot is shown in each image. Each Figure also shown the bright intensity ring which is used for the quantitative analysis of the endothelial cell pattern size distributions.

The human endothelial cell border patterns with higher cell densities, more endothelial cells per square millimeter, show corresponding shifts in the position of the first bright ring in the two dimensional Fourier transform image. The cell patters with the higher cell densities and the higher spatial frequencies show the position of the first bright intensity ring in the Fourier transform shifted to higher spatial frequencies.

The analysis of the intensity distributions in the two dimensional Fourier transforms is as follows. Please refer to Fig.. 4, and to Figs. 5-8. These image may be related to the drawing in Fig. 10. In Fig 10 the letter **A** is the magnitude of the the center of the first bright ring in the Fourier transform. The average endothelial area is proportional to the quantity: one divided by **A**. **The endothelial cell patterns with higher cell densities contain cells of smaller cell areas.** The width of the first bright ring is given by the letter **B**. **The ratio of the quantity B to the quantity A is proportional to the coefficient of variation of the average cell area in the endothelial input pattern.**

This paper shown how the optical Fourier transform patterns of binary human endothelial cell patterns can be quantitatively analyzed. The two quantities that are immediately determined from the analysis of the Fourier transforms are the following: (1) the average endothelial cell area, and (2) the coefficient of variation of the average endothelial cell area.

The determination of endothelial cell shape, the distribution of endothelial cell shapes, and the extraction of other cellular features from the endothelial cell patterns is more difficult. Work is in progress to automate the the collection of data from the angular and radial intensity distributions of the Fourier transform, the extraction of features to be used for cell pattern recognition, and the use of neural networks for automated pattern recognition.

While this investigation is concerned with the automated analysis of human corneal endothelial cell patterns and their quantitative analysis it is clear that the methods and techniques have a wide application to biology and medicine. These methods can be useful in automated pattern recognition in biological screening, automated Pap tests, automated pathology, and cell biology.

4. ACKNOWLEDGEMENTS

This work was supported by a grant from the National Institutes of Health, National Eye Institute, EY-06958.

5 REFERENCES

1. D.J. Mayer, **Clinical Wide-Field Specular Microscopy,** Bailliere Tindall, London, 1984.

2. B.R. Masters "Characterization of corneal specular endothelial photomicrographs by their Fourier transforms.".*Digital and Optical Shape Representation and Pattern Recognition*, Richard D. Juday, Editor, Proc. SPIE 938, 246-252, (1988)

3. B.R. Masters, Y.-K Lee, W.T. Rhodes, Fourier Transform Method for Statistical Evaluation of Corneal Endothelial Morphology, In: **Noninvasive Diagnostic Techniques in Ophthalmology,** Ed. B.R. Masters, Springer-Verlag, New York, 122-141, 1990.

4. Y.-K Lee, W.T. Rhodes, "Feature detection and enhancement by a rotating kernel min-max transformation", *Hybrid Image and Signal Processing II*, D.P Casasent and A.G. Tescher, Editors, Proc. SPIE 1297, pp. 154-159, 1990.

5. Y.-K. Lee, "Nonlinear Image Processing and Pattern Analysis by Rotating Kernal Transformation and Optical Fourier Transform," Ph.D Thesis, Georgia Institute of Technology, December, 1990

6. Y.-K. Lee, and W.T. Rhodes, "Nonlinear image processing by rotating kernal transformations," Optics Letters, vol. 15(23), pp. 1383-1385, 1990.

7. B.R. Masters, "Diagnostic digital image processing of human corneal endothelial cell patterns," Visual Communications and Image Processing'90, Murat Kunt, Editor, SPIE Vol. 1360, 676-689, 1990.

8. B.R. Masters, Y-K. Lee, W.T. Rhodes, "Fourier transform method to determine human corneal endothelial morphology," Halina Podbielska, M.D., Editor, Proc. SPIE 1429, 82-94, 1991.

9. H. Lipson, **Optical Transforms**, Academic Press, London, 1972.

10. R.N. Bracewell, **The Fourier Transform and its Applications**, 2ed., McGraw-Hill, New York, 1986.

11. H. Stark, **Applications of Optical Fourier Transforms**, Academic Press, New York, 1982,

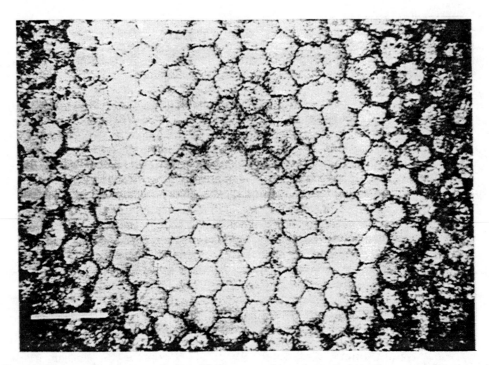

Fig.1. The cell patterns of rabbit corneal endothelial cells at the posterior surface of the endothelial cells. This image was made with a confocal microscope in the backscattered light mode. The scale bar is 50 microns. The corneal endothelial cells are polygonal, nonuniformly oriented, and show various numbers of sides and different cell areas. In the clinic, human endothelial cell patterns are images with a device called a specular microscope which images the specular reflection of the cells and their cell boundaries to form the image. These images are called specular photomicrographs.

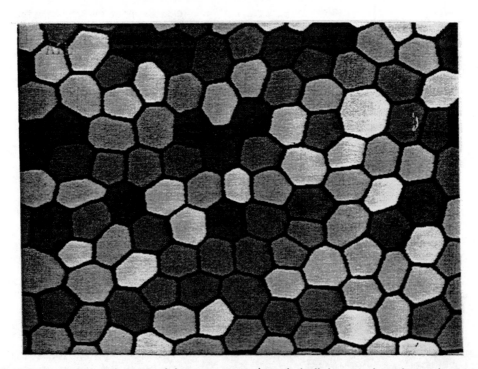

Fig. 2. A digitized image of human corneal endothelial specular photomicrographs made with a specular microscope. This central region of the human cornea has about 1000 corneal endothelial cells in each square millimeter. The various cell shapes and cell orientations are shown in the figure.

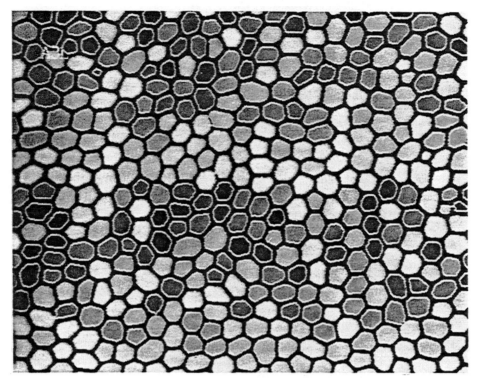

Fig. 3. A digitized image of human corneal endothelial specular photomicrographs made with a specular microscope. This central region of the human cornea has about 3000 corneal endothelial cells in each square millimeter. The various cell shapes and cell orientations are shown in the figure.

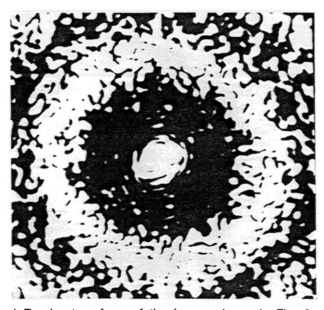

Fig. 4. An optical Fourier transform of the image shown in Fig. 3. A HeNe laser was the light source and a lens produced the optical Fourier transform which was imaged onto the film plane of a camera. This image shows the center bright spot and the wide circular annulus of intensity. The distance in the image between the center of the central bright spot and the center of the annulus correlates with the average cell density of the endothelial cell pattern that was placed in the optical system to form the Fourier transform. It was further found that the average width of the annulus divided by the distance between the central region and the center of the annulus corresponds to the coefficient of variation of the average cell area.

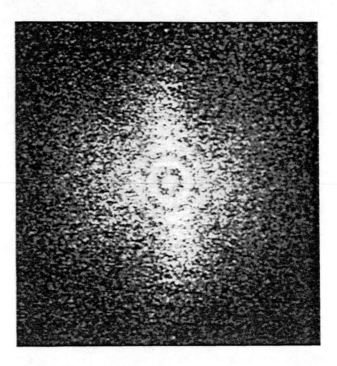

Fig. 5. An example of the digital Fourier Transform of a binary image of endothelial cell patterns. The input cell pattern has 1000 cells per millimeter squared. The input pattern was digitized with CCD camera into a frame grabber and the resulting image was digitally transformed into the two dimensional Fourier transform. The image is the logarithm of the intensity of the Fourier Transform.
The central spot is shown as well as the first bright ring of intensity.

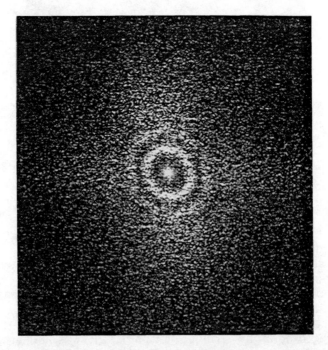

Fig. 6. An example of the digital Fourier Transform of a binary image of endothelial cell patterns. The input cell pattern has 1500 cells per millimeter squared. The methods are the same as described in Fig. 5.

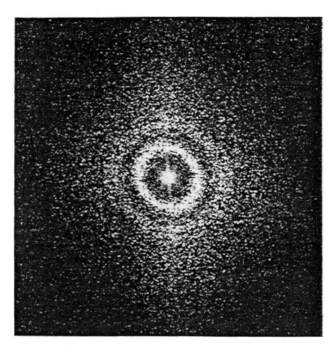

Fig. 7. An example of the digital Fourier Transform of a binary image of endothelial cell patterns. The input cell pattern has 2500 cells per millimeter squared. The methods are the same as described in Fig. 5.

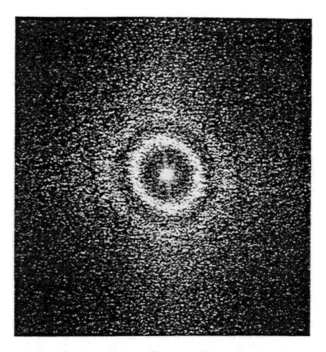

Fig. 8. An example of the digital Fourier Transform of a binary image of endothelial cell patterns. The input cell pattern has 3000 cells per millimeter squared. The methods are the same as described in Fig. 5.

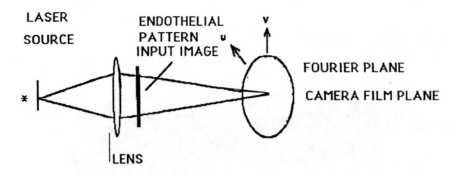

Fig. 9. A diagram of the optical system to produce the optical Fourier transforms of the endothelial image patterns.

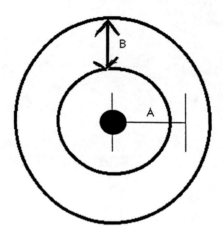

fig. 10. A diagram of how the Fourier transform of the binary endothelial cell patterns can be analyzed to determine the average cell area and the coefficient of variation of the average cell area.

The magnitude of the line segment from the center of the central intensity spot to the center of the the first bright ring of intensity is labeled **A.** The width of the first bright ring is labeled **B**. Compare this diagram with Fig. 3. which shows an actual optical Fourier transforms of the binary human endothelial cell pattern.

Reprinted with permission from *IEEE Transactions on Biomedical Engineering*,
Vol. 36(12), pp. 1210-1221 (December 1989). ©1989 IEEE.

Chrono-Coherent Imaging for Medicine

KENNETH G. SPEARS, JENIFER SERAFIN, NILS H. ABRAMSON, XINMING ZHU,
AND HANS BJELKHAGEN

(Invited Paper)

Abstract—We describe a new method for imaging with visible and near visible light inside media, such as tissues, which have strong light scattering. The chrono-coherent imaging (CCI) method is demonstrated in this paper for a transmission geometry where an absorbing object is completely hidden from normal visual observation by light scattering of the media. The resultant images are most similar to X rays, with cumulative transmission showing absorption features and refractive index differences in the media. We discuss laser coherence properties, coherence measurements, the relation of CCI to light-in-flight holography, holographic film properties relevant to CCI, a particular optical setup for CCI, the results of a demonstration experiment imaging an absorbing object hidden by light scattering, and an experiment to estimate the clinical applicability of CCI.

Introduction

THE idea of imaging inside the body with optical wavelengths is appealing, but light scattering of tissues and other optical distortion creates severe practical problems. The field of transillumination has developed as a specialized diagnostic method, especially in pediatric transillumination [1], despite the formidable problems of light scattering. The diffuse nature of the image quality in transillumination has been characterized by the word diaphanography, which is apparently becoming synonymous with transillumination. The application of transillumination (TI) in clinical medicine has been most extensive in pediatric medicine, which suggests that many diagnostic problems are sensitive to optical imaging methods. Cranial TI in infants has been used for hydrocephalus, subdural hygroma, subdural effusion and hematoma, and various intracranial pathologies [2]-[10]. The TI of chest areas in infants has been used for diagnosing neonatal pneumothorax [11] and for aiding surgeons [12]. Abdominal diagnostics have been done for congenital abnormality of the mesenteric vein [13] and various abdominal masses [8], [14], [15]. Additional applications of TI in

nonpediatric medicine have been developed for sinuses [16], basal carcinoma [17], and cardiac anomalies [18].

The early work by Cutler [19] on breast lesions has recently been extended into breast cancer detection [20]-[28]. The transmission geometry of diaphanography and the need for better diagnostics of breast tumors has resulted in clinical instruments which use electronic video imaging in the near infrared [21], [24]. Clinical tests of breast diaphanography [24], [29]-[31] suggest that the method is not adequate for a single screening technique. The potential for tissue selectivity in the red and near infrared spectral regions has been recognized and quantitatively characterized for breast tissue specimens [32].

The diaphanography method has been studied [33] as a candidate for tomographic improvements, although the diffuse nature of the images makes this approach difficult. Comparisons of different imaging methods [30], [31] for breast tumors including sonography, thermography and X-ray mammography have suggested that X-ray mammography is currently superior. The medical applications of TI (diaphanography) seem to be limited by the resolution rather than the mechanism of tissue interaction and its relevance to diagnosis.

This paper gives a simple discussion of coherent imaging and chrono-coherent imaging (CCI) techniques which explains the basic concepts and identifies the problems which require further attention. We discuss experimental aspects such as laser coherence properties, coherence measurements for lasers, holographic film properties under conditions of CCI, and a particular geometry for CCI. We present results of an experiment which records the image of a hidden object and conclude with a discussion of tissue properties and a summary of the potential of CCI for medical imaging.

Coherent Imaging

The possibility of removing scattered light from imaging was discussed early in the development of picosecond lasers [34]. This first suggestion used a laser pulse in a liquid media to create a transient optical photographic shutter for imaging a time slice from an object illuminated with a picosecond pulse where the light scatter from earlier and later times was reduced. This idea has some practical problems of shutter technology, and rather than using a picosecond shutter or streak camera for conventional imaging the idea of using time coincident detection of a

Manuscript received September 26, 1988; revised February 27, 1989. This work was supported by the Medical Free Electron Laser Program of the Strategic Defense Initiative Organization through the Midwest Biolaser Institute.

K. G. Spears, J. Serafin, and H. Bjelkhagen are with the Departments of Chemistry and Biomedical Engineering, Northwestern University, Evanston, IL 60208.

N. H. Abramson is with the Royal Institute of Technology, Industrial Metrology, S-100 44 Stockholm, Sweden.

X. Zhu is with the Department of Chemistry and Biomedical Engineering, Northwestern University, Evanston, IL 60208, on leave from Shanghai Institute of Optics and Fine Mechanics, Academia Sinica, Peoples Republic of China.

IEEE Log Number 8931107.

light pulse by direct time overlap with a reference pulse has evolved.

The method of nonlinear summing of reference and object light frequencies in crystals is routinely used by picosecond spectroscopists [35], [36] to characterize pulse durations. This method [37], [38] was directly used in optical ranging measurements in order to obtain depths of well defined structures inside tissues of the eye and skin [38]. The reference pulse in this case serves to time the reflection delay with an accuracy controlled by the pulse duration. At a particular time delay the apparatus records an intensity proportional to the overlap of reflected signals and the reference pulse. The method maps all reflections in some solid angle, including scatter, and can observe natural enhancements above the scatter.

The intrinsic image possibilities of a two beam interference pattern was invented by Gabor [39] and is known as holographic image formation [40]. Recent research combining the properties of short duration pulses and holography have suggested new ways to capture images with good spatial resolution [41]–[45]. These methods have been described as light-in-flight recording, and they provide the basis for our research. Other nonlinear optical methods may be possible, but they are somewhat more speculative [46].

The idea behind holography is that image information in the optical waves reflected from the object to a photographic plate is contained in the phase of light arriving at the plate. This phase information can be captured by creating an interference pattern on the plate with a reference optical beam. If the phases are coherent over a distance greater than the object, then three-dimensional information is recorded in the interference pattern. Later viewing of the developed plate by a coherent laser will reconstruct the image due to diffraction. A key point about coherence lengths (spatial extent of phase coherence) of the original illuminating laser beam is that short coherence lengths can only create holographic images for a restricted spatial extent of an object. Coherence length l_c and pulse duration t_d are related to the speed of light in one limit; for example, a nominal 1 ps pulse has a coherence length of 0.3 mm in vacuum where $l_c \sim ct_d$ and $c = 3 \times 10^{10}$ cm/s. However, coherence lengths can be much shorter than the pulse duration, and even continuous lasers can have coherence lengths of 100 ps; therefore, we need to define a coherence time τ_c where $l_c = c\tau_c$. With special arrangements even white light can be used to make holographic records of absorption features in a transparency by using a transmission geometry and diffraction gratings to match dispersion on the plate [47], [48].

Light-in-flight recording by holography [42]–[45] can be understood by the basics in the prior paragraph. In this method, a short coherence length pulse is split into two parts and geometrically arranged to both illuminate an object and scan a reference beam across a holographic plate so that holographic images can be formed in a continuous time sequence across the plate. In Fig. 1 we schematically illustrate light-in-flight holography by showing how the

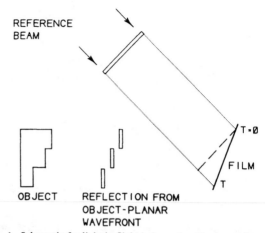

Fig. 1. Schematic for light-in-flight holography. For image formation the pulse reflection must arrive at the plate at the same time as some part of the reference beam.

reflections from the object arrive at the plate so that different slices (defined by the coherence length) arrive at delay times corresponding to the object geometry. These image slices are recorded in a time sequence because the reference beam is sweeping the plate with increasing time delay. The result is a continuous series of holographic images along the plate, each of which is a two-dimensional slice of the object.

CHRONO-COHERENT IMAGING

Introduction

Chrono-coherent imaging is an adaptation of light-in-flight recording to medical imaging. As in light-in-flight holography, the reference pulse and image pulse must arrive at the photographic plate within the coherence time in order to create an image. All other light arriving at a specific area of the plate will not create an image, so very intense scattered light which takes paths leading to a slight shift in arrival time will not affect the image. Short pulse duration freezes motion, but the coherence time of a pulse defines the spatial depth of resolution. Consequently, an intense long duration (~ 1 ms) and a short coherence time (0.1 ps = 0.03 mm) laser pulse can freeze biological motion and resolve short distances defined by the short coherence length.

Unlike light-in-flight recording which is done in air, medical imaging applications have a liquid medium and do not emphasize reflectivity of solid objects. The imaging modality is differential reflectivity or absorption, and it involves the effects of shadows from differential absorption (or differential scattering). In some cases, differential time delay from different refractive indexes in tissue could be important. For example, in a simple transmission geometry each time delayed image is a cumulative result of all effects leading to that time delay. This is a unique type of real image which might use techniques for image reconstruction or deconvolution to create very detailed views of internal objects. Of course, scattered light will increase at later time delays and add more noise to these images. Unlike X rays, one exposure gives a series of different images of the same transmission path, which greatly increases the information content. Also, the method allows research into an optical, lens based, method of selecting a sequence of depth zones; although tomographic techniques are also possible. In addition, the use of tunable lasers in the near infrared allows tuning the image selectivity for types of molecules, such as oxy or deoxy hemoglobin, which can give tissue selectivity and the possibility of cancer screening based on blood enriched cancer types. The major obstacles of CCI are the possible image distortions from refractive index heterogeneity in tissue structures and the low transmission of light through substantial thicknesses of tissue. CCI will remove light scattering as the major barrier in the application of optical wavelengths to imaging inside the body. However, the tissue thickness limits and possible resolution limits of CCI must be determined before estimates of clinical applicability of the method can be made.

Experimental Technique

The experimental arrangement of CCI is very simple. Abramson and Spears [49] have described how single laser pulses can be used for light-in-flight holography. That work used relatively long pulse coherence times of 7 ps to demonstrate the possibilities of a transmission geometry for rejecting scattered light due to differential time delays inside objects.

Fig. 2(a) shows the transmission geometry for clear objects, such as blocks of plastic, to illustrate how the object transmission and coherent reference beam are arranged on the photographic film (or glass plate). A scattering medium, composed of a single diffusing plate on either side of the objects, simulates the problem of recording information about transparent objects inside a scattering medium. In this illustration the reference beam wavefront will impact the holographic recording plate first on one edge and then sweep across the plate. This is how we crate coherent images at successive times. The time delays of the object and reference beam in Fig. 2(a) must be synchronized sufficiently to create a time overlap somewhere on the plate. The pulse length is less than the object thickness and only a very small fraction of the entering pulse intensity arrives at the photographic plate without distortion by scattering. Fig. 2(b) illustrates how unscattered remnants of the original wavefront are delayed by the different object thicknesses to provide three distinct pieces separated by time delays. In a typical experiment with diffuser plates, only a *very small fraction* of the incident laser is not scattered by the plates. The human eye only sees a red, diffuse glow when the combination of two diffuser plates and the objects are illuminated by a He–Ne laser. Absolutely no solid object, let alone transparent objects, can be discerned between the diffuser plates by the human eye under these conditions. The wavefronts of Fig. 2(b) clearly show that the first image at time $T1$ should be interpreted as a shadow of the objects. The next image should be of the upper section of plastic at time $T2$ and the lower object thickness (two thicknesses of plastic) should arrive last at time $T3$. An

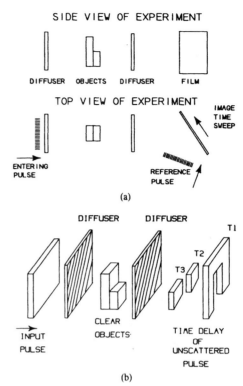

Fig. 2. (a) Transmission geometry for clear objects. The reference beam sweeps across the film coherently recording the wavefront transmitted through the object. (b) Time delay of the planar unscattered wavefront created by different thicknesses of clear objects.

experiment based on this type of geometry [49] confirmed that image information can be recorded in the presence of *overwhelming scattered light*, the image is clear enough to maintain edge boundaries, and time delays of objects only slightly longer than the pulse coherence time can clearly discriminate the object thickness and shape. In water-based tissues the refractive index difference between water and other tissues can be small, consequently the differential time delay going through an object of thickness x with a refractive index difference from water of δn can be calculated as $\delta t = \delta n x / c$ where c is the speed of light. This suggests that subpicosecond coherence times will be required to resolve objects separated only by refractive index time delays. Such short coherence times also will be required to remove scattered light interference from the image formation in a nearly constant refractive index media. However, the tunability of the CCI wavelength allows selective absorption by objects to form absorption shadows. In this application of CCI the scattered light rejection is the main function of a short coherence time.

In the experiments described in this work we emphasize the imaging of absorbing objects inside scattering media. This problem is similar to reading a newspaper in a bottle of milk. In Fig. 3(a) we illustrate the simplest case of an absorbing object creating a "shadow" in the transmitted wavefront. The absorbing object should be considered as an absorption on a diffuse wavefront created by very slight scattering prior to the object. Large scattering angles prior

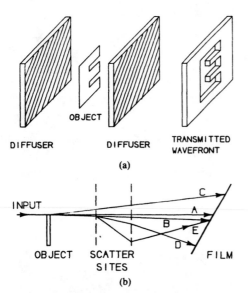

(a)

(b)

Fig. 3. (a) Unscattered planar wavefront transmitted through an absorber between diffusers. (b) Object definition by edge scattering and media scattering. Rays *A*, *B*, and *C* are only scattered by the object edge and rays *D* and *E* are alternative paths for ray *B* which are scattered by the media. Only rays arriving ''simultaneously'' at the film with a reference beam will be coherently recorded.

to the object will not contribute to the coherent image formation because they arrive at different times on the plate. Unfortunately, the picture in Fig. 3(a) distorts the concept of holographic image formation in that the recording of an absorption is not as simple as drawn there. Essentially the coherent recording method will record what your eye would see, but not as a real shadow image, which is what exists in normal photography. In Fig. 3(b) we demonstrate how an object edge is defined by three rays *A*, *B*, and *C*; however, only rays *A* and *B* arrive at the plate within the coherence time of the reference pulse. All three of these rays will define a single point of the object edge in a coherent image formation process; similar to holography, more rays for every point will give a better image. However, because of the short coherence time of the reference beam we reject some useful rays such as *C*. In addition, multiple scattered light such as rays *D* and *E* are no longer defining the object edge, and they serve as background noncoherent exposure. In CCI the reference beam is the equivalent of a fast shutter synchronized to eliminate rays taking different delay times than the desired time. Rays could be scattered prior to encountering the object and still be useful if they all have similar time delay (i.e., coherence) at the object edge so that a diffuse illumination front is created.

From this description we see that three main problems must be addressed:

1) Attenuation of the initial laser intensity.

2) Sufficiently short coherence time to reject scattered light, but still retain object resolution.

3) Extraction of a coherent image from a recording medium which also records the intensity of the scattered light as an incoherent film blackening. We will be discussing details of these points in later sections.

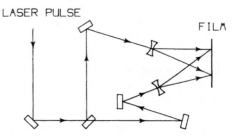

Fig. 4. Schematic for measuring the coherence time of laser pulses in a holographic method.

EXPERIMENTAL APPARATUS

Lasers and Coherence Measurements

The measurement of coherence time for laser pulses, especially single pulse lasers, has not been a common method of laser characterization. We have recently developed a simple holographic method [50] for measurement of single pulse coherence or multiple pulse average coherence, which we use in this work. We have used four types of lasers in our preliminary work on CCI. The lasers vary widely in their pulse durations and coherence properties. We require that the laser pulse coherence be short, although the actual pulse duration can be very long.

The creation of femtosecond pulse durations with equivalent, transform limited pulse coherence is a recent area of technological development. Such femtosecond pulses with perfectly controlled phase would be an ideal light source for coherent imaging; however, in CCI we need a laser with very large energy because there will be great attenuation of laser by the tissue scattering. Consequently, we need to examine the coherence properties of nontransform limited lasers; and in particular we need to control the coherence properties of long duration lasers (~ 1 ms) so that large energies can be transmitted through tissues without risk of damage.

The coherence measurement method uses a setup much like CCI to split a beam into two identical beams and record the time resolved interference between these two beams in a geometry where the reference beam sweeps the film with as much time dispersion as required to accurately record the coherent interference. Fig. 4 shows a schematic drawing of this setup. In typical setups for measuring pulses greater than 3 ps in coherence time we use a crossing angle of $2\beta = 50°$ and two -35 mm focal length lenses to expand the beams large enough to cover the film 60 cm from the lenses. Pulse energies are controlled to ensure exposure in the linear region of the film, which requires 5 $\mu J/cm^2$. The pattern is measured after developing by scanning a 5 mW He–Ne laser on the film. In this geometry the diffraction efficiency versus displacement on the film Δx relate to the relative coherence versus time by

$$\Delta t = 2\Delta x \sin \beta / c \qquad (1)$$

where c is the speed of light in air.

Some results for different lasers are shown in Fig. 5 where the solid line curves represent a Gaussian fit to the

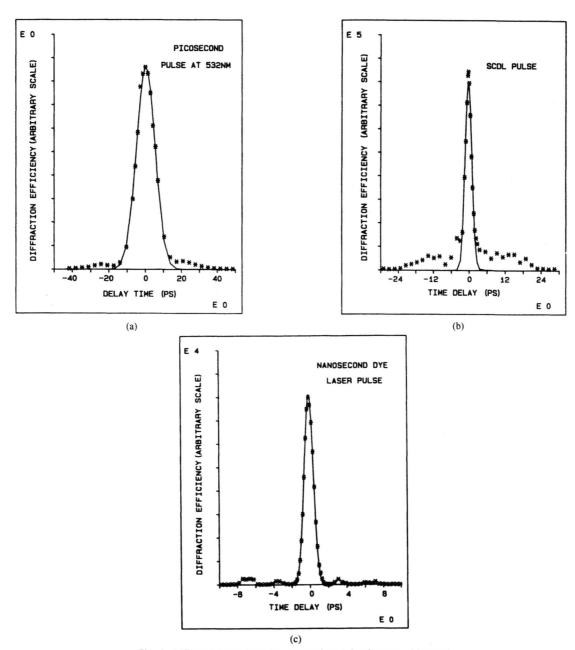

Fig. 5. Diffracted beam intensity versus time delay between object and reference beam. (a) Nd : YAG laser pulse at 532 nm. FWHM of 15 ps with extra coherence wings obtained at full laser power. (b) Short cavity dye laser pulse with a coherence time of 2.6 ps. (c) Five nanosecond dye laser pulse with added time broadening from a diffraction grating which gives an effective coherence time of 1.1 ps.

data. Fig. 5(a) is for the second harmonic of a Nd : YAG laser of Gaussian spatial profile and 9 mJ output energy. The pulse duration of this laser was measured as 28 ps by second harmonic autocorrelation. The coherence time of a single pulse measured by the FWHM of Fig. 5(a) was 15 ps, and fluctuations of ±3 ps were observed on different single shots. The two small bumps to either side of the main coherence peak were observed at the largest laser powers, and demonstrate how pulse coherence relates to laser operation. In this case, the side bumps appear at high power and probably relate to spectral changes due to gain

saturation at high power. We can demonstrate different background effects in a short cavity dye laser (SCDL) pumped by the Nd : YAG laser. Fig. 5(b) demonstrates a narrow coherence time of 2.6 ps for a 22 ps pulse duration. In this case the background coherence fluctuations are not so regular in spacing as the Nd : YAG laser, but they are significant. For the case (not shown) of a CW mode-locked dye laser of 4 ps duration the observed coherence FWHM for an average of 2×10^6 pulses was 2.6 ps, and little background was present.

Fig. 5(c) shows the coherence properties of a 5 ns

pulsed dye laser pumped by a Nd : YAG laser which was operated with no tuning element at 560 nm. This laser had a sufficiently short coherence time that a diffraction grating was necessary to tilt the wavefront of the reference beam, thereby creating a smaller crossing angle between the reference and object wavefronts at the film. This technique is similar to Fig. 4 and was used for the CCI experiments which are described later (see Figs. 8, 9). Interestingly, this laser and our measurement setup show a 1.1 ps effective coherence time for a nominal 5 ns pulse duration. The background coherence noise is not very large, but much larger than the nominal prediction of τ_c/t_d obtained if ideal fourth-order coherence was a dominant effect [50], [51]. This result confirms an earlier suggestion [52] that a dye laser of nanosecond duration can be used to create ultrashort coherence times. Our measurements have shown that the noise under the coherence spike is small; and we have demonstrated CCI with this nanosecond dye laser and the CW mode-locked dye laser (see later section).

It is important to better understand the coherence properties of long duration lasers and how these properties control CCI image limitations, and we are just beginning this process. The spectral width of a laser pulse only can be quantitatively related to its coherence properties for idealized assumptions; consequently, the measurement method we have developed is an important experimental tool. Fig. 6 schematically illustrates how a long duration pulse can be composed of very short coherent subpulses. Here we show two long duration pulses of time t_d composed of N subpulses of coherence time τ_c. Each subpulse effectively acts as a short pulse and the final interference pattern is a cumulative effect of N pulses. Long duration pulses in CCI make it possible for large energies to be transmitted through tissues without damage.

Holographic Film and Developer

We have used Agfa Gevaert holographic film in a 70 mm flexible film format with emulsion 10E56 for 532 and 560 nm lasers and emulsion BC75 for 600 nm lasers. The exposure was in the linear range of the H & D curves of the respective film, which required multiple pulses for some cases. The exposed film had optical density between 0.5 and 2.5. The development chemistry, designated SM-6, was designed by one of us to reduce the reciprocity failure of holograms recorded with short pulses [54].

Film Resolution and Sensitivity Under CCI Conditions

The holographic recording of images in CCI forms a coherent diffraction pattern in the presence of incoherent film blackening by delayed scattered light from tissue. These conditions are not normal holographic conditions, and one expects to lose resolution of the coherent image because of noise from scattered light on the film. In the case of extreme plate blackening one may need to use bleaching chemistry to convert the amplitude hologram into a phase hologram so that enough light can go through the film during reconstruction. We have done one simple

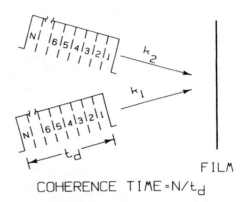

Fig. 6. Laser pulses of duration t_d composed of N coherent subpulses overlapping on film. Subpulses with the same index are coherent.

study to investigate a range of conditions for film illumination.

A single 0.5 mJ pulse at 532 nm and about 8 ps coherence time was used to create an interference pattern from the coherence of the pulse in a geometry like Fig. 4. The object and reference beam intensities were quantitatively measured using a photodiode. We used 70 mm holographic film of type 10E56. Object beam energies were varied from 1.48 $\mu J/cm^2$ down to 0.0041 $\mu J/cm^2$. The reference beam energy was approximately constant at 18.5 $\mu J/cm^2$, this energy was not varied in these preliminary tests. By attenuation of the object beam with neutral density filters the ratio of reference to object energies ranged from 10 : 1 to 4500 : 1. At reference beam to object beam ratios of 10 : 1, 50 : 1, 375 : 1, and 1400 : 1, a range of incoherent scatter levels was tested by using additional pulses from the reference beam alone. Scatter to object ratios of up to 8500 : 1 were tested.

The holograms were developed and then bleached over half of the area to create a clear film with a phase hologram of the coherent image next to an amplitude hologram. The phase hologram was measured in these experiments and agreed with those amplitude holograms which could be directly compared. The bleached film was then scanned with an 8 mW He–Ne laser of 0.5 mm diameter and the diffracted beam intensity was measured over the length of the film with a photodiode and picoammeter. The image recorded is a pulse shape which is related to the coherence time of the laser and geometry of recording, much like Fig. 5(a). Increasing amounts of incoherent light, analogous to scattered light in CCI, cause progressive reduction in our peak amplitude compared with the background noise, which is approximately constant from the particular bleaching chemistry. The width of the image is maintained even up to our largest amounts of scattered light. As we expected, the effects of background scattered light depend on the ratio of reference to object intensity. A weak object beam is similar to expected conditions of CCI where we will have only a small amount of transmitted light; however, in this test we have not done the important optimization of reference intensity which we know will improve the resolution for a given object intensity.

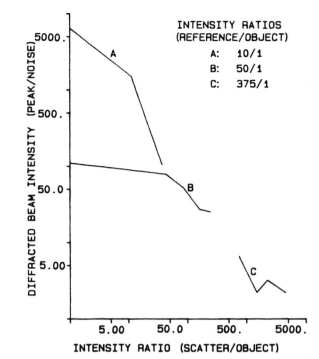

Fig. 7. The ratio of peak intensity to noise in the background as a function of scattered light intensity divided by object intensity. For weaker object beams larger amounts of scatter can be tolerated with reduced values of peak / noise ratio.

In Fig. 7 we have plotted the ratio of peak amplitude to background noise in the image as a function of scattered light. We can observe reasonable values of the amplitude/ background noise ratio for large amounts of scattered light compared to the object light. Interestingly, the human eye can discriminate the image better than our crude method of measurement so that larger amounts of scattered light than shown in Fig. 7 gave discernible diffraction. For the largest amounts of scattered light we measured, the equivalent CCI procedure should give images of absorbing features in the transmission path without requiring signal enhancement techniques.

We have presented some initial film measurements that demonstrate the following relevant points about CCI:

1) Coherent image discrimination above background can be maintained with weak object beam exposures in the presence of high levels of scattered light exposure (1 : 8400 ratio of object to scattered light).

2) The spatial region of coherent interference on the film does not undergo unusual changes when a large amount of background exposure is present.

3) The absolute energy required for an object exposure is very small; however, we have yet to demonstrate *image quality* rather than coherent interference at levels as small as 0.004 $\mu J / cm^2$.

The importance of these data also are reflected in the absolute values of energy/area, even without optimization of the reference beam intensity. For eventual clinical application we might consider using a laser energy of 0.8 J / cm^2 for object exposure. This energy might be attenuated by the object to our currently measured level of

0.004 $\mu J / cm^2$, which is a transmission loss of 9 orders of magnitude. The significance of this dynamic range for estimating tissue thickness limits of CCI are discussed later. Although these data indicate that large levels of scattered light can be tolerated, our initial measurements suggest that scattered light diminishes along with the useful object light so that plate blackening may not be a problem (see next section). Future experiments in tissue models will test this tentative observation and determine the importance of scattered light for particular CCI geometries.

CCI Experiments

Geometry

The geometry of CCI requires that the spread of the coherence time on the film provide a viewing aperture large enough to record a finite object. If the reference beam is to intersect the film at a convenient angle with respect to the object beam, then a simple calculation of the sweep speed of a planar wavefront [see (1)] demonstrates that a very small angle between the object and reference wavefront is required. Due to geometric constraints this is difficult to achieve without additional optical setup or tilting one of the wavefronts relative to its propagation direction. We have chosen to leave the wavefront entering the object at normal incidence to its propagation direction so that scattered light is clearly defined as delayed relative to all points of the wavefront which intersect the object. The reference beam can be tilted by the well known properties of a diffraction grating, which we arrange to increase the sweep speed of the reference beam rather than slow it down as was suggested by other workers for light-in-flight holography [55]. Fig. 8(a) demonstrates how a reflection grating can be used to tilt the wavefront of a beam. The reflection grating formula is given by (2) and the tilt angle by (3).

$$\frac{n\lambda}{d} = \sin \theta_1 + \sin \theta_2 \qquad (2)$$

$$\tan \alpha = \frac{\cos \theta_2}{\sin \theta_1 + \sin \theta_2} \qquad (3)$$

where n is the diffraction order, d is the groove spacing of the grating, and the tilt angle α is defined by the grating properties and geometry. For example, a 1200 1/mm grating with an input wavelength of 560 nm and 40° will have an exit angle θ_2 of 1.67° and a tilt angle of 56.1°.

Fig. 8(b) shows the film position and crossing of the two wavefronts on the film. We can compute the effective sweep speed of the coherent intersection in terms of the film angle relative to each wavefront. This result is given in (4) in terms of F, the distance on the film, and the angles χ_1 and χ_2 which are the wavefront to film angle for object and reference beams, respectively.

$$\frac{F}{\tau_e} = c / \left(\frac{\sin \chi_2}{\sin \alpha} - \frac{\sin \chi_1}{\sin \alpha'} \right). \qquad (4)$$

The effective coherence time τ_e of the pulse then defines the spatial extent of the interference region on the film.

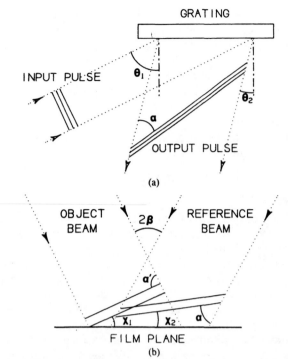

(a)

(b)

Fig. 8. (a) Wavefront tilting with respect to the propagation direction after diffraction by a grating. (b) Object and reference beam wavefronts crossing at the film. The sweep speed on the film can be calculated in terms of the film angle relative to each wavefront.

We define τ_e as an effective coherence time measured in a calibration experiment with a known time delay in half of the object beam. The FWHM of the interference patterns (see Fig. 5) from this measurement define τ_e. For example, for a coherence time of 1 ps, $\chi_1 = 29°$, and $\chi_2 = 33.9°$, the interference region would be 1.6 mm wide using the tilt angle calculated above.

Fig. 9 demonstrates the overall setup of our experiment, with beam expansion occurring before the grating; it was observed that beam expansion after the grating with a large, multielement lens removes the tilt from the wavefront leaving only the dispersive effects. The position of the grating is important for controlling the effects of grating dispersion on the necessarily large frequency bandwidth of the laser pulse. The angle of dispersion σ is given by $\sigma = n \Delta\lambda / d \cos\theta_2$, and the spread at a distance z from the grating is therefore σz. The dispersion occurs perpendicular to the direction of propagation of the beam and therefore at an angle α to the tilted wavefront. This results in an increase in the coherence time of the reference beam $\Delta\tau_c = \sigma z / \tan\alpha$. For example, for a half-bandwidth of 3.4 nm and a 1200 1/mm grating there will be a 10 ps increase in coherence time due to dispersion for a grating placed 1100 mm from the film. Since it is necessary to work in the subpicosecond coherence range for the CCI method, we desire a minimum dispersion by selection of the grating parameters and a grating placement close to the film. In our case we have used a grating of 1200 1/mm in first order with a distance from the film of 110 mm, resulting in an increase in coherence time of 1 ps. The effective coherence time was measured to be 1.1 ps in this geom-

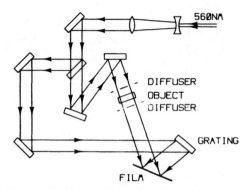

Fig. 9. Geometry for Chrono-Coherent Imaging which minimizes the dispersive effects of the reflection grating.

etry indicating that the majority of the coherence spread is due to dispersion and not the intrinsic laser coherence which could be ~ 0.1 ps. It would obviously be advantageous to eliminate the diffraction grating and therefore significantly reduce our coherence time. In future experiments, the reference beam either will arrive from behind the film (similar to reflection holographic recording) or will reflect from a beamsplitter placed between the object and the film. These methods will achieve the small angle between reference and object beam necessary to spread out the interference pattern without the use of the grating.

In the geometry of Fig. 9 the spread of the coherence length on the film controls the size of the object which can be recorded on the film, while the effective coherence length controls the degree of scattered light rejection. The relationship between object size, coherence length on the film, and viewing size is demonstrated in Fig. 10(a) and in (5) and (6).

$$\cos\delta = L/(L + c\tau_e) \tag{5}$$

$$V = F + 2(L + c\tau_e)\sin\delta. \tag{6}$$

For example, in our experiment $\tau_e = 1.1$ ps, $L = 30$ cm, and $F = 2$ mm. This would result in a maximum object size of 3.0 cm. However, since the interference pattern on the film F acts as an aperture through which the image is viewed by the observer, the actual maximum object size V' is determined by the point of observation. This is shown in Fig. 10(b), and calculations use (6) with V', δ' instead of V, δ, where δ' is defined by (7) and $\delta' \leq \delta$.

$$\tan\delta' = F/2Y. \tag{7}$$

The observation point Y has a minimum value which can include the complete region F on the film and the object size V. This minimum value is computed from (7) with $\delta' = \delta$. Larger values of Y give a smaller object size V' when viewed through a region F on the film. Equation (8) can be used to compute V' if Y is understood to be greater than the minimum value.

$$V' = F(1 + L/Y) \tag{8}$$

Absorbing Objects Inside Scattering Media

The objective of our first experiment was to demonstrate that a coherence time on the order of 1 ps will ef-

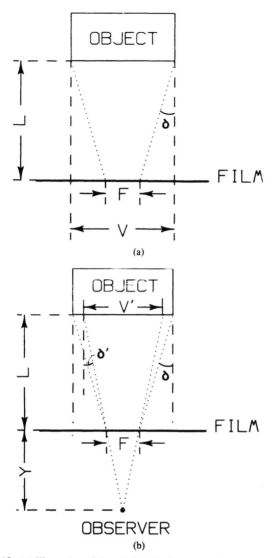

Fig. 10. (a) Illustration of the relationship between coherence spread on the film F object size V and object distance from the film L. (b) The position of the observer further limits the maximum object size for a given coherence spread on the film. The dimension Y is the distance from the observers eye to the film.

ficiently remove scattered light from a transmission geometry in which an absorbing object is completely unresolved by normal visual methods. We will also show that multiple pulses, each of coherence time much shorter than the pulse length and of very low energy will additively form a useful hologram in the CCI method. Fig. 9 shows that two ground glass diffuser plates are used to obscure a black letter E (8 mm high with a linewidth of 2.5 mm) which is mounted between them. We used a 560 nm nanosecond dye laser at 10 Hz with an effective coherence time (FWHM of the overlap pattern) after the grating of 1.1 ps. The laser energy was about 10 mJ per pulse; after beam expansion, the object was illuminated with approximately 0.7 mJ/cm^2/pulse, and the reference beam was approximately 0.1 μJ/cm^2/pulse at the film. The object beam intensity was slightly less than the reference beam intensity at the film, indicating a 10^4 loss due

to scatter through the diffuser plates. The film was Agfa Gevaert 10E56 and the exposure was 1 s or 10 pulses. The scattered light which gave an incoherent plate blackening was not severe and no bleaching was required.

The results of this experiment are shown in Fig. 11. Fig. 11(a) shows a photograph of the object as it appears to the eye illuminated with white light. Absolutely no sign of the object is visible. Fig. 11(b) is a photograph of the CCI image of the letter E as viewed with an expanded He–Ne laser. The image is clearly the letter E, now quite visible by the CCI method. A similar experiment was completed using a CW mode-locked dye laser with only 2.4 mW/cm^2 power and a coherence time of 2.1 ps. The longer coherence time and lower energy resulted in longer exposure times and a dimmer image covered with more scatter.

From this experiment, we can conclude that CCI removes scattered light which normally obscures object information. We have demonstrated how to tilt the reference wavefront, and thereby spread out the interference pattern on the film to image objects whose spatial extent is much larger than the coherence length of the laser. Also, we have used a pulse train of weak pulses to create a hologram additively. This is important because longer duration pulsed lasers or a series of pulses with short coherence times are practical directions for technical development of a clinical system.

A second experiment was performed to estimate the maximum tissue thickness through which CCI can be performed. To do this, we used a tissue phantom of known optical properties. We then experimentally determined the maximum thickness of this phantom through which a coherent image could be formed with our low laser energy. The diffuse transmittance of this thickness was then calculated and related to actual tissue data. Extrapolation to larger laser energies yields an estimate of the tissue thickness limits of CCI.

The tissues phantom was 0.133 mm thick slabs of paraffin (Parafilm) pressed together to act as a continuous medium. Grossweiner *et al.* measured the optical properties of the Parafilm for us. They previously have measured optical constants of animal and plant tissues [56] and used tissue models [57] to determine losses due to scattering and absorption. The model uses the one-dimensional diffusion approximation to determine scattering and absorption coefficients (s and k, respectively) from measured reflectance and transmittance. The computer program also performs the inverse calculation of diffuse transmittance and reflectance for various thicknesses and a given s and k. This allows comparison of tissue types or comparison of phantoms to actual tissue thicknesses. The scattering and absorption coefficients of Parafilm were measured for a three slab (0.399 mm) thickness. The diffuse transmittance was calculated and then expanded to any thickness by $t^{n/3}$ where n is the number of slabs of parafilm.

In our experiment, an absorbing object was placed in the center of the Parafilm layers and a holographic image

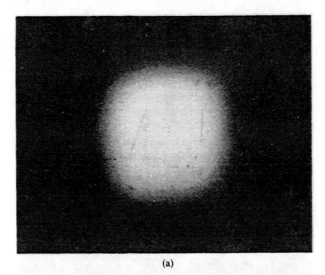

(a)

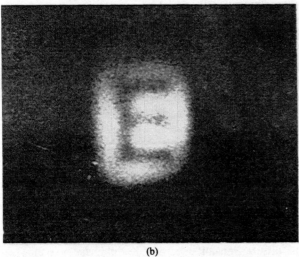

(b)

Fig. 11. (a) Photograph of absorbing object through diffuser plates illuminated from behind with white light. The object is a letter *E* and it is obscured by scattered light. (b) Photograph of a hologram of the object prepared by the CCI method. Object is visible due to scattered light rejection.

was formed using the CCI method. Additional layers of Parafilm were added until the image became very dim. The object was a black letter "*C*" 1 cm high with a 0.2 cm linewidth. The laser was a modelocked CW dye laser with the tuning element removed. The energy of the object beam was 0.08 mJ/cm^2 with a 0.2 s exposure time. The image was clearly the letter "*C*" but was somewhat dimmer than the "*E*" in Fig. 11(b). This was due to the short exposure time which was required to prevent vibrational stability problems. We were unable to do any resolution tests, such as a resolution chart, because of the extremely low energy available. The final Parafilm thickness was 28 slabs of Parafilm with the "*C*" at the center of the medium.

The diffuse transmittance of this Parafilm thickness was then calculated using the measured optical properties. The diffuse transmittance of 28 slabs of Parafilm was computed to be 2.4×10^{-2}. The optical constants for leg dermis [58] and breast tissue [32] were used to determine equivalent tissue thicknesses. These were calculated to be 2.6 mm and 1.8 cm for leg dermis and normal breast tissue, respectively.

In order to extrapolate these data to determine the limits of CCI, the possibility of damage to the skin must be considered. The American National Standards Institute (ANSI Z136.1-1986) indicates that no damage will occur to skin from a 1 ms duration, 694.3 nm pulse with 0.2 J/cm^2 energy, or from a 1 ms duration, 1064 nm pulse with 1.0 J/cm^2 energy. Since we will be working at wavelengths where absorption is low, we will assume 0.8 J/cm^2 as our safe limit for these calculations. Theoretically, this would make imaging possible through 6.4 cm of breast tissue, or 2.6 mm of leg dermis plus 4.6 cm of breast tissue. However, this extrapolation does not consider the ultimate resolution because we have only used a coarse object rather than a resolution chart. Tests using full thickness phantoms are required to define CCI limits.

In summary, CCI will give useful images over significant thicknesses of tissue. A single laser pulse of less than 1 ms duration can be used to freeze biological motion and give a two-dimensional image which is easy to analyze by direct visual observation. Imaging through several centimeters of breast tissue could be very useful in clinical applications; however, our initial experiments could not determine resolution for thick tissue phantoms. Resolution losses could further limit the potential of CCI for thick samples. In the event that only thin tissue samples are possible when high resolution is required, reflection geometries could be used. Reflection geometries also might be used to image over 3 cm deep with lower resolution, which would make many more applications possible.

CONCLUSIONS

CCI has been demonstrated as a new method of imaging objects inside a scattering medium. In our development of chrono-coherent imaging we have analyzed transmission image formation in a particular geometric set up of CCI, and also characterized some properties of lasers and holographic media for this application. For a test experiment we formed an image of a normally unobservable letter *E* positioned between scattering plates. The successful image recording of the letter by CCI demonstrates that CCI can overcome strong attenuation of a laser beam by scattering and create a coherent image of light transmission through absorbing objects in the presence of strong scattered light. Tissue estimates indicate that CCI could be quite useful in many clinical situations. The main features of a new imaging technique for medicine have been identified and tested in this work. Further development of medical applications will now be directed to more exact tissue simulations and actual tissue samples.

ACKNOWLEDGMENT

We would like to thank Prof. B. Sullivan of Northwestern for comments on image formation models.

REFERENCES

[1] S. M. Donn and L. R. Kuhns, *Pediatric transillumination*. Chicago, IL: Year Book Medical, 1983.

[2] L. Calliauw, "The value of transillumination of the skull in neurological examination of neonates and infants," *Acta Neurochir*, vol. 10, pp. 75-91, 1961.

[3] R. A. W. Lehman *et al.*, "Cystic intracranial teratoma in an infant," *J. Neurosurg.*, vol. 33, pp. 334-338, 1970.

[4] J. N. Rozovski *et al.*, "Cranial transillumination in early and severe malnutrition," *Brit. J. Nutr.*, vol. 25, pp. 107-111, 1971.

[5] G. W. Nixon, "Congenital porencephaly," *Pediatrics*, vol. 54, pp. 43-50, 1974.

[6] J. S. Haller, "Skull transillumination," in *Neonatal Neurology*, M. C. Coleman. Baltimore, MD: University Park, 1981.

[7] S. M. Donn *et al.*, "Rapid detection of neonatal intracranial hemorrhage by transillumination," *Pediatrics*, vol. 64, pp. 843-847, 1979.

[8] A. J. Martin *et al.*, "Production of a permanent radiographic record of transillumination of the neonate," *Radiol.*, vol. 122, pp. 540-541, 1977.

[9] M. Johns, "Transillumination of the infant skull," *J. Audiovisual Media Med.*, vol. 2, pp. 140-149, 1979.

[10] S. R. Arridge, M. Cope, P. van der Zee, P. J. Hillson, and D. T. Delpy, "Visualization of the oxygenation state of brain and muscle in newborn infants by near infra-red transillumination," *Information Processing in Medical Imaging*, S. L. Bacherach, Ed. Dordrecht: Martinus Nijhoff, 1985, pp. 155-176.

[11] L. R. Kuhns *et al.*, "Diagnosis of pneumothorax or pneumomediastinum in the neonate by transillumination," *Pediatrics*, vol. 56, pp. 355-360, 1975.

[12] J. R. Buck *et al.*, "Fiberoptic transillumination—A new tool for the pediatric surgeon," *J. Pediat. Surg.*, vol. 12, pp. 451-463, 1977.

[13] D. B. Shurtleff *et al.*, "Clinical use of transillumination," *Arch. Dis. Child.*, vol. 41, pp. 183-187, 1966.

[14] H. C. Mofenson and J. Greensher, "Transillumination of the abdomen in infants," *Amer. J. Dis. Child.*, vol. 115, pp. 428-431, 1968.

[15] J. J. Wedge *et al.*, "Abdominal masses in the newborn: 63 cases," *J. Urol.*, vol. 106, pp. 770-775, 1971.

[16] F. O. Evans *et al.*, "Sinusitis of the maxillary antrum," *New Eng. J. Med.*, vol. 293, pp. 735-739, 1975.

[17] L. Goldman, "Transillumination as a diagnostic aid," *Arch. Dermatol.*, vol. 112, p. 262, 1976.

[18] A. Daneshwar *et al.*, "Transventricular illumination," *Ann. Thorac. Surg.*, vol. 28, pp. 94-95, 1979.

[19] M. Cutler, "Transillumination as an aid in the diagnosis of breast lesions, Surgery," *Gynecol. Obstet.*, vol. 48, pp. 721-729, 1929.

[20] B. Ohlsson, J. Gunderson, and D. G. Nilsson, "Diaphanography: A method for evaluation of the female breast," *World Journal Surg.*, vol. 4, pp. 701-707, 1980.

[21] E. Carlsen, "Transillumination light scanning," *Diagnostic Imaging*, vol. 4, pp. 28-60, 1982.

[22] D. J. Watmough, "Transillumination of breast tissues: Factors governing optimal imaging of lesions," *Radiol.*, vol. 147, pp. 89-92, 1983.

[23] M. F. McIntosh, "Breast light scanning: A real time breast imaging modality," *Journal de l'Association Canadienne des Radiologistes*, vol. 34, pp. 288-290, 1983.

[24] R. J. Bartrum and H. C. Crow, "Transillumination lightscanning to diagnose breast cancer: a feasibility study," *Amer. J. Roentgenol.*, vol. 142, pp. 409-414, 1984.

[25] V. Marshall, D. C. Williams, and K. D. Smith, "Diaphanography as a means of detecting breast cancer," *Radiol.*, vol. 150, pp. 339-343, 1984.

[26] C. R. B. Merritt, M. A. Sullivan, A. Segaloff, and W. P. McKinnon, "Real time transillumination light scanning of the breast," *Radiograph.*, vol. 4, pp. 989-1009, 1984.

[27] B. Drexler, J. L. Davis, and G. Schofield, "Diaphanography in the diagnosis of breast cancer," *Radiol.*, vol. 157, pp. 41-44, 1985.

[28] G. E. Geslien, J. R. Fisher, and C. Delaney, "Transillumination in breast cancer detection: screening failures and potential," *Amer. J. Roentgenol.*, vol. 144, pp. 619-622, 1985.

[29] H. Wallberg, A. Alveryd, P. Sundelin, and S. Troell, "The value of diaphanography as an adjunct to mammography in breast diagnostics," *Acta-Chir-Scand, (Suppl)*, vol. 530, pp. 83-87, 1986.

[30] F. L. Greene, C. Hicks, V. Eddy, and C. Davis, "Mammography, sonomammography, and diaphanography (lightscanning). A comparative study with histologic correlation," *Amer. Surg.*, vol. 51, pp. 58-60, 1985.

[31] R. F. Girolamo and J. V. Gaythorpe, "Clinical diaphanography—its present perspective," *CRC-Crit. Rev. Oncol. Hematol.*, vol. 2, pp. 1-31, 1984.

[32] S. Ertefai and A. E. Profio, "Spectral transmittance and contrast in breast diaphanography," *Med. Phys.*, vol. 12, pp. 393-400, 1985.

[33] P. C. Jackson, P. H. Stevens, J. H. Smith, D. Kear, H. Key, and P. N. T. Wells, "The development of a system for transillumination computed tomography," *Brit. J. Radio.*, vol. 60, pp. 375-380, 1987.

[34] M. A. Duguay and A. T. Mattick, "Ultrahigh speed photography of picosecond light pulses and echoes," *Appl. Opt.*, vol. 10, pp. 2162-2170, 1971.

[35] H. Park, M. Chodorow and R. Kompfner, "High resolution optical ranging system," *Appl. Opt.*, vol. 20, pp. 2389-2394, 1981.

[36] H. Mahr and M. D. Hirsch, "An optical up-conversion light gate with picosecond resolution," *Opt. Comm.*, vol. 13, pp. 96-99, 1975.

[37] A. P. Bruckner, "Picosecond light scattering measurements of cataract microstructure," *Appl. Opt.*, vol. 17, pp. 3177-3183, 1978.

[38] J. G. Fujimoto, S. De Silvestri, E. P. Ippen, C. A. Puliafito, R. Margolis, and A. Oseroff, "Femtosecond optical ranging in biological systems," *Opt. Lett.*, vol. 11, pp. 150-152, 1986.

[39] D. Gabor, "A new microscopic principle," *Nature*, vol. 161, p. 77-1948; D. Gabor, "Microscopy by reconstructed wavefronts," *Proc. Roy. Soc.*, A197, p. 454, 1949.

[40] R. J. Collier, C. B. Burckhardt, and L. H. Lin, *Optical Holography*, New York: Academic, 1971.

[41] D. I. Staselko, Y. N. Denisyuk, and A. G. Smirnov, "Holographic recording of the time-coherence pattern of a wave train from a pulsed laser source," *Opt. Spectroscopy Eng.*, vol. 26, pp. 225-229, 1969.

[42] N. Abramson, "Light-in-flight recording: High-speed holographic motion pictures of ultrafast phenomena," *Appl. Opt.*, vol. 22, pp. 215-231, 1983.

[43] ——, "Light-in-flight recording by holography," *Opt. Lett.*, vol. 3, pp. 121-123, 1978.

[44] ——, "Light-in-flight recording. 2: Compensation for the limited speed of the light used for observation," *Appl. Opt.*, vol. 23, pp. 1481-1492, 1984.

[45] ——, "Light-in-flight recording. 4: Visualizing optical relativistic phenomena," *Appl. Opt.*, vol. 24, pp. 3323-3329, 1985.

[46] H. J. Gerritsen, "Holography and four-wave mixing to see through the skin," SPIE, vol. 519; *Anal. Opt. Proc.*, pp. 128-131, 1984.

[47] E. N. Leith and B. J. Chang, "Space-invariant holography with quasi-coherent light," *Appl. Optics*, vol. 12, pp. 1957-1963, 1973.

[48] E. N. Leith, D. Angell, and C. P. Kuei, "Superresolution by incoherent-to-coherent conversion," *J. Opt. Soc. Amer. A*, vol. 4, pp. 1050-1054, 1987.

[49] N. H. Abramson and K. G. Spears, "Single pulse light-in-flight recording by holography," *Appl. Opt.*, to be published.

[50] X. Zhu, K. G. Spears, and J. Serafin, "Ultrashort pulsed laser coherence measurements by single pulse holography and four-wave mixing," *J. Opt. Soc. Amer. B*, to be published.

[51] H. J. Trebino, E. K. Gustafson, and A. E. Siegman, "Fourth-order partial-coherence effects in the formation of integrated-intensity gratings with pulsed light sources," *J. Opt. Soc. Amer. B*, vol. 3, pp. 1295-1304, 1986.

[52] H. Nakatsuka, M. Tomita, M. Fujiwara, and S. Asaka, "Subpicosecond photon echoes by using nanosecond laser pulses," *Optics Comm.*, vol. 52, pp. 150-152, 1984.

[53] J. E. Golub and T. W. Mossberg, "Studies of picosecond collisional dephasing in atomic sodium vapor using broad-bandwidth transient four-wave mixing," *J. Opt. Soc. Amer. B*, vol. 3, pp. 554-559, 1986.

[54] H. Bjelkhagen, private communication from prior work.

[55] N. Abramson, S.-G. Pettersson, and H. Bergstrom, "Light-in-flight recording 5: theory on slowing down the faster-than-light motion of the light-shutter," *Appl. Opt.*, 1988.

[56] J. L. Karagiannes, Z. Zhang, B. Grossweiner, and L. I. Grossweiner, "Applications of the one-dimensional diffusion approximation to the optics of tissues and tissue models," *Appl. Opt.*, to be published.

[57] S. L. Jacques and S. A. Prahl, "Modeling optical and thermal distributions in tissue during laser irradiation," *Laser Surg. Med.*, vol. 6, p. 494, 1987.

[58] S. L. Jacques, C. A. Alter, and S. A. Prahl, "Angular dependence of HeNe laser light scattering by human dermis," *Laser Life Sci.*, vol. 1, p. 309, 1987.

Kenneth G. Spears received the Ph.D. degree in physical chemistry in 1970 from the University of Chicago, Chicago, IL.

He is currently an Associate Professor of Chemistry and Biomedical Engineering at Northwestern University, Evanston, IL. He has developed picosecond lasers, near infrared lasers, and has worked on laser interactions with molecules since 1972. He was awarded an Alfred P. Sloan Foundation Fellowship in 1974 and has authored over 60 peer-reviewed papers in a variety of fields. He is also a laser research consultant to Illinois Masonic Hospital and the Chicago Institute of Neuroscience and Neuroresearch.

Dr. Spears is a board member of the Midwest Biolaser Institute.

Jenifer Serafin received the B.S. degree in chemical engineering from the University of Boulder, CO, and the Master's degree in biomedical engineering from Northwestern University, Evanston, IL in May 1989. Her research was concentrated on medical applications of lasers.

Nils H. Abramson is currently a Professor with the Royal Institute of Technology, Industrial Metrology, Stockholm, Sweden. He has published over 100 papers on holography and holds 20 patents.

Xinming Zhu, photograph and biography not available at the time of publication.

Hans Bjelkhagen received the Ph.D. degree in industrial metrology from the Royal Institute of Technology, Stockholm, Sweden in 1978.

He is an Associate Professor of Biomedical Engineering at Northwestern University, Evanston, IL, and serves as a consultant to the Wenske Laser Center, Ravenswood Hospital. He has authored over 50 papers and holds a number of patents.

EXPERIMENTAL VERIFICATION OF IMAGE DETECTION IN HIGHLY SCATTERING MEDIA USING ANTENNA PROPERTIES OF OPTICAL HETERODYNE MICROSCOPE SCHEME

Indexing terms: Image processing, Microscopes and microscopy

The spatial resolution capability for image detection in the presence of strong scattering inside a medium is verified by virtue of the antenna properties of the optical heterodyne method. The image formation of test microletters in a highly scattering solution is successfully achieved using an optical heterodyne scanning microscope.

An optical heterodyne system is recognised to be both a receiver and an antenna.[1,2] Its antenna properties can provide not only high spatial resolution for detection and image formation but also excellent directivity to distinguish between specific directions. The technology proposed utilises the optical heterodyne method to achieve image detection in highly scattering absorptive media. The conventional direct detection technique can not be employed because of the presence of widely dispersive multiple scattering. This heterodyning method offers advantages for the application to highly scattering absorptive media like biological tissues, systems and substances as well as various objects and environments surrounded or covered by smoke, fog, cloud, etc. No experimental study of these features of the optical heterodyne method have been reported. We are pursing the basic studies on image detection in highly scattering absorptive media, aimed the optical computed tomography (OCT) or laser sensing tomography (LST) for noninvasive and noncontact biological measurements.[3,4]

This letter reports the detection principle and experimental results of the evaluation of the spatial resolution capability and the image detection of a test sample in highly scattering media based on the antenna properties of the optical heterodyne method.

Fig. 1 shows the experimental arrangement. The output beam of a single-wavelength He–Ne laser at 632·8 nm with

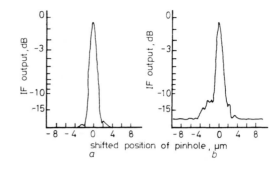
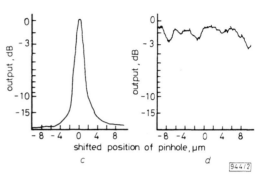

Fig. 2 *Relative intensity distribution of IF output*

  a Without ground glass
  b With ground glass
  c Conventional technique without ground glass
  d Conventional technique with ground glass

about 2 mW output power is divided in two paths by a beam splitter. One passes through an acousto-optic modulator to cause a frequency shift by 80 MHz. This signal beam is then focussed on the sample by a microscope objective lens. The other one serving as a local oscillator beam passes through an acousto-optic modulator and is shifted in frequency by 81 MHz. A pinhole of 2 μm in diameter is installed in the signal beam path so that it can be shifted across the beam by means of a PZT pusher. An IF output signal from the photomultiplier tube is amplified and electronically filtered. It is then recorded as a function of the shifted position of the

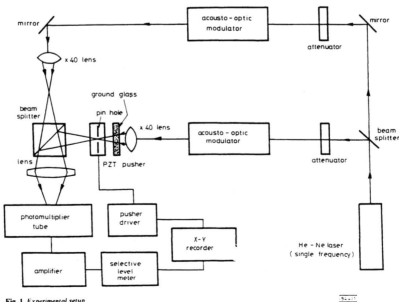

Fig. 1 *Experimental setup*

pinhole with respect to the optical beam axis. To disturb the wavefront of signal beam, a ground glass is placed in front of the pinhole.

In Fig. 2, the results measured by this optical heterodyne microscope method are presented to evaluate the capability of spatial resolution. Before the ground glass, an objective lens of magnification ×40 was used for the signal beam and the estimated value of signal beam spot size was approximately 1·3 μm. In the direct detection, only the signal beam frequency-shifted by an acousto-optic modulator was employed. In Fig. 2a, the intensity distribution of the IF output without the ground glass is depicted. Fig. 2b shows the IF output with the ground glass. Fig. 2c shows the intensity distribution measured by the direct detection method without the ground glass. Fig. 2d is the result with the ground glass.

In both the cases of Figs. 2a and b, the FWHM was measured to be 1·45 μm and are equal to the theoretical value in this heterodyning scheme. The FWHM for the intensity profile of Fig. 2c was about 2 μm which is almost the same with the pinhole diameter. No signal was detected by the direct detection technique when the ground glass had been placed as seen in Fig. 2d. These results demonstrate that the optical heterodyne method realises the ability to distinguish the original beam in the presence of strong scattering or migration in the propagating medium.

We performed an image detection experiment employing a setup similar to that shown in Fig. 1 except for the scanning and image display operations. A sample transmitting the focused laser beam was scanned using a X–Y PZT pusher. The driving signal of the PZT pusher was a X–Y scanning signal from an oscilloscope, and the Z input to the oscilloscope was modulated by an envelope signal on the IF output. The test sample was a photographic film on which three micro-letters 'BIO' had been arranged. The original size of this image was about 70 μm in length and about 30 μm in height. This image film was inserted in a glass cell filled with a milk–water mixed solution. The thickness of solution was kept at 1 mm both in front and at the back of the film.

Fig. 3a shows an original photograph of the sample image taken with a conventional microscope. This image is not so clear because a green filter was usually used in the microscope. In Fig. 3b, the image detected by the optical heterodyne microscope method without the solution in the cell is illustrated for comparison. Figs. 3c and d show the detected images by the same method for the mixed solutions of 20% and 33% milk in water, respectively. Fig. 3e is the result for a 20% milk solution measured by a conventional microscope. No image is detected. These optical heterodyne microscope images, Fig. 3c and d, can achieve similar quality with resolution as good as the detected image without a strong light-scattering medium like Fig. 3b.

In conclusion, we have evaluated the spatial resolution capability for image formation in highly scattering media utilising the optical heterodyne method. The conventional direct detection technique creates severe practical problems. The

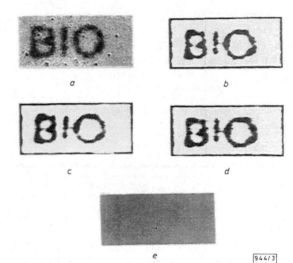

Fig. 3 *Comparison of detected images*

a Original image
b No solution
c 20% milk solution
d 33% milk solution
e Conventional technique with 20% milk solution

successful image detection of the test sample by the optical heterodyne scanning scheme demonstrates that this method can overcome the diffuse nature of an image in the presence of strong scattering and even large attenuation in the medium.

M. TOIDA*   12th March 1990
M. KONDO†
T. ICHIMURA†
H. INABA*,†

* INABA Biophoton Project
Research Development Corporation of Japan
Yagiyama-Minami 2-1-1, Taihaku-ku, Sendai 982, Japan

† Research Institute of Electrical Communication
Tohoku University, Katahira 2-1-1, Aoba-ku, Sendai 980, Japan

References

1 CORCORAN, V. J.: 'Directional characteristics in optical heterodyne detection processes', *J. Appl. Phys.*, 1965, **36**, pp. 1819–1825
2 SIEGMAN, A. E.: 'The antenna properties of optical heterodyne receivers', *Appl. Opt.*, 1966, **5**, pp. 1588–1594
3 TOIDA, M., KONDO, M., and INABA, H.: 'Optical heterodyne technique for achieving excellent image detection in highly sealtering media such as biological substances and tissues'. OSA Annual Meeting, 1989 Tech. Dig. Series, Vol. 18, Paper F16, p. 223
4 TOIDA, M., KONDO, M., ICHIMURA, T., and INABA, H.: 'Research and development for optical computer tomography based on optical heterodyne detection scheme as a new measurement method of biological tissues and systems', *J. Japan Soc. Laser Medicine*, 1989, **10**, pp. 51–54 (in Japanese)

Reprinted from *Photon Migration and Imaging in Random Media and Tissues,* Proc.
SPIE Vol. 1888, pp. 69-75 (1993). ©1993 SPIE.

Imaging of oblique structures in scattering media by time-gated viewing and coherence imaging (CI)

Jürgen Beuthan, Klaus Dörschel, Gerhard Müller, Olaf Minet, Bernd Messer

Laser-Medizin-Zentrum an der Freien Universität Berlin, Krahmerstr. 6-10, D 1000 - Berlin 45

ABSTRACT

Comperative measurements were undertaken in imaging of oblique structures in scattering media.

First: An experimental set-up is described for an optically switched ps-radar. Hereby, laser pulses with duration of 3 ps are used to illuminate the object and an optically switched Kerr-gate which is selecting the light pulses scattered by the object (blood-vessel-phantom). The power of the set-up is demonstrated by the identification of this phantom embedded in several kinds of human tissue. The depth of observation was found in the range of 2 mm to 5 mm.

Second: The coherence imaging (CI) is a new technique for non-invasive cross-sectional imaging of biological structure based on low coherence interferometry. In a modified Mach-Zehnder-Interferometer we positioned a phantom (tray with Intralipid solution with test structure inside). The transmitted photons were optically modulated. These marked "coherent photons" were detected during an on-dimensional scan through the test structure in the scattering media.

1. INTRODUCTION

Light propagation in biological tissue specially in the near infrared (600 to 1300 nm) has become a field of evergrowing interest. The improving the curacy in measuring the optical tissue parameters yields improve possibilities to develop optical imaging techniques in medical diagnostics. The goal is not simply to replace traditional X-ray imaging, but also to gain new additional diagnostic informations based on the results of tissue optics. It has been shown for example that in case on inflammation or soft tissues the value of the scattering coefficient is increased whilst X-ray and MRI is not able to provide such sensitive results as well.[1] This paper therefore will discuss various possibilities of optical imaging and their limitations.

2. OPTICALLY SWITCHED ps-RADAR

Ultrafast optical gates have been realized with gate times down to 10^{-13} s by using various effects of non-linear optics and ps- and fs-laser pulses.[2,3] First results have been reported by Duguay et al.[4] and Diels et al..[5] Because of their two-dimensional switching behaviour Kerr-gates are most preferable. Therefore we developed an experimental set-up using ps-laser pulses to switch the gate and hence to immage oblique structures in tissue.[6] To reduce the scattering halo for imaging of oblique structures in tissue an experimental set-up as shown in Fig. 1 has been developed. The ultra fast light pulse has been generated by a Nd:glass laser system. The light of the pulse is splitting in two parts of the beam now. One part of the beam switches the Kerr-gate whilst the second beam illuminates the sample. The scattered and reemitted light from the sample is imaged through the Kerr-gate onto an image intensifier module. Using an optical delay line the trigger to switch the Kerr-gate can be varied.

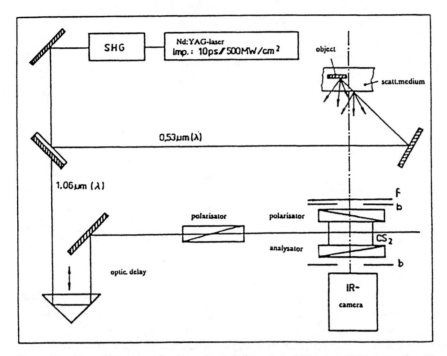

Fig. 1. Experimental set-up for imaging in biological tissue. b - diaphragm, f - filter.

As a light source a Nd:phosphate-glass laser (mode-lock regime) has been used. The repetition-frequence was 0,1 Hz with 40 mode-locking pulses each. Using an electro-optic gate single pulses will be extracted. For further reduction of the pulse length this pulse passed an absorber, which is composed out of AlCl-Tetrazaporphin, Nitrobenzine and Lewis acid. The resulting pulse length is approximately 3 ps. Each invidual pulse has an energy of 12 mJ. Using a KDP crystal the first harmonic (λ = 527 nm) is generated to illiminate the sample. The fundamental pulse λ = 1054 nm switches the Kerr-gate. The Kerr-gate itself is nothing else than a cuvette with CS_2 with a thickness of 5 mm placed between cross polarizes. Furthermore two diaphragms have been aligned which fit the diameter of the birefringenous zone (approx. 8 mm ϕ). A combination of a low-pass filter (BG 18) and a dielectric mirror supresses the switching pulse sufficiently with respect to the image intensifier. The optical delays are managed by use of a triple-prism. The timing behaviour of the optical gate determines the quality of the image. Therefore the system response function T(r,t) has been calculated.

$$T(r,t) = T_0 \cdot \sin^2 [\delta\varphi (r,t)/2]$$

whereby the phase delay function is given by:

$$\delta\varphi(r,t) = \delta\varphi(t) \exp-(r^2/w^2)$$

and the time-depending phase delay can be written as

$$\delta(t) = \frac{2\pi L n_2}{\lambda_T \tau} \int_{-\infty}^{t} [E_s^2 (t')] \exp \left(\frac{t-t'}{\cdot \tau} \right) dt'$$

Furthermore as we taken into account:
- the beam profile is gaussian
- $[E_s^2 (t)]$: the time-averaged value of the electric field of the gate pulse
- T_0 - maximum transmission of the gate
- L - interaction, w - beam radius, n_2 - non-linear refractive index, τ - relaxation time of the Kerr-medium

Fig. 2 shows the system function T(t) at various positions within the aperture.

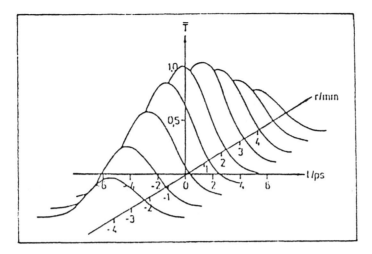

Fig. 2. T(t) of the optical gate (OCS) at various points within the aperture (the graph is normalized to T(t,r=0)).

Table 1 shows the results of the optimal parameters of the optical controlled switch (OCS):

Table 1   Parameter of the OCS

gate time	~ 5 ps
dynamic range D_{max}	400
transmission T_{0max}	0.04
T of the closed OCS	10^{-4}
intensity of the switching pulse	~ 350 MW/cm^2

The recording of the images has been performed by use of a high sensitive photographic film NP 27. For alignment of the experimental set-up a CCD-array of an optical multi channel analyzer has been used.

Fig. 3 shows a sketch of the sample. In a closed Quartz-cuvette a blood vessel (1,5 mm u PE-catheter filled with heparinized blood) is embedded between two 5 mm thick slices of brain tissue. The optical delay line has been adjusted in two different positions, first to detect the reemitted light out of bulk tissue, and second to image the slice where the blood vessel is located (Fig. 4).

Due to scattering this technique can be used for angiography or small blood vessels (or other structures) only for limited depths of a few millimeters. Table 2 shows the maximal depths for imaging for various tissues where spatial frequency of the image of 0.5 Lp/mm still may be yielded.

Table 2

Type of tissue	Depth of imaging
brain tissue	5 mm
muscle tissue	4 mm
skin	3 mm
connective tissue	3 mm

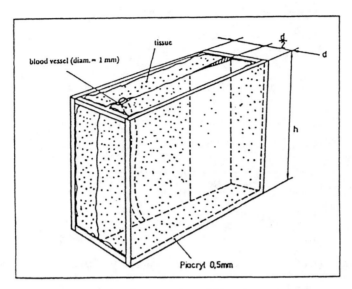

Fig. 3. Principle sketch of the phantom to investigate the optical ps-radar.[7]

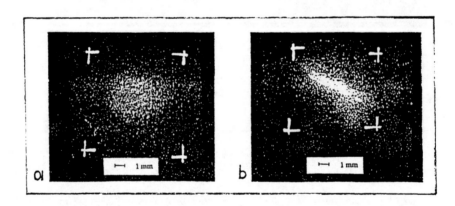

Fig. 4a. Imaging in non-structured slice of bulk tissue.
Fig. 4b. Imaging in determined slice with a blood vessel located 5 mm inside brain tissue.[7]

3. COHERENCE IMAGING

The number of ballistic photons is reduced exponentially when transilluminating high scattering media with a collimated laser beam. The pathway of these photons is governed by the laws of geometric optics provided no further interaction takes place. The transmitted intensity (I_b/I_0) of these ballistic photons therefore depends on the thickness, the absorption and scattering probability of the scattered medium only. This small number of ballistic photons is superimposed by a tremendous higher amount of scattered photons at the detector behind the sample.

We used a modified Mach-Zehnder-Interferometer to select ballistic and scattered photons. Within this Mach-Zehnder-Interferometer one beam has been modulated with an accousto-optic modulator and is superimposed at the detector with the beam which has been transmitted through the scattering medium. Because of the statistic phase distribution of the scattered photons these will generate with the reference beam only an constant offset signal, whereby the ballistic photons will generate a modulated signal with the difference frequency between probe and reference beam.

Fig. 5 shows the experimental set-up for the detection of small structures in scattered media. For a better local resolution within the sample a confocal imaging technique was used.

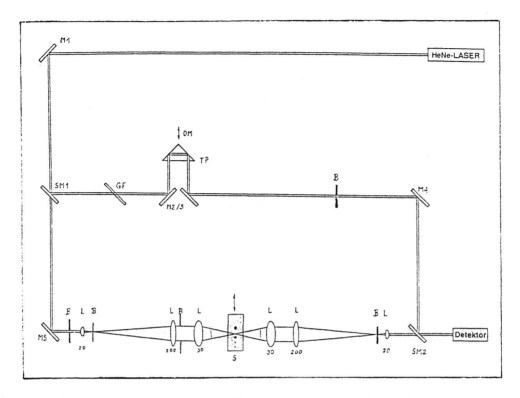

Fig. 5. Experimental set-up for detection of oblique structures in scattering medium by coherent imaging (with confocal imaging).

The advantage of the confocal technique is gained by the fact that all illuminated areas within the scattering sample which are outside the beam waist will only behave like a constant attenuator. By moving the beam waist through the sample a tomographic image can be built up step by step. Due to this experimental set-up in a first experiment the sampling diaphragm had a diameter of 10 μm and the valuation of the beam waist starting at the object plane has been detected using a sampling chamber S of 15 mm thickness filled with water. Fig. 6 shows the measured intensity distribution of beam waist at different positions near the focal plane. From the size of the measured beam waist we can estimate that a lateral resolution of 20 μm and in z-direction of about 0.5 mm is possible.

In a second step the sample chamber was filled with a 10 % solution of Intralipid with three different mixtures, 1:100, 1:80 and 1:60. At the object plane a 60 μm ϕ wire has been placed. The results are shown in Fig. 7.

4. DISCUSSION

Comparative investigations show the advantage and disadvantage of optical methods for imaging in strongly scattering media.

With the optical ps-radar the detection of structures up to 2 mm to a depth of 4 mm and with a contrast of 4 % was possible. The ps-radar technique could be useful to improve the contrast for fluorescence angiograpghy.

The coherent detection imaging technique is able to resolve microsturctures up to a depth of 4 mm. The most progress should be important in diagnostic of skin and eye.

For large depths the use of scattered photons is necessary because for example in breast we need 10 photons to transmit only non-scattered 1 photon for sample of 50 mm thickness. May be phase modulation combined with optical synthetic aperture ranging opens new possibilities in future.

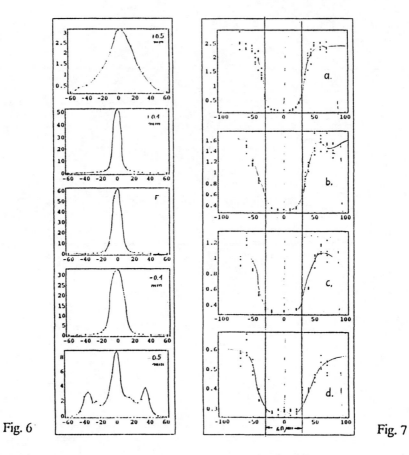

Fig. 6

Fig. 7

Fig. 6. Beam waist intensity distribution using a sampling aperture of 10 μm ϕ. In addition detection planes ± 0.1 mm and ± 0.5 mm have been detected.

Fig. 7. Intensity profile of a 60 μm thick wire in scattering media (10 % Intralipid):
a = water, b = 1:100 %, c = 1:80 %, d = 1:60.

REFERENCES

1. J. Beuthan and G. Müller, Infrarotdiaphanoskopie, MEDTECH 1, pp. 13-17, 1992.
2. G. Moron, B. Drowin and M.M. Denariez-Roberge, Appl. Phys. Letter 20, pp. 453, 1972.
3. H. Mahr and M.D. Hirsch, Optics Commun. 13 (2), pp. 96, 1975.
4. M.A. Duguay, J.W. Hansen, Appl. Phys. Letters 15, pp. 192, 1969.
5. J.C. Diels, J.J. Fontaine and W. Rudolph, Revue de Physique Appliquée 22, pp. 113, 1987.
6. F. Fink, J. Beuthan and E. Klose, "Ein optisches ps-Radar zur bildhaften Darstellung von Objektstrukturen in menschlichen Geweben," Exp. Techn. d. Physik 38, 3, pp. 197-206, 1990.
7. J. Beuthan, Grundlagenuntersuchungen zur Infrarotdiaphanoskopie (IRD), Diss. MMA, pp. 101, 1982.

Section Five
Applications in Diagnostics and Therapy

Reprinted with permission from *Analytical Biochemistry*, Vol. 195, pp. 330-351 (1991). ©1991 Academic Press, Inc.

Quantitation of Time- and Frequency-Resolved Optical Spectra for the Determination of Tissue Oxygenation

E. M. Sevick,[1] B. Chance,[2] J. Leigh, S. Nioka, and M. Maris

Department of Biochemistry and Biophysics, School of Medicine, University of Pennsylvania, Philadelphia, Pennsylvania 19104-6089

Received October 29, 1990

The recent development of near-infrared time- and frequency-resolved tissue spectroscopy techniques to probe tissue oxygenation and tissue oxygenation kinetics has led to the need for further quantitation of spectroscopic signals. In this paper, we briefly review the theory of light transport in strongly scattering media as monitored in the time and frequency domains, and use this theory to develop algorithms for quantitation of hemoglobin saturation from the photon decay rate ($\partial \log R/\partial t$) obtained using time-resolved spectroscopy, and from the phase-shift (θ) obtained from frequency-resolved, phase-modulated spectroscopy. To test the relationship of these optical parameters, we studied the behavior of $\partial \log R/\partial t$ and θ as a function of oxygenation in model systems which mimicked the optical properties of tissue. Our results show that deoxygenation at varying hemoglobin concentrations can be monitored with the change in the photon decay kinetics, $\Delta \partial \log R/\partial t$ in the time-resolved measurements, and with the change in phase-shift, $\Delta \theta$, in the frequency-resolved technique. Optical spectra of the adult human brain obtained with these two techniques show similar characteristics identified from the model systems.

© 1991 Academic Press, Inc.

The attenuation of light over a known path length, L, provides a quantitative description of the concentration of light absorbing species via a Beer–Lambert relationship,[3]

$$\mu_a = -\frac{1}{L} \log_e \frac{I}{I_0} = \epsilon[C], \qquad [1]$$

where ϵ is the extinction coefficient (cm^{-1} mM^{-1}); [C] is the concentration of absorber (mM); I and I_0 are the detected and incident light intensity, respectively; and μ_a is the absorption coefficient of the sample in units of cm^{-1}. When the sample does not scatter light, the path length that light travels before detection is L and is taken to be the dimension of the cuvette holding the sample. However, if the sample multiply scatters light, then a distribution of path lengths results that may be significantly longer than the dimension of the cuvette. Thus, quantitative description via equation (1) of concentrations in a strongly scattering medium or tissue becomes complicated. Despite this, oximetry and other near-infrared tissue continuous-wave spectroscopy (CWS)[4] techniques attempt to assess relative oxy- and deoxyhemoglobin concentrations by monitoring the attenuation of light in tissue.

Recently, Chance and co-workers introduced the concept of using time- and frequency-resolved spectroscopic techniques to monitor the total path lengths, L, in order to quantitatively detect changes in tissue absorption (1–6). In time-resolved spectroscopy, the distribution of path lengths traveled in tissue is directly measured by monitoring the intensity of light emitted as a function of time after an incident impulse (Fig. 1a). Assuming the light travels a constant speed, c, within the scattering medium or tissue, the path lengths traveled are found directly from the "time-of-flight," t, such that $L = c \cdot t$. Measurement of light intensity versus

---

[1] Current address: Department of Chemical Engineering, Vanderbilt University, Nashville, TN 37235.

[2] To whom correspondence should be directed.

[3] It is important to note that Eq. [1] and the extinction coefficient are based upon the Napierian log expression. Thus, unless otherwise noted, ϵ is 2.303 times the $\log_{10}$ value usually used by biochemists.

[4] Abbreviations used: CWS, continuous wave spectroscopy; DPF, differential path length factor; AICD, automatic implanted cardioventricular defibrillator.

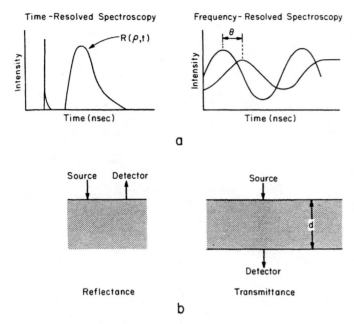

FIG. 1. (a) The techniques of time- and frequency-resolved spectroscopy consist of detecting light a distance ρ away from a source which emits an impulse of light (time-resolved spectroscopy), or a steady light with sinusoidally modulated intensity (frequency-resolved spectroscopy). In time-resolved spectroscopy, the impulse response gives the distribution of pathlengths traveled by photons. In phase frequency-resolved spectroscopy, the phase-shift of the detected light with respect to the incident light gives a statistical description of the path length distribution. (b) Both reflectance and transmittance geometries of the source and detector are used in time- and frequency-resolved tissue spectroscopies.

"time-of-flight" therefore describes the distribution of total path lengths traveled by light. In frequency-resolved spectroscopy, the phase-shift, θ, of light intensity emitted a known distance away from a sinusiodally modulated light source (Fig. 1a) can be used to monitor changes in an effective mean of the distribution of path lengths. The rapid development of these two techniques to monitor changes in total path lengths as a function of tissue oxygenation has led to the need for a precise method to quantify hemoglobin saturation from such measurements. Specifically, these measurements consists of monitoring the time- or frequency-resolved components of reflectance or transmittance at a distance ρ away from the light source (Fig. 1b).

In this paper, we present the basis by which both time- and frequency-resolved measurements can be used to quantitate absorption, and thereby hemoglobin saturation in tissues. Specifically we will present (i) the diffusive theory for light transport to predict the distribution of path lengths in strongly scattering media such as tissue; (ii) experimental measurements which monitor the distribution of pathlengths from time- and frequency-resolved techniques; (iii) the basis of dual-wavelength measurements for the quantitation of

hemoglobin saturation; and (iv) actual time- and frequency-resolved measurements in strongly scattering media with added hemoglobin to simulate the optical properties of tissue. These *in vitro* simulations demonstrate the potentials of time- and frequency-resolved spectroscopic techniques to detect changes in tissue oxygenation *in vivo*.

1. TRANSPORT OF LIGHT IN STRONGLY SCATTERING MEDIA

An understanding of the theory of light transport is required in order to understand the parameters which govern the distribution of path lengths traveled by light in a strongly scattering medium. There are both particle and wave descriptions of light transport, which are congruent to one another (see, for example, see Ref. (7)). The equations for the particle description are more tractable than those for the wave description. For this reason, most investigators employ the particle descriptions to describe light transport in strongly scattering media. Herein, we use the particle description and describe the transport of light through scattering media in terms of light "particle" migration, or "photon migration."

The process of photon migration can be described as follows: In any continuous medium, "particles" of light, or photons, travel at a constant speed dependent upon the refractive index of the medium (i.e., the speed of light (cm/sec) = $3.0 \times 10^{10}/n$, where n is the refractive index of the medium). In a sample which scatters light, photons travel with constant direction and speed until a "scatterer" is encountered. In simple terms, a scatterer can be considered to be a particle or position at which photons change momentum elastically (i.e., change direction, yet maintain speed). Depending upon the properties of the scatterer, the photons may scatter in random directions, or in a preferential forward or backward direction. The distance traveled by photons between scattering "events" is called the scattering length, l^*, and is dependent upon the nature and the concentration of scatterers in the medium. The total path length, L, traveled by photons when migrating from a source to a detector is simply the scattering length times the number of scattering events, n: $L = n \, l^*$. In the absence of scatterers, the total path length traveled by photons before detection is simply the geometric distance between source and detector. Therefore, L is known and Eq. [1] is valid. On the other hand, as the number of scatterers increase, the total path length, L, that one photon travels before detection becomes increasingly greater than the geometric distance between source and detector. In addition, since the change in direction at each scattering event is random, or at least semirandom, there is a distribution of total path lengths traveled by photons that successfully migrate from the source to detector.

In addition to scattering properties of the medium, the absorption properties also affect the total path lengths traveled by photons that successfully migrate to the detector. Qualitatively, as the absorbance of the medium increases, the probability that photons survive as they encounter consecutive scattering events decreases. Thus, the probability of detecting photons that have traveled longer path lengths diminishes and the distribution of path lengths is shortened. On the other hand, as the absorbance of the medium decreases, the distribution of path lengths is again lengthened as the probability of detecting photons that travel long path lengths is increased. The change in total path length distributions as a function of the absorbance is the key for spectroscopy and imaging (8–11) using methods of time- and frequency-resolved techniques.

1.1. Diffusion Approximation to Photon Migration in Strongly Scattering Media

The description above for photon migration can be combined with Monte Carlo simulation techniques to model the trajectories of migrating photons in scattering media and to compute the distribution of total path lengths traveled as a function of the scattering and absorbance (for example, see (10, 12–14)). These computational methods are often intractible, requiring significant computer times for statistically accurate results.

Alternatively, one can describe the migration of photons as a diffusional process in which there is a gradient in the number of photons, or alternatively in the photon fluence rate, $\phi(r, t)$, distributed from the source. The fluence rate is equal to $N_a \times c$, or the product of the number of photon at position r and time, t, and the speed of photons through the medium. The fluence rate, or the effective "concentration" of photons at position r and time t, in a tissue or turbid media may be obtained from the solution of the general diffusion equation (for review, see (7, 15–16))

$$\frac{1}{c}\frac{\partial}{\partial t}\phi(r, t) - D\nabla^2\phi(r, t) + \mu_a\phi(r, t) = S(r, t), \quad [2]$$

where D is the diffusion coefficient and S a source term. For photon migration, the diffusion coefficient is equal to

$$D = \frac{1}{3\{\mu_a + (1 - g)\mu_s\}}, \quad [3]$$

where μ_s is the scattering coefficient (cm^{-1}) and g is the mean cosine of scattering angle. The term $(1 - g)\mu_s$ is referred to as the effective scattering coefficient and is equal to the reciprocal of the isotropic, mean scattering length, l^* (i.e., when the direction of scatter is completely random). The absorption coefficient μ_a is based upon the Napierian extinction coefficient. Equation [2] is a general heat and mass transfer diffusion equation and,

for the application of light propagation in highly scattering media, has been derived from the radiative transfer equation for the transport of neutral particles (17). The analogy between heat transfer and photon migration is a powerful one allowing one to use solution and solution techniques for temperature distributions and apply them to find fluence rate distributions in similar problems. For example, the solution for the fluence distribution following an impulse of light is directly analogous to the solution for temperature distributions in an infinite medium following a short pulse of energy. The solution for the fluence distributions in an infinite media with a point source of a steady-state periodic fluctuation in $S(r, t)$ is directly analogous to the solution for temperature distributions in an infinite media with steady state fluctuation in energy deposition at a point source. The application of the diffusion approximation to describe light transport in turbid media has been discussed by numerous investigators including Ishimaru (7) and Profio and Dorion (16).

1.2. Diffusion Approximation to Predict Time-Resolved Spectra in Reflectance and Transmittance Geometries

As described in the Introduction and Fig. 1, time-resolved spectroscopy consists of monitoring the intensity of light or number of photons that successfully migrate to and arrive at position ρ at time, t, following an impulse of light at $\rho = 0$. Depending upon the source and detector configuration, the intensity of detected light is referred to as the reflectance, $R(\rho, t)$, or the transmittance, $T(\rho, d, t)$. Both $R(\rho, t)$ and $T(\rho, d, t)$ are measures of the number of photons that have traveled a time-of-flight, t, and a total path length, $L(=ct)$, through the sample.

Recently, Patterson et al. (15) have solved for temporal reflectance, $R(\rho, t)$, and transmittance, $T(\rho, d, t)$, following an impulse of light using the solution for the fluence distribution in an infinite media solution as a Green's function with realistic boundary conditions. Their equations are written

$$R(\rho, t) = (4\pi Dc)^{-3/2}z_0 t^{-5/2}\exp(-\mu_a ct)\exp\left(-\frac{\rho^2 + z_0^2}{4Dct}\right) \quad [4]$$

and

$$T(\rho, d, t) = (4\pi Dc)^{-3/2}t^{-5/2}\exp(-\mu_a ct)\exp\left(-\frac{\rho^2}{4Dct}\right)$$

$$\times \left\{(d - z_0)\exp\left[-\frac{(d - z_0)^2}{4Dct}\right]\right.$$

$$- (d + z_0)\exp\left[-\frac{(d + z_0)^2}{4Dct}\right]$$

$$+ (3d - z_0)\exp\left[\frac{(3d - z_0)^2}{4Dct}\right]$$

$$\left.- (3d - z_0)\exp\left(-\frac{(3d - z_0)^2}{4Dct}\right)\right\}, \quad [5]$$

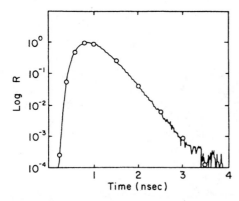

FIG. 2. The log R versus time obtained from time-resolved spectroscopy of human calf muscle (2). The solid line denotes the regression to Eq. [4]. Parameter estimates for this spectra yielded $\mu_a = 0.176$ cm^{-1} and $(1 - g)\mu_s = 8.3$ cm^{-1} (15).

where z_0 is the equal to $[(1 - g)\mu_s]^{-1}$ and ρ and d are the radial and depth cylindrical coordinates for the radial distance of light source and detector. In the case of transmittance, d is the thickness of the tissue or media. Regardless of the measurement geometry, the intensity of the detected light at response time t is proportional to $\exp(-\mu_a ct)$ as predicted by the analogous solution for the temperature or fluence distribution in an infinite medium at a specified distance away from the source. Again, since (i) t is the time-of-flight of photons arriving at point $(\rho, 0)$ for reflectance and (ρ, d) for transmittance following an impulse of light at $\rho = 0$; and (ii) R and T represent the flux of photons reaching that point; Eqs. [4] and [5] essentially describe the distribution of photons that have traveled path length, $L(=ct)$, for the two measurement configurations. From the inspection of these equations, one can see that the distribution of photon time-of-flights or photon path lengths, L, is dependent upon the values of μ_a and μ_s for a known source and detector configuration. Thus, time-resolved spectroscopy gives an opportunity to directly measure the distribution of photon path lengths from the reflectance (or transmittance) intensity versus time measurements.

Indeed, eq. [4] has been fit to experimental time-resolved spectra obtained from reflectance measurements made of a turbid media with independently measured scattering and absorption coefficients (18) as well as of a human calf muscle (2, 15). Figure 2 shows that the experimental curve of log $R(\rho, t)$ versus time obtained from time-resolved spectroscopy of the human calf muscle can be described by Eq. [4]. Figure 2 also illustrates the features of the impulse response which is a direct measurement of the distribution of path lengths: (i) the time of maximum signal is delayed with respect to the time of the input impulse of light, and (ii) the decay rate at long response times follow a simple exponential. From Eq. [4] the slope of the $\log_e R$ versus time can be expressed as (15)

$$\frac{\partial}{\partial t} \log_e R(\rho, t) = -\frac{5}{2t} - \mu_a c + \frac{\rho^2}{4Dct^2}. \quad [6]$$

Furthermore, $\partial \log_e R/\partial t$ asymptotically approaches the quantity $-\mu_a c$ at long response times,

$$\lim_{t \to \infty} \frac{\partial}{\partial t} \log_e R(\rho, t) = -\mu_a c. \quad [7]$$

In addition, from the time of maximum detected signal, t_{max}, $(1 - g)\mu_s$ can be determined,

$$(1 - g)\mu_s = \frac{1}{3\rho^2} (4\mu_a c^2 t_{max}^2 + 10 c t_{max}) - \mu_a. \quad [8]$$

For the human calf data shown in Fig. 2, $\mu_a = 0.176$ cm^{-1} and $(1 - g)\mu_s = 8.3$ cm^{-1} (15). Thus, from the distribution of path lengths directly monitored via time-resolved spectroscopy, the absorption and effective scattering (μ_a and $(1 - g)\mu_s$) coefficients can be obtained.

In addition, the speed of light in tissue can be obtained from time-resolved spectroscopy by monitoring the earliest photon arrival time as the geometric distance between the source and detector is altered. While microspectroscopists have studied index matching in tissue studies, it is unlikely that their study of microscopic thickness is representative of the 1-meter photon migration path lengths studied herein. At the same time, the attenuation of the direct beam from input to output makes "optical ranging" difficult since the number of photons making the direct path with negligible scattering in the human brain is small. Nevertheless, we can measure the time delay of the earliest photons detectable. Figure 3 shows the earliest arrival time measured with respect to the instrument function versus the geometric separation distance in a human adult brain (BC). If it is assumed that the photons with the earliest arrival time are minimally influenced by the scattering and absorption properties in the tissue and retain directionality, then geometric distance between the source and detector should be proportional to the arrival time. The constant of proportionality should approach the speed of light through the tissue. The slope of the least-squares regression in Fig. 3 shows that $c = 22 \pm 1.3$

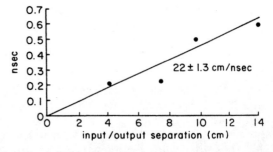

FIG. 3. The earliest arrival time (ns) versus the geometric distance between the source and detector on an adult human brain (BC 66). The slope of the least-squares regressed line gives $c = 22 \pm 1.3$ cm/ns which translates to a refractive index for tissue = 1.36 ± 0.08.

cm/ns within brain tissue. This translates into a refractive index of 1.36 ± 0.08 which is within the range of refractive indices previously reported for tissue (19).

1.3. Diffusion Approximation to Predict Frequency-Resolved Spectra in Reflectance and Transmittance Geometries

In frequency-resolved spectroscopy, instead of an impulse of light, the source at $\rho = 0$ consists of light whose intensity is sinusoidally modulated at frequency, f. The detected light intensity at distance ρ away from the source is both amplitude demodulated and phase-shifted with respect to the incident source intensity (Fig. 1b). The measured phase-shift, θ, and the modulation, M, of the emitted light with respect to that of the incident light are related to the sine and cosine Fourier transforms of the impulse response function (20). In the case of reflectance and transmittance, the impulse response is given by Eqs. [4] and [5], respectively or the time-resolved spectra. Furthermore, since the impulse response functions are descriptions of the photon path length distributions then θ is a description of the path length distributions measured in the frequency domain. Indeed, in Appendix A1.1 we show that θ can be directly related to the mean of the distribution of path lengths traveled by photons before detection. The modulation of the detected intensity also varies with the absorbance and path length distributions in a strongly scattering medium. However, since our emphasis in this paper is to show how changes in the distribution of path lengths can be used to detect changes in absorption in strongly scattering media, we do not discuss here the quantitation of absorption from measurements of M. Nevertheless, modulation may also be important measurement to detect changes in absorption in a strongly scattering medium. Expressions of the phase-shift and modulation of the detected intensity may also be directly found from Eq. [2] with the source term representing a sinusoidally modulated photon flux at point $\rho=0 : S(\rho=0, t) = A + M \times \sin(2\pi f \cdot t)$.

Recently, Patterson et al. (18) obtained analytical solution for θ from the sine and cosine Fourier transforms of eq. [4]. Their equation for θ can be rewritten

$$\theta(\rho, f) = -\Psi \sin\frac{\Theta}{2} - \tan^{-1}\frac{-\Psi \sin\dfrac{\Theta}{2}}{1 + \Psi \cos\dfrac{\Theta}{2}}, \quad [9]$$

where

$$\Psi = \sqrt{3(1-g)\mu_s\rho^2\{(\mu_a c)^2 + (2\pi f)^2\}^{1/2} c^{-1}}$$

$$\Theta = \tan^{-1}\left\{\frac{2\pi f}{\mu_a c}\right\}.$$

One can show that for the strongly scattering media, i.e., $(1-g)\mu_s \gg \rho$ or d, Eq. [9] describes phase-shift measure-

ments using either transmittance or reflectance geometries.

Patterson et al. (18) have suggested that at low modulation frequencies, the phase-shift describes a delay time and the mean of the distribution of path lengths, $\langle L \rangle$, traveled before detection via the relationship

$$\theta = \tan^{-1}2\pi f \langle t \rangle = \tan^{-1}\frac{2\pi f \langle L \rangle}{c} \sim \frac{2\pi f \langle L \rangle}{c}. \quad [10]$$

Appendix A1.1 shows when the expression in Eq. [9] is expanded in powers of f, at low modulation frequencies, the phase-shift becomes equal to $2\pi f \cdot \langle t \rangle$, where $\langle t \rangle$ of the mean time-of-flight. Since photons travel at constant speed, c, then one can express the mean time-of-flight in terms of a mean path length traveled before detection, $\langle L \rangle$. However, as the modulation frequency becomes larger, the phase-shift does not describe the true mean path length. In fact, as the modulation frequency increases, the $\langle L \rangle$ derived from Eq. [10] becomes less than the true mean path length. In this study, we refer to $\langle L \rangle$ as an "effective" mean path length and report measurements of phase-shift in terms $\langle L \rangle$ to illustrate that phase-shift measurements can be used to monitor the distribution of path lengths traveled by photons before detection.

Using intralipid/india ink solutions of varying concentration and scattering coefficients as well as polystyrene microsphere suspensions of known $(1-g)\mu_s$, we have verified that Eq. [9] accurately describes the phase-shift at measured in reflectance geometry (21) and when absorption is small. Figures 4a–4c summarize experiments in which phase shift was measured as a function of absorber concentration, scatterer concentration, as well as source-detector separation, ρ, and modulation frequency, f. Figures 4a and 4b show that at 200 MHz, the effective mean path length (i) decreases with increased absorption due to added india ink in intralipid solution, yet (ii) increases with added concentration of polystyrene microspheres which act as Mie scatterers. Furthermore, the magnitude of effective mean path length, $\langle L \rangle$, change due to absorption increases with the scattering capacity of the medium. Indeed, Eq. [9] quantitatively predicts the changes in phase-shift or effective mean path length shown in Figs. 4a and 4b (21). Figure 4c shows the measurement of phase-shift at modulation frequencies of 39 and 220 MHz as a function of source-detector separation on two different concentrations of intralipid solution. As described by the Eq. [9] and the experimental data in Fig. 4, phase-shift increases with scatterer concentration and source-detector separation, ρ; the magnitude of phase-shift change due to $(1-g)\mu_s$ or ρ increases with modulation frequency. In summary, our measurements

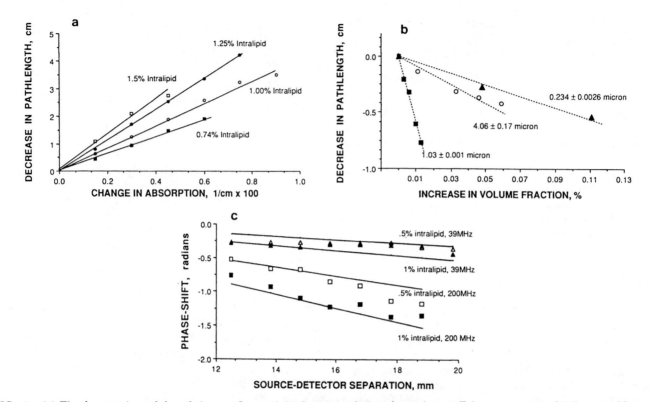

FIG. 4. (a) The decrease in path length (cm, $-\Delta L = -\Delta\theta c/2\pi f$) versus solution absorption coefficient, μ_a, measured following addition of 0.1% india ink aliquots to solutions of 0.74, 1.0, 1.25, and 1.50% intralipid (20% solution, Kabi Vitrum, Inc., Clayton, NC). The symbols denote the average of three to five reflectance measurements with source–detector separation, ρ, equal to 3 cm. Standard error bars cannot be distinguished from the symbols in the figure. As predicted from the diffusion approximation, the effective, mean path length decreases with increasing absorption. In addition, the magnitude of the path length change increases with the scattering coefficient of the medium. Reproduced from Ref. (21). (b) The decrease in pathlength (cm, $-\Delta L = \Delta\theta c/2\pi f$) measured with increasing volume fraction, ϕ (%), of 0.234, 1.03, and 4.06 μm diameter polystyrene microspheres suspensions (Polysciences, Inc., Warrington, PA, and Dow Medical Products, Midland, MI). As predicted by the diffusion approximation increased scattering causes the effective, mean path length to increase. Since the microspheres act as Mie scatterers, one can compute the scattering efficiency for each suspension. For suspensions of polystyrene with $d = 0.234$ μm, $(1 - g)\mu_s$ = 47.6 ϕ cm^{-1}; with $d = 1.03$ μm, $(1 - g)\mu_s = 306.8$ ϕ cm^{-1}; and with $d = 4.6$ μm, $(1 - g)\mu_s = 82.4$ ϕ cm^{-1}. This is consistent with the experimental data showing the greatest increase in effective, mean path length per volume percentage change for microspheres with $d = 1.03$ μm and the smallest increase for microspheres with $d = 0.234$ μm. Reproduced from Ref. (21). (c) The phase-shift (radians) monitored at modulation frequencies of 39- and 200-MHz as a function of intralipid concentration and source–detector separation. The solid lines denote the theoretical values calculated from Eq. [9] for assumed values of $\mu_a = 0$ and $(1 - g)\mu_s = 14.5$ and 7.25 cm^{-1} (35). The differences between theoretical and experimental points may be due to the error in approximating $(1 - g)\mu_s$ and μ_a for the two concentrations of intralipid. As predicted from the diffusion approximation, the magnitude of the phase-shift increases with source–detector separation, ρ; scattering coefficient of the medium, $(1 - g)\mu_s$; and the modulation frequency, f.

of changing phase-shift or effective, mean path length are in quantitative agreement with that predicted by Eq. [9].

1.4. Relationship of Time- and Frequency-Resolved Spectroscopy with CWS

From the previous two sections, it is apparent that time-resolved spectroscopy monitors changes in the distribution of path lengths with change in absorption, and the phase-shift of frequency-resolved spectroscopy can be used to detect changes in the mean of the distribution of path lengths. As described in the equations summarized above, the change in the distribution of

path lengths or the mean of the distribution can be due to changes in scattering and/or absorption.

In continuous wave systems, changes in detected light attenuation (I/I_0) due to absorption are accompanied by changes in the distribution of photon path lengths. Yet this spectroscopic technique does not provide measurement of path lengths traveled before detection. As discussed in the previous section, increased absorption decreases $\langle L \rangle$. While, Delpy et al. (12) have developed a modified Beer–Lambert equation with a differential path length factor (DPF) to account for the difference between the geometric distance between source and detector, ρ, and the mean path length, $\langle L \rangle$, continuous wave tissue spectroscopy nevertheless continues to be subject to significant errors. Indeed, we find the equivalent to the DPF in terms of the diffusion approximation to be functions of μ_a and $(1 - g)\mu_s$ (see Appendix A1.2 for derivation)

$$\text{DPF} = \frac{\sqrt{3}}{2} \sqrt{\frac{(1 - g)\mu_s}{\mu_a}}. \qquad [11]$$

Alternatively, Groenhuis et al. (22, 23) have determined a method by which optical properties of μ_a and $(1 - g)\mu_s$ can be estimated from a series of radial measurements of reflectance obtained from continuous wave spectroscopy.

Nevertheless, only time- and frequency-resolved spectroscopic techniques are self calibrating, affording measurements which can be used to provide optical information of μ_a and $(1 - g)\mu_s$. In Section 2.0, we describe the basis of dual-wavelength measurements using time- and frequency-resolved spectroscopy to assess the μ_a and specifically, the hemoglobin saturation in tissues. However, before that we briefly comment upon the applicability of the theory for photon migration in strongly scattering media to describe photon migration in tissues.

1.5. Applicability of the Diffusion Approximation to Detecting Absorption in Tissues

The applicability of the diffusion approximation to describe experimental time- and frequency-resolved measurements in well-characterized model systems has been documented (18, 21) and fitted to tissue measurements (15, 18). Indeed the existence of these fits suggests that tissue can be treated as a homogeneous medium. Tissue homogeneity is central to the diffusion description of tissue photon migration and inhomogeneities may prevent quantitation of absorbance from measurements of photon migration using time- and frequency-resolved techniques. Yet when the length scale of inhomogeneity is smaller than the scattering lengths, l^*, such as may be the case for brain cortex and skeletal muscle, diffusion theory may provide an excellent description of photon migration. The scattering lengths for these tissues are on the order of 1 mm. In the case of a superficial layer of differing scattering and absorption properties, such as the skin in skeletal muscle, or the skull in brain measurements, analysis of the diffusion approximation and Monte Carlo simulation have shown that quantitation of the absorption in underlying tissues may still be obtained (14, 24). Thus, we restrict our discussion to those tissues and tissue measurements in which the migrating photons sample tissue volumes that can be treated as a continuous, homogeneous medium.

On the other hand, it should also be recognized that there are cases where inhomogeneities in tissue absorption or scattering predominate, such as in the presence of a tumor or subdural or epidural brain hemorrage. In these cases, the problem of spectroscopy is replaced by one of imaging or localization. The problem of using measurement of photon migration for the localization of absorbing objects constitutes a separate, but equally important application of time- and frequency-resolved techniques. The analysis of photon migration by the diffusion approximation does not apply to localization studies.

2.0. TIME- AND FREQUENCY-RESOLVED SPECTROSCOPY FOR THE DETERMINATION OF TISSUE HEMOGLOBIN SATURATION

The capacity to monitor path lengths in homogeneous tissue volumes suggests the use of time- and frequency-resolved spectroscopy to noninvasively quantitate tissue hemoglobin saturation and tissue oxygenation on the basis of hemoglobin absorbance. In the mammalian brain, absorbance is due to water, cytochrome iron and copper, and oxy- and deoxygenated forms of hemoglobin. Investigators (12, 25) have shown that in the near-infrared region, absorbance due to water and cytochrome is negligible compared to that due to the oxy- and deoxygenated forms of hemoglobin.

Thus, at two near-infrared wavelengths, λ_1 and λ_2, the absorption coefficient in units of cm^{-1} can be written in terms of the Beer–Lambert relationship

$$\mu_a^{\lambda_1} = \epsilon_{Hb}^{\lambda_1}[Hb] + \epsilon_{HbO_2}^{\lambda_1}[HbO_2]$$
$$\mu_a^{\lambda_2} = \epsilon_{Hb}^{\lambda_2}[Hb] + \epsilon_{HbO_2}^{\lambda_2}[HbO_2], \qquad [12]$$

where ϵ is the extinction coefficient ($\text{cm}^{-1}\ \text{mM}^{-1}$) and $[HbO_2]$ and $[Hb]$ are the tissue concentrations of oxy- and deoxygenated forms of hemoglobin. If the hemoglobin saturation is $Y = HbO_2/(Hb + HbO_2)$, the one can combine the equations for tissue absorption,

$$\frac{\mu_a^{\lambda_1}}{\mu_a^{\lambda_2}} = \frac{\epsilon_{Hb}^{\lambda_1} + Y(\epsilon_{HbO_2}^{\lambda_1} - \epsilon_{Hb}^{\lambda_1})}{\epsilon_{Hb}^{\lambda_2} + Y(\epsilon_{HbO_2}^{\lambda_2} - \epsilon_{Hb}^{\lambda_2})}. \qquad [13]$$

Furthermore, if λ_2 is the isosbestic wavelength of hemoglobin (i.e., 800 nm), then Eq. [13] can be rewritten

$$\frac{\mu_a^{\lambda_1}}{\mu_a^{\lambda_2}} = \frac{\epsilon_{Hb}^{\lambda_1}}{\epsilon_{Hb}^{\lambda_2}} + \frac{\Delta\epsilon_{HbO_2-Hb}^{\lambda_1}}{\epsilon_{Hb}^{\lambda_2}}\ Y. \qquad [14]$$

Thus, inspection of Eqs. [13] and [14] show that the ratio of absorption due to hemoglobin measured at two near-infrared wavelengths is (i) a unique function of tissue hemoglobin saturation, and (ii) independent of total hemoglobin concentration, $[Hb + HbO_2]$, or cerebral blood volume.

On the other hand, when the background absorbance is not negligible, as may be the case in skeletal muscle, methods must be found to distinguish between background absorbance and that due to hemoglobin. In the dog gastrocnemius, both hemoglobin and myoglobin contribute 75 and 25%, respectively, to the total tissue absorbance. While the spectra for hemoglobin and myoglobin clearly overlap, the respective high and low oxygen affinities cause the two oxygen carriers to deoxygenate sequentially (26). Furthermore, since the concentration of myoglobin is not generally a variable in tissues, the absorbance due to myoglobin is essentially a constant in the clinically relevant range of tissue pO$_2$. In addition, melanin has a flat absorption in the near-infrared region and is localized in the thin layer of skin. Thus, hemoglobin is the optically active absorbing component for "early warning" detection of tissue oxygenation. For tissue with background absorbance, α^λ, the following Beer–Lambert relationship describes tissue absorption in the clinically relevant range of tissue pO$_2$:

$$\mu_a^{\lambda_1} = \epsilon_{Hb}^{\lambda_1}[Hb] + \epsilon_{HbO_2}^{\lambda_1}[HbO_2] + \alpha^{\lambda_1}$$

$$\mu_a^{\lambda_2} = \epsilon_{Hb}^{\lambda_2}[Hb] + \epsilon_{HbO_2}^{\lambda_2}[HbO_2] + \alpha^{\lambda_2}. \qquad [15]$$

Sections 2.1 and 2.2 below discuss approaches to monitor hemoglobin absorbance in the brain, as well as in skeletal tissues, using time- and frequency-resolved techniques. Appendices A1.3 and A1.4 discuss how time- and phase frequency-resolved measurements can be used to monitor hemoglobin saturation in the presence of background absorption.

The objective of dual-wavelength optical measurements is to maximize changes in the ratio of absorption coefficients with physiologically relevant changes in Y through the appropriate choice of λ_1 and λ_2. Figure 5 illustrates that the dual-wavelength combinations that "straddle" the isosbestic point afford greater sensitivity of $\mu_a^{\lambda_1}/\mu_a^{\lambda_2}$ to Y (27). For the wavelength combination of 754 and 816, which is the combination employed in our phase-modulated spectrophotometers (4, 28), we assume literature values based upon decadice extinction coefficients of $\Delta\epsilon_{HbO_2-Hb}^{754} = -0.025$ cm^{-1} mM^{-1}; $\epsilon_{Hb}^{754} = 0.38$ cm^{-1} mM^{-1}; $\Delta\epsilon_{HbO_2-Hb}^{816} = 0.03$ cm^{-1} mM^{-1}; $\epsilon_{Hb}^{816} = 0.18$ cm^{-1} mM^{-1} (29). From Eq. (13) and these values, the hemoglobin saturation can be calculated from ratio of absorption coefficients measured at 754 and 816 nm,

$$Y(\times100\%) = \frac{38 - 18\ (\mu_a^{754}/\mu_a^{816})}{25 + 3\ (\mu_a^{754}/\mu_a^{816})}. \qquad [16]$$

The goal of any optical measurement of tissue oxygenation is therefore to obtain the ratio of absorption coefficients for quantitation of tissue hemoglobin saturation. As described in Section 1, changes in the distribution of path lengths as well as the mean of the distribution measured may be used to detect changes in tissue absorption. We have previously discussed the shortcom-

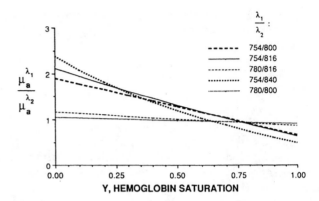

FIG. 5. The ratio of absorption coefficients for various wavelength combinations that straddle the isosbestic point of hemoglobin (800 nm) as a function of hemoglobin saturation.

ings of CWS to quantitate absorption in strongly scattering media. In the following two sections we describe how dual-wavelength measurements from time- and frequency-resolved may be used to obtain the ratio absorption coefficients and to therefore provide quantitative measurement of cerebral oxygenation.

2.1. Hemoglobin Saturation from Time-Resolved Spectroscopy

From Eq. [7], one can see that the ratio of $\partial \log_e R/\partial t$ monitored at the two wavelengths should asymptotically approach the ratio of absorption coefficients when $t \gg t_{max}$,

$$\frac{\partial \log_e R(\rho, t)^{\lambda_1}/\partial t}{\partial \log_e R(\rho, t)^{\lambda_2}/\partial t} \rightarrow \frac{\mu_a^{\lambda_1}}{\mu_a^{\lambda_2}} \quad \text{when } t \gg t_{max}, \qquad [17]$$

when the first and third terms of the right hand side of Eq. [6] contribute insignificantly to $\partial \log_e R/\partial t$. For the case of $\mu_a \sim 0.07$ cm^{-1}, and $(1-g)\mu_s \sim 8$ cm^{-1}, at 10 ns this assumption leads to an overestimation of μ_a by about 10%. Thus, quantitation of cerebral tissue hemoglobin saturation using the algorithm in Eq. [16] leads to an error of 10%. Figures 6a and 6b illustrate the simulated family of curves $(\partial \log_e R^{754}/\partial t)/(\partial \log_e R^{816}/\partial t)$ for various saturations of a medium with 43 and 100 μM total hemoglobin concentration and with $(1-g)\mu_s = 8$ cm^{-1}. The values depicting the ratios of absorbance at the two wavelengths are also graphically represented for comparison of error associated with Eq. [17]. From the asymptotic value of $(\partial \log_e R^{754}/\partial t)/(\partial \log_e R^{816}/\partial t)$ obtained at 43 μM at 5 ns the ratio of absorption coefficients can be obtained to within 10% of the true value and the hemoglobin saturation determined. At higher total hemoglobin concentrations, such as 100 μM as shown in Fig. 6b, an even smaller error is obtained due

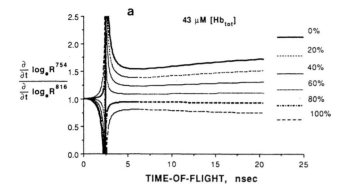

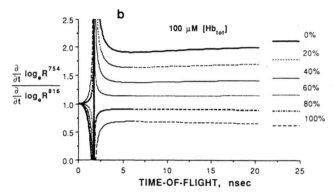

FIG. 6. The ratio of $(\partial(\log_e R^{754})/\partial t)/(\partial(\log_e R^{816})/\partial t)$ versus time as calculated from Eq. [4] as a function of hemoglobin saturation when (a) $[Hb_{tot}] = 43$ μM and when (b) $[Hb_{tot}] = 100$ μM. The asymptotic value of $(\partial(\log_e R^{754})/\partial t)/(\partial(\log_e R^{816})/\partial t)$ gives the ratio of absorption coefficients from which the hemoglobin saturation can be obtained from Eq. [16]. The values for the true ratio of absorption coefficients at varying saturation is given in the right of each figure. The data simulates a highly scattering medium with $(1 - g)\mu_s = 8$ cm^{-1}, $\rho = 3$ cm, and shows increasing error associated with the determination of tissue hemoglobin saturation at low saturations and low $[Hb_{tot}]$.

to the increasing accuracy of assuming $\partial \log_e R^{\lambda}/\partial t \to (-\mu_a c)$ at time t.

On the other hand, the errors due to (i) background absorbance and (ii) assuming $\partial \log_e R^{\lambda}/\partial t$ approaches the quantity $(-\mu_a c)$ at times on the order of t_{max} may be rendered negligible if one considers the difference in the photon decay rates as a function of wavelength. Since scattering is a very weak function of wavelength over the small range employed in these techniques, then inspection of Eq. [6] shows the difference in $\partial \log_e R^{\lambda}/\partial t$ at response time, t, equals the change in absorption, $\Delta\mu_a$,

$$\frac{\partial}{\partial t} \log_e R(\rho, t)\bigg|_{\mu_a^1} - \frac{\partial}{\partial t} \log_e R(\rho, t)\bigg|_{\mu_a^2} = c(\mu_a^2 - \mu_a^1), \quad [18]$$

where the superscripts denote measurements during states of differing absorption, as in the case of dual-wavelength measurement or measurement across states of differing oxygenation. The assumption that tissue scattering properties are constant over the small range

of wavelengths employed is borne by experimental time-resolved measurements in blood-free perfused cat and dog brain (3). In these measurements we find that t_{max} is wavelength insensitive. Inspection of Eq. (8) indicates that in the absence of absorption, t_{max} is a function of the effective scattering coefficient, $(1 - g)\mu_s$. In addition, there are no changes found in transcranial optical densities measured using both continuous wave and time-resolved spectroscopies in living and postmortem animal brains perfused free of hemoglobin (1, 2, 12, 25). Again, these results suggest no change in $(1 - g)\mu_s$. In Section 3.0 we detail experimental measurements in model systems which mimic tissue which verify this behavior.

For determination of hemoglobin saturation, the ratio of differences between $\partial \log_e R^{\lambda}/\partial t$ measured at two wavelengths is related to the ratio of absorption difference. Therefore the tissue hemoglobin saturation can also be determined. Furthermore, this method will account for background absorption. Appendix A1.3 outlines how the ratio of $\partial \log_e R^{\lambda}/\partial t$ differences measured at two wavelengths can be used to determine tissue hemoglobin saturation.

2.2. Hemoglobin Saturation from Measurements of Phase-Shift at Single- and Double-Modulation Frequencies Using Frequency-Resolved Spectroscopy

Typically, single- and double-frequency phase modulation spectrometers are preferred because their duty-ratio approaches one while that of time-resolved spectrometers is about 10^{-3}. In frequency-resolved spectroscopy, measurements of phase-shift are made at high modulation frequencies, whereby changes in absorption are manifested in significant and accurate measureable changes in phase-shift (see, for example, the frequency dependence in Fig. 4c). It should be stressed, that at these higher modulation frequencies, the phase-shift does not measure the mean of the distribution of path lengths traveled by photons before detection as it does at low modulation frequencies (see, for example, Appendix A1.1). In the following, we outline the method by which we use measurements of θ, or alternatively, of the effective mean path length, $\langle L \rangle$, to calculate the hemoglobin saturation at dual-wavelength measurements at high modulation frequencies.

In the case that the modulation frequency is large such that $2\pi f \gg \mu_a^{\lambda_1} c, \mu_a^{\lambda_2} c$ Eq. [9] can be simplified to (see Appendix A1.3)

$$|\theta^{\lambda}| = a\rho \sqrt{(1 - g)\mu_s f} \left\{ 1 - \frac{\mu_a c}{4\pi f} \right\} \quad [19]$$

Figures 4a through 4c show that experimental measurements of θ as a function of μ_a, $(1 - g)\mu_s$, ρ, and f follow the behavior predicted by Eq. [19]. Furthermore, since the effective tissue scattering coefficient is wavelength insensitive (see above in Section 2.1), the ratio of θ measured at two wavelengths can be written

$$\frac{\theta^{\lambda_1}}{\theta^{\lambda_2}} = \frac{1 - (\mu_a^{\lambda_1}c/4\pi f)}{1 - (\mu_a^{\lambda_2}c/4\pi f)} . \qquad [20]$$

If background absorbance is negligible as in the case of the brain, Eq. [20] shows that the ratio of phase-shifts is a function of hemoglobin saturation and independent of the tissue scattering properties. However, since μ_a^λ is dependent on the total concentration of hemoglobin, then the ratio of phase-shifts cannot be used to quantitate tissue oxygenation independently of cerebral blood volume. If θ_0^λ is taken to be equal to the phase-shift at wavelength λ due to tissue scattering and background absorption, as in the case of skeletal muscle, then Eq. [20] can be rewritten

$$\frac{\theta^{\lambda_1} - \theta_0^{\lambda_1}}{\theta^{\lambda_2} - \theta_0^{\lambda_2}} = \frac{\mu_a^{\lambda_1}}{\mu_a^{\lambda_2}} . \qquad [21]$$

Therefore, the relative ratio of phase-shift can be used for determination of hemoglobin saturation independently of blood volume and in the presence of background absorption. Equations [20] and [21] are equally valid for transmittance as well as reflectance measurements. Appendix A1.4 describes the derivation of Eqs. [19]–[21].

As discussed in Section 2.1, tissue scattering is wavelength insensitive over the small range employed in near-infrared studies. Thus in the absence of background absorption, θ_2^λ can be expected to be a constant for the two wavelengths employed. Therefore, either independent measurement of θ_0^λ, obtained by perfusing experimental tissues free of hemoglobin, or a priori estimates of the tissue scattering properties must be known to use Eq. [21] in order to quantitatively detect changes in hemoglobin saturation. In the presence of background absorption, experimental measurement of θ_0^λ may be required. Nevertheless, for brain tissues, $(1 - g)\mu_s$ and θ_0 are not expected to vary and phase frequency-resolved spectroscopic tissue measurements should be transferable. Table 1 summarizes the values of θ_0 calculated from Eq. [9] due to tissue scattering alone (μ_a is set to zero). The value of tissue scattering, $(1 - g)\mu_s$ is assumed to be 6.8 cm^{-1}, which has been obtained from the value of t_{max} (cf. Eq. [8]) measured using time-resolved methods in cat brains perfused free of hemoglobin. For comparison, the least-squares fit of Eq. [5] of time-resolved spectra of human brain and skeletal muscle (18) yields the values of $(1 - g)\mu_s$ to be approximately 8 cm^{-1}.

As described earlier, we derived Eqs. [19] through [21] under conditions of high modulation frequency, i.e., $2\pi f$

TABLE 1

Values of θ_0 for the Dog Head as a Function of Source–Detector Separation, ρ, at 200-MHz Modulation Frequency

Source–detector separation (cm)	θ_0 (radians)
1.0	−0.36
1.5	−0.67
2.0	−1.0
2.5	−1.4
3.0	−1.7
4.0	−2.4

Note. Values are estimated from Eq. [9] (μ_a is taken to be zero and $\Theta = 1.571$ radians) with $(1 - g)\mu_s$ taken to be 6.8 cm^{-1} as determined from time-resolved spectroscopy (taken from Ref. (21)).

$\gg \mu_a^\lambda c$. Previously, the effective lifetime of the decay of the time-resolved spectra or of the distribution of total path lengths traveled has been described as $1/\mu_a^{\lambda_1}c$ (30). In the frequency domain, when the modulation frequency is high such that $2\pi f \gg \mu_a^{\lambda_1}c$, we are effectively sampling at rates faster that the effective lifetime. For these optimal conditions, Eqs. [19] through [21] are derived. However, as the absorption or the concentration of hemoglobin increases, the effective lifetime decreases and the impulse response decays more rapidly. Under these conditions, if a greater modulation frequency is not employed, error will be associated with hemoglobin saturations determined from Eq. [21] to determine hemoglobin saturation. Figure 7 illustrates the behavior of Eq. [21] for a family of phase-shifts with varying concentrations of hemoglobin at a modulation frequency of 200 MHz. The relationship described by Eq. [21] is valid at physiological pO$_2$s, but gives lower values during extreme hypoxia and/or increased blood volumes when the tissue absorption is maximal due to deoxyhemoglobin. Again, the use of appropriate modulation frequencies can minimize the errors in approximating the hemoglobin saturation at low pO$_2$s using equation [21]. Typically, tissue hemoglobin concentrations are reported from 0 to 100 μM and the clinically relevant range of tissue pO$_2$ is between 15 and 50 mm Hg. From Fig. 7 one can see that for a tissue with an effective hemoglobin concentration of 30 μM, which is typical of a microvascular bed, modulation frequencies should be 300 MHz or greater for accurate clinical detection of tissue oxygenation. For tissue hemoglobin concentrations of 50 μM, modulation frequencies should be 400 MHz or greater.

As shown in Fig. 4, we have demonstrated the capacity of the diffusion theory and measurement of phase-shift for the quantitative detection of absorption in a strongly scattering sample. We have also used Eq. [21] to monitor the hemoglobin saturation in isolated perfused tumors perfused alternately with crystalloid and red blood cell suspensions (14, 31). Experimentally we

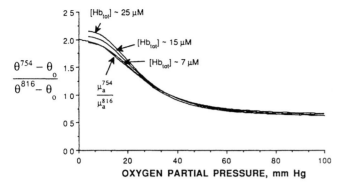

FIG. 7. The ratio of phase-shift differences relative to θ_0 at wavelengths of 754 and 816 nm as a function of hemoglobin concentration (7, 15, and 25 μM) and solution of pO_2 (mm Hg). The curves were calculated from Eq. [9] and the hemoglobin saturation curve ($n = 2.8$, $P_{50} = 25$ mm Hg) with an effective scattering coefficient of 8 cm^{-1} and $\rho = 3$ cm. The bold curve denotes the curve of the ratio of absorption coefficients, μ_a^{754}/μ_a^{816} versus solution pO_2 calculated from Eq. [16] and the hemoglobin saturation curve. As is the case for time-resolved spectroscopy (see Fig. 6), the error in approximating hemoglobin saturation increases at very low saturations.

have found that θ_0 is larger than θ^λ when measured in the presence of hemoglobin. Since the mean of the path length distribution is expected to decrease with absorption, this result is expected. Furthermore, our results are in agreement with those obtained by Delpy et al. (12) showing that physiological changes in the absorption due to tissue deoxygenation contribute small, yet significant changes to the distribution of path lengths. In Section 5.0 we also show that the phase-shift measured at 200 MHz can be used to detect changes in brain oxygenation.

In the following, we present experimental evidence which suggests that the distribution of total path lengths traveled before detection as well as the mean of the distribution can be used to assess the absorption in strongly scattering media using time- and frequency-resolved spectroscopy. Specifically, we present results from *in vitro* experiments employing a respiring cell suspension of *Saccharomyces cerevisiae* and dilute solutions of intralipid (i) to verify the diffusion approximation for the description of $\partial(\log R)/\partial t$, and θ, as outlined in Section 1.0, and (ii) to demonstrate the potential use of the algorithms described above to determine hemoglobin saturation in tissue. Finally, in light of the methodologies presented herein to quantify tissue oxygenation, we briefly review a limited number of time- and frequency-resolved spectroscopic measurements *in vivo* in order to evaluate these technologies as new tissue spectroscopic tools.

3.0. TIME- AND FREQUENCY-RESOLVED SPECTROSCOPY OF *IN VITRO* MODEL SYSTEMS

In vitro studies to verify the use of the diffusion approximations to quantify hemoglobin saturations in tissues requires (i) a scattering media with optical properties similar to that of tissue; (ii) the addition of hemoglobin in concentrations which mimic the effective concentrations in tissues; and (iii) a method by which oxygen consumption and oxygen addition can be controlled in order to monitor changes in hemoglobin saturation. For these studies, we have chosen *in vitro* models since for this first approximation they provide homogeneous scattering and absorption characteristics which are the basis of the diffusion approximations described in Section 1.0. While a perfused tissue or organ has been used in this and other laboratories for these studies, the difficulties of removing and replenishing RBCs in the tissue vasculature limits their use for verifying time- and frequency-resolved spectroscopic measurements.

3.1. Experimental Measurements of R(ρ, t) and θ in a Strongly Scattering Hemoglobin Solution

In the following we present time- and frequency-resolved spectroscopic results obtained with a yeast cell and Intralipid (Kabi Vitrum, Inc., Clayton, NC) suspensions (*S. cerevisiae*) to which hemoglobin was added in known, variable amounts. The cell intralipid suspensions mimicked the light-scattering properties of tissue and the yeast provided a sink for oxygen consumption allowing measurement of the distributions of path lengths and the monitoring of the mean path length during oxygenation and deoxygenation. Measurements were made when the mixture was initially oxygenated and then deoxygenated a short time later by the respiring yeast cells. Hemoglobin, obtained from lysed, outdated human red blood cells (American Red Cross) was added in aliquots resulting in total hemoglobin concentrations ranging from 10–60 μM. Repetitive responses were obtained by bubbling oxygen into the yeast–blood model after complete deoxygenation (6).

3.1.1 Distribution of Photon Path Lengths from Time-Resolved Measurements

Figure 8 shows block diagram of the experimental apparatus containing the cylindrical vessel with the yeast/blood mixture. In order to simulate the adult human head and to minimize optical interaction with the top and bottom of the vessel, we have employed a 14 cm diameter cylinder 10 cm in height. The source and detectors were positioned symmetrically about the circumference at the mid-height of the vessel. Various source/detector configurations were possible with the geometric separations ranging from 3 to 10 cm in circumference. Time-resolved spectra were obtained as described in Ref. (1) prior to the addition of hemoglobin, and successively with each addition of a known volume of hemoglobin. Following each addition, the solution was sparged with oxygen to raise solution pO_2.

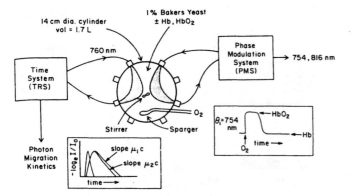

FIG. 8. The yeast/blood *in vitro* model for measurements of time-resolved and frequency-resolved phase modulated spectroscopy presented in Figs. 9–14.

Figure 9 illustrates the time-resolved spectra, or the distribution of path lengths, presented as log R versus time for the source–detector separation of 6 cm on the 14 cm diameter yeast/blood model. There are two points to note: (i) the impulse response reaches a maximum quickly (3 ns) after the impulse input and (ii) the impulse response attenuates three log units over 6–7 ns following the impulse input. Herein, we also present results in terms of $\log_{10} R$ instead of $\log_e R$. For this case, the change in slope, $\Delta \partial(\log R)/\partial t$ is used to detect changes in the absorption coefficient, $\Delta\mu_a^{10}$ based on $\log_{10}$ extinction coefficients,

$$\Delta\mu_a^{10} = \Delta\mu_a \cdot 2.303. \qquad [22]$$

Path length distributions: Effect of absorption on $\partial(\log R)/\partial t$. In the absence of hemoglobin, the distribution of photon path lengths extended beyond 7.5 ns or 165 cm (=7.5 ns × 22 cm/ns). When hemoglobin was added under oxygenated conditions, the distribution of path lengths was shortened: the values did not extend beyond 7.0 ns or 154 cm. As described in Eq. [6], the slope of the log R versus time at time, t, or $\partial(\log R)/\partial t$, is comprised of $-\mu_a^{10}c$ and two other terms which are a function of t, $(1-g)\mu_s$, and ρ. As described by Eq. [18], the change in $\partial(\log R)/\partial t$ with added HbO_2 in Fig. 9 corresponds to the addition of an absorber to the medium resulting in $\Delta\mu_a^{10} = 0.0029$ cm^{-1} (i.e., = 0.0320–0.0291 cm^{-1}). For the addition of 16 μM HbO_2, μ_a^{10} from the Beer–Lambert relationship should increase by 0.0021 cm^{-1} (=$\epsilon_{HbO_2}^{760} \times$ [HbO$_2$] = 0.13 cm^{-1} mM^{-1} × .016 mM). Thus, the time-resolved spectra can be used to assess added absorber in strongly scattering media which mimic tissue.

When the hemoglobin became deoxygenated as the delivery of oxygen was stopped, the distribution of path lengths was further shortened to ~6.2 ns or 136 cm due to the increased absorption of the deoxyhemoglobin at

760 nm. Since the yeast respiration assured deoxygenation, the addition of 16 μM of Hb should cause an increase in the magnitude of $\partial(\log R)/\partial t$ by 0.0061 cm^{-1} (=$\epsilon_{Hb}^{760} \times$ [Hb] = 0.38 cm^{-1} mM^{-1} × 0.016 mM^{-1}). The slope of the log R versus time, or $\partial(\log_e R)/\partial t$, with added Hb should be equal to 0.0352 cm^{-1} (i.e., =0.0291 cm^{-1} + 0.0061 cm^{-1}). However, the slope of the experimental log R versus time corresponded to 0.0412 cm^{-1}. We attribute the difference between experiment and expected slope in this latter case to experimental error of incomplete oxygenation.

Figure 10 further illustrates that the change in $\partial \log_e R/\partial t$ with deoxygenation is linearly related to the hemoglobin concentration. Equation [18] shows that the difference in slopes, $\partial \log_e R/\partial t_{deoxy} - \partial \log_e R/\partial t_{oxy}$, should to be approach the difference in absorption coefficients times the speed of light. Since $\{\mu_{adeoxy} - \mu_{aoxy}\}c = \Delta\epsilon_{Hb-HbO_2}[Hb_{tot}]c$, the plot of $(\partial \log_e R/\partial t_{deoxy} - \partial \log_e R/\partial t_{oxy})/c$ versus total hemoglobin concentration, [Hb$_{tot}$], should yield a straight line with zero intercept and slope equal to $\Delta\epsilon_{Hb-HbO_2}$. For the difference in $\log_e R$ versus [Hb$_{tot}$] shown in Fig. 10, the slope is equal to 2.303 × $\Delta\epsilon_{Hb-HbO_2}$(=2.303 × 0.25 cm^{-1} mM = 0.52 cm^{-1} mM^{-1}). Thus, the slope of the $\log_e R$ versus time curve obtained from time-resolved spectroscopy are functions of tissue absorption properties as described by Eqs. [6] and [18].

Furthermore from the plot of $\partial \log R/\partial t$ versus ρ at constant [Hb$_{tot}$] in Fig. 11, one can see from the parallel curves for the deoxy- and oxygenated yeast/blood system that $\mu_{adeoxy} - \mu_{aoxy}$ or $\partial \log R/\partial t_{deoxy} - \partial \log R/\partial t_{oxy}$ is not a function of ρ, as predicted by Eq. [18]. However, as predicted by Eq. [6], $\partial \log R/\partial t$ at short and moderate response times t, increases with ρ. When the slope of the log R versus time is taken at late response times, $t \gg t_{max}$,

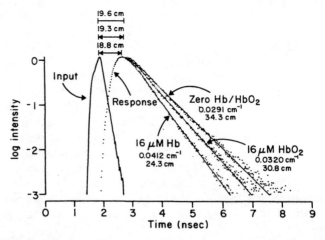

FIG. 9. The impulse response with (i) 1% yeast, (ii) 1% yeast with 16 μM HbO$_2$, and (iii) 1% yeast with 16 μM Hb as a function of time following impulse of incident light at 760 nm. The separation between source–detector was 6 cm and the wavelength employed was 760 nm; cylinder diameter, 14 cm. Shown are the values for t_{max} as well as $\partial \log R/\partial t$ taken at times t.

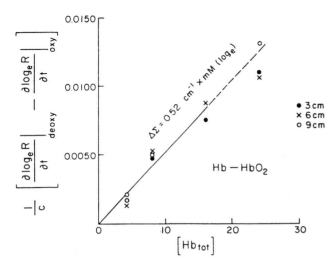

FIG. 10. The change in absorption (cm^{-1}) upon deoxygenation versus total hemoglobin concentration, [Hb$_{tot}$] (μM). The change in absorption was obtained from the difference of $(1/c)\partial \log_e R/\partial t$ taken at $t \gg t_{max}$ under oxy- and deoxygenated conditions. The symbols denote measurements at varying source–detector separations and the solid line represents the least squares regression. As suggested by Eq. [7] at $t \gg t_{max}$, $\partial \log_e R/\partial t$ becomes insensitive to changes in ρ.

the dependence of $\partial \log R/\partial t$ upon ρ is lost as suggested by Eq. [7].

Path length distributions: Effect of ρ. The typical impulse responses for varying source–dectector separations, ρ, from 3 to 6 cm with 24 μM oxyhemoglobin are shown in Fig. 12. From the slope of the terminal portions of the impulse response curves at $t \gg t_{max}$, it can be found that the $\partial \log R/\partial t$ at the two separations is similar. As suggested by Eq. [7], the slope of the terminal portion of the log R versus time curve should approach $-\mu_a^{10}c$. Experimentally, for $\rho = 3$ cm, we find $\mu_a^{10} = 0.039$ cm^{-1}; for $\rho = 6$ cm, $\mu_a^{10} = 0.036$ cm^{-1}. From the Beer–Lambert relationship, μ_a^{10} is expected to be 0.031 cm^{-1}. As expected, at $t \gg t_{max}$ the source–detector separation

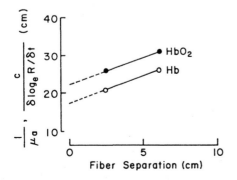

FIG. 11. The effect of fiber separation, ρ (cm), upon μ_a as measured from $(1/c)\partial \log R/\partial t$ at early response times for oxy- and deoxygenated blood/yeast model containing 16 μM [Hb$_{tot}$]. The ordinate is plotted as $(1/\mu_a)$ or the mean free absorption path length (cm).

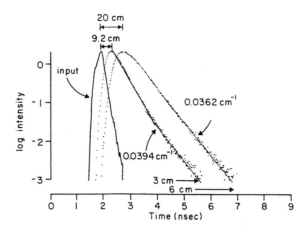

FIG. 12. The effect of input/output fiber separation upon $\partial \log R/\partial t \gg t_{max}$ in the yeast/blood model with 1% yeast and 24 μM [HbO$_2$] as shown in the plot of log R versus time; cylinder diameter, 14 cm. The values for $\partial \log R/\partial t$ and t_{max} are indicated for the source–detector separations of 3 and 6 cm. The input function is also indicated as well.

in this model system has minimal effect upon $\partial \log R/\partial t$. The discrepancies between measured and theoretical values of the time-resolved spectra may be due to experimental error. Nevertheless, we provide exemplary evidence for (i) the validity Eqs. [6] and [18] to describe photon migration in highly scattering media such as tissue, and (ii) the potential to derive information of absorption properties from the path length distributions measured from time-resolved spectroscopy.

Time of maximum detected signal. As described in Eq. [8], the time for maximum detected signal in the impulse response, t_{max}, is related strongly to $(1 - g)\mu_s$ and ρ; and since $\mu_a \ll (1 - g)\mu_s$, to a lesser extent upon μ_a. As shown in Fig. 13, we experimentally investigated the effect of the time for maximum signal measured with respect to the impulse instrument function as shown in Fig. 9. Figure 13 shows t_{max} (ns) versus concentration of added hemoglobin (2–30 μM) for source–detector separations of 3, 6, and 9 cm. At each source–detector separation, time-resolved measurements are made when the yeast/blood mixture was completely oxygenated and subsequently, deoxygenated. As expected, t_{max} increased with increasing ρ. As predicted by Eq. [8], small increases in t_{max} were observed with increased abosrption due to the deoxygenation of hemoglobin. These changes were within the error of determining t_{max}, yet increased with the separation of the source and detector, ρ, from 6 to 9 cm. Thus the effect of deoxygenation could not be observed in t_{max} at small ρ, but was observed at larger ρ. As shown in Eq. [8], when μ_a is comparable to $(1 - g)\mu_s$ and ρ is large, t_{max} becomes sensitive to changes in absorption properties of the media. Nevertheless, this study shows that for $\rho \leqslant 3$ cm, $(1 - g)\mu_s$ can be determined from t_{max}. Once $(1 - g)\mu_s$ is known, then the slope

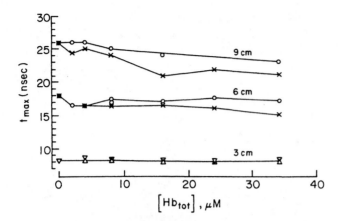

FIG. 13. The effect of hemoglobin concentration (μM) and source–detector fiber separation (cm) upon t_{max} (ns) in a 1% yeast model. Fiber source–detector geometries were varied so that separations of 3, 6, and 9 cm were obtained as the system was repeatedly oxygenated and deoxygenated. At separations of 6 and 9 cm, measurements made following deoxygenation are denoted by the open circles. As shown in the figure, increases in t_{max} are noted with the increased absorption due to deoxyhemoglobin at 760 nm. At 3 cm, there was no difference in t_{max} in the oxy- and deoxygenated states.

of the log R can be used to determine μ_a directly as suggested by Eq. [6].

Summary of time-resolved spectra with changes in hemoglobin saturation. The time-resolved data presented above behave consistently as a function of $(1 - g)\mu_s$ and ρ as predicted from diffusion approximation for photon migration reviewed in Section 1.0. The results in Fig. 9–13 emphasize the validity of attributing the shifts in the distribution of path lengths and specifically, the rate of decay at long response times, $\partial \log R/\partial t$, to the absorption properties of hemoglobin. Since the data presented herein represent time-resolved measurements made at a single wavelength, the terminal slope was taken as an indicator of absorption. The ratio of reflectance measurements at dual wavelengths (Section 2.1), $(\partial \log_e R^{\lambda_1}(\rho, \text{t}))/(\partial \log_e R^{\lambda_2}(\rho, \text{t})) \rightarrow \mu_a^{\lambda_1}/\mu_a^{\lambda_2}$ should enable determination of hemoglobin saturation as shown in Fig. 6. Nevertheless, in these initial results using a single wavelength in the model system, we have demonstrated the capacity for spectroscopic determination of μ_a using time-resolved measurements. In addition, we have shown that for smaller separations, (i.e., $\rho \leq 3$ cm in the current model), t_{max} also becomes a sensitive indicator of $(1 - g)\mu_s$ when $(1 - g)\mu_s \gg \mu_a$.

3.1.2. "Effective" Mean Path Length from Frequency-Resolved Measurements

Simultaneously to the time-resolved measurements, a dual-wavelength phase modulation system (220 MHz) (4,28) was employed to measure the effective mean path lengths, $\langle L \rangle$, at 754 and 816 nm for the yeast/blood system. The advantage of phase-modulation spectroscopy

is that it gives continuous recording as in CWS yet gives a statistical measure of the distribution of path lengths. Figure 14 shows that phase, frequency-resolved spectroscopy and CWS give similar signal to noise (since both have a duty ratio that approaches one) in the yeast/blood model as it is allowed to deoxygenate completely from the oxygenated state.

To investigate quantitatively the behavior of θ obtained from phase frequency-resolved spectroscopy, the relationship between total hemoglobin concentrations and oxygenation status was investigated similarly to those studies presented above for time-resolved spectroscopy. The wavelength employed by the laser diode of the phase modulated spectrometer differed slightly from that of the time-resolved studies (i.e., 754 and 840 instead of 760 nm) in order to obtain maximum sensitivity. Figure 15 shows change in the effective, mean path length measured upon deoxygenation $\Delta\langle L \rangle_{\text{oxy-deoxy}}$ for the two wavelengths at 200 MHz with added hemoglobin concentrations ranging from 0 to 40 μM. The values of mean path lengths were computed from measured small angle phase-shift via the relationship described in Eq. [11]. The scattering medium consisted of 0.5% intralipid (with an approximate, effective scattering coefficient, $(1 - g)\mu_s \sim 7.25$ cm^{-1}) with 2% yeast added to consume oxygen via respiration. The source–detector fiber arrangement consisted of two 8-mm fiber optic

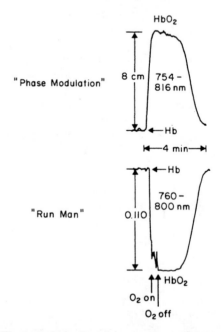

FIG. 14. The typical kinetics of oxygenation and deoxygenation of hemoglobin in the yeast/blood model as detected by phase modulated spectroscopy and continuous wave spectroscopy. The model contained 1% yeast with 34 μM [Hb$_{tot}$]. The top trace depicts the phase-shift difference ($\theta^{754}-\theta^{816}$) and the bottom trace shows the intensity difference ($I^{760}-I^{800}$) from the continuous wave machine, Runman. The arrows denote when oxygen sparing started and stopped. $\rho = 6$ cm.

bundles 6 cm apart for the detection of light and a 3-mm fiber optic source midpoint between the two fiber detectors. This configuration afforded maximum sensitivity to changes in hemoglobin saturation at the greatest possible signal intensity. Assuming that the yeast mixture did not significantly absorb light at 754 or 840 nm, we found that the addition of 2% yeast to intralipid increased the effective scattering coefficient to approximately 8 cm^{-1}. The solid lines in Fig. 15 are calculated from Eqs. [11] and [19] for the specified [Hb$_{tot}$], $(1 - g)\mu_s$, and the source–detector separation. The symbols denote individual measurements. It is noteworthy that the change in effective mean path length derived from the measured phase-shift tends to increase linearly with total absorber concentration, as predicted from Eq. [19].

In order to verify that Eq. [9] can be used to describe the phase-shift (or alternatively, the effective mean path length as described in Eq. [11] due to hemoglobin deoxygenation in a highly scattering media, we have simultaneously monitored solution pO$_2$ and θ at 754 nm in an Intralipid solution with an assumed $(1 - g)\mu_s$ equal to 7.25 cm^{-1}, and containing 0.01% yeast, and 27 μM of hemoglobin. Deoxygenation occurred over a period of 2 h over which time measurement of solution pO$_2$ and θ were continually made. Figure 16 shows the effective, mean path length calculated from Eq. [11] using experimental values of θ versus solution pO$_2$. The solid line denotes that predicted from a combination of the hemoglobin saturation curve and Eqs. [9] and [10]. The discrepancy between experimental and theoretically derived values of path length change is due probably to the left shifting of the hemoglobin saturation curve of our blood samples caused by accumulations of DPG during blood baking. Nevertheless, Fig. 16 shows the unique

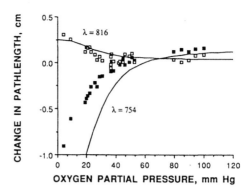

FIG. 16. The mean photon path length, (cm), measured at 754 and 816 nm versus pO$_2$ (mm Hg) with 27 μM [Hb$_{tot}$] in a 0.5% intralipid solution (μ_s = 7.25 cm^{-1}) with 0.01% yeast added to consume oxygen. The symbols denote actual measurements while the solid line denotes the path length changes predicted by the extinction coefficients cited, the hemoglobin saturation curve (P_{50} = 25 mm Hg, n = 2.8), and Eqs. [9] and [11].

behavior of phase-shift, or effective mean path length changes measured simultaneously at 754 and 816 nm as a function of solution pO$_2$. The lack of significant changes in effective path length monitored at 816 nm is due to the closeness to the hemoglobin isosbestic point at 800 nm.

Appendix A1.8 describes the use of dual-wavelength, dual frequency phase frequency-resolved spectroscopy for the determination of absorbance in strongly scattering media.

4.0. CHARACTERISTICS OF TIME-RESOLVED AND PHASE-MODULATED SPECTROSCOPY *IN VIVO*

In the previous section, the characteristics of time-resolved and phase frequency-resolved spectroscopy were investigated in an *in vitro* model taken to approximate the dimensions and optical properties of the adult human head. In the following, we present preliminary measurements of oxygenation of adult human brain for spectroscopic measurements of $\partial \log_e R/\partial t$ and θ which show characteristics which we have identified in the *in vitro* models described above.

4.1. Time-Resolved Measurements in the Human Adult Brain

Figure 17 shows the product $\partial \log_e R/\partial t \cdot 1/c$ evaluated at $t \gg t_{max}$ as a function of source–detector separation, ρ, for a series of studies using both streak camera and single photon counting technologies to monitor photon migration in human adult heads. Overall, the variation of $\partial \log_e R/\partial t/c$ is small from 8- to 16-cm source–detector separations in accord with studies of rat brain (12) and the model study presented in Section 3.1.1. As described by Eq. [7], $\partial \log_e R/\partial t \cdot 1/c$ should approach μ_a at long response times. Using Monte Carlo simulations of a

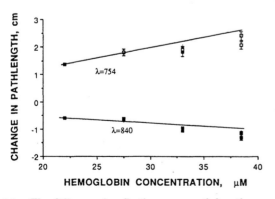

FIG. 15. The difference in effective mean path lengths measured during oxy- and deoxygenation, $\Delta \langle L \rangle_{oxy-deoxy}$ (cm) versus total hemoglobin concentration, [Hb$_{tot}$] (μM) measured in a 0.5% intralipid solution ($(1 - g)\mu_s$ = 7.25 cm^{-1}) and with source–detector separation distance of 3 cm. The dual-wavelength measurements were performed at 754 and 840 nm. The symbols and error bars denote actual measurements and the solid line represents the pathlength changes predicted by the change in extinction coefficients and Eq. [9].

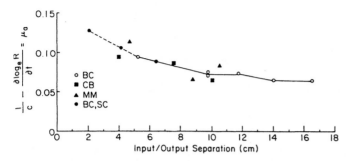

FIG. 17. The absorption coefficient at 760 nm, μ_a, calculated from $(1/c) \cdot \partial \log_e R/\partial t$ for a variety of source–detector fiber separations on eight human adult heads. The legend identifies the symbols for each individual. At greater separations, μ_a approaches 0.075 cm^{-1}.

model skull with three times greater scattering capacity and smaller absorption than the underlying brain tissue, we have shown that the skull contribution to photon migration becomes smaller as the source–detector separations in increase, and $\partial \log_e R/\partial t \cdot 1/c$ approaches that obtained from simulations without the skull present (14). Figure 17 shows that this behavior may occur *in vivo*, with the absorption coefficient of human brain measured from $\partial \log_e R(\rho, t)/\partial t$ at 760 nm approaching approximately 0.075 cm^{-1} at $\rho > 3$ cm. The scatter of all individuals is ±8% with respect to the open circle data (BC). A much larger population is required to quantify human subject variability.

As would be expected from the discussion in Section 1.0, the direct application of time-resolved spectroscopy to the human forehead should enable determination of hemoglobin saturation from characteristics of the path length distribution via Eq. [17]. The asymptotic values of $\partial \log_e R/\partial t \cdot 1/c$ measured for three individuals is listed in Table 2. Assuming that $\partial \log_e R/\partial t \cdot 1/c$ approaches μ_a for two wavelengths at 3- and 5-cm source–detector separation distances, then the ratio of $\partial \log_e R/\partial t \cdot 1/c$ at each wavelength should provide a description of the hemoglobin saturation via Eq. [17]. For the two individuals, the hemoglobin saturation is calculated to be 65, 57, and 50%, consistent with the known arteriovenous saturations values for brain of 66% (32). The calculation of hemoglobin saturation for the two subjects is found in the Appendix A1.5.

4.2 Phase Frequency-Resolved Spectroscopy Measurement of Changing Oxygenation Conditions in the Human Adult Brain

Similar spectroscopic responses to deoxygenation are expected with phase-modulation spectroscopy *in vivo* as occurred in the yeast/blood model. If $\mu_a^{760} = 0.075$ cm^{-1} as measured from time-resolved spectra (See Section 4.1; Fig. 17), then assuming $(1 - g)\mu_s \sim 8$ cm^{-1}, one should obtain effective, mean path length of 17 cm from

a source–detector separation of 3 cm at a 220-MHz modulation frequency. Indeed, the values of the effective mean path length for the adult human brain measured using a 220-MHz phase frequency-resolved spectrophotometer are 23.2 ± 1.6 cm for 8 normal controls between the ages of 20 and 76 years. The discrepancy between the measured and predicted value of mean photon path length may be due to (i) the assumptions of μ_a and $(1 - g)\mu_s$, and (ii) that the potential effect of a more strongly scattering skull will further increase the phase-shift (14). Appendix A1.6 shows an example calculation for $\langle L \rangle$ measured at 760 nm and at a modulation frequency of 220 MHz.

In order to demonstrate the changes in deoxygenation in the adult brain, measurement of phase-shift and therefore $\langle L \rangle$ were made at 754 and 816 nm during breath holding for a period of 1 min. As shown in Fig. 18, similar changes were noted with *in vivo* deoxygenation as measured in the *in vitro* yeast/blood model system. Due to circulatory delay, the maximum deoxygenation was reached 10 s after the cessation of breath holding, followed by a rapid recovery with a half-time of 15 s. The deoxygenation is only a small portion of the change that would have occurred in the case of complete deoxygenation.

Figure 19 illustrates the use of phase frequency-resolved spectroscopy in the study of cardiac arrest. Here we illustrate the transient deoxygenation of the human adult brain in AICD (automatic implanted cardioventricular defibrillator) implant procedure in which cardiac arrest and defibrillation occurs. Brain hemoglobin deoxygenation occurs rapidly with a half-time of 4 s, and a recovery with a half-time of 10 s at 760 nm. The change shown at 816 nm is delayed until the restart of the heart. Since 816 nm is close to the isosbestic point and changes little with deoxygenation (i.e., see Fig. 16), this is evidence of no change in the total blood volume of

TABLE 2

Dual-Wavelength Determination of Hemoglobin Saturation in the Adult Human Brain Using Time-Resolved Spectroscopy

	Subject					
	1		2		3	
λ (nm)	760	800	760	800	760	800
ρ (cm)	5.5		5.5		3.0	
μ_a (cm^{-1}) $\times 10^3$ ($=1/c \cdot \partial \log_e R/\partial t$)	57	48	41	32	75	69
μ_a^{760}/μ_a^{800}	1.19		1.28		1.09	
$Y \times 100\%$ (see appendix)	57%		50%		65%	

the tissue sampled by the migrating photons. Assuming that the tissue oxygenation of the patient prior to arrest was similar to that described from the time-resolved studies presented in Section 4.1 (i.e., $\mu_a = 0.075$ cm^{-1} at Hb saturation $\sim 70\%$), then an approximate 40% deoxygenation occurred upon arrest as computed from the phase-shift. Appendix A1.7 outlines the approximations for this study.

5.0. SUMMARY

In conclusion, we have shown that the photon migration characteristics, more specifically, the distribution of photon path lengths traveled before detection may be determined from time-resolved and phase frequency-resolved spectroscopy and can be used to assess hemoglobin oxygenation in an *in vitro* model as well as *in vivo*. Quantitation of hemoglobin saturation for time-resolved spectroscopy requires information of the slope of $\log_e R$ versus t, or $\partial \log_e R / \partial t$, at long response times ($t \gg t_{max}$) measured at two wavelengths, or alternatively information of $\partial \log_e R / \partial t$ at multiple wavelengths at shorter response times (Appendix A1.3). In contrast, additional information of tissue scattering is required for the dual-wavelength measurement of hemoglobin saturation from phase modulated spectroscopy.

While it is clear that dual-wavelength, time-resolved spectroscopy offers the greatest potential for the determination of hemoglobin saturation independent of assumptions of tissue scattering and total blood volume, the instrument is slow (>30 s is required) and no direct readout is provided. The availability of laser diodes in the infrared wavelength range makes time-resolved spectroscopy more portable. Equipment requirements also include the photon counting system, for which single channel operation is not prohibitively large, as well as a microchannel plate detector. To date, this system has not been programmed to give the time course of

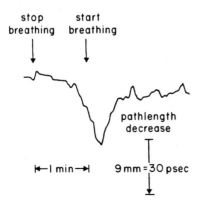

FIG. 18. The real-time tracing of the phase-shift difference (θ^{754}–θ^{816}) in the human adult brain (MM) during breath holding. The phase-shifts were monitored at 220 MHz and the time and path length changes are as noted in the figure.

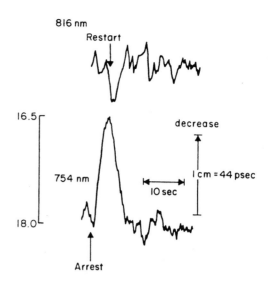

FIG. 19. AICD study. The real-time tracing of the dual-wavelength phase-shifts measured at 220 MHz at 754 and 816 nm during cardiac arrest and resuscitation. The arrows denote the state of cardiac arrest and resuscitation. The time and path length changes are noted in the figure. The lack of changes at 816 nm, which is close the hemoglobin isosbestic point, reflects little change in the tissue blood volume.

dual-wavelength signal changes vital for the study of oxygenation kinetics in tissues such as exercising muscle. Measurement of time-resolved spectroscopic signals requires time scales for adequate signal collection that are on the order of the time scale for tissue oxygenation kinetics.

On the other hand, phase frequency-resolved spectroscopy is highly economical and portable and can readily operate at multiple wavelengths and multiple frequencies and still remain convenient to use. It can also provide dynamic measurements over the time scales required for tissue oxygenation kinetics. However, dual-wavelength, single-frequency phase spectroscopy may require an additional assumption or a measurement of tissue scattering properties, presumably measured from time-resolved spectroscopy. It may be that the scattering properties of certain tissues, such as the human head, do not vary considerably facilitating the use of single-frequency, dual-wavelength measurement of *in vivo* hemoglobin saturation. If on the other hand, scattering may be expected to vary, as in disease, then calibration of $(1-g)\mu_s$ with time-resolved spectroscopy or dual-wavelength, dual-frequency phase spectroscopy would provide economical and convenient measure of *in vivo* hemoglobin saturation (see, for example, Appendix A1.8).

Finally, continuous wave spectroscopic measurements offers no information of the distribution of path lengths and thereby can be expected to vary with experimental conditions. Furthermore, since absorption itself affects the distribution of path lengths in tissues, determination of hemoglobin saturation is difficult. Correction for the unknown path length by the DPF renders quantitation difficult without independent time- or frequency-resolved spectroscopy measurement of the distribution of path lengths. While the great simplicity of continuous wave spectroscopy is attractive, especially if correction factors for path lengths changes are constant and transferable, it should not be used in clinical situations where both scattering and hemoglobin absorption change (for example, a cancer patient undergoing radiation therapy; an Alzhemier's patient; or a rapidly growing or healing tissue, such as a neonate brain). In these cases, it is mandatory that path length changes be monitored simultaneously if quantitation of tissue oxygenation is to be achieved.

In this paper, we have presented the algorithms and experimental measurements of (i) dual-wavelength, time-resolved spectroscopy and (ii) dual-wavelength, phase frequency-resolved spectroscopy. In addition we have briefly commented upon and detailed in Appendixes A1.3 and A1.8 the multiwavelength and dual-frequency algorithms for time- and frequency-resolved measurements which would eliminate or minimize the assumptions due to background absorbance and tissue scattering. Future research is required to ascertain the optimal algorithm and technique for accurate determination of *in vivo* hemoglobin saturation in various clinical situations.

APPENDIX A1

A1.1 Relationship between $\langle L \rangle$ and Phase-Shift as Measured Using Phase-Modulated Spectroscopy

One can show that at low modulation frequencies, i.e., as $2\pi f \ll \mu_a c$, the phase-shift is a direct measure of the mean time-of-flight, $\langle t \rangle$. Furthermore, since photons travel at a constant speed, then the phase-shift at low modulation frequencies describes the effective, mean path length, $\langle L \rangle$, traveled by photons migrating from a source to a detector. In the following we mathematically show that at low modulation frequencies expressions for the mean time-of-flight, $\langle t \rangle$, and the phase-shift, θ, and are equivalent.

To derive the expression for θ as the modulation frequency becomes small, one can expand the sine and cosine terms in Eq. [9] to the first power of f. In the limit of small f, $\psi = \sqrt{3\mu_a(1-g)\mu_s\rho^2}$. The expression for θ can be written

$$\theta \rightarrow -\sqrt{3\mu_a(1-g)\mu_s\rho^2} \cdot \frac{\pi f}{\mu_a c}$$
$$- \tan^{-1}\left\{\frac{-\sqrt{3\mu_a(1-g)\mu_s\rho^2} \cdot (\pi f/\mu_a c)}{1 + \sqrt{3\mu_a(1-g)\mu_s\rho^2}}\right\}. \quad [A1]$$

When the arc tangent term is expanded to the first power of f, Eq. [A1] becomes

$$\theta \rightarrow \frac{-3\mu_a(1-g)\mu_s\rho^2}{1 + \sqrt{3\mu_a(1-g)\mu_s\rho^2}} \cdot \frac{\pi f}{\mu_a c}, \quad [A2]$$

which is similar to the expression given by Patterson *et al.* (18). In the strongly scattering regime, i.e., $(1-g)\mu_s$ is large, and at large ρ, Eq. [A2] can be written

$$\theta \rightarrow \frac{\sqrt{3}\rho}{2c} \sqrt{\frac{(1-g)\mu_s}{\mu_a}} \cdot 2\pi f. \quad [A3]$$

An expression for the mean time-of-flight, $\langle t \rangle$, can be found from expressions of the $R(\rho, t)$ describing time-resolved spectra and the distribution of path lengths traveled before detection,

$$\langle t \rangle = \frac{\int_0^\infty R(\rho, t)t\partial t}{\int_0^\infty R(\rho, t)\partial t}. \quad [A4]$$

Using the integral forms of Gradshteyn and Ryzhik (34), expression [A4] was evaluated to give

$$\langle t \rangle = \frac{\sqrt{3}\rho}{2c} \sqrt{\frac{(1-g)\mu_s}{\mu_a}}. \quad [A5]$$

Comparison of Eqs. [A3] and [A5] show that the phase-shift is equal to $\langle t \rangle \cdot 2\pi f$:

$$\theta \rightarrow 2\pi f \cdot \langle t \rangle \rightarrow 2\pi f \cdot \frac{\langle L \rangle}{c}, \quad [A6]$$

which is analogous to the expression given in Eq. [10] in the limit of small $\langle L \rangle$.

It is important to note that this expression exists strictly as the modulation frequency becomes small. In this case, change in the phase-shift represents change in the mean of the distribution of path lengths. Thus, all path lengths are equally weighted in measurement of phase-shift at low modulation frequency. As the modulation frequency becomes higher, then shorter path lengths become more heavily weighted than longer path lengths. To explore this, we have used Monte Carlo analysis of layered media to simulate time-resolved spectra and fast Fourier transforms to arrive at the frequency-resolved spectra of phase-shift versus modulation frequency (14). Our results show that the presence of a superficial layer, which predominantly affects the number of photons which travel shallow penetration depth, or shorter total path lengths (33), causes little change in the measured phase-shift at low modulation frequencies, but dramatic changes at higher frequencies. Application of Eq. [10] to describe the effective mean path lengths at all frequencies, indicate that shorter and shorter penetration depths and total path lengths are more heavily weighted in measurement of phase-shift at greater frequency.

Throughout the text, we refer to the phase-shift as the effective mean photon path length since at larger modulation frequencies, it is not the mean path length measured, but rather an approximate description of the distribution of photon path lengths traveled before detection.

A1.2. Derivation of the DPF Using Photon Migration Theory

Previously, to correct for the distribution of path lengths traveled in tissue CWS measurements, Delpy *et al.* (12) introduced the DPF such that the Beer's law expression becomes

$$\text{absorbance} = \text{DPF}\rho\epsilon[C] \qquad [A7]$$

and the factor $\text{DPF} \cdot \rho$ is equal to the mean path length traveled before detection. Upon inspection Eqs. [A5] and [A7], the expression described by Eq. [11] can be found.

A1.3. Determination of Hemoglobin Saturation from Multiwavelength Measurement of Time-Resolved Spectra

Since the scattering properties of tissue are insensitive to wavelength, the difference in $\partial(\log_e R)/\partial t$ measured at different wavelengths at time, t, is equal to $(\mu_a^{\lambda_2} - \mu_a^{\lambda_1})c$ as described in Eq. [18]. Thus, since μ_a^λ can be described by the Beer–Lambert relationship (Eq. [15]), one can write.

$$\frac{\partial \log_e R^{\lambda_1}|_t - (\partial/\partial t)\log_e R^{\lambda_2}|_t/\partial t}{\partial \log_e R^{\lambda_3}|_t - (\partial/\partial t)\log_e R^{\lambda_2}|_t/\partial t}$$
$$= \frac{(\epsilon_{\text{Hb}}^{\lambda_1} - \epsilon_{\text{Hb}}^{\lambda_2}) + Y(\epsilon_{\text{HbO}_2}^{\lambda_1} - \epsilon_{\text{HbO}_2}^{\lambda_2} - \epsilon_{\text{Hb}}^{\lambda_1} + \epsilon_{\text{Hb}}^{\lambda_2}) + ((\alpha^{\lambda_1} - \alpha^{\lambda_2})/[\text{Hb}_{\text{tot}}])}{(\epsilon_{\text{Hb}}^{\lambda_3} - \epsilon_{\text{Hb}}^{\lambda_2}) + Y(\epsilon_{\text{HbO}_2}^{\lambda_3} - \epsilon_{\text{HbO}_2}^{\lambda_2} - \epsilon_{\text{Hb}}^{\lambda_3} + \epsilon_{\text{Hb}}^{\lambda_2}) + ((\alpha^{\lambda_3} - \alpha^{\lambda_2})/[\text{Hb}_{\text{tot}}])}. \qquad [A8]$$

In the event that the background absorbance, α^λ, is negligible or changes little over the small range of wavelengths employed, then the ratio of the difference in $\partial(\log_e R)/\partial t$ measured at different wavelengths at time, t, can be used to assess tissue hemoglobin saturation.

Inspection of Eq. [A5] indicates that the ratio of the difference in $\langle t \rangle$ could also be used to determine the hemoglobin saturation from multiple-wavelength measurement. However, since small changes in $\langle t \rangle$ would occur due to the relative small changes in μ_a, it is improbable that $\langle t \rangle$ could provide accurate determination of hemoglobin saturation.

A1.4. Dual-Wavelength Measurements of Phase-Shift at Single Modulation Frequencies

The derivation of Eq. [17] for single-frequency measurements of phase-shift at two wavelengths depends first upon the assumption that the modulation frequency is high such that $2\pi f \gg \mu_a c$. Under these conditions, the arc tangent term in the expression for Θ given in Eq. [9] can be expanded to yield $\Theta = \pi/2 - \mu_a c/2\pi f$. Using standard trigonometric identities to (i) expand the terms of $\sin(\pi/2 - \mu_a c/2\pi f)/2$ and $\cos(\pi/2 - \mu_a c/2\pi f)/2$ and (ii) to approximate sine and cosine of small angle, $(\mu_a c/2\pi f)/2$, Eq. [9] can be rewritten

$$\theta^\lambda = -\sqrt{\frac{6\pi(1-g)\mu_s\rho^2 f}{c}}\sin\frac{\pi}{4}\left\{1 - \frac{\mu_a^\lambda c}{4\pi f}\right\}$$
$$-\tan^{-1}\left\{\frac{-\sqrt{(6\pi(1-g)\mu_s\rho^2 f/c)}\sin(\pi/4)\{1 - \mu_a^\lambda c/4\pi f\}}{1 + \sqrt{(6\pi(1-g)\mu_s\rho^2 f/c)}\sin(\pi/4)\{1 - \mu_a^\lambda c/4\pi f\}}\right\}. \qquad [A9]$$

Further expansion of the arc tangent term of Eq. [A9] to the first-order yields

$$\theta^\lambda = -\sqrt{\frac{6\pi(1-g)\mu_s\rho^2 f}{c}}\sin\frac{\pi}{4}\left(1 - \frac{\mu_a^\lambda c}{4\pi f}\right)$$
$$\times\left\{1 - \frac{1}{1 + \sqrt{(6\pi(1-g)\mu_s\rho^2 f/c)}\sin(\pi/4)(1 - \mu_a^\lambda c/4\pi f)}\right\}. \qquad [A10]$$

In the strongly scattering regime (i.e., large $(1-g)\mu_s$) and at large ρ, Eq. [A10] becomes

$$\theta^\lambda = -\sqrt{\frac{6\pi(1-g)\mu_s\rho^2 f}{c}}\sin\frac{\pi}{4}\left\{1 - \frac{\mu_a^\lambda c}{4\pi f}\right\}, \qquad [A11]$$

which is that described in Eq. [19] in the text. From Eq. [9] one can determine that the phase-shift in the absence of absorption is expressed by

$$\theta_0 = -\sqrt{\frac{6\pi(1-g)\mu_s\rho^2 f}{c}}\sin\frac{\pi}{4}. \qquad [A12]$$

In the presence of background absorbance, α^λ, θ_o is given by

$$\theta_0^\lambda = -\sqrt{\frac{6\pi(1-g)\mu_s\rho^2 f}{c}}\sin\frac{\pi}{4}\left\{1 - \frac{\alpha^\lambda c}{4\pi f}\right\}. \qquad [A13]$$

Thus the relative phase shift at wavelength, λ, with respect to θ_o is given by

$$\theta^\lambda - \theta_0^\lambda = -\sqrt{\frac{6\pi(1-g)\mu_s\rho^2 f}{c}}\sin\frac{\pi}{4}\left\{\frac{\mu_{a_{Hb/HbO2}}^\lambda c}{4\pi f}\right\}. \quad [A14]$$

If the scattering properties of tissue are wavelength-insensitive (see discussion in Section 2.1) then ratio of relative phase-shifts measured at two wavelengths, λ_1 and λ_2 is equal to the ratio of absorbance due to tissue hemoglobin as described in Eq. [21].

A1.5. Calculation of Hemoglobin Saturation from Time-Resolved Measurements

We assume that at source–detector separations greater than 3 cm on the human head, $\partial \log_e R/\partial t$ curve gives the quantity, $-\mu_a c$. From the discussion in Section 2.0, we can write

$$\frac{(1/c)(\partial/\partial t)\log_e R^{760}}{(1/c)(\partial/\partial t)\log_e R^{800}} = \frac{\mu_a^{760}}{\mu_a^{800}} = \frac{\epsilon_{Hb}^{760}}{\epsilon_{Hb}^{800}} - \frac{\Delta\epsilon_{HbO2-Hb}^{760}}{\epsilon_{Hb}^{800}}Y. \quad [A15]$$

Thus, from values of the extinction coefficient (ϵ_{Hb}^{760} = 0.38 cm^{-1} mM^{-1}; ϵ_{HbO2}^{760} = 0.16 cm^{-1} mM^{-1}; $\epsilon_{Hb}^{800} = \epsilon_{HbO2}^{800}$ = 0.20 cm^{-1} mM^{-1} (29), the ratio of slopes at 760 and 800 nm will be equal to

$$\frac{\partial/\partial t \log_e R^{760}}{\partial/\partial t \log_e R^{800}} = 1.90 - 1.25\,Y, \quad [A16]$$

where Y is the hemoglobin saturation expressed as a fraction. Since $\partial \log R/\partial t$ was measured from the terminal slope of the $\log R$ versus t curve (i.e., at $t \gg t_{max}$), this algorithm should entail minimal error as indicated from the simulations presented in Fig. 6.

A1.6. Calculation of $\langle L \rangle$ for Normal Human Adult Brain.

The combination of Eqs. [9] and [10] can be used to give the effective mean of the distribution of path lengths, $\langle L \rangle$. For the parameters: c = 22 cm/s; f = 220 MHz, $(1-g)\mu_s$ = 8 cm^{-1}, ρ = 3 cm, and μ_a = 0.075 cm^{-1} (as shown from the time-resolved data shown in Fig. 17), one can find that $\langle L \rangle$ is predicted to be 17.5 cm. The actual measurement of phase-shift at 760 nm gives $\langle L \rangle$ = 23.2 ± 1.6 cm in eight human adults. From Monte Carlo simulations of a model head with a 3-mm annulus with scattering properties three times that of the brain, we have estimated that the skull causes an additional $\langle L \rangle$ of approximately 15 cm at ρ = 1.2 cm (14).

From Eq. [A5] one can find that the true mean of the distribution of path lengths is 26 cm. As described in Appendix A1.1, the effective mean path length is less than the true mean path length.

A1.7. Determination of Percentage Deoxygenation during Cardiac Arrest in Figure 19

We assume that the scattering properties in the brain are constant between state 1, denoted as the prearrest state, and state 2, denoted as the arrest state. Furthermore, since the 816-nm signal does not change until after the restart of the heart, we assume the total blood volume is constant for the short arrest. Therefore, changes in $\langle L \rangle$ are due to deoxygenation alone. In Appendix A1.1, Eqs. [A9] and [A11] show that in the event that $2\pi f > \mu_a c$, then the first term of Eq. [9] predominates. Thus, if one combines Eqs. [9] and [10], one can write the following expression for the ratio of effective, mean path lengths:

$$\frac{\langle L\rangle_1}{\tan\sin(1/2)\tan^{-1}(2\pi f/\mu_a^{760_1}c)}$$
$$= \frac{\langle L\rangle_2}{\tan\sin(1/2)\tan^{-1}(2\pi f/\mu_a^{760_2}c)}. \quad [A17]$$

The parameters utilized are $\mu_a^{760_1}$ = 0.075 cm^{-1} (from the time-resolved data shown in Fig. 17), Y_1 = 70% (32), f = 220 MHz. $\langle L\rangle_1$ and $\langle L\rangle_2$ are equal to 18 and 16.5 cm as described in Fig. 19. From Eq. [A18] we find that the ratio, $\mu_a^{760_1}/\mu_a^{760_2}$ is equal to 0.67.

From the Beer–Lambert relationship, one can see that from the ratio of absorption coefficients, the saturation in state 2 can be solved for

$$\frac{\mu_a^{760_1}}{\mu_a^{760_2}} = \frac{\epsilon_{Hb}^{760} + \Delta\epsilon_{HbO2-Hb}^{760}Y_1}{\epsilon_{Hb}^{760} + \Delta\epsilon_{HbO2-Hb}^{760}Y_2}. \quad [A18]$$

Using the extinction coefficients for 760 nm previously discussed in Section 2.0, we find Y_2 to correspond to an approximate 40% deoxygenation upon cardiac arrest.

A1.8. Hemoglobin Saturation Determination from Dual-Wavelength, Dual-Frequency Phase-Shift Measurements

As briefly described in Section 3.0, tissue hemoglobin saturation can also be determined from dual-wavelength, dual-frequency measurements of phase-shift. We denote the two modulation frequencies, f_1 and f_2 and restrict ourselves to the optimal case of using high frequencies such that $2\pi f_{1,2} \gg \mu_a^{\lambda_1\lambda_2}c$. From Eq. [A11] one can find the differences in phase-shift measured at one wavelength and two frequencies can be expressed as

$$\frac{\theta_{f_1}^{\lambda_1}}{\sqrt{f_1}} - \frac{\theta_{f_2}^{\lambda_1}}{\sqrt{f_2}} = \sqrt{\frac{6\pi(1-g)\mu_s\rho^2 f}{c}}\sin\frac{\pi}{4}\frac{\mu_a^{\lambda_1}}{4\pi}\left\{\frac{1}{f_2} - \frac{1}{f_1}\right\}.$$
$$[A19]$$

The ratio of this difference measured at two wavelengths can thus be written

$$\frac{(\theta_{f_1}^{\lambda_1}/\sqrt{f_1}) - (\theta_{f_2}^{\lambda_1}/\sqrt{f_2})}{(\theta_{f_1}^{\lambda_2}/\sqrt{f_1}) - (\theta_{f_2}^{\lambda_2}/\sqrt{f_2})} = \frac{\mu_a^{\lambda_1}}{\mu_a^{\lambda_2}}. \qquad [A20]$$

Since the scattering function is a wavelength-insensitive over the near-infrared range employed, one can see immediately that dual-frequency, dual-wavelength phase modulated spectroscopy can be used to obtain the ratio of absorption coefficients. As described in Sections A1.3 and A1.4, if background absorbance is negligible or wavelength insensitive, then dual-frequency, dual-wavelength phase modulated spectroscopy in the near-infrared range can give measures of tissue hemoglobin saturation via Eqs. [13] or [16].

APPENDIX 2A: NOMENCLATURE

c	speed of light in the media (cm/s)
$[C]$	concentration of absorber (mM)
d	thickness of tissue slab from transmittance measurements
D	effective diffusion coefficient for the transport of light ($= \{3(\mu_a + (1-g)\mu_s)\}^{-1}$, cm^{-1})
g	the mean cosine of anisotropic scattering angle
f	modulation frequency (MHz)
I, I_0	detected and incident light intensity, respectively
l^*	isotropic, mean scattering length between consecutive scattering lengths
L	path length of light ($= c \cdot t$) traveled before detection (cm)
n	number of scattering events taken for a photon to travel total path length, L
r	radial position (cm)
$R(\rho, t)$	reflectance of light at a tissue surface at time, t, and distance, ρ, away from the source light source term
t	time (s)
$T(\rho, d, t)$	transmittance of light across a slab of tissue of thickness d, and fiber separation, ρ, at time t
t_{max}	time of maximum detected $R(\rho, t)$ in time-resolved spectroscopy (s)
Y	hemoglobin saturation expressed as a function
z_0	equal to $\{(1-g)\mu_s\}^{-1}$ (cm)
α	the absorption coefficient due to non-hemoglobin constituents of tissue (cm^{-1})
ϵ	extinction coefficient of an absorber (cm^{-1} mM^{-1}) based upon Napierian log terms unless otherwise noted
$\phi(r, t)$	photon fluence rate or flux of photon at position r and time t
ρ	distance between source and detector in reflectance or transillumination measurements (cm)
μ_a	absorption coefficient (cm^{-1})
μ_a^{10}	absorption coefficient (cm^{-1}) based upon decadice extinction coefficients
$(1-g)\mu_s$	scattering coefficient (cm^{-1})
θ	phase-shift of light detected distance ρ away from a source of sinusoidally modulated light intensity (radians)
θ_0	phase-shift due to scattering or absorption other than hemoglobin (radians)

ACKNOWLEDGMENTS

This work was supported by NIM, Inc.; American Cancer Society, BE-13; NS-27346; and HL44124. E.M.S. was a recipient of a postdoctoral fellowship, NCI-CA08783. We thank M. Osbaken and M. Patterson for their reviews of this work.

REFERENCES

1. Chance, B., Leigh, J., Miyake, H., Smith, D., Nioka, S., Greenfield, R., Finlander, M., Kaufmann, K., Levy, W., Young, M., Cohen, P., Yoshioka, H., and Boretsky, R. (1988) *Proc. Natl. Acad. Sci. USA* **85**, 4971–4975.
2. Chance, B., Nioka, S., Kent, J., McCully, K., Fountain, K., Greenfield, M., and Holtom, G. (1988) *Anal. Biochem.* **174**, 698–707.
3. Chance, B., Smith, D. S., Nioka, S., Miyake, H., Holtom, G., and Maris, M. (1989) *in* Photon Migration in Tissues (Chance, B., Ed.), pp. 121–135, Plenum, New York, NY.
4. Chance, B., Maris, M., Sorge, J., and Zhang, M. Z. (1990) *Proc. SPIE–Int. Soc. Opt. Eng.* **1204**, 481–491.
5. Chance, B., Leigh, J. S., and Holtom, G. (1988) MRI/MRS Identification of Hemoglobin Species: Use of Time Resolved Spectroscopy. 7th Annual Meeting for the Society of Magnetic Resonance in Medicine, p. 585, August 20–26.
6. Chance, B., and Sevick, E. M. (1991) *Biophys. J.* **59**, 378a.
7. Ishimaru, A. (1978) Wave Propagation and Scattering in Random Media, pp. 175–188, Academic Press, San Diego.
8. Berndt, K. W., and Lakowicz, J. R. (1991) *Proc. SPIE–Int. Soc. Opt. Eng.* **1431**, 149–160.
9. Fishkin, J., Gratton, E., van de Ven., M. J. and Mantulin, W. W. (1991) *Proc. SPIE–Int. Soc. Opt. Eng.* **1431**, 122–135.
10. Haselgrove, J., Leigh, J., Yee, C., Wang, N. G., Maris, M., and Chance, B. (1991) *Proc. SPIE–Int. Soc. Opt. Eng.* **1431**, in press.
11. Hebden, J. C., and Kruger, K. A. (1991) *Proc. SPIE–Int. Soc. Opt. Eng.* **1431**, 30–41.
12. Delpy, D. T., Cope, M., van der Zee, P., Arridge, S., Wray, S., and Wyatt, J. (1988) *Phys. Med. Biol.* **33**, 1433–1442.
13. Nossal, R., Bonner, R. F., and Weiss, G. H. *J. Appl. Opt.* **28**, 2238–2244.
14. Sevick, E. M., and Chance, B. (1991) *Proc. SPIE–Int. Opt. Soc. Eng.* **1431**, 84–96.
15. Patterson, M. S., Chance, B., and Wilson, B. C. (1989) *J. Appl. Opt.* **28**, 2331–2336.

16. Profio, A. E., and Dorion, D. R. (1987) *Photochem. Photobiol.* **46,** 591–599.
17. Duderstadt, J. J., and Hamilton, L. J. (1976) Nuclear Reactor Analysis, pp. 140–144, Wiley, New York.
18. Patterson, M. S., Moulton, J. D., Wilson, B. C., and Chance, B. (1990) *Proc. SPIE–Int. Soc. Opt. Eng.* **1203,** 62–75.
19. Bolin, F. P., Pruess, L. E., Taylor R. C., and Ference, R. J. (1989) *Appl. Opt.* **28,** 2297–2303.
20. Weber, G. J. (1977) *Chem. Phys.* **66,** 4081–4091.
21. Sevick, E. M., Weng, J., Maris, M., and Chance, B. (1991) *Proc. SPIE–Int. Soc. Opt. Eng.* **1431,** 264–275.
22. Groenhuis, R. A. J., Bosch J. J. T., and Ferwerda, H. A. (1983) *Appl. Opt.* **22,** 2463–2467.
23. Groenhuis, R. A. J. Ferwerda, H. A., and Bosch, J. J. T. (1983) *Appl. Opt.* **22,** 2456–2462.
24. Nossal, R. J., and Bonner, R. F. (1991) *Proc. SPIE–Int. Soc. Opt. Eng.* **1431,** 21–29.
25. Miyake, H., Nioka, S., Zaman, A., Smith, D., and Chance, B. (1991) *Anal. Biochem.* **192,** 149–155.
26. Wang, Z., Noyszewski, E. A., and Leigh, J. (1990) *Magn. Reson. Med.* **14,** 562–567.
27. Theorell, H., and Chance, B. (1951) *Acta Chem. Scand.* **5,** 1127–1144.
28. Weng, J., Zhang, M. Z., Simmons, K., and Chance, B. (1991) *Proc. SPIE–Int. Soc. Opt. Eng.* **1431,** 161–170.
29. Lemberg, R., and Legg, J. W. (1949) Hematin Compounds and Bile Pigments, Interscience, New York.
30. Lakowicz, J. R., and Berndt, K. (1990) *Chem. Phys. Lett.* **166,** 1130–1133.
31. Sevick, E., Maris, M., and Chance, B. (1990) *J. Cancer Res. Clin. Oncol.* **116,** S514.
32. Nioka, S., Chance, B., Smith, D. S., Mayevsky, A., Reilly, M. P., Alter, C., and Asakura, T. (1990) *Pediatr. Res.* **28,** 54–62.
33. Weiss, G. H., Nossal, R., and Bonner, R. F. (1989) *J. Mod. Opt.* **36,** 349–359.
34. Gradshteyn, I. S., and Ryzhik, I. M. (1965) Tables of Integrals, Series, and Products, p. 340, Academic Press, New York.
35. Wilson, B. C., Patterson, M. S., and Burns, D. M. (1986) *Laser Med. Sci.* **1,** 235–244.

TOWARDS HUMAN BRAIN NEAR INFRARED IMAGING: TIME RESOLVED AND UNRESOLVED SPECTROSCOPY DURING HYPOXIC HYPOXIA

M. Ferrari[*], R.A. De Blasi[+], F. Safoue[+], Q. Wei[^], and G. Zaccanti[^]

[*]Dipartimento di Scienze e Tecnologie Biomediche, Università dell'Aquila, Italy and Laboratorio di Biologia Cellulare, Istituto Superiore di Sanità, [+]Istituto di Anestesiologia e Rianimazione, I Università di Roma, Roma Italy; [^]Dipartimento di Fisica, Università di Firenze, Firenze, Italy

INTRODUCTION

Near infrared (IR) spectroscopy (NIRS) on animals and humans originated from the work of Jobsis (1977). Early cerebral and muscle NIRS measurements using multi-wavelength photometers were utilized for a better spectral analysis and quantification purposes (Ferrari et al., 1989). Only pulse time and phase modulation spectroscopies can calculate pathlength in brain and muscle. Optical imaging in the near IR using these time-resolved methods is currently pursued by different groups (Chance, 1991 for a review). There are however significant technical and clinical problems related to the imaging technique yet to be solved before it can become truly a routine clinical tool.

When transmitting picosecond laser pulses and detecting photons on the opposite side of the object, the contrast can be strongly enhanced by detecting only the photons with the shortest traveling time. Short time resolution would restrict the scattering path and could provide further amelioration in image definition. Recently, Hitachi research laboratories (Shinohara et al., 1991, and this volume) obtained images of rat brain oxygenation during middle cerebral artery ischemia using dual wavelength picosecond near IR laser technique combined with conventional back projection image reconstruction. The aim of this paper was to investigate human brain oxygenation changes during hypoxic hypoxia using two wavelength picosecond near IR laser spectroscopy. Pathlengths were mapped on the human forehead. By combining spectral information obtained by a fast scanning spectrometer with pathlength data it was possible to quantify oxy- and deoxy-hemoglobin (Hb) concentration changes during hypoxic hypoxia.

METHODS

All measurements were obtained on adult volunteers. Each subject was submitted to graded steps of hypoxic hypoxia (FiO$_2$ 21, 10, 7, 6%). Arterial Hb saturation was measured by pulse oximetry. The brain was illuminated using an optic fiber (70 cm length, 0.3 cm active diameter) by ultrashort light pulses (duration 4 ps, repetition rate 76 MHz, wavelengths 760 and 800 nm) from a Coherent 700 dye laser (Fig. 1).

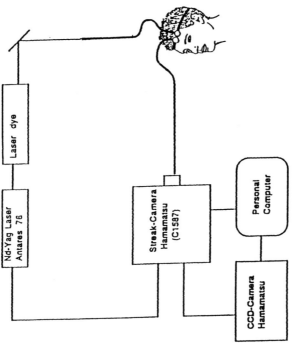

FIGURE 1. Experimental set-up used in human brain time-resolved spectroscopy.

The average power was 50-100 mW at the tip of the fiber. The light emerging from tissue was collected with an optic fiber (70 cm length, 0.5 cm active diameter) positioned at 3-5 cm distance. Light was measured over a 5 sec period by a syncroscan streak camera (Hamamatsu Photonics). The resolution of this equipment is a few picoseconds and the temporal window 1500 psec. Measurements were collected every 30 sec. Using this equipment the time of flight and temporal dispersion of light pulses through a multiple scattering medium can be studied. Optical density changes were calculated from the integral of the measured received pulses. The transit times (t) of the IR photons can be converted into distance travelled through the medium (d) using the formula d=ct/n (n=1.4, tissue refractive index). The mean path length was calculated from the weighted average of time in the pulse shape. The differential pathlength factor (DPF) was calculated dividing the mean pathlength by the interfiber distance. The slope of the logarithmic curve was calculated fitting the signal over a time

The tissue absorption coefficient spectra ($\Delta \mu_a$) were split into $\Delta[Hb]$ and $\Delta[HbO_2]$ using multilinear regression analysis (Cope et al., 1988) of the Hb- and HbO_2- spectra (Wray et al., 1988). The regression analysis was performed over the wavelength region 750 to 900 nm with data points at 2 nm intervals.

interval of about 300 psec starting from the time of half peak amplitude. The slope changes are associated with the variations of the absorption coefficient σ (cm^{-1}) of the medium. This time interval was chosen taking into account the linearity of this portion.

Spectral measurements were made using a fast scanning spectrophotometer (mod. 6500, NIRSystems, Silver Spring, MD). The spectral analysis procedure has been recently described (Ferrari et al., 1989). Two optic fibers (200 cm length and 0.5 cm active diameter) were applied 3-4 cm apart by a black rubber support so that a stable

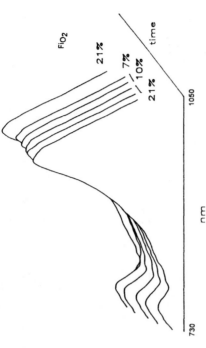

FIGURE 3. Successive near IR spectra from forehead of a representative subject during hypoxic hypoxia. Hypoxia caused an increase of the peak at 755 nm more consistent at the most severe tested hypoxia level (FiO$_2$ 7%). The last spectrum was collected 1 min after recovery in air.

RESULTS

Near IR spectra of human brain are very similar to previously published cat and dog spectra. Fig. 2 shows a spectrum measured on the human forehead compared to the spectrum of an apple. Both spectra, obtained with comparable optic fiber geometry, showed the water peak. The 755 nm deoxy-Hb peak is the only notable spectral feature which differentiates brain and apple spectra. When a volunteer is subjected to hypoxic hypoxia as shown in Fig, 3, the 755 nm peak rises constantly with increasing hypoxic hypoxia. Fig.4 shows typical pulse shapes measured on the forehead with different distances of the optic fibers. Small changes of the DPF were found when the DPF was mapped on the forehead (Fig. 5).

Fig.6 shows typical pulses measured at 760 nm before and during 10 min hypoxic hypoxia. Consistent changes of the pulse amplitude and slope were observed only at the most severe tested hypoxic hypoxia level. Fig.7 shows the time course of σ measured from a light pulse at 760 nm and 800 nm during graded hypoxic hypoxia and recovery. Using 760 nm light, σ increased gradually during hypoxia. No changes were observed using 800 nm light suggesting that no consistent blood volume changes occur during moderate hypoxia. σ measured at 760 nm rapidly recovered with room air ventilation.

By combining spectral information with pathlength data it was possible to quantify oxy and deoxy Hb-concentration changes during hypoxic hypoxia. Fig. 8 shows

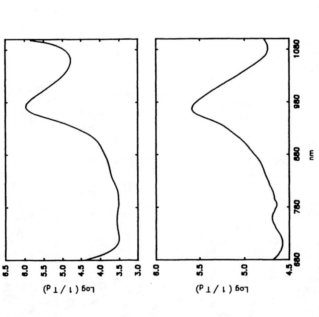

FIGURE 2. Typical near IR spectra of an human forehead (lower panel) and an apple (upper panel). The absorption band centered around 960 nm is attributable to water overtones. Brain presents also a band centered at around 755 nm attributable to deoxy Hb. T, diffuse transmittance.

fiber geometry was achieved. NIRSystems software was utilized to automatically collect a scan every 5 sec. Spectra were analyzed according to a modified Lambert-Beer law in order to obtain quantification of Hb changes during the experimental procedures. Difference spectra (ΔA) of the brain tissue were calculated relative to the pre-hypoxic period. These were converted into brain absorption coefficient ($\Delta \mu_a$) using $\Delta \mu_a = \Delta A/(Bd)$ where d was the physical separation of the optodes on skin surface and B was the DPF. Changes in brain absorption coefficient were assumed to result only from changes in the concentration of oxy- and deoxy-Hb (Wray et al., 1988). The results were expressed as micromoles per liter of tissue ($\mu M/L$).

the time course of Hb-saturation, Hb-content and cytochrome oxidase (cyt a-a₃) redox changes during hypoxic hypoxia. Hb-content and cytochrome redox state did not change during hypoxia. Hb-content transiently raised only when FiO_2 returned to 21%.

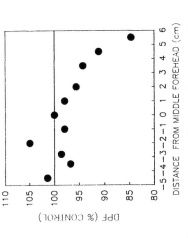

FIGURE 5. Differential pathlength factor (DPF) changes in the human forehead. The optic fibers, positioned at 3 cm distance, were moved along a plane perpendicular to the body sagittal axis. The reference plane was positioned at the level of the forehead center.

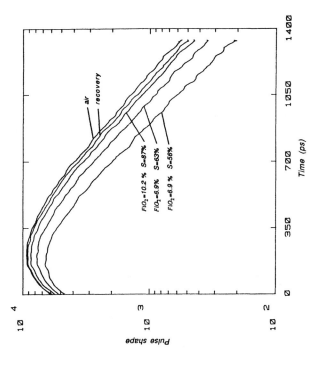

Figure 6. Pulse shape (arbitrary units) measured at 760 nm before and during 10 min hypoxic hypoxia. Consistent changes of pulse amplitude and slope were observed at the most severe tested hypoxic hypoxia level. Pulse slope recovered when the volunteer returned to air ventilation.

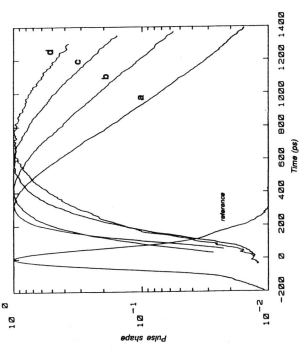

FIGURE 4. Pulse shape measured with the optic fibers at different distances (d) on the forehead. The maximum of each pulse was normalized to 1. Curves a-d correspond to d=2.0, 2.5, 3.0, and 4.0 cm respectively. The reference pulse was obtained with fibers aligned in air. For any curve the time t=0 corresponds to the arrival time for the unscattered transmitted beam. Differential pathlength factor for curves a-c was 5.9, 5.9 and 6.4 respectively.

CONCLUSIONS

NIRS has been developed experimentally and clinically to non-invasively monitor brain and muscle Hb/myoglobin-oxygenation and cytochrome a-a₃ redox state. Relevant human brain clinical applications are summarized in Table 1. Optical imaging in the near IR using time-resolved methods is currently pursued by different groups. Using these methods, at the Hitachi research laboratories (Shinohara et al., 1991, and this volume) images of rat brain oxygenation were obtained. To the best of our knowledge, the present results constitute the first report of human brain oxygenation monitoring by optic fiber time resolved spectroscopy on volunteers during graded hypoxic hypoxia. These results and the reported recent findings on time gate imaging of phantoms (Chance, 1991) suggest that human brain IR imaging might be performed in the near future using new tools such as ultrafast lasers, tunable over a wide spectral range, and ultrafast electronics.

583

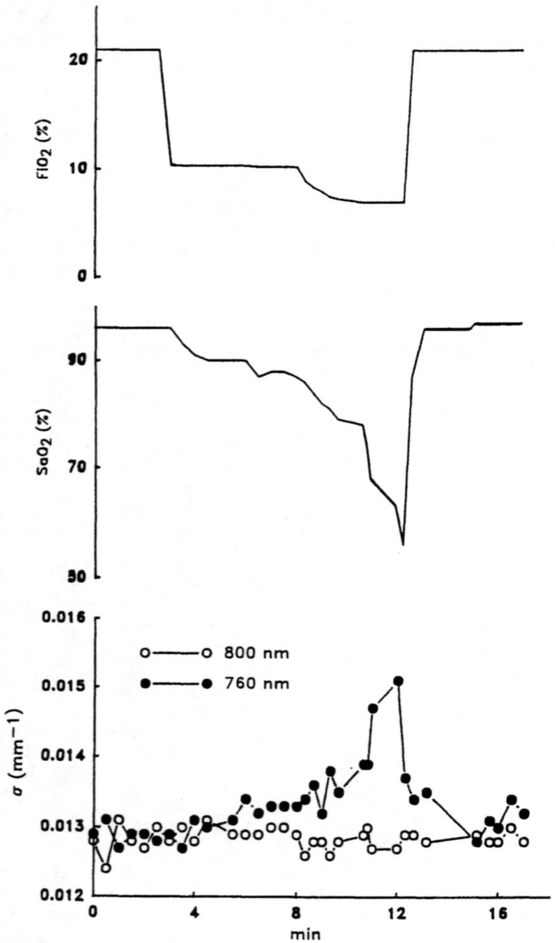

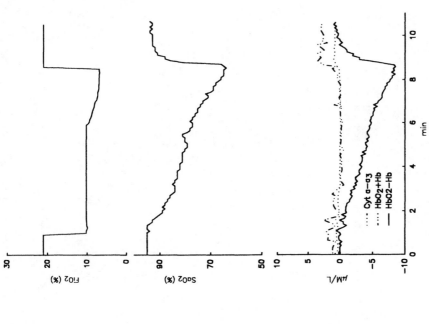

FIGURE 8. Time course of Hb saturation, Hb content and cytochrome oxidase (cyt a-a_3) redox changes during hypoxic hypoxia. Hb volume and cytochrome redox state did not change during hypoxia. Hb volume raised when FiO_2 returned to 21%. Symbols as Fig. 7.

ACKNOWLEDGEMENTS

We wish to thank Prof. S. Califano, Director of the European Laboratory for Non-linear spectroscopy, University of Florence. This research was supported in part by CNR contribution 91.00253.04. This research has been performed in the framework of the "Centro di ricerca interuniversitario: studio dei meccanismi molecolari coinvolti nel danno tissutale da ipossia e iperossia e di molecole che modificano tali lesioni".

FIGURE 7. Time course of σ measured from the slope of the light pulse at 760 nm and 800 nm during graded hypoxic hypoxia and recovery. Using 760 nm light, σ increased gradually during hypoxia. No changes were observed using 800 nm light suggesting that no consistent blood volume changes occurred during moderate hypoxia. σ measured at 760 nm rapidly recovered with room air ventilation. FiO_2 (inspired oxygen fraction); SaO_2 (Hb saturation measured by pulse oximetry on the nose).

Table 1. Main clinical applications of NIRS

FIELD OF APPLICATION	INVESTIGATED PARAMETER	AUTHORS
ADULT		
HYPOXIC HYPOXIA IN HEALTHY VOLUNTEERS	HbV, HbS, blood flow, transit time	Elwell et al.,1992, Hampson et al.,1990 McCormick et al.,1991
GENERAL ANESTHESIA	HbV, HbS	(Fox et al, 1985)
VASCULAR PATIENTS	HbV, HbS	(Ferrari et al., 1987)
CARDIAC SURGERY	HbS during cardio-pulmonary bypass	(Tamura,1991)
	HbS during surgery	(Koorn and Silvay,1991)
CARDIAC ARREST	Hyperoxia-reperfusion	(Smith,1990)
CENTRIFUGAL ACCELERATION	HbV, HbS	(Glaister and Jöbsis,1988)
CHILDREN		
CARDIAC SURGERY	HbV, HbS during Cardiopulmonary bypass	(Steven et al,1990)
NEWBORN		
INTENSIVE CARE	HbS monitoring during spontaneous hypoxia	(Brazy et al,1985)
	HbV, HbS	(Wyatt et al,1986)
	Blood flow, volume	(Edwards et al,1988, 1990)
	Blood volume changes during hypercapnia	(Wyatt et al,1991)
	Crying influence on HbV	(Brazy,1988)
	HbV changes during hypertension	(Brazy et al,1986)
	Hypoxia, bradicardia effects on HbS	(Livera et al,1991)
CARDIAC SURGERY	HbS during extracorporeal circulation	(Liem et al,1992)
FETUS		
LABOUR	Oxytocin effects on HbV, HbS	(Peebles et al,1991)

Hemoglobin content, HbV; Hemoglobin saturation, HbS

REFERENCES

Brazy J.E., Lewis D.V., Mitnick M.H., Jobsis F.F. (1985) Non invasive monitoring of cerebral oxygenation in preterm infants: preliminary observations. Pediatrics 75:217-225.

Brazy J.E., Lewis D.V. (1986) Changes in cerebral blood volume and cytochrome aa_3 during hypertensive peaks in preterm infants. J Pediatr 108:983-987.

Brazy J.E. (1988). Effects of crying on cerebral blood volume and cytochrome aa_3. J Pediatr 112:457-461.

Chance B. (1991) In: Time Resolved Spectroscopy and Imaging of Tissue, B. Chance, Editor, Proc. SPIE 1431.

Cope M., Delpy D.T., Reynolds E.O.R., Wray S., Wyatt J., van der Zee P. (1988) Methods of quantitating cerebral near infrared spectroscopy data. Adv Exp Med Biol. 222:183-189.

Edwards A.D., Richardson C., Cope M., Wyatt J.S., Delpy D. T., Reynolds E.O.R. (1988). Cotside measurement of cerebral blood flow in ill newborn infants by near infrared spectroscopy. Lancet 2:770-771.

Edwards A.D, Wyatt J.S., Richardson C.E., Potter A., Cope M., Delpy D.T., Reynolds E.O.R. (1990) Effects of indomethacin on cerebral haemodynamics and oxygen delivery investigated by near infrared spectroscopy in very preterm infants. Lancet 2:1491-1495.

Elwell C.E, Cope M., Edwards A.D., Wyatt J.S., Reynolds E.O.R., Delpy D.T. (1992) Measurement of cerebral blood flow in adult humans using near infrared spectroscopy - methodology and possible errors. Adv Exp Med Biol (in press).

Ferrari M, Zanette E, Sideri G., Giamini I, Fieschi C., Carpi, A. (1987) Effects of carotid compression, as assessed by near infrared spectroscopy, upon cerebral blood volume and hemoglobin O_2 saturation. J Royal Soc Med 80:83-87.

Ferrari M., Wilson D.A., Hanley D.F., Hartman J.F., Traystman R.J., Rogers M.C. (1989) Non invasive determination of venous hemoglobin saturation in the dog by derivative near infrared spectroscopy. Am J Physiol 256:H1493-H1499.

Fox E., Jobsis F.F., Mitnick M.H. (1985) Monitoring cerebral oxygen sufficiency in anesthesia and surgery. Adv Exp Med Biol 191:849-854.

Glaister D.H, Jobsis F.F. (1988) A near-infrared spectro-photometric method for studying brain O_2 in man during +G_z acceleration. J Aerospace Med 59:199-207.

Hampson N.B., Camporesi E.M., Stolp B.W., Moon R.E., Shook J.E., Grebel J.A., Piantadosi C.A. (1990) Cerebral oxygen availability by NIR spectroscopy during transient hypoxia in humans. J Appl Physiol 69:907-913.

Jobsis F.F. (1977) Non invasive infrared monitoring of cerebral and myocardial oxygen sufficiency and circulatory parameters. Science 198:1264-1267.

Koorn R., Silvay G. (1991) Evaluation of the Somanetics[R] Invos[R] 3100 cerebral oximeter during cardiac surgery. 13th Ann Meet Soc Cardiovascular Anesthesiol p.176.

Liem K.D., Hopman J.C.W., Kollée L.A.A., Oeseburg B. (1992) Assessment of cerebral oxygenation and hemodynamics by near infrared spectrophotometry during induction of ECMO. Adv Exp Med Biol (in press).

Livera L.N., Spencer S.A., Thorniley M.S, Wickramasinghe Y.A., Rolfe P.(1991) Effects of hypoxemia and bradycardia on neonatal cerebral haemodynamics. Arch Dis Child 66:376-380.

McCormick P.W., Stewart M., Goetting M.G., Balakrishnan G. (1991) Regional cerebrovascular oxygen saturation measured by optical spectroscopy in humans. Stroke 22:596-602.

Peebles D.M., Edwards A.D., Wyatt J.S., Bishop A.P., Cope M., Delpy D.T., Reynolds E.O.R.(1991) Effect of oxytocin on fetal brain oxygenation during labour. Lancet 338:254-255.

Shinohara Y., Haida M., Kawaguchi F., Ito Y., Takeuchi H. (1991) Hemoglobin oxygen-saturation image of rat brain using near infrared light. J Cerebral Blood Flow Metab 11:S459.

Smith D.S., Levy W., Maris M., Chance B. (1990) Reperfusion hyperoxia in brain after circulatory arrest in humans. Anesthesiology. 73:12-19.

Steven J.M., Kurth C.D., Nicholson S.C., Phoon C., Chance B. (1990) Continuous non invasive assessment of brain oxygenation and blood volume during cardiopulmonary bypass in children undergoing ADS closure. Anesthesiology 73:A457.

Tamura M.(1991) Non-invasive monitoring of brain oxygen metabolism during cardiopulmonary bypass by near infrared spectrophotometry. Jap Circ J 55:330-335.

Wray S., Cope M., Delpy D.T., Wyatt J.S., Reynolds E.O.R. (1988) Characterization of the near infrared absorption spectra of cytochrome $a.a_3$ and haemoglobin for the non invasive monitoring of cerebral oxygenation. Biochem Biophys Acta 933:184-192.

Wyatt J.S., Cope M., Delpy D.T., Wray S., Reynolds E.O.R. (1986) Quantification of cerebral oxygenation and hemodynamics in sick newborn infants by near infrared spectrophotometry, Lancet. 2:1063-1066.

Wyatt J.S., Edwards A.D., Cope M., Delpy D.T., McCormick D.C., Potter A., Reynolds E.O.R. (1991) Response of cerebral blood volume to changes in arterial carbon dioxide tension ir preterm and term infants. Ped Res 29:553-557.

van der Zee P., Cope M., Arridge S.R., Essenpreis M., Potter L.A., Edwards A.D., Wyatt J.S., McCormick D.C., Roth S.C., Reynolds E.O.R., Delpy D.T. (1992) Experimentally measured optical pathlengths for the adult head, calf and forearm and the head of the newborn infant as a function of inter optode spacing. Adv Exp Med Biol (in press).

Polarized Light Examination and Photography of the Skin

R. Rox Anderson, MD

• **Light reflected from skin has two components: regular reflectance, or "glare" arising from the surface, and light backscattered from within the tissue. The regular reflectance contains the visual cues related to surface texture, whereas the backscattered component contains the cues related to pigmentation, erythema, infiltrates, vessels, and other intracutaneous structures. Unlike the backscattered component, regular reflectance preserves the plane of polarization of polarized incident light. Thus, viewing skin through a linear polarizer, under linearly polarized illumination, separates the two components of tissue reflectance. Thirty patients were examined and photographed in this manner. When the planes of polarization are parallel, images with enhanced surface detail are obtained. When the planes are orthogonal, wrinkles and surface detail disappear, and an enhanced view of vasculature and pigmented lesions is obtained. Simple, clinically useful techniques are presented.**

(Arch Dermatol. 1991;127:1000-1005)

The optical properties of skin are complex and dynamic,[1,2] and determine its appearance. What one views is the image of two basic components that comprise all reflected light from the skin (Fig 1).

Approximately 4% to 7% of incident light at all wavelengths undergoes reflectance on encountering the air-skin boundary because of the large change in the refractive index between the air and the stratum corneum.[1] This component is also called regular, or Fresnel, reflectance, because it follows Fresnel's equations relating reflectance to the angle of incidence, plane of polarization, and refractive index.[3,4] For regular reflectance, the angle of reflectance is equal to the angle of incidence. This component accounts for the "glare," or "shine," from skin, and is the major cue by which surface texture is judged. Even when there is no obvious glare from the skin, this component is present. Changes in surface texture due to aging, altered keratinization, hydration, and other factors affect regular reflectance, making the skin look rough, smooth, wrinkled, oily, dry, or wet.

The 93% to 96% of incident light not reflected at the skin surface enters the tissue, where it is absorbed and/or scattered.[1] Scattering causes a change in the direction of light propagation, and is the only physical process by which this light can be returned through the skin surface to participate in skin reflectance. In white skin, multiple scattering from the dermis accounts for the majority of visible light reflectance, and is caused predominantly by collagen fibers.[1,5] Variations in epidermal thickness and melanin content, blood content, oxygen saturation, carotenoids, and abnormal pigments such as hemosiderin or dermal melanin account for the hues of skin by attenuating this backscattered component.[1,2,5,6] The backscattered light component carries few or no visual cues related to the surface texture, yet it carries all visual cues related to internal skin structures such as vessels or infiltrates.

Multiple scattering scrambles the polarization of incident light. In contrast, regular reflection preserves the plane of polarized incident light. This allows a simple technique for the separation of these two components in photography or examination of skin. This study was conducted using linearly polarized light photography and examination of normal and abnormal skin and nail conditions. Enhancement of the surface (regular) reflectance component is useful for examination of texture, elevation, and scale. Complete elimination of regular reflectance by "crossed" polarizers yielded unique images of the skin, which are useful for enhanced examination of pigmented, vascular, and inflammatory

Accepted for publication February 28, 1991.

From the Department of Dermatology, Harvard Medical School, Massachusetts General Hospital, Boston.

Reprint requests to Department of Dermatology, Harvard Medical School, Massachusetts General Hospital, Boston, MA 02114 (Dr Anderson).

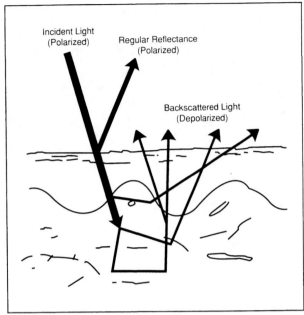

Fig 1.—Schematic representation of the two components of skin reflectance.

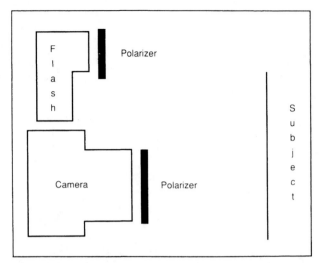

Fig 2.—Schematic arrangement of camera, flash, and polarizing filters.

lesions. The methods are simple and easily adapted to routine clinical use.

METHODS

The general method used was photography and examination of skin in vivo, through a linear polarizer, using a linearly polarized light source. When the incident and detected planes of polarization are parallel, the regular (Fresnel) reflectance component is attenuated less than the depolarized backscattered component. This causes relative enhancement of the regular reflectance component. When the incident and detected planes of polarization are perpendicular (crossed), the regular reflectance is entirely eliminated from detection (Fig 2).

Gray plastic linear polarizer sheets (Edmund Scientific 71940) were cut for use over light sources, including camera flash sources. This material is not perfectly spectrally neutral, although it is gray and did not greatly affect color balance. A linear polarizing filter (Hoya PL) was placed over the camera lens. The spectral transmittance was measured from 400 to 700 nm of the sheet polarizer and filter and placed with parallel and perpendicular planes of polarization. A diode array spectrophotometer (Hewlett-Packard) was used.

A pair of clip-on gray sunglasses (Polaroid) was worn for the clinical examinations, during which a bright polarized light source was used. A standard slide carousel projector (Kodak), into which a 2-inch-square piece of the polarizer material was inserted, served as the light source. Equivalent results were obtained when a polarizer was placed over several standard incandescent illumination sources in the dermatology clinic.

A camera (Yashica SLR, model FX-D) with a flash unit (CS-220) and a 50-mm lens was used. Antireflection-coated +4- or +2-diopter close-up lenses were used for close-up photography. Before the polarizing sheet was cut and mounted onto the output face of the flash unit, the sheet was precisely oriented relative to the camera polarizing filter such that the orientation mark on the polarizing filter was "up" for parallel planes of polarization and horizontal for perpendicular planes of polarization. This camera system uses an automatic flash control that operates from a photocell mounted on the flash unit. To maintain automatic exposure operation, a small piece of the polarizing material was taped over the flash-controlling photocell, to mimic the light loss due to the polarizer over the camera lens. With systems using through-the-lens metering, this step is unnecessary because the light entering the camera is used to control the flash output. Equivalent photographs were obtained with both a through-the-lens system (Nikon) and an inexpensive portable camera (Minolta Freedom Tele) fitted with similar polarizer filters. Thirty-five-millimeter slide film (ASA 100 Agfa or Kodachrome) was used and processed routinely. Photographs were taken at f/4 or f/5.6 (with the Yashica system) for this study.

Thirty patients with various dermatologic conditions were examined and photographed in this manner during normal clinical activity. This included normal skin of various skin types; photoaged skin; epidermal and dermal pigmented lesions including nevi, lentigines, seborrheic keratoses, nevi of Ota, melasma, and poikiloderma; papular lesions including papular mucinosis, acne, and granuloma annulare; scaling lesions including psoriasis, ichthyosis, dermatitis, and exfoliative erythroderma; "connective tissue" disorders including morphea and dermatomyositis with calcinosis cutis; vascular lesions including portwine stains, rosacea, essential telangiectasia, and phlebectasia of the leg; tattoos; erythema annulare centrifugum; necrobiosis lipoidica diabeticorum; longitudinal melanonychia; nail pitting and dystrophy; Muerke's nails; and scalp lesions of psoriasis, alopecia areata, and discoid lupus erythematosus.

RESULTS

Transmission spectra of the sheet polarizer, the polarizing camera filter, and the two filters together in parallel and perpendicular orientation are shown in Fig 3.

Figures 4 through 8 are paired photographs taken with parallel and crossed planes of polarization. The rotation of the camera's polarizing filter by 90° was the only change between these paired photographs; in no case was the light source moved or the exposure conditions changed.

Parallel Planes of Polarization

There was a striking difference in the appearance of skin, nails, and hair when they were viewed or photographed with the polarizers crossed vs parallel. The ability to discern details of surface texture was enhanced with parallel polarized light examination. The net effect was to somewhat accentuate glare from the skin surface. This made the examination of scale, nail dystrophy and pitting, elevation or depression, loss of skin markings due to atrophy, and wrinkling more apparent than by normal examination. The ability to discern pigmentation, vascularity, and color was lessened, owing to greater glare from the skin surface. Visualization of scalp lesions was somewhat more difficult owing to regular reflection (shine) from the hair and scalp.

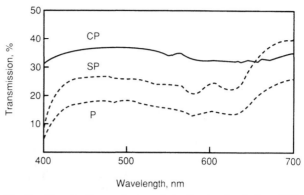

Fig 3.—Spectral transmission of plastic sheet polarizer (SP) and camera (Hoya) polarizing (CP) filters, singly and together in parallel (P) orientations. With perpendicular orientation, the transmission was less than 1% across the visible spectrum.

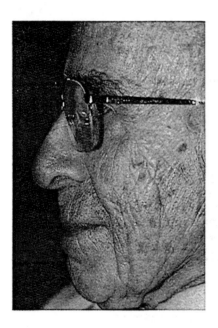 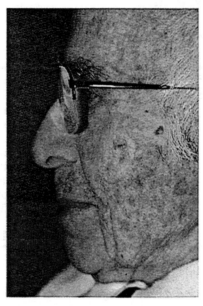

Fig 4.—An octagenarian skin scientist with wrinkles and actinic and seborrheic keratosis. Left, Parallel polarization image, emphasizing wrinkles and scale. Right, Crossed polarization image, showing loss of wrinkles and well-defined pigmented lesions.

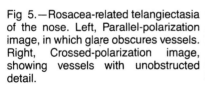

Fig 5.—Rosacea-related telangiectasia of the nose. Left, Parallel-polarization image, in which glare obscures vessels. Right, Crossed-polarization image, showing vessels with unobstructed detail.

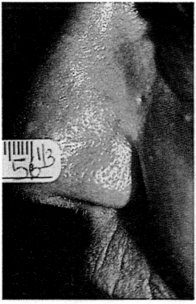 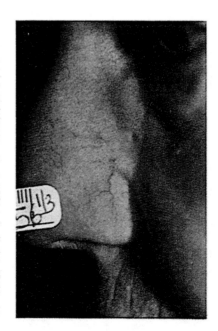

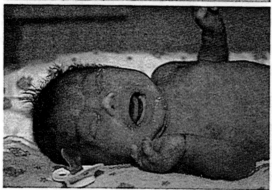

Fig 6.—Ten-day-old collodion baby with recessive ichthyosis. Top, Parallel-polarization image, showing tight, smooth membrane with scale. Bottom, Crossed-polarization image, eliminating surface details but emphasizing inflammatory changes and areas of local vasoconstriction on the face.

Perpendicular (Crossed) Planes of Polarization

With the planes of polarization crossed, essentially all surface detail and glare were eliminated. The appearance was strikingly different than during conventional examination of the skin. All wrinkles and skin markings disappeared, with the exception of very deep furrows, which appeared as dusky lines (Fig 4). Elimination of surface details gave the skin a soft, diffuse, almost "air-brushed" appearance, but without loss of true focus, as evidenced by sharply defined pigmented hairs. In polarized light photography, the need to use a larger camera aperture to compensate for light attenuation by the polarizers results in a more limited depth of field, which is apparent in Fig 4. In psoriatic plaques, the white appearance of dense scale was reduced, emphasizing the inflammatory component. It was essentially impossible to discern whether lesions were raised or depressed.

The ability to view internal structures such as vessels, pigmentation, and infiltrates was greatly enhanced under crossed polarization. Individual vessels of portwine lesions, rosacea, periungual telangiectasia, and necrobiosis lipoidica diabeticorum were much more easily seen (Fig 5). The response of portwine stains or tattoos and pigmented lesions to treatment with pulsed dye or Q-switched ruby lasers, respectively, was more easily evaluated. With ×10 magnification, the detailed structure of pigmented lesions and ectatic microvessels was apparent, similar to that obtained with skin microscopy after application of mineral oil. Areas of inflammation, infiltrate, or calcium were more easily seen and demarcated in figurate erythemas, ichthyosis, lupus erythematosus, psoriasis, and dermatomyositis with calcinosis cutis. The subtle yellow-greenish hue of gran-

Fig 7.—Longitudinal melanonychia due to a benign nevus in a patient with acquired immunodeficiency syndrome. Top, Parallel-polarization image, in which glare obstructs the view of nail plate pigmentation. Bottom, Crossed-polarization image, without glare.

Fig 8.—Face of patient with rosacea. Left, Parallel-polarization image shows skin surface detail. Right, Crossed-polarization image clearly shows vascular changes and a peculiar dark cross in the eyes due to birefringence of the cornea.

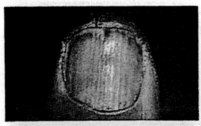
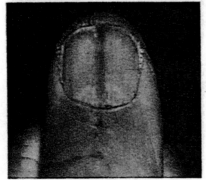
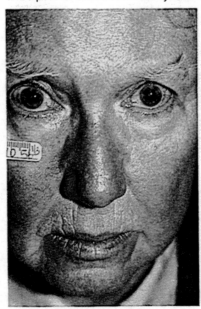
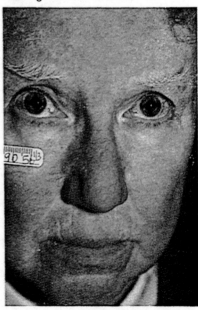

uloma annulare lesions was more easily seen under diascopy with this technique than under conventional lighting. Pigmented lesions were strikingly better demarcated under crossed-polarization examination, and it was easier to discern variegation of both pigmentation and color.

The typical glare in nail plate photos was entirely absent, allowing an unobstructed view of nail bed abnormalities and longitudinal melanonychia (Fig 7). The "sheen" from hair was also absent, allowing better photographs of inflammatory scalp lesions. The iris and sclera were also somewhat more easily seen and photographed owing to the absence of corneal reflex, and there was a peculiar dark "cross" induced over the iris (Fig 8), presumably because of birefringence of the corneal stroma.[7]

COMMENT

Polarizers are widely used in photography and daily life to reduce glare. Common polarizing sunglasses are oriented such that regular reflection from horizontal glossy or wet surfaces, which is partially or fully polarized depending on the angle of incidence, is reduced. Circular polarizers are widely used to reduce glare from computer and video screens. Polarization photography as a means of reducing or eliminating glare in normal skin has been reported,[8] but lesional skin was not examined. A conceptually similar technique has been reported for ocular photography.[9] The use of a single polarizing filter to reduce glare is well known in photography, but polarized light sources are not in general studio or commercial use. The results obtained in this study strongly suggest that polarized light photography would be a useful photographic studio technique to emphasize or eliminate, eg, skin wrinkles. The direct examination of skin lesions using polarized light techniques has, to my knowledge, not been previously reported.

The use of a linearly polarized light source, and a second polarizer over the camera or examiner's eye, is a simple and clinically useful tool for examination and photography of the skin. When the primary interest is surface morphology, parallel orientation of the polarizers enhances the appearance of wrinkles, depression, elevation, scale, and nail or hair shaft dystrophies. When the primary interest is inflammatory, infiltrative, pigmented, or vascular lesions, crossed (perpendicular) orientation eliminates all glare from the surface, and an enhanced, unobstructed view of internal skin structure and color is obtained. In fact, a full range of control over the amount of surface detail to be seen can be obtained by variation of the angle between the two planes of polarization. At 45° orientation, conventional images are obtained. One can therefore emphasize surface or subsurface detail for the best examination or illustration of skin lesions. With crossed polarization, a view of skin strikingly different from that seen on normal examination occurs.

Polarization photography can be done simply, without much extra time or equipment. Essentially any camera system can be modified for use with this technique. With the polarized flash unit mounted on the camera, the relative polarizer orientation does not vary as the camera is moved about. Once one is accustomed to orienting the polarizers, it is easy to take pictures that are identical to normal photographs (polarization planes at 45°), surface enhanced (parallel planes of polarization) or glare eliminated (perpendicular planes of polarization), by simply rotating the camera's polarizer. With through-the-lens camera metering systems, a circular rather than linear polarizer should be used over the camera lens, to maintain proper exposure control.

Two problems associated with use of polarizers should be noted. First, if large apertures are needed because of the attenuation of light by the polarizers, a limited depth of field occurs. The two polarizers used produce a net attenuation of approximately 10:1, which necessitates opening the camera aperture by approximately three stops if no other compensation is made. This is generally not a problem in close-up photographs, because there is ample exposure from most flash units. Using faster speed film minimizes the problem. For whole-body polarized photographs, secondary flash units would probably be needed. A second potential problem is some loss of color balance, if the polarizing sheet placed over the flash unit is not sufficiently neutral. The gray (not green or brown) sheet polarizers are best.

Crossed-polarization examination appears to be clinically useful for a limited number of specific purposes. The need to wear polarizing glasses, and to orient either the source or one's head to achieve the required perpendicular orientation of the polarizers, was quite distracting in this study. Placing a polarizer on a head-mounted examination lamp, however, solves the orientation problem, such that a glare-free view can be obtained from any viewing angle. Although examination of inflammatory, infiltrative, vascular, and pigmented lesions is clearly enhanced, only rarely would use of this technique alter diagnosis. Certain procedures, however, may be more easily performed without glare from the skin, hair, or nail surface. These include sclerotherapy, in which visualization of small vessels is essential; demarcation of pigmented or inflammatory lesions prior to biopsy or excision, especially in the presence of scale; and treatment of vascular or pigmented lesions, eg, with lasers.

As noted by Gould,[10] presentation of one's "best" data or results can be irresistible, even by steadfastly objective scientists. "Trick" photography, whether intentional or not, is probably common in dermatologic literature. The techniques presented here could be used either to eliminate such tricks or to enhance them. A recent report in the ARCHIVES[11] made the point that inflammatory and pigmented lesions could be photographically "cured" simply by arranging the glare from the skin surface to coincide with the lesional skin. Such "cures" would be impossible using crossed-polarization photography, because glare is eliminated regardless of source or camera position. In contrast, photographs taken with parallel polarization enhance the appearance of surface texture, and would be useful in controlled studies related to aging, photoaging, and wrinkling. If used with digital image acquisition, in which images may be subtracted from one another, a high-contrast image of only the skin surface would be produced.

Finally, a configuration of some potential use, or at least amusement, would utilize a lighted mirror. If separate polarizers are placed over both the lights and the mirror face, an unobstructed view of one's face is seen in the mirror, without the need to wear polarizing glasses. By rotating either polarizer, one's own face can be seen with, or without, wrinkles! As in the tale of Snow White, the potential for such a mirror shall herewith be left to the imagination.

This work was supported by grant RO1-AR25395 from the National Institutes of Health, Bethesda, Md.

I thank Jeffrey Dover, MD, for helpful discussions and Irvin H. Blank, PhD, for his photogenicity.

References

1. Anderson RR, Parrish JA. The optics of human skin. *J Invest Dermatol*. 1981;77:13-19.

2. Tregear RT. Photons and molecules. In: *Physical Functions of the Skin*. Orlando, Fla: Academic Press Inc; 1966:96-112.

3. Bennett JM, Bennett HE. Polarization. In: Driscoll WG, Vaughan W, eds. *Handbook of Optics*. New York, NY: McGraw-Hill International Book Co; 1978:6-13.

4. Jenkins FA, White HE. *Fundamentals of Optics*. 4th ed. New York, NY: McGraw Hill International Book Co; 1976:523-527.

5. Anderson RR, Hu J, Parrish JA. Optical radiation transfer in human skin and applications in in vivo remittance spectroscopy. In: Marks R, Payne PA, eds. *Proceedings of Symposium on Bioengineering and the Skin*. Lancaster, England: MTP Press Ltd; 1981:245-254.

6. Edwards EA, Duntley SQ. The pigments and color of human skin. *Am J Anat*. 1939;65:1-33.

7. Cope WT, Wolbarsht ML, Yamanashi BS. The corneal polarization cross. *J Opt Soc Am [A]*. 1978;68:1139-1141.

8. Philip J, Carter NJ, Lenn CP. Improved optical discrimination of skin with polarized light. *J Soc Cosmet Chem*. 1988;39:121-132.

9. Fariza E, O'Day T, Jalkh AE, Medina A. Use of cross-polarized light in anterior segment photography. *Arch Ophthalmol*. 1989;107:608-610.

10. Gould SJ. *The Mismeasure of Man*. New York, NY: WW Norton & Co Inc; 1983.

11. Slue WE Jr. Photographic cures for dermatologic disorders. *Arch Dermatol*. 1989;125:960-962.

Reprinted from *Optical Engineering*, Vol. 32(2), pp. 222-226 (February 1993).
©1993 SPIE.

Two-channel fiber optic skin erythema meter

Harri Kopola, MEMBER SPIE
University of Oulu
Department of Electrical Engineering
Linnanmaa
SF-90570 Oulu, Finland

Arto Lahti
University of Oulu
Clinic of Dermatology
Kajaanintie 52A
SF-90220 Oulu, Finland

Risto A. Myllylä, MEMBER SPIE
Technical Research Centre of Finland
Optoelectronics Laboratory
P.O. Box 202
SF-90571 Oulu, Finland

Matti Hannuksela
University of Oulu
Clinic of Dermatology
Kajaanintie 52A
SF-90220 Oulu, Finland

Abstract. The skin erythema meter is a fiber optic, dual-wavelength reflectance meter that measures the reflectance of the skin on two wavelengths, one the blood/hemoglobin absorption band (555 nm) and another a reference (660 nm). The instrument consists of a fiber optic sensor head, a microprocessor-based control and analysis unit, and a plotter, and it presents the relation between the measured reflectance results in terms of a reflectance index [R(555 nm):R(660 nm)]. The measurement cycle, including printing, takes 5 s. Stability tests on the erythema meter (constant distance, reference object) showed the standard deviation of the reflectance index to be ±0.1%, whereas that in repeatability tests was less than ±0.5% for skin and less than ±0.2% for paper with hand-held positioning and repetition. The dynamic change in the reflectance index was about 30% with strong irritation. Results of various irritation test series on human skin are also presented. Finally, the performance and applicability of the skin erythema meter with respect to allergy test procedures, irritancy testing, and measurement of uv-induced erythema are discussed.

Subject terms: biomedical optics; skin reflectance; erythema; fiber optic sensors; irritancy testing; optical sensing; color recognition.

Optical Engineering 32(2), 222-226 (February 1993).

1 Introduction

Erythema is one of most important visible changes in the inflammatory response of skin. Hitherto it has been possible to quantify it only subjectively by eye, using rough scales. Its objective quantification would be of importance for both research and clinical work, however, e.g., for allergy test procedures, irritancy testing, and the measurement of ultraviolet radiation (UV)-induced erythema.

The first major attempt[1-3] at the objective measurement of erythema employed laser Doppler velocimetry (LVD) to assess the microvascular blood flow rate in the skin. One skin-color-quantifying method is tristimulus colorimetry.[4] Westerhof et al.[5] present results on the quantification of UV-induced erythema with a portable chromameter (Minolta) and compares a* readings of the Commission Internationale de l'Eclairage L*a*b* color space obtained with the chromameter, which has the best correlation with visual grading and the largest dynamic range. A more accurate method for measuring skin color or its reflectance spectrum employs a recording spectrophotometer equipped with an integrating sphere.[6-8]

Narrow-band spectrophotometers using selected wavelengths already give sufficient information on erythema occurrences, but cannot be extended to the measurement of pigmentation. A portable dual-wavelength (546 and 672 nm) instrument for quantifying erythema has been described.[9,10]

Paper BM-052 received July 1, 1992; revised manuscript received Sep. 15, 1992; accepted for publication Sep. 22, 1992. This paper is a revision of a paper presented at the SPIE conference on Optical Fibers in Medicine V, Jan. 1990, Los Angeles. The paper presented there appears (unrefereed) in SPIE Proceedings Vol. 1201.

This instrument employs the normal filter spectrophotometer principle, a fiber optic probe, and ratio measurement. Mendelow et al.[11] report the use of a haemelometer for erythema measurement. This instrument has 45-deg lighting and 0-deg viewing geometry, LED sources (wavelengths 566 and 640 nm), a hemispheric measurement head, and ratio measurement. New instruments are still under development, however, and although they have a resolution of up to 1:150, no repeatability or stability results have been mentioned.

A description is given here of a new skin erythema meter developed recently. This instrument is based on LED light sources, a fiber optic measurement head, and advanced signal processing. The construction of the instrument, its performance, and test measurements are discussed.

2 Reflectance of the Skin

Normal human skin is illustrated in Fig. 1(a), and a simplified layered model is given in Fig. 1(b). It is assumed to comprise a system of uniformly and randomly distributed light absorbing and scattering particles, the dimensions of which are much less than the thickness of the layer. Approximations and formulas in the literature[9,12] show that the reflectance of monochromatic light is

$$R_\lambda = R/\phi_0$$
$$= R_S + (1 - R_S)(R_1 + T_1^2 R_2 + T_1^2 T_2^2 R_3 + T_1^2 T_2^2 T_3^2 R_4) , \quad (1)$$

where R_S is the specular reflectance from the surface; T_1, R_1, T_2, R_2, T_3, R_3, and R_4 are the transmittance and diffuse reflectance of different layers, and ϕ_0 is the diffuse reflectance of a white reference surface.

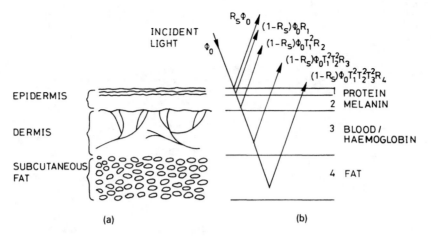

Fig. 1 (a) Schematic diagram of the human skin and (b) simplified layered model of the skin.

If we assume that $R_S \ll 1$, $R_1 \ll 1$, $R_2 \ll 1$, and $R_3 \ll 1$ and approaches zero, then Eq. (1) can be simplified to

$$R_\lambda = T_1^2 T_2^2 T_3^2 R_4 \ . \tag{2}$$

This means that the protein, melanin, and hemoglobin layers obey the Beer-Lambert law of radiation absorption and the fat layer is perfectly reflecting. However, the absorption and scattering coefficients for each layer are wavelength dependent. This simple model cited[9] illustrates the phenomena, and more detailed descriptions of skin optics and light and skin interactions are provided by several authors,[13–17] including verifications of measurements and theoretical results.[17]

Figure 2 shows the absorption spectra of different skin pigments. The color of the skin is determined largely by the melanin and the quantity of blood. The absorption of hemoglobin within the 520- to 580-nm wavelength range is high, falling rapidly in the red part of the visible spectrum. Thus, the amount of blood modulates the reflectance effectively at wavelengths from 520 to 580 nm but has hardly any effect at wavelengths over 630 nm. Melanin has a gently decreasing absorption coefficient within the range 520 to 700 nm, causing visual differences. In the comparison measurements of the normal skin of a patient with irritated skin, the differences in the amount of melanin, which is not constant over the body, can be minimized by ensuring that the selected test site (irritated) is adjacent to the reference site (normal). We can thus assume that the melanin is "constant" over our test area.

The basic feature to be considered in skin reflectance measurement is the ratio of green to red wavelengths. We calculate the reflectance index as follows:

$$R_i = R_g / R_r \ , \tag{3}$$

where the subscripts g and r denote green and red.

3 Construction and Operation

A rough block diagram of the skin erythema meter is shown in Fig. 3. As can be seen, the system is composed of a microprocessor-based control and analysis unit with program switches, a four-digit display and plotter interface,

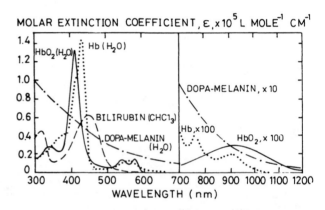

Fig. 2 Absorption spectra for major human skin pigments.

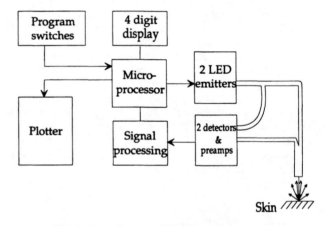

Fig. 3 Block diagram of the skin erythema meter.

two LEDs, a fiber optic probe, two photodiode detectors, and signal processing electronics.

The microprocessor-based control logic feeds time-multiplexed chopping pulses (Fig. 4) to two LEDs. The fiber optic bundle leads the emitted radiant flux to the measurement end of the probe and a portion of it to the reference detector. The light reflected from the skin is led to the measurement detector. The two pulse chains received from the preamplifiers are amplified, filtered, sampled, and con-

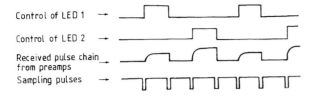

Control of LED 1 →

Control of LED 2 →

Received pulse chain
from preamps

Sampling pulses →

Fig. 4 Control pulse diagram of the light sources and sampling.

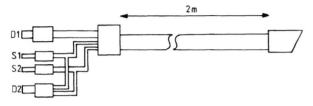

Fig. 5 Fiber optic probe.

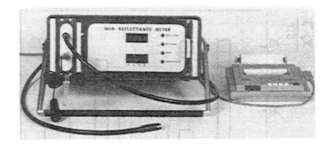

Fig. 6 Skin erythema meter.

verted to binary words in the signal-processing unit. Samples are taken synchronously during one sampling sequence from both the measurement signal modulated by the object and the reference signal led directly from the LEDs to the reference detector, from each group of two pulses and from each background between the pulses, giving a total of eight samples. The relative reflectance program developed for use with the instrument calculates, displays, and prints the ratio $R(555 \text{ nm}):R(660 \text{ nm})$ as a measurement result.[18–20]

The optical part of the instrument consists of two LEDs (peak wavelengths 555 and 660 nm), two PIN photodiode detectors, a fiber optic probe, and a mechanical fastening construction. Figure 5 shows the construction of the fiber optic probe. It is composed of two transmitting bundles (S1 and S2) and two receiving bundles (D1 and D2). Bundles S1, S2, and D1 are gathered together and mixed randomly in the common measurement end. The active diameter of the measurement end is 5 mm. A small part of both transmitting bundles forms the reference bundle D2. The sensor head can be equipped with two different mechanical parts to apply to optimal measurement distances with a 45-deg or perpendicular geometry (0 deg). A photograph of the skin erythema meter is shown in Fig. 6.

A typical measurement procedure with this instrument is as follows. The device is first calibrated against a reference surface (e.g., $BaSO_4$ white standard, MgO, reference skin). This takes 7 s and is automatic, being activated by pushing a switch. The program starts by plotting a heading, after which the instrument is ready to perform measurements. After positioning the sensor head ''near'' the skin surface, the measurement function is activated with a hand-held switch. Measurement takes 2.5 s (averaging 4096 individual measurement events) and the result is plotted immediately. A new measurement can be started while plotting is still in progress, providing a measurement sequence of about 5 s. All this can be done in normal lighting (daylight, artificial light) without touching the skin.

4 Measurements and Results

We report here on some tests performed using the erythema meter and other commercial instruments (spectroradiometer, chromameter, laser Doppler flowmeter). Stability tests on the erythema meter (constant distance, reference object) showed the standard deviation (SD) of the reflectance to be $\pm 0.3\%$ during the first 30 min and $\pm 0.1\%$ after that (test period 8 h). Thus, the drifts in the electronics and radiant flux of the sources and the sensitivity differences between the detectors allow a reasonable resolution. Repeatability tests using paper and skin showed the standard deviation of the reflectance index to be less than $\pm 0.5\%$ for skin and less than $\pm 0.2\%$ for paper (45-deg measurement) with hand-held positioning and repetition.

Thirty successive *in vivo* repeatability measurements were performed on UV-induced erythema sites [one patient, three test sites: minimal erythema dose (MED) 1 MED, dose 4 MEDs, and nonirradiated skin site] 20 to 22 h after irradiation using the skin erythema meter, chromameter, spectroradiometer, and laser Doppler flowmeter. The dynamic range of the equipment was calculated as follows: $X_4 - X_N$, where X_4 is the mean of the measurements (30) from the 4 MED test site (marked erythema) and X_N the mean from the nonirradiated test site. The SD represents the repeatability of successive measurements for each test site and instrument. Figure 7 shows the relation between the dynamic range and the SD (for each test site and instrument). This relation shows the number of quantification levels (''steps'') of the size of the SD that fit into the dynamic range. The skin erythema meter gives a fairly equal number of quantification steps independent of the strength of the reaction (4 MEDs marked erythema, 1 MED weak erythema, N nonirradiated normal skin), whereas the laser Doppler flowmeter shows an increasing standard deviation as the erythema becomes more pronounced. This test illustrates the repeatability of sampling (position, touch, etc.) carried out by means of different instruments in the case of ''stable'' UV-induced erythema sites, but not the responses of different skin types.

Figure 8 shows reflectance spectra for human skin measured with a Rofin-Sinar spectroradiometer in different positions on the human body (Caucasian). White typing paper was used as the calibration standard. It is seen that the absolute reflectance, highest at about 620 nm, varied from 52% (lip) to 85% (forehead). The spectra are quite similar in shape in all cases except the arm. The erythema meter measures reflectances in the hemoglobin absorption range (555 nm, bandwidth 30 nm) and plain reference range (660 nm, bandwidth 30 nm) and prints the ratio of these values as the result.

An irritation test was evaluated using methyl nicotenate in concentrations of 0.5, 2, 10, and 50 mM and an alcohol blank. Figure 9 shows the reflectance index measured as a

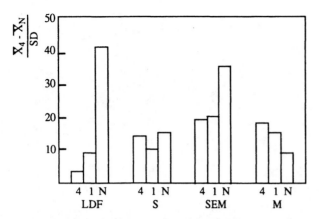

Fig. 7 *In vivo* repeatability of measurements (30) of UV erythema produced by four MEDs (4), one MED (1), and a normal skin site (N). Instruments are LDF = laser Doppler flowmeter, S = spectroradiometer, SEM = skin erythema meter, and M = Minolta chromameter. The relation of the dynamic range ($X_4 - X_N$) of the instruments to the SD is shown.

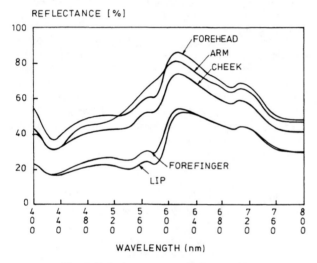

Fig. 8 Reflectance spectra for human skin.

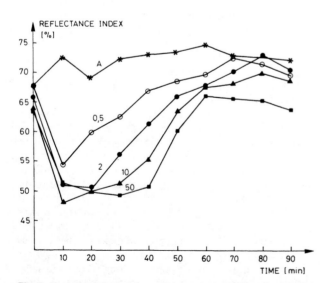

Fig. 9 Nonimmunological immediate contact reactions to a methyl nicotenate dilution series at five measurement sites on human skin.

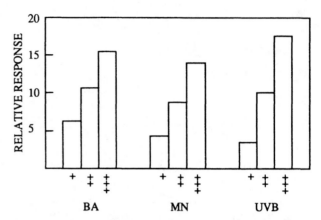

Fig. 10 Comparison of visual grading and erythema meter values for reactions elicited by benzoic acid (BA), methyl nicotinate (MN), and UV irradiation (UVB).

function of time from the five given test points. The measurements were performed with 0-deg geometry. The dynamic change in the reflectance index was about 30% at strong concentrations and the response time was concentration dependent (from 10 to 40 min). The reflectance index value is saturating to the 50% level when using 2 mM concentrations or stronger, and returns to the basic level (as before irritation) in 80 to 90 min. Comparison of the reflectance indices obtained with the erythema meter with the spectra generated by the Rofin-Sinar spectroradiometer shows that the erythema meter indicated equal dynamic changes to those of the spectroradiometer. The responses of the skin erythema meter are compared with visual grading [+ (weak), + + (moderate), + + + (marked erythema)] in Fig. 10. Irritation was induced by benzoic acid (BA), methyl nicotinate (MN), and UV irradiation.

5 Conclusion

This meter developed for skin erythema determination uses the ratio between two reflected wavelengths (555 and 660 nm) as an erythema indicator. The instrument is microprocessor controlled and includes advanced signal processing for background light elimination. The fiber optic probe enables 45- and 0-deg measurement without touching the skin. The resolution of the instrument in stability tests proved to be ±0.1% (reflectance index), and the SD of the reflectance index with hand-held positioning for measurements from "living skin" was less than ±0.5%. Irritation reaction measurements performed with the erythema meter and a commercial spectroradiometer showed equal dynamic changes of 30% in the reflectance index. Also the erythema induced by benzoic acid, methyl nicotenate, and UV irradiation showed good correspondence compared to visual grading. The erythema meter developed here nevertheless allows rapid measurements (<5 s) and enables the monitoring of time-dependent reactions (several parallel test points) conveniently and repetitively.

References

1. G. Nilsson, T. Tenland, and P. Oberg, "A new instrument for continuous measurement of tissue blood flow by light beating spectroscopy," *IEEE Trans. Biomed. Eng.* **27**(1), 12–19 (1980).
2. T. Tenland, "On laser Doppler flowmetry methods and microvascular applications," PhD Dissertation, Linkoping University (1982).

3. R. Blanken, P. van der Valk, and J. Nater, "Laser-Doppler flowmetry in the investigation of irritant compounds on human skin," *Dermatosen* **34**, 5–9 (1986).

4. J. Serup and T. Agner, "Colorimetric quantification of erythema—a comparison of two colorimeters (Lange Micro Color and Minolta Chroma Meter CR-200) with a clinical scoring scheme and Laser Doppler flowmetry," *Clin. Exp. Dermatol.* **15**, 267–272 (1990).

5. W. Westerhof, B. van Hasselt, and A. Kammeijer, "Quantification of uv-induced erythema with a portable computer controlled chromameter," *Photodermatology* **3**, 310–314 (1986).

6. W. Buckley and F. Grum, "Reflection spectrophotometry," *Arch. Dermatol.* **83**, 249–261 (1961).

7. C. Skegg, "The external integrating sphere: an instrument for objective surface color measurements," *Int. Lab.* **11**, 68–74 (April 1981).

8. S. Wan, J. Parrish, and F. Jaenicke, "Quantitative evaluation of ultraviolet induced erythema," *Photochem. Photobiol.* **37**(6), 643–648 (1983).

9. B. Diffey, R. Oliver, and P. Farr, "A portable instrument for quantifying erythema induced by ultraviolet radiation," *Br. J. Dermatol.* **III**, 663–672 (1984).

10. P. Farr and B. Diffey, "Quantitative studies on cutaneous erythema induced by ultraviolet radiation," *Br. J. Dermatol.* **III**, 673–682 (1984).

11. A. Mendelow, A. Forsyth, J. Feather, A. Baillie, and A. Florence, "Skin reflectance measurements of patch test responses," *Contact Dermat.* **15**, 73–78 (1986).

12. J. Dawson, D. Barker, D. Ellis, E. Grassam, J. Cotterill, G. Fisher, and J. Feather, "A theoretical and experimental study of light absorption and scattering by in vivo skin," *Phys. Med. Biol.* **25**(4), 695–709 (1980).

13. S. Takatani and M. Graham, "Theoretical analysis of diffuse reflectance from a two-layer tissue model," *IEEE Trans. Biomed. Eng.* **26**(12), 656–664 (1979).

14. S. Wan, R. Anderson, and J. Parrish, "Analytical modeling for the optical properties of the skin with in vitro and in vivo applications," *Photochem. Photobiol.* **34**, 493–499 (1981).

15. R. Anderson and J. Parrish, "The optics of human skin," *J. Invest. Dermatol.* **77**(1), 13–19 (1981).

16. A. Welch, C. Denham, G. Yoon, and M. van Gemert, "Seven flux model for light distribution in laser irradiated tissue," in *Proc. ICALEO'85, L.I.A.* **49**, 43–48 (1985).

17. M. J. C. van Gemert, S. L. Jacques, H. J. C. M. Sterenborg, and W. M. Star, "Skin optics," *IEEE Trans. Biomed. Eng.* **36**(12), 1146–1154 (1989).

18. H. Kopola, R. Kaijansaari, and R. Myllylä, "An eight channel fiber optical spectrophotometer for industrial applications," in *Fiber Optic Sensors*, H. Arditty and L. Jeunhomme, Eds., *Proc. SPIE* **586**, 204–209 (1986).

19. H. Kopola, "Intensity-modulated fibre optic sensors for robotic, medical and industrial applications," *Acta Univ. Oul.* **C45** (1988).

20. H. Kopola, A. Lahti, R. Myllylä, and M. Hannuksela, "A skin erythema meter," in *Optical Fibers in Medicine V*, A. Katzir, Ed., *Proc. SPIE* **1201**, 345–352 (1990).

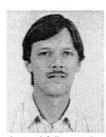

Harri Kopola received the Dipl. Engineering, Licentiate of Technology, and Doctor of Technology degrees in electrical engineering from the University of Oulu, Finland, in 1980, 1982, and 1988, respectively. He has been working with intensity-modulated fiber optic sensors for robotic, medical, and industrial applications; electrically controlled optical attenuators; and optical polatization measurement at the University of Oulu. In 1989, he was a postdoctoral fellow at the University of Ottawa, Canada, developing a fiber optic electric field sensor. His current research interests are in the areas of optical sensor technology and colorimetry.

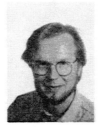

Arto Lahti received his MD in 1975 from the University of Helsinki, Finland, and he finished his doctoral thesis on nonimmunologic contact urticaria in 1980. In 1981, he became a specialist in dermatology. From 1983 to 1985 he worked as a postdoctoral fellow at the University of California, San Francisco, developing animal models for chemically induced immediate type contact reactions in the skin. Since 1986 he has worked as a senior lecturer in the Department of Dermatology, University of Oulu, Finland. His main research interest has been the standardization of measurement techniques for both allergic and nonallergic skin test reactions.

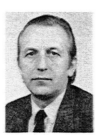

Risto A. Myllylä received the Dipl. Engineering, Licentiate of Technology, and Doctor of Technology degrees in electronics engineering from the University of Oulu, Finland, in 1970, 1973, and 1976, respectively. From 1971 to 1973 he was a laboratory engineer and from 1974 to 1977 was an acting associate professor in the Department of Electrical Engineering, University of Oulu. In 1978, he became an associate professor of electronics. From 1977 to 1978, he worked as a visiting scientist with the support of a Humboldt Scholarship at the University of Stuttgard, Germany. In 1988 he joined the Technical Research Centre of Finland's Electronics Laboratory as a research professor. His research interests include industrial instrumentation development, particularly in electro-optical measurements. He is the author of more than 150 papers.

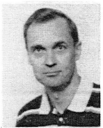

Matti Hannuksela received his MD in 1966 and his PhD in 1971 from the University Helsinki, Finland. He is a specialist in dermatology, dermatological allergology, and occupational dermatology. From 1971 to 1972 he headed the outpatient department of the Department of Dermatology, University Central Hospital, Helsinki; from 1972 to 1976 he headed the allergy unit of the Department of Dermatology, University Central Hospital, Helsinki; and from 1976 to 1991 he was professor, chairman, and doctor-in-chief in the Department of Dermatology, University Central Hospital, Oulu. Since 1991, he has been medical director at South Karelia Central Hospital, Lappeenranta. Hannuksela has published about 250 original and review articles on dermatological allergology, UV-light therapies, and skin diseases.

Reprinted with permission from *Optics Letters,* Vol. 15(21), pp. 1179-1181
(November 1, 1990). ©1990 Optical Society of America.

Time-resolved transillumination for medical diagnostics

S. Andersson-Engels, R. Berg, and S. Svanberg

Department of Physics, Lund Institute of Technology, P.O. Box 118, S-221 00, Lund, Sweden

O. Jarlman

Department of Diagnostic Radiology, Lund University Hospital, S-221 85, Lund, Sweden

A time-gated technique to improve the possibility of localizing spatial differences in absorption when transilluminating a turbid, highly scattering medium, such as human tissue, is demonstrated. When transmitting picosecond laser pulses and detecting photons on the opposite side of the object, the contrast can be strongly enhanced by detecting only the photons with the shortest traveling time. Measurements on a 35-mm-thick tissue phantom with 5-mm-diameter absorbing objects inside are reported with data for a human hand *in vivo*. Implications for optical mammography (diaphanography) are discussed.

Today mammography is the golden standard in breast cancer diagnosis. However, tumors sometimes cannot be seen, especially in a dense breast, and the use of ionizing radiation is also a matter of concern since there is a hypothetical risk of cancer induction, especially in young women. Tissue transillumination is a diagnostic modality based on the characteristic absorption of light in malignant tumors owing to the surrounding neovascularization.[1–3] In optical transillumination, wavelengths with low absorption in tissue, i.e., red or near-infrared light, have to be used.[4] The main problem is that in this wavelength region the dominating attenuating effect is not absorption but scattering.[5] The scattering coefficient is of the order of 10 mm^{-1}, while the absorption coefficient is of the order of 0.1 mm^{-1}.[6] The large scattering coefficient induces pronounced multiple scattering in the tissue.[7,8] This effect causes a decreased contrast when breast transillumination is performed.[9] Different methods to reduce the effect of light scattering have been suggested.[10–12] In this Letter a time-gating technique to do this is demonstrated.

The time-gating technique is based on the concept that light which leaves the transilluminated breast earlier has traveled a shorter and straighter path in the tissue than light exiting later. This early light is less scattered and thus contains more information about the spatial localization of the absorption, which in this case means the localization of the tumor. Such a technique has been analyzed theoretically by Maarek *et al.*[13]

In this Letter we describe experiments on a tissue-like phantom and a hand *in vivo* to investigate the increase in contrast when the time-gating technique is used in a highly scattering medium. The first demonstration using a solid object in a scattering liquid was presented in Ref. 14.

Figure 1 shows the experimental setup. The light source was a mode-locked Coherent CR-3000K Ar-ion laser pumping a Coherent CR-599 dye laser equipped with a cavity dumper. The pulses from the dye laser

were measured and evaluated to be 8 psec (FWHM) wide by using an autocorrelator. The average output power was 50 mW at the chosen wavelength of 630 nm, and the repetition frequency was approximately 5 MHz. The laser pulses irradiated the object, and the light was detected on the opposite side. The detector assembly consists of a small (<1-mm) aperture and a lens that focuses the light onto a 600-μm optical fiber. The acceptance angle for the detector is 2°, i.e., the light can enter the detector only if the angle is less than 1° off the optical axis. To achieve time-resolved detection, delayed coincidence techniques were used. The detector fiber is connected to a photon-counting multichannel plate (Hamamatsu 1564U-07), and the

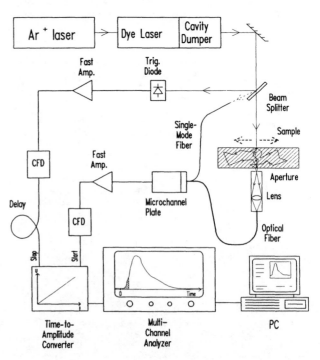

Fig. 1. Experimental setup.

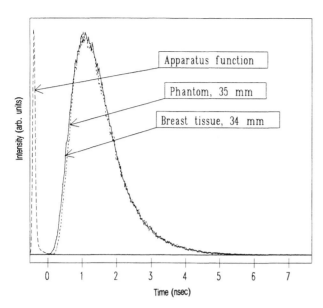

Fig. 2. Typical detected time-dispersion curves. The dotted curve shows the dispersion curve obtained when transilluminating the 35-mm-thick paraffin phantom. The solid curve shows the result when transilluminating a 34-mm-thick breast sample *in vitro* 1 h postmastectomy.. The impulse response function of the system (apparatus function) is also given.

signal is fed through a fast amplifier and a constant fraction discriminator (CFD) to a time-to-amplitude converter. This signal is the start signal for the time-to-amplitude converter. The stop signal comes from a diode triggering on the incident pulse. The trigger pulse is also fed through a fast amplifier and a CFD. The output signal from the time-to-amplitude converter is fed to a multichannel analyzer in which a histogram of arrival time for the photons is formed, i.e., the temporal dispersion curve. The curves can be transferred to a computer (PC) for evaluation. The impulse response function for this system is approximately 80 psec (FWHM). The impulse response is shown in Fig. 2. The experimental setup and the evaluation procedure are discussed in more detail in Ref. 15.

In order to ensure a well-defined measurement situation, experiments were performed on a tissue phantom, which was a block of paraffin. The dimensions of the paraffin were 150 mm × 55 mm × 35 mm, and thus the minimum optical path length was 35 mm. In Fig. 2 a comparison between the temporal dispersion curves for real breast *in vitro* and the phantom tissue can be seen. The solid curve shows the result when transilluminating a 34-mm-thick sample of breast tissue 1 h postmastectomy. The dotted curve shows the temporal dispersion curve obtained with the 35-mm-thick phantom. As can be seen, the curves are similar, and thus the phantom should be a good substitute for real tissue in this experiment. A considerable fraction of the light exits more than 3 nsec after the first transmitted light, which corresponds to an effective path length of more than 60 cm owing to heavy multiple scattering. Five holes were drilled into the phantom perpendicularly to the laser beam–detector plane.

Pieces of black rubber cord were inserted into the holes to simulate ideal totally absorbing tumors. Figure 3 (top) shows the phantom. The cords are 5 mm in diameter and located 5.5, 11.5, 17.5, 23.5, and 29.5 mm from the surface that is closest to the laser beam. The phantom can be translated across the beam–detector axis, and scanning can thus be performed. A temporal dispersion curve was sampled for 60 sec for every millimeter from 0 to 100 mm. To permit comparison of the different dispersion curves, a time-reference peak was obtained with every curve. That is, a single-mode optical fiber of suitable length was connected to the multichannel plate to detect a small part of the input pulse and thus create an impulse response peak in front of every dispersion curve, and this peak thus formed a reference in time. Before evaluation the curves were deconvoluted with the impulse response function to increase the effective time resolution. Figure 3 (bottom) shows the result of the scanning. The dashed curve shows all the detected light, i.e., the integral of the dispersion curves. The solid curve shows the amount of light detected early. The early light is the light detected during the first 100 psec of the dispersion curve. This corresponds to five channels in the multichannel analyzer. The width of the early light window is a compromise between the contrast and the signal-to-noise ratio. The wider the window the better the signal-to-noise ratio but the lower the contrast. A window of 100 psec corresponds to a distance 0.6 times the thickness of the phantom,

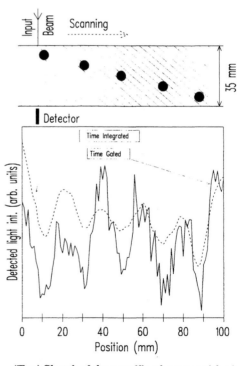

Fig. 3. (Top) Sketch of the paraffin phantom with pieces of black rubber cord inserted into it. (Bottom) Detected light intensity when scanning over the phantom with a resolution of 1 mm. The solid curve shows the result when light is detected the first 100 psec of every dispersion curve, i.e., the time-gated technique. The dashed curve shows the total amount of light detected at each point. The curves are arbitrarily normalized.

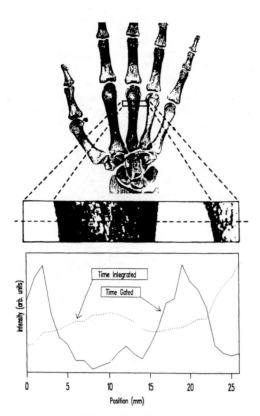

Fig. 4. Detected light intensity when scanning across a hand *in vivo*. The solid curve corresponds to the light detected during the first 80 psec, and the dotted curve is the total detected light.

calculated with a medium refractive index of 1.4. Thus the light detected with the time-gated technique is determined by a weighted average absorption over a volume of the phantom. The difference is that with the time-gated technique this volume is much smaller and more localized. The probability of detecting light that has traveled across the phantom without being scattered at all is almost zero, since the mean free path length for the photons is of the order of 100 μm. A test with polarization as a discriminating criterion verified this. If some of the light is not scattered, there should be a difference in the amount of vertically and horizontally polarized light exiting since the input pulse is vertically polarized, but the light exiting the phantom was totally unpolarized, even the detected early photons.

As can be seen in Fig. 3, there is an increase in contrast when the early light method is utilized. The contrast is defined as $C = (I_2 - I_1)/(I_1 + I_2)$, where I_1 is the amount of light detected with a cord between the laser beam and the detector and I_2 is the amount of light detected with no cord between the laser beam and the detector. The contrast varies for the time-gated case between approximately 0.5 and 0.8. The contrast for the total detected light is 0.1–0.3. The improvement in contrast is better than 2.5 times for all the pieces of cord. The figures also show that the contrast is much less dependent on the position of the cord in the phantom.

A similar scan was also carried out across a human hand *in vivo*. The results are shown in Fig. 4. The solid curve corresponds to the light intensity detected during the first 80 psec, and the dotted curve shows the total amount of light detected. The scan was performed approximately 10 mm below the knuckle of the middle finger. As can be seen in Fig. 4 there is a significant demarcation of the bones. It can also be seen that the two curves are out of phase. This phenomenon still needs to be investigated.

In summary, when performing transillumination of a turbid, highly scattering medium such as tissue for the purpose of detecting spatial variations in absorption, we have shown that the time-gating technique can be used to improve the result. To be able to use this technique for malignant tumor detection in the female breast, an imaging system should be used. We are planning the development of such a technique as well as spectroscopic recordings for evaluating optimal wavelengths to obtain the best contrast between malignant tumors and healthy breast tissue. Such spectral differences are much enhanced when using the time-gated technique since the attenuation due to absorption is then favored over attentuation due to scattering.

Valuable discussions with L. O. Svaasand and skillful help from Jonas Johansson are gratefully acknowledged. This research was supported by the Swedish Board for Technical Developments.

References

1. B. Ohlsson, J. Gundersen, and D.-M. Nilsson, World J. Surg. **4,** 701 (1980).
2. D. J. Watmough, Radiology **147,** 89 (1983).
3. B. Drexler, J. L. Davis, and G. Schofield, Radiology **157,** 41 (1985).
4. S. Ertefai and A. E. Profio, Med. Phys. **12,** 393 (1985).
5. B. C. Wilson, M. S. Patterson, S. T. Flock, and D. R. Wyman, in *Photon Migration in Tissue*, B. Chance, ed. (Plenum, New York, 1989).
6. R. Marchesini, A. Bertoni, S. Andreola, E. Melloni, and A. E. Sichirollo, Appl. Opt. **28,** 2318 (1989).
7. M. S. Patterson, B. Chance, and B. C. Wilson, Appl. Opt. **28,** 2331 (1989).
8. D. T. Delpy, M. Cope, P. van der Zee, S. Arridge, S. Wray, and J. Wyatt, Phys. Med. Biol. **33,** 1433 (1988).
9. G. A. Navarro and A. E. Profio, Med. Phys. **15,** 181 (1988).
10. K. G. Spears, J. Serafin, N. H. Abramson, X. Zhu, and H. Bjelkhagen, IEEE Trans. Biomed. Eng. **36,** 1210 (1989).
11. P. P. Ho, P. Baldeck, K. S. Wong, K. M. Yoo, D. Lee, and R. R. Alfano, Appl. Opt. **28,** 2304 (1989).
12. M. Toida, T. Ichimura, and H. Inaba, in *Conference on Lasers and Electro-Optics*, Vol. 7 of OSA Technical Digest Series (Optical Society of America, Washington, D.C., 1990), pp. 548–550.
13. J. M. Maarek, G. Jarry, J. Crowe, M.-H. Bui, and D. Laurent, Med. Biol. Eng. Comput. **24,** 407 (1986).
14. S. Andersson-Engels, R. Berg, J. Johansson, K. Svanberg, and S. Svanberg, in *Laser Spectroscopy IX*, M. Feld, ed. (Academic, New York, 1989), pp. 500–504.
15. R. Berg, M.S. thesis, Lund Reports on Atomic Physics LRAP-106 (Lund Institute of Technology, Lund, Sweden, 1989).

Reprinted from *Time-Resolved Laser Spectroscopy in Biochemistry III,* Proc. SPIE
Vol. 1640, pp. 254-261 (1992). ©1992 SPIE.

Frequency Domain Imaging of Thick Tissues Using a CCD

T. French, J. Maier and E. Gratton.

Laboratory for Fluorescence Dynamics, Department of Physics, University of Illinois at
Urbana-Champaign, 1110 W. Green Street, Urbana, Illinois 61801.

ABSTRACT

Imaging of thick tissue has been an area of active research during the past several
years. Among the methods proposed to deal with the high scattering of biological
tissues, the time resolution of a short light probe traversing a tissue seems to be the
most promising. Time resolution can be achieved in the time domain using correlated
single photon counting techniques or in the frequency domain using phase resolved
methods. We have developed a CCD camera system which provides ultra high time
resolution on the entire field of view. The phase of the photon diffusion wave traveling
in the highly turbid medium can be measured with an accuracy of about one degree at
each pixel. The camera has been successfully modulated at frequencies on the order of
100 MHz. At this frequency, one degree of phase shift corresponds to about 30 ps
maximum time resolution. Powerful image processing software displays in real time
the phase resolved image on the computer screen.

1. INTRODUCTION

We have sought to produce an instrument for the imaging of thick biological tissue:
a non-invasive, non-destructive two dimensional imaging station for real time analysis.
Our instrument is essentially a cross correlated phase fluorometer that includes a
modulated, intensified CCD camera to collect data across its entire field of view and a
modulated laser diode to deliver probing short light pulses to the turbid sample. All
data are collected in the frequency domain owing to the simplicity in this domain of the
diffusion model of photons in highly scattering, highly absorbing media. Two
dimensional projections of the internal details of a sample are created when the camera
obtains the wave front information of the photon diffusion waves emerging from the
sample. The details can be resolved currently with a resolution of several millimeters.
The system can be set to continuously acquire frequency domain images at a rate of
about one phase resolved image per minute making time evolution studies possible.
Others[1,2,3] have developed similar procedures for acquiring data in the time domain but
none of these can acquire data in two dimensions simultaneously.

2. THEORY

In the time domain, Patterson *et al.*[1] were able to show the diffusion model correctly
describes photon transport through media with high scattering and high absorption.
The corresponding frequency domain work has been done by Fishkin and Gratton[4].

Although light pulses diffuse through turbid media, the diffusional wave front
remains coherent for each modulation frequency component. Unfortunately, each
frequency component propagates at a different rate and the diffusional waves are
exponentially attenuated as they pass through the medium. For time domain methods,
the dispersion of the medium makes it necessary to use photodetectors with ultra fast
gating abilities in order to see the coherent emerging wave front. In the frequency
domain, phase synchronously modulated photodetectors can be used to select a single
frequency component of the emerging wave front. Usable thickness of a sample is
determined by the noise limits of the light detection scheme. We estimate the thickness
limit of our system to be about 10 cm.

Another result of the diffusion model is that the wavelength of the photon diffusional
wave will decrease with increasing modulation frequency (i.e. higher modulation
frequencies allow examination of finer details). The corresponding way to increase the
spatial resolution in the time domain is to decrease the gating time of the CCD to a speed
that a CCD camera is currently unable to handle or to resort to a different imaging
system such as a streak camera that is unable to acquire two dimensional data
simultaneously.

601

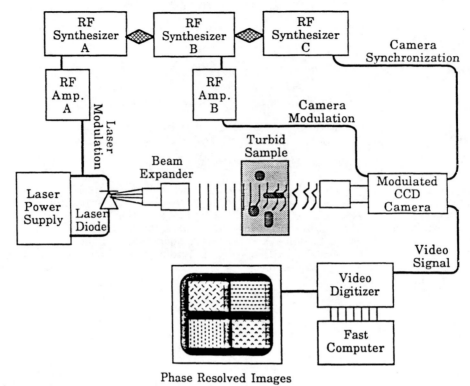

Phase Resolved Images

Fig. 1. Experimental set up.

3. MATERIALS AND METHODS

The camera system was created to replace an older imaging system that was based on a phase fluorometer. The precursor created phase resolved images by calculating the phase and modulation of light in the area to be imaged one point at a time. An image was created by scanning the detector across the field of view in a raster fashion. Although time consuming, the images created had well known attributes such as spatial resolution and dynamic range. The mechanics of the system were also known to operate well because they were based on an operating instrument.

The new imaging instrument consists of three basic elements: the laser, the camera, and the digitizer/computer. The complete system is shown schematically in fig. 1.

The laser light is amplitude modulated and the beam is expanded to illuminate the sample with plane waves. The diode laser (Spectra Diode Labs, SDL-2431-H2) operates at 810 nm and can emit about 250 mW of optical power. A typical power level is about 30 mW. Light is delivered to the sample via an optical fiber with a 100 mm diameter. Amplitude modulation of the laser beam is achieved by controlling the electrical power the diode receives. A high power radio frequency (RF) signal produced by an external synthesizer and amplifier provide the modulation control.

Light pulses entering the highly scattering sample diffuse through the object emerging with a distorted wave front that is recorded with the CCD. By studying the wave front in the frequency domain, internal details of the sample become evident. The camera is a high resolution monochrome video CCD camera (Cohu Inc. model 4812-2000/ER) with a dual stage image intensifier (ITT type F4144) attached. The CCD is a 2/3" format imager with 754 x 244 active pixels (11 mm x 27 mm each). Camera electronics read the CCD sixty times a second and transmit the video in standard RS-170 format. Synchronization of the frame rate is necessary and is achieved by sending the appropriate phase locked signals to the electronics from an external synthesizer.

The image intensifier is a dual stage microchannel plate (MCP) that serves two purposes. First, with a luminous gain of up to one million, the MCP is used to increase the gain of the camera. More importantly for our system the MCP is used to modulate the gain of the camera at rates up to 100 MHz.

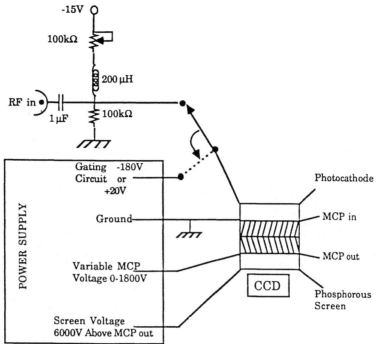

Fig. 2. Modulation circuit used to deliver an RF signal to the MCP.

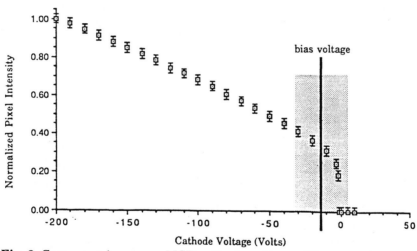

Fig. 3. Camera gain versus MCP cathode voltage. The grayed area represents the amplitude of the RF signal used to modulate the camera.

The circuit that delivers the RF signal to the MCP is a simple one (shown in fig. 2). The RF signal is sent to the cathode of the image intensifier mainly because this is where the smallest voltage can be applied and still obtain good modulation. The reasonable RF signals that can be externally generated force the cathode to be operated at low voltages. Unfortunately, the voltage from the cathode to the MCP determines to a great extent the best focus the camera can achieve. Thus our system never has great focus meaning we do not necessarily have a resolution of 754 x 244 pixels at the CCD. The gain of the MCP as a function of cathode voltage was found and is given in fig. 3 and was used to determine the amplitude and DC offset of the RF signal that would be appropriate to modulate the gain of the camera. The current circuit responds up to 100 MHz. Minor revisions in the circuit could improve its frequency response. Furthermore, a resonant circuit could be installed to provide excellent response at a given frequency. This would allow us to modulate the MCP with a greater amplitude RF signal than we are presently using resulting in better spatial resolution.

603

Fig. 4. Phase resolved images of the model system created by the raster scanning instrument. Shading of the images is based on a linear scale that assigns the lightest shade (white) to the maximum values and the darkest shade (black) to the minimum values.

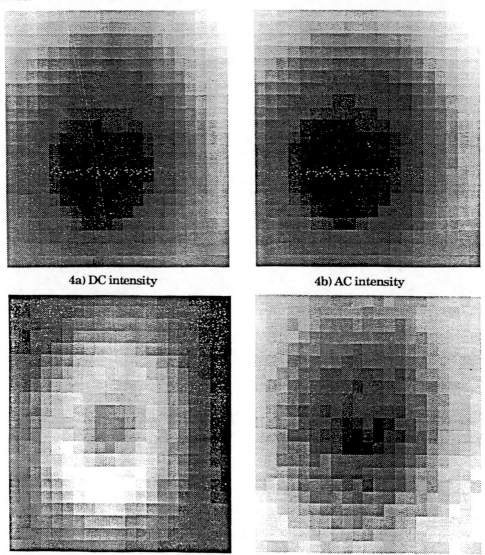

4a) DC intensity

4b) AC intensity

4c) phase shift

4d) modulation

To bring the light emerging from the sample to the CCD, a standard macro / zoom lens (D. O. Industries, Zoom 7000) is used. We have found the lens to have good light collecting ability and good field of view. The versatility the lens adds to the system in accommodating various sized objects and various object distances has proved helpful. The front focal plane of the lens has always been set to the outer surface of the sample in successful images.

The laser and camera form the heart of a cross correlation spectrometer. Since the laser is modulated at radio frequencies, the camera must also have a method to gate the light at radio frequencies. As stated above, the MCP provides the camera this ability. The MCP is modulated at a frequency just slightly different than that of the laser. Through the process of heterodyning the incoming light appears to the CCD to be arriving at the difference in frequencies called the cross correlation frequency. This frequency down conversion of the transmitted light is essential to the operation of the system because the camera has a limited response time and would otherwise be unable to image the transmitted light in a meaningful way. The cross correlated signal is sampled several times per wave form. Our specific system uses a cross correlation

Fig. 5. Phase resolved images of the model system created by the camera based instrument. Shading of the images is based on a linear scale that assigns the lightest shade (white) to the maximum values and the darkest shade (black) to the minimum values.

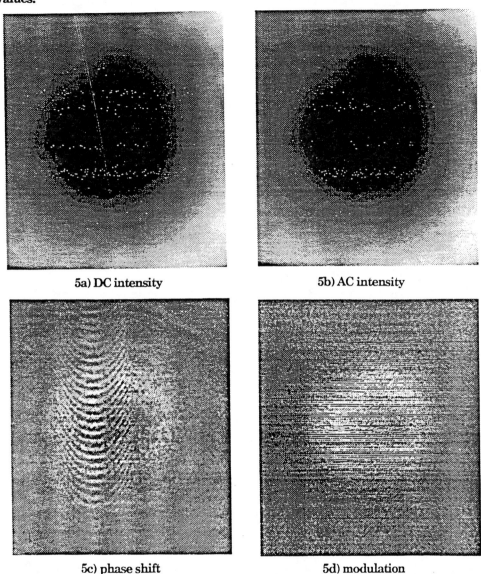

5a) DC intensity

5b) AC intensity

5c) phase shift

5d) modulation

frequency of 15 Hz and a sampling rate of 60 Hz for four samples per wave form. Each sample is digitized and stored and then integrated by summing corresponding samples of each wave form. Resulting images have a greater dynamic range and a better signal to noise ratio than without integration.

For the data processing our system has a video rate digitizer (MATROX Electronic Systems Ltd., Image-1280) installed in a PC compatible computer (Gateway 2000, 486/25). The digitizer is able to transform analog data to eight bit digital data at 15 MHz and can perform simple image manipulation functions (such as image addition) simultaneous to data acquisition. The digitizer also has 8 Mb of VRAM to store incoming images. Working in parallel to the digitizer, the computer can be used to compute the frequency domain images.

Data is prepared for analysis by Fourier transforming the samples to their frequency domain representation and calculating the modulation. The only image processing generally used at this stage is clipping the range of the data for display to eliminate extraneous points.

4. RESULTS AND DISCUSSION

To show that the instrument based on the camera operates correctly, images of a model biological system were created using both the new and the old instruments. The model system was a blackened washer immersed half deep in a high scattering solution of Intralipid®-20% and water. Intralipid®-20% is solution of fat emulsion that when diluted appears very similar to milk. The washer was blackened to absorb incoming light rather that reflect it. The washer was about 3 cm in diameter with a 1 cm diameter hole. These images are shown in figs. 4 and 5.

The raster scan system collected 400 data points equally spaced (2 mm spacing) about a 4 cm by 4 cm imaging area. The scattering solution contained 20 ml of Intralipid®-20% per 1000 ml of water. In this experiment, the thickness of the solution was 3.5 cm. The laser was operated at a modulation frequency of 120 Mhz and at an optical power of 70 mW. This instrument took about 40 minutes to created the phase resolved images presented.

The camera system created phase resolved images that had dimensions of 230 by 256 pixel. This corresponds to an image size of about 4 cm by 4 cm composed of 59,000 equally spaced points with a spacing of 0.2 mm. The scattering solution contained 12 ml of Intralipid®-20% per 1000 ml of water. This time the thickness of the solution was 2.5 cm. The laser was modulated at 90 Mhz and at an optical power of 10 mW. The camera system spent only about one minute to create the given images. Because there was a non-uniform phase background, the background was subtracted from the phase shift image presented in fig. 4c.

There are still many questions to be answered about the operation of this system. These include questions of minimum resolvable object size and inherent image contrast factors (wavelength of illumination, modulation frequency, inhomogeneous absorption and inhomogeneous scattering). In spite of these, the system has shown itself to be viable as a method of probing the internal structures of turbid media.

Presently, the system can repeat images at about once a minute due to the algorithm that performs the acquisition. In the future, we will be able to decrease the image acquisition time and thereby increase the duty cycle of the instrument as we understand the workings of the digitizer better. We would also like to see the system used to create volumetric images using techniques such as computer aided tomography.

5. ACKNOWLEDGEMENTS

This work was performed at the Laboratory for Fluorescence Dynamics (LFD) in the Department of Physics at the University of Illinois at Urbana-Champaign (UIUC). This work and the LFD are supported jointly by the Division of Research Resources of the National Institutes of Health (RR03155) and the UIUC.

6. REFERENCES

1. M. S. Patterson, B. Chance and B. C. Wilson, *Appl. Opt.* 28, 2331-2336 (1989).
2. J. C. Hebden, R. A. Kruger, and K. S. Wong, *Appl. Opt.* 30, 788-794 (1991).
3. S. Andersson-Engels, J. Johansson, U. Stenram, K. Svanberg and S. Svanberg, *J. of Photochem. Photobiol. B*, 363-369 (1990).
4. J. B. Fishkin and E. Gratton, *Phys. Rev. B*, submitted (1991).

Reprinted from *Physiological Monitoring and Early Detection Diagnostic Methods,*
Proc. SPIE Vol. 1641, pp. 21-34 (1992). ©1992 SPIE.

Imaging of Diffusing Media by a Progressive Iterative Backprojection Method Using Time-Domain Data

R. L. Barbour[†], H. L. Graber, and J. Lubowsky
Departments of Pathology and Biophysics, SUNY Health Science Center at Brooklyn, 450 Clarkson Ave.,
Brooklyn, NY 11203

R. Aronson
Department of Physics, Polytechnic University, 333 Jay St. Brooklyn, NY 11201

B. B. Das, K. M. Yoo, and R. R. Alfano
Institute for Ultrafast Spectroscopy and Lasers, Departments of Electrical Engineering and Physics,
City College of the City University of New York, NY, NY 10031

[†]Author to whom inquiries should be addressed.

Abstract

A method for the reconstruction of 3-D images of the interior of dense scattering media, based on the analysis of time-resolved backscattered signals is described. The method evaluates a linear perturbation equation by a progressive iterative backprojection scheme. A key feature of the method is the use of weighting functions which estimate the impact that absorption of photons in the interior have on the response of detectors located at the surface. Examples of reconstructed images shown are based on the analysis of simulated data for multilayered media and simulated and experimental data for media containing finite-volume absorbers. These results contain features which indicate that images having high resolution are obtainable even in the limiting case where the view angle is restricted to only backscattered signals and the absorption contrast across an interior boundary is 1%. A general scheme, similar to a layer-stripping approach, is described for the case where signals emerging about a target are measured.

1.0 Introduction

A common theme among almost all imaging technologies used to examine tissue, including X-ray CT, PET, SPECT, acoustic tomography, and others, is their reliance on the detection of coherent (i.e., straight line paths) or nearly coherent signals. This observation is not a coincidence; in many cases the dominant signal is coherent, and because the paths of the detected radiation are well-defined, this acts to greatly simplify the computational effort required for image reconstruction. Even MRI can be considered a coherent imaging method, as the volume of target medium contributing to the detector response is well-defined.

While many useful applications based on this scheme have been identified, for many types of media the ability to detect coherent signals represents a special case. That is, the fact that such signals exist at all means that the penetrating radiation interacts only weakly with the target medium. In addition, even under these conditions, if the thickness of the target medium is large relative to the scattering pathlength, then at large depths in the medium the intensity of the coherent component becomes vanishingly small while that of the diffusely scattered signal can become dominant. Moreover, there are many instances where the incident radiation interacts strongly with the target medium and is intensely scattered (e.g., tissue at optical frequencies). Here the measurable penetration depth of coherent radiation is very small. Thus, in a general sense, the ability to detect coherent signals becomes a matter of scale.

For many practical applications, imaging schemes based on the analysis of diffusely scattered radiation would permit use of a much broader frequency range of penetrating radiation, while also potentially allowing for imaging to much greater depths than currently is achievable. Further, although scattering significantly complicates the imaging problem, it affords the capacity for remote sensing (i.e., detection of backscattered signals). Thus, diffusion-based imaging schemes could potentially have a much broader application range than current imaging methods.

The practical development of diffusion-based imaging schemes will not be easy. Models of the forward problem are incomplete, necessitating use of approximations of questionable validity. Moreover, the computational complexity of the inversion schemes will, invariably, be much greater than those encountered for methods based on coherent signals. This observation indicates that, as a practical matter, progress in developing suitable algorithms could be significantly slowed unless attention to issues common to large-scale computing problems are addressed[1,2]. These added difficulties are, however, partially compensated for by the expectation that in many applications even low-resolution images could prove useful. We believe this is the likely case for many of the potential applications for imaging of tissues at NIR frequencies.

Our starting point for considering a diffusion-based imaging scheme, and in particular for the optical imaging problem, is the assumption that the intensity of any coherent signal is sufficiently small as to be undetectable. We have previously described a perturbation approach as a model for image recovery[3-6] of media which diffusely scatter penetrating radiation. The spirit of this approach is similar to the compensation theorem method used in electrical impedance tomography[7]. Both iteratively adjust a current estimate until the readings calculated for the estimated medium match with those detected. Also, both methods are confronted with the added difficulty that there is significant uncertainty as to the path of the detected signal, which may make the problem underdetermined. In the case of the optical method, however, this uncertainty can be reduced by employing time-resolved methods in either the time[8-12] or frequency[13-15] domain. Alfano and co-workers[9-11], for example, have proposed imaging schemes that exploit the existence of photons having traversed even large thickness of tissue along quasi-straight line paths.

In this report, we have extended our studies of the perturbation model to include the evaluation of time-resolved data obtained by simulation and by backscatter experiment using a femtosecond (fs) colliding pulse laser. To maximize the spatial selectivity in the simulation studies, tightly collimated receivers (~0.095 sr cone of acceptance) were modeled using Monte Carlo methods, and the backscattered signals were recorded as a function of distance and orientation of the receivers about each source location. In addition, to further enhance spatial selectivity, several early discrete time intervals, rather than the value for the mean time-of-flight[16], were selected as input data for the reconstruction algorithm. Time-gated images based on evaluation of calculated data examined media having either a layered structure, in which the contrast or thickness of intermediate layers were varied, or a medium containing a finite absorber in the shape of the letter 'T'. Images derived from experimental data examined media containing a finite black absorber in the shape of a sphere. A more thorough examination of the perturbation approach and its application to steady-state measurements is presented in an accompanying paper[17].

2.0 Methods

2.1 Monte Carlo Simulations

The computational platform[2] used for running Monte Carlo codes and the techniques that were employed to increase the efficiency of the calculation[15] are described in accompanying papers. Results from two types of simulations were evaluated by the reconstruction algorithms. The first type modeled the responses of collimated detectors on the surface of a dense scattering medium, by estimating the contribution of photons propagating within the medium to the photon flux at the surface after every scattering event. The estimator is a function of the probabilities that a photon can reach the detector without another collision, and that it can survive to the present collision site without being absorbed or escaping from the medium[15]. The second type counted the collisions occurring in each voxel of the medium, and weighted each of these scoring events by the probability of a photon surviving all of its preceding collisions to arrive at an estimate of the spatial distribution of collisions. In all cases the media modeled here were infinite in length and width and 10 mean free pathlengths (MFP) thick; scattering was isotropic.

Some of the media modeled in the simulations were heterogeneous in all three spatial dimensions, while others were heterogeneous in only the z-dimension. Additionally, simulations were conducted to model both the steady-state and the time-resolved illumination schemes. In all, five different detector configurations were required. These configurations, and the situations for which each was appropriate are:

1. <u>Steady-State, 'T' absorber</u>. Heterogeneous in three spatial dimensions, see Legend of Figure 4 for description of absorber. The surface of the medium was divided into a 100 x 100 cell square grid centered at the point of entry of the injected photons, with each cell 1 MFP^2 in area. Each detector received photons exiting the medium in one of the grid cells. Photon fluxes were recorded in units of no. photons emerging/ incident photon/ sr/ MFP^2.

2. <u>Time-resolved, 'T' absorber</u>. Photons exiting in the grid cells were binned according to the total distance they had propagated within the medium. The bins corresponded to all photons that emerged after a total distance of between n and n + 1 MFP, n =

0,1,...,99. Photon fluxes were recorded in units of no. photons emerging/ incident photon/ sr/ MFP^3.

3. Time-resolved, 2- and 3-layer media. Heterogeneous in one spatial dimension, see Results for description of absorbers. The photon flux at the surface has cylindrical symmetry about the source. The surface of the medium was divided into 15 circular rings centered at the point of entry of the injected photons, with a 1-MFP difference between the inner and outer radii of each ring. The outer radius was n MFP, n = 1,2,...,15. Time resolution and photon flux units were the same as in the preceding case.

4. Steady-state, collision density. The medium was homogeneous, and divided into a 41x41x10 grid of cubical cells, with each cell 1 MFP^3 in volume. Each detector measured the collision density in one of the voxels, with the result reported in units of collisions/ incident photon/ MFP^3.

5. Time-resolved, collision density. Medium and cells were as in the previous case. The collisions were binned according to the total distance a photon had propagated in the medium prior to the current collision. The bins corresponded to all collisions occurring after a total distance between .5n and .5(n + 1) MFP, n = 0,1,...143. The results were recorded in units of collisions/ incident photon/ MFP^4.

2.2. Experimental Methods

The data used in image reconstructions from experimental measurements were obtained by directing 100 fs light pulses generated by a colliding pulse modelocked laser to a vessel containing diluted whole milk and a submerged aluminum sphere with a matte black paint surface. The temporal profiles of the backscattered light were measured by a streak camera. A description of the experiment and sketch of the set-up is given in Graber et al.[15].

2.3 Weight Function Calculation

The weight in a given voxel for a particular source-detector pair is equal to $-\partial I_{jk}/\partial \Sigma a_i$, the partial derivative of the detected photon flux with respect to the macroscopic absorption cross-section in the voxel. Here, i, j and k are the indices of the voxel, source and detector, respectively. As was shown previously[4], radiation transport theory can be used to derive an expression for the weight in the case of steady-state illumination. The formula reported there is:

$$w_{ijk} = \frac{S_j F_{ij} F_{ik}}{4\pi V_i \Sigma_t^2} \tag{1}$$

where S_j is the strength of source j (photons/ unit time); V_i is the volume of voxel i (MFP^3, cm^3,...) ; Σ_t is the total macroscopic cross-section (distance^{-1}); F_{ij} and F_{ik} are the collision densities in voxel i due to a single photon launched from source j and detector k, respectively. There is flexibility in the expression for weight; the particular expression in equation 1 is based on the assumption that Σ_t is constant throughout the medium and the unknown quantity sought in each voxel is the difference in macroscopic absorption cross-section, Σ_a, relative to a known reference medium. In many practical situations Σt will also be variable, and it will be appropriate to remove the factor of $1/\Sigma_t^2$ from the weight and let the change in the ratio Σ_a/Σ_t^2 be the unknown.

When time-resolved measurements are performed, the weight in a given voxel is a function of time. The weight at a particular time is not proportional to a simple product of two collision densities; rather, the correct expression must account for all possible combinations of source-to-voxel time (τ) and voxel-to-detector time $(t - \tau)$ that sum to the same total source-to-detector time (t). The expression for time-dependent weight has the product in equation 1 replaced by a convolution integral:

$$w_{ijk}(t) = \frac{S_j}{4\pi V_i \Sigma_t^2} \int_0^t F_{ij}(\tau)F_{ik}(t - \tau)d\tau \tag{2}$$

The right-hand side of equation 2 is the instantaneous weight at time t. To find the weight in a time window of finite extent, this expression is integrated over the time interval of interest:

$$w_{ijk}(t_1 - t_2) = \frac{S_j}{4\pi V_i \Sigma_t^2} \int_{t_1}^{t_2} \int_0^t F_{ij}(\tau)F_{ik}(t - \tau)d\tau dt \tag{3}$$

609

Because the Monte Carlo simulations that calculated the collision densities accumulated them in bins of finite width (i.e., finite time intervals), it was necessary to approximate the integral in equation 3 by a sum. In doing so, it was assumed that the weight could not be accurately calculated to at time resolution better than twice as coarse as that in the collision density data. The discretized version of equation 3 that was used to calculate the weights used in the image reconstructions is:

$$w_{ijk}(N) = \frac{1}{2}\sum_{t_1=1}^{2N} F_{ij}(t_1)\left\{ \left[\sum_{t_2=1}^{M-1} F_{ik}(2N-M+1-t_1+t_2) \right] \right.$$
$$\left. + \frac{1}{2}[F_{ik}(2N+1-t_1) + F_{ik}(2N-M+1-t_1)] \right\}$$

(4)

where N = time window index and M = number of collision density bins in weight function time window. If continuous functions for $F_{ij}(t)$ and $F_{ik}(t)$ were available, equation 4 would be equivalent to using the trapezoidal rule to approximate the double integral in equation 3.

2.4 Image reconstruction

The image reconstruction algorithms were based on a perturbation model in which the structure of the test medium is assumed to be close to that of a known reference medium. In that case, the reconstruction reduces to a problem of solving a system of linear equations[3-5]. The successive stages of development of this system are:

$$(I - I_0)_{ijk} = w_{ijk}(\Sigma_a - \Sigma_a^0)_i \tag{5a}$$

$$(I - I_0)_{jk} = \sum_i w_{ijk}(\Sigma_a - \Sigma_a^0)_i \tag{5b}$$

$$\Delta I = \mathbf{W}\Delta\Sigma_a \tag{5c}$$

Equation 5a shows that the change in photon flux at the surface for source j and detector k, due to an absorption difference in voxel i, is the product of $\Delta\Sigma_a$ and the weight for that voxel, source, and detector. In equation 5b, we use the approximation that these effects are simply additive, with the net difference ΔI_{jk} equal to the sum of the changes due to $\Delta\Sigma_a$ in all the voxels. Each source-detector pair contributes an equation of the form of 5b to the system in 5c. Equation 5c is fully determined if the number of photon flux measurements is equal to the number of voxels in the medium.

For reasons discussed by Barbour et al.[4] and Wang et al.[17], iterative numerical methods for solving equation 5c are preferable to direct methods. The varieties of reconstruction algorithms used in this study, which are described in the following section, were applicable to both the steady-state and time-resolved situations. The quantities ΔI and $\mathbf{W}$ in equation 5c may refer to the detector readings and weights for either type of measurement. In practice, the time-resolved reconstructions yielded faster convergence, and required significantly less time for each iteration, than those employing steady-state data (see Results for quantitative comparison). This is a consequence of the smaller number of calculations performed, which in turn is due to the fact that steady-state weight functions encompass the entire volume involved in the reconstruction, while time-resolved weight functions, at early time intervals, are non-zero in only a small fraction of this volume.

2.5 Variations of the reconstruction algorithm

Several different evaluation schemes have been formulated and tested for the solution of equation 5c. These have included substituting related quantities for ΔI and $\mathbf{W}$, as well as varying the order in which the data were evaluated. All of the images presented in this study were obtained using the progressive iterative backprojection algorithm described in Barbour et al[4]. The two parts of each iteration step are:

$$s_i^n = \frac{\sum_j \sum_k w_{ijk}\left[-c_{jk}^{n-1} + \left(\frac{\Delta I}{I_0}\right)_{jk} \right]}{\sum_j \sum_k w_{ijk}} + s_i^{n-1} \tag{6a}$$

$$c_{jk}^n = \frac{\sum_i w_{ijk} s_i^n}{\sum_i w_{ijk}} \qquad (6b)$$

with $n \geq 1$, and letting $s_i^0 = 0$ for all i and $c_{jk}^0 = 0$ for all j and k. s_i^n is the nth-iteration estimate of the image density in the ith voxel, c_{jk}^n is the nth-iteration estimate of the relative darkening, $\Delta I/I_0$, for the measurement made with the source j and detector k. Detector readings were evaluated as normalized differences, $\Delta I/I_0$, rather than their absolute differences, ΔI, as the former quantity can more easily account for expected fluctuations in source intensity and detector sensitivity. Answers derived from the two quantities, although different, will be correlated. For steady-state and time resolved measurements, the algorithms employed were progressive in distance or time and distance, respectively. In the latter case, where both time and distance were parameters, the iteration initially incorporated only detector readings corresponding to the smallest source-detector separation r, and earliest time window. Data from the same set of detectors at later times and the next larger r were subsequently included.

For the reconstructions of two- and three-layer media, the assumed knowledge was that the medium was heterogeneous in only the depth dimension, so that ΔI_{jk} was a function of only r and detector orientation. After each application of equation 6a the average value of s_i^n was calculated in each layer, and this was taken to be the image density of all voxels at that depth. The absolute values of the weights were employed in these reconstructions.

Reconstructions of the medium used in the experiments were done with the assumptions that the scattering was isotropic, that the scattering medium had the same refractive index as water, and that the absorber was known to be symmetric about the two major axes of the grid on which the source fiber was scanned.

3.0 Results

3.1 Comparison of Weight Functions for Time-Independent and Time-Gated Measurements

We have previously shown that by evaluating a linear perturbation equation (equation 5c) for backscattered signals, images of subsurface structures can be obtained[3-5]. A key aspect in this approach is the use of estimates of the site-dependent effect of absorption on detected photon flux for each source-detector pair considered. An example of these gradients, referred to here as weights, for time-independent backscattered measurements is shown in Figure 1. These results were calculated, as described in Methods, by evaluating equation 1 for a medium having finite thickness (10 MFP), isotropic scattering, $\Sigma_a/\Sigma_t = .01$ and detectors located 1 (Panel A) and 5 (Panel B) MFP from the source. For illustration purposes, the value of the function in equation 1 has been displayed as a contour plot (X-Z slice) by ranking voxels in order of descending weight by the indicated percentiles. Thus voxels located within the first 10% contour contain the greatest weight and, correspondingly, occupy the smallest total volume (directly beneath the source and detector).

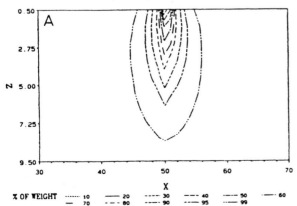 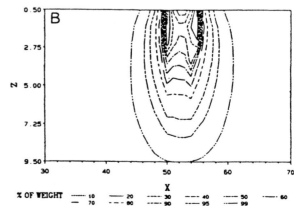

Legend to Figure 1: Contour Plots of vertical sections through steady-state weight functions. Plane of section is y = 50, with light

source directed normal to surface at $(x,y,z) = (50,50,0)$. Detector is located at $(51,50,0)$ (Panel A) or $(55,50,0)$ (Panel B), and is inclined 10° from normal, so that axes of source and detector intersect at a point below the surface $(z > 0)$. Weights were calculated by eq. 1 in Methods, and voxels were ranked in order of descending weight. Contours are the intersections of the plane $y = 50$ with the surfaces bounding the indicated percentiles of the total weight.

One of the difficulties encountered when evaluating steady-state signals is that detected photons have the opportunity to propagate throughout the target medium. At a given detector location, signals from shallow and deep regions are detected simultaneously. Since the latter always have weights much less than voxels located nearer the surface in the vicinity of the source and detector, especially for small source-detector separation distances, it becomes increasingly more difficult to detect the presence of excess absorption in deeper regions. At these depths, the reconstruction problem can become severely underdetermined.

One approach to isolating signals having a given pathlength is to employ time-resolved methods. At early time intervals, the maximum distance the detected photons may have propagated in the medium is sharply limited. Examples of weight functions calculated by using equation 4 for time-gated signals are shown in Figure 2. Results shown are expressed as in Figure 1. At early time intervals (Panel A, $t = 9$-10 mean free times (MFT) (i.e., time for photons to travel a total distance of 9-10 MFP), $r = 5$ MFP) all of the detected photons are restricted within a small finite volume. At later times (Panel B, $t = 69$-70 MFT, $r = 5$ MFP), this volume has increased greatly, and the volume corresponding to any given contour contains voxels at a greater depth than in the case of time-independent observations (cf., Figure 1, Panel B). In terms of the reconstruction problem, relative to the time-independent case, use of early time signals can greatly reduce the number of voxels which must be scored. Related to this is the observation that, at early times, the uncertainty of paths of detected photons is also less.

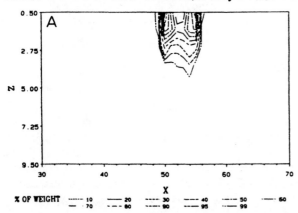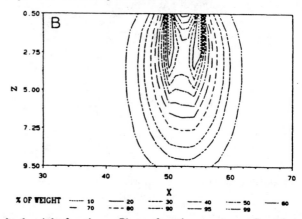

Legend to Figure 2: Contour plots of vertical sections through time-resolved weight functions. Plane of section, source configuration, and detector configuration are the same as in Figure 1B. Detector accepted photons after traveling a total distance between 9 and 10 (Panel A) or between 69 and 70 (Panel B) MFP in the medium. Weights were calculated by eq. 4 in Methods, and presented in the same manner as in Figure 1.

It is of interest to estimate the degree of advantage time-gated measurements should have over time-independent measurements in the reconstruction problem. While this will likely depend on several factors (e.g., selection of source-detector positions, order in which data are evaluated[4], geometry of target medium, spatial location of absorbing regions, type of algorithm employed) a comparison of the value of the weight functions obtained for the same source-detector pair using the different measurement schemes is instructive. Data in Figure 3 shows this comparison for detectors positioned 1 and 10 MFP from the source. Results shown represent a contour plot of the ratio of relative weights (i.e., the fraction of the total weight) in each voxel (time-gated/ time-independent, X-Z slice) at the indicated time intervals. Values of this ratio greater than one indicate a greater sensitivity by time-gated measurements to excess absorption in the medium, while values less than one indicate a greater sensitivity by time-independent measurements. In all three examples a consistent triphasic trend is observed. The value of the ratio of weights for voxels located in the vicinity of the source and detector is less than one. At intermediate distances, the ratio becomes greater than one, followed by a precipitous decline at greater distances. This behavior, although complex, is not unexpected. Interestingly, at early time intervals and for detectors located close to the source (Panel A, $r = 1$ MFP, $t = 19$-20 MFT), the position of the region of greater sensitivity for time-gated measurements is located not in between, but outside of, the region between the source and detector, and forms a truncated bowl-shaped structure. In the example shown, the value of the ratio in this region reaches a maximum of approximately 3. At later time intervals, for the same detector location (Panel B, t = 69-70 MFT), the maximum value of the ratio increases to greater than 14 and occurs at greater depths. Thus, for this particular source-detector pair and in the indicated region, a time-gated measurement affords a considerable advantage over a time-independent measurement. The advantage gained by time-gating in a particular region, however, is highly sensitive to which source-detector pair is examined. When a comparison is made for a similar time interval (t = 65-70 MFT) but at a greater source-detector separation (r = 10 MFP, Panel C), the maximum value of this ratio is reduced to only approximately 1.35. In this case it is apparent that, at least for the example shown, little advantage is gained by employing a time-gated measurement.

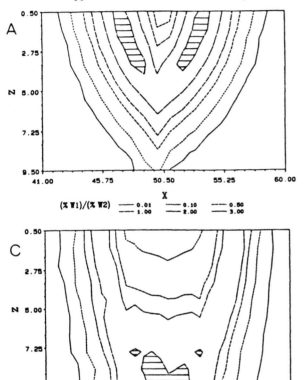

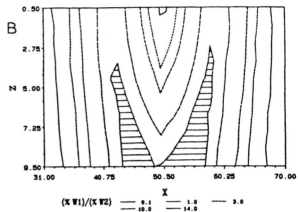

Legend to Figure 3: Contour plots of ratios of time-resolved (tr) relative weights to steady-state (ss) relative weights, i.e., $(w_i^{tr} \sum_{i'} w_{i'}^{ss})/(w_i^{ss} \sum_{i'} w_{i'}^{tr})$ Plane of section, source configuration, detector configuration are the same as in Figures 1 and 2. Detector is located at (x,y,z) = (51,50,0) (Panel A and B) or (60,50,0) (Panel C). Detector accepted photons that exited after traveling a total distance between 19 and 20 (Panel A), 69 and 70 (Panel B), or 65 and 70 (Panel C) MFP in the medium. Shaded areas are regions of greatest sensitivity enhancement due to time-gating.

3.2 Image Reconstruction by Progressive Backprojection for Time-Independent and Time-Gated Signals

Representative plots of reconstructed images obtained by evaluating steady-state and time-resolved data for media containing the "T" shaped absorber are shown in Figures 4 and 5, respectively. A strict comparison is not entirely valid as the number and locations of the source-detector pairs and number of iterations performed are not identical. Steady-state data were evaluated using a scheme progressive in distance (i.e., D_1, D_1D_2, $D_1D_2D_3$, ..., where the family of detectors D_1, D_2, D_3,..., are located at successively greater distances from the source). A similar approach was used to evaluate time-resolved data. An analysis progressive in distance was accomplished by simultaneously considering all time windows for a given family of source-detector pairs (i.e., $D_1(\sum_{t1}^{tn})$, $D_1D_2(\sum_{t1}^{tn})$, $D_1D_2D_3(\sum_{t1}^{tn})$,...., (Figure 5, panel A and B)). An analysis progressive in time and distance sequentially considered each time window for a particular family of source-detector pairs (i.e., D_{1t1}, D_{1t1t2}, ..., $D_{1t1...tn}$, $D_{1t1...tn}D_{2t1}$, $D_{1t1...tn}D_{2t1t2}$, ..., (Figure 5, Panels C and D)). In order to reduce the computation time and to test the robustness of the algorithm, only a portion of the available data was evaluated. This had the effect of making the problem underdetermined, as the number of observations evaluated were between 18-63% of the number of unknowns. Inspection of Figure 4 shows that whereas the region of greatest darkening coincides reasonably well with the actual location of the absorber, the quality of the image is not good. It should be noted, however, that the detectors whose values were used in the reconstruction were all within 2 transport MFP from a source. At this distance, more than 85% of the total weight lies in voxels less deep than the absorber. Thus, only a small portion of the incident signal had the opportunity to interact with the target. Despite these limitations, and that the problem was determined to an extent of only 9%, the reconstructed image correctly identifies the existence of asymmetry in the shape of the absorber, and its approximate location.

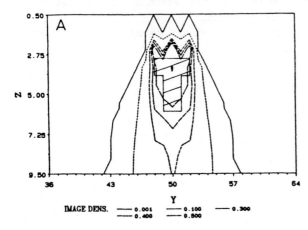 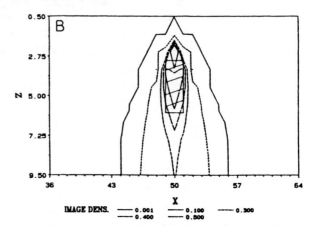

Legend to Figure 4: Contour plots of vertical sections through image of T, reconstructed by equations 6a and 6b, and using steady-state weight functions and reflectance measurements. The planes of section are x = 50 (Panel A) and y = 50 (Panel B), with the true sections through the absorber in these planes shaded in. The medium is infinitely long and wide, 10 MFP thick, scatters photons isotropically, and has $\Sigma_a = .01\Sigma_t$. The absorber is a black body ($\Sigma_a = \infty$) with nonreflective planar boundaries. Reconstruction program employed only readings for detectors at r = 1 in the first 200 iterations, readings for detectors at r = 1 and r = $\sqrt{2}$ in the next 200, and readings for detectors at r = 1, r = $\sqrt{2}$, and r = 2 in the final 200. Readings were obtained at 19 locations of the source beam relative to the absorber, all lying within a circle of radius 6 MFP about the point (50,50,0) on the surface. The symmetry of the absorber effectively increases the number of source positions to 61. Two detector orientations were used at each detector location, one inclined 10° from the normal, the other inclined 80° from the normal.

With the above caveats noted, comparison of Figures 4 and 5 reveals that images of much higher resolution can be achieved using time-resolved data. Comparison of Panel A and B to C and D in Figure 5 also indicates that an analysis progressive in time and distance appears to yield an answer having a slightly better edge detection than when the analysis is progressive only in distance, even though the former was less determined (24 vs. 63% respectively) and required approximately 10% less cpu time to evaluate. The maximum depth in the medium to which the image was calculated is less than for the time-independent case, as the longest time window examined (12 MFT) restricted all photons detected to within 6 MFP of the surface. It should also be noted that because of an interpolation routine inherent in the graphics package used to plot the data, the apparent image density gradient observed in the reconstructed images in some cases underestimated the actual gradient. In particular, for Panel D of Figure 5, the horizontal gradient between z = 4 and z = 6 is infinite, indicating that perfect edge detection was achieved.

In the above example, the data used for image reconstruction was based on the presence of a black absorber against a weakly

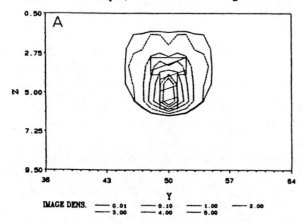 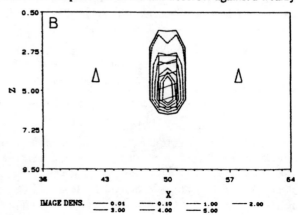

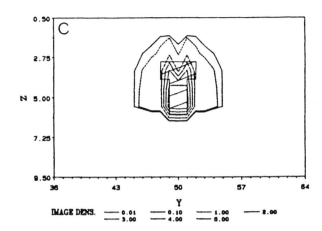
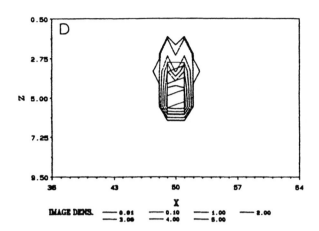

IMAGE DENS. ── 0.01 ── 0.10 ── 1.00 ── 2.00
── 3.00 ── 4.00 ── 5.00

Legend to Figure 5: Contour plots of vertical sections through image of T, reconstructed by equations 6a and 6b, and using time-resolved weight functions and reflectance measurements. Three time windows were employed, corresponding to photons exiting after traveling a total distance in the ranges 0-4, 4-8, and 8-12 MFP in the medium. Progression to the next larger set of detector readings occurred automatically when the rate of decrease of the rms error of the calculated detector readings fell below a preset threshold. Source and detector configurations for the reflectance measurements are the same as in Figure 4, except that only 12 of the 19 source locations were used in this reconstruction (symmetry of absorber increases number to 42). In the reconstruction whose result is shown in Panels A and B, detector readings from all three time windows were brought into the reconstruction at the same time. Program used only readings for detectors at r = 1 in the first 117 iterations, readings for detectors at r = 1 and r = √2 in the next 171, readings for detectors at r = 1, r = √2, and r = 2 in the next 157, and readings for detectors at r = 1, r = √2, r = 2, and r = √5 in the final 50. For the reconstruction whose result is shown in Panels C and D, program first used only readings for the smallest value of r and first time window, then added the data from the remaining time windows sequentially, before considering readings obtained at the next larger value of r. The number of iterations performed at each stage were: 2 for r = 1, t1; 244 for r = 1, t1, t2; 163 for r = 1, t1, t2, and t3; 500 for r = 1, t1, t2, t3, and r = √2, t1; 110 for r = 1, t1, t2, t3, and r = √2, t1, t2.

absorbing background. For many practical applications, especially for optical measurements of tissue at NIR frequencies, the absorption contrast between different layers of tissue, or the capillary tree and tissue, will be much less. For this reason it was of interest to examine heterogeneous media having low contrast (1-7%). Results shown in Tables 1 and 2 are based on simulations of 3-layer media in which the thickness or absorption, respectively, of the intermediate layer was varied. In all cases a layered structure was assumed, reducing the number of unknowns to 10. A total of 7 time windows was considered, between 0 and 28 MFT in steps of 4 MFT, for a detector located 1 MFP from the source and oriented 10° from vertical. For the first study, the absorption contrast was held constant at 1:5:1% in the top, intermediate and bottom layers respectively; the thickness of the intermediate layer varied from 1-4 MFP, beginning at z = 4. Inspection of the Table reveals that in all cases the algorithm correctly identified the presence of an intermediate layer. The observation that no absorption was detected at depths below z = 7 indicates that the algorithm was able to "see through" the intermediate layer and correctly determine the lack of excess absorption

Table 1: Three Layer Absorber Problem - Variable Boundary (Σ_a/Σ_t = .01: .05: .01)

Layer	Orig	20	1000	7200	Layer	Orig	20	1000	7200
		Iteration Number					Iteration Number		
			Image Density					Image Density	
1	O	0	0	9.33E-5	1	O	0	0	1.44E-4
2	O	0	0	0	2	O	0	0	0
3	O	0.0389	0	0	3	O	0.0365	0	0
4	X	0.319	0.267	0.201	4	X	0.428	0.262	0.186
5	O	0.587	0.944	1.29	5	X	0.825	1.36	1.70
6	O	0.711	1.10	0.688	6	O	1.04	1.88	1.83
7	O	0.755	0.729	0	7	O	1.14	1.62	0
8	O	0.743	0.0124	0	8	O	1.15	0.767	0
9	O	0.722	0	0	9	O	1.13	0	0
10	O	0.694	0	0	10	O	1.10	0	0

Layer	Orig	20	1000	7200	Layer	Orig	20	1000	7200
			Image Density					Image Density	
1	O	0	0	1.83E-4	1	O	0	0	1.93E-4
2	O	0	0	0	2	O	0	0	0
3	O	0.0331	0	0	3	O	0.0321	0	0
4	X	0.457	0.241	0.164	4	X	0.463	0.233	0.161
5	X	0.898	1.48	1.80	5	X	0.916	1.50	1.80
6	X	1.16	2.21	2.34	6	X	1.19	2.30	2.47
7	O	1.28	2.10	0.076	7	X	1.32	2.29	0.373
8	O	1.31	1.34	0	8	O	1.35	1.60	0
9	O	1.30	0.320	0	9	O	1.35	0.618	0
10	O	1.27	0	0	10	O	1.33	0	0

Legend to Table 1: Values of reconstructed image densities of three-layer media. Media were infinitely long and wide, 10 MFP thick, and scattered photons isotropically. They were heterogeneous in only the depth dimension, with the ratio Σ_a/Σ_t in the three layers fixed at .01:.05:.01, the superficial layer boundary fixed at z = 3, and the thickness or the intermediate layer varied between 1 and 4 MFP. Detector readings from seven time windows were employed, ranging from 0-4 MFT to 24-28 MFT in steps of 4 MFT, and all for detectors at r = 1. Due to the layered structure, there were only ten unknowns in the reconstruction problem.

in the deeper layers. The reconstructed images shown are, however, clearly imperfect. The image density is not uniform, and for media having thinner inclusions edge blurring is evident and the depth of maximum density is incorrect by one layer.

Results of reconstructed images of media in which the contrast of the intermediate layer was varied between 1% and 7% are shown in Table 2. In these studies, the thickness of the intermediate layer was held constant at 4 MFP, beginning at layer 4. Inspection of the Table 2 shows that even in the case where the absorption contrast is only 1% above background, the reconstructed image correctly identified the presence of the intermediate layer. In addition, the lack of excess absorption in the

Table 2: Three Layer Absorber Problem - Variable Contrast (Boundary Z = 4 - 7)

$\Sigma_a/\Sigma_t(.01: .02: .01)$ — Iteration Number $\Sigma_a/\Sigma_t(.01: .04: .01)$ — Iteration Number

Layer	Orig	20	1000	5000	Layer	Orig	20	1000	5000
			Image Density					Image Density	
1	O	0	0	1.46E-4	1	O	0	0	1.44E-4
2	O	0	0	1.25E-4	2	O	0	0	0
3	O	0.0772	0	2.14E-6	3	O	0.023	0	0
4	X	0.130	0.053	0.0384	4	X	0.360	0.170	0.120
5	X	0.264	0.423	0.472	5	X	0.719	1.17	1.37
6	X	0.350	0.722	0.794	6	X	0.938	1.86	1.99
7	X	0.398	0.827	0.516	7	X	1.05	1.95	0.709
8	O	0.416	0.766	0	8	O	1.09	1.54	0
9	O	0.422	0.619	0	9	O	1.09	0.925	0
10	O	0.419	0.406	0	10	O	1.08	0.149	0

$\Sigma_a/\Sigma_t(.01: .06: .01)$ — Iteration Number $\Sigma_a/\Sigma_t(.01: .08: .01)$ — Iteration Number

Layer	Orig	20	1000	5000	Layer	Orig	20	1000	5000
			Image Density					Image Density	
1	O	0	0	2.12E-4	1	O	0	0	2.66E-4
2	O	0	0	0	2	O	0	0	0
3	O	0.042	0	0	3	O	0.062	0	0
4	X	0.556	0.302	0.211	4	X	0.724	0.441	0.313
5	X	1.09	1.78	2.17	5	X	1.40	2.30	2.87
6	X	1.40	2.66	2.79	6	X	1.77	3.21	3.14
7	X	1.55	2.55	0.209	7	X	1.94	2.77	0
8	O	1.59	1.65	0	8	O	1.96	1.29	0
9	O	1.58	0.453	0	9	O	1.93	0	0
10	O	1.54	0	0	10	O	1.87	0	0

Legend to Table 2: Values of reconstructed image densities of three-layer media. Media were infinitely long and wide, 10 MFP thick, and scattered photons isotropically. They were heterogeneous in only the depth dimension, the superficial layer boundary fixed at z = 3, the deep boundary fixed at z = 7, and the ratio Σ_a/Σ_t in the three layers variable from .01:.02:.01 to .01:.08:.01. Source and detector configurations, time windows, and number of unknowns all were the same as in Table 1.

deeper region was also correctly identified. At higher contrast, the calculated image density increased as would be expected, but showed signs of instability for media in which the absorption in the intermediate layer exceeded the background by ≥7%. This finding is not surprising, in view of the assumption of linearity for the perturbation equation. In effect, this assumption implies that an absorbing region does not cast a shadow.

It was further desirable to evaluate the perturbation model using experimental data. Time-resolved backscattered measurements were acquired as described in Methods by directing 100-fs pulses of light at 620 nm to a vessel containing diluted whole milk in which a 1-cm-diameter black aluminum sphere was positioned 5 mm below the surface. The transport MFP of the medium, as determined by transmission measurements[18], was 0.82 mm, while the absorption length was 253 mm. A raster-type scan was performed, involving 9 source locations. At each one, the backscattered flux was measured at five points along a straight line, between 2.5 and 12.5 mm from the source at 2.5 mm intervals. Thus, a total of 45 separate measurements were made. After accounting for symmetry, this number increased to 300 which served as the primary data for the reconstruction problem (i.e., although the absorber has infinitely many axes of symmetry, only three were used in the reconstruction). The location of these relative to the position of the target are shown in Figure 6 Panel A. Representative plots of normalized temporal profiles, $(\Delta I/I_0)$ vs. t, from which data were sampled are shown in Figure 6 Panel B. For a given profile, a total of 3 time intervals were selected; one just prior to departure of the ordinate value from zero, one in the middle of the rising phase and one in the plateau region. The time intervals over which these values were sampled are indicated by the dotted lines.

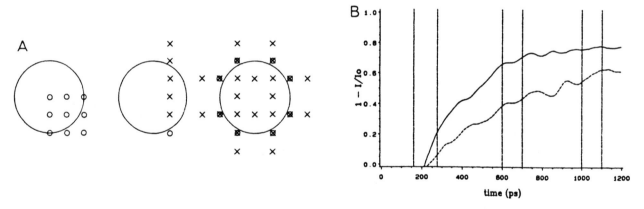

Legend for Figure 6: Panel A: Locations of source and detector fibers relative to spherical absorber in the experimental setup. Left, the nine relative positions of the source fiber (small circle); reconstruction program allowed symmetry of absorber (large circle) to increase the number to twenty five. Middle, the five positions of the detector fiber (cross) relative to the source, for a single source fiber location. Right, reconstruction program allowed symmetry of absorber to increase the number of source and detector fibers from one and five to eight and forty, respectively. Panel B: Reduction of intensity of measured backscattered light, relative to absorberless reference medium, vs. time. Data were smoothed by calculating at 31-point moving average prior to graphing. For both curves shown, the fibers are separated by 12.5 mm; in both cases the source fiber is placed over an edge of the absorber. The top (solid) curve is the result when the source-detector line bisects the absorber; the bottom (dashed) curve is the result when the absorber lines on one side of the source-detector line. The three pairs of dashed vertical lines show the time intervals from which the three data points used in the reconstruction were selected for all measurements made at r = 12.5 mm.

In an effort to reduce computation time and the complexity of the algorithm, simplifications were introduced. The first involved a rescaling of the problem to a more coarse grid. Data corresponding to a given time interval were assigned to time-resolved weight functions calculated for a half-space medium with isotropic scattering and $\Sigma_a = .01\Sigma_t$, with detectors oriented normally to the medium and positioned between 1 and 5 MFP from the source in steps of 1 MFP. The time intervals over which the weight functions were calculated were 0-4, 4-8, 8-12 MFT for each detector location. In this manner, the weight functions for detectors r = 1, r = 2,..., r = 5, for each time interval, were assigned to detectors positioned 2.5, 5, ..., 12.5 mm from a source. Thus a total of 15 different time-resolved weight functions were used in the reconstruction calculation.

The second simplification was the use of a given weight function to cover a range of time points in the temporal profiles. Overall, both approximations introduce an averaging effect which will serve to reduce the recoverable resolution. In addition, the problem was underdetermined, as the amount of input data was only 15% of the number of unknowns. The resultant calculated image, using a scheme progressive in position and time, is shown in Figure 7. Inspection reveals that whereas the image obtained is very crude, evidence for a structure having a curved surface located below the surface of the medium is present.

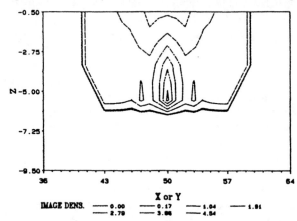

Legend to Figure 7: Contour plot of vertical section through image of spherical absorber, reconstructed by equations 6a and 6b, and using time-resolved weight functions and experimental reflectance measurements. Data from three hundred source detector pairs (see Figure 6A) and three time windows (see Figure 6B) were used in the reconstruction. Weight functions employed were those for a half-space medium with $\Sigma_a = .01\Sigma_t$, with the weight functions for r = 1,2,3,4, and 5 MFP assigned to the detector fibers placed, respectively, 2.5, 5.0, 7.5, 10.0, and 12.5 mm from the source. The time windows 0-4, 4-8, and 8-12 MFT were assigned to the three data points chosen for the reconstruction from each of the temporal profiles.

4.0 Discussion

The current report extends our studies on the backscattering imaging problem in dense scattering media to include use of time-resolved signals. While no attempt was made to preform a systematic survey, evidence obtained does indicate the following. Evaluation of the linear perturbation equation with time-resolved signals permits the recovery of images having higher resolution than is achieved with steady-state signals. At this point it is not clear whether this represents a fundamental property of the measurement schemes or is more of a function of the computational effort employed to evaluate the problems.

While a less rigorous approach was used here to evaluate the perturbation equation than described by Wang et al.[17], the observation that portions of the reconstructed image contained evidence of high resolution is very encouraging. This optimistic interpretation is further supported when it is noted that, in all cases, the images obtained were based on underdetermined problems in which the view angle of measurement was severely restricted (i.e., only backscattered measurements were performed). Results of evaluation of the three-layer problem also support an optimistic perspective. The calculated images showed that, in many cases, both the top and bottom boundaries were well-resolved, even in the case of only 1% absorption contrast between layers.

A heuristic strategy introduced in the evaluation of the perturbation equation is the idea of evaluating the data in a progressive manner. This scheme appears analogous to a layer-stripping approach and makes use of the *a priori* knowledge that whatever the interior gradient of detected photons is, it will always be steepest for detectors located closest to the source, and decline for more distant detectors. When extended to the time domain, a scheme progressive in time can also be considered. The limited evidence obtained suggest that this may also be helpful.

Another heuristic strategy we have recently begun to consider has been to express the value of a weighting function in a given voxel as the fraction of the total weight for a particular source-detector pair instead of its absolute value. The idea here is that whereas the absolute value of the weight in a given voxel will always decrease with increasing distance separating source and detector, the fraction of the total weight for the voxel when compared to other source-detector configurations need not vary monotonically. The reason for this is that the weight gradient varies with the source-detector configuration and as a function of time. Thus the fractional value of the weight for a source-detector pair in a voxel may be several times greater than for the same voxel but different source-detector pair, even though its absolute value is less. The significance of this is that it potentially allows for a differential weighting of the weight functions in a manner which serves to improve discrimination of the contribution of the signals from greater depths from those originating predominately from more shallow depths.

As is the case for the results presented by Wang et al[17], data shown here constitute only one step of the perturbation equation. An iterative solution would require that output from the inverse solution be used as input for the forward problem.

Evaluation of the latter will require the use of numerical methods such as Monte Carlo methods or a relaxation solver described by Schlereth et al.[1,2], among others. While hard evidence is lacking, we believe that an iterative solution of the perturbation equation in a progressive manner might well prove a more effective approach to image recovery, particularly for the case in which signals about the target are evaluated. The idea here is that before any reasonable assessment of the optical properties of the interior of a diffusing media is possible, good assessment of the more superficial layers must first be made. This assertion is based partly on a practical consideration of the size of the computation required for a problem in which all detector readings are evaluated simultaneously. A schematic of this approach is depicted in Figure 8. Image recovery would proceed by considering first the family of detectors that lie closest to a source, for all source positions. Iterative solution of the forward and inverse problems would result in a scoring of voxels which lie near the surface. Consideration of more distant detectors (and/or at later times) would lead to determination of deeper layers.

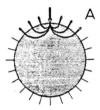
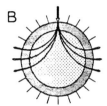
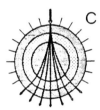
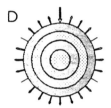

Legend to Figure 8: Proposed "layer-stripping" approach for improved resolution of interior regions of a highly scattering medium. Method considers a progressive iterative analysis of the inverse and forward problem. Data yielding the most reliable information about near surface structures are first considered (A). This information is used to update the forward problem which is then used to evaluate detector values which preferentially probe to successively greater depths (B). Transmission measurements serve to best define properties of the most interior regions (C), yielding the final image (D).

The approach described here is one of several our group is evaluating for the image recovery problem. A satisfactory solution will require the consideration of several factors: use of *a priori* data to constrain permissible values[15,19], appropriate modeling of the forward problem to account for refraction and reflection of photons across internal boundaries[20], iterative updates of the forward problem[1,2], efficient error-minimization protocols[17], and consideration of a suitable computing platform[1,2], among others. Although our emphasis has been on examining backscattered signals, this has been based largely on consideration of practical constraints likely encountered in any acute care setting. It seems likely that measurements about an object will prove best. Recent reports by Arridge et al.[16], Singer et al.[21] and Grünbaum et al.[22] support this view. While much more development is required to optimize the imaging algorithms, results reported here indicate that fairly high resolution images can be obtained for simple structures, using only backscattered signals, to a depth of at least 7 transport MFP.

5.0 References

1. F. H. Schlereth, J. M. Fossaceca, A. D. Keckler and R. L. Barbour, "Multicomputer based neural networks for imaging in random media", in *IEEE Proc. Nuclear Science Symposium*, Nov. 1991, In Press.

2. F. H. Schlereth, J. M. Fossaceca, A. D. Keckler and R. L. Barbour, "Imaging in diffusing media with a neural net formulation: A problem in large scale computation". SPIE, vol 1641, accompanying paper in these proceedings, 1992.

3. R. Aronson, R. L. Barbour, J. Lubowsky and H. Graber, "Application of Transport Theory to NIR Medical Imaging," in *Modern Mathematical Models in Transport Theory; Advances and Applications*, Vol. 51, pp 64-75, Birkhauser Press, 1991.

4. R. L. Barbour, H. L. Graber, R. Aronson and J. Lubowsky, "Imaging of subsurface regions in random media by remote sensing", in *Proc. Time-Resolved Spectroscopy and Imaging of Tissues*, SPIE Vol. 1431, pp 192-203, 1991.

5. R. L. Barbour, H. Graber, R. Aronson and J. Lubowsky, "Model for 3-D Optical Imaging of Tissue", in 10th *Annual International Geoscience and Remote Sensing Symposium* (IGARSS), Vol. II, pp. 1395-1399, 1990.

6. R. L. Barbour, H. Graber, J. Lubowsky and R. Aronson, "Monte Carlo Modeling of Photon Transport in Tissue. V. Model for 3-D Optical Imaging of Tissue", Biophys. J., 57, p. 382a, abst. no. 603, 1990.

7. J. G. Webster, ed., *Electrical Impedance Tomography*. Adam Hilger, Bristol, England,1990.

8. B. Chance, et al. "Comparison of time-resolved and unresolved measurements of deoxyhemoglobin in brain", in Proc. Nat. Acad. Sci. vol. 85, 4971-4975, 1988.

9. K. M. Yoo, Q. Xing, and R. R. Alfano, "Imaging object hidden in highly scattering media using femtosecond second harmonic generation cross-correlation time-gating", Opt. Lett., 16, 1019, 1991.

10. R. R. Alfano, P. P. Ho, and K. M. Yoo, "Photons for prompt tumor detection", Physics World, 5, 37, 1991.

11. L. M. Wang, P. P. Ho, C. Liu, G. Zhang and R. R. Alfano, "Ballistic 2-D imaging through scattering walls using an ultrafast optical Kerr gate", Science, 253, 769, 1991.

12. G. Hebden and R. A. Kruger, "A time-of-flight breast imaging system: spatial resolution performance," in *Proc. Time Resolved Spectroscopy and Imaging of Tissues*", SPIE Vol. 1431, pp 225-231, 1991.

13. J. Fishkin, E. Gratton, M. J. vandeVen and W. W. Mantulin, "Diffusion of Intensity Modulated Near-Infrared Light in Turbid Media", ibid, pp 122-135, 1991.

14. E. M. Sevick, B. Chance, J. Leigh, S. Nioka and M. Maris, "Quantitation of Time- and Frequency-Resolved Optical Spectra for the Determination of Tissue Oxygenation", Anal. Biochem., 195, 330-351, 1991.

15. H. L. Graber, R. L. Barbour, J. Lubowsky, R. Aronson, B. B. Das, K. M. Yoo and R. R. Alfano, "Evaluation of Steady-State, Time- and Frequency-Domain Data for the Problem of Optical Diffusion Tomography", SPIE Vol. 1641, accompanying paper in these proceedings, 1992.

16. S. R. Arridge, P. van der Zee, M. Cope, and D. T. Delpy, "Reconstruction methods for infra-red absorption imaging", in *Proc.Time Resolved Spectroscopy and Imaging of Tissues*", SPIE Vol. 1431, pp 204-215, 1991.

17. Y. Wang, J. H. Chang, R. Aronson, R. L. Barbour, H. L. Graber and J. Lubowsky, "Imaging of Scattering Media by Diffusion Tomography: An Iterative Perturbation Approach", SPIE Vol. 1641, accompanying paper in these proceedings, 1992.

18. K. M. Yoo, F. Liu, R. R. Alfano, "When Does the Diffusion Approximation Fail to Describe Photon Transport in Random Media?", Phys. Rev. Lett., 64, pp 2647-2650, 1990. Erratum: op. cit., 65, p 2210, 1990.

19. R. L. Barbour, H. L. Graber, R. Aronson and J. Lubowsky, "Determination of Macroscopic Optical Properties of Multilayer Random Media by Remote Sensing", in *Proc. Time Resolved Spectroscopy and Imaging of Tissues*", SPIE Vol. 1431, pp 52-62, 1991.

20. R. Aronson, "Exact Interface Conditions for Photon Diffusion", SPIE Vol. 1641, accompanying paper in these proceedings, 1992.

21. J. R. Singer, F. A. Grünbaum, P. Kohn and J. P. Zubelli, "Image reconstruction of the interior of bodies that diffuse radiation", Science, vol. 248, pp. 990-993. 1990.

22. F. A. Grünbaum, P. Kohn, G. A. Latham, J. R. Singer and J. P. Zubelli, "Diffuse tomography", in *Proc. Time-Resolved Spectroscopy and Imaging of Tissues*, SPIE Vol. 1431, pp 232-238, 1991.

Reprinted with permission from *Journal of Laser Applications,* Vol. 5(2,3), pp. 43-60
(Fall 1993). ©1993 Laser Institute of America, Toledo, Ohio.

Laser Light Scattering in Biomedical Diagnostics and Therapy

Valery V. Tuchin
Chernyshevsky Saratov State University
Astrakhanskaya 83, 410071 Saratov, Russia

Key Words: *Laser Light Biotissue Interaction, Diagnostics and Therapy, Laser Applications*

ABSTRACT

The description of special features of laser light interaction with biotissues, such as the skin, eye and dental tissues etc., with respect to laser diagnostics and therapy methods development is done. Optical models of transparent and turbid biotissues are analyzed. The role of static and dynamic light scattering in the light dosimetry, tissue heating, and receiving information of biotissue optical parameters, its structure, movements, and vibrations is considered.

INTRODUCTION

LASER APPLICATION in biology and medicine is based on the usage of a great number of phenomena connected with different types of coherent and noncoherent light interaction with biotissues and cells [1-11]. Laser radiation can be absorbed, reflected, scattered and remitted by biological medium and each of the mentioned processes carries information about micro- and macrostructure of this medium, the movement and shape of its components. Laser radiation has a nonspecific thermal effect, i.e. it acts like electromagnetic radiation of any range of wavelengths. Thermal effects, unlike nonlaser light sources, can be realized in very small volumes (within a cell and even its partials), and during very short periods of time. Other mechanisms of low-intensity laser radiation interaction with biotissues, the basis of which are the photodynamic and phototoxic effects in sensitized tissues as well as effects of stimulation and inhibition of a number of metabolic processes within the cells of nonsensitized tissues, are also possible.

Considered in the paper are effects of laser radiation interaction with biotissues that mainly belong to static and dynamic light scattering. These effects are the basis of some methods of laser diagnostics and therapy, including the problems of light dosimetry, tissue heating, and receiving information of biotissue optical parameters, its structure and vibrations.

BIOTISSUE STRUCTURE AND MODELS OF LIGHT PROPAGATION

Optics of Tissue with Basic Multiple Scattering

Biological tissues are optically inhomogeneous absorbing media and have a higher refractive index than air. Therefore, by the incidence of a laser beam at the boundary bio-object-air some part of it is reflected and penetrates the rest into the depth of the object. The laser beam broadens and decays due to multiple scattering and absorption. Volume scattering is the cause of the propagation of rather considerable part of radiation

> **❝**
>
> *Prof. Tuchin's very useful overview concerns mostly eye and skin but the basic principles can apply to other areas of laser diagnostics . . .*
>
> **❞**

in reverse direction (back scattering). The energy of the absorbed light transforms into heat, that increases the temperature of the biological object. Absorption spectra are defined by the type of dominating absorbing centers and the water contained in biotissues. Absolute values of the absorption coefficients are in the range from 10^{-2} to $10^4 cm^{-1}$. In UV and IR ($\lambda \geq 2$ μm) spectral bands prevails absorption and therefore the scattering contribution is small and the light penetrates not deeply, only within several cell layers. Optical thickness (penetration depth) of the typical biotissue is from 0.5 to 2.5 mm for the visible region. Both scattering and absorption take place and about 15-40% of the incident beam are reflected at these wavelengths. Scattering prevails over absorption and the penetration depth raises to 8-10 mm in the region 0.6-1.5 μm. The back scattering increases considerably and the intensity of the light, reflected from the biotissue, reaches 35-70% of the incident beam.

The light interaction with the skin is rather complicated owing to the multilayer structure [9-12]. The stratum corneum reflects about 5-7% of the incident radiation. The collimated beam of the incident light transforms into diffused one by reflection due to the microscopic inhomogeneity of the boundary air-stratum corneum. The greater part of the light reflected from the skin is formed owing to the back scattering by different layers of the skin (stratum corneum, epidermis, and dermis). The absorption of the scattered light by the skin pigments provides quantitative information about concentration of bilirubin, oxygen saturation, and contents of drugs in tissue or blood, which is the basis of a number of diagnostic methods for different diseases. Considerable penetration of the light in the range of the wavelengths of the so-called therapeutic window into the depth of the man's organism is the basis of phototherapy [13].

" ——————————————

. . . important applications here for cataract diagnostics and for psoriasis and for photodynamic therapy . . .

—————————————— "

Analyzing scattering and absorption of light by tissues, uniform distribution of absorbing and scattering centers is assumed (excluding some special cases, e.g., optical media of eye). If attenuation of laser beams (UVB, UVC, and IR, $\lambda \geq 2$ μm) occurs mainly due to specular reflection and absorption, then in accordance with Beer's law, intensity of transmission through biological object light is described by the expression:

$$I(z)=(1-R)I_0 \exp(-\mu_t z), \qquad (1)$$

where R is the coefficient of specular reflection (when incident beam is directed normally to medium surface, $R=((n-1)/(n+1))^2$; n is the relative refractive index of tissue and environment; I_0 is the intensity of incident light; $\mu_t=\mu_a+\mu_s$, μ_a is the absorption coefficient, μ_s is the scattering coefficient; z is the depth. Mean free path length of photons in tissue is defined as $l_{ph}=1/\mu_t$, $\mu_a \gg \mu_s$.

For UVA, visible, and near IR the case of anisotropic scattering, which is characterized by strong directness of scattering, is more typical. Description of anisotropic scattering meets great difficulties, because there are no simple relations between measured reflection and transmission coefficients, and the parameters, which characterize absorption and scattering in theory. Mathematical description of process of light propagation in tissues and in turbid media can be done with the help of the Maxwell's equations or using the theory of radiative energy transfer. Solution of Maxwell's equations should be performed, taking into consideration the statistical nature of unhomogeneous medium, and would include all kinds of diffractive effects. This way is mostly common, and it is applied in many studies of tissues [1-4,14].

Radiative transfer theory is much simpler from a mathematical point of view. It is correct for ensemble of sufficiently distant scatterers, and it is successfully applied for solution of various

practical problems related to the optics of tissues [14-23]. The main equation of radiative transfer theory looks like [4,14]:

$$\frac{\partial I(r,s)}{\partial s} = -\mu_t I(r,s) + \frac{\mu_s}{4\pi} \int_{4\pi} I(r,s')p(s,s')d\Omega', \qquad (2)$$

where p(s,s') is the scattering phase function, $d\Omega'$ is the unit solid angle around direction s', I(r,s) is the radiance in point r at direction s [W cm^{-2}sr^{-1}].

Phase function p(s,s') describes scattering properties of medium and represents probability density function of photon scattering from direction s to direction s'. If scattering is symmetrical relative to direction of incident wave, then phase function depends only on angle θ between directions s and s', i.e.

$$p(s,s')=p(\theta), \qquad \int_0^\pi p(\theta)2\pi\sin\theta d\theta=1,$$

that corresponds to assumption of random distribution of scatterers in tissue volume and expresses the fact that structure of tissue is not spatially correlated.

In many practical cases phase function is well approximated by the Henyey-Greenstein function (corresponding to forward directed Mie scattering):

$$p(\theta)= \frac{(1-g^2)}{(1+g^2-2g\cos\theta)^{3/2}}, \qquad (3)$$

$$g \equiv \langle\cos\theta\rangle = \int_0^\pi p(\theta)\cos\theta \, 2\pi\sin\theta d\theta, \qquad (4)$$

θ is the scattering angle, g is the mean scattering cosine (parameter of anisotropy). Value of g varies from -1 to 1: g = 0 corresponds to the case of isotropic scattering; g=1 corresponds to total forward scattering, when p(θ) is proportional to δ-function in direction of incident beam; g=-1 relates to total backward scattering.

When multiple scattering plays the major role, the method of discrete ordinates or multi-flux theory can be applied. Two-flux Kubelka-Munk model, 3-, 4-, and 7-flux models are the special cases of the multi-flux theory [3,4,10,15,16]. Applying to the laser-tissue interactions, 3-flux model includes two diffuse fluxes (forward and backward) and collimated forward flux, and 7-flux model consists of six diffuse fluxes in 3D space and collimated forward flux. Random walk model using the quantity of the probability density for photons path length distribution is also applied for description of anisotropic light scattering in biotissues [24].

Multiple scattering in the conditions of arbitrary geometry of the sample and of complicated angular distribution of incident beam can be taken into account, using the Monte Carlo method, based on numerical simulation of photon transport in scattering medium [4,5,10,17-21]. Random walk of photon inside the sample of tissue is traced from its entrance point until its absorption or exit medium. Fluence rate distribution inside the medium is calculated using the function of absorbed photons distribution obtained in numerical simulation. The Monte Carlo method is applied for solution of wide range of problems. In particular, it is useful for modeling of propagation of the narrow beams with Gaussian and flat distributions of incident light and of diverging beams, formed after fiber tips.

For strongly scattering media, its diffuse component is almost isotropic, and it can be presented as the sum of spherical harmonics series. The first two terms are the base for diffusion theory [4,14]. Diffuse flux rate Ψ_d is determined by the diffusion equation, containing diffusion parameter $\mu_d^2 = 3 \mu_a \delta$, where $\delta = \mu_s (1-g) + \mu_a$ is the transport coefficient, $1_d = 1/\mu_d$ is the diffusion length. Transport coefficient is considerably less than coefficient μ_t, therefore, mean transport length $1_\delta = 1/\delta$ is significantly larger than mean free path length $1_{ph} = 1/\mu_t$. The studies showed that if value of g is near to 1 (g $\approx$ 0.9), diffusion approximation gives reasonable results for the optical density $\tau = \int \mu_t dl = 1-20$. Typical values of g for tissues are in the range 0.6-0.9.

Attenuation of wide laser beam with incident intensity I_o in conditions of multiple scattering may be described by the expression, close to (1):

$$I(z) = I_0 q \exp(-\mu_d z), \qquad (5)$$

where q is a parameter assuming not only reflection of light at the interface air-tissue, but additional irradiation of upper layers of tissue due to backscattering, too. This approximate expression is only accurate away from the tissue surface, at depths $z \rangle 1_d$. Typical values of q parameter for tissues are 1-5, and mainly dependent on beam diameter (1-20 mm) [22]. The depth of light penetration into the tissue is given by the expression

$$1_e = 1_d [1nq + 1]. \qquad (6)$$

The fluence rate distribution inside tissue is a complex function of μ_a, μ_s, anisotropy parameter g, and of the size of laser beam. This fact brings the essential difficulties to the quantitative dosimetry of radiation for laser therapy [22,23]. The investigation of light propagation within tissues with complex structure (e.g., multi-layered tissue) may be done for simplification using 1D theory, when the size of laser beam is much more than the radiation penetration depth [12]. The typical examples of multi-layered tissues are the skin and the urinary bladder wall. While irradiating these tissues by visible and near IR laser light, sufficiently powerful collimated component exists even at large depths, because each layer is thin enough to transmit laser beam. Light transmission in this case can be described in the framework of three-flux model, with the help of which the fluence rate distribution inside each layer, depending on the thickness of the layer d, absorption coefficient μ_{ai}, scattering coefficient μ_{si}, scattering phase function $p_i(\theta)$, and refractive index n_j, is calculated [12]. For four-layer model of the skin (epidermis, upper dermis, blood plexus, lower dermis) [10,12] the calculations showed that fluence rate in epidermis at $\lambda = 577$ nm is approximately 2 times higher than incident fluence rate, in upper dermis it decreases from the value $1.75I_0$ to $0.3I_0$, and in the region of blood plexus fast falls to zero.

Using the conception of multiple scattering in densely-packed random media, which is valid for most biotissues, we can pre-

dict radiant energy transport in turbid tissues with the help of the Monte Carlo simulating techniques [10,17-19,25]. The Monte Carlo simulations are based on macroscopic optical properties that are assumed to extend uniformly over small units of tissue volume. The simulations do not treat the details of radiant energy distribution within individual cells. Our Monte Carlo program is based on using the Green's function of medium's response to unit external action. The algorithm allows to account the presence of several layers with different optical properties, finite size of incident beam, reflection of light at the interface between layers [17,21,26,27].

Using stationary radiative transfer theory (2), suitable boundary conditions for each of the layers and surfaces, the calculations have been performed for 2-, 5- or 7-layered media, consisting of epidermis and dermis (for UVA light); epidermis, dermis, subcutaneous fat, vein wall and blood (for red laser light biostimulation of vein blood); and epidermis, upper dermis, blood plexus, lower dermis, subcutaneous fat, vein wall and blood (for calculating of tissue hyperthermia accompanying blood biostimulation). The thickness and optical parameters of the skin and underlying tissues are presented in Tables 1 and 2 [9,10,18,21,27,28,29]. As scattering phase function $p_i(\theta)$ for all layers Henyey-Greenstein functions (3) with anisotropy factor g_i for i-th layer were accepted. It was considered collimated and directed normally to the skin surface incident laser beam with Gaussian and flat (on the tip of fiber) initial profiles. In Figure 1 one can see the calculated fluence rate distribution U(r,z) inside the skin for Gaussian and flat red and UVA laser beam.

Table 1. Optical parameters of tissues at $\lambda = 633$ nm

N	Layer	μ_{ai}, cm^{-1}	μ_{si}, cm^{-1}	g_i	n	Thickness, mm
1	Epidermis	25	480	0.79	1.50	0.065
2	Upper dermis	2.7	187	0.82	1.40	0.565
3	Blood plexus	25	400	0.98	1.35	0.09
4	Lower dermis	2.7	187	0.82	1.40	0.565
5	Subcutaneous fat	0.2	20	0.80	1.45	0.32
6	Vessel wall	6	414	0.91	1.37	0.61
7	Blood	25	400	0.98	1.35	6.38

Table 2. Optical parameters of normal (psoriatic) skin at $\lambda = 337$ nm

N	Layer	μ_{ai}, cm^{-1}	μ_{si}, cm^{-1}	g_i	n	Thickness, mm
1	Epidermis	32 (20)	165 (311)	0.72	1.55	0.065
2	Upper dermis	23	145	0.12	1.55	1.25

Structure variety of biotissues defines the different character of light penetration through them. As the laser radiation is rather effectively used in stomatology the structure features of the dental tissues are discussed elsewhere [30,31] from the point of view of the light penetration through it. The dental tissues – enamel and dentine – are bundles of natural diffusing lightguides matched to each other [30]. Experimental and

FIGURE 1. *Total fluence rate distribution in the skin (Monte-Carlo simulation) z is the skin depth, r is the distance from beam axis:*

a) – power 1 mW, λ = 633nm, Gaussian beam with radius 1 mm | *b) – power 1 W, λ = 337 nm, flat beam with radius 1 mm, 1 – normal skin, 2 – psoriatic skin*

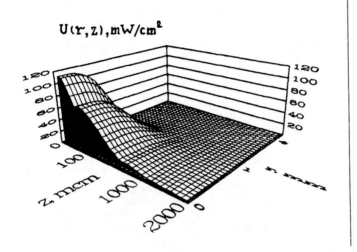

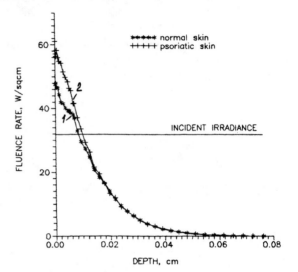

Table 3. Optical characteristics of human biotissues

Biotissue	λ, nm	μ_a, cm⁻¹	μ_{s1}, cm⁻¹	μ_a', cm⁻¹	g	l_{ph}, μm	$l_{\delta'}$, μm	$l_{d'}$, μm	References and remarks.
Stratum corneum	351	300	2200	220	0.9	4	19	15	
	400	230	2000	200	0.9	5	23	18	Data from [10] Values for dermis are changed in accordance to experimental data for λ=633 nm.
Epidermis	351	100	1100	306	0.722	8	25	29	
	488	50	600	143	0.761	15	52	59	
	633	35	450	88	0.804	21	81	88	$g_E = g_0 = 0.62+0.29\ 10^{-3}\lambda$ (nm),
	800	40	420	62	0.852	22	98	90	$l_{ph}=1/(\mu_a+\mu_s)$, $l_\delta=1/(\mu_a'+\mu_s')$, $l_d=1/(3\mu_a(\mu_a+\mu_s'))]^{1/2}$, $\mu_s'=\mu_s(1-g)$.
Dermis	351	5.2	458	127	0.722	22	76	220	
	488	2.6	250	60	0.761	40	160	452	
	633	2.0	187	37	0.804	53	256	654	
	800	1.7	175	30	0.852	57	315	786	
Dermis leg	635	1.8	244	78	0.68	41	125	482	
Bareast (skin et al)	635	0.2	395	-	-	25	-	-	Data from [4], p.2324, the sliced samples, thickness from 20 to 100 μm.
Lung (parenchymatous tissue)	515	25.5	356	-	-	26	-	-	
	635	8.1	324	81	0.75	30	112	215	
Muscle (striated)	515	11.2	530	-	-	18	-	-	
Uterus (inner wall)	635	0.35	394	122	0.69	25	82	882	Vein *Saphena Magna* [26].
Skin and vein wall (from the leg)	633	3.1	70.7	11	0.8	135	690	861	
Normal aorta: media	351	22	690	55	0.92	14	130	140	
	488	6	460	46	0.90	21	192	327	
	633	2.3	340	34	0.90	29	275	632	
	800	1.6	250	30	0.88	40	316	812	Data for μ_a, μ_s and g from [32].
intima	351	33	450	72	0.84	21	95	98	
	488	13	270	43	0.84	35	179	214	
	633	3.5	200	32	0.84	49	282	518	
	800	2.0	150	24	0.84	66	385	801	
adventitia	351	50	440	110	0.75	20	62	64	
	488	17	300	66	0.78	31	120	154	
	633	6	240	49	0.81	41	182	318	
	800	4	180	29	0.84	54	303	502	
Dental dentine	633	6.0	1200	72	0.44	8	15	91	Data for μ_a, μ_s and g from [31].
Dental enamel	633	0.97	1.1	-	-	-	-	-	
Brain tissues: white matter	488	1.0	-	60	-	-	164	740	
	630	0.2	-	32	-	-	311	2275	
	800	0.2	-	40	-	-	249	2036	
grey matter	514	19.5	-	85	-	-	96	128	Samples thickness 1.3-5.8 mm measurements using spectrophotometer with integrating sphere, data for μ_a and μ_s from graphs of [33].
	585	14.5	-	63	-	-	129	172	
	630	4.3	-	52	-	-	178	371	
	800	1.0	-	45	-	-	217	851	
miligant glioma	488	12.5	-	3	-	-	645	415	
	630	3.0	-	3	-	-	1667	1361	
melanotic melanoma	585	2	-	158	-	-	54	82	
	630	20.0	-	75	-	-	105	132	
	800	8.0	-	40	-	-	208	295	

calculated data of optical characteristics for some human biotissues with principle multiple scattering are represented in Table 3.

Optical Models of Eye Tissues: Transmission Spectra

Optical models of biotissues are defined by the dimensions and form of the scatterers, by their spatial distribution, the values of refraction and absorption indices of scatterers and the ground substance, the degree of material anisotropy. For eye tissues the distances between scatterers and their dimensions are comparable with the wavelength, the absorption for visible region is weak, the relative refraction index of scatterers material is small ("soft" particles). The typical eye biotissues models are long dielectric circular cylinders (cornea, sclera) or balls (lens) distributed in the isotropic ground material chaotically (sclera, turbid lens) or according to a certain law (transparent cornea and lens) [1,34-44].

Analysis of scattering for the eye tissues can be carried out on the basis of the model of a single scattering due to the small scattering cross-section [1,36-44]. When the scatterers location is nonordered, the resulting field intensity is the sum of the scattering field intensities of the individual particles. In other cases we need the summing of scattering field amplitudes of the individual particles corresponding interference effects which take place at presence of the near-order scatterers [1,36-44]. Integrally the indicatrix for the symmetric scattering of the particles with a pair correlation is described by the equation

$$I(\theta)=I_0(\theta)\left\{1+\rho\int_0^\infty [g(R)-1]\exp[i(\bar{s}_1-\bar{s}_0)\bar{R}]d^3R\right\}=I_0(\theta)F, \quad (7)$$

where $I_0(\theta)$ is the indicatrix of an isolated particle, θ is the scattering angle, $g(R)$ is the radial distribution function of the scatterers centers, $\bar{s}_0$ and $\bar{s}_1$ are unit vectors showing the direction of incident and scattered waves respectively, $\bar{R}$ is the scatterer radius-vector, d_3R is its volume and the integral F allows for the interference effects. $g(R)$ is the ratio of local density to mean density of scattering centers [36]. The character of scattering by a separately taken particle is to be known to use this equation allowing for the interference effects of scattered light by ensemble of particles. The calculation for the eye tissues are to be carried out with Mie theory because the wavelength is of the same order as the dimensions of nonuniformities. Such calculations for the eye tissues can be found in [1,37-39,42-44].

In the case of cataractous lens and other turbid biotissues the scatter system becomes a polydispersive system, which is characterized by the distribution function of the scatterers radii $f(r)$. For cataractous lens it is possible to use the model of binary mixture of hard spheres with small r_1 and large r_2 radii. The expression for scattered light intensity can be found using four structural functions $g_{11}(R)$, $g_{22}(R)$, $g_{12}(R)$ and $g_{21}(R)$, which are the own and mutual radial distribution functions for the particles of the first and the second fractions [45]. For disordered structures such as sclera ($g(R)=1$) the gamma radii distribution function being applicable [40].

$$f(r)=r^{\mu}exp(-\mu\beta), \tag{8}$$

where $\Delta r/r_0 = 2.35/\sqrt{\mu}$, $\beta = r/r_0$, Δr is a halfwidth of distribution and r_0 is the more probable scatterer radius.

The intensity of the light, penetrated through the layer of the scattering tissue of the thickness d, is defined by the equation:

$$I=I_0exp(-\rho\sigma_s d), \tag{9}$$

where ρ is the mean density of the scattering centers, σ_s is the scattering cross section

$$\sigma_s = \frac{1}{\rho}\int_{4\pi}(I(\theta)/I_0)d\Omega. \tag{10}$$

For eye tissues $\rho\sigma_s d \langle\langle 1$. Calculated and experimental transmission spectra of cornea, crystalline lens and sclera show high transmittance of the cornea and crystalline lens and the absence of this for the normal sclera as well as the transmission loss for a turbid crystalline lens for visible wavelength range [1,2,44]. The following data were used for calculations of transmission spectra of the eye tissues. The cornea fibrils diameter is ≈ 26 nm, the refractive index of their matter $n\approx1.470$, the ground substance has the reflective index $n \approx 1.345$, the cornea thickness in the center is 0.46 mm, the mean density of fibril centers is $3\cdot10^{10}cm^{-2}$, $g(R)$ function was taken from [36]. The sclera consists of analogous collagen fibrils but their interorientation is random ($g(R) = 1$) and the diameter changes in the wide range ($\mu = 0.33$, $\beta = 1000$). The sclera thickness is ≈ 1 mm; the mean density of fibril centers is $6\cdot10^{10}cm^{-2}$. The transparent crystalline lens is an optically homogeneous ground substance with $n \approx 1.345$ in which spherical inhomogeneities with $n \approx 1.380$ are definitely distributed; $g(R)$ function was determined from experimental indicatrix, using Eq. (7) [1,40]. The thickness of the crystalline lens is 5 mm, the scatterers density is of order of $10^{11}cm^{-3}$. In the tissue of the turbid crystalline lens there appear new inhomogeneities (conglomerates of high-molecular proteins) with the refractive index $n \approx 1.50$, the sphere diameters of which are within the range 2-6 μm and the scatterers density reaches $10^{12}cm^{-3}$.

The calculated and experimental sclera transmission spectra show that it considerably scatters the light all over the range from 300 to 800 nm. The sclera was effectively brightened up being effected by 76% *Verographyn* solution with the refraction index of 1.46 and being transparent in the visible range. The cornea transparence is explained by the high degree of its fibrils arrangement, so the light intensity decreases due to interference along all directions except the incident light direction. The effect of scattering is the most essential in a short wavelength region and defines small UV radiation transmittance of the cornea, approximately 50% for $\lambda = 320$ nm. Disordering of the fibrils distribution (for example after Keratomy) results in decreasing of cornea transmission, especially in the short wavelength region (Purkinier's effect) [42]. Another essential feature of the cornea is the presence of a preferable direction of the fibrils alignment. The results of such anisotropy are birefringence and dichroism of the cornea [39,44]. The transmission spectrum substantially depends on the orientation of polarization vector of the linear polarized light relative to the collagen fibrils; the light polarized along fibrils is scattered more effectively. The cornea polarization sensitivity in UV spectrum region ($\lambda = 320$ nm) is about 5 higher than in the red one ($\lambda = 630$ nm). The comparison of the experimental and calculated spectra shows that high transparency of normal crystalline lens is explained by its high degree of ordering and by the absence of the strong absorption bands lying in the visible region. The lens transparency decreases with the structure disturbances growth [1].

Taking into account the multiple scattering gives a slight razing of sclera and cornea transparency [45,46]. For cornea irradiated by normally incident polarized light of visible range ($\lambda = 700$ nm) the discrepancy is equal to 1%, and for UV light ($\lambda = 300$ nm) it reaches 8%. The transmittance of light polarized along fibrils growths and of orthogonal polarized light goes down, so the multiple scattering leads to decreasing of cornea anisotropy.

Presented in [1,2,44] calculations of the eye tissues spectra do not include some specific features of absorbing species, such as kynurenine, age-related chromophors leading to generalized yellowing of the lens proteins [47], and water absorbing bands in IR range. The main idea of discussing calculations was to show the important role of scattering in forming of the eye tissue spectra. Of course, absorbing species, besides those mentioned above, these may be hemoglobin, bilirubin, melanin, porphyrin etc.; must be included in calculations, but it is not simple to consider absorbing accurately, because of unknown distribution of absorbing centers.

Biotissues Optical Characteristics Control

The character of reflection, absorption and scattering by biotissue can be effectively changed with the help of different artificial methods. For example, reflection and absorption spectra can be changed by dyeing. Such biological objects are called dyed or sensitized ones. Sensitization of biological material is widely used for examination of the mechanism of light interaction with separate components of this material as well as in practical biomedicine for diagnostics and selective photodestruction of separate components of a biological object. Diagnostics and therapy of a cancerous tumor as well as PUVA therapy of psoriasis and other skin diseases are based on this.

One can increase considerably, up to 40 times, the transmission of soft blood-filled biological tissues by light-weight pressure. Puncture and stretching of the tissue provide analogous effects. Brightening of live tissue is bound up with the increase of its optical homogeneity due to the density growth of scattering centers (collagen fibrils of muscular tissue) and forcing blood out of the pressed region, that assists to increasing the ground substance refraction index, which becomes comparable with the refractive index of the muscular tissue. The other method of considerable light scattering decreasing is the matching of the refractive indices of light scattering centers and of the ground substance owing to the injection of suitable drugs into the tissue. Methods and techniques of biotissues optical characteristics control are presented in Table 4.

Table 4. Biotissues optical characteristics control [1,2,9,44,45,48,49,50,51,89]

Method	Technique	Tissue	The main result
Addition of absorbers (dyeing, sensitization, irradiation et. al)	Adding of dyes, drugs and "sunscreen" creams	All types	Increasing of selectivity and sensitivity for photochemical and photo-destructive reactions, decreasing of transmittance, changing of reflection
	UV-irradiation (erythema melanogenesis, radiation dyeing)	Skin, eye lens	
Addition of scatterers	Adding "sunscreen" creams	Skin	Decreasing of transmittance
	Reducing of temperature (9-12°C)	Eye lens	Decreasing of transmittance (cold revezible cataract)
Extraction of absorbers and scatters	Adding of water and aqueous lactic acid (during 0.5 - 4 hrs)	Skin	Increasing of transmittance, changing of reflection
	Compression and stretching	Blooded soft tissues	
Immersion	**Adding of oils, creams, water, drugs (matching of refractive index)**	Skin, sclera	
		Cornea	Changing of polarization anisotropy
Decreasing of thickness	Compression, stretching, and puncture	Soft tissues skin, sclera	Increasing of transmittance
Increasing of thickness	UV-irradiation (hyperplaisia)	Skin	Decreasing of transmittance

DETERMINATION OF THE SKIN OPTICAL, STRUCTURAL, AND DYNAMIC PARAMETERS

Spectrophotometry and Angular Measurements

The investigations of the optical parameters of the skin are of great use in perfection of photo- and photochemical methods for treatment of skin diseases, and of diffuse optical tomography [2,9,10,21-29,51-56]. In order to receive reliable results it is essential to take into account the radiation scattered in the skin, particularly in the epidermis. Besides, the ways of preparation of the skin (epidermal) samples exert considerable influence on the results of measurements. For making samples we use the very promising technique of skin surface glue strippings, some kind of tissue biopsy [29]. The skin surface stripping contains only upper layers with the total thickness varied from 30 to 50 μm. The transmission and reflection spectra of the samples in the range from 240 to 400 nm can be obtained using the commercially available spectrophotometers with integrating sphere [29,56,57]. The samples, obtained from the internal surface of the forearm of healthy tanless volunteers and from the skin areas occupied by psoriatic eruption of the same localization in progressive dermatosis stage, were investigated [29]. Total coefficients of transmission and diffuse reflection of the epidermal stripping (ES) are defined by the epidermal linear absorption (μ_a) and scattering (μ_s) coefficients. To obtain the ES spectra $\mu_a(\lambda)$ and $\mu_s(\lambda)$ the Kubelka-Munk approximation of radiative transfer theory, accounting Fresnel reflection at the boundaries of the three layer sample (epidermal stripping-glue-guartz glass), was used [10,11,29,51].

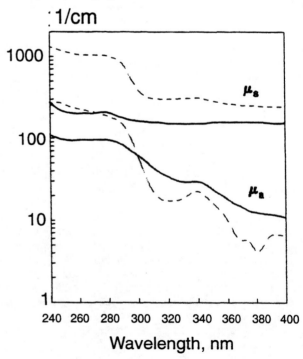

FIGURE 2. Calculated on the base of diffuse transmission and reflection measurement spectra of absorption and scattering coefficients of epidermis strippings for normal (———) and psoriatic (– – –) skin [29].

Spectra of absorption and scattering coefficients of ES are presented in Figure 2. Absorption of UV-radiation by the upper epidermal layers qualitatively looks like absorption spectrum of the protein solution [9]. The main contributions to the epidermis absorption of UV-radiation in the range from 240 to 300 nm are given by nuclear acids, aromatic aminoacids (tryptophane, tyrosine, phenylalanine) and urocanic acid [9,57,59]. Besides, in this wavelength range some lipids, contained in the cell membranes, have considerable absorption.

The differences in the absorption of the short wavelength (240-300 nm) radiation of healthy people and the samples taken from psoriatic nidi (see Figure 2) become explicable when considering the metabolic homeostasis in the skin. It is noted [60], that maintenance of nucleoproteins (DNA and RNA) in parakeratotic scales of psoriatic skin is 10-12 times higher than their concentration in normal stratum corneum. With psoriasis maintenance of the main "endogenous screen", urocanic acid also increases. In the UVA wavelength range (315-400 nm) the melanin plays the leading role in photoprotection. With psoriasis (on the progressive stage) the accumulation of sulfhydryl groups in the psoriatic nidi is observed; they make depressing influence on melanogenesis, by blocking the transport and inclusion of copper in the enzyme tyrosinase [61].

The refractive index of stratum corneum is equal to 1.55 [9], and so when the specular reflection occurs at the interface "air-skin" about 4% of the normally incident light is reflected. Deeper layers of epidermis play an important role in diffuse light reflection; they scatter a part of radiation in the direction of the skin surface and form the diffuse component R, increasing the total reflectance to 6-10%. With psoriasis, by increasing the inhomogeneities of the psoriatic nidi, presenting of filled-by-air micro spaces between parakeratotic scales, UVA reflection increases to 10-15%, that is connected with increasing of backscattering.

Also developed was the 4-flux Kubelka-Munk theory (2 collimated and 2 diffuse fluxes formed by incident and specular reflected laser beams, and volume scattering), taking into account Fresnel reflection at the sample boundaries which allows defining of the total transmittance, diffuse reflectance, scattering and absorption coefficients spectra of ES from experimental reflection and transmission spectra of the samples [62].

The angular dependencies of the intensity of scattered laser light ($\lambda = 633$ nm) give information of differences in structure of successive strippings and allow the determination of parameter of scattering anisotropy [54,62]. It was found that for successive strippings $g_1 = 0.89$, $g_2 = 0.88$, $g_3 = 0.90$ [62].

Frequency Domain Approach

Recently, time dependent methods of spectroscopy of turbid media attracted attention of many researchers [63-72], particularly as a tool for *in vivo* applications. Description of the propagation of short laser pulses in tissues with multiple scattering in the framework of rigorous Maxwell's theory meets serious mathematical difficulties [14]. For this reason, the radiative transfer theory (RTT) is widely used. In many cases diffusion approximation of RTT can be applied [14,65-71]. Thus, Patterson et al [70] have obtained the expressions, allowing calculation of the optical parameters of scattering

tissues from measurements of time profile of pulses of diffusely scattered light. Good agreement of their theory with experimental data has been reported [69,70]. On the other hand, recently the method of frequency domain measurements has been suggested [63-69, 71,72] for investigation of photon migration in scattering media. The results of measurements in frequency domain seem to be more convenient for interpretation and can be obtained, using less sophisticated apparatus, than ones in time domain [67,71,73]. For example, NIM Inc. has developed a dual wavelength frequency domain spectro-photometer for non-invasively quantifying hemoglobin saturation [73].

Based on the time dependent RTT, it is possible to describe dependences of modulation coefficient M and phase shift $\Delta\Phi$ of scattered light on modulation frequency ω for sinusoidally modulated initial radiation [63]. Assuming that angular distribution of time dependent and time independent parts of diffuse radiation coincide (this assumption is much weaker, than usually used diffusion approximation [69,70]), for detector placed on the tissue surface out of initial beam it was found

$$M = \exp\left(-\frac{\tau\mu_s\omega^2 t_1^2}{1+\omega^2 t_1^2}\right), \qquad \Delta\Phi = \omega\left(\frac{\tau\mu_s t_1}{1+\omega^2 t_1^2}+t_r\right) \quad (11)$$

where t_1 is the life time of photon in absorbed state, $t_r = \tau n/c_0$. Parameter τ can be considered as mean path length of photons in tissue, depending on geometry of experiment and absorbing and scattering parameters of tissue (μ_a, μ_s, g). Using Eqs.(11) and the least squares method it was performed processing of the results of frequency domain measurements, which have been done *in vivo* for human finger [71]. Scattering coefficient μ_s, life time t_1 and mean path length L have been calculated. We have obtained the following values: $\mu_s = 2.49$ cm^{-1}, $t_1 = 5.76 \cdot 10^{-11}$ sec, L = 2.23 cm.

Epidermis Structure Diagnostics

Static and dynamic diffraction methods, using unfocused and focused laser beams, are of great interest for biotissue structure diagnostics [74-77]. Focused laser beam scanning of the skin surface in principle allows one to receive information about skin structure. Nevertheless, because of the skin surface movements and very complicated optical response [77], laser profilometry was realized only for silicone replicas of the skin surface [76]. In order to work out objective methods of the skin structure diagnostics allowing some skin diseases monitoring, theoretical and experimental investigations of the Gaussian focused laser beam scattering by thin layers of epidermis [78] was done. For experimental investigations of the amplitude-phase transmission functions of the epidermis strippings (ES), coherent optical analyzer (COA) has been designed (see Fig.3,a). In the process of a mechanical scanning of a diffraction pattern in the direction being orthogonal to the system's optical axis the spatial power spectrum instantaneous values on various spatial frequencies were recorded. Because of a small size of the ES surface's illuminated area, partially developed speckle field is formed in the Fourier plane of COA. The statistical properties of this field are correlated with the structural features of the object at the

FIGURE 3. Coherent optical analyzer. a) – optical scheme: 1 –
He-Ne laser, 2 – beam expander, 3 – focusing microobjective, 4
– epidermis stripping, 5 – step – moving platform, 6 – Fourier-
transform objective, 7 – photodetector, 8 – signal processor. b) –
probability density functions of the instantaneous signal values
for epidermal stripping samples of normal (□ □ □) and
psoriatic (■ ■ ■) skin.

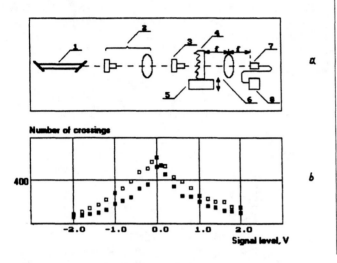

FIGURE 4. Differential speckle – interferometer for pulse wave
monitoring. a) – optical scheme: 1 – He-Ne laser, 2 – lens, 3 –
prism, 4 – skin surface, 5 – beam splitter prism, 6 – fiber, 7 –
photomultiplier, 8 – recorder b – a – d) experimental
pulsegrams, radial pulse of 28 year old male (b – pulse point
"tson," c – "khan," d – "chug").

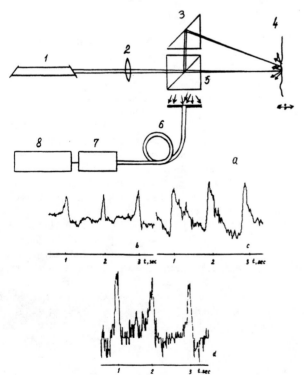

low spatial frequencies (about 10^3-10^4 m^{-1}). This gives the
possibility to reveal some skin pathologies, concerned with the
epidermis structure changes, such as psoriasis, eczema, etc.

The measured probability density functions of the
instantaneous COA signal values obtained during the scanning
of ES samples of normal and psoriatic skin are presented in
Figure 3, b. These preliminary results show the rise of the light
scattering, caused by structural changes of psoriatic epidermis,
and are in a qualitative agreement with spectrophotometric
measurements and Monte Carlo simulation (see Figures 1, 2).

**Pulse-wave Monitoring Using Skin Surface
Dynamic Light Scattering**

Laser heterodyne interferometric vibrometer was successfully
applied for measurement of the inner ear basilar membrane
vibrations [79]. These vibrations are small and membrane
surface quality is good enough to receive a specular reflection.
For rough surface, such as the skin surface, where oscillations
are large (at pulse points) more simple homodyne speckle-
interferometer was used [80]. It was shown that homodyne
speckle-interferometer output signal amplitude is random and
defined by scattering surface profile realization and conditions
of speckle-field observation. For measurement of high
amplitude vibrations interferometer output signal distribution is
near to Rayleigh's one and transformed into unilateral Gaussian
distribution for the small amplitudes. If vibration amplitude is
not small, one can observe amplitude-phase modulation of
interferometer output signal, caused by small mutual lateral
shifts of interfering speckle-fields, induced by angular
vibrations, which are characteristic for the living objects. It was
found that for measurement of biovibrations with not small
amplitude, it is useful to apply differential schemes of speckle-
interferometer [80]. Using the differential speckle-
interferometer, shown in Figure 4, a, pulse waves monitoring
was carried out. Pulse waves were observed at the points of skin
surface on wrist (in Tibetan pulse diagnostics these points are
called "tson", "khan" and "chug"). Optical signal was detected
at the point of space, where speckle-fields were matched. In this
region interferometer's output signal is maximal. Pulsegrams are
shown in Figure 4,b,c. In order to exclude the influence of the
volume scattering on the results, a metal-glue composition was
applied, which forms a thin layer on the skin surface. Note that
the volume scattering can be partially excluded by using UVA
irradiation with low penetration depth.

The space-time projection of normalized human skin surface
oscillations were analyzed, based on the data of spectra and
phase relations of the cardiovibration signal, received for norm
and stenosis of the mitral valve, with the use of acoustical
sensors [80,81]. Increasing the degree of disease seriousness
leads to topological changing in space-time projection structure.
At a certain stage in projection a loop appears, and the size of
this loop is determined by disease seriousness. As the outcome
vibration amplitude is small for the differential speckle-
interferometer, so the non-linear effects distort the output signal
just a little, so there are very small differences between the
space-time projections of the skin vibration function and the
output signal of interferometer. Note that the lateral shifts of
vibrating skin surface may essentially distort the structure of the
space-time projection of interferometer signal. In the output

signal, noise, caused by these lateral shifts, appeared. As a result, the projection trajectories become chaotic [80,81]. Many peculiarities of the phase portrait appear after the filtration of the output signal of the interferometer. So, the cardiodiagnostic method based on the studies of speckle-interferometer output signal space-time projection topology seems very promising.

On the other hand, the detailed analysis of the influence of inclined and tangent human skin surface oscillations on the accuracy of the interferometrical biovibration measurement serves as the basis of the new methods of laser cardio-diagnostics. Two schemes of speckle-interferometer (without the reference wave), allowing one to investigate inclined and lateral skin surface vibrations, have been performed [81]. Besides the thin metal layer, a thin rubber membrane was attached to the skin, which also allows avoidance of the influence of the volumetric scattering in the skin.

DETERMINATION OF THE EYE OPTICAL PARAMETERS

Measurement of the Scattering Matrix

Propagation of the light through biotissue is characterized not only by absorption and scattering coefficient, and scattering anisotropy factor (phase function), but also by changes of the polarization properties of the scattered light, depending on the size, refractive index, morphology, internal structure, and optical activity of the scatterer [1,44,45,82-85]. The elastic light scattering by biotissue is the most completely described by a light scattering matrix (S-matrix), the so-called Mueller's matrix, each of its 16 elements being a function of the wavelength, scatterers sizes, their form and material [1,82-85].

For the measurements of the S-matrix of the biological tissues and fluids, the computer controlled scattering matrix meter (polarization laser nephelometer) was developed (see Fig. 5) [1,35,37-39,43,44]. A scheme was realized with the rotating retarders (phase plates), which has a comparatively simple processing electronics software and allows avoidance of many of the experimental artifacts peculiar to DC measurements and to methods utilizing electrooptic modulators [83]. The S-matrix meter has the fixed polarizer P and A analyzer, and two rotating phase plates F and F' before and after the bio-object. The polarizer and analyzer are aligned in parallel with each other and their transmission planes are orthogonal to the scattering plane; the fast axis of the phase plates F and F' form the angles with the scattering plane φ and φ', and introduced phase differences δ and δ' respectively.

If $S_o \left\{ I_o, Q_o, U_o, V_o \right\}$ – is a Stokes vector-parameter of the incident light, and $S \left\{ I, Q, U, V \right\}$ – Stokes vector-parameter of the scattered light, then the matrix equation for total optical system can be written as [82]

$$S = \overline{A} \times \overline{F}' \times M \times \overline{F} \times \overline{P} \times \overline{S}_o \qquad (12)$$

where $\overline{A}, \overline{F}', \overline{F}, \overline{P}$, and M are the matrices of optical elements and bio-object. The ratio of the rotation rates of the phase plates $\overline{F}, \overline{F}'$ was taken equal to 1:5, i.e. $\varphi' = 5\varphi$, because all of 16 S-matrix elements are uniquely determined in this case [86]. Using (12) the intensity of scattered light can be represented in

the form of Fourier series expansion [86]

$$I = a_0 + \sum_{k=1}^{12} \left(a_{2k} \cos 2k\varphi + b_{2k} \sin 2k\varphi \right), \qquad (13)$$

where

$$a_{2k} = \sum_{i=1}^{N} I(\varphi_i) \cos 2k\varphi_i ; \qquad b_{2k} = \sum_{i=1}^{N} I(\varphi_i) \sin 2k\varphi_i , \qquad (14)$$

$I(\varphi)$ is the intensity of scattered light detected by photoreceiver for certain orientation of the fast axis of the first retarder.

Fourier coefficients (14) are defined by polarization characteristics of bio-object and optical elements of the set-up. The most simple expressions they have for retarders phase difference $\delta-\delta'$ equal exactly to $\pi/2$. These and more complicated expressions of M matrix elements usable for arbitrary phase differences $\delta-\delta'$ can be found in [40,43,44].

The computer controlled S-matrix meter provides the scattering angle scanning in the range $0 \div \pm 175°$ with the minimal step of 4' and accuracy of 5". The He-Ne laser (633 nm) with stable intensity was used as a light source. Microcomputer driven retarders allowed 256 indications per one rotation cycle of the first phase plate, i.e. in Eq. (14) N = 256. A photon counting electronic scheme was used with photomultiplier, amplitude discriminator (clipping amplifier), and counter, coupled with computer. Applications of the fast Fourier analysis allowed to measure and calculate all 16 S-matrix elements for the fixed scattering angle during the time about 1 sec with the accuracy of 3-5%. Digital correlator (100 channels, time delay of 1 μs) was used for the quasi-elastic light scattering experiments. Usually the incident on the bio-object laser beam had a spot size about 0.1 mm with the total power not higher than 0.1 mW.

It must be noted that there are some other possibilities to reduce experimental artifacts in measuring of polarization characteristics of the scattered light. Simpler and requiring only few optical components for its realization is "phase differential scattering" technique [83]. This technique is based on the usage of the two-frequency Zeeman laser with two lines having orthogonal polarization as a light source. The main advantage of such approach is in the possibility of direct measurement of the amplitude scattering matrix elements, which contain more "pure" information about scatterers then Mueller's matrix elements, which contain seriously mixed information. The phase differential scattering approach was successfully applied for investigation of pure aqueous suspensions of different viable bacteria [83].

Possibilities of Cataract Diagnostics

The angular dependence measurement of intensity S-matrix elements of the transparent and turbid eye crystalline lenses were carried out using S-matrix meter (Fig. 5) [1,37-40,43,44]. The measured angular S-matrix characteristics of the cataractous lens considerably differ from those of the transparent one (Figure 6), and indicate the appearance of the large

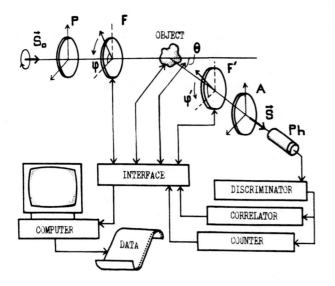

FIGURE 5. *Scheme of S-matrix meter.*

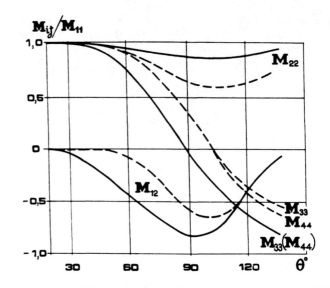

FIGURE 6. *Experimental indicatrices of normal (———) and cataractous (– – –) human crystalline lens S-matrix elements.*

nonspherical scattering particles in the turbid lens media (due to formation of high-molecular protein conglomerates). The transparent lens is characterized by the presence of a fine dispersive scatterer fraction with sizes near 0.5 μm only. The turbid lens contains a large dispersive fraction of scatterer size distribution function f(r), analytical view of which was approximated by a gamma – distribution (8) [87]. Calculations show not high sensitivity of elastic scattering to changes of the distribution parameters μ and β for fraction of the small scatterers. This low sensitivity hampers the solution of inverse problem on extraction of the size distribution function for the fine dispersive fraction and causes the need for using quasi-elastic scattering measurements, which are very sensitive just for ensembles of the small particles [1,38,88,89].

The elastic scattering method has the desirable sensitivity for determination of the large particle fractions of the size distribution, so it can be the base of the early cataract diagnostics technique [1,40,43-45]. Results of the direct model experiments illustrating this point are shown in Figure 7. The measurements were done for the solution of the α-crystallins (quasi-monodispersive fraction of particles with diameter about 0.02 μm), extracted from fresh calf lens,** and high-molecular protein conglomerates (mean diameter about 0.8 μm), extracted from the turbid crystalline lens [45]. It is clear that the measurement of S-matrix elements allows detection of the appearance of large dispersion fraction of the scatterers, when the transparency of the solution is changed only on 1%.

For *in vivo* cataract diagnostics, laser radiation is directed on the crystalline lens by some angle, passes through the cornea (M_{c2}) and aqueous humor chamber (M_{ch}), then, the radiation having been scattered by the lens (M_{1s}) along the direction of the eye optical axis passes back through the aqueous humor

FIGURE 7. *Indicatrices of S-matrix elements for the solutions of α-crystalline and large particles dispersive fraction extracted from the eye lens [45]. α-crystalline concentration $w_1 = 0.3$, large dispersive concentration w_2: $1 – w_2 = 0$ (τ = 99%); $2 - w_2 = 5 \cdot 10^{-5}$ (τ = 98%); $3 – w_2 = 1.4 \cdot 10^{-4}$ (τ = 94%); $4 – w_2 = 2.5 \cdot 10^{-4}$ (τ = 90%), τ is the solution transmittance for λ = 633nm, the thickness of solution layer is 5 mm.*

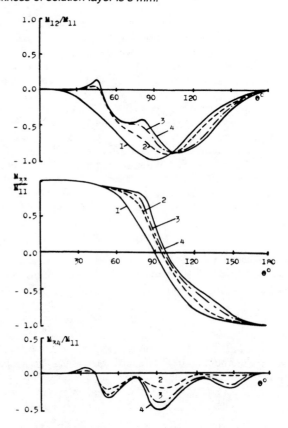

**α-crystalline specimen was given by Prof. J. Clauwaert from the Antwerp University

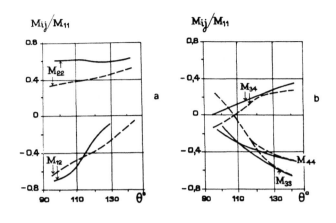

FIGURE 8. *In vivo measured indicatrices of S-matrix elements for normal (solid lines) and cataractous (dashed lines) rabbit eyes.*

chamber (M_{ch}) and cornea center (M_{c1}) and gets into S-matrix meter. The full S-matrix has the view

$$M = M_{c1} \times M_{ch} \times M_{1s} \times M_{ch} \times M_{c2}.$$ (15)

M_{c1} and M_{ch} do not introduce considerable distortions into M_{1s} extraction as far as they are matrices near isotropic bodies. M_{c2} requires statistical data on a great number of cornea to eliminate its influence on results. In addition, for clear cornea matrix, elements of M_{c2} are well defined and their influence on cataract informative elements of M is not high. *In vivo* measurements of S-matrix elements were realized for rabbits with normal and artificially induced naphthalene cataract [35,40,44] (Figure 8).

The possibility of early cataract diagnostics is opening the way for the medicamental therapy of this widespread disease. An introduction of such a diagnostic method into the clinical practice depends at present on a S-matrix meter time-response. The achieved time-response equal to 1sec is to be improved only by the order to exclude the effect of patient eye oculmotor reaction. The required time-response can be achieved by the increasing S-matrix meter fast-action or constructing the system of automatic tracking of the eye angular position. Typical values of the eye movement parameters (interval between sequential movement phases $\Delta t \approx 0.2$ sec and amplitude not exceeding 8°) allow use of both approaches. The first of these approaches seems to be the most simple technically by the application of the optoelectronic polarization control units, but in accordance with [83] gives some additional artifacts. The second approach can be realized without any building of the tracking system, only by using computer software excluding the complicated behavior of the eye ball position. Note that the meter and measurement technique are to be maximally simplified to be introduced in clinic (the measurement can be achieved for several recorded scattering angles only; the intensity of the scattered light can be increased by use of the stable green He-Ne laser [$\lambda = 543.3$ nm].

Examples of S-matrix Meter Application

S-matrix meter can be used for *in vitro* investigation of polarization characteristics of the different eye tissues from cornea to retina; in future it will be possible to take *in vivo* measurements for the whole eye with extraction of structural information about separate tissues. The last will be possible after careful *in vitro* investigation of separate eye tissues. According to (15), the S-matrix of aqueous humor M_{ch} can be found for known matrices of the cornea and lens. It has been shown for rabbit eye that aqueous humor is a transparent isotropic medium, some scattering (whole scattered light intensity does not exceed 1.5-2.0% of the incident one) of which is caused by the components of organic origin dissolved in it [40,44].

The vitreous humor's S-matrix looks like S-matrix of the transparent crystalline lens [40,44]. However, the presence of larger scatterers with lower refractive index as well as amorphous structure of the vitreous humor provide some differences. As with the aqueous humor, the vitreous humor does not change polarization characteristics of directly passed radiation. It gives the possibility of studying eye bottom polarization characteristics. On the other hand, different vitreous humor pathologies are to be revealed in S-matrix elements indicatrices variation. Particularly, small hemorrhages can influence the indicatrices notably having the view near to that obtained for erythrocytes [40,44].

The angular distribution of the S-matrix elements of monolayer of disk-shaped and spherulized erythrocytes (optically soft particles) during a change in their packing density have been studied by authors of [90]. The influence of packing density on the angular dependence of element M_{11} at $\theta = 15\text{-}16°$ for disks as well as spheres has been determined. The factor determining the angular variation of elements M_{11}, M_{22}, M_{33}, M_{21} in the range of angles $\theta = 110°\text{-}170°$ is the shape of the particles, not their packing density. The possibility of determining the refractive index of erythrocytes from the magnitude element M_{12} at scattering angles $\theta = 140°\text{-}160°$ is indicated.

S-matrix measurement approach was also used for investigation of the vesicle-capsular plague antigen complex formation [91]. The presence of optical activity of the scatterers was confirmed by non-equality of the normalized M_{33} and M_{44} elements, non-zero magnitudes of M_{23} (M_{32}) and M_{13} (M_{31}) elements, with the relations $M_{23} = -M_{32}$ and $M_{13} = -M_{31}$ being fulfilled with good accuracy. The calculations under the assumption that the scattering system is monodispersive with the particles diameter of 0.03 μm gave for initial vesicle suspension the refractive index magnitudes $n_L = 1.39$ and $n_R = 1.41$ for the left and right circular polarization. The results of S-matrix measurement for the vesicle-capsular plague antigen complex shows the increasing in optical activity of liposomes due to the interaction with the antigen. In that case calculation gave $n_L = 1.38$ and $n_R = 1.42$.

Applications of S-matrix elements measurement for investigations of suspensions of different particles, including the helical sperm head, several species of bacteria are overviewed in [83,84]. These measurements are not simple because of small magnitudes of informative matrix elements, such as M_{34}, due to random orientation of scatterers in an aqueous suspension. The angle dependence of normalized M_{34} element for different bacteria is oscillating function (similar to that represented in Figure 7), and the positions of maxima are very sensitive to changes of bacteria size [84].

Sensitive polarization-modulation system based on photo-elastic modulator capable of measuring small fraction of circular polarized light in a depolarized background (1:1000) was successfully used for discriminating short- and long-path photons transmitted through a multiply scattering medium [92].

The Small Angle Scattering

The measurement of the small angle scattering is very important for ophthalmology, for small amounts of laser size pollutants finding in pure liquids, and for transparent tissue tomography (see, for example, [64,85,93]. Small angle scattering recording is quite difficult for weak scattering and weak absorbing eye tissues because of the influence of an intensive directly passed coherent laser beam. The coherent component of the light beam can be suppressed by using coherence phenomena. Polarization interferometer developed by the authors of [94] serves these purposes effectively and was used for the analysis of the small angle scattering in liquid crystals. The more simple method was proposed for the small angle indicatrix measurement, which does not require precise tuning and continuous control [95]. Experimental set-up is shown schematically in Figure 9. The investigated sample is placed into one of the Mach-Zender interferometer arms. The angle of 0.5° is adjusted between interfering beams. The system consisting of the slit with the width of 10μm and photomultiplier operating in photon counting mode is used to record an interference pattern for the given direction (θ angle). That allows determination of the local visibility υ, the intensity of each beam I_1 and I_2 in the same direction, and intensity of scattered light

$$I_s = I_1 - \frac{\upsilon^2(I_1 + I_2)^2}{4 \cdot I_2}. \qquad (16)$$

Unit angular resolution is defined by the width of the interference band, which can be decreased to the limits of receiving system resolution. This method is applicable for different types of biotissue. It was successfully used for investigation of the human eye cornea small angle scattering [40].

APPLICATION IN LASER THERAPY

UVA Laser Therapy

The success of laser therapy mainly depends on correct dosimetry of laser light inside biotissues. The precision of laser light intensity determination inside tissue is defined by absorbing and scattering coefficients, and scattering anisotropy parameter g measurement accuracy. So, the developing of methods of μ_a, μ_s and g determination is very important not only for some kinds of tissue pathology diagnostics, but also for laser light dosimetry and controlling of tissues transparency.

The investigation of the normal and psoriatic skin absorption and scattering spectra (see Figure 2) makes it possible to

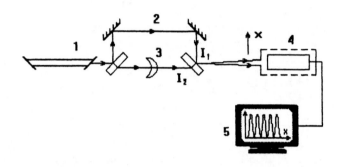

FIGURE 9. Experimental set-up for investigation of the small – angle laser light scattering by biotissues. 1 – laser; 2 – interferometer; 3 – bio-object; 4 – photomultiplier; 5 – monitor.

FIGURE 10. Fiber-mirror unit for percutaneous irradiation of blood: 1 – optical fiber; 2 – unit body; 3 – mirror reflecting surface; 4 – immersion liquid; I – epidermis; II – dermis; III – subcutaneous fat; IV – vessel wall; V – blood.

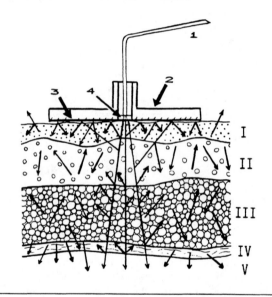

explain some photobiological effects and to choose the ways of optimization of photo- and photochemical therapy, including laser PUVA therapy [29,53,60]. The coefficients μ_a and μ_s were used for calculation of UVA radiation distribution within the skin during laser PUVA treatment of psoriasis [53]. Calculations have been performed using the Monte Carlo method. Detailed description of Monte Carlo program has been done elsewhere [17,21,27]. The laser treatment was realized by means of nitrogen laser (337 nm). Optical parameters of dermis at this wavelength were taken from [28] (see Table 2). As scattering phase functions of epidermis and dermis the Henyey-Greenstein functions were used. The calculated results are shown in Figure 1b.

To optimize the phototherapy it was suggested to decrease the backscattering with the help of application of mineral oils, which have the refractive index equal to 1.46-1.48, on the skin [9]. It was shown that dimethylsulfoxide and glycerin may be

FIGURE 11. Temperature distribution in the skin irradiated by visual CW laser (633 nm, power 25 mW)

(a) and by UV quasi-continuous laser (337 nm, power 150 mW)

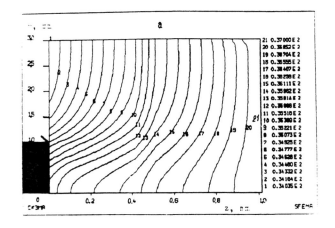

(b). z is the depth, r is the radial coordinate (for center of laser beam r = o), beam radius 1 mm.

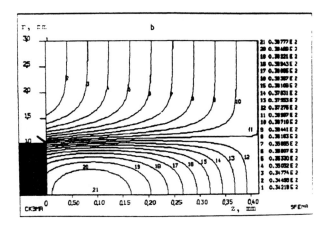

used for the same purpose [29]. The volume reflection coefficient of UV radiation decreases also, when photosensitizing cream "Puvaderm" is embracated in the skin. Application of these preparations does not influence dramatically the optical parameters of normal skin, but increases essentially penetration of UV radiation into psoriatic nidi.

The PUVA therapy is widely used in medical practice for treatment of psoriasis, vitiligo and many other skin diseases. The idea of selective phototherapy can be easily realized by using the lasers having high monochromaticity and radiation intensity [53,96,97]. It is advantageous to transfer into UVA band due to the essential depth of radiation penetration (see Figure 1), its low pigmentation efficiency and smaller danger of inducing cancerous diseases [98]. By using narrow-band UVA laser radiation one can employ photosensitization of the biological tissue by more suitable furocoumarine. In particular,

N_2 – laser radiation ($\lambda = 337$ nm) is very effective for interaction with psoralen, which has an absorption band $\lambda = 335$ nm, high level of quantum efficiency of DNA binding and skin sensitization [53].

For laser PUVA (LPUVA) laser-fiber-optical system was used, based on N_2- laser ($\lambda = 337$ nm, the mean power – 170 mW, the pulse power – 15 kW, pulse duration – 10 ns), which contains fiber-optical irradiator of the skin and dosimetry unit (power meter, timer, shutter and controlling microprocessor) [53]. The exposure of separate psoriatic elements (the diameter – up to 7 mm) with a single dose of 0.1 J/cm^2 with a preliminary photosensitization of the nidi caused the regress of psoriatic papule already by the total dose about 1 J/cm^2.

The potential patients for the LPUVA are persons suffering from psoriasis with the area of nidi – up to 25% cutaneous covering (e.g. psoriasis of palms and soles, of the hairy part of a head, single disseminated patches, and so on). The application field of the LPUVA can be spread on the other forms of skin pathology, by which it is necessary to provide the locality of exposure and it is desirable not to expose the parts of obviously unchanged skin to extra UVA radiation: vitiligo, neurodermatitis, lichen ruber planus, alopecia.

The designed UVA laser system is rather universal and can be used in wide range of disease diagnostics and therapy. For example, it was successfully used in realization of universal method of disease diagnostics, based on the measuring of the migration rate of polymorphonuclear leucocytes, mononuclears and lymphocytes to the focus of an aseptic inflammatory reaction caused by local laser beam irradiation (10-12 J/cm^2, skin photosensitization) [53].

Just the same techniques and doses were used for realization of the prolonged photochemo-reflexo-puncture therapy. In that case the long-term conservation of the focus of an aseptic inflammatory reaction in the exposure zone (biologically active points) allows one to obtain prolonged effect (up to two weeks) on the puncture points [99].

Laser Photodynamic, Biostimulation, and Hyperphermic Therapy

The red light irradiation of tissues and blood also gives some possibilities for disease treating [13,22,23,25-27,99-106]. Experimental optical and morphometrical investigations were done, and computer simulations of light penetration through the skin and adjacent tissues (see Figure 1,a), suggesting a method of noninvasive laser irradiation of blood in vessels. This method allows increasing space irradiance in the volume of interaction of laser light with blood due to return of a part of backscattered light into the tissue using reflecting coating, slight compression of tissue and immersion in the area of contact of optical fiber tip with the skin surface. Mentioned principles have become the basis for design of the fiber-mirror unit for percutaneous laser irradiation of blood (PLIB) (see Figure 10).

Vein *Saphena Magna* of the level of medical malleolus and vein *Cubiti* in cubital fossa were chosen as objects for topographic, anatomical, and optical investigations, which were necessary for justification of PLIB techniques [27,102]. PLIB was successfully used for treating of atopic dermatitis and renal diseases of children, and tropical ulcers of lower extremities. Designed laser-optical system for PLIB, which contains fiber-mirror irradiator and dosimetry system (power meter, timer, regulated light attenuator, and controlling microprocessor)*[†] may be applied for irradiating of rather large areas of the skin and whole organs, used in some biostimulating techniques, for photodynamic and hyperthermic therapy of small skin tumors [100-106].

Thermal Response

Laser therapy and biostimulation are the promising directions of modern photomedicine. Many methods of phototherapy, including above mentioned percutaneous irradiation of blood in the visible range and LPUVA therapy, are under very intensive investigations by many authors [9,13,19,21,27,48,53,97,103]. Nevertheless, the biotissue thermal response usually does not include phototherapy technology. Moreover, the well-known investigations of biotissue laser induced hyperthermia can be used for this purpose only partially, because they were done for another light dosage and experimental geometry (see for example [4,104]). So, the influence of laser induced tissue hyperthermia on the therapeutic effect of LPUVA and percutaneous irradiation of blood was not yet analyzed. For example, in [105] it was noted that tissue's thermal response leads to the synergistic effect of photodynamic therapy and accompanying hyperthermia, but uncontrolled hyperthermia leads to some complication in light dosimetry.

In order to analyze the influence of temperature rising on LPUVA therapy and percutaneous irradiation of blood in vessels, the stationary temperature fields inside the skin, irradiated by laser beams of visible (λ = 633 nm) and UVA (λ = 337 nm) wavelengths [21] were calculated. Heat generation in biotissue is a function of the product of the absorption coefficient μ_a and the total fluence rate U(r,z). To examine the influence of the optical and geometrical parameters on the thermal response of multi-layer tissue such as the skin, the heat conduction equation was solved using an adaptive finite element model with boundary conditions of convective heat exchange with environment at the skin surface.*[‡]. For stationary solution, about 2000 triangular elements over area of 12 mm^2 and results of Monte Carlo simulation for total light fluence rate inside tissue were used [21].

The optical parameters which are shown in Tables 1 and 2 for two models of the skin were used in a Monte Carlo simulation of irradiation of skin by red (λ = 633 nm) and UV (λ = 337 nm) laser beams. The first model is important for transcutaneous irradiation of blood in large veins and the second relates to UVA laser photochemotherapy. Simulations were made for CW laser beams with flat profile, beam radius equal to 1 mm, and total power equal to 25 mW for 633 nm and 150 mW for 337 nm. Calculations of temperature fields were made using thermal parameters taken from [28,107-109]: thermal conductivity k_T = 1.06 and 0.62 W/m • K, specific heat C = 3.35 • 10^3 and 3.50 • 10^3 J/kg•K, density ρ = 1.09•10^3 and 1.00•10^3 kg/m^3 for the skin and blood, respectively. Temperature distributions were

calculated for constant initial skin surface temperature T_c = = 34°C, which corresponds to invironmental temperature T_e = 22°C, and internal body temperature T_b = 37°C without laser irradiation influence (see Figure 11).

For this low intensive and high penetrating red laser beam, and six times more intensive and low penetrating UVA beam, both power density and temperature distributions are quite different. Maximal change of the skin surface temperature in the central part of the red beam is slightly more than 1.5°C, and across the beam from central part to its radius, the skin surface temperature changes uniformly (goes down) in the limits about 1.1°C.

The UVA laser beam inside tissue is not widely spread in transverse direction. That's why the skin surface temperature changes rapidly in the region at the boundary of laser beam, where $\partial T/\partial r$ = 7.5°C/mm. High temperature region (39.8°C) is located on the beam axis on the distance about 0.1 mm under the skin surface. The high temperature region localization for given laser beam, optical and thermal tissue parameters depend on boundary conditions for temperature on the skin surface and inside body.

As the nitrogen laser with λ = 337 nm is the pulse laser it is important to estimate an additional rising of temperature at the time of pulse duration. For determination of nonsteady temperature distribution in biotissue, the 1-D finite element model was used, taking into account spatial thermal flux spreading too [21]. For typical nitrogen laser with pulse duration 10 nsec and pulse repetition rate 100 Hz it was found that temperature additional rise should be equal to 3.5°C. It should be pointed out that calculations [21] do not include the local thermal processes, which have to raise temperature in a small area around melanin granules or in epidermal layers, where molecules of photosensitizer are located. So the local temperature may be some degrees higher.

The intensities of visual and UVA laser beams used in laser therapy produce such values of temperature rise in the skin layers which are much lower than the thresholds of epidermal necrosis ($\simeq$ 70°C) or explosive vaporization ($\simeq$ 160°C) [28]. Nevertheless, the calculated rising of temperature is quite enough to influence therapeutic effects [104].

CONCLUSION

This overview concerns only some aspects of the problem of light interaction with biological tissues bound up with light scattering by random and organized tissue structures. Of course, this paper mainly reflects the author's scientific interests, and could not be considered as the overview representing all directions of investigation of this very wide area.

The presented methods and results allow some conclusions and suggestions concerning further investigations.

1. The traditional spectrophotometric technique is very promising for biotissue investigations and needs of developing more perfect biotissue models taking into account spatial and radii distributions of absorbers and scatterers, that is necessary for the accurate determination of absorbing and scattering parameters of biotissue and its structure.

---

*[†]The apparatus was developed by Yu. P. Sinichkin.
*[‡]This method was developed by A.N. Yakunin and Yu. N. Scherbakov.

2. The angular measurements for many wavelengths should also give new information about scattering anisotropy of bio-media with basic multiple scattering and about polarization anisotropy of the form and scatterers medium optical activity and birefringence for bio-objects with principle single or low-step scattering.

3. It is necessary to develop methods for solving the inverse scattering problem taking into account geometry of the sample and light beam, valid for arbitrary ratio of the scattering and absorbing coefficients. In many cases, very promising is the inverse Monte Carlo method, but for fast calculations different methods would be useful based on radiative transfer theory.

4. Nowdays the intensive study of the frequency-domain methods of biotissue optical characteristics investigation takes place, nevertheless, this problem is not closed and needs developing.

5. The coherent optical methods are very promising for bio-tissue structure, vibration and motility analysis. The development of these methods requires the elaboration of fundamentals of speckle-optics and laser beam interference in the volumetric scattering media.

6. The S-matrix method has been well-known in optics for many years, and recently used by many authors for investigation of biological tissues and cell suspensions. It was usually used only in intensity matrix – Mueller's matrix, but application of the two frequency Zeeman laser allows measuring elements of amplitude matrix and opens the way to simplify solving of the inverse problem for some biological structures.

7. The dosimetry of laser light and accompanying thermal action is a very important direction of investigation in photo-therapy. Nowadays, many authors have worked out basic dosimetry principles. Nevertheless, it is necessary to develop 3-D tissue models dosimetry taking into account individual features of man's tissues, therapy technology and optical characteristics of treating apparatus.

ACKNOWLEDGEMENTS

I am very grateful to my former student, friend and colleague Dr. L. P. Shubochkin, who introduced me into laser bio-medicine, and who suddenly died on 20 January 1992.

Many thanks to all my colleagues for their cooperation, especially to Drs. I. L. Maksimova, S. R. Utz, Yu. P. Sinichkin, S. S. Ul'yanov, D. A. Zimnyakov, I. A. Utz, V. I. Kochubey, V. P. Ryabukho, students I. V. Yaroslavsky, A. Yu. Barabanov, S. N. Tatarintsev, S. V. Romanov, A. N. Yaroslavskaya, I. V. Meglinsky, V. G. Kukavsky.

REFERENCES

1. A. V. Priezzhev, V. V. Tuchin, L. P. Shubochkin, *Laser Diagnostics in Biology and Medicine*, Nauka, Moscow, 1989.

2. V. V. Tuchin, *Lasers and Fiber Optics In Biomedicine*, Saratov State University Publishers, Saratov, 1992.

3. *Special Issue on Lasers in Biology and Medicine*, IEEE J. Quantum Electr., vol. 20, pp. 1342-1532, 1984; vol. 23, pp. 1701-1855; vol. 26, 1990.

4. *Special Issue on Optical Properties of Mammalian Tissues*, Appl. Optics, vol. 28, pp. 2207-2357, 1989.

5. *Dosimetry of Laser Radiation In Medicine and Biology*, SPIE Proc. vol. IS 5, 1989.

6. *Biomedical Optics '91, Proc. SPIE, vols. 1420-1423, 1427, 1429, 1991.*

7. Biomedical Optics '92, Proc. SPIE, vols. 1640-1650, 1992; Biomedical Optics '93, Proc. SPIE, vols. 1876-1890.

8. *Laser and Medicine,* Academy of Sciences of the USSR. Bulletin Physical series, vol. 54, N8, N10, 1990.

9. R. R. Anderson, J. A. Parrish, "Optical properties of human skin," in *The Science Photomedicine,* Plenum Press, N.Y., 1982.

10. M.J.C. van Gemert, S. L. Jacques, H.J.C.M. Sterenborg, W. M. Star, "Skin optics," *IEEE Trans. Biomedical Eng.,* vol. 36, pp. 1146-1154, 1989.

11. W.-F. Cheong, S. A. Prahl, A. J. Welsh, "A review of the optical properties of biological tissues," *IEEE J. Quantum Electr.,* vol. 26, pp 2166-2185, 1990.

12. M.J.C. van Gemert, G.A.C.M. Schets, M. S. Bishop et al., "Optics of tissue in multi-layer slab geometry," *Lasers Life Sci.,* vol. 2, pp. 1-18, 1988.

13. J.-L. Boulnois, "Photophysical processes in recent medical laser developments: a review," *Lasers in Medical Science,* vol. 1, pp. 47-66, 1985.

14. A. Ishimaru, *Wave propagation and scattering in random media,* Academic Press, NY, 1978.

15. M.J.C. van Gemert, W. M. Star, "Relations between the Kubelka-Munk and the transport equation models for anisotropic scattering," *Lasers in Life Science,* vol. 1, pp. 287-298, 1987.

16. A. J. Welch, G. Yoon, M.J.C. van Gemert, "Practical models for light distribution in laser – irradiated tissue," *Lasers in Surgery and Medicine,* vol. 6, pp. 488-493, 1987.

17. I. V. Yaroslavsky and V. V. Tuchin, "Light penetration through multi-layered turbid media: a Monte Carlo simulation," *Opt. and Spectrosc.,* vol. 72, pp. 134-139, 1992.

18. S. L. Jacques, "Monte-Carlo modeling of light transport in tissues," *Tissue Optics,* Academic Press, N.Y., 1992.

19. B. A. Medvedev, V. V. Tuchin and I.V. Yaroslavsky, "Mathematical model of laser PUVA psoriasis treatment," *Proc. SPIE,* vol. 1403, pp. 682-689, 1990.

20. S. A. Prahl, M. Keijzer, S. L. Jacques, A. J. Welch, "Monte Carlo model of light propagation in tissue," In: *Dosimetry of Laser Radiation in Medicine and Biology,* eds G. J. Muller, D. H. Sliney, SPIE Optical Eng. Press, vol. IS5, pp. 102-113, 1989.

21. A. N. Yakunin, Yu. N. Scherbakov, V. V. Tuchin, S. R. Utz, I. V. Yaroslavsky, "Temperature distribution in biotissues under CW low intensity laser irradiation," *Proc. SPIE,* vol. 1646-23, 1992.

22. W. M. Star, B. C. Wilson, M. S. Patterson, "Light delivery and opti-cadosimetry in photodynamic therapy of solid tumors," *Photodynamic Therapy, Basic Principles* and *Clinical Applications,* eds B. W. Henderson, T. J. Dougherty, Marcel Dekker, Inc, N.Y., pp. 335-368, 1992.

23. S. L. Jacques, "Simple optical theory for light dosimetry during PDT," *Proc. SPIE,* vol. 1645-18, 1992.

24. R. Nossal, R. F. Bonner, G. H. Weiss, "Influence of path length on remote optical sensing of properties of biological tissue," *Appl. Optics,* vol. 28, N12, pp. 2238-2244, 1989; Statistics of penetration depth of photons re-emitted from irradiated tissue," J. Modern Optics, vol. 36(3), pp. 3419-359, 1989.

25. S. L. Jacques, "The role of skin optics in diagnostic and therapeutic uses of lasers," *in Lasers in Dermatology,* Springer-Verlag Berlin, Heidelberg, pp. 1-21, 1991.

26. V. V. Tuchin, S. R. Utz, I. V. Yaroslavsky, D. A. Kedrov, V. A. Tscukanov, E. J. Osyncev, "Blood Lasers Irradiation Through Skin. Justification of Method," In Proc. 5th Intern. Congress European Laser Association on Laser in Medicine, Graz, 1990.

27. S. R. Utz, V. V. Tuchin, I. V. Yaroslavsky et al., "Percutaneous blood laser biostimulation. First clinical results," *SPIE*, vol. 1643-41, 1992.

28. S. L. Jacques, M. Keijzer, "Dosimetry for lasers and light in dermatology: Monte Carlo simulations of 577-nm pulsed laser penetration into cutaneous vessels," *Proc. SPIE*, vol. 1422-01, 1991.

29. V. V. Tuchin, I. V. Yaroslavsky, S. R. Utz, A. Yu. Barabanov et al., "Skin optical parameters determination for laser photochemotherapy," *Proc. SPIE*, vol. 1645-55, 1992.

30. G. B. Al'tschuler, V. N. Grisimov, "Waveguide effect of light transport into a human dental," *Dokl. Akad. Nauk USSR*, vol. 310, pp. 1245-1248, 1990.

31. J. R. Zijp, J. J. ten Bosch, "Angular dependence of He-Ne-laser light scattering by bovine and human dentine," *Archs Oral Biol.*, vol. 36, pp. 283-289, 1991.

32. M. Keijzer, R. R. Richards-Kortum, S. L. Jacques, M. S. Feld, "Fluorescence Spectroscopy of Turbid Media: Autofluorescence of the Human Aorta," *Appl. Optics*, vol. 28, pp. 4286-4292, 1989.

33. H. J. C.M. Sterenborg, M. J. C. van Gemert, W. Kamphorst, J. G. Wolbers, W. Hogervorst, "The Spectral Dependence of the Optical Properties of Human Brain," *Lasers Med. Sci.*, vol. 4, pp. 221-227, 1989.

34. F. A. Bettelheim, S. Ali, "Light scattering of normal human lens. 3. Relationship between forward and back scatter of whole excised lenses," *Exp. Eye Res.*, vol. 41, pp. 1-9, 1985.

35. L. P. Shubochkin, V. V. Tuchin, "*In vivo* laser scattering spectroscopy of human eye tissues," in *Spectroscopy of Biological Molecules. State of the Art*, eds. A. Bertoluzza, C. Fagnano, and P. Monti, Societa Editrice Esculapio, Bologna, pp. 421-424, 1989.

36. D. E. Freund, R. L. McCally, R. A. Farrell, "Direct summation of fields for light scattering by fibrils with applications to normal corneas," *Applied Optics*, vol. 25, pp. 2739-2746, 1986; R. L. McCally, R. A. Farrell, "Light scattering from cornea and corneal transparency," in *New Developments in Noninvasive Studies to Evaluate Ocular Function*, B. Masters, ed., Springer-Verlag, N.Y., 1990.

37. V. V. Tuchin, L. P. Shubochkin and I. L. Maksimova, "Laser light scattering by anisotropic binary biological objects (Eye medium treatment)," in *Laser Scattering Spectroscopy of Biological Objects* (Studies in Phys. and Theor. Chemistry), vol. 45, eds. J. Stepanek, P. Auzenbacher, B. Sedlacek, Elsevier, Amsterdam-Oxford-N.Y.-Tokyo, pp. 611-620, 1987.

38. I. L. Maksimova, S. V. Romanov, L. P. Shubochkin, V. V. Tuchin, "Structural diagnostics of biological objects by elastic and quasi-elastic laser light scattering," in *Proc. 2nd International Conference on Laser Scattering Spectroscopy of Biological Objects*, ed. B. Nemet, Pecs, Hungary, pp. 216-227, 1988.

39. I. L. Maksimova, V. V. Tuchin, and L. P. Shubochkin, "Scattering effects in laser radiated biological tissue," in *Lasers and Applications*, International School, Sayanogorsk, East Siberia, pp. 107-127, Krasnoyarsk, 1991.

40. L. P. Shubbochkin, V. V. Tuchin, "New results in human eye laser diagnostics," *Proc. SPIE*, vol. 1403, pp. 720-731, 1990.

41. F. A. Bettelheim, "Physical basis of lens transparency," in *The Ocular Lens. Structure, Function, and Pathology*, ed. H. Maisel, N.Y., Basel: Marcel Dekker, Inc., pp. 265-300, 1985.

42. I. L. Maksimova, V. V. Tuchin and L. P. Shubochkin, "Polarisation characteristics of human cornea," *Opt. Spectrosc. USSR*, vol. 60, pp. 801-806, 1986.

43. I. L. Maksimova, V. V. Tuchin, L. P. Shubochkin, "Light scattering matrix of the eye lens," *Opt. Spectrosc. USSR*, vol. 65, pp. 615-620, 1988.

44. L. P. Shubochkin, *Light Scattering Features of Biological Structures in Application to Laser Diagnostics in Ophthalmology*. Saratov State University (Thesis), 1987.

45. I. L. Maksimova, *Concentration Effects on Light Scattering by the Bioparticles Systems*. Saratov State University (Thesis), 1991; I. L. Maksimova, L. P. Shubochkin, "Light scattering matrices of densely packed binary system of hard spheres," *Proc. SPIE*, vol. 1403, Pt. 2, pp. 749-751, 1990; *Opt. Spectrosc.*, vol. 70, N6, pp. 1276-1281, 1991.

46. T. B. Smith, "Multiple scattering in the cornea," *J. Modern Optics*, vol. 35, pp. 93-101, 1988.

47. J. Dillon, "The photophysics and photobiology of the eye," *J. Photochem. Photobiol. B: Biology*, vol. 10, pp. 23-40, 1991.

48. N. Mueller – Stolzenburg, G. J. Mueller, "Transmission on 308 nm excimer laser radiation for ophthalmic microsurgery – medical, technical and safety aspects," in *Advances in Laser Medicine II. Safety and Laser Tissue Interaction*, eds. H.-P. Berlin, G. Biamino, G. J. Mueller et.al, Laser-Medizin-Zentrum, pp. 133-147, 1989.

49. G. A. Askar'yan, "The increasing of laser and other radiation transport through soft turbid physical and biological media," *Quantum Electronics*, vol. 9, N7, pp. 1379-1383, 1982.

50. M. Bando, N.-T. Yu, J. F. R. Kuck, "Fluorophors and chromophors from rat lens crystallins in UV with hydroxykynurenine," *Invest. Ophthalmol. Vis. Sci.*, vol. 25, pp. 581-585, 1984.

51. M. Seyfried, "Optical radiation interaction with living tissue," in *Radiation Measurement in Photobiology*, Ch. 9, pp. 191-223, Academic Press Ltd., 1989.

52. W. A. J. Bruls, J. C. van der Leun, "Forward scattering properties of human epidermal layers," *Photochemistry and Photobiology*, vol. 40, pp. 231-242, 1984.

53. V. V. Tuchin, S. R. Utz, A. Yu. Barabanov et al., "Laser photochemotherapy of psoriasis," *Proc. SPIE*, vol. 1422, pp. 85-96, 1991.

54. S. L. Jacques, C. A. Alter, S. A. Prahl, "Angular dependence of He-Ne laser light Scattering by human dermis," *Lasers in the Life Sciences*, vol. 1, pp. 309-333, 1987.

55. P. Kini, A. P. Dhawan, "Reconstruction of ambedded absorbes in random media with applications in non-invasive 3D imaging of skin lesions," *Proc. SPIE*, vol. 1767-37, 1992.

56. J. M. Schmitt, G. X. Zhou, E. C. Walker, R. T. Wall, "Multilayer model of photon diffusion in skin," *J. Opt. Soc. Am. A.*, vol. 7, pp. 2141-2153, 1990.

57. K. F. Kolmel, B. Sennhenn, K. Giese, "Investigation of skin by UV remittance spectroscopy," *British J. Dermatology*, vol. 122, N2, pp. 209-216, 1990.

58. M. A. Everett, E. Yeargers, R. M. Sayre and R. L. Olson, "Penetration of epidermis by ultraviolet rays," *Photochem. Photobiol.*, vol. 5, pp. 533-542, 1966.

59. D. I. Cripps, *Solar damage to the skin, Current concepts*, Upjohn Company, Kalamazoo, Michigan 1990.

60. S. I. Dovgansky and S. R. Utz, *Psoriasis, or Psoriatic Disease*, University Press, Saratov, 1992 (in Russian).

61. N. B. Zlatkov. *Psoriasis*, Sofia, Med. and Physcult., 1988.

62. V. V. Tuchin, "Light interaction with biological tissues (overview)," *Proc. SPIE*, vol. 1884-19, 1993.

63. I. V. Yaroslavsky, V. V. Tuchin, "Frequency domain measurements of tissue optical parameters: a theoretical analysis," *Proc. SPIE*, vol. 1981-07, 1993.

64. B. Chance, "Optical Method," *Annu. Rev. Biophys. Biophys. Chem.*, vol. 20, pp. 1-28, 1991.

65. E. M. Sevick, B. Chance, J. Leigh et al., "Quantitation of time-and frequency-resolved optical spectra for determination of tissue oxygenation," *Anal. Biochem*, vol. 195. pp. 330-351, 1991.

66. K. M. Yoo, Feng Liu, and R. R. Alfano, "Photon migration in random media: angle and time resolved studies," *Proc. SPIE*, vol. 1204, pp. 492-497, 1990.

67. A. H. Gandjbakhche, J. M. Schmitt, R. Bonner, R. Nossal, "Random walk theory applied to noninvasive *in vivo* optical measurements of human tissue," IEEE Trans Biomedical Eng., vol. 39. pp. 332-333, 1992.

68. W. Cui, L. E. Ostrander, "Effect of local absorption changes on phase shift measurement using phase modulation spectroscopy, *Proc. SPIE*, vol. 1888-32, 1993.

69. S. R. Arridge, P. van der Zee, M. Cope, D. T. Delpy, "Reconstruction methods for infra-red absorption imaging," *Proc. SPIE*, vol. 1431-23, 1991; S. R. Arridge, M. Cope, D. T. Delpy, "The theoretical basis for the determination of optical pathlengths in tissue: temporal and frequency analysis," *Phys. Med. Biol.*, vol. 37, pp. 1531-1560, 1992.

70. M. S. Patterson, B. Chance, B. C. Wilson, "Time-resolved reflectance and transmittance for the non-invasive measurement of tissue optical properties," *Appl. Opt.*, vol. 28, pp. 2331-2336, 1989; S. J. Madsen, M. S. Patterson, B. S. Wilson et al., "Time resolved diffuse reflectance and transmittance studies in tissue simulating phantoms: a comparison between theory and experiment," *Proc. SPIE*, vol. 1431-06, 1991.

71. J. R. Lakowicz, K. W. Berndt, "Frequency-domain measurements of photon migration in tissues," *Chem. Phys. Lett.*, vol. 166, pp. 246-252, 1990; J. R. Lakowicz, K. W. Berndt, M. L. Johnson, "Photon migration in scattering media and tissue," *Proc. SPIE*, vol. 1204, pp. 468-480, 1990.

72. M. S. Patterson, J. D. Moulton, B. C. Wilson, K. W. Berndt, J. R. Lakowicz, "Frequency domain reflectance for the determination of the scattering and absorption properties of tissue," *Appl. Optics*, vol. 30, N31, pp. 4474-4476, 1991.

73. PMD 3000 b, Phase Modulation Device, NIM Inc. Preliminary Technical Specification, 9/91-2.

74. L. Luciano, E. Reale, H. Konitz, U. Boseck, S. Bosek, "Alignment of cholesterol in the membrane bilayer," *The J. Histochemistry and Cytochemistry*, vol. 37, N9, pp. 1421-1425, 1989.

75. B. R. Masters, Y.-K. Lee, W. T. Rhodes, "Fourier transform method for statistical evaluation of corneal endothelial morphology," in *Noninvasive Diagnostic Techniques in Ophthalmology*, ed. B. R. Masters, Springer-Verlag, N. Y., pp. 122-141, 1990.

76. R. Saur, U. Schramm, R. Steinhoff, H. H. Wolff, "Strukturanalyse der hautoberflache durch computergestutzte laser-profilometerie," *Hautarzt*, vol. 42, pp. 499-506, 1991.

77. S. S. Ul'yanov, V. P. Ryabukho, V. V. Tuchin, "Focused laser beam scattering on moving non-smooth surfaces with one dimensional profile," *Proc. SPIE*, vol. 1723, pp. 138-142, 1991.

78. V. V. Tuchin, D. A. Zimnyakov, S. R. Utz et al., "Laser light scattering in epidermis structure diagnostics," *Proc. SPIE*, vol. 1884-34, 1993.

79. S. M. Khanna, R. Dandliker, J.-K. Willemin et al., "Cellular vibration and motility in the organ of corti," *Acta oto-Laryngologica*, Suppl. 467, 1989.

80. V. V. Tuchin, V. P. Ryabukho, S. S. Ul'yanov, "Speckle interferometry in the measurements of biotissue vibrations," *Proc. SPIE*, VOL. 1647, 1992.

81. S. S. Ul'yanov, V. V. Tuchin, "Pulse-wave monitoring by means of focused laser beams scattered by skin surface and membrances," *Proc. SPIE*, vol. 1884-35, 1993; "The analysis of space-time projection of differential and Michelson – type speckle interferometers output signal for cardiovibration measurement," *Proc. SPIE*, vol. 1981, 1993.

82. C. V. Bohren, D. R. Huffman, *Absorption and Scattering of Light by Small Particles*, N.Y., John Wiley and Sons, 1986.

83. R. G. Johnston, S. B. Singham, G. C. Salzman, "Polarized light scattering," in *Comments on Molecular and Cellular Biophysics*, vol. 5, N3, pp. 171-192, Gordon and Breach, Science Publ. Inc., 1988; G. C. Salzman, S. B. Singham, R. G. Johnston, "Light scattering and cytometry," in *Flow Cytometry and Sorting*, pp. 81-107, Wiley-Liss, Inc., 1990.

84. W. P. van de Merwe, D. R. Huffman, B. V. Bronk, "Reproducibility and sensitivity of polarized light scattering for indentifying bacterial suspension," *Appl. Optics*, vol. 28, pp. 5052-5057; B. V. Bronk, W. P. van de Merwe, M. Stanley, "*In vivo* measure of average bacterial cell size form a polarized light scattering function," Cytometry, vol. 13, pp. 155-162, 1992.

85. M. Hofer, O. Glatter, "Mueller matrix calculations for randomly oriented rotationally symmetric objects with low contrast," *Appl. Optics*, vol. 28, N12, pp. 2389-2400, 1989.

86. P. S. Hauge, "Recent Developments in Instruments in Instrumentation in Ellipsometry," Surface Science, vol. 96, pp. 108-140, 1980.

87. O. N. Kozina, I. L. Maksimova, S. V. Romanov and S. N. Tatarintsev, "Investigations of the biological particles polydispersity by the nephelometry techniques," in *Laser and Fiber Optic Diagnostics*, ed. V. V. Tuchin, Saratov, pp. 46-50, 1989.

88. M. van Laethem, J.-Z. Xia and J. Clauwaert, "The use of photon-correlation spectroscopy to detect early changes in the eye-lens." in *Proc. 2nd International Conference on Laser Scattering Spectroscopy of Biological Objects*, ed. B. Nemet, Pecs, Hungary, pp. 228-232, 1988.

89. R. R. Ansari, H. S. Dhadwal, M. C. W. Campbell, M. A. Dellavecchia, "A fiber optic sensor for ophthalmic refractive diagnostics," *proc. SPIE*, vol. 1648, pp. 83-105, 1992.

90. A. N. Korolevich, A. Ya. Khairullina, L. P. Shubochkin, "Scattering matrix of monolayer of optically soft close-packed particles," *Opt. Spectrosc. USSR*, vol. 68, N2, pp. 236-239, 1990.

91. N. P. Guseva, I. L. Maksimova, S. V. Romanov, L. P. Shubochkin, S. N. Tatarintsev, "Investigation of vesicle-capsular plague antigen complex formation by elastic laser radiation scattering," *Proc. SPIE*, vol. 1403, pp. 332-334, 1990.

92. J. M. Schmitt, A. H. Gandjbakhche, R. F. Bonner, "Use of polarized light to discriminate short-path photons in a multiply scattering medium;" *Appl. Optics*, vol. 31, pp. 6535-6546, 1992.

93. R. P. Hemenger, "Small-angle intraocular light scatter: a hypothesis concerning its source," *J. Opt. Soc. Am.*, vol. A5, pp. 577-582, 1988.

94. S. M. Arakelian, L. E. Arushanian and Yu. S. Chilingarian, "Fluctuations in nematic liquid crystal in light scattering experiments," *Soviet J. Exp. and Theor. Phys.*, vol. 80, pp. 1186-1198, 1981.

95. I. L. Maksimova, L. P. Shubochkin and V. V. Tuchin, "Method of scattering indicatrix measurement," *Soviet patent* N1323927 Al, 5.02.86.

96, H. Trönnier, "Antipsoriascher effect monochromatischer lasersstrahlungen," Z. Hautkr., Bd. 57, ss. 17-23, 1982.

97. J. A. Parrish, K. F. Jaenicke, R. R. Anderson, "Erythema and melanogenesis action spectra of normal human skin," *Photochem. Photobiol.*, vol. 36, pp. 187-191, 1982.

98. L. Roza, R. A. Baan, I. C. van der Leun and R. Kligman, "UVA hazards in skin associated with the use of tanning equipment," *Photochem. Photobiol. B: Biol.*, vol. 3, pp. 281-287, 1989.

99. V. V. Mokretsov, S. R. Utz, N. V. Vinichenko et al., "Laser reflexotherapy in UV and IR wavelengths," *Proc. SPIE*, vol. 1981, 1993.

100. F. Asencio-Arana, V. Garcia-Fons, V. Torres-Gil et al., "Effects of a low-power He-Ne laser on the healing of experimental colon anastomoses: our experience," *Optical Engineering*, vol. 31, pp. 1452-1457, 1992.

101. J. J. Anders, R. C. Borke, S. K. Woolery, W. P. van de Merve, "Low power laser irradiation alters the rate of regeneration of the rat facial nerve," *Laser Surgery Med.*, vol. 13, pp. 72-82, 1993.

102. S. R. Utz, Yu. P. Sinichkin, V. V. Tuchin, I. V. Yaroslavsky, et. al, "Method and apparatus for percutaneous laser irradiation of blood and tissues," *Proc. SPIE,* vol. 1981, 1993.

103. S. L. Jacques, S. A. Prahl, "Modelling optical and thermal distributions in tissue during laser irradiation," *Lasers in Surgery and Medicine,* vol. 6, pp. 494-503, 1987.

104. L. O. Svaasand, C. J. Gomer, E. Morinelli. "On the physical rationale of laser induced hyperthermia," *Laser Med. Sci.,* vol. 5, N2, pp. 121-127, 1990.

105. W. M. Star, "Light delivery and light dosimetry for photodynamic therapy," *Laser Med. Sci.,* vol. 5, N2, pp. 107-113, 1990.

106. S. R. Utz, I. A. Utz, V. V. Tuchin, "Effect of low-energy laser biostimulation on rheological properties of blood," *Proc. SPIE,* vol. 1883-13, 1993.

107. D. Decker-Dunn, D. A. Cristensen, W. Mackie, J. Fox, G. M. Vincet, "Optothermal mathematical model and experimental studies for laser irradiation of arteries in the presence of blood flow," *Appl. Optics,* vol. 28, N12, pp. 2263-2272, 1989.

108. V. P. Zharov, B. V. Zubov, V. I. Lostchilov, "Investigations of optical and thermal properties of biotissues by means of pulse photothermal radiometry," Preprint N146, Moscow, Institute of General Physics, 1987.

109. F. A. Duck, Physical properties of tissue a comprehensive reference look," *Acad. Press.,* 1990.

Editor's Note:

Accepted for publication: May 27, 1993

Reprinted with permission from *Lasers in Medical Science,* Vol. 2,
pp. 235-242 (1987). ©1987 Academic Press Inc. (London) Ltd.

Quantitative Light Dosimetry in Vitro and in Vivo

JOHANNES P.A. MARIJNISSEN, WILLEM M. STAR

Dr Daniel den Hoed Cancer Centre, P.O. Box 5201, 3008 AE Rotterdam, The Netherlands

Abstract. Knowledge of the radiant energy fluence rate in tissues during laser irradiation is important for the understanding and improvement of the results of preclinical as well as clinical treatments. Quantitative data are extremely rare, however. In this paper, quantitative measurements of energy fluence rates are reported, in vitro as well as in vivo, with emphasis on light dosimetry for photodynamic therapy. Examples are given of fluence rate distributions that may occur during surface irradiation, intracavity irradiation of hollow organs (bladder) and interstitial irradiation. For the same incident irradiance, the energy fluence rate in tissue may vary considerably, depending on type of tissue, wavelength and geometry. During experimental and clinical interstitial PDT-treatments a considerable decrease in light penetration into tumours was observed, apparently indicating changes in optical properties as a result of treatment. This demonstrates the importance of in vivo light dosimetry.

INTRODUCTION

A qualitative illustration of the importance of light dosimetry is given in Fig. 1. Obviously, red light penetrates much deeper than green light and beef attenuates more than chicken muscle. In the human body, the bladder may have optical properties similar to chicken muscle, whereas tissues containing myoglobin may be optically similar to beef. Interstitial irradiation for PDT with green light is apparently not feasible, at least not for tissues like beef. More sophisticated light dosimetry requires quantitative measurements, of course.

The radiant energy fluence rate (in W/m^2) at a point in a medium is the total energy of the photons incident per second on a small sphere centred at that point, divided by the cross-sectional area of the sphere. When this quantity is multiplied by the absorption coefficient (in m^{-1}) of a chromophore in the tissue (tissue pigment or photosensitizer) the energy absorbed per second and per unit volume is obtained (in W/m^3). The latter is the quantity of interest in all medical laser applications.

Calculations of light energy fluence rates and energy absorption in tissues have been published, but the values of the optical constants used were often uncertain and incomplete and the theoretical models inadequate (1–5). Measurements of the energy fluence rate have rarely been reported, because proper instrumentation was not available. The purpose of the present paper is to briefly describe the type of probe required for such measurements and to show some experimental results, which illustrate the importance of quantitative measurements of energy fluence rate in vitro as well as in vivo. Examples will bear on methods of irradiation encountered in photodynamic therapy (PDT).

LIGHT DOSIMETRY PROBE: CONSTRUCTION AND CALIBRATION

According to the definition of the radiant energy fluence rate a suitable probe must have an isotropic response. The fluence rate in the medium of interest should vary little over the dimensions of the probe, which restricts its diameter to a millimetre or less. An example of such a probe is shown in Fig. 2. An isotropic probe is obtained (Fig. 3) when the end of the fibre is at the centre of a nearly spherical bulb and the photon mean free path in the bulb is short compared with its diameter, so that each photon is scattered several times before it enters the fibre. Our first model had a diameter of 1.5 mm (6) which was later reduced to about 0.8 mm (7). A similar probe of 2.5 mm diameter has recently been described by McKenzie (8). In our first models (6, 7) we used an epoxy, mixed with a light scattering material (obtained from a fluorescent light tube). Our latest models

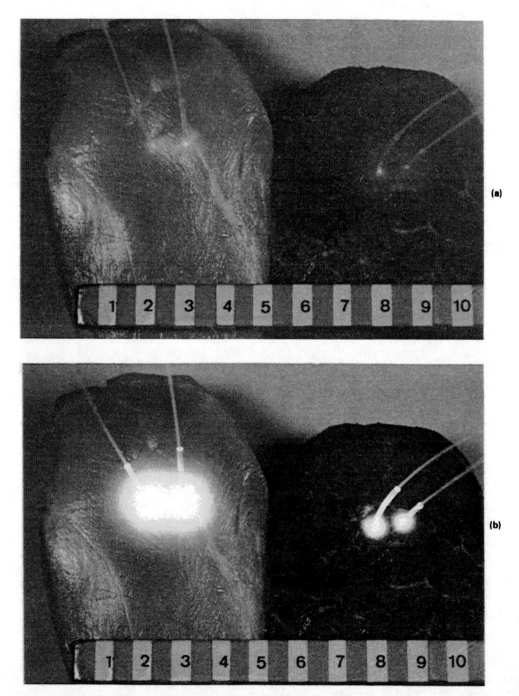

Fig. 1. Two diffusing fibres of 2 cm length inserted through transparent catheters 1 cm apart into 'chicken muscle' (left) and beef (right). The numbers indicate centimetres. (a), Both meats irradiated with 14 mW per fibre at a wavelength of 630 nm (red). (b), Both meats irradiated with 14 mW per fibre at a wavelength of 514.5 nm (green).

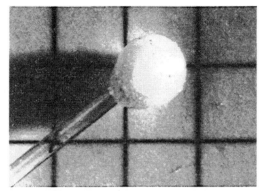

Fig. 2. Isotropic probe, i.e. a bulb of light scattering material mounted on an optical fibre. The distance between the lines is 1 mm.

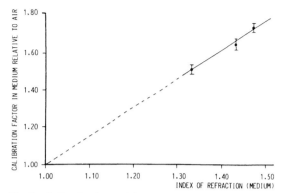

Fig. 4. Calibration factor of the isotropic probe as a function of the index of refraction of the medium, relative to the calibration in air. The reading of the detector in a medium, after calibration in air, must be multiplied by the calibration factor to obtain the fluence rate in the medium.

have been turned on a lathe out of a suitable white plastic. (We used polyetheneterephthalate, trade name Arnite.)

The distal end of the fibre is connected to a photomultiplier or photodiode with appropriate amplification and read out electronics. Calibration of the probe (in W/m^2) can be done in a collimated light beam of known irradiance. It is important to perform the calibration of the probe in a (clear) medium with the same index of refraction as the (turbid) medium in which the measurements will be made.

For example: if calibration is done in air, the reading of the same irradiance in water is reduced by a factor of 1.52 so that the calibration has to be multiplied by this factor. The physical explanation of this effect is that part of the diffuse light within the probe that is totally reflected at the bulb-air interface, can leave the

probe when air (index of refraction $n = 1$) is replaced by water ($n = 1.33$). We have established a calibration curve as a function of n from calibrations in various clear media with n up to 1.47 (glycerin) which is shown in Fig. 4. For measurements in tissues the appropriate index of refraction was estimated.

RESULTS

External surface irradiation

The data shown in Fig. 5 were taken in one of the tissues of Fig. 1. A glass vessel was filled with large chunks of tissue and a flat surface was created, which was irradiated with a per-

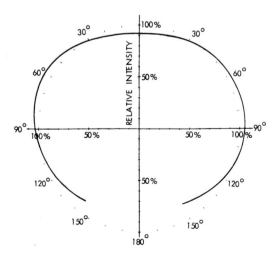

Fig. 3. Polar diagram of light detector response, which is isotropic ±10%. The detector bulb is at the origin and the fibre lies in the plane of the paper, along the axis towards 180°.

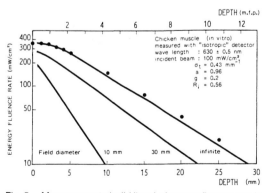

Fig. 5. Measurements (solid lines) of energy fluence rate in chicken muscle as a function of depth at the axis of a parallel incident light beam of circular cross section. The black circles show results of calculations for infinite beam diameter using diffusion theory (7) and the optical constants given in the figure: σ_t, absorption + scattering coefficient; a, (scattering coefficient)/σ_t; g, average cosine of the scattering angle; R_i, internal reflection factor for diffuse light at the tissue–air boundary; m.f.p., photon mean free path.

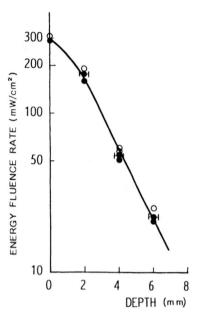

Wave length: 630 ± 0.5 nm
Field diameter: 15 mm

Fig. 6. Energy fluence rate in rat rhabdomyosarcoma in vitro (volume 5.7 cm³), from a perpendicularly incident collimated light beam of 100 mW/cm² and 15 mm diameter. Different symbols indicate different sets of measurements.

pendicularly incident beam of light. The quantitative agreement between theoretical calculations using measured optical constants (7) and measured fluence rate confirms the calibration of the probe. Two phenomena should be noted. First, the energy fluence rate just below the surface for the largest diameter is 3.5 times the irradiance of the incident beam. This is due to the strong scattering of light within tissue and to total reflection back into the tissue (factor R_i) of that fraction of the diffuse light that is incident at the tissue-air boundary at an angle larger than the critical angle. The second phenomenon is the dependence of the fluence rate in tissue on the beam diameter, which is also the result of strong light scattering.

Fig. 6 shows measurements similar to Fig. 5 on a rat rhabdomyosarcoma. The ratio (R) between the energy fluence rate at the surface and the irradiance of the incident beam is 3 in this case, but would have been still larger for a larger beam diameter. The fluence rate de-

creases more rapidly upon increasing depth when compared with chicken muscle in Fig. 5, even when the difference in beam diameter is taken into account. This may have been caused by the limited volume of the tumour (25 × 30 × 15 mm) which limits the amount of scattered light. Another possibility is, of course, that the optical properties of the rat rhabdomyosarcoma are different from chicken muscle. As the ratio R, defined above, is not much different for both tissues, it is expected that σ_a/σ_s (σ_s = scattering coefficient, σ_a = absorption coefficient) is not much different either. This expectation is based on the fact that theoretically the ratio R depends only on σ_a/σ_s, if g (the average cosine of the scattering angle) is the same. Therefore, both σ_a and σ_s may be larger for the rhabdomyosarcoma than for chicken muscle.

Another interesting feature is shown in Fig. 7. At 4.5 mm depth at the edge of a 15 mm diameter beam the fluence rate is only half its value at the axis of the beam. Such effects must be taken into account if a nonsuperficial tumour is to be treated effectively by PDT using surface irradiation.

Irradiation of bladder

Fig. 8 shows light energy fluence rates as a function of depth in bladder, for various irradiation conditions. When the whole bladder wall is irradiated with water or Intralipid (a highly

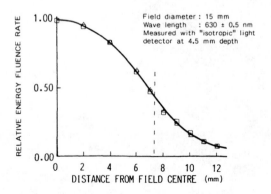

Field diameter : 15 mm
Wave length : 630 ± 0.5 nm
Measured with "isotropic" light detector at 4.5 mm depth

Fig. 7. Radial profile of energy fluence rate measured at 4.5 mm depth, relative to the value at the beam axis, in a rat rhabdomyosarcoma (same as in Fig. 6).

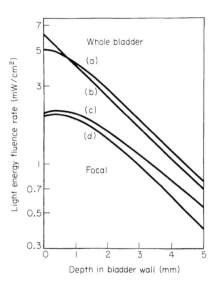

Fig. 8. Energy fluence rate as a function of depth in the wall of a spherical model bladder of 8 cm internal diameter, wall thickness 1 cm, irradiated by an isotropic light source at the centre emitting 0.2 W, which yields 1 mW/cm² unattenuated incident light at the bladder surface. The data were calculated mathematically with diffusion theory, and were confirmed by measurements in optical phantoms (9) with the same optical constants (Table 1). (a), Whole bladder irradiated with water in the bladder cavity. (b), Whole bladder irradiated with Intralipid in the bladder cavity. (c), Focal irradiation with water in the bladder and an incident beam of 40 mm diameter, 1 mW/cm². (d), Same as (c), with 10 mm beam diameter.

scattering fat emulsion) in the bladder cavity, the ratio between the fluence rate at the tissue surface and the incident irradiance is 5 or 6, respectively which is even larger than the ratio in Figs 5 and 6. This large ratio was confirmed

Table 1. Optical constants used for phantom mixtures and for energy fluence rate calculations in a model study for dosimetry in PDT of bladder

Material	Scattering coefficient σ_s (mm^{-1})	Absorption coefficient σ_a (mm^{-1})	Average cosine of scattering angle (g)
Intralipid (0.2%)	1.1	0.00019	0.83
Bladder tissue (dog)	5.9	0.06	0.85

Data measured with red light (wavelength 630 nm).

by measurements in vivo in dog bladder (9). It can be explained by the fact that with surface irradiation some back scattered light is lost, whereas in the bladder all back scattered light re-enters the bladder wall elsewhere. With focal irradiation of a limited area of the bladder again some back scattered light is lost. Furthermore, there is now only a very small difference in index of refraction at the boundary between tissue and water, so that R_i (Fig. 5) is nearly zero. This explains why in the case of focal irradiation with water in the bladder the ratio between the fluence rate in tissue at the surface and the irradiance of the primary beam is only 2.

Interstitial irradiation

In order to optimize energy fluence rate distributions in a preclinical study of interstitial PDT (10) 'optical isodoses' were measured about a diffusing fibre used in this study (Fig. 9a). Comparing these data with isodoses about a linear radioactive source commonly used in interstitial radiotherapy (Fig. 9b) it appeared that the patterns were quite similar. For this particular type of tumour it was therefore possible to apply interstitial PDT in much the same way as interstitial radiotherapy.

In our experimental study of interstitial PDT the energy fluence rate at the tumour boundary was monitored with an isotropic probe during each treatment and the integrated value was in fact used to determine if the prescribed light dose had been delivered. Fig 10 shows that during treatment, with constant input power per fibre, the probe measured a continuously decreasing energy fluence rate. Apparently the effects of the treatment, possibly haemorrhage (11), cause changes in the optical properties of the tumour. A decrease in light penetration during treatment has also been observed in an experimental study of PDT for ocular tumours (12).

We have established a dose response relationship for interstitial PDT of a transplantable rat rhabdomyosarcoma (Marijnissen et al unpublished data). With an optimized protocol it was possible to achieve a 100% cure rate (follow-up 100 d) for this tumour model. This prompted us to start a pilot study of interstitial PDT for human tumours. In this clinical study we have also measured the light energy fluence rate by inserting an isotropic detector in one of the transparent plastic catheters implanted into the tumour for insertion of light delivering

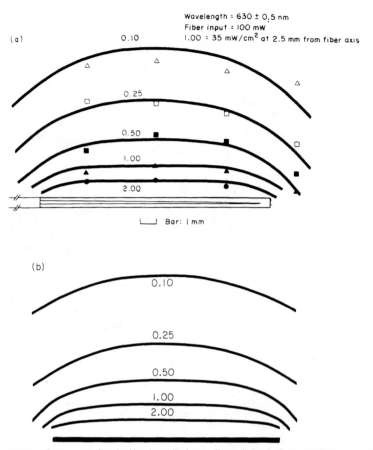

Wavelength : 630 ± 0.5 nm
Fiber input : 100 mW
1.00 : 35 mW/cm² at 2.5 mm from fiber axis

(a)

0.10

0.25

0.50

1.00

2.00

Bar: 1 mm

(b)

0.10

0.25

0.50

1.00
2.00

Fig. 9. (a), Lines of constant energy fluence rate ('optical isodoses') about a linear light applicator (diffusing fibre) of 17 mm length. Points were measured in vitro in a rat rhabdomyosarcoma (24 × 16 × 15 mm). Lines represent empirical model calculations fitting the data and normalized to 1 at 2.5 mm from the source axis. (b), Lines of constant radiation dose (isodoses) about a linear radioactive source (iridium-192) of 17 mm length, normalized to 1 at 2.5 mm from the source axis.

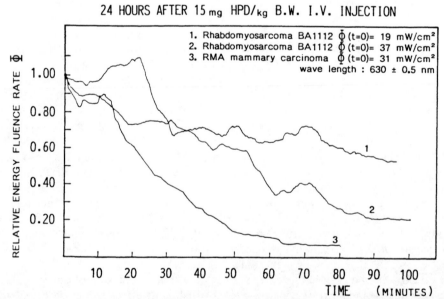

24 HOURS AFTER 15 mg HPD/kg B.W. I.V. INJECTION

1. Rhabdomyosarcoma BA1112 Φ (t=0)= 19 mW/cm²
2. Rhabdomyosarcoma BA1112 Φ (t=0)= 37 mW/cm²
3. RMA mammary carcinoma Φ (t=0)= 31 mW/cm²
   wave length : 630 ± 0.5 nm

RELATIVE ENERGY FLUENCE RATE Φ

TIME (MINUTES)

Fig. 10. Energy fluence rate measured during interstitial PDT of transplantable rat tumours with four linear light applicators (diffusing fibres), normalized to the value at the start of irradiation. Only 100 mW per fibre was delivered, keeping the tumor temperature below 40 °C. The isotropic light detector was placed under the skin overlying the tumour about 4 mm away from the nearest fibre.

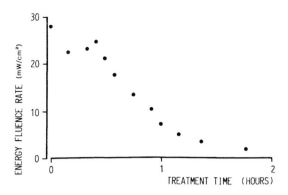

Fig. 11. Energy fluence rate measured during interstitial PDT of a neck node in a patient. A power of 65 mW was delivered through each of four diffusing fibres of 3 cm length. Treatment 72 h after i.v. administration of 2 mg/kg Photofrin II. An istotropic light detector was inserted into the tumour approximately 5 mm away from the nearest fibre. The planned treatment time was 2 h, to deliver approximately 150 J per cm of diffusing fibre, assuming light penetration into the tumour remained constant.

fibres. The result of such a measurement is shown in Fig. 11. A dramatic decrease of the measured fluence rate was observed, showing that the planned total light dose could in fact not be delivered in a reasonable time.

The phenomena shown in Figs 10 and 11 are not caused by thermal effects, such as charring. The power delivered was always less than 100 mW per cm length of diffusing fibre. The plastic catheters used for insertion of both the light delivering fibres and the light dosimetry probe were clear and uncharred upon removal after treatment. Temperature measurements within the experimental tumours during PDT-treatment yielded values not exceeding 40 °C.

DISCUSSION AND CONCLUSION

We have shown that for the same incident irradiance quantitative measurements of light energy fluence rate yield quite different results depending on the geometry considered. We have shown the influence of a finite beam diameter on the effective depth of penetration and on the profile of the fluence rate at a few mm depth in tissue. We have demonstrated the effect of a difference in index of refraction between the tissue and the medium at its boundary (air or water) where internal reflection of diffuse light within the tissue affects the energy fluence rate. We have also shown that in vivo measurements of energy fluence rate during interstitial PDT indicate changes in tissue properties which even more complicate light dosimetry.

This is by no means a complete study. It rather is a brief survey of phenomena that are observed when quantitative measurements of light energy fluence rate are performed in vitro and in vivo. To the best of our knowledge, such data have never been published before. Yet, they are essential. The purpose of this paper therefore should be to indicate the amount of

work still to be done to bring light dosimetry to a level where it may help us to better understand and further improve the results of experimental and clinical laser treatments.

REFERENCES

1 Van Gemert MJC, de Kleijn WJA, Hulsbergen-Henning JP. Temperature behaviour of a model port-wine stain during argon laser coagulation. *Phys Med Biol* 1982, **27**:1089–104

2 Wan S, Anderson RR, Parrish JA. Analytical modeling for the optical properties of the skin with in vitro and in vivo applications. *Photochem Photobiol* 1981, **34**:493–9

3 Gijsbers GHM, Breederveld D, van Gemert MJC et al. In vivo fluorescence excitation and emission spectra of hematoporphyrin derivative. *Lasers Life Sci* 1986, **1**:29–48

4 Van Gemert MJC, Welch AJ, Star WM et al. Tissue optics for a slab geometry in the diffusion approximation. *Lasers Med Sci* 1987, **2**:295–302

5 Grossweiner LI. Optical dosimetry in photodynamic therapy. *Lasers Surg Med* 1986, **6**:462–6

6 Marijnissen JPA, Star WM. Phantom measurements for light dosimetry using isotropic and small aperture detectors. In: Doiron DR, Gomer CJ (eds) *Porphyrin localization and treatment of tumors*. New York: Alan Liss, 1984:133–48

7 Marijnissen JPA, Star WM, van Delft JL, Franken NAP. Light intensity measurements in optical phantoms and in vivo during HPD-photoradiation treatment, using a miniature light detector with isotropic response. In: Jori G, Perria C (eds) *Photodynamic therapy of tumours and other diseases*. Padova: Libreria Progetto, 1985:387–90

8 McKenzie AL. Can diffusion be assumed in correcting for oblique incidence in laser photodynamic therapy? *Phys Med Biol* 1986, **31**:285–90

9 Star WM, Marijnissen JPA, Jansen H et al. Light dosimetry for photodynamic therapy by whole bladder wall irradiation. *Photochem Photobiol* 1987, **46**:619–24

10 Marijnissen JPA, Star WM, Versteeg AAC, Franken NAP. Pilot study on interstitial HPD-PDT in rats bearing solid mammary carcinoma or rhabdomyosarcoma. In: Jori G, Perria C (eds) *Photodynamic therapy of tumours and other diseases*. Padova: Libreria Progetto, 1985:243–46

11 Star WM, Marijnissen JPA, van den Berg-Blok AE et al. Destruction of rat mammary tumor and normal tissue microcirculation by hematoporphyrin derivative photoradiation observed in vivo in sandwich observation chambers. *Cancer Res* 1986, **46**:2532–40

12 Franken NAP, van Delft JL, Dubbelman TMAR et al. Hematoporphyrin derivative photoradiation treatment of experimental malignant melanoma in the anterior chamber of the rabbit. *Curr Eye Res* 1985, **4**:641–54

Key words: Photodynamic therapy; Light dosimetry; Isotropic detector

Reprinted with permission from *Applied Optics,* Vol. 28(12), pp. 2280-2287
(June 15, 1989). ©1989 Optical Society of America.

Laser-induced hyperthermia of ocular tumors

Lars O. Svaasand, Charles J. Gomer, and A. Edward Profio

Experimental results for the optical distribution and temperature rise during laser irradiation of tumors are presented. The experimental conditions are chosen to simulate laser irradiation of ocular tumors. The tumor models are human retinoblastoma heterotransplanted in athymic mice, murine mammary carcinoma in C3H/HEJ mice, and B16 melanotic melanoma in C57/BL6 mice. The experimental results are discussed in terms of a mathematical model where the thermal distribution is calculated from the bioheat transfer equation, and the optical distribution is determined according to diffusion theory.

I. Introduction

Approximately 2000 new cases of primary intraocular tumors (uveal melanoma in adults and retinoblastoma in children) are diagnosed each year in the United States. Conventional treatments for these tumors include enucleation, external beam radiation, brachytherapy, photocoagulation, and cryotherapy. Recently, the use of intraocular hyperthermia has been proposed as an adjunct to radiation therapy using scleral plaque brachytherapy. Methods for inducing intraocular hyperthermia include microwave, ultrasound, and rf applicators.[1] Each of these procedures can produce efficient thermal gradients in ocular tumors, but unfortunately the thermal gradients are not specifically localized to the tumor tissue. The absorption of visible and near IR light is, on the other hand, tissue specific. The use of lasers emitting within the region of transparency of the cornea and lens has the potential to initiate a localized elevation of the tumor temperature.

The normal human eye has a transmission of more than 80% in the 500–950-nm wavelength region. In the near IR the transmission has a minimum value of 40% between 950 and 1000 nm. But the transmission increases to ~80% again at a 1100-nm wavelength and then drops off to ~10% in the 1200–1300-nm region. The eye is opaque for wavelengths larger than 1400 nm as well as for wavelengths shorter than 400 nm.[2,3]

The absorption in the pigmented epithelium and choroidal layer, is dominated by melanin absorption and drops linearly with the wavelength from ~70% at 450 nm to 10% at 1000 nm. The absorption in the 1000–1150-nm region is typically 10%, and it goes further down to <5% at 1200 nm.

The reflectance of the pigmented epithelium and choroidal layer increases linearly with the wavelength from 10% at 500 nm to 40% at 900 nm. The reflectance maintains a value of 40–45% up to 1300 nm, and it drops to 15% at a 1450-nm wavelength.[2,3]

The present work emphasizes an experimental evaluation of relevant optical and thermal properties related to laser-induced ocular hyperthermia. Properties of nonpigmented tumors were analyzed in terms of human retinoblastoma heterotransplanted in athymic mice and a mouse mammary carcinoma transplanted in C3H/HEJ mice. The corresponding properties of pigmented tumors were investigated using a B16 melanotic melanoma transplanted in C57/BL6 mice.

The accessible physical data of the tumor structure, geometry, and vasculature are, in the case of noninvasive clinical procedures, very limited. The mathematical description of the thermal distribution is, therefore, expressed in terms of a simplified analytical model that only requires input of some characteristic data of the tumor and its surroundings. The experimental results reveal, however, that this model predicts the temperature rise with reasonably good accuracy.

II. Reflectance Measurements

The total reflectance, i.e., both specular and diffuse, was measured for the tumors at several wavelengths. The optical sources were an argon-ion laser emitting simultaneously at 488- and 515-nm wavelengths, a

Lars Svaasand is with University of Trondheim, Trondheim, Norway; Charles Gomer is with Clayton Ocular Oncology Center Childrens Hospital of Los Angeles USC School of Medicine Los Angeles, CA 90027, and A. E. Profio is with University of California, Santa Barbara, Department of Chemical & Nuclear Engineering, Santa Barbara, California 93106.

Received 27 November 1988.
0003-6935/89/122280-08$02.00/0.
© 1989 Optical Society of America.

DCM dye laser for red light and a Nd:YAG laser at a 1064-nm wavelength. The reflected light was collected by a 60-mm diam integrating sphere. The light was measured with a silicon photodiode, and a barium oxide target was used as a unity reflectance reference. The mice were anesthetized with an intraperitoneally injection of Nembutal (0.45 μg/gm), and the normal skin covering the tumor was resected. The laser light was coupled through a 200-μm diam fused silica fiber, and the exposed tumor surface was irradiated in a 4-mm diam region. The results are given in Table I.

The wavelength dependence of the reflection coefficients is determined by the spectral properties of the hemoglobin and melanin absorption. The highest values for the reflectance are found in the near IR where absorption in both hemoglobin and melanin is at a minimum.[4]

III. Optical Penetration Depth

Analytical evaluation of the optical distribution in highly scattering media, such as most tissues, is very complex. Solutions based on the exact form of the electromagnetic equations are unobtainable, and most analyses are based on an approximate description in terms of a photon transport equation.[5,6] However, for several applications the optical field may be adequately approximated with optical diffusion theory.[7–9] The local radiance is then assumed to be almost isotropic, and the optical distribution will be characterized by a diffuse radiant energy fluence rate. The optical distribution can then be expressed as

$$\mathrm{div}\mathbf{j}_0 = -\beta\phi + q_0, \qquad (1a)$$

$$\mathbf{j}_0 = -\zeta\,\mathrm{grad}\phi, \qquad (1b)$$

where $\mathbf{j}_0$ is the diffuse energy flux vector and ϕ is the radiant energy fluence rate. The diffusion constant is ζ, and the optical absorption coefficient is β. The diffuse optical energy source density q_0 represents the energy which is scattered directly into a diffuse distribution from an incoming collimated beam.

Equations (1a) and (1b) can be expressed in the form

$$\nabla^2(\beta\phi) - \frac{\beta\phi}{\delta^2} = -\frac{q_0}{\delta^2}, \qquad (2a)$$

where the optical penetration depth δ is given by

$$\delta = \sqrt{\frac{\zeta}{\beta}}. \qquad (2b)$$

The general solution for the absorbed optical power density $\beta\phi$ in a uniform medium can then be expressed as

$$\beta\phi = \frac{1}{4\pi\delta^2} \iiint \frac{q_0}{r} \exp\left(-\frac{r}{\delta}\right) dv, \qquad (3)$$

where the integral shall be taken over all space. The distance from the source density q_0 contained in an element of volume dv is given by r.

The optical distribution for a nonuniform case, such as when the plane surface of a tissue is irradiated with a collimated beam, can be approximated by assuming that all light is scattered to a diffuse distribution in the surface layer.[9,10] The absorbed power density in the tissue can then be expressed as

$$\beta\phi = \frac{(1-\gamma)}{2\pi\delta^2} \iint \frac{I}{r} \exp\left(-\frac{r}{\delta}\right) dA, \qquad (4)$$

where I is the incident optical power density, γ is the reflection coefficient, and r is the distance from each element dA of the irradiated surface. The integral will be taken over the entire irradiated spot.

This type of approximation usually gives a reasonably good description of the optical distribution. The approximation is adequate in regions distal to the irradiated surface, whereas the description might be of limited validity in regions close to the surface. The light distribution in the proximal region might have important contributions from nonscattered incident light and there might be a tendency to forward scattering.

In such cases the description might be improved by expressing the emission from each irradiated surface element by a semiempirical relationship of the form

$$d(\beta\phi) = \frac{(1-\gamma)}{2\pi\delta^2} \frac{I}{r} \exp\left(-\frac{r}{\delta}\right)(1+n)\cos^n\theta\, dA, \qquad (5)$$

where θ is the angle between r and the direction of the incident collimated beam. The parameter n characterizes the deviation from the diffuse isotropic case; the isotropic case corresponds to a value of n equal to zero. The value of n for the almost isotropic case will be in the range between 0 and 1, and the more forward scattering dominated cases can be approximated with higher values of n. The factor $(1+n)$ ensures that the totally absorbed power is the same for all values of n.

The light intensity of an infinite broad plane beam will, in accordance with Eq. (4), be attenuated exponentially with the distance from the irradiated surface. The penetration depth, i.e., the distance corresponding to a reduction of a fluence rate by a factor $1/e = 0.37$, was measured in the murine tumor models.

The tumor surface was pressed slightly against the plane surface of a glass cuvette as shown in Fig. 1. The plane surface of the tumor, which had a diameter of typically 10–15 mm, was irradiated through the cuvette with a broad beam of uniform power density.

Table I. Total Reflection Coefficient (Specular and Diffuse); Measured in vivo

Tumor	Wavelength (nm)			
	488/514	630	665	1064
B16 melanotic melanoma in C57/BL6 mice	0.05	0.06	0.08	0.23
Human retinoblastoma in athymic mice				
(Typical tumor)	0.12	0.23	0.19	0.17
(Hemorrhage region)	0.07	0.19	0.21	0.19
Mammary carcinoma in C3H/HEJ mice	0.09	0.25	0.35	0.35
Greene's amelanotic melanoma in anterior chamber, rabbit	0.09	—	0.26	0.26

Typical individual and local variations ±12%.

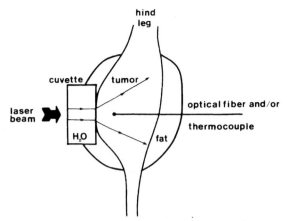

Fig. 1. Experimental setup. A cylindrical water filled cuvette of 20-mm diameter and 10-mm height was pressed slightly against the tumor surface. The normal skin covering the tumor was resected, and the nonexposed surface of the tumor was thermally insulated with a thick layer of grease. The light is irradiated onto the tumor through the cuvette. The temperature rise was monitored with a 200-μm diam Chromel-Alumel microthermocouple mounted coaxially with the optical beam. The optical distribution is measured with an optical fiber terminated with a 1-mm diam sphere of highly scattering material. This omnidirectional detector fiber was mounted either coaxially with the optical beam, as shown in the figure, or orthogonal to the beam axis.

The fluence rate was measured at various depths with an inserted optical fiber. An incision was made with a hypodermic needle, and the fiber was inserted after retraction of the needle. There was minimal bleeding. The detector fiber, which was mounted coaxially with the incident beam, was positioned to various distances from the irradiated surface with use of a micropositioning device. The tip of this fiber was covered with a 1-mm diam sphere of highly scattering material which enabled the collection of light arriving from all directions (Laserguide, Inc., Santa Barbara). The detected light was guided through the fiber and measured by a silicon photodiode.

The fluence rate vs distance from the irradiated tumor surface is shown in Fig. 2. The tumor in this case was a human retinoblastoma transplanted in the hind leg of an athymic mouse. Corresponding measurements were also performed on the other two tumor models. The results are summarized in Table II.

These values are in agreement with previously reported postmortem values for human brain tumors.[10] The measured value of 2.0 mm for the melanotic melanoma indicates that, although the melanin absorption is significantly reduced in the near IR compared with the visible, it is still an important chromophore at these wavelengths. However, the observation that the penetration depth at a 1064-nm wavelength in strongly pigmented tumors has about the same value as that for red light in nonpigmented tissues, might be important for clinical procedures. The value indicates that the Nd:YAG laser might be an important thermal source for the treatment of ocular tumors. The low absorption reduces the probability for local hot spots in pigmented regions such as the pigmented epithelium and

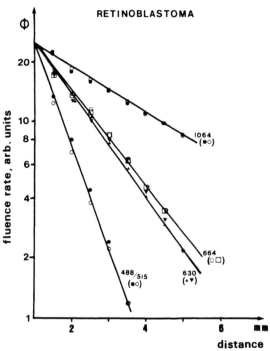

Fig. 2. Optical fluence rate vs distance from irradiated surface. *In vivo* measurements in a 10-mm diam human retinoblastoma growing in athymic mice. The 10-mm diam tumor was inoculated in one hind leg. The tumor surface was irradiated by a broad beam with uniform power density. Measurements are given for irradiations at a 488/515-nm wavelength (simultaneous emission of the two lines from a continuous argon-ion laser) at a 630- and a 664-nm wavelength (continuous DCM dye laser) and at a 1064-nm wavelength (continuous Nd:YAG laser). All results are normalized to the same extrapolated value at the tumor surface. The two sets of data points for each wavelength correspond to subsequent insertions of the detector fiber in the same region of the tumor.

choroid, and it ensures an adequate penetration in pigmented tumors.

The light distributions in a direction transversel to the axis of the incident beam are shown in Fig. 3. The omnidirectional detector fiber was here oriented normal to the beam and again positioned to the various locations by the micropositioning device. The results for the mammary carcinoma are shown by the dashed lines in Fig. 3. Figures 3(a) and 3(b) show transversal light distribution at 2.5-mm depth for two different diameters of the irradiated spot, i.e., respectively 2

Table II. Optical Penetration Depth, Measured *In Vivo*

| Tumor | Wavelength (nm) | | | |
	488/515	630	665	1064
Human retinoblastoma in athymic mice	1.6	3.3	3.6	7.5
Mammary carcinoma in C3H/HEJ mice	1.1	2.0	2.3	3.7
B16 melanotic melanoma in C57/BL6 mice	—	0.5	0.5	2.0

Penetration depth in millimeters.
Typical individual and local variations ±25%.

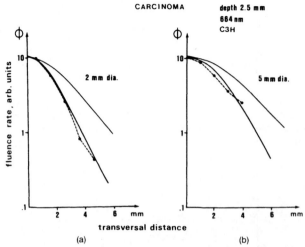

CARCINOMA depth 2.5 mm
664 nm
C3H

(a)   (b)

Fig. 3. Optical fluence rate vs distance from the axis of the incident beam. The distribution is measured in a plane 2.5 mm below the irradiated surface. *In vivo* measurements on mammary carcinoma in C3H/HEJ mice at a 664-nm wavelength: (a) and (b) correspond, respectively, to a 2- and 5-mm diam irradiated spot. The experimental results are given by dashed lines. The upper solid lines in both figures correspond to theoretical predictions from Eq. (4) with an optical penetration depth $\delta = 2.3$ mm. The lower solid lines correspond to calculations in accordance with Eq. (5), where $n = 1$ and $\delta = 2.3$ mm. All values are normalized to the same value at the axis of the beam.

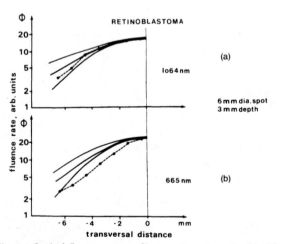

RETINOBLASTOMA

(a)

1o64 nm

6 mm dia. spot
3 mm depth

665 nm   (b)

Fig. 4. Optical fluence rate vs distance from the axis of incident beam. The distribution is measured in a plane 3 mm below the irradiated surface, and the diameter of the irradiated spot is 6 mm. *In vivo* measurements on human retinoblastoma in athymic mice: (a) and (b) correspond, respectively, to 1064- and 665-nm wavelength irradiation. The experimental results are given by dashed lines. The upper solid lines in both figures correspond to calculations in accordance with Eq. (4) with $\delta = 7.5$ mm in (a) and $\delta = 3.6$ mm in (b). The middle and lower solid lines correspond, respectively, to calculations from Eq. (5) with $n = 1$ and $n = 2$. The values for the optical penetration depth are the same as used for the upper solid lines. All values are normalized to the same value at the axis of the beam.

and 5 mm. The upper solid curves in both figures correspond to the theoretically expected distributions in accordance with Eq. (4) where the incident beam is assumed to be scattered to an isotropic distribution in the surface layer itself. The solid lower curves give the corresponding distribution in the case of a moderate forward scattering where the parameter n in Eq. (5) has been put equal to $n = 1$.

Corresponding results for the retinoblastoma are shown by the dashed lines in Fig. 4. The upper solid curves, middle solid curves, and lower solid curves correspond, respectively, to $n = 0$, $n = 1$, and $n = 2$. The measurements of the transversal light distributions thus indicate that the light proximal to the irradiated surface is not completely isotropically scattered. This tendency is more pronounced for the retinoblastoma than for the carcinoma.

The difference in the scattering properties might also explain the significant higher values for the penetration depth in the retinoblastoma. A reduced scattering will, in the case of the same absorption coefficient, reduce the probability for absorption and, therefore, enhance the penetration.

IV. Thermal Distribution in a Perfused Medium

The fundamental properties of heat transport in a perfused medium may be approximated with the bioheat transfer equation.[9,11–13]

A simple form of this equation yields

$$\text{div}\mathbf{j} = -\frac{\partial}{\partial t}(\rho^{CT}) - (T - T_a)\rho_b C_b Q + q, \quad (6a)$$

$$\mathbf{j} = -\kappa\,\text{grad}T, \quad (6b)$$

where $\mathbf{j}$ is the heat flux vector, T is the local temperature, and T_a is the arterial blood temperature. The time is given by t, q is the heat source density, κ is the thermal conductivity, and Q is the blood perfusion rate given in the volume of perfused blood per unit volume of tissue in unit time. The specific gravity and specific heat of the tissue are, respectively, ρ and C. The corresponding quantities for blood are ρ_b and C_b. The differences in these quantities between tissue and blood are usually quite insignificant. The heat source density q represents the heat generated by metabolic activity as well as heat delivered by absorption of optical power. If, however, the temperature T is interpreted as the local temperature rise above a normal uniform temperature distribution, q can be taken as the absorbed optical power density only. The arterial blood temperature T_a should, in accordance with this interpretation of T, be equated to zero.

It the solutions are expressed in terms of thermal waves of the form

$$T \propto \exp[j(\omega t - \mathbf{k}\mathbf{r})], \quad (7)$$

where ω and $\mathbf{k}$ are, respectively, the frequency and wave vector, Eq. (6) can be written

$$\nabla^2 T + k^2 T = -\frac{q}{\kappa}. \quad (8)$$

The magnitude of the wave vector is given by

$$k^2 = -\left(\frac{1}{\delta_v^2} + \frac{j\omega}{\chi}\right), \qquad (9)$$

where the thermal diffusivity χ is given by

$$\chi = \frac{\kappa}{\rho C} \qquad (10)$$

and where the thermal penetration depth δ_v is expressed by

$$\delta_v = \sqrt{\frac{\chi}{Q}}. \qquad (11)$$

The steady state solution of Eq. (6) can, in the case of a uniform medium, be expressed in the form

$$T = \frac{1}{4\pi\kappa} \iiint \frac{q}{r} \exp\left(-\frac{r}{\delta_v}\right) dv, \qquad (12)$$

where the integral will be taken over all space.

The cooling from blood perfusion is insignificant if the optical power is absorbed in a region of linear dimensions much less than the thermal penetration depth. The resulting thermal gradients will in such cases be sufficiently steep to yield a heat transport completely dominated by thermal conduction. A relevant irradiated spot size during laser-induced hyperthermia of ocular tumors will be 3–6 mm in diameter. The vascularity of the bulk of the tumor mass is usually quite limited. It is, therefore, reasonable to anticipate a thermal penetration depth in the tumorous mass of the order of 10 mm.[9] The thermal penetration depth of the tumor surroundings, the vitreous, the sclera, and the orbital fat are all expected to be larger than 10 mm. An exception is the choroidal layer where the high blood perfusion rate in the $Q = 0.1\text{-s}^{-1}$ range corresponds to a thermal penetration depth of the order of 1–2 mm. But the total thickness of the human choroidal layer, 125 μm, is, on the other hand, only a fraction of a thermal penetration depth. The contribution to the steady state cooling by perfusion in, for example, a 7-mm diam choroidal region below the heated tumor is, according to Eq. (6), of the order of 20 mW for a 10°C temperature rise. It might, therefore, be reasonable to neglect the contribution to heat transfer from blood perfusion, except perhaps in cases of thin extensive choroidal tumor surrounded by intact vasculature. The heat transfer by the choroidal flow is also usually negligible if the exposure time is less than the reciprocal blood perfusion rate, i.e., less than typically 10 s.[13,14]

The thermal conductivity of tumors was evaluated by measuring the steady state temperature rise from an inserted local heat source. The heat source was 488/515-nm irradiation from an optical fiber inserted in the center of 10–15 mm diam tumors. The temperature distribution was measured with an inserted 200-μm diam Chromel-Alumel microthermocouple, and the thermocouple junction was positioned with a micromanipulator device. The contributions to the temperature readings from optical power absorbed by the metallic thermocouples were insignificant. The temperature rise at distances much larger than the optical

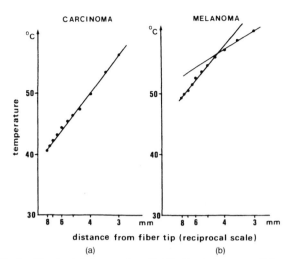

Fig. 5. Steady state temperature distribution in tumors vs distance from the tip of the inserted optical fiber (reciprocal scale on horizontal axis). Irradiated power of 500 mW at a 488/515-nm wavelength: (a) and (b) (right) give, respectively, the temperature rise measured *in vivo* in mammary carcinoma, in C3H/HEJ mice and B16 melanotic melanoma in C57/BL6 mice. The solid line in (a) corresponds to thermal conductivity $\kappa = 0.52$ W/m·K. The data points in (b) are fitted to two lines; the line valid for the 4–8 mm region from the fiber tip corresponds to $\kappa = 0.61$ W/m·K, and the line valid for the 3–4-mm region from the fiber corresponds to $\kappa = 1.1$ W/m·K.

penetration depth is here only due to thermal conduction from the region proximal to the fiber tip. Typical results for mammary carcinoma and melanoma are given in Figs. 5(a) and 5(b), respectively. The temperature rise vs reciprocal distance from the source will, in the case of spherically symmetric geometry in a tissue with insignificant blood perfusion, form a straight line [Eq. (12)]. The thermal conductivity of the mammary carcinoma varied little with distance, as follows from the proximity of the data points to the straight line shown in Fig. 5(a). This line corresponds to a thermal conductivity $\kappa = 0.52$ W/m·K. The corresponding results for the melanoma shown in Fig. 5(b) give a thermal conductivity $\kappa = 0.61$ W/m·K in the 4–8-mm region from the fiber tip. The results for melanoma revealed, however, a higher effective thermal conductivity proximal to the fiber tip. The measured conductivity, which in this region was higher than the value for pure water, indicates a contribution from convective cooling. The difference between the thermal distributions in the case of the melanoma and carcinoma is believed to be due to the structure of the tumors. The carcinoma had a solid firm structure which limited any convective cooling to a minimum, whereas the melanoma exhibited a more loose and aqueous structure. There was no *a priori* liquefactive necrosis, but it is possible that the temperature of more than 60°C was initiating some proximal to the fiber tip. A reduction of the irradiated power to correspond to a maximum temperature of ~50°C resulted in a reduction of the effective thermal conductivity in the proximal region to 0.66 W/m·K. The average values measured in the 4–8-mm region from the source were $\kappa =$

0.52 W/m · K and $\kappa = 0.54$ W/m · K for, respectively, the mammary carcinoma and melanoma. These parameters are in agreement with previously reported values for thermal conductivities of tissues.[15]

The temperature distribution in externally irradiated tumors was evaluated in the experimental setup shown in Fig. 1. The normal skin covering the tumor was resected, and the exposed tumor surface was pressed slightly against the glass cuvette. To simulate the thermal surroundings of a retinal or choroidal tumor, the cuvette was filled with water. The remaining part of the tumor was thermally insulated with a thick layer of grease. The temperature of the surrounding air was kept close to the normal body temperature of the animals. The laser beam was passed through the cuvette, and the temperature distribution was evaluated with a microthermocouple array consisting of five individual junctions each separated by 2 mm. The array was mounted in a 1-mm diam Teflon tube. The temperature distribution was measured along the axis of the incident optical beam. The steady state temperature distributions are shown by the dashed lines in Fig. 6. The observation that the difference between the *in vivo* and postmortem measurements is insignificant indicates that the contribution to the cooling from blood perfusion is negligible. The tumor is in the present experimental setup surrounded by media with approximately the same thermal properties. It is, therefore, adequate to calculate the temperature rise from Eq. (12), which is only strictly valid for a thermally uniform medium of infinitely large extent. The solid curve in Fig. 6 gives the temperature rise calculated in accordance with this equation. The absorbed optical power density is, however, calculated in accordance with a further simplification of Eqs. (4) and (5). The absorbed energy density is taken to be constant over the cross-sectional area of a cone. Two radii of this cone correspond to the distances from the beam axis where the absorbed power density, as determined from Eq. (5), has dropped down to $1/e$ compared to the values at the axis. The two radii of some of the cone are determined at the distances from the surface corresponding to $\delta/2$ and $3 \cdot \delta/2$. This model thus assumes a spatial distribution of the absorbed power density of the form

$$\beta\phi = \frac{(1-\gamma)I}{\delta}\left(\frac{r_0}{r_{\text{eff}}}\right)^2 \exp\left(-\frac{x}{\delta}\right), \qquad (13)$$

where r_0 is the radius of the irradiated spot and r_{eff} is the radius of the cone at distance x from the surface. The optical parameters are in Fig. 6: reflection coefficient $\gamma = 0.23$, optical penetration depth $\delta = 2$ mm, and scattering parameters $n = 1$. The thermal conductivities in the tumor and the cuvette are both taken equal to $\kappa = 0.6$ W/m · K. The thermal penetration depth is, since the blood perfusion is insignificant, infinitely large. The solid curves shown in Figs. 7–9 are all calculated according to Eqs. (12) and (13). The corresponding optical and thermal parameters are given in the figure legends.

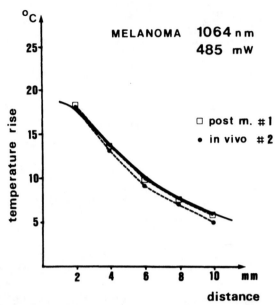

Fig. 6. Steady state temperature rise vs distance from the irradiated surface, measured along the axis of the incident beam. The dashed lines give results from *in vivo* measurements on B16 melanotic melanoma in C57/BL6 mice. Irradiated power 485 mW at a 1064-nm wavelength with a 6-mm diam irradiated spot. Optical power measured after transmission through cuvette (~75% transmission). The lower and upper broken lines correspond, respectively, to *in vivo* and *postmortem* measurements in the same tumor. The solid curve corresponds to calculations in accordance with Eqs. (5), (12), and (13) together with the scattering parameter $n = 1$, reflection coefficient $\gamma = 0.23$, optical penetration depth $\delta = 2$ mm, and thermal conductivity $\kappa = 0.6$ W/m · K.

The corresponding results for the mammary carcinoma are shown in Fig. 7, where the three dashed lines give results for different animals. To improve the spatial resolution the thermocouple array was substituted by the single 200-μm diam thermocouple. Temperature distributions measured with this setup are shown in Fig. 8. The two dashed lines correspond to subsequent insertions in the same region of a retinoblastoma. Corresponding results for the retinoblastoma at another wavelength, 630 nm, are shown in Fig. 9. The dashed lines correspond, in the same manner as in Fig. 8, to subsequent insertions in the same region of the tumor.

Experimental results for retinoblastoma are summarized in Fig. 10. The steady state temperature rise due to irradiation at various wavelengths has been normalized to 10°C rise at the tumor apex. The numbers in parentheses in Fig. 10 are the optical power required to obtain this temperature rise in the case of uniform irradiation over a 6-mm diam spot size. These results demonstrate that the high optical penetration depth at a 1064-nm wavelength in the retinoblastoma results in a very acceptable temperature distribution; the temperature rise is above 7°C up to a distance of 7 mm from the irradiated surface. The corresponding distance for red light is about half of

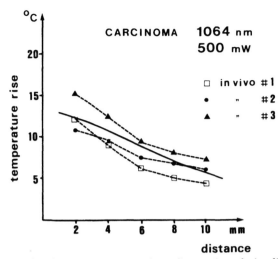

Fig. 7. Steady state temperature rise vs distance from the irradiated surface, measured along the axis of the incident beam. The three dashed lines give results from *in vivo* measurements on mammary carcinoma in C3H/HEJ mice on different animals. Power irradiated onto a 500-mW tumor at a 1064-nm wavelength with a 6-mm diam irradiated spot. The solid curve corresponds to calculations [Eqs. (5), (12), (13)] with the following parameters: $n = 1$, $\gamma = 0.35$; $\delta = 3.7$ mm; and $\kappa = 0.6$ W/m · K.

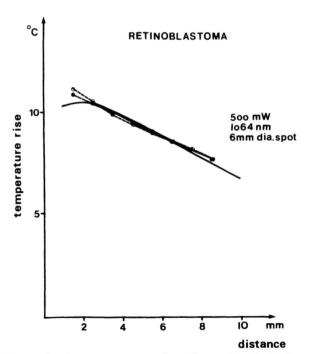

Fig. 8. Steady state temperature rise vs distance from the irradiated surface, measured along the axis of the incident beam. The dashed lines give results from *in vivo* measurements on human retinoblastoma in athymic mice. The two lines correspond to subsequent insertions of a 200-μm diam thermocouple in the same region of the tumor. Power irradiated onto the 500-mW tumor at a 1064-nm wavelength with a 6-mm diam irradiated spot. The solid curve corresponds to calculation [Eqs. (5), (12), (13)] with the following parameters: $n = 1$; $\gamma = 0.18$; $\delta = 7.5$ mm; and $\kappa = 0.6$ W/m · K.

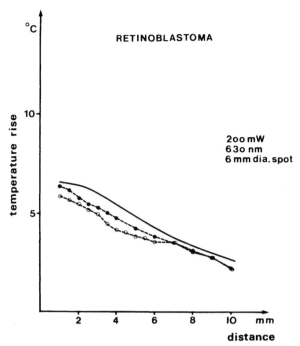

Fig. 9. Steady state temperature rise vs distance from the irradiated surface, measured along the axis of the incident beam. The dashed lines give results from *in vivo* measurements on human retinoblastoma in athymic mice. The two lines correspond to subsequent insertions of a 200-μm diam thermocouple in the same region of the tumor. Power irradiated onto tumor 200 mW at a 630-nm wavelength with a 6-mm diam irradiated spot. Transmission in the cuvette is ∼95% at this wavelength. The solid curve corresponds to calculations [Eqs. (5), (12), (13)] with the following parameters: $n = 1$; $\gamma = 0.21$; optical penetration depth $\delta = 3.3$ mm; and $\kappa = 0.6$ W/m · K.

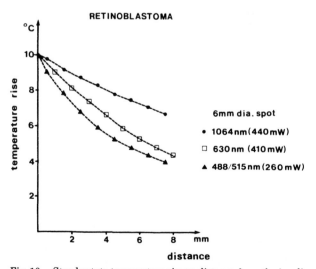

Fig. 10. Steady state temperature rise vs distance from the irradiated surface, measured along the axis of the incident beam. The three dashed lines give results from *in vivo* measurements on human retinoblastoma in athymic mice at different wavelengths. The diameter of the irradiated spot is 6 mm. All results have been normalized to a 10°C temperature rise at the tumor apex. The corresponding required incident optical power onto the tumor at the different wavelengths is as follows: 440 mW at 1064 nm; 410 mW at 630 nm; and 260 mW at 488/515 nm.

this value, and the value in the case of blue/green light is reduced to ~2 mm.

The work has in part been supported by grants from the Royal Norwegian Council for Scientific and Industrial Research and from Fokus bank, Trondheim. The work was performed in conjunction with the Clayton Foundation for Research and supported in part by USPHS grants CA-44733, CA-31230 and CA-43087 awarded by the National Cancer Institute, NIH.

References

1. J. A. Dickson and S. K. Calderwood, "Thermosensitivity of Neoplastic Tissues *In Vivo*," in *Hyperthermia in Cancer Therapy*, F. K. Storm and G. K. Hall, Eds. (Boston, 1983), p. 63.
2. W. J. Geeraets and E. R. Berry, "Ocular Spectral Characteristics as Related to Hazards from Lasers and Other Light Sources," Am. J. Ophthalmol. **66**, 15–26 (1968).
3. S. Lerman, *Radiant Energy and the Eye* (Macmillan, New York, 1980).
4. F. Hillenkamp, "Interaction Between Laser Radiation and Biological Systems," in *Lasers in Biology and Medicine*, F. Hillenkamp, R. Pratesi, and C. A. Sacci, Eds. (Plenum, New York, 1980), p. 37.
5. A. E. Profio and D. R. Doiron, "Dosimetry Considerations in Phototherapy," Med. Phys. **8**, 190–198 (1981).
6. B. C. Wilson and G. Adam, "A Monte Carlo Model for the Absorption and Flux Distributions of Light in Tissue," Med. Phys. **10**, 824–831 (1983).
7. C. C. Johnson, "Optical Diffusion in Blood," IEEE Trans. Biomed. Eng. **BME-17**, 129–134 (1970).
8. A. Ishimaru, *Wave Propagation and Scattering in Random Media* (Academic, New York, 1978), p. 157.
9. L. O. Svaasand, "Photodynamic and Photohyperthermic Response of Malignant Tumors," Med. Phys. **12**, 445–449 (1985).
10. L. O. Svaasand and R. Ellingsen, "Optical Penetration in Human Intracranial Tumors," Photochem. Photobiol. **41**, 73–78 (1985).
11. H. H. Pennes, "Analysis of Tissue and Arterial Blood Temperatures in the Resting Human Forearm," J. Appl. Physiol. **1**, 93–97 (1948).
12. R. K. Jain, "Bioheat Transfer, Mathematical Models of Thermal Systems," in *Hyperthermia in Cancer Therapy*, F. K. Storm and G. K. Hall, Eds. (Boston, 1983), p. 9.
13. R. Birngruber, "Thermal Modeling in Biological Tissues," in *Lasers in Biology and Medicine*, F. Hillenkamp, R. Pratesi, and C. A. Sacci, Eds. (Plenum, New York, 1980), p. 37.
14. A. J. Welch, E. H. Wissler, and L. A. Priebe, "Significance of Blood Flow in Laser Irradiated Tissue," IEEE Trans. Biomed. Eng. **BME-27**, 164–168 (1980).
15. A. J. Welch, "The Thermal Response of Laser Irradiated Tissue," IEEE J. Quantum Electron. **QE-20**, 1471–1482 (1984).

Reprinted from *Optical Methods for Tumor Treatment and Detection: Mechanisms and Techniques in Photodynamic Therapy,* Proc. SPIE Vol. 1645, pp. 155-165 (1992).

Simple optical theory for light dosimetry during PDT.

Steven L. Jacques

Laser Biology Research Laboratory
University of Texas M. D. Anderson Cancer Center
1515 Holcombe Blvd., Houston, Texas 77030

1. ABSTRACT

The relationship between light dosimetry and the photodynamic process is outlined.

2. INTRODUCTION

Photons are one of the 3 major reactants in the photodynamic reaction that yields toxic photoproduct for cell killing. Dosimetry of light is a major concern when planning a photodynamic therapy (PDT) protocol. This paper presents a very simple approach toward the tissue optics with a practical conclusion about how tissue optics affects planning of day-to-day PDT dosimetry. The paper does not address all the complexities of real tissue dosimetry, such as heterogeneous tissues, variable absorption due to changing tissue blood content, and variable tissue oxygen levels. The paper outlines the optical behavior in a homogeneous tissue, which is a starting point for understanding light dosimetry.

3. SIMPLIFIED TISSUE OPTICS

3.1 Tissue optical properties

The first step is to understand the three intrinsic optical properties that specify tissue optics. The absorption coefficient, μ_a, in cm^{-1} determines the probability of absorption events as a photon propagates in a tissue. For a pathlength L, the probability that a photon will not be absorbed is $\exp(-\mu_a L)$, and the mean pathlength before absorption is $1/\mu_a$. A typical value for μ_a in the visible (especially the red) spectrum is 1 cm^{-1} and the mean free path is 1 cm. Similarly, the scattering coefficient, μ_s, in cm^{-1} determines the probability that a photon scatters during propagation. For a pathlength L, the probability that a photon will not be scattered is $\exp(-\mu_s L)$, and the mean free path between scattering events is $1/\mu_s$. A typical value for μ_s is 100 cm^{-1} and the mean free path is 100 μm. Therefore, there are typically 100 scattering events before a photon is absorbed. For each scattering event, the photon's trajectory is deflected by an angle θ. The average value $\langle\cos\theta\rangle$ determines the effectiveness of scattering, and is called the anisotropy of scattering, g. For tissues, the average of g is about 0.9, which corresponds to a deflection of 26°. Approximately, the photon must scatter $1/(1-g)$ or 10 times before the photon loses its orientation with respect to the initial direction of irradiation and migrates as a random walk. During the first 10 scattering events, the photon is penetrating into the tissue and the subsequent 90 scattering events before absorption occurs are a random walk. Calculations of photon propagation often use the reduced scattering coefficient, μ_s', equal to $\mu_s(1-g)$. Table 1 summarizes these properties for the case of rat muscle at 630 nm.

3.2 Measurement of tissue optical properties using video camera

The optical properties of Table 1 refer to *in vivo* rat muscle. The measurements were conducted by measuring the lateral spread of light in the tissue using a video camera while irradiating with a narrow 1-mm diameter laser beam (helium-neon). The skin was surgically retracted to expose the muscle of the rear leg flank of an anesthetized rat. The laser beam was directed onto the muscle and a video camera recorded the spatial pattern of escaping reflectance, $R(r, \theta)$. Also, a distant detector sampled the total diffuse reflectance, R_d, escaping from the leg (calibrated against standard reflector). Four attenuation filters were used at the laser output to span three orders of magnitude of power output, which allowed the camera to collect four sets of $R(r, \theta)$ data covering a large dynamic range. An image analysis program (Image, by W. Rasband, NIH) digitized individual $R(r)$ data for various θ. The images showed no variation with θ. After correcting for the attenuation filters, the four sets of individual $R(r)$ data were fit to the approximate expression: $R(r) = A\, r^{-m} \exp(-r/\delta)$, yielding values for the scaling constant A, a variable number m between 1 and 2, and the penetration depth δ (see Eq. 2 below).[1] Although this expression is slightly inaccurate and further work on improved expressions for $R(r)$ are in progress, the results yielded a reasonable value for δ.

Therefore, two measurements were made: δ based on the lateral spread of light seen by the camera and R_d based on the distant detector. These two measurements specified the two unknowns, μ_a and μ_s', as illustrated by Wilson and Jacques.[1] The anisotropy, g, was assumed to equal about 0.9, a typical value, for the sake of completeness, but we shall not rely on that assumption in this paper. The optical properties of rat muscle are summarized in Table 1.

Table 1: Optics of rat muscle at 633 nm.		
optical properties:		
absorption	μ_a	0.3 cm^{-1}
scattering	μ_s	40 cm^{-1}
anisotropy	g	0.9
reduced scattering	μ_s' = $\mu_s(1\text{-}g)$	4 cm^{-1}
propagation parameters:		
penetration depth	δ	5.1 mm
diffuse reflectance	R_d	0.34
backscatter term	k	4.4
depth of 1/e of irradiance	z_e	12.7 mm

3.3 Light penetration

The penetration of light into a tissue is specified by the tissue optical properties. First consider a clear solution with an absorption, μ_a, of 0.3 cm^{-1} (the same as rat muscle, Table 1). There is no scattering in this solution, so the only attentuation is due to absorption. Figure 1 shows the penetration of a broad uniform beam of light into such a clear solution. After 30 mm of propagation, the irradiance (1 W/cm^2) has dropped to 407 mW/cm^2.

Second, consider the addition of scattering to this solution until the scattering matches that of rat muscle, μ_s equals 40 cm^{-1} and g equals 0.9, or μ_s' equal 4 cm^{-1} (calculated by Monte Carlo simulation). The scattering causes light to be reflected back toward the tissue surface where it accumulates. The light is less penetrating and the fluence, $\psi(0)$, of light within the tissue at the surface is 3.2 W/cm^2, which is more than the 1 W/cm^2 delivered irradiance, ψ_o. The backscattered light has augmented the delivered irradiance to yield a higher fluence within the tissue at the surface.

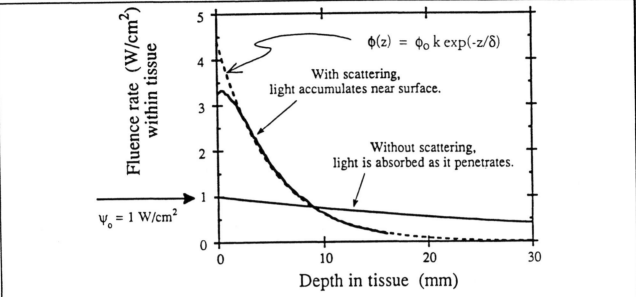

Fig. 1: Penetration of a broad laser beam into clear vs turbid media. The clear medium has the absorption of rat muscle (Table 1) but no scattering. The light decays by simple exponential attenuation. The solid line for the medium with scattering was calculated by Monte Carlo simulation using the optical properties of rat muscle, Table 1. The dashed line is an approximate expression which is inaccurate near the surface but accurate at depth in the tissue.

A simple expression describes the penetration of a broad beam of light:

$$\psi(z) = \psi_o\, k\, \exp(-z/\delta) \quad \text{for } z > \delta \tag{Eq. 1}$$

The factor δ is the so-called *penetration depth* which describes the pathlength that causes a 1/e attenuation of light. The value of δ depends on the optical properties:

$$\delta = \frac{1}{\sqrt{3\,\mu_a\,(\mu_a + \mu_s(1\text{-}g))}} \tag{Eq. 2}$$

Equation 1 is only an approximation that is accurate at deeper depths. Near the surface, Eq. 1 is inaccurate. Figure 1 compares the $\psi(z)$ predicted by Eq. 1 (dashed line) and the true $\psi(z)$ based on Monte Carlo calculations (solid line).

The values of δ for a variety of tissues and tumors are shown in Fig. 2, based on literature values compiled by Cheong et al.[2] in their review and unpublished data by this author. The δ falls with increasing wavelength until the near infrared spectral range, 700-1300 nm, where optical properties are roughly constant and light is most penetrating. This range is called the *therapeutic window*.[3] Note that the values of δ for tissues (Fig. 2A) versus tumors (Fig. 2B) are not significantly different. Although a particular tumor may have slightly different optical properties than the surrounding normal tissue, after all if one can *see* the tumor then the optics must be different, in general there is not a systematic difference between tissues and tumors. Typical values of δ are in the range of 2-7 mm.

The factor k is the backscatter term that accounts for the augmentation of the irradiance, ψ_0, by backscattered light. The value of k is directly related to the diffuse reflectance, R_d, that one observes from the tissue. (Diffuse reflectance equals the total reflectance minus the specular reflectance from the air/tissue interface.) Figure 3A illustrates the behavior of k as a function of R_d.[4] Typical values of R_d for tissues at 630 nm are 30-40% which indicates k values of 4-5. The relation between k and R_d for a tissue with refractive index of 1.37 (typical for a tissue with 70-80% water content) can be summarized, based on Monte Carlo calculations:[1]

$$k = 3 + 5.1 R_d - 2\exp(-9.7 R_d) \qquad\qquad \text{(Eq. 3)}$$

The value of diffuse reflectance, R_d, depends on the ratio of effective scattering to absorption, $\mu_s(1-g)/\mu_a$. This relation is shown in Fig. 3B. A simple approximation for R_d is:

$$R_d \approx \exp(-7\delta\mu_a) \qquad\qquad \text{(Eq. 4)}$$

In other words, the apparent effective pathlength, L, for photons that escape as reflected light is 7δ.

One important point deserves emphasis. The term *penetration depth* is often quoted in discussions of tissue optics. To many people, the term δ denotes the depth, z_e, where light has fallen to 1/e of the irradiance. For a clear solution, this is true. The δ equals $1/\mu_a$ and is identical with z_e. However, for a turbid tissue z_e does not equal δ. The factor k becomes important. The depth where light falls to 1/e of the irradiance is given:

$$z_e = \delta(1 + \ln(k)) \qquad\qquad \text{(Eq. 5)}$$

For k equal 4-5, z_e is 2.4-2.6 times greater than δ. So if a rat muscle has a δ of 5.1 mm and a k of 4.4, then the value of z_e is 12.7 mm.

In summary, the simple light dosimetry along the central z axis within a tissue during irradiation with a broad uniform beam is given by Eqw. 1-4, executed in the following order:

Simplest light dosimetry for a broad beam of irradiance:	
(1) calculate δ	(Eq. 2)
(2) calculate R_d	(Eq. 4)
(3) calculate k	(Eq. 3)
(4) calculate $\psi(z)$	(Eq. 1).

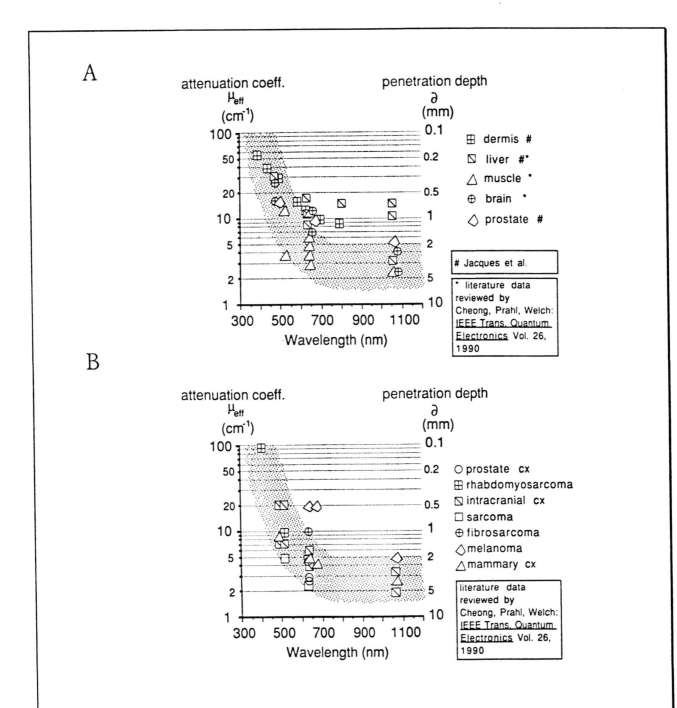

Fig. 2: Optical properties of various tissues and tumors. The effective attenuation coefficient, μ_{eff}, equals $1/\delta$ where δ is the optical penetration depth. (A) Normal tissues. (B) Tumors. Note that there is generally little difference between normal tissue and tumors. Data from Cheong et al. (Ref. 2) and Jacques (unpublished).

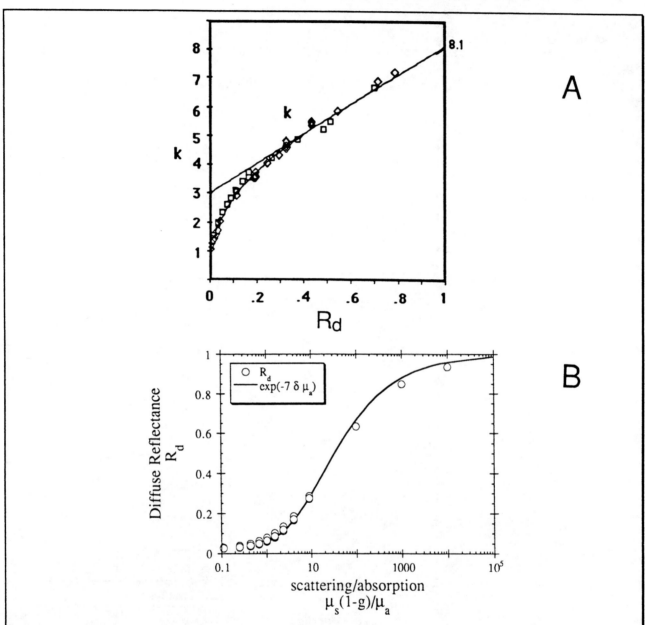

Fig. 3: (A) The backscatter parameter, k, vs diffuse reflectance, R_d. The various data points are for various μ_a, μ_s, and g, as calculated by Monte Carlo simulations (Ref 4). See Eq. 3. (B) R_d as a function of optical properties expressed as $\mu_s(1-g)/\mu_a$. The circles represent exact values of R_d computed by the adding-doubling method as implemented by Prahl[5] for various values of μ_a, μ_s, and g. The solid line represents $R_d = \exp(-7 \delta \mu_a)$. See Eq. 4.

3.3 Geometry of irradiation affects light penetration

The above simple light dosimetry is true for a broad beam, but if the irradiance is narrow then the situation is different. Figure 4 illustrates the effect that the geometry of irradiance exerts on the light dosimetry. Figure 4A and 4B compare the same total beam energy when delivered by a broad beam vs a narrow beam (uniform flat-field beams). The narrow beam achieves a greater penetration (iso-irradiance curve for 1 W/cm² reaches 14 mm depth), but note that the fluence at the point of light injection is very concentrated, exceeding 400 W/cm². This is sufficient to cause burning and/or ablation of the tissue. In contrast, the broad beam achieves comparable although slightly less penetration (1 W/cm² iso-irradiance curve reaches 8 mm depth) but involves only a moderate surface fluence, just over 3 W/cm². By broadening the beam one avoids excessive irradiance yet still achieves significant depth of penetration.

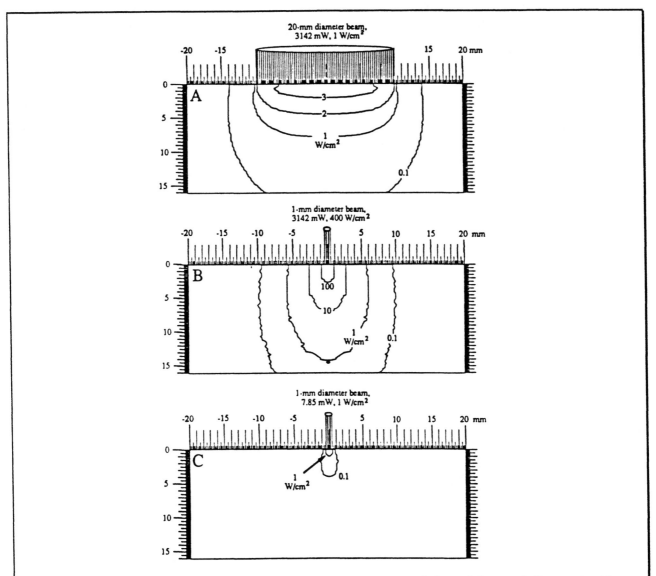

Fig. 4: Effect of geometry on light penetration into tissue. A broad beam delivers significanct energy without excessive irradiance. A narrow beam with the same total energy as the broad beam causes excessive irradiance at the surface, which can cook or ablate tissue. A narrow beam with the same irradiance as the broad beam has too little total energy to achieve significant light penetration. (A) Broad beam, 20-mm dia., 3.142 W, 1 W/cm². (B) Narrow beam, 1-mm dia., 3.142 W, 400 W/cm². (C) Narrow beam, 1-mm dia., 0.00785 W, 1 W/cm².

One could easily increase the irradiance of the broad beam several fold without overheating the tissue surface and consequently deliver more total light into the tissue. One would achieve a depth of penetration as deep as the narrow beam and certainly much wider. A broad beam is definitely advantageous over a narrow beam for PDT.

Figure 4C shows a narrow beam with the same irradiance as the broad beam of Fig. 4A (1 W/cm^2) but much less total energy because the beam is so small. The amall amount of total energy prevents significant light penetration.

4. HOW OPTICS AFFECT PDT DOSIMETRY

4.1 Dosimetric equation for PDT

Figure 5 shows a simplified schematic diagram of PDT. The dosimetric equation that describes PDT can be summarized:

$$P_{th} = \Phi \, \mu_{a.dye} \, b \, \psi_o \, t \, k \, \exp(-z_{necrosis}/\delta) \qquad \text{(Eq. 6)}$$

where ψ_o is irradiance in W/cm^2, t is the exposure time in s, and k is the backscatter term. P_{th} is the threshold production of singlet oxygen (moles/cc) that causes cell death and $z_{necrosis}$ is the depth of PDT-induced necrosis within a tissue. The other factors are listed in Table 2, which outlines a typical PDT protocol using a hypothetical photosensitizer. Note that the term $\psi_o \, t \, k \, \exp(-z_{necrosis}/\delta)$ represents the amount of light that has reached the deep boundary of necrosis. The factor b is a conversion constant. For red light at 630 nm, there are 3.15×10^{18} photons per J of energy, or 5.23×10^{-6} moles of photons per J.

The factor $\mu_{a.dye}$ indicates the absorption coefficient due to dye in the tissue:

$$\mu_{a.dye} = \varepsilon \, C \, \log_e(10) \qquad \text{(Eq. 7)}$$

where ε is the dye extinction coefficient and C is the dye concentration in the tissue. The relationship between the delivered dosage of dye (eg. mg/kg body weight) and the amount of dye in the tissue ($\mu g/g$ tissue) is an important variable, but shall here be approximated by the following example. A delivered dye dosage of 5 mg/kg body weight is assumed to yield a mass concentration, m, in the tissue of $2 \times 10^{-6} \text{ g/cm}^3$ tissue.

The only photons that contribute to PDT are those photons that are absorbed by photodynamic dye. The rate of light absorption by the tissue is specified by the product $\mu_a \psi$ in W/cm^3, where μ_a is the tissue absorption:

$$\text{light absorbed} = \mu_a \psi \qquad \text{(Eq. 8)}$$

But the light absorption by the photodynamic dye is $\mu_{a.dye}\psi$, where $\mu_{a.dye}$ is the absorption coefficient of the dye:

$$\text{light absorbed by dye} = \mu_{a.dye}\psi \qquad \text{(Eq. 9)}$$

The value of $\mu_{a.dye}$ is usually much less than the total μ_a. Consider a photodynamic dye, such as a hypothetical but typical porphyrin, which has achieved a mass concentration, m, of about 2 $\mu g/cm^3$ in the tissue, has an extinction coefficient, ε, of about 4000 $(cm^{-1})/(L\ mole^{-1})$, and a molecular weight, MW, of about 600 g/mole. The molar concentration, C, in moles/L equals 1000m/MW. The absorption coefficient due to dye, $\mu_{a.dye}$, is calculated:

$$\mu_{a.dye} = \varepsilon\ C \log_e(10) = \varepsilon \frac{1000\ m}{MW} \log_e(10) \qquad (Eq,\ 10)$$

$$= \frac{4000\ cm^{-1}}{mole/L} \frac{(1000\ cm^3/L)(2 \times 10^{-6}\ g/cm^3)}{600\ g/mole} \log_e(10)$$

$$= 0.031\ cm^{-1}$$

which is about 10 times lower than the typical tissue absorption of ~0.3 cm^{-1}. So only about 10% of all the absorbed photons are absorbed by photodynamic dye.

Rearranging Eq. 6 yields:

$$z_{necrosis} = \delta \log_e(\frac{\Phi\ \mu_{a.dye}\ b\ \psi_o\ t\ k}{P_{th}}) \qquad (Eq.\ 11)$$

Note that $z_{necrosis}$ is equal to the penetration depth, δ, times the logarithm of all the other factors.

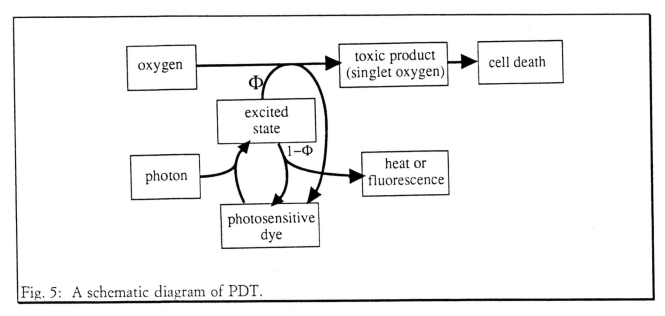

Fig. 5: A schematic diagram of PDT.

In the example of Table 2, a typical PDT dosimetry is hypothetically summarized. Red light (0.2 W/cm^2 at 630 nm) is delivered for 20 minutes. The *photodynamic threshold dose,* which we shall call D_{th}, that is required for necrosis is estimated to be about 1 x 10^{18} photons absorbed by dye per cc of tissue, based on the work of Patterson et al.[6] The quantum efficiency, Φ, for excited dye to react with oxygen and yield toxic photoproduct is assumed to be 0.2. The threshold value for cell death (P_{th}) is equal to $D_{th}/(\Phi\ 6.02 \times 10^{23})$ which equals 8.3×10^{-6} moles/cm^3. Therefore, Eq. 11 predicts a depth of necrosis of 7.2 mm.

TABLE 2: Typical PDT dosimetry with red light.

Name	Symbol	Value	Units
Photons:			
wavelength	λ	630	nm
irradiance	ψ_0	0.2	W/cm^2
exposure time	t (min)	20	min
optical penetration depth	δ (mm)	5.1	mm
optical backscatter constant	k	4.4	---
conversion constant	b	5.23×10^{-6}	moles/J
Photosensitive dye:			
delivered dose	---	5	mg/kg b.w.
tissue concentration	m	2×10^{-6}	g dye/cm^3 tissue
dye molecular weight	MW	600	g/mole
extinction coefficient	ε	4000	cm^{-1}/(mole/liter)
dye absorption in tissue	$\mu_{a.dye}$	0.031	cm^{-1}
quantum efficiency	Φ	0.2	---
Tissue necrosis:			
threshold photodynamic dose	---	1×10^{-18}	photons/cm^3 absorbed by dye
threshold toxic product	P_{th}	8.3×10^{-6}	moles/cm^3
zone of necrosis	$z_{necrosis}$	7.2	mm

(These are hypothetical values in the typical range for PDT, chosen to demonstrate Eqs. 6 and 11. Oxygen is assumed to be in excess.)

We have ignored the effect that oxygen concentration has on the PDT process by assuming that oxygen is in exess. If oxygen is not in excess, then the value of the apparent quantum yield Φ will drop. Excited-state dye molecules will become less likely to react with oxygen and produce toxic photoproduct.

4.2 How to use all this optics in day-to-day PDT dosimetry

The depth of necrosis caused by PDT can be adjusted by changing the dosimetry factors. Equation 11 indicates that if either the irradiance (ψ_0), the exposure time (t), the dye concentration in the tissue ($\mu_{a.dye}$), the quantum yield (Φ), or the backscatter term (k) increases by a factor of 2, then the $z_{necrosis}$ will increase by the amount $\log_e(2)\delta$. In general, if the product of these terms increases by a factor X, then $z_{necrosis}$ will increase by $\log_e(X)\delta$:

$$\text{new } z_{necrosis} = \text{initial } z_{necrosis} + \log_e(X)\delta \qquad \text{(Eq. 12)}$$

For our example of Table 2, the depth of necrosis is 7.2 mm. The value of δ is 5.1 mm. If one increases the irradiance by a factor of 2, then the $z_{necrosis}$ is expected to increase by $\log_e(2)\delta$ or 3.5 mm to yield a new $z_{necrosis}$ of 10.7 mm.

In other words, $z_{necrosis}$ is linearly related to δ and logarithmically related to all other factors. The optical penetration depth of a tissue is of central importance for PDT dosimetry. If one observes a particular $z_{necrosis}$ for a specific set of experimental conditions, then one can predict how a change in parameters will increase or decrease $z_{necrosis}$. Knowledge of the tissue optical properties and δ will allow prediction of how adjustment of treatment parameters will alter the $z_{necrosis}$.

5. DISCUSSION

This paper provides a first approximation for PDT dosimetry. There are many factors and effects which can complicate this simple approach. Tissue hemorrhage can change the penetration depth δ, oxygen levels can drop which lowers the quantum yield Φ, the efficacy of the photosensitive dye can vary with time thereby affecting the value of P_{th}, the light exposure can "photobleach" dye which alters $\mu_{a.dye}$. These and other effects can complicate the situation. The purpose of this paper is to outline the simple baseline relationships as a starting point for understanding PDT dosimetry.

6. REFERENCES

1   Wilson, B.C., S. L. Jacques: Optical reflectance and transmittance of tissues: Principles and applications. *IEEE J. Quantum Electronics*, 26(12):2186-2199, 1991.

2   Cheong WF, SA Prahl, AJ Welch: A review of the optical properties of biological tissues. *IEEE J. Quantum Electronics*, 26(12):2166-2185, 1991.

3   Parrish JA: New comcepts in therapeutic photomedicine: Photochemistry, optical targeting and the therapeutic window. *J. Invest. Dermatol.* 77:45-50, 1981.

4   Jacques SL: Simple theory, measurements, and rules of thumb for dosimetry during photodynamic therapy. *Proceedings of SPIE, Photodynamic Therapy: Mechanisms*, 1065: 100-108, 1989.

5   Prahl SA: Light transport in tissue. Ph.D. dissertation, University of Texas at Austin, 1988.

6   Patterson, Wilson, Graff: *In vivo* tests of the concept of photodynamic threshold dose in normal rat liver photosensitized by aluminum chlorosulphonated phthalocyanine. *Photochem. Photobiol.* 51:343-349, 1990.

Author Index

Subject Index